ALTERNATE SOURCES

SECOND EDITION

KINK, INK
TORONTO

Publisher & Editor
Trevor Jacques

Graphic Design
Trevor Jacques & Dan Bowers

Editorial Assistants
PBVF & MSOH

Advertising & Book Sales
Trevor Jacques

Distribution Worldwide
Kink, Ink, P. O. Box 19591-255, 55 Bloor Street West,
Toronto, Ontario M4W 3T9. Canada
(416) 962 1040, Facs.: (416) 962 1044

Distribution United Kingdom
Turnaround Distributors, 27 Horsell Road, London N5.
(171) 609 7638, Facs.: (171) 700 1205

Distribution Australasia
Edition Habit Press, 112 Bondi Beach, New South Wales 2000.
2 387 4339, Facs.: 2 389 2966

Wholesale North America
Marginal Distribution, Unit 102, 277 George Street,
Peterborough, Ontario K9J 3G9.
(705) 745 2326, Facs.: (705) 745 2326
Alamo Square Distributors, P. O. Box 14543, San Francisco, California. 94114.
(415) 252 0643, Facs.: 415 863 7456
Baker & Taylor, 652 East Main Street, Bridgewater, New Jersey 08807.
(908) 218 0400
Bookpeople, 7900 Edgewater Drive, Oakland, California 94621.
(510) 632 4700, Facs.: (510) 632 1281
Xclusiv Distributors, 451 50th. Street, Brooklyn, New York 11220.
(718) 439 1271, Facs.: (718) 439 1272

Kink, Ink
P. O. Box 19591-255, 55 Bloor Street West,
Toronto, Ontario. M4W 3T9. Canada.
(416) 962 1040, Facs. (416) 962 1044
Editor@Alternate.com
SAN: S1196111

Single copies may be ordered directly from:
Alternate Sources, P. O. Box 19591-255, 55 Bloor Street West,
Toronto, Ontario M4W 3T9. Canada

Canadian Cataloguing in Publication Data

Alternate Sources
1994-
Annual.
ISSN 1201-2823
ISBN 1-895857-09-0
1. Fetishism—Directories. 2. Sadomasochism—Directories.
3. Bisexuality—Directories. 4. Transvestism—Directories.
5. Leather life style (Sexuality)—Directories.
HQ1.A58 306.77'025 C95-900146-8

First printing, January, 1996
Typeset in Toronto, Canada. Printed in Canada.

DISCLAIMER

This book is designed to give information in regard to the subject matter covered. It is sold under the understanding that the publisher, author, and editor are not engaged in rendering professional services. If legal or other expert assistance is required, the services of a competent professional should be sought.

It is not the purpose of this directory to reprint all the information that is otherwise available to the author, editor, and/or publisher, but to complement and extend other texts. You are urged to read all the available material, learn as much as possible about SM play, sado-masochism, transexuality, transvesticism, and other alternate sexual expressions, and to tailor the resultant information to your own needs.

Every effort has been made to make this book as complete and accurate as possible. However, there may be mistakes both typographical and of content. Therefore, this text should be used only as a guide and not as the ultimate source of information. Furthermore, this text only contains information up to the time of printing.

The author, editor, and Kink, Ink shall have neither liability nor responsibility to any person or entity with respect to loss or damage caused, or alleged to be caused, directly or indirectly, by the information contained in this book.

If you do not wish to be bound by the above, you may return this book to the publisher for a full refund.

None of the businesses in Alternate Sources is necessarily owned or operated by people of a particular sexual orientation; nor do any of them specifically welcome only a particular kind of client. The symbols used in this book are for the reader's guidance only. They should not be taken as a formal indication of the sexuality of the owners or operators of the listed organization, its staff, or models.

The listing of any organization in this book is not in any way an endorsement by the publisher of said organization; nor is the inclusion of an advertisement paid for by the advertiser to be construed in any manner as an endorsement by the publisher of the advertiser or the advertiser's products or services.

Alternate Soures is intended for adults of legal majority. The nature of the book is such that a minor could use it to gain access to the places that provide adult goods and services. For that reason, the publisher does not knowingly distribute Alternate Sources to minors.

Welcome

Welcome to the second edition of *Alternate Sources*. With over 10,000 listings and five indexes, it's the most complete global resource for the alternate sexuality communities. Over 2 years of work and verification have gone into *Alternate Sources*.

We produced *Alternate Sources* because we could not find a single, global resource directory for all the alternate sexes and sexualities. For instance, there were many listings of gay and lesbian bars around the world, but no global listings of BDSM bars for all sexes and sexualities. Many of the listings lacked information we wanted, such as Internet e-mail and World-Wide Web addresses.

We have included resources that further a healthy exploration and/or expression of an alternate sexuality itself. Hence, a gay and lesbian student or support organization or a BDSM toy supplier would be listed, but not, say, a flower shop catering to the gay and lesbian community. The latter shop caters to daily life, rather than specifically to the expression of an alternate sexuality (our apologies to those with flower fetishes). Some of the listings are included because, while in and of themselves they would not be included, they are known to provide a gateway to more information about the alternate sexuality communities (such as local gay newspapers which list local BDSM meetings & events). We have also included more mainstream resources that are known to be friendly to the alternate sexuality communities (such as national newspapers that have published balanced articles about these communities.

A great deal of effort has gone into ensuring that all the listings in *Alternate Sources* are as accurate as we can make them. You'll also notice that the information provided by the listees varies, so not all of the listings have quite as much detail as the rest. We know that people change address and may do so between completion of our manuscript and your purchasing the book. Please tell us of any inaccuracies or omissions you notice, so that we can continue to keep *Alternate Sources* the best global resource for kinky folk.

We hope you find *Alternate Sources* of use as you explore the world's alternate sexualities.

About This Guide & How to Use It

Alternate Sources is a global directory of resources, sorted by country, province, town, and type of organization.

For the purposes of the directory, we have used *alternate* to mean anything to do with the leather/BDSM/fetish world and other alternate sexual expressions, such as homosexuality and bisexuality, transgender and transsexual, transvestitism and cross dressing, as well as adult baby play and other activities that might interest you. We found an enormous variety in people's interests, so, if you have a "kink," it's almost certainly listed here (if not, please tell us).

Depending on the country and its customary use of provinces, states, counties, or regions, we have used the same divisions. So, you'll find Canada divided by province and then town, England by county and then town, Italy by region and then town, and the U. S. A. by state and then town. France, Germany, and others do not use their regional divisions, so neither did we. These countries are sorted directly by town.

There is a table of contents at the front of the directory that shows the order in which listings occur. For instance, if you wanted to find Toronto, you'd look it up under: Canada, Ontario, Toronto in the table of contents. The table of contents is followed immediately by an alphabetical listing of town names, so that you can look up a town if you're unsure of which province (or state, region, or county) it is in. In this index of towns, it would be listed as: Toronto, Canada, followed by the page number.

At the beginning of the directory listing, you'll find the resources that are international in scope. These are sorted by type of organization and name. So are the national resources that you'll find at the top of each country, and the provincial (or state, region, or county, as appropriate) resources at the top of each province (or state, region, or county). Listings in the international, national, and regional sections are *not* repeated in the local sections.

For each country, we have included a quick summary of national information, where it is available:

- The name of the capital;
- The official language(s);
- The national holiday(s);
- The country's major religions;
- The phone access code for international calls to outside the country (use this to call out of the country and then add the city/area code of the country you are calling);
- The international country code for when you want to call that country from another country (usually two digits);
- The number of times zones in the country and how many hours from GMT they are;
- The age(s) of consent for sexual activities. Where possible, we will indicate for heterosexual, gay male, and lesbian activities;
- The legal age for consumption of alcohol; and
- The type of electricity provided in the country.

Where possible, at the top of the regional listings we list:

- The population;
- The capital/county town/city;
- The time zone, where relevant;
- Information about the sodomy laws; and
- The legal drinking age.

Each town or city has been divided into the types of organization. For example, if you're looking for a book store, look for it under Stores: Books.

Each entry in the book has been structured for easy access to the data. The same type of information, when it is available, is always in the same place in the entry's block of text. Please note that due to space considerations some entries have only one line of information at either the start *or* end of their entry; the rest is in the next or previous column. Here are the things you might find:

- The name of the organization or publication;
- The mailing address of the organization (or street address, if there is no separate postal address);
- The main 'phone number, followed by the facsimile number (if there is one);
- A second 'phone phone number followed by the cellular 'phone number;
- The BBSs telephone number and maximum modem speed for the organization;
- The e-mail address of the organization;
- The Internet Uniform Resource Location (URL): World-Wide Web (http), file transfer protocol (ftp), and gopher addresses are provided, as applicable;
- The hours of business;
- The forms of payment that the establishment accepts, where applicable;
- A contact name, if applicable;
- A few words about the organization;
- The price of their catalogue, where relevant (n.b. please remember to add something for postage, packing, and taxes);
- The frequency of publication, where applicable;
- Any languages spoken, other than the local language; and
- Any notes about addressing of envelopes to ensure the privacy of the addressee.

The page headings throughout the directory work just like those in a telephone directory, to indicate where you are. The countries are sorted by their English name, but, beyond that, we have used the local spelling of town and province wherever possible. Where there are two known *local* spellings of the name, we have used the one in most common local usage first, for example: Bruxelles / Brussel. So, in this example, since Brussels is predominantly French speaking, even though it's in the Flemish part of Belgium, we've put the French spelling before the Flemish.

At the back of the listings, we've put an index by name of organization, so if you want to look up an organization, publication, or business by name, it's right there. We've included the town name and telephone number where these are known, with the index entry.

After the index by names, we've put an index by type of organization. So if you want to look up all the whip manufacturers, they're all in one place for you. This index has each type category divided by the primary clientele for the organization. This will allow you to find, say, all the magazine publishers that serve the lesbian community.

After the index by type, we've put a list of medical and counselling professionals who have been identified as understanding the special needs of people with alternate sexualities. They are prepared for the questions of, say, transsexuals or BDSMers, depending on the counsellor.

Categories

Each entry in Alternate Sources is categorized by the type of organization. We have included types of organizations that we feel can be of use to anyone interested in the alternate scene, be they provider or user of the goods and/or services. So, an author or researcher may want to know where to get research material and where to find publishers; publishers will want access to distributors, newspapers, and magazines for book distribution and reviews, but also to printers who may print alternate subjects; consumers will read books and magazines and want to know where to get them. We have taken a similar approach to sexual aids, health, and sexuality. We have listed the categories below and summarized some of the reasoning behind their inclusion in Alternate Sources

Note that many of the listings include a subdivision of *General*. This means that they usually serve the general population, but that they may have information you seek, or that they may provide a service you need. For instance, Printers: General are general book printers who *may* be prepared to print books about alternate sexualities; Stores: Leatherwork Supplies: General are everyday leatherwork supply shops that may have the tools you need. Please use your discretion when contacting these stores. They may not want to know what you do in bed. Also, some of the categories have not needed the extra breakdown into a General subdivision. Again, please use your discretion to determine whether to talk with them about sexual matters, for example: a Store: Clothing: Uniforms may not cater specifically to the alternate sexuality community, but they may have just the military cap you seek.

Accommodation Only places that provide for BDSM and fetish needs have been listed. For example: "bed and breakfast and shackles." (There are plenty of directories of gay and lesbian accommodations, so there is no need to duplicate them here. We have listed these directories, however.)

Archives Any archive relevant to alternate sexual expressions. Useful mainly for research.

Bars We have included BDSM/fetish, transvestite,

and transsexual bars. (As for accommodation, there are directories with this information. We have listed the directories. Please tell us if you'd like to see gay, lesbian, and bisexual bars in future editions.)

BBSs Computer bulletin boards relevant to alternate expressions. The advantage of these boards is that they can, like the rest of the Internet, be reached from anywhere, and they offer the user a certain anonymity. (This anonymity is also one of their downfalls since people can leave insults anonymously, unless the board is very well policed by its operators. That could lay the operators open to accusations of censorship. It's a difficult line....)

Book Services Book services are, for the most part, mail order houses that allow people to buy books without fear of being spotted buying "one of those books," thereby performing a useful service to those who are just starting to explore their alternate sexuality.

Book Shops The listed book shops are sources of literature on alternate sexualities, and can often be used as a starting point as one explores a new town. Very often these book shops stock free local magazines that will list local organizations and events of interest to you. (N.b. these are listed under Stores: Books.)

Counsellors Counsellors have been included because there are many counsellors who are sympathetic to alternate sexual expressions. Those who have been specifically identified as being "kink-aware" are noted with a Κ (the Greek kappa) symbol, and are listed in the separate index of Kink-Aware Professionals (KAP) in the back of the directory.

Distributors Included for manufacturers, stores, publishers, and self-published authors.

Helplines Help for anyone with concerns about HIV, sexuality, and some other issues.

Mail order Included for producers and consumers of books, erotica, videos, and safer sex products.

Manu-facturers These listings include the original manufacturer of the basic goods, such as leather and rubber manufacturers, and the manufacturers of finished goods, such as toys and clothing made of the basic goods.

Organi-zations Organizations relevant to alternate sexual expressions, such as academic institutions concerned with sexuality, AIDS organizations, and family and youth support organizations set up to help those with issues related to alternate sexualities.

Piercers For those interested in body modification.

Publishers Publishers have been subdivided into several subgroups, depending on whether the product is a book, magazine, video, listing, etc. They have been further divided by the basic content and intent of the publication.

Radio There are many programs and some complete radio stations devoted to sexuality. These have been included to help, say, an author get publicity, and an individual to find out more about alternate sexual expressions.

Stores Shops retailing books, clothing, adult toys, and literature are included for anyone buying or selling goods useful to members of the alternate sexuality communities.

Suppliers There are some suppliers who do not fit any of the major categories, so they have been included in this catch-all category. This category is subdivided where appropriate.

Television There are many programs devoted to homosexual and BDSM issues being broadcast, particularly in North America. These are included here as possible sources of information or as a means to promote your work or product.

Symbol Definitions

Primary clientele of the organization:

- ☺ All sexes and sexualities
- ⚥ Bisexual, both sexes
- ♀ Female, all sexualities
- ⚣ Gay male
- 👫 Heterosexual, male and female
- 🚺 Heterosexual, female only
- 🚹 Heterosexual, male only
- ⚢ Lesbian
- ⚧ Lesbian, gay, bisexual, and transgender
- ♂ Male, all sexualities
- 🦋 Transgender (also transsexual), all sexes and sexualities
- ⌂ Transvestite (also known as cross dressing), all sexes and sexualities

Type of business:

- ▽ A non-profit organization (irrespective of tax status) intended mainly for the lesbian, gay and bisexual community, but others may be welcome

- ☐ A non-profit organization (irrespective of tax status) not intended mainly for the lesbian, gay and bisexual community
- ▼ A for-profit organization that wants to be listed as wholly owned or operated by members of the lesbian, gay and bisexual community. Other clients may be welcome
- ■ A for-profit organization that does not want to be listed as owned or operated by members of the lesbian, gay and bisexual community, but they are welcome

Wheelchair access to the premises of the listed organization:

- Accessible by wheel chair. Lavatory accessibility unknown
- Premises and lavatory accessible by wheelchairs
- Access to both premises and lavatory possible with help
- Premises accessible with help by wheelchair
- Premises accessible by wheelchair, but lavatory access requires help
- Call ahead for accessibility

The following symbols are used to identify phone and e-mail numbers:

- Phone
- Cellular
- Facsimile (Facs./Fax)
- Modem
- E-mail
- Web URL
- Opening hours

When the organization accepts payment for goods and services, the following symbols are used to indicate the types of payment accepted. Most organization accept cash.

- Cash
- ✓ Cheques
- $ Money Order
- Traveller's Cheques
- Visa
- Master Card
- American Express
- Diner's Club
- Discover
- ¢ Electronic funds transfer

Where to get more copies

Alternate Sources is available through most good book shops and adult stores. If you have trouble finding it, please contact the publisher for your copy.

Safe, Sane, & Consensual Definitions

In the last few years, a creed of sorts has been adopted by the BDSM communities around the world. We'd like you to know what it is, so that you can help spread the word about healthy play, too. By the way, we'd also like to add the word *fun* to the list. If it's not fun, don't do it. You can probably think of many better things to do and ways to spend your money. The following definitions were taken from *On The Safe Edge, A Manual for SM Play* by Trevor Jacques, Dr. Dale, Michael Hamilton, and Sniffer (used with permission of the copyright holder):

Safe All players have taken the necessary precautions to prevent psychological and physical damage to themselves, including the transmission of disease.

Sane All players are in full possession of their mental faculties and are fully aware of the risks involved in the play they intend.

Consensual All players fully understand the potential risks of their intended play and have consented to the activities. This consent can be withdrawn or modified by any player at any time.

Border crossing descriptions

Much has been said and feared about crossing borders between countries with items used for alternate sexual practices such as BDSM and transvestitism. The best summary that we can come up with is that, provided none of the items you intend to carry across the border is a prohibited item in the country to which you are going and you are not carrying so many of them that you might be construed as trying to sell them once you arrive, it is unlikely that you will be detained at any border. It is possible, however, that customs or immigration officials may ask you what you are doing with the items. The best answers are the real ones: "They're sex toys," "I give safer sex lectures, and these are some of my props," "I herd animals with this whip, in my spare time" (true; they just happen to be human animals herded during play...).

Customs and immigration are only interested if you look like you're going to be breaking the law. (For example, carrying more than six dildos in Texas can be construed as "trafficking in dildos....") Check out the laws before you travel, then be honest at the border. If you're just going to visit friends, say so. There's no need to say more. Many people feel compelled to tell border officials all the details of their trip. Don't bother; if your intentions are legal, they're not interested.

Table of Contents

International Resources 1

Australia 24

NATIONAL RESOURCES 24
AUSTRALIAN CAPITAL TERRITORY 25
Canberra 25
Coffs Harbour 25
NEW SOUTH WALES 25
Albury 25
Armidale 25
Callaghan 25
Castle Hill 25
Lismore 25
Milsons Point 25
Newcastle 25
Penrith 25
Petersham 25
Rozelle 25
Sydney 26
Tweed Heads 27
Wagga Wagga 27
Wollongong 27
NORTHERN TERRITORY 28
Alice Springs 28
Darwin 28
QUEENSLAND 28
Annerley 28
Brisbane 28
Bundaberg 29
Cairns 29
New Farm 29
Noosa 29
Nundah 29
Rockhampton 29
Surfer's Paradise 29
Toowooba 29
Townsville 29
SOUTH AUSTRALIA 29
State Resources 29
Adelaide 30
Daw Park 31
Elizabeth Vale 31
Ingle Farm 31
Lobethal 31
Plympton 31
TASMANIA 31
Hobart 31
Wivenhoe 31
VICTORIA 31
State Resources 31
Bendigo 31
Melbourne 31
Northcote 33
WESTERN AUSTRALIA 33
State Resources 33
Bentley 33
Cloverdale 33
Doublview 33
Gosnells 33
Morley 33
Murdoch 33
Northbridge 33
Perth 33
Victoria Park 34

Austria 34

NATIONAL RESOURCES 34
Bregenz 34
Dornberg 34
Dornbirn 34
Graz 34
Innsbruck 34
Klagenfurt 34
Linz 34
Salzburg 34
Wien 35

Belgium 35

NATIONAL RESOURCES 35
Aalst / Alost 36
Antwerpen / Anvers 36
Bruxelles / Brussel 36
Charleroi 38
Deurne 38
Gent / Gand 38
Hainault 38
Herentals 38
Kortrijk / Courtrai 38
Leuven / Louvain 38
Liège / Luik / Luttich 38
Lovendegem 38
Mechelen / Malines 38
Namur / Namen 39
Oostende / Ostende 39
Schoten 39
Sint Niklaas 39
Veerle-Laakdal 39
Wilrijk 39
Wondelgem 39

Brazil 39

Rio de Janeiro 39
São Paulo 39

Bulgaria 40

NATIONAL RESOURCES 40

Byelorussia 40

Minsk 40

Canada 40

NATIONAL RESOURCES 40
ALBERTA 42
Provincial Resources 42
Banff 42
Calgary 42
Edmonton 43
Grande Prairie 44
Jasper 44
Lethbridge 44
Okotoks 44
Red Deer 44
BRITISH COLUMBIA 44
Provincial Resources 44
Burnaby 44
Coquitlam 44
Grand Forks 44
Kamloops 44
Kelowna 44
Kootnays 44
Ladner 44
Langley 44
Nanaimo 44
New Westminster 44
Prince George 44
Squamish 45
Terrace 45
Vancouver 45
Victoria 46
MANITOBA 47
Provincial Resources 47
Brandon 47
Dugald 47
Winnipeg 47
NEW BRUNSWICK 48
Fredricton 48
Moncton 48
Riverview 48
Saint John 48
NEWFOUNDLAND 48
Saint John's 48
NORTH WEST TERRITORIES 48
Yellowknife 48
NOVA SCOTIA 48
Halifax 48
New Glasgow 48
Sydney 49
ONTARIO 49
Provincial Resources 49
Barrie 49
Belleville 49
Bonfield 49
Burlington 49
Cooksville 49
Don Mills 49
Erin 49
Guelph 49
Haliburton 50
Hamilton 50
Kingston 50
Kitchener 50
Lindsay 51
London 51
MacTier 51
Mississauga 51
Niagara Falls 51
North Bay 52
North York 52
Orillia 52
Oshawa 52
Ottawa 52
Owen Sound 53
Peterborough 54
Saint Catharines 54
Saint Thomas 54
Sault Saint Marie 54
Scarborough 54
Stratford 54
Sudbury 54
Thornhill 54
Thunder Bay 54
Timmins 55
Toronto 55
Waterloo 60
Whitby 61
Windsor 61
PRINCE EDWARD ISLAND 61
Charlottetown 61
QUÉBEC 61
Provincial Resources 61
Athelstan 61
Beaconsfield 61
Chicoutimi 61
Gatineau 61
Hull 61
Joliette 61
Laval 61
Montréal 61
Noranda 63
Outremont 63
Québec 63
Saint Antoine des Laurentides 63
Sherbrooke 63
Trois-Rivières 63
Victoriaville 63
SASKATCHEWAN 63
Regina 64
Saskatoon 64
YUKON 64
Whitehorse 64

Channel Islands 64

GUERNSEY 64
County Resources 64
JERSEY 64
Saint Helier 64

Chile 64
Santiago 64
Costa Rica 65
San José 65
Czech Republic 65
Praha 65
Denmark 65
NATIONAL RESOURCES 65
Ålborg 65
Århus 65
Broenshoej 65
Frederiksberg 66
Greve 66
Holbæck 66
København 66
Kolding 66
Odense 66
Silkeborg 66
Sønderborg 67
Viborg 67
England 67
NATIONAL RESOURCES 67
AVON 70
Bath 70
Bristol 70
Weston-Super-Mare 70
BEDFORDSHIRE 70
County Resources 70
Bedford 70
Leighton Buzzard 70
Luton 71
BERKSHIRE 71
County Resources 71
Maidenhead 71
Reading 71
Slough 71
Thatcham 71
Wokingham 71
BUCKINGHAMSHIRE 71
High Wycombe 71
Milton Keynes 71
CAMBRIDGESHIRE 71
Cambridge 71
Peterborough 71
CHESHIRE 71
Chester 71
Crewe 71
Liverpool 71
Macclesfield 72
Runcorn 72
Sandbach 72
Stalybridge 72
Stockport 72
Warrington 72
Windsford 72
CORNWALL 72
Cambourne 72
Launceston 72
Penryn 72
Penzance 72
Saint Austell 72
Truro 72
CUMBRIA 72
Carlisle 72
Kendal 72
Penrith 72
Seascale 72
DERBYSHIRE 72
Chesterfield 72
Derby 72
Heanor 73
Middleton 73
DEVON 73
County Resources 73
Barnstaple 73
Exeter 73
Newton Abbot 73
Plymouth 73
Torquay 73
DORSET 73
County Resources 73
Bournemouth 73
Ferndown 73
Stoke Abbot 73
DURHAM 73
Darlington 73
Durham 74
EAST SUSSEX 74
Brighton 74
Eastbourne 74
Hailsham 74
Hastings 74
Hove 74
ESSEX 74
Basildon 74
Braintree 75
Buckhurst Hill 75
Chelmsford 75
Chigwell 75
Colchester 75
Hadleigh 75
Harlow 75
Leytonstone 75
Romford 75
Southend 75
Stanford-Le-Hope 75
Thornton Heath 75
Westcliff On Sea 75
GLOUCESTERSHIRE 75
Gloucester 75
Nailsworth 75
GREATER MANCHESTER 75
County Resources 75
Beswick 75
Manchester 75
Oldham 76
Prestwich 76
Rochdale 76
Wigan 76
HAMPSHIRE 76
Andover 76
Northam 76
Portsmouth 76
Southampton 77
HEREFORD & WORCESTER 77
County Resources 77
Hereford 77
Kidderminster 77
HERTFORDSHIRE 77
Letchworth 77
Saint Albans 77
HUMBERSIDE 77
Bridlington 77
Grimsby 77
Hull 77
Scunthorpe 77
ISLE OF MAN 77
Douglas 77
ISLE OF WIGHT 77
County Resources 77
Freshwater 77
Sandown 77
KENT 78
Ashford 78
Canterbury 78
Chatham 78
Chislehurst 78
Folkestone 78
Gravesend 78
Maidstone 78
Margate 78
Near Marden 78
Royal Tunbridge Wells 78
LANCASHIRE 78
County Resources 78
Blackpool 78
Bolton 78
Burnley 78
Darwen 78
Lancaster 78
Leyland 79
Preston 79
White Cross 79
LEICESTERSHIRE 79
County Resources 79
Leicester 79
LINCOLNSHIRE 79
County Resources 79
Boston 79
Grantham 79
Lincoln 79
LONDON 79
County Resources 79
London 79
MERSEYSIDE 87
County Resources 87
Birkenhead 87
Liverpool 87
Saint Helens 87
MIDDLESEX 87
Feltham 87
Teddington 87
Twickenham 87
Uxbridge 87
NORFOLK 88
Great Yarmouth 88
King's Lynn 88
Norwich 88
NORTH YORKSHIRE 88
Harrogate 88
Middlesbrough 88
Scarborough 88
York 88
NORTHAMPTONSHIRE 88
County Resources 88
Northampton 89
West Haddon 89
NOTTINGHAMSHIRE 89
County Resources 89
Mansfield 89
Nottingham 89
OXFORDSHIRE 89
County Resources 89
Oxford 89
SHROPSHIRE 90
County Resources 90
Hollinswood 90
Shrewsbury 90
Telford 90
SOMERSET 90
Bridgwater 90
Bristol 90
Burnham-on-Sea 90
Evercreech 90
Taunton 90
SOUTH YORKSHIRE 90
County Resources 90
Sheffield 90
STAFFORDSHIRE 91
County Resources 91
Hanley 91
SUFFOLK 91
County Resources 91
Bury Saint Edmund's 91
Ipswich 91
Lowestoft 91
Woodbridge 91
SURREY 91
Camberley 91
Croydon 91
East Molesley 91

Egham 91
Godlaming 91
Guildford 91
Kew Gardens 91
SUSSEX 91
Chichester 91
Hastings 91
Worthing 92
TEESIDE 92
Stockton-on-Tees 92
TYNE & WEAR 92
Gateshead 92
Newcastle upon Tyne 92
Sunderland 92
WARWICKSHIRE 92
Kenilworth 92
Nuneaton 92
Royal Leamington Spa 92
Stratford-upon-Avon 92
Warwick 92
WEST MIDLANDS 92
County Resources 92
Birmingham 93
Coventry 93
Hockley 93
Solihull 93
Stourbridge 93
Walsall 93
Wolverhampton 94
WEST YORKSHIRE 94
Bradford 94
Halifax 94
Hebden Bridge 94
Huddersfield 94
Leeds 94
Wakefield 94
WILTSHIRE 94
Salisbury 94
Swindon 94

Finland 95

NATIONAL RESOURCES 95
HÄMEEN LÄÄNI 95
Lahti 95
Oulu 95
Tampere 95
KESKISUOMEN LÄÄNI 95
Jyväskylä 95
KUOPION LÄÄNI 96
Kuopio 96
LAPPIN LÄÄNI 96
Rovaniemi 96
OULUN LÄÄNI 96
Oulu 96
POHJOIKARJALAN LÄÄNI 96
Joenssun 96
TURUNPORIN LÄÄNI 96
Turku 96
UUDENMAAN LÄÄNI 96
Helsinki 96
Hyvinkää 97
Oulu 97
VAASAN LÄÄNI 97
Kokkola 97
Vaasa 97

France 97

NATIONAL RESOURCES 97
Aix-en-Provence 97
Alençon 97
Amiens 97
Angers 98
Annecy 98
Antibes 98
Argenteuil 98
Auxerre 98
Beauvais 98
Besançon 98
Béziers 98
Biarritz 98
Blanquefort 98
Bordeaux 98
Boulogne-sur-Mer 98
Brest 99
Caen 99
Cahors 99
Cannes 99
Carcassone 99
Châlons 99
Chambéry 99
Cherbourg 99
Clermont-Ferrand 99
Corse 99
Courcouronnes 99
Créteil 99
Dammarie les Lys 99
Didenheim 99
Dijon 99
Dunkerque 99
Epinal 99
Gap 99
Grenoble 100
Guéret 100
Issy Les Moulineaux 100
La Rochelle 100
Laval 100
Le Mans 100
Lille 100
Limoges 100
Lyon 100
Marseille 101
Meaux 101
Metz 101
Mons 101
Montpellier 101
Montréal La Cluse 101
Mulhouse 101
Nancy 102
Nantes 102
Nice 102
Nîmes 102
Orléans 102
Palaiseau 102
Paris 102
Pau 104
Perpignan 105
Poitiers 105
Poussan 105
Quimper 105
Rennes 105
Riems 105
Rochefort 105
Roissy 105
Rosny sous Bois 105
Rouen 105
Saint Denis 105
Saint Etienne 105
Saint Lô 105
Saint Louis 105
Saint Malo 105
Saint Michel 105
Saintes 106
Soissons 106
Strasbourg 106
Thionville 106
Toulon 106
Toulouse 106
Tours 106

French Guiana 106

Cayenne 106

Germany 106

NATIONAL RESOURCES 107
Aachen 108
Aalen 109
Ahaus 109
Ahlen 109
Allmendingen 109
Altenkirchen 109
Arnsberg 109
Arnstadt 109
Aschaffenberg 109
Augsburg 109
Bamberg 109
Bayreuth 109
Bergkirchen 109
Berlin 109
Bernberg 111
Biberach 111
Biedenkopf 111
Bielefeld 111
Bitterfeld 112
Bocholt 112
Bochum 112
Bonn 112
Bottrop 112
Brandenburg 112
Braunschweig 112
Bremen 113
Bremerhaven 113
Celle 113
Chemnitz 113
Clausthal-Zellerfeld 113
Cottbus 114
Darmstadt 114
Dillenburg 114
Dinslaken 114
Dollnstein 114
Donaueschingen 114
Dortmund 114
Dresden 114
Duisberg 114
Duisburg 114
Düsseldorf 115
Eckernförde 115
Eichstätt 115
Eisenach 115
Elmshorn 115
Emden 116
Erfurt 116
Erlangen 116
Essen 116
Esslingen 116
Finnentrop 116
Flensburg 116
Frankfurt am Main 117
Freiburg 117
Fremdingen 117
Freudstadt 117
Fulda 117
Fürth 118
Gaggenau 118
Geldern 118
Gelnhausen 118
Gelsenkirchen 118
Gera 118
Germersheim 118
Gießen 118
Gladbeck 118
Görlitz 118
Göttingen 118
Greifswald 118
Güdingen 119
Gummersbach 119
Hagen 119
Halberstadt 119
Halle (Saale) 119
Hamburg 119
Hameln 121
Hamm 121
Hannover 121
Hattersheim 122
Heide 122
Heidelberg 122

Heilbronn 122
Herne 122
Hildesheim 122
Hirschhorn 122
Hohenmölsen 122
Holzminden 122
Hoyerswerda 122
Ilmenau 122
Ingolstadt 122
Insel 122
Ispringen 122
Ittlingen 122
Jena 122
Kaarst 123
Kaiserlautern 123
Karlsruhe 123
Kassel 123
Kiel 123
Kitzingen 123
Kleve 123
Koblenz 123
Köln 124
Konstanz 125
Krefeld 125
Lahr 125
Landau 125
Leipzig 125
Leverhusen 125
Limburg 125
Lingen 125
Lübeck 126
Lüdenscheid 126
Ludwigsburg 126
Ludwigshafen 126
Lüneburg 126
Magdeburg 126
Mainz 126
Mannheim 126
Marburg 127
Menden 127
Minden 127
Moers 127
Mölln 127
Mönchengladbach 127
Mülhausen 127
Mülheim 127
München 127
Münster 128
Neubrandenburg 129
Neumünster 129
Neuss 129
Neustadt 129
Neustrelitz 129
Nordhorn 129
Nürnberg 129
Oberhausen 130
Offenbach 130
Offenburg 130
Oldenburg 130
Olpe 130
Osnabrück 130
Paderborn 130
Passau 131
Pforzheim 131
Plauen 131
Potsdam 131
Preetz 131
Putbus 131
Recklinghausen 131
Regensburg 131
Rendsburg 131
Reutlingen 131
Rheine 131
Rosenheim 131
Rostock 131
Rottweil 131
Saarbrücken 132
Salzwedel 132
Schatthausen 132
Schwalmstadt 132
Schwerin 132
Siegen 132
Soest 132
Solingen 132
Stuttgart 132
Suhl 134
Thürmsdorf 134
Trier 134
Troisdorf 134
Tübingen 134
Tuttlingen 134
Uelzen 134
Ulm 134
Unna 134
Viersen 134
Villingen-Schwenningen 134
Weimar 134
Wesel 135
Westerland 135
Wiesbaden 135
Wilhelmshaven 135
Wilnsdorf 135
Witten 135
Wolfsburg 135
Worms 135
Wupperthal 135
Würzburg 135
Zwickau 136

Hong Kong 136
Hong Kong 136

Iceland 136
Reykjavik 136

Ireland 136
NATIONAL RESOURCES **136**
CAVAN **136**
Cavan 136
CORK **136**
County Resources 136
Cork 137
Wilton 137
DUBLIN **137**
County Resources 137
Dublin 137
GALWAY **137**
County Resources 137
Galway 137
KILDARE **138**
Maynooth 138
LIMERICK **138**
County Resources 138
Limerick 138
MEATH **138**
Drogheda 138
TIPPERARY **138**
Clonmel 138
Waterford 138

Israel 138
Tel-Aviv 138

Italy 138
NATIONAL RESOURCES **138**
ABRUZZO **139**
Chieti 139
L'Aquila 139
Pescara 139
Rieti 139
Teramo 139
BASILICATA **139**
Matera 139
Potenza 139
CALABRIA **139**
Catanzaro 139
Cosenza 139
Crotone 140
CAMPANIA **140**
Avellino 140
Capri 140
Caserta 140
Napoli 140
EMILIA ROMAGNA **140**
Bologna 140
Bolzano 140
Ferrara 140
Forli 140
Modena 140
Parma 141
Ravenna 141
Riccione 141
Rimini 141
FRIULI-VENEZIA GIULIA **141**
Gorizia 141
Pordenone 141
Trieste 141
Udine 141
LAZIO **141**
Roma 141
LIGURIA **142**
Genova 142
La Spezia 142
LOMBARDIA **142**
Bergamo 142
Brescia 142
Cremona 142
Milano 142
Pavia 143
Sondrio 143
Varese 143
MARCHE **143**
Ancona 143
Macerata 143
Pesaro 143
MOLISE **143**
Campobasso 143
PIEMONTE **143**
Regional Resources 143
Alessandria 144
Asti 144
Biella 144
Cuneo 144
Torino 144
PUGLIA **144**
Bari 144
Brindisi 144
Foggia 144
Lecce 144
Taranto 145
SARDEGNA **145**
Alghero 145
Cagliari 145
Sassari 145
SICILIA **145**
Caltanissetta 145
Catania 145
Masalucia 145
Messina 145
Palermo 145
Ragusa 145
TOSCANA **145**
Empoli 145
Firenze 145
Pisa 146
Siena 146
TRENTINO **146**
Bolzano 146
Trento 146
UMBRIA **146**
Perugia 146
Terni 146
VALLE D'AOSTA **146**
Aosta 146
VENETO **146**
Belluno 146

Legnano 146
Mestre 146
Padova 146
Rovigo 147
Treviso 147
Venezia 147
Verona 147
Vicenza 147

Japan 147

NAGOYA-SHI 147
Makamura-Ku 147
Mizuho-Ku 147
OSAKA 147
Nishi-Ku 147
TOKYO 147
Adachi-Ku 147
Bunkyo-Ku 147
Kita-Ku 147
Koto-Ku 147
Minato-Ku 148
Shibuya-Ku 148
Shinjuku-Ku 148

Liechtenstein 148

NATIONAL RESOURCES 148

Luxembourg 148

Crauthem 148
Luxembourg 148

Malaysia 148

Kuala Lumpur 148

Martinique 148

Fort-de-France 149

Mexico 149

NATIONAL RESOURCES 149
BAJA CALIFORNIA NORTE 149
Tijuana 149
D. F. 149
Mexico City 149
JALISCO 149
Guadalajara 149
Puebla 149

Namibia 149

Swakopmund 149
Windhoek 149

The Netherlands 149

NATIONAL RESOURCES 150
Aalsmeer 151
Akmaar 151
Alkmaar 151
Almelo 151
Amstelveen 151
Amsterdam 151
Apeldoorn 153
Arnhem 153
Baarle Nassau 154
Bergen op Zoom 154
Breda 154
Bussum 154
Capelle a/d Ijssel 154
Delft 154
Delfzijl 154
Den Haag 154
Den Helder 154
Doetinchem 154
Dordrecht 154
Eindhoven 155
Emmen 155
Enschede 155
Gemert 155
Gorinchem 155
Gouda 155
Groningen 155
Haarlem 155
Heereveen 156
Heerlen 156
Hendrik Ido Ambacht 156
Hertogenbosch, 's / Den Bosch 156
Hilversum 156
Hoogeveen 156
Hoogland 156
Hoorn 156
Leeuwarden 156
Leiden 156
Maastricht 156
Middleburg 156
Nieuw-Vennep 156
Nijmegen 156
Oss 157
Pijnakker 157
Renkum 157
Roermund 157
Roosendaal 157
Rotterdam 157
Terheijden 158
Terneuzen 158
Tiel 158
Tilburg 158
Uden 158
Uithoorn 158
Utrecht 158
Valkenswaard 158
Veghel 158
Venlo 158
Venray 158
Vlissingen 159
Voorburg 159
Wageningen 159
Weert 159
Woerden 159
Zoetermeer 159
Zwolle 159

New Zealand 159

NATIONAL RESOURCES 159
Auckland 160
Blenheim 161
Christchurch 161
Dunedin 161
Gisborne 162
Hamilton 162
Hastings 162
Invercargill 162
Kapiti / Horowhenua 162
Napier 162
Nelson 162
Palmerston North 162
Rotorua 163
Tauranga 163
Timaru 163
Wellington 163
Whangarei 163

Northern Ireland 163

NATIONAL RESOURCES 163
ANTRIM 164
Belfast 164
LONDONDERRY 164
Derry 164

Norway 164

NATIONAL RESOURCES 164
AKERSHUS 164
Hebekk 164
Oslo 164
BUSKERUD 165
Drammen 165
Hønefoss 165
Kongsberg 165
FINNMARK 165
Kirkenes 165
HEDMARK 165
Hamar 165
HORDALAND 165
Bergen 165
MØRE OG ROMSDAL 165
Ålesund 165
Kristiansund 165
Molde 165
NORDLAND 165
Bodø 165
Mo 165
Rana 165
OPPLAND 165
Gjøvik 165
Lillehammer 165
ØSTFOLD 165
Fredrikstad 165
Moss 166
ROGALAND 166
Sandnes 166
Sogndal 166
Stavanger 166
SOGN OG FJORDANE 166
Førde 166
SØR TRONDELAG 166
Trandheim 166
Tromdheim 166
Trondheim 166
TROMS 166
Tromsø 166
VEST-AGDER 166
Kristiansand 166
VESTFOLD 166
Larvik 166
Sandefjord 166
Tønsberg 167

Portugal 167

NATIONAL RESOURCES 167
Lisboa 167

Puerto Rico 167

San Juan 167

Scotland 167

NATIONAL RESOURCES 167
BORDERS 167
County Resources 167
CENTRAL 167
Stirling 167
DUMFRIES & GALLOWAY 167
County Resources 167
FIFE 168
Buckhaven 168
Kirkcaldy 168
Saint Andew's 168
GRAMPIAN 168
Aberdeen 168
Lumphanan 168
HIGHLAND 168
Inverness 168
Wick 168
LOTHIAN 168
Edinburgh 168
STRATHCLYDE 169
County Resources 169
Ayr 169
Glasgow 169
Greenock 170
Paisley 170
TAYSIDE 170
Dundee 170
Perth 170

South Africa 170

NATIONAL RESOURCES 170
CAPE PROVINCE 170
Cape Town 170
East London 171
Johannesburg 171
Kimberly 171
NATAL 171
Durban 171
Pietermaritzburg 171
ORANGE FREE STATE 171
Bloemfontein 171
TRANSVAAL 171
Johannesburg 171
Pretoria 172

Spain 172

NATIONAL RESOURCES 172
Barcelona 172
Madrid 172
Zaragoza 172

Sweden 172

NATIONAL RESOURCES 173
BOHUSLÄN 173
Göteborg 173
BORG 173
Alingsås 173
DALARNA 173
Falun 173
GÄSTRIKLAND 173
Gävle 173
GOTLAND 173
Visby 173
HALLAND 173
Halmstad 173
JÄMTLAND 173
Östersund 173
MALMÖHUS IÄN 173
Malmö 173
MEDELPAD 174
Sundsvall 174
NARKE 174
Örebro 174
NORRBOTTEN 174
Luleå 174
Piteå 174
ÖSTERGÖTLAND 174
Linköping 174
Norrköping 174
SKÅNE 174
Helsingborg 174
Karlstad 174
Lund 174
SMÅLAND 175
Jönköping 175
Växjö 175
SÖDERMANLAND 175
Eskilstuna 175
Nyköping 175
STOCKHOLM 175
Regional Resources 175
Stockholm 175
UPPLAND 176
Uppsala 176
VÄRMLAND 176
Karlstad 176
VÄSTERBOTTEN 176
Skellefteå 176
Umeå 176
VÄSTERGÖTLAND 176
Borås 176
Trollhättan 176
VÄSTMANLANDS IÄN 176
Västerås 176

Switzerland 176

NATIONAL RESOURCES 176
Aarau 177
Baden 177
Basel / Bâle 177
Bern 177
Berne 178
Biel 178
Chur 178
Frauenfeld 178
Fribourg / Freiburg 178
Genève / Genf 178
Hinwil 178
Lausanne 178
Liestal 178
Lugano 178
Luzern / Lucerne 178
Mammern 178
Neuchâtel / Neuenburg 178
Neuenhof 178
Rothrist 178
Saint Gallen 179
Saint Moritz 179
Schaffhausen 179
Sion 179
Solothurn 179
Ticino 179
Viganello 179
Visp 179
Winterthur 179
Zug 179
Zürich 179

Turkey 180

Istanbul 180

U.S.A. 180

NATIONAL RESOURCES 180
ALABAMA 191
State Resources 191
Anniston 191
Auburn 191
Birmingham 191
Florence 191
Hoover 191
Huntsville 191
Mobile 192
Montgomery 192
Pelham 192
Tuscaloosa 192
ALASKA 192
Anchorage 192
Chugiak 193
Juneau 193
ARIZONA 193
State Resources 193
Chloride 193
Clarkdale 193
Flagstaff 193
Phœnix 193
Saint Paul 194
Tempe 194
Texarkana 194
Tucson 194
ARKANSAS 195
State Resources 195
Avoca 195
El Dorado 195
Fayetteville 195
Jonesboro 195
Little Rock 195
North Little Rock 196
CALIFORNIA 196
State Resources 196
Agnew 196
Agoura Hills 196
Albany 196
Alpine 196
Arcata 196
Auburn 196
Bakersfield 196
Ben Lomand 196
Berkeley 196
Beverly Hills 197
Buena Park 197
Burbank 197
Camarillo 197
Canoga Park 197
Cathedral City 198
Chico 198
Chula Vista 198
Claremont San Dimas 198
Compton 198
Concord 198
Corona 198
Corte Madera 198
Culver City 198
Cypress 198
Daly City 198
Danville 198
Davis 199
Desert Hot Springs 199
El Cajon 199
El Cerrito 199
El Toro 199
Emeryville 199
Encino 199
Escondido 199
Eureka 199
Fairfield 199
Forestville 199
Fort Bragg 199
Fountain Valley 199
Fresno 199
Fullerton 200
Garden Grove 200
Glendale 200
Gualala 200
Guernville 200
Hawthorne 200
Hayward 201
Healdsburg 201
Hollywood 201
Huntington Beach 201
Irvine 201
Jenner 201
Laguna Beach 201
Lake Tahoe 202
Lakewood 202
Laytonville 202
Livermore 202
Long Beach 202
Los Angeles 203
Marina Del Rey 206
Mendocino 206
Menlo Park 206
Mill Valley 206
Milpitas 206
Mission Hills 206
Modesto 206
Monrovia 206
Mountain View 206
Napa 207
Newport Beach 207
North Hollywood 207
Oakland 207
Orange 208
Pacific Beach 208
Pacific Grove 208
Pacifica 208
Palm Springs 208
Palmdale 209
Palo Alto 209
Pasadena 209
Petaluma 209
Pomona 209
Redwood City 209
Riverside 209
Sacramento 209

San Anselmo 210
San Bernardino 210
San Diego 210
San Dimas 212
San Francisco 212
San José 219
San Juan Capistrano 220
San Luis Obispo 220
San Marcos 220
San Mateo 220
San Rafael 220
Santa Ana 221
Santa Barbara 221
Santa Clara 221
Santa Cruz 221
Santa Monica 222
Santa Rosa 222
Santee 222
Seal Beach 222
Sonora 222
Soquel 222
Stanford 222
Stockton 222
Studio City 223
Sunnyvale 223
Sylmar 223
Tarzana 223
Topanga 223
Travis 223
Tucson 223
Tujunga 223
Tulare 223
Tustin 223
Ukiah 223
Universal City 223
Upland 224
Valencia 224
Vallejo 224
Valley Village 224
Van Nuys 224
Ventura 224
Victorville 224
Visalia 224
Walnut Creek 224
Walnut 224
West Hollywood 224
Whittier 225
Woodland Hills 225
Yorba Linda 226
COLORADO **226**
State Resources 226
Arvada 226
Aspen 226
Aurora 226
Boulder 226
Colorado Springs 226
Denver 227
Durango 229
Englewood 229
Fort Collins 229
Grand Junction 229
Greeley 229
Lakewood 229
Thornton 229
CONNECTICUT **229**
State Resources 229
Bridgeport 229
Bristol 229
Colchester 230
Danbury 230
Darien 230
Dayville 230
East Hartford 230
Enfield 230
Fairfield 230
Greenwich 230
Haddam 230
Hartford 230
Manchester 231
Meriden 231
Middletown 231
New Britain 231
New Haven 231
New London 231
New Preston 232
Norwich 232
Rocky Hill 232
South Windsor 232
Southington 232
Stamford 232
Thompson 232
Torrington 232
Trumbull 232
Unionville 232
Waterbury 232
Weston 232
Willimantic 232
Windsor 232
DELAWARE **232**
Claymont 232
Newark 232
Rehoboth Beach 233
Willmington 233
Wilmington 233
DISTRICT OF COLUMBIA **233**
State Resources 233
Washington 233
FLORIDA **235**
State Resources 235
Aventura 235
Boca Raton 235
Bradenton 236
Brandon 236
Cape Coral 236
Clearwater 236
Coral Springs 236
Crystal Springs 236
Daytona 236
Fort Lauderdale 236
Fort Myers 237
Fort Pierce 237
Gainesville 237
Hernando 237
Hollywood 237
Jacksonville 238
Key West 238
Lakeland 238
Land 'O Lakes 238
Largo 238
Lithis 238
Lutz 238
Margate 238
Miami 238
Miami Beach 239
Naples 239
North Miami Beach 240
Ocala 240
Olaca 240
Orlando 240
Panama City 241
Pensacola 241
Pompano Beach 241
Saint Petersburg 241
Sarasota 241
South Beach 242
Sunrise 242
Tallahassee 242
Tampa 242
West Palm Beach 243
Winter Park 243
Zephyrs Hills 243
GEORGIA **243**
State Resources 243
Athens 243
Atlanta 243
Buford 245
Decatur 245
Doraville 245
Lithonia 245
Macon 245
Marietta 245
Norcross 245
Rosewell 246
Savannah 246
Valdosta 246
HAWAII **246**
State Resources 246
Hawaii (Big Island) 246
Maui 246
Oahu 246
IDAHO **247**
State Resources 247
Boise 247
Caldwell 247
Moscow 247
Pocatello 247
ILLINOIS **247**
Alton 247
Arlington Heights 247
Aurora 248
Belleville 248
Bloomington 248
Carbondale 248
Champaign / Urbana 248
Chicago 248
De Kalb 252
Des Plaines 252
Edwardsville 252
Galesburg 252
Glen Ellyn 252
Highland Park 252
Lake Bluff 252
Lake Villa 252
Monticello 252
Peoria 252
Riverside 252
Rock Island 253
Rockford 253
South Bend 253
Springfield 253
Villa Park 253
Washington 253
Wheaton 253
Winfield 253
Winnetka 253
Wood Dale 253
Woodridge 253
INDIANA **253**
State Resources 253
Bloomington 253
Eldridge 254
Evansville 254
Fishers 254
Fort Wayne 254
Goshen 254
Greenwood 254
Indianapolis 254
Lafayette 255
Michigan City 255
Mishawaka 255
Muncie 255
Richmond 255
South Bend 255
Terre Haute 255
IOWA **255**
State Resources 255
Ames 256
Cedar Rapids 256
Council Bluffs 256
Davenport 256
Des Moines 256
Dubuque 256
Evansdale 256
Grinnell 256
Iowa City 256
Iowa Falls 257
Mason City 257
Mount Vernon 257
Waterloo 257

KANSAS **257**
State Resources 257
Kansas City 257
Kechi 257
Lawrence 257
Leavenworth 258
Lindsborg 258
Manhattan 258
Overland Park 258
Shawnee Mission 258
Topeka 258
Wichita 258
KENTUCKY **258**
State Resources 258
Bowling Green 258
Lexington 259
Louisville 259
Newport 259
Owensboro 260
LOUISIANA **260**
State Resources 260
Alexandria 260
Baton Rouge 260
Gretna 260
Lafayette 260
Lake Charles 260
Monroe 260
New Orleans 260
Shreveport 261
Thibodaux 261
MAINE **261**
State Resources 261
Auburn 262
Augusta 262
Bangor 262
Biddleford 262
Brunswick 262
Damariscotta 262
East Waterboro 262
Ellsworth 262
Gardiner 262
Hallowell 262
Lewiston 262
Portland 262
Waterville 263
MARYLAND **263**
State Resources 263
Annapolis 263
Baltimore 263
Bethesda 265
Charlestown 265
Chicopee 265
College Park 265
Columbia 265
Deer Park 265
Fort Meade 265
Frederick 265
Gaithersburg 265
Glen Burnie 265
Greenbelt 265
Hyattsville 265
Langley Park 265
Lanham 265
Laurel 265
Rockville 266
Salisbury 266
Silver Spring 266
Temple Hills 266
Walkersville 266
Wheaton 266
MASSACHUSETTS **266**
State Resources 266
Allston 266
Amherst 266
Andover 267
Attleboro Falls 267
Avon 267
Belmont Center 267
Boston 267
Boylston 270
Bridgewater 270
Burlington 270
Charlestown 270
Dennisport 270
Dorchester 270
East Dedham 270
Framingham 270
Gloucester 270
Great Barrington 270
Greenfield 270
Hadley 270
Haverhill 271
Lowell 271
Malden 271
Marblehead 271
Marlborough 271
Medfield 271
Middleboro 271
Millis 271
Natick 271
Needham Heights 271
Newburyport 271
Newton Centre 271
Nonantum 271
Northampton 271
Orleans 272
Palmer 272
Pittsfield 272
Provincetown 272
Randolph 272
Shawseen 272
Springfield 272
Swansea 272
Thorndike 272
Vineyard Haven 272
Waltham 273
Watertown 273
Wayland 273
West Medford 273
West Newton 273
Westford 273
Weymouth 273
Williamstown 273
Woburn 273
Worcester 273
MICHIGAN **273**
State Resources 273
Allendale 274
Ann Arbor 274
Bay City 274
Benton Harbor 274
Berkeley 274
Chelsea 274
Dearborn 274
Detroit 274
Dexter 275
Douglas 275
Dowagiac 275
East Landing 275
Ferndale 275
Flint 275
Grand Rapids 276
Holland 276
Jackson 276
Kalamazoo 276
Keego Harbor 276
Lansing 277
Livonia 277
Madison Heights 277
Marquette 277
Mount Morris 277
Mount Pleasant 277
Muskegon 277
New Baltimore 277
Novi 277
Petosky 277
Pontiac 277
Portage 277
Redford 278
Royal Oak 278
Saginaw 278
Saline 278
Southfield 278
Southgate 278
Traverse City 278
Warren 278
Ypsilanti 278
MINNESOTA **278**
State Resources 278
Albert Lea 279
Brooklyn Center 279
Concord 279
Duluth 279
Eagan 279
Eden Prairie 279
Mankato 279
Marsall 279
Minneapolis / Saint Paul 279
Moorhead 281
Northfield 281
Reno 281
Rochester 281
Saint Cloud 282
Waseca 282
Winona 282
MISSISSIPI **282**
State Resources 282
Biloxi 282
Greenville 282
Hattiesburg 282
Jackson 282
MISSOURI **282**
State Resources 282
Ava 282
Cape Giradeau 282
Columbia 283
Ferguson 283
Independence 283
Kansas City 283
Marceline 284
Saint Charles 284
Saint Louis 284
Springfield 284
Wentzville 285
MONTANA **285**
State Resources 285
Billings 285
Bozeman 285
Butte 285
Missoula 285
NEBRASKA **285**
State Resources 285
Lincoln 285
Omaha 285
NEVADA **286**
State Resources 286
Henderson 286
Las Vegas 286
Reno 287
Sparks 287
NEW HAMPSHIRE **287**
State Resources 287
Amherst 287
Bartlet 287
Campton 287
Concord 287
Conway 287
Durham 287
Francestown 287
Hanover 287
Keene 287
Manchester 288
Merrimack 288
Nashua 288
Plymouth 288
Portsmouth 288
Salem 288
Sanbornville 288
Weirs Beach 288
West Franklin 288

NEW JERSEY	**288**
State Resources	288
Asbury Park	289
Atlantic City	289
Berlin	289
Blackwood	289
Blairstown	289
Brick	289
Brick Town	289
Bridgewater	290
Butler	290
Chatham	290
Cherry Hill	290
Denville	290
Dover	290
Dunellen	290
East Rutherford	290
Edison	290
Egg Harbor City	290
Fort Lee	290
Hackensack	290
Hawthorne	290
Highland	290
Hoboken	290
Howell	290
Huntington	290
Irvington	290
Jersey City	290
Linden	291
Lyndhurst	291
Mays Landing	291
Metuchen	291
Middlesex	291
Millburn	291
Montclair	291
Moorestown	291
Morristown	291
Neptune	291
New Brunswick	291
New Providence	292
Newark	292
North Bergen	292
North Brunswick	292
North Haledon	292
Oakland	292
Piscataway	292
Plainfield	292
Princeton	292
Red Bank	292
River Edge	292
Roselle	292
Sewell	293
Somerville	293
Stone Harbor	293
Sussex	293
Teaneck	293
Titusville	293
Toms River	293
Trenton	293
Union City	293
Washington Township	293
Wayne	293
Westmount	293
Wildwood	293
Woodbridge	293
Woodcliff Lake	293
NEW MEXICO	**293**
State Resources	293
Albuquerque	294
Clovis	294
Las Cruces	294
Santa Fe	295
Serafina	295
Taos	295
Tesuque	295
University Park	295
NEW YORK	**295**
State Resources	295
Albany	295
Amityville	296
Annandale on Hudson	296
Babylon	296
Bay Shore	296
Bayside	296
Binghamton	296
Brentwood	297
Bronx	297
Brooklyn	297
Buffalo	298
Centereach	298
Chatham	298
Coram	298
Cortland	298
Deer Park	299
East Hampton	299
East Meadow	299
East Setauket	299
Elmhurst	299
Elmira	299
Fairport	299
Far Rockaway	299
Fayetteville	299
Forest Hills	299
Fredonia	299
Great Neck	299
Hampstead	299
Huntington Station	299
Island Park	299
Ithaca	299
Kingston	299
Mattydale	299
Nassau	299
New Paltz	299
New York	300
Niagara Falls	310
Oneonta	310
Oswego	310
Pelham	310
Plattsburgh	310
Port Chester	310
Potsdam	310
Poughkeepsie	310
Rego Park	310
Rochester	310
Ronkonkoma	311
Saranac Lake	311
Saratoga Springs	311
Schenectady	311
Stony Brook	311
Syracuse	312
Teaneck	312
Troy	312
Utica	312
Vestal	312
Webster	312
Williamsville	312
Woodside	312
Woodstock	312
NORTH CAROLINA	**313**
State Resources	313
Asheville	313
Boone	313
Chapel Hill	313
Charlotte	313
Dallas	314
Durham	314
Fayetteville	315
Flat Rock	315
Gastonia	315
Greensboro	315
Hickory	315
Raleigh	315
Ramseur	316
Salisbury	316
Sanford	316
Wilmington	316
Winston-Salem	316
NORTH DAKOTA	**316**
Fargo	316
Grand Forks	317
Minot	317
OHIO	**317**
State Resources	317
Akron	317
Ashland	317
Athens	317
Bowling Green	317
Cincinnati	317
Cleveland	318
Columbus	319
Dayton	321
Euclid	321
Greenville	321
Ironton	321
Kent	321
Lakewood	321
Leipsic	321
Lima	321
Lorain	321
Mansfield	322
Marion	322
Mentor	322
Oberlin	322
Oxford	322
Parma	322
Reynoldsburg	322
Sheffield Lake	322
Springfield	322
Steubenville	322
Toledo	322
Yellow Springs	322
Youngstown	322
OKLAHOMA	**322**
State Resources	323
Lawton	323
Muskogee	323
Oklahoma City	323
Tulsa	323
OREGON	**324**
State Resources	324
Aloha	324
Ashland / Medford	324
Astoria	324
Baker City	324
Bend	324
Central Point	324
Clackamas	324
Coos Bay	325
Corvallis	325
Eugene	325
Klamath Falls	325
La Grande	325
Lake Oswego	325
Newport	325
Pacific City	326
Portland	326
Roseburg	327
Salem	327
Springfield	327
PENNSYLVANIA	**327**
State Resources	327
Allentown	327
Altoona	327
Bensalem	327
Blacklick	328
Bryn Mawr	328
Buckingham	328
Carlisle	328
Castle Shannon	328
Clarion	328
Easton	328
Edinboro	328
Erie	328
Gettysburg	328
Harrisburg	328
Havertown	328
Huntington Valley	328
Jenkintown	329
King of Prussia	329
Lancaster	329

Lansdowne 329
Lehigh Valley 329
Levittown 329
Lewisburg 329
Malvern 329
Meadville 329
Morrisville 329
New Hope 329
Norristown 329
Philadelphia 329
Pittsburgh 331
Pocono Summit 332
Reading 333
State College 333
Stroudsburg / Poconos 333
Tionesta 333
Wayne 333
West Chester 333
West Point 333
Wilkes-Barre 333
Williamsport 333
Willow Grove 333
York 333
RHODE ISLAND 334
State Resources 334
East Greenwich 334
East Providence 334
Kingston 334
Providence 334
Riverside 334
SOUTH CAROLINA 334
State Resources 334
Aiken 334
Charleston 334
Clemson 335
Columbia 335
Greenville 335
Greenwood 335
North Augusta 335
Pawleys Island 335
Spartanburg 335
West Columbia 335
SOUTH DAKOTA 335
State Resources 335
Brookings 335
Hill City 335
Rapid City 335
Sioux Falls 336
TENNESSEE 336
State Resources 336
Brentwood 336
Chattanooga 336
Cookeville 336
Johnson City 336
Kingsport 336
Knoxville 336
Lavergne 336
Liberty 336
Memphis 336
Millington 337
Murfreesboro 337
Nashville 337
Saint Bethlehem 338
Woodlawn 338
TEXAS 338
State Resources 338
Abilene 338
Amarillo 338
Arlington 338
Austin 338
Bellaire 339
Bryan 339
Bulverde 339
College Station 339
Corpus Christi 339
Dallas / Fort Worth 339
Del Valle 341
Denton 341
El Paso 341
Galveston 342
Helotes 342
Houston 342
Huntsville 343
Irving 343
Jersey Village 343
Lewisville 343
Longview 343
Lubbock 344
Manchaca 344
Merkel 344
New Waverly 344
Richland Hills 344
Rosebud 344
San Angelo 344
San Antonio 344
Tyler 344
Waco 345
Wichita Falls 345
UTAH 345
State Resources 345
Logan 345
Midvale 345
Orem 345
Park City 345
Pleasant Grove 345
Salt Lake City 345
VERMONT 345
State Resources 346
Bennington 346
Brattleboro 346
Burlington 346
Manchester Center 346
Montpelier 346
Plainfield 346
Rutland 346
Saint Albans 346
Saint Johnsbury 346
Worcester 346
VIRGINIA 346
State Resources 347
Alexandria 347
Annandale 347
Arlington 347
Blacksburg 347
Charlottesville 347
Chesapeake 348
Danville 348
Denbigh 348
Fairfax 348
Falls Church 348
Fredericksburg 348
Gloucester Point 348
Lynchburg 348
Newport News 348
Norfolk 348
Radford 348
Richmond 349
Roanoke 349
Springfield 349
Staunton 349
Tysons Corner 349
Virginia Beach 349
Williamsburg 349
Woodbridge 350
Woodstock 350
WASHINGTON 350
State Resources 350
Belleview 350
Bellingham 350
Chehalis 350
Everett 350
Kirkland 350
Montesano 350
Mount Vernon 350
Olympia 350
Pullman 350
Seattle 350
South Renton 353
Spokane 354
Tacoma 354
Vancouver 354
Walla Walla 354
Wenatchee 354
Yakima 354
WEST VIRGINIA 354
State Resources 354
Berkeley Springs 354
Charleston 354
Dunbar 354
Huntington 354
Martinsburg 355
Morgantown 355
Parkersburg 355
Shepherdstown 355
Wheeling 355
WISCONSIN 355
State Resources 355
Ashland 355
Beloit 355
Cazenovia 355
Fox Valley 355
Green Bay 356
Janesville 356
La Crosse 356
Madison 356
Menasha 356
Milwaukee 356
Portage 357
Racine 358
Rhinelander 358
River Falls 358
Sheboygan 358
Stevens Point 358
Superior 358
Waukesha 358
Wausau 358
West Allis 358
Whitewater 358
WYOMING 358
Casper 358
Jackson 358
Laramie 358

Wales 358

NATIONAL RESOURCES 359
CLWYD 359
Wrexham 359
DYFED 359
Aberystwyth 359
Carmarthen 359
GLAMORGAN 359
Cardiff 359
Swansea 359
GWENT 359
Newport 359
Trellech 359
GWYNEDD 359
Bangor 359
POWYS 359
Llandrindod Wells 359
Welshpool 359

Index of Place Names

Aachen, Germany 🕮 108
Aalen, Germany 🕮 109
Aalsmeer, The Netherlands 🕮 151
Aalst / Alost, Belgium 🕮 36
Aarau, Switzerland 🕮 177
Aberdeen, Scotland 🕮 168
Aberystwyth, Wales 🕮 359
Abilene, U.S.A. 🕮 338
Abruzzo, Italy 🕮 139
Adachi-Ku, Japan 🕮 147
Adelaide, Australia 🕮 30
Agnew, U.S.A. 🕮 196
Agoura Hills, U.S.A. 🕮 196
Ahaus, Germany 🕮 109
Ahlen, Germany 🕮 109
Aiken, U.S.A. 🕮 334
Aix-en-Provence, France 🕮 97
Akershus, Norway 🕮 164
Akmaar, The Netherlands 🕮 151
Akron, U.S.A. 🕮 317
Alabama, U.S.A. 🕮 191
Alaska, U.S.A. 🕮 192
Albany, U.S.A. 🕮 196, 295
Albert Lea, U.S.A. 🕮 279
Alberta, Canada 🕮 42
Ålborg, Denmark 🕮 65
Albuquerque, U.S.A. 🕮 294
Albury, Australia 🕮 25
Alençon, France 🕮 97
Alessandria, Italy 🕮 144
Ålesund, Norway 🕮 165
Alexandria, U.S.A. 🕮 260, 347
Alghero, Italy 🕮 145
Alice Springs, Australia 🕮 28
Alingsås, Sweden 🕮 173
Alkmaar, The Netherlands 🕮 151
Allendale, U.S.A. 🕮 274
Allentown, U.S.A. 🕮 327
Allmendingen, Germany 🕮 109
Allston, U.S.A. 🕮 266
Almelo, The Netherlands 🕮 151
Aloha, U.S.A. 🕮 324
Alpine, U.S.A. 🕮 196
Altenkirchen, Germany 🕮 109
Alton, U.S.A. 🕮 247
Altoona, U.S.A. 🕮 327
Amarillo, U.S.A. 🕮 338
Ames, U.S.A. 🕮 256
Amherst, U.S.A. 🕮 266, 287
Amiens, France 🕮 97
Amityville, U.S.A. 🕮 296
Amstelveen, The Netherlands 🕮 151
Amsterdam, The Netherlands 🕮 151
Anchorage, U.S.A. 🕮 192
Ancona, Italy 🕮 143
Andover, England 🕮 76
Andover, U.S.A. 🕮 267
Angers, France 🕮 98
Ann Arbor, U.S.A. 🕮 274
Annandale on Hudson, U.S.A. 🕮 296
Annandale, U.S.A. 🕮 347
Annapolis, U.S.A. 🕮 263
Annecy, France 🕮 98
Annerley, Australia 🕮 28
Anniston, U.S.A. 🕮 191
Antibes, France 🕮 98
Antrim, Northern Ireland 🕮 164
Antwerpen / Anvers, Belgium 🕮 36
Aosta, Italy 🕮 146
Apeldoorn, The Netherlands 🕮 153
Arcata, U.S.A. 🕮 196
Argenteuil, France 🕮 98
Århus, Denmark 🕮 65
Arizona, U.S.A. 🕮 193
Arkansas, U.S.A. 🕮 195
Arlington Heights, U.S.A. 🕮 247
Arlington, U.S.A. 🕮 338, 347
Armidale, Australia 🕮 25
Arnhem, The Netherlands 🕮 153
Arnsberg, Germany 🕮 109
Arnstadt, Germany 🕮 109
Arvada, U.S.A. 🕮 226
Asbury Park, U.S.A. 🕮 289
Aschaffenberg, Germany 🕮 109
Asheville, U.S.A. 🕮 313
Ashford, England 🕮 78
Ashland / Medford, U.S.A. 🕮 324
Ashland, U.S.A. 🕮 317, 355
Aspen, U.S.A. 🕮 226
Asti, Italy 🕮 144
Astoria, U.S.A. 🕮 324
Athelstan, Canada 🕮 61
Athens, U.S.A. 🕮 243, 317
Atlanta, U.S.A. 🕮 243
Atlantic City, U.S.A. 🕮 289
Attleboro Falls, U.S.A. 🕮 267
Auburn, U.S.A. 🕮 191, 196, 262
Auckland, New Zealand 🕮 160
Augsburg, Germany 🕮 109
Augusta, U.S.A. 🕮 262
Aurora, U.S.A. 🕮 226, 248
Austin, U.S.A. 🕮 338
Australia 🕮 24
Australian Capital Territory, Australia 🕮 25
Austria 🕮 34
Auxerre, France 🕮 98
Ava, U.S.A. 🕮 282
Avellino, Italy 🕮 140
Aventura, U.S.A. 🕮 235
Avoca, U.S.A. 🕮 195
Avon, England 🕮 70
Avon, U.S.A. 🕮 267
Ayr, Scotland 🕮 169
Baarle Nassau, The Netherlands 🕮 154
Babylon, U.S.A. 🕮 296
Baden, Switzerland 🕮 177
Baja California Norte, Mexico 🕮 149
Baker City, U.S.A. 🕮 324
Bakersfield, U.S.A. 🕮 196
Baltimore, U.S.A. 🕮 263
Bamberg, Germany 🕮 109
Banff, Canada 🕮 42
Bangor, U.S.A. 🕮 262
Bangor, Wales 🕮 359
Barcelona, Spain 🕮 172
Bari, Italy 🕮 144
Barnstaple, England 🕮 73
Barrie, Canada 🕮 49
Bartlet, U.S.A. 🕮 287
Basel / Bâle, Switzerland 🕮 177
Basildon, England 🕮 74
Basilicata, Italy 🕮 139
Bath, England 🕮 70
Baton Rouge, U.S.A. 🕮 260
Bay City, U.S.A. 🕮 274
Bay Shore, U.S.A. 🕮 296
Bayreuth, Germany 🕮 109
Bayside, U.S.A. 🕮 296
Beaconsfield, Canada 🕮 61
Beauvais, France 🕮 98
Bedford, England 🕮 70
Bedfordshire, England 🕮 70
Belfast, Northern Ireland 🕮 164
Belgium 🕮 35
Bellaire, U.S.A. 🕮 339
Belleview, U.S.A. 🕮 350
Belleville, Canada 🕮 49
Belleville, U.S.A. 🕮 248
Bellingham, U.S.A. 🕮 350
Belluno, Italy 🕮 146
Belmont Center, U.S.A. 🕮 267
Beloit, U.S.A. 🕮 355
Ben Lomand, U.S.A. 🕮 196
Bend, U.S.A. 🕮 324
Bendigo, Australia 🕮 31
Bennington, U.S.A. 🕮 346
Bensalem, U.S.A. 🕮 327
Bentley, Australia 🕮 33
Benton Harbor, U.S.A. 🕮 274
Bergamo, Italy 🕮 142
Bergen op Zoom, The Netherlands 🕮 154
Bergen, Norway 🕮 165
Bergkirchen, Germany 🕮 109
Berkeley Springs, U.S.A. 🕮 354
Berkeley, U.S.A. 🕮 196, 274
Berkshire, England 🕮 71
Berlin, Germany 🕮 109
Berlin, U.S.A. 🕮 289
Bern, Switzerland 🕮 177
Bernberg, Germany 🕮 111
Berne, Switzerland 🕮 178
Besançon, France 🕮 98
Beswick, England 🕮 75
Bethesda, U.S.A. 🕮 265
Beverly Hills, U.S.A. 🕮 197
Béziers, France 🕮 98
Biarritz, France 🕮 98
Biberach, Germany 🕮 111
Biddleford, U.S.A. 🕮 262
Biedenkopf, Germany 🕮 111
Biel, Switzerland 🕮 178
Bielefeld, Germany 🕮 111
Biella, Italy 🕮 144
Billings, U.S.A. 🕮 285
Biloxi, U.S.A. 🕮 282
Binghamton, U.S.A. 🕮 296
Birkenhead, England 🕮 87
Birmingham, England 🕮 93
Birmingham, U.S.A. 🕮 191
Bitterfeld, Germany 🕮 112
Blacklick, U.S.A. 🕮 328
Blackpool, England 🕮 78
Blacksburg, U.S.A. 🕮 347
Blackwood, U.S.A. 🕮 289
Blairstown, U.S.A. 🕮 289
Blanquefort, France 🕮 98
Blenheim, New Zealand 🕮 161
Bloemfontein, South Africa 🕮 171
Bloomington, U.S.A. 🕮 248, 253
Boca Raton, U.S.A. 🕮 235
Bocholt, Germany 🕮 112
Bochum, Germany 🕮 112
Bodø, Norway 🕮 165
Bohuslän, Sweden 🕮 173
Boise, U.S.A. 🕮 247
Bologna, Italy 🕮 140
Bolton, England 🕮 78
Bolzano, Italy 🕮 140, 146
Bonfield, Canada 🕮 49
Bonn, Germany 🕮 112
Boone, U.S.A. 🕮 313
Borås, Sweden 🕮 176
Bordeaux, France 🕮 98
Borders, Scotland 🕮 167
Borg, Sweden 🕮 173
Boston, England 🕮 79
Boston, U.S.A. 🕮 267
Bottrop, Germany 🕮 112
Boulder, U.S.A. 🕮 226
Boulogne-sur-Mer, France 🕮 98
Bournemouth, England 🕮 73
Bowling Green, U.S.A. 🕮 258, 317
Boylston, U.S.A. 🕮 270
Bozeman, U.S.A. 🕮 285
Bradenton, U.S.A. 🕮 236
Bradford, England 🕮 94
Braintree, England 🕮 75

Brandenburg, Germany 🕮 112
Brandon, Canada 🕮 47
Brandon, U.S.A. 🕮 236
Brattleboro, U.S.A. 🕮 346
Braunschweig, Germany 🕮 112
Brazil 🕮 39
Breda, The Netherlands 🕮 154
Bregenz, Austria 🕮 34
Bremen, Germany 🕮 113
Bremerhaven, Germany 🕮 113
Brentwood, U.S.A. 🕮 297, 336
Brescia, Italy 🕮 142
Brest, France 🕮 99
Brick Town, U.S.A. 🕮 289
Brick, U.S.A. 🕮 289
Bridgeport, U.S.A. 🕮 229
Bridgewater, U.S.A. 🕮 270, 290
Bridgwater, England 🕮 90
Bridlington, England 🕮 77
Brighton, England 🕮 74
Brindisi, Italy 🕮 144
Brisbane, Australia 🕮 28
Bristol, England 🕮 70, 90
Bristol, U.S.A. 🕮 229
British Columbia, Canada 🕮 44
Broenshoej, Denmark 🕮 65
Bronx, U.S.A. 🕮 297
Brookings, U.S.A. 🕮 335
Brooklyn Center, U.S.A. 🕮 279
Brooklyn, U.S.A. 🕮 297
Brunswick, U.S.A. 🕮 262
Bruxelles / Brussel, Belgium 🕮 36
Bryan, U.S.A. 🕮 339
Bryn Mawr, U.S.A. 🕮 328
Buckhaven, Scotland 🕮 168
Buckhurst Hill, England 🕮 75
Buckingham, U.S.A. 🕮 328
Buckinghamshire, England 🕮 71
Buena Park, U.S.A. 🕮 197
Buffalo, U.S.A. 🕮 298
Buford, U.S.A. 🕮 245
Bulgaria 🕮 40
Bulverde, U.S.A. 🕮 339
Bundaberg, Australia 🕮 29
Bunkyo-Ku, Japan 🕮 147
Burbank, U.S.A. 🕮 197
Burlington, Canada 🕮 49
Burlington, U.S.A. 🕮 270, 346
Burnaby, Canada 🕮 44
Burnham-on-Sea, England 🕮 90
Burnley, England 🕮 78
Bury Saint Edmund's, England 🕮 91
Buskerud, Norway 🕮 165
Bussum, The Netherlands 🕮 154
Butler, U.S.A. 🕮 290
Butte, U.S.A. 🕮 285
Byelorussia 🕮 40
Caen, France 🕮 99
Cagliari, Italy 🕮 145
Cahors, France 🕮 99
Cairns, Australia 🕮 29
Calabria, Italy 🕮 139
Caldwell, U.S.A. 🕮 247
Calgary, Canada 🕮 42
California, U.S.A. 🕮 196
Callaghan, Australia 🕮 25
Caltanissetta, Italy 🕮 145
Camarillo, U.S.A. 🕮 197
Camberley, England 🕮 91
Cambourne, England 🕮 72
Cambridge, England 🕮 71
Cambridgeshire, England 🕮 71
Campania, Italy 🕮 140
Campobasso, Italy 🕮 143
Campton, U.S.A. 🕮 287
Canada 🕮 40
Canberra, Australia 🕮 25
Cannes, France 🕮 99
Canoga Park, U.S.A. 🕮 197
Canterbury, England 🕮 78
Cape Coral, U.S.A. 🕮 236
Cape Giradeau, U.S.A. 🕮 282
Cape Province, South Africa 🕮 170
Cape Town, South Africa 🕮 170
Capelle a/d Ijssel, The Netherlands 🕮 154
Capri, Italy 🕮 140
Carbondale, U.S.A. 🕮 248
Carcassone, France 🕮 99
Cardiff, Wales 🕮 359
Carlisle, England 🕮 72
Carlisle, U.S.A. 🕮 328
Carmarthen, Wales 🕮 359
Caserta, Italy 🕮 140
Casper, U.S.A. 🕮 358
Castle Hill, Australia 🕮 25
Castle Shannon, U.S.A. 🕮 328
Catania, Italy 🕮 145
Catanzaro, Italy 🕮 139
Cathedral City, U.S.A. 🕮 198
CAvan, Ireland 🕮 136
Cayenne, French Guiana 🕮 106
Cazenovia, U.S.A. 🕮 355
Cedar Rapids, U.S.A. 🕮 256
Celle, Germany 🕮 113
Centereach, U.S.A. 🕮 298
Central Point, U.S.A. 🕮 324
Central, Scotland 🕮 167
Châlons, France 🕮 99
Chambéry, France 🕮 99
Champaign / Urbana, U.S.A. 🕮 248
Channel Islands 🕮 64
Chapel Hill, U.S.A. 🕮 313
Charleroi, Belgium 🕮 38
Charleston, U.S.A. 🕮 334, 354
Charlestown, U.S.A. 🕮 265, 270
Charlotte, U.S.A. 🕮 313
Charlottesville, U.S.A. 🕮 347
Charlottetown, Canada 🕮 61
Chatham, England 🕮 78
Chatham, U.S.A. 🕮 290, 298
Chattanooga, U.S.A. 🕮 336
Chehalis, U.S.A. 🕮 350
Chelmsford, England 🕮 75
Chelsea, U.S.A. 🕮 274
Chemnitz, Germany 🕮 113
Cherbourg, France 🕮 99
Cherry Hill, U.S.A. 🕮 290
Chesapeake, U.S.A. 🕮 348
Cheshire, England 🕮 71
Chester, England 🕮 71
Chesterfield, England 🕮 72
Chicago, U.S.A. 🕮 248
Chichester, England 🕮 91
Chico, U.S.A. 🕮 198
Chicopee, U.S.A. 🕮 265
Chicoutimi, Canada 🕮 61
Chieti, Italy 🕮 139
Chigwell, England 🕮 75
Chile 🕮 64
Chislehurst, England 🕮 78
Chloride, U.S.A. 🕮 193
Christchurch, New Zealand 🕮 161
Chugiak, U.S.A. 🕮 193
Chula Vista, U.S.A. 🕮 198
Chur, Switzerland 🕮 178
Cincinnati, U.S.A. 🕮 317
Clackamas, U.S.A. 🕮 324
Claremont San Dimas, U.S.A. 🕮 198
Clarion, U.S.A. 🕮 328
Clarkdale, U.S.A. 🕮 193
Clausthal-Zellerfeld, Germany 🕮 113
Claymont, U.S.A. 🕮 232
Clearwater, U.S.A. 🕮 236
Clemson, U.S.A. 🕮 335
Clermont-Ferrand, France 🕮 99
Cleveland, U.S.A. 🕮 318
Clonmel, Ireland 🕮 138
Cloverdale, Australia 🕮 33
Clovis, U.S.A. 🕮 294
Clwyd, Wales 🕮 359
Coffs Harbour, Australia 🕮 25
Colchester, England 🕮 75
Colchester, U.S.A. 🕮 230
College Park, U.S.A. 🕮 265
College Station, U.S.A. 🕮 339
Colorado Springs, U.S.A. 🕮 226
Colorado, U.S.A. 🕮 226
Columbia, U.S.A. 🕮 265, 283, 335
Columbus, U.S.A. 🕮 319
Compton, U.S.A. 🕮 198
Concord, U.S.A. 🕮 198, 279, 287
Connecticut, U.S.A. 🕮 229
Conway, U.S.A. 🕮 287
Cookeville, U.S.A. 🕮 336
Cooksville, Canada 🕮 49
Coos Bay, U.S.A. 🕮 325
Coquitlam, Canada 🕮 44
Coral Springs, U.S.A. 🕮 236
Coram, U.S.A. 🕮 298
Cork, Ireland 🕮 136, 137
Cornwall, England 🕮 72
Corona, U.S.A. 🕮 198
Corpus Christi, U.S.A. 🕮 339
Corse, France 🕮 99
Corte Madera, U.S.A. 🕮 198
Cortland, U.S.A. 🕮 298
Corvallis, U.S.A. 🕮 325
Cosenza, Italy 🕮 139
Costa Rica 🕮 65
Cottbus, Germany 🕮 114
Council Bluffs, U.S.A. 🕮 256
County Resources
  Bedfordshire, England 🕮 70
  Berkshire, England 🕮 71
  Borders, Scotland 🕮 167
  Cork, Ireland 🕮 136
  Devon, England 🕮 73
  Dorset, England 🕮 73
  Dublin, Ireland 🕮 137
  Galloway, Scotland 🕮 167
  Galway, Ireland 🕮 137
  Greater Manchester, England 🕮 75
  Guernsey, The Channel Islands 🕮 64
  Hereford & Worcester, England 🕮 77
  Isle of Wight, England 🕮 77
  Lancashire, England 🕮 78
  Leicestershire, England 🕮 79
  Limerick, Ireland 🕮 138
  Lincolnshire, England 🕮 79
  London, England 🕮 79
  Merseyside, England 🕮 87
  Northamptonshire, England 🕮 88
  Nottinghamshire, England 🕮 89
  Oxfordshire, England 🕮 89
  Shropshire, England 🕮 90
  South Yorkshire, England 🕮 90
  Staffordshire, England 🕮 91
  Strathclyde, Scotland 🕮 169
  Suffolk, England 🕮 91
  West Midlands, England 🕮 92
Courcouronnes, France 🕮 99
Coventry, England 🕮 93
Crauthem, Luxembourg 🕮 148
Cremona, Italy 🕮 142
Créteil, France 🕮 99
Crewe, England 🕮 71
Crotone, Italy 🕮 140
Croydon, England 🕮 91
Crystal Springs, U.S.A. 🕮 236
Culver City, U.S.A. 🕮 198
Cumbria, England 🕮 72

Cuneo, Italy 144
Cypress, U.S.A. 198
Czech Republic 65
D. F., Mexico 149
Dalarna, Sweden 173
Dallas / Fort Worth, U.S.A. 339
Dallas, U.S.A. 314
Daly City, U.S.A. 198
Damariscotta, U.S.A. 262
Dammarie les Lys, France 99
Danbury, U.S.A. 230
Danville, U.S.A. 198, 348
Darien, U.S.A. 230
Darlington, England 73
Darmstadt, Germany 114
Darwen, England 78
Darwin, Australia 28
Davenport, U.S.A. 256
Davis, U.S.A. 199
Daw Park, Australia 31
Dayton, U.S.A. 321
Daytona, U.S.A. 236
Dayville, U.S.A. 230
De Kalb, U.S.A. 252
Dearborn, U.S.A. 274
Decatur, U.S.A. 245
Deer Park, U.S.A. 265, 299
Del Valle, U.S.A. 341
Delaware, U.S.A. 232
Delft, The Netherlands 154
Delfzijl, The Netherlands 154
Den Haag, The Netherlands 154
Den Helder, The Netherlands 154
Denbigh, U.S.A. 348
Denmark 65
Dennisport, U.S.A. 270
Denton, U.S.A. 341
Denver, U.S.A. 227
Denville, U.S.A. 290
Derby, England 72
Derbyshire, England 72
Derry, Northern Ireland 164
Des Moines, U.S.A. 256
Des Plaines, U.S.A. 252
Desert Hot Springs, U.S.A. 199
Detroit, U.S.A. 274
Deurne, Belgium 38
Devon, England 73
Dexter, U.S.A. 275
Didenheim, France 99
Dijon, France 99
Dillenburg, Germany 114
Dinslaken, Germany 114
District of Columbia, U.S.A. 233
Doetinchem, The Netherlands 154
Dollnstein, Germany 114
Don Mills, Canada 49
Donaueschingen, Germany 114
Doraville, U.S.A. 245
Dorchester, U.S.A. 270
Dordrecht, The Netherlands 154
Dornberg, Austria 34
Dornbirn, Austria 34
Dorset, England 73
Dortmund, Germany 114
Doublview, Australia 33
Douglas, England 77
Douglas, U.S.A. 275
Dover, U.S.A. 290
Dowagiac, U.S.A. 275
Drammen, Norway 165
Dresden, Germany 114
Drogheda, Ireland 138
Dublin, Ireland 137
Dubuque, U.S.A. 256
Dugald, Canada 47
Duisberg, Germany 114
Duisburg, Germany 114
Duluth, U.S.A. 279
Dumfries & Galloway, Scotland 167
Dunbar, U.S.A. 354
Dundee, Scotland 170
Dunedin, New Zealand 161
Dunellen, U.S.A. 290
Dunkerque, France 99
Durango, U.S.A. 229
Durban, South Africa 171
Durham, England 73, 74
Durham, U.S.A. 287, 314
Düsseldorf, Germany 115
Dyfed, Wales 359
Eagan, U.S.A. 279
East Dedham, U.S.A. 270
East Greenwich, U.S.A. 334
East Hampton, U.S.A. 299
East Hartford, U.S.A. 230
East Landing, U.S.A. 275
East London, South Africa 171
East Meadow, U.S.A. 299
East Molesley, England 91
East Providence, U.S.A. 334
East Rutherford, U.S.A. 290
East Setauket, U.S.A. 299
East Sussex, England 74
East Waterboro, U.S.A. 262
Eastbourne, England 74
Easton, U.S.A. 328
Eckernförde, Germany 115
Eden Prairie, U.S.A. 279
Edinboro, U.S.A. 328
Edinburgh, Scotland 168
Edison, U.S.A. 290
Edmonton, Canada 43
Edwardsville, U.S.A. 252
Egg Harbor City, U.S.A. 290
Egham, England 91
Eichstätt, Germany 115
Eindhoven, The Netherlands 155
Eisenach, Germany 115
El Cajon, U.S.A. 199
El Cerrito, U.S.A. 199
El Dorado, U.S.A. 195
El Paso, U.S.A. 341
El Toro, U.S.A. 199
Eldridge, U.S.A. 254
Elizabeth Vale, Australia 31
Ellsworth, U.S.A. 262
Elmhurst, U.S.A. 299
Elmira, U.S.A. 299
Elmshorn, Germany 115
Emden, Germany 116
Emeryville, U.S.A. 199
Emilia Romagna, Italy 140
Emmen, The Netherlands 155
Empoli, Italy 145
Encino, U.S.A. 199
Enfield, U.S.A. 230
England 67
Englewood, U.S.A. 229
Enschede, The Netherlands 155
Epinal, France 99
Erfurt, Germany 116
Erie, U.S.A. 328
Erin, Canada 49
Erlangen, Germany 116
Escondido, U.S.A. 199
Eskilstuna, Sweden 175
Essen, Germany 116
Essex, England 74
Esslingen, Germany 116
Euclid, U.S.A. 321
Eugene, U.S.A. 325
Eureka, U.S.A. 199
Evansdale, U.S.A. 256
Evansville, U.S.A. 254
Evercreech, England 90
Everett, U.S.A. 350
Exeter, England 73
Fairfax, U.S.A. 348
Fairfield, U.S.A. 199, 230
Fairport, U.S.A. 299
Falls Church, U.S.A. 348
Falun, Sweden 173
Far Rockaway, U.S.A. 299
Fargo, U.S.A. 316
Fayetteville, U.S.A. 195, 299, 315
Feltham, England 87
Ferguson, U.S.A. 283
Ferndale, U.S.A. 275
Ferndown, England 73
Ferrara, Italy 140
Fife, Scotland 168
Finland 95
Finnentrop, Germany 116
Finnmark, Norway 165
Firenze, Italy 145
Fishers, U.S.A. 254
Flagstaff, U.S.A. 193
Flat Rock, U.S.A. 315
Flensburg, Germany 116
Flint, U.S.A. 275
Florence, U.S.A. 191
Florida, U.S.A. 235
Foggia, Italy 144
Folkestone, England 78
Førde, Norway 166
Forest Hills, U.S.A. 299
Forestville, U.S.A. 199
Forli, Italy 140
Fort Bragg, U.S.A. 199
Fort Collins, U.S.A. 229
Fort Lauderdale, U.S.A. 236
Fort Lee, U.S.A. 290
Fort Meade, U.S.A. 265
Fort Myers, U.S.A. 237
Fort Pierce, U.S.A. 237
Fort Wayne, U.S.A. 254
Fort-de-France, Martinique 149
Fountain Valley, U.S.A. 199
Fox Valley, U.S.A. 355
Framingham, U.S.A. 270
France 97
Francestown, U.S.A. 287
Frankfurt am Main, Germany 117
Frauenfeld, Switzerland 178
Frederick, U.S.A. 265
Fredericksburg, U.S.A. 348
Frederiksberg, Denmark 66
Fredonia, U.S.A. 299
Fredricton, Canada 48
Fredrikstad, Norway 165
Freiburg, Germany 117
Fremdingen, Germany 117
French Guiana 106
Freshwater, England 77
Fresno, U.S.A. 199
Freudstadt, Germany 117
Fribourg / Freiburg, Switzerland 178
Friuli-Venezia Giulia, Italy 141
Fulda, Germany 117
Fullerton, U.S.A. 200
Fürth, Germany 118
Gaggenau, Germany 118
Gainesville, U.S.A. 237
Gaithersburg, U.S.A. 265
Galesburg, U.S.A. 252
Galveston, U.S.A. 342
Galway, Ireland 137
Gap, France 99
Garden Grove, U.S.A. 200
Gardiner, U.S.A. 262
Gastonia, U.S.A. 315
Gästrikland, Sweden 173

Gateshead, England 📖 92
Gatineau, Canada 📖 61
Gävle, Sweden 📖 173
Geldern, Germany 📖 118
Gelnhausen, Germany 📖 118
Gelsenkirchen, Germany 📖 118
Gemert, The Netherlands 📖 155
Genève / Genf, Switzerland 📖 178
Genova, Italy 📖 142
Gent / Gand, Belgium 📖 38
Georgia, U.S.A. 📖 243
Gera, Germany 📖 118
Germany 📖 106
Germersheim, Germany 📖 118
Gettysburg, U.S.A. 📖 328
Gießen, Germany 📖 118
Gisborne, New Zealand 📖 162
Gjøvik, Norway 📖 165
Gladbeck, Germany 📖 118
Glamorgan, Wales 📖 359
Glasgow, Scotland 📖 169
Glen Burnie, U.S.A. 📖 265
Glen Ellyn, U.S.A. 📖 252
Glendale, U.S.A. 📖 200
Gloucester Point, U.S.A. 📖 348
Gloucester, England 📖 75
Gloucester, U.S.A. 📖 270
Gloucestershire, England 📖 75
Godlaming, England 📖 91
Gorinchem, The Netherlands 📖 155
Gorizia, Italy 📖 141
Görlitz, Germany 📖 118
Goshen, U.S.A. 📖 254
Gosnells, Australia 📖 33
Göteborg, Sweden 📖 173
Gotland, Sweden 📖 173
Göttingen, Germany 📖 118
Gouda, The Netherlands 📖 155
Grampian, Scotland 📖 168
Grand Forks, Canada 📖 44
Grand Forks, U.S.A. 📖 317
Grand Junction, U.S.A. 📖 229
Grand Rapids, U.S.A. 📖 276
Grande Prairie, Canada 📖 44
Grantham, England 📖 79
Gravesend, England 📖 78
Graz, Austria 📖 34
Great Barrington, U.S.A. 📖 270
Great Neck, U.S.A. 📖 299
Great Yarmouth, England 📖 88
Greater Manchester, England 📖 75
Greeley, U.S.A. 📖 229
Green Bay, U.S.A. 📖 356
Greenbelt, U.S.A. 📖 265
Greenfield, U.S.A. 📖 270
Greenock, Scotland 📖 170
Greensboro, U.S.A. 📖 315
Greenville, U.S.A. 📖 282, 321, 335
Greenwich, U.S.A. 📖 230
Greenwood, U.S.A. 📖 254, 335
Greifswald, Germany 📖 118
Grenoble, France 📖 100
Gretna, U.S.A. 📖 260
Greve, Denmark 📖 66
Grimsby, England 📖 77
Grinnell, U.S.A. 📖 256
Groningen, The Netherlands 📖 155
Guadalajara, Mexico 📖 149
Gualala, U.S.A. 📖 200
Güdingen, Germany 📖 119
Guelph, Canada 📖 49
Guéret, France 📖 100
Guernsey, The Channel Islands 📖 64
Guernville, U.S.A. 📖 200
Guildford, England 📖 91
Gummersbach, Germany 📖 119
Gwent, Wales 📖 359
Gwynedd, Wales 📖 359
Haarlem, The Netherlands 📖 155
Hackensack, U.S.A. 📖 290
Haddam, U.S.A. 📖 230
Hadleigh, England 📖 75
Hadley, U.S.A. 📖 270
Hagen, Germany 📖 119
Hailsham, England 📖 74
Hainault, Belgium 📖 38
Halberstadt, Germany 📖 119
Haliburton, Canada 📖 50
Halifax, Canada 📖 48
Halifax, England 📖 94
Halland, Sweden 📖 173
Halle (Saale), Germany 📖 119
Hallowell, U.S.A. 📖 262
Halmstad, Sweden 📖 173
Hamar, Norway 📖 165
Hamburg, Germany 📖 119
Hämeen Lääni, Finland 📖 95
Hameln, Germany 📖 121
Hamilton, Canada 📖 50
Hamilton, New Zealand 📖 162
Hamm, Germany 📖 121
Hampshire, England 📖 76
Hampstead, U.S.A. 📖 299
Hanley, England 📖 91
Hannover, Germany 📖 121
Hanover, U.S.A. 📖 287
Harlow, England 📖 75
Harrisburg, U.S.A. 📖 328
Harrogate, England 📖 88
Hartford, U.S.A. 📖 230
Hastings, England 📖 74, 91
Hastings, New Zealand 📖 162
Hattersheim, Germany 📖 122
Hattiesburg, U.S.A. 📖 282
Haverhill, U.S.A. 📖 271
Havertown, U.S.A. 📖 328
Hawaii (Big Island), U.S.A. 📖 246
Hawaii, U.S.A. 📖 246
Hawthorne, U.S.A. 📖 200, 290
Hayward, U.S.A. 📖 201
Healdsburg, U.S.A. 📖 201
Heanor, England 📖 73
Hebden Bridge, England 📖 94
Hebekk, Norway 📖 164
Hedmark, Norway 📖 165
Heereveen, The Netherlands 📖 156
Heerlen, The Netherlands 📖 156
Heide, Germany 📖 122
Heidelberg, Germany 📖 122
Heilbronn, Germany 📖 122
Helotes, U.S.A. 📖 342
Helsingborg, Sweden 📖 174
Helsinki, Finland 📖 96
Henderson, U.S.A. 📖 286
Hendrik Ido Ambacht, The Netherlands 📖 156
Hereford & Worcester, England 📖 77
Hereford, England 📖 77
Herentals, Belgium 📖 38
Hernando, U.S.A. 📖 237
Herne, Germany 📖 122
Hertfordshire, England 📖 77
Hertogenbosch, 's / Den Bosch, The Netherlands 📖 156
Hickory, U.S.A. 📖 315
High Wycombe, England 📖 71
Highland Park, U.S.A. 📖 252
Highland, Scotland 📖 168
Highland, U.S.A. 📖 290
Hildesheim, Germany 📖 122
Hill City, U.S.A. 📖 335
Hilversum, The Netherlands 📖 156
Hinwil, Switzerland 📖 178
Hirschhorn, Germany 📖 122
Hobart, Australia 📖 31
Hoboken, U.S.A. 📖 290
Hockley, England 📖 93
Hohenmölsen, Germany 📖 122
Holbæck, Denmark 📖 66
Holland, U.S.A. 📖 276
Hollinswood, England 📖 90
Hollywood, U.S.A. 📖 201, 237
Holzminden, Germany 📖 122
Hønefoss, Norway 📖 165
Hong Kong 📖 136
Hoogeveen, The Netherlands 📖 156
Hoogland, The Netherlands 📖 156
Hoorn, The Netherlands 📖 156
Hoover, U.S.A. 📖 191
Hordaland, Norway 📖 165
Houston, U.S.A. 📖 342
Hove, England 📖 74
Howell, U.S.A. 📖 290
Hoyerswerda, Germany 📖 122
Huddersfield, England 📖 94
Hull, Canada 📖 61
Hull, England 📖 77
Humberside, England 📖 77
Huntington Beach, U.S.A. 📖 201
Huntington Station, U.S.A. 📖 299
Huntington Valley, U.S.A. 📖 328
Huntington, U.S.A. 📖 290, 354
Huntsville, U.S.A. 📖 191, 343
Hyattsville, U.S.A. 📖 265
Hyvinkää, Finland 📖 97
Iceland 📖 136
Idaho, U.S.A. 📖 247
Illinois, U.S.A. 📖 247
Ilmenau, Germany 📖 122
Independence, U.S.A. 📖 283
Indiana, U.S.A. 📖 253
Indianapolis, U.S.A. 📖 254
Ingle Farm, Australia 📖 31
Ingolstadt, Germany 📖 122
Innsbruck, Austria 📖 34
Insel, Germany 📖 122
Invercargill, New Zealand 📖 162
Inverness, Scotland 📖 168
Iowa City, U.S.A. 📖 256
Iowa Falls, U.S.A. 📖 257
Iowa, U.S.A. 📖 255
Ipswich, England 📖 91
Ireland 📖 136
Ironton, U.S.A. 📖 321
Irvine, U.S.A. 📖 201
Irving, U.S.A. 📖 343
Irvington, U.S.A. 📖 290
Island Park, U.S.A. 📖 299
Isle Of Man, England 📖 77
Isle of Wight, England 📖 77
Ispringen, Germany 📖 122
Israel 📖 138
Issy Les Moulineaux, France 📖 100
Istanbul, Turkey 📖 180
Italy 📖 138
Ithaca, U.S.A. 📖 299
Ittlingen, Germany 📖 122
Jackson, U.S.A. 📖 276, 282, 358
Jacksonville, U.S.A. 📖 238
Jalisco, Mexico 📖 149
Jämtland, Sweden 📖 173
Janesville, U.S.A. 📖 356
Japan 📖 147
Jasper, Canada 📖 44
Jena, Germany 📖 122
Jenkintown, U.S.A. 📖 329
Jenner, U.S.A. 📖 201
Jersey City, U.S.A. 📖 290
Jersey Village, U.S.A. 📖 343
Jersey, The Channel Islands 📖 64
Joenssun, Finland 📖 96
Johannesburg, South Africa 📖 171

Index of Place Names

Johnson City, U.S.A. 🕮 336
Joliette, Canada 🕮 61
Jonesboro, U.S.A. 🕮 195
Jönköping, Sweden 🕮 175
Juneau, U.S.A. 🕮 193
Jyväskylä, Finland 🕮 95
Kaarst, Germany 🕮 123
Kaiserlautern, Germany 🕮 123
Kalamazoo, U.S.A. 🕮 276
Kamloops, Canada 🕮 44
Kansas City, U.S.A. 🕮 257, 283
Kansas, U.S.A. 🕮 257
Kapiti / Horowhenua, New Zealand 🕮 162
Karlsruhe, Germany 🕮 123
Karlstad, Sweden 🕮 174, 176
Kassel, Germany 🕮 123
Kechi, U.S.A. 🕮 257
Keego Harbor, U.S.A. 🕮 276
Keene, U.S.A. 🕮 287
Kelowna, Canada 🕮 44
Kendal, England 🕮 72
Kenilworth, England 🕮 92
Kent, England 🕮 78
Kent, U.S.A. 🕮 321
Kentucky, U.S.A. 🕮 258
Keskisuomen Lääni, Finland 🕮 95
Kew Gardens, England 🕮 91
Key West, U.S.A. 🕮 238
Kidderminster, England 🕮 77
Kiel, Germany 🕮 123
Kildare, Ireland 🕮 138
Kimberly, South Africa 🕮 171
King of Prussia, U.S.A. 🕮 329
King's Lynn, England 🕮 88
Kingsport, U.S.A. 🕮 336
Kingston, Canada 🕮 50
Kingston, U.S.A. 🕮 299, 334
Kirkcaldy, Scotland 🕮 168
Kirkenes, Norway 🕮 165
Kirkland, U.S.A. 🕮 350
Kita-Ku, Japan 🕮 147
Kitchener, Canada 🕮 50
Kitzingen, Germany 🕮 123
Klagenfurt, Austria 🕮 34
Klamath Falls, U.S.A. 🕮 325
Kleve, Germany 🕮 123
Knoxville, U.S.A. 🕮 336
København, Denmark 🕮 66
Koblenz, Germany 🕮 123
Kokkola, Finland 🕮 97
Kolding, Denmark 🕮 66
Köln, Germany 🕮 124
Kongsberg, Norway 🕮 165
Konstanz, Germany 🕮 125
Kootnays, Canada 🕮 44
Kortrijk / Courtrai, Belgium 🕮 38
Koto-Ku, Japan 🕮 147
Krefeld, Germany 🕮 125
Kristiansand, Norway 🕮 166
Kristiansund, Norway 🕮 165
Kuala Lumpur, Malaysia 🕮 148
Kuopio, Finland 🕮 96
Kuopion Lääni, Finland 🕮 96
L'Aquila, Italy 🕮 139
La Crosse, U.S.A. 🕮 356
La Grande, U.S.A. 🕮 325
La Rochelle, France 🕮 100
La Spezia, Italy 🕮 142
Ladner, Canada 🕮 44
Lafayette, U.S.A. 🕮 255, 260
Laguna Beach, U.S.A. 🕮 201
Lahr, Germany 🕮 125
Lahti, Finland 🕮 95
Lake Bluff, U.S.A. 🕮 252
Lake Charles, U.S.A. 🕮 260
Lake Oswego, U.S.A. 🕮 325
Lake Tahoe, U.S.A. 🕮 202
Lake Villa, U.S.A. 🕮 252
Lakeland, U.S.A. 🕮 238
Lakewood, U.S.A. 🕮 202, 229, 321
Lancashire, England 🕮 78
Lancaster, England 🕮 78
Lancaster, U.S.A. 🕮 329
Land 'O Lakes, U.S.A. 🕮 238
Landau, Germany 🕮 125
Langley Park, U.S.A. 🕮 265
Langley, Canada 🕮 44
Lanham, U.S.A. 🕮 265
Lansdowne, U.S.A. 🕮 329
Lansing, U.S.A. 🕮 277
Lappin Lääni, Finland 🕮 96
Laramie, U.S.A. 🕮 358
Largo, U.S.A. 🕮 238
Larvik, Norway 🕮 166
Las Cruces, U.S.A. 🕮 294
Las Vegas, U.S.A. 🕮 286
Launceston, England 🕮 72
Laurel, U.S.A. 🕮 265
Lausanne, Switzerland 🕮 178
Laval, Canada 🕮 61
Laval, France 🕮 100
Lavergne, U.S.A. 🕮 336
Lawrence, U.S.A. 🕮 257
Lawton, U.S.A. 🕮 323
Laytonville, U.S.A. 🕮 202
Lazio, Italy 🕮 141
Le Mans, France 🕮 100
Leavenworth, U.S.A. 🕮 258
Lecce, Italy 🕮 144
Leeds, England 🕮 94
Leeuwarden, The Netherlands 🕮 156
Legnano, Italy 🕮 146
Lehigh Valley, U.S.A. 🕮 329
Leicester, England 🕮 79
Leicestershire, England 🕮 79
Leiden, The Netherlands 🕮 156
Leighton Buzzard, England 🕮 70
Leipsic, U.S.A. 🕮 321
Leipzig, Germany 🕮 125
Letchworth, England 🕮 77
Lethbridge, Canada 🕮 44
Leuven / Louvain, Belgium 🕮 38
Leverhusen, Germany 🕮 125
Levittown, U.S.A. 🕮 329
Lewisburg, U.S.A. 🕮 329
Lewiston, U.S.A. 🕮 262
Lewisville, U.S.A. 🕮 343
Lexington, U.S.A. 🕮 259
Leyland, England 🕮 79
Leytonstone, England 🕮 75
Liberty, U.S.A. 🕮 336
Liechtenstein 🕮 148
Liège / Luik / Luttich, Belgium 🕮 38
Liestal, Switzerland 🕮 178
Liguria, Italy 🕮 142
Lille, France 🕮 100
Lillehammer, Norway 🕮 165
Lima, U.S.A. 🕮 321
Limburg, Germany 🕮 125
Limerick, Ireland 🕮 138
Limoges, France 🕮 100
Lincoln, England 🕮 79
Lincoln, U.S.A. 🕮 285
Lincolnshire, England 🕮 79
Linden, U.S.A. 🕮 291
Lindsay, Canada 🕮 51
Lindsborg, U.S.A. 🕮 258
Lingen, Germany 🕮 125
Linköping, Sweden 🕮 174
Linz, Austria 🕮 34
Lisboa, Portugal 🕮 167
Lismore, Australia 🕮 25
Lithis, U.S.A. 🕮 238
Lithonia, U.S.A. 🕮 245
Little Rock, U.S.A. 🕮 195
Livermore, U.S.A. 🕮 202
Liverpool, England 🕮 71, 87
Livonia, U.S.A. 🕮 277
Llandrindod Wells, Wales 🕮 359
Lobethal, Australia 🕮 31
Logan, U.S.A. 🕮 345
Lombardia, Italy 🕮 142
London, Canada 🕮 51
London, England 🕮 79
Londonderry, Northern Ireland 🕮 164
Long Beach, U.S.A. 🕮 202
Longview, U.S.A. 🕮 343
Lorain, U.S.A. 🕮 321
Los Angeles, U.S.A. 🕮 203
Lothian, Scotland 🕮 168
Louisiana, U.S.A. 🕮 260
Louisville, U.S.A. 🕮 259
Lovendegem, Belgium 🕮 38
Lowell, U.S.A. 🕮 271
Lowestoft, England 🕮 91
Lubbock, U.S.A. 🕮 344
Lübeck, Germany 🕮 126
Lüdenscheid, Germany 🕮 126
Ludwigsburg, Germany 🕮 126
Ludwigshafen, Germany 🕮 126
Lugano, Switzerland 🕮 178
Luleå, Sweden 🕮 174
Lumphanan, Scotland 🕮 168
Lund, Sweden 🕮 174
Lüneburg, Germany 🕮 126
Luton, England 🕮 71
Lutz, U.S.A. 🕮 238
Luxembourg 🕮 148
Luxembourg, Luxembourg 🕮 148
Luzern / Lucerne, Switzerland 🕮 178
Lynchburg, U.S.A. 🕮 348
Lyndhurst, U.S.A. 🕮 291
Lyon, France 🕮 100
Maastricht, The Netherlands 🕮 156
Macclesfield, England 🕮 72
Macerata, Italy 🕮 143
Macon, U.S.A. 🕮 245
MacTier, Canada 🕮 51
Madison Heights, U.S.A. 🕮 277
Madison, U.S.A. 🕮 356
Madrid, Spain 🕮 172
Magdeburg, Germany 🕮 126
Maidenhead, England 🕮 71
Maidstone, England 🕮 78
Maine, U.S.A. 🕮 261
Mainz, Germany 🕮 126
Makamura-Ku, Japan 🕮 147
Malaysia 🕮 148
Malden, U.S.A. 🕮 271
Malmö, Sweden 🕮 173
Malmöhus län, Sweden 🕮 173
Malvern, U.S.A. 🕮 329
Mammern, Switzerland 🕮 178
Manchaca, U.S.A. 🕮 344
Manchester Center, U.S.A. 🕮 346
Manchester, England 🕮 75
Manchester, U.S.A. 🕮 231, 288
Manhattan, U.S.A. 🕮 258
Manitoba, Canada 🕮 47
Mankato, U.S.A. 🕮 279
Mannheim, Germany 🕮 126
Mansfield, England 🕮 89
Mansfield, U.S.A. 🕮 322
Marblehead, U.S.A. 🕮 271
Marburg, Germany 🕮 127
Marceline, U.S.A. 🕮 284
Marche, Italy 🕮 143
Margate, England 🕮 78
Margate, U.S.A. 🕮 238
Marietta, U.S.A. 🕮 245
Marina Del Rey, U.S.A. 🕮 206
Marion, U.S.A. 🕮 322
Marlborough, U.S.A. 🕮 271
Marquette, U.S.A. 🕮 277

Marsall, U.S.A. 📖 279
Marseille, France 📖 101
Martinique 📖 148
Martinsburg, U.S.A. 📖 355
Maryland, U.S.A. 📖 263
Masalucia, Italy 📖 145
Mason City, U.S.A. 📖 257
Massachusetts, U.S.A. 📖 266
Matera, Italy 📖 139
Mattydale, U.S.A. 📖 299
Maui, U.S.A. 📖 246
Maynooth, Ireland 📖 138
Mays Landing, U.S.A. 📖 291
Meadville, U.S.A. 📖 329
Meath, Ireland 📖 138
Meaux, France 📖 101
Mechelen / Malines, Belgium 📖 38
Medelpad, Sweden 📖 174
Medfield, U.S.A. 📖 271
Melbourne, Australia 📖 31
Memphis, U.S.A. 📖 336
Menasha, U.S.A. 📖 356
Menden, Germany 📖 127
Mendocino, U.S.A. 📖 206
Menlo Park, U.S.A. 📖 206
Mentor, U.S.A. 📖 322
Meriden, U.S.A. 📖 231
Merkel, U.S.A. 📖 344
Merrimack, U.S.A. 📖 288
Merseyside, England 📖 87
Messina, Italy 📖 145
Mestre, Italy 📖 146
Metuchen, U.S.A. 📖 291
Metz, France 📖 101
Mexico 📖 149
Mexico City, Mexico 📖 149
Miami Beach, U.S.A. 📖 239
Miami, U.S.A. 📖 238
Michigan City, U.S.A. 📖 255
Michigan, U.S.A. 📖 273
Middleboro, U.S.A. 📖 271
Middleburg, The Netherlands 📖 156
Middlesbrough, England 📖 88
Middlesex, England 📖 87
Middlesex, U.S.A. 📖 291
Middleton, England 📖 73
Middletown, U.S.A. 📖 231
Midvale, U.S.A. 📖 345
Milano, Italy 📖 142
Mill Valley, U.S.A. 📖 206
Millburn, U.S.A. 📖 291
Millington, U.S.A. 📖 337
Millis, U.S.A. 📖 271
Milpitas, U.S.A. 📖 206
Milsons Point, Australia 📖 25
Milton Keynes, England 📖 71
Milwaukee, U.S.A. 📖 356
Minato-Ku, Japan 📖 148
Minden, Germany 📖 127
Minneapolis / Saint Paul, U.S.A. 📖 279
Minnesota, U.S.A. 📖 278
Minot, U.S.A. 📖 317
Minsk, Byelorussia 📖 40
Mishawaka, U.S.A. 📖 255
Mission Hills, U.S.A. 📖 206
Mississauga, Canada 📖 51
Mississipi, U.S.A. 📖 282
Missoula, U.S.A. 📖 285
Missouri, U.S.A. 📖 282
Mizuho-Ku, Japan 📖 147
Mo, Norway 📖 165
Mobile, U.S.A. 📖 192
Modena, Italy 📖 140
Modesto, U.S.A. 📖 206
Moers, Germany 📖 127
Molde, Norway 📖 165
Molise, Italy 📖 143
Mölln, Germany 📖 127
Mönchengladbach, Germany 📖 127
Moncton, Canada 📖 48
Monroe, U.S.A. 📖 260
Monrovia, U.S.A. 📖 206
Mons, France 📖 101
Montana, U.S.A. 📖 285
Montclair, U.S.A. 📖 291
Montesano, U.S.A. 📖 350
Montgomery, U.S.A. 📖 192
Monticello, U.S.A. 📖 252
Montpelier, U.S.A. 📖 346
Montpellier, France 📖 101
Montréal La Cluse, France 📖 101
Montréal, Canada 📖 61
Moorestown, U.S.A. 📖 291
Moorhead, U.S.A. 📖 281
Møre og Romsdal, Norway 📖 165
Morgantown, U.S.A. 📖 355
Morley, Australia 📖 33
Morristown, U.S.A. 📖 291
Morrisville, U.S.A. 📖 329
Moscow, U.S.A. 📖 247
Moss, Norway 📖 166
Mount Morris, U.S.A. 📖 277
Mount Pleasant, U.S.A. 📖 277
Mount Vernon, U.S.A. 📖 257, 350
Mountain View, U.S.A. 📖 206
Mülhausen, Germany 📖 127
Mülheim, Germany 📖 127
Mulhouse, France 📖 101
München, Germany 📖 127
Muncie, U.S.A. 📖 255
Münster, Germany 📖 128
Murdoch, Australia 📖 33
Murfreesboro, U.S.A. 📖 337
Muskegon, U.S.A. 📖 277
Muskogee, U.S.A. 📖 323
Nagoya-shi, Japan 📖 147
Nailsworth, England 📖 75
Namibia 📖 149
Namur / Namen, Belgium 📖 39
Nanaimo, Canada 📖 44
Nancy, France 📖 102
Nantes, France 📖 102
Napa, U.S.A. 📖 207
Napier, New Zealand 📖 162
Naples, U.S.A. 📖 239
Napoli, Italy 📖 140
Narke, Sweden 📖 174
Nashua, U.S.A. 📖 288
Nashville, U.S.A. 📖 337
Nassau, U.S.A. 📖 299
Natal, South Africa 📖 171
Natick, U.S.A. 📖 271
National Resources
  Australia 📖 24
  Austria 📖 34
  Belgium 📖 35
  Bulgaria 📖 40
  Canada 📖 40
  Denmark 📖 65
  England 📖 67
  Finland 📖 95
  France 📖 97
  Germany 📖 107
  Ireland 📖 136
  Italy 📖 138
  Liechtenstein 📖 148
  Mexico 📖 149
  New Zealand 📖 159
  Northern Ireland 📖 163
  Norway 📖 164
  Portugal 📖 167
  Scotland 📖 167
  South Africa 📖 170
  Spain 📖 172
  Sweden 📖 173
  Switzerland 📖 176
  The Netherlands 📖 150
  U.S.A. 📖 180
  Wales 📖 359
Near Marden, England 📖 78
Nebraska, U.S.A. 📖 285
Needham Heights, U.S.A. 📖 271
Nelson, New Zealand 📖 162
Neptune, U.S.A. 📖 291
Netherlands 📖 149
Neubrandenburg, Germany 📖 129
Neuchâtel / Neuenburg, Switzerland 📖 178
Neuenhof, Switzerland 📖 178
Neumünster, Germany 📖 129
Neuss, Germany 📖 129
Neustadt, Germany 📖 129
Neustrelitz, Germany 📖 129
Nevada, U.S.A. 📖 286
New Baltimore, U.S.A. 📖 277
New Britain, U.S.A. 📖 231
New Brunswick, Canada 📖 48
New Brunswick, U.S.A. 📖 291
New Farm, Australia 📖 29
New Glasgow, Canada 📖 48
New Hampshire, U.S.A. 📖 287
New Haven, U.S.A. 📖 231
New Hope, U.S.A. 📖 329
New Jersey, U.S.A. 📖 288
New London, U.S.A. 📖 231
New Mexico, U.S.A. 📖 293
New Orleans, U.S.A. 📖 260
New Paltz, U.S.A. 📖 299
New Preston, U.S.A. 📖 232
New Providence, U.S.A. 📖 292
New South Wales, Australia 📖 25
New Waverly, U.S.A. 📖 344
New Westminster, Canada 📖 44
New York, U.S.A. 📖 295, 300
New Zealand 📖 159
Newark, U.S.A. 📖 232, 292
Newburyport, U.S.A. 📖 271
Newcastle upon Tyne, England 📖 92
Newcastle, Australia 📖 25
Newfoundland, Canada 📖 48
Newport Beach, U.S.A. 📖 207
Newport News, U.S.A. 📖 348
Newport, U.S.A. 📖 259, 325
Newport, Wales 📖 359
Newton Abbot, England 📖 73
Newton Centre, U.S.A. 📖 271
Niagara Falls, Canada 📖 51
Niagara Falls, U.S.A. 📖 310
Nice, France 📖 102
Nieuw-Vennep, The Netherlands 📖 156
Nijmegen, The Netherlands 📖 156
Nîmes, France 📖 102
Nishi-Ku, Japan 📖 147
Nonantum, U.S.A. 📖 271
Noosa, Australia 📖 29
Noranda, Canada 📖 63
Norcross, U.S.A. 📖 245
Nordhorn, Germany 📖 129
Nordland, Norway 📖 165
Norfolk, England 📖 88
Norfolk, U.S.A. 📖 348
Norrbotten, Sweden 📖 174
Norristown, U.S.A. 📖 329
Norrköping, Sweden 📖 174
North Augusta, U.S.A. 📖 335
North Bay, Canada 📖 52
North Bergen, U.S.A. 📖 292
North Brunswick, U.S.A. 📖 292
North Carolina, U.S.A. 📖 313
North Dakota, U.S.A. 📖 316
North Haledon, U.S.A. 📖 292
North Hollywood, U.S.A. 📖 207
North Little Rock, U.S.A. 📖 196
North Miami Beach, U.S.A. 📖 240

Index of Place Names

North West Territories, Canada 48
North York, Canada 52
North Yorkshire, England 88
Northam, England 76
Northampton, England 89
Northampton, U.S.A. 271
Northamptonshire, England 88
Northbridge, Australia 33
Northcote, Australia 33
Northern Ireland 163
Northern Territory, Australia 28
Northfield, U.S.A. 281
Norway 164
Norwich, England 88
Norwich, U.S.A. 232
Nottingham, England 89
Nottinghamshire, England 89
Nova Scotia, Canada 48
Novi, U.S.A. 277
Nundah, Australia 29
Nuneaton, England 92
Nürnberg, Germany 129
Nyköping, Sweden 175
Oahu, U.S.A. 246
Oakland, U.S.A. 207, 292
Oberhausen, Germany 130
Oberlin, U.S.A. 322
Ocala, U.S.A. 240
Odense, Denmark 66
Offenbach, Germany 130
Offenburg, Germany 130
Ohio, U.S.A. 317
Oklahoma City, U.S.A. 323
Oklahoma, U.S.A. 322
Okotoks, Canada 44
Olaca, U.S.A. 240
Oldenburg, Germany 130
Oldham, England 76
Olpe, Germany 130
Olympia, U.S.A. 350
Omaha, U.S.A. 285
Oneonta, U.S.A. 310
Ontario, Canada 49
Oostende / Ostende, Belgium 39
Oppland, Norway 165
Orange Free State, South Africa 171
Orange, U.S.A. 208
Örebro, Sweden 174
Oregon, U.S.A. 324
Orem, U.S.A. 345
Orillia, Canada 52
Orlando, U.S.A. 240
Orléans, France 102
Orleans, U.S.A. 272
Osaka, Japan 147
Oshawa, Canada 52
Oslo, Norway 164
Osnabrück, Germany 130
Oss, The Netherlands 157
Östergötland, Sweden 174
Östersund, Sweden 173
Østfold, Norway 165
Oswego, U.S.A. 310
Ottawa, Canada 52
Oulu, Finland 95, 96, 97
Oulun Lääni, Finland 96
Outremont, Canada 63
Overland Park, U.S.A. 258
Owen Sound, Canada 53
Owensboro, U.S.A. 260
Oxford, England 89
Oxford, U.S.A. 322
Oxfordshire, England 89
Pacific Beach, U.S.A. 208
Pacific City, U.S.A. 326
Pacific Grove, U.S.A. 208
Pacifica, U.S.A. 208
Paderborn, Germany 130
Padova, Italy 146
Paisley, Scotland 170
Palaiseau, France 102
Palermo, Italy 145
Palm Springs, U.S.A. 208
Palmdale, U.S.A. 209
Palmer, U.S.A. 272
Palmerston North, New Zealand 162
Palo Alto, U.S.A. 209
Panama City, U.S.A. 241
Paris, France 102
Park City, U.S.A. 345
Parkersburg, U.S.A. 355
Parma, Italy 141
Parma, U.S.A. 322
Pasadena, U.S.A. 209
Passau, Germany 131
Pau, France 104
Pavia, Italy 143
Pawleys Island, U.S.A. 335
Pelham, U.S.A. 192, 310
Pennsylvania, U.S.A. 327
Penrith, Australia 25
Penrith, England 72
Penryn, England 72
Pensacola, U.S.A. 241
Penzance, England 72
Peoria, U.S.A. 252
Perpignan, France 105
Perth, Australia 33
Perth, Scotland 170
Perugia, Italy 146
Pesaro, Italy 143
Pescara, Italy 139
Petaluma, U.S.A. 209
Peterborough, Canada 54
Peterborough, England 71
Petersham, Australia 25
Petosky, U.S.A. 277
Pforzheim, Germany 131
Philadelphia, U.S.A. 329
Phœnix, U.S.A. 193
Piemonte, Italy 143
Pietermaritzburg, South Africa 171
Pijnakker, The Netherlands 157
Pisa, Italy 146
Piscataway, U.S.A. 292
Piteå, Sweden 174
Pittsburgh, U.S.A. 331
Pittsfield, U.S.A. 272
Plainfield, U.S.A. 292, 346
Plattsburgh, U.S.A. 310
Plauen, Germany 131
Pleasant Grove, U.S.A. 345
Plymouth, England 73
Plymouth, U.S.A. 288
Plympton, Australia 31
Pocatello, U.S.A. 247
Pocono Summit, U.S.A. 332
Pohjoikarjalan Lääni, Finland 96
Poitiers, France 105
Pomona, U.S.A. 209
Pompano Beach, U.S.A. 241
Pontiac, U.S.A. 277
Pordenone, Italy 141
Port Chester, U.S.A. 310
Portage, U.S.A. 277, 357
Portland, U.S.A. 262, 326
Portsmouth, England 76
Portsmouth, U.S.A. 288
Portugal 167
Potenza, Italy 139
Potsdam, Germany 131
Potsdam, U.S.A. 310
Poughkeepsie, U.S.A. 310
Poussan, France 105
Powys, Wales 359
Praha, The Czech Republic 65
Preetz, Germany 131
Preston, England 79
Prestwich, England 76
Pretoria, South Africa 172
Prince Edward Island, Canada 61
Prince George, Canada 44
Princeton, U.S.A. 292
Providence, U.S.A. 334
Provincetown, U.S.A. 272
Provincial Resources
  Alberta, Canada 42
  British Columbia, Canada 44
  Manitoba, Canada 47
  Ontario, Canada 49
  Québec, Canada 61
Puebla, Mexico 149
Puerto Rico 167
Puglia, Italy 144
Pullman, U.S.A. 350
Putbus, Germany 131
Québec, Canada 61, 63
Queensland, Australia 28
Quimper, France 105
Racine, U.S.A. 358
Radford, U.S.A. 348
Ragusa, Italy 145
Raleigh, U.S.A. 315
Ramseur, U.S.A. 316
Rana, Norway 165
Randolph, U.S.A. 272
Rapid City, U.S.A. 335
Ravenna, Italy 141
Reading, England 71
Reading, U.S.A. 333
Recklinghausen, Germany 131
Red Bank, U.S.A. 292
Red Deer, Canada 44
Redford, U.S.A. 278
Redwood City, U.S.A. 209
Regensburg, Germany 131
Regina, Canada 64
Regional Resources
  Piemonte, Italy 143
  Stockholm, Sweden 175
Rego Park, U.S.A. 310
Rehoboth Beach, U.S.A. 233
Rendsburg, Germany 131
Renkum, The Netherlands 157
Rennes, France 105
Reno, U.S.A. 281, 287
Reutlingen, Germany 131
Reykjavik, Iceland 136
Reynoldsburg, U.S.A. 322
Rheine, Germany 131
Rhinelander, U.S.A. 358
Rhode Island, U.S.A. 334
Riccione, Italy 141
Richland Hills, U.S.A. 344
Richmond, U.S.A. 255, 349
Riems, France 105
Rieti, Italy 139
Rimini, Italy 141
Rio de Janeiro, Brazil 39
River Edge, U.S.A. 292
River Falls, U.S.A. 358
Riverside, U.S.A. 209, 252, 334
Riverview, Canada 48
Roanoke, U.S.A. 349
Rochdale, England 76
Rochefort, France 105
Rochester, U.S.A. 281, 310
Rock Island, U.S.A. 253
Rockford, U.S.A. 253
Rockhampton, Australia 29
Rockville, U.S.A. 266
Rocky Hill, U.S.A. 232
Roermund, The Netherlands 157
Rogaland, Norway 166
Roissy, France 105

Roma, Italy 🕮 141
Romford, England 🕮 75
Ronkonkoma, U.S.A. 🕮 311
Roosendaal, The Netherlands 🕮 157
Rosebud, U.S.A. 🕮 344
Roseburg, U.S.A. 🕮 327
Roselle, U.S.A. 🕮 292
Rosenheim, Germany 🕮 131
Rosewell, U.S.A. 🕮 246
Rosny sous Bois, France 🕮 105
Rostock, Germany 🕮 131
Rothrist, Switzerland 🕮 178
Rotorua, New Zealand 🕮 163
Rotterdam, The Netherlands 🕮 157
Rottweil, Germany 🕮 131
Rouen, France 🕮 105
Rovaniemi, Finland 🕮 96
Rovigo, Italy 🕮 147
Royal Leamington Spa, England 🕮 92
Royal Oak, U.S.A. 🕮 278
Royal Tunbridge Wells, England 🕮 78
Rozelle, Australia 🕮 25
Runcorn, England 🕮 72
Rutland, U.S.A. 🕮 346
Saarbrücken, Germany 🕮 132
Sacramento, U.S.A. 🕮 209
Saginaw, U.S.A. 🕮 278
Saint Albans, England 🕮 77
Saint Albans, U.S.A. 🕮 346
Saint Andew's, Scotland 🕮 168
Saint Antoine des Laurentides, Canada 🕮 63
Saint Austell, England 🕮 72
Saint Bethlehem, U.S.A. 🕮 338
Saint Catharines, Canada 🕮 54
Saint Charles, U.S.A. 🕮 284
Saint Cloud, U.S.A. 🕮 282
Saint Denis, France 🕮 105
Saint Etienne, France 🕮 105
Saint Gallen, Switzerland 🕮 179
Saint Helens, England 🕮 87
Saint Helier, The Channel Islands 🕮 64
Saint John's, Canada 🕮 48
Saint John, Canada 🕮 48
Saint Johnsbury, U.S.A. 🕮 346
Saint Lô, France 🕮 105
Saint Louis, France 🕮 105
Saint Louis, U.S.A. 🕮 284
Saint Malo, France 🕮 105
Saint Michel, France 🕮 105
Saint Moritz, Switzerland 🕮 179
Saint Paul, U.S.A. 🕮 194
Saint Petersburg, U.S.A. 🕮 241
Saint Thomas, Canada 🕮 54
Saintes, France 🕮 106
Salem, U.S.A. 🕮 288, 327
Saline, U.S.A. 🕮 278
Salisbury, England 🕮 94
Salisbury, U.S.A. 🕮 266, 316
Salt Lake City, U.S.A. 🕮 345
Salzburg, Austria 🕮 34
Salzwedel, Germany 🕮 132
San Angelo, U.S.A. 🕮 344
San Anselmo, U.S.A. 🕮 210
San Antonio, U.S.A. 🕮 344
San Bernardino, U.S.A. 🕮 210
San Diego, U.S.A. 🕮 210
San Dimas, U.S.A. 🕮 212
San Francisco, U.S.A. 🕮 212
San José, Costa Rica 🕮 65
San José, U.S.A. 🕮 219
San Juan Capistrano, U.S.A. 🕮 220
San Juan, Puerto Rico 🕮 167
San Luis Obispo, U.S.A. 🕮 220
San Marcos, U.S.A. 🕮 220
San Mateo, U.S.A. 🕮 220
San Rafael, U.S.A. 🕮 220
Sanbornville, U.S.A. 🕮 288
Sandbach, England 🕮 72
Sandefjord, Norway 🕮 166
Sandnes, Norway 🕮 166
Sandown, England 🕮 77
Sanford, U.S.A. 🕮 316
Santa Ana, U.S.A. 🕮 221
Santa Barbara, U.S.A. 🕮 221
Santa Clara, U.S.A. 🕮 221
Santa Cruz, U.S.A. 🕮 221
Santa Fe, U.S.A. 🕮 295
Santa Monica, U.S.A. 🕮 222
Santa Rosa, U.S.A. 🕮 222
Santee, U.S.A. 🕮 222
Santiago, Chile 🕮 64
São Paulo, Brazil 🕮 39
Saranac Lake, U.S.A. 🕮 311
Sarasota, U.S.A. 🕮 241
Saratoga Springs, U.S.A. 🕮 311
Sardegna, Italy 🕮 145
Saskatchewan, Canada 🕮 63
Saskatoon, Canada 🕮 64
Sassari, Italy 🕮 145
Sault Saint Marie, Canada 🕮 54
Savannah, U.S.A. 🕮 246
Scarborough, Canada 🕮 54
Scarborough, England 🕮 88
Schaffhausen, Switzerland 🕮 179
Schatthausen, Germany 🕮 132
Schenectady, U.S.A. 🕮 311
Schoten, Belgium 🕮 39
Schwalmstadt, Germany 🕮 132
Schwerin, Germany 🕮 132
Scotland 🕮 167
Scunthorpe, England 🕮 77
Seal Beach, U.S.A. 🕮 222
Seascale, England 🕮 72
Seattle, U.S.A. 🕮 350
Serafina, U.S.A. 🕮 295
Sewell, U.S.A. 🕮 293
Shawnee Mission, U.S.A. 🕮 258
Shawseen, U.S.A. 🕮 272
Sheboygan, U.S.A. 🕮 358
Sheffield Lake, U.S.A. 🕮 322
Sheffield, England 🕮 90
Shepherdstown, U.S.A. 🕮 355
Sherbrooke, Canada 🕮 63
Shibuya-Ku, Japan 🕮 148
Shinjuku-Ku, Japan 🕮 148
Shreveport, U.S.A. 🕮 261
Shrewsbury, England 🕮 90
Shropshire, England 🕮 90
Sicilia, Italy 🕮 145
Siegen, Germany 🕮 132
Siena, Italy 🕮 146
Silkeborg, Denmark 🕮 66
Silver Spring, U.S.A. 🕮 266
Sint Niklaas, Belgium 🕮 39
Sion, Switzerland 🕮 179
Sioux Falls, U.S.A. 🕮 336
Skåne, Sweden 🕮 174
Skellefteå, Sweden 🕮 176
Slough, England 🕮 71
Småland, Sweden 🕮 175
Södermanland, Sweden 🕮 175
Soest, Germany 🕮 132
Sogn og Fjordane, Norway 🕮 166
Sogndal, Norway 🕮 166
Soissons, France 🕮 106
Solihull, England 🕮 93
Solingen, Germany 🕮 132
Solothurn, Switzerland 🕮 179
Somerset, England 🕮 90
Somerville, U.S.A. 🕮 293
Sønderborg, Denmark 🕮 67
Sondrio, Italy 🕮 143
Sonora, U.S.A. 🕮 222
Soquel, U.S.A. 🕮 222
Sør Trondelag, Norway 🕮 166
South Africa 🕮 170
South Australia, Australia 🕮 29
South Beach, U.S.A. 🕮 242
South Bend, U.S.A. 🕮 253, 255
South Carolina, U.S.A. 🕮 334
South Dakota, U.S.A. 🕮 335
South Renton, U.S.A. 🕮 353
South Windsor, U.S.A. 🕮 232
South Yorkshire, England 🕮 90
Southampton, England 🕮 77
Southend, England 🕮 75
Southfield, U.S.A. 🕮 278
Southgate, U.S.A. 🕮 278
Southington, U.S.A. 🕮 232
Spain 🕮 172
Sparks, U.S.A. 🕮 287
Spartanburg, U.S.A. 🕮 335
Spokane, U.S.A. 🕮 354
Springfield, U.S.A. 🕮 253, 272, 284, 322, 327, 349
Squamish, Canada 🕮 45
Staffordshire, England 🕮 91
Stalybridge, England 🕮 72
Stamford, U.S.A. 🕮 232
Stanford, U.S.A. 🕮 222
Stanford-Le-Hope, England 🕮 75
State College, U.S.A. 🕮 333
State Resources
  Alabama, U.S.A. 🕮 191
  Arizona, U.S.A. 🕮 193
  Arkansas, U.S.A. 🕮 195
  California, U.S.A. 🕮 196
  Colorado, U.S.A. 🕮 226
  Connecticut, U.S.A. 🕮 229
  District of Columbia, U.S.A. 🕮 233
  Florida, U.S.A. 🕮 235
  Georgia, U.S.A. 🕮 243
  Hawaii, U.S.A. 🕮 246
  Idaho, U.S.A. 🕮 247
  Indiana, U.S.A. 🕮 253
  Iowa, U.S.A. 🕮 255
  Kansas, U.S.A. 🕮 257
  Kentucky, U.S.A. 🕮 258
  Louisiana, U.S.A. 🕮 260
  Maine, U.S.A. 🕮 261
  Maryland, U.S.A. 🕮 263
  Massachusetts, U.S.A. 🕮 266
  Michigan, U.S.A. 🕮 273
  Minnesota, U.S.A. 🕮 278
  Mississipi, U.S.A. 🕮 282
  Missouri, U.S.A. 🕮 282
  Montana, U.S.A. 🕮 285
  Nebraska, U.S.A. 🕮 285
  Nevada, U.S.A. 🕮 286
  New Hampshire, U.S.A. 🕮 287
  New Jersey, U.S.A. 🕮 288
  New Mexico, U.S.A. 🕮 293
  New York, U.S.A. 🕮 295
  North Carolina, U.S.A. 🕮 313
  Ohio, U.S.A. 🕮 317
  Oklahoma, U.S.A. 🕮 323
  Oregon, U.S.A. 🕮 324
  Pennsylvania, U.S.A. 🕮 327
  Rhode Island, U.S.A. 🕮 334
  South Australia, Australia 🕮 29
  South Carolina, U.S.A. 🕮 334
  South Dakota, U.S.A. 🕮 335
  Tennessee, U.S.A. 🕮 336
  Texas, U.S.A. 🕮 338
  Utah, U.S.A. 🕮 345
  Vermont, U.S.A. 🕮 346
  Victoria, Australia 🕮 31
  Virginia, U.S.A. 🕮 347
  Washington, U.S.A. 🕮 350
  West Virginia, U.S.A. 🕮 354
  Western Australia, Australia 🕮 33
  Wisconsin, U.S.A. 🕮 355

Staunton, U.S.A. 🕮 349
Stavanger, Norway 🕮 166
Steubenville, U.S.A. 🕮 322
Stevens Point, U.S.A. 🕮 358
Stirling, Scotland 🕮 167
Stockholm, Sweden 🕮 175
Stockport, England 🕮 72
Stockton, U.S.A. 🕮 222
Stockton-on-Tees, England 🕮 92
Stoke Abbot, England 🕮 73
Stone Harbor, U.S.A. 🕮 293
Stony Brook, U.S.A. 🕮 311
Stourbridge, England 🕮 93
Strasbourg, France 🕮 106
Stratford, Canada 🕮 54
Stratford-upon-Avon, England 🕮 92
Strathclyde, Scotland 🕮 169
Stroudsburg / Poconos, U.S.A. 🕮 333
Studio City, U.S.A. 🕮 223
Stuttgart, Germany 🕮 132
Sudbury, Canada 🕮 54
Suffolk, England 🕮 91
Suhl, Germany 🕮 134
Sunderland, England 🕮 92
Sundsvall, Sweden 🕮 174
Sunnyvale, U.S.A. 🕮 223
Sunrise, U.S.A. 🕮 242
Superior, U.S.A. 🕮 358
Surfer's Paradise, Australia 🕮 29
Surrey, England 🕮 91
Sussex, England 🕮 91
Sussex, U.S.A. 🕮 293
Swakopmund, Namibia 🕮 149
Swansea, U.S.A. 🕮 272
Swansea, Wales 🕮 359
Sweden 🕮 172
Swindon, England 🕮 94
Switzerland 🕮 176
Sydney, Australia 🕮 26
Sydney, Canada 🕮 49
Sylmar, U.S.A. 🕮 223
Syracuse, U.S.A. 🕮 312
Tacoma, U.S.A. 🕮 354
Tallahassee, U.S.A. 🕮 242
Tampa, U.S.A. 🕮 242
Tampere, Finland 🕮 95
Taos, U.S.A. 🕮 295
Taranto, Italy 🕮 145
Tarzana, U.S.A. 🕮 223
Tasmania, Australia 🕮 31
Taunton, England 🕮 90
Tauranga, New Zealand 🕮 163
Tayside, Scotland 🕮 170
Teaneck, U.S.A. 🕮 293, 312
Teddington, England 🕮 87
Teeside, England 🕮 92
Tel-Aviv, Israel 🕮 138
Telford, England 🕮 90
Tempe, U.S.A. 🕮 194
Temple Hills, U.S.A. 🕮 266
Tennessee, U.S.A. 🕮 336
Teramo, Italy 🕮 139
Terheijden, The Netherlands 🕮 158
Terneuzen, The Netherlands 🕮 158
Terni, Italy 🕮 146
Terrace, Canada 🕮 45
Terre Haute, U.S.A. 🕮 255
Tesuque, U.S.A. 🕮 295
Texarkana, U.S.A. 🕮 194
Texas, U.S.A. 🕮 338
Thatcham, England 🕮 71
Thibodaux, U.S.A. 🕮 261
Thionville, France 🕮 106
Thompson, U.S.A. 🕮 232
Thorndike, U.S.A. 🕮 272
Thornhill, Canada 🕮 54
Thornton Heath, England 🕮 75
Thornton, U.S.A. 🕮 229
Thunder Bay, Canada 🕮 54
Thürmsdorf, Germany 🕮 134
Ticino, Switzerland 🕮 179
Tiel, The Netherlands 🕮 158
Tijuana, Mexico 🕮 149
Tilburg, The Netherlands 🕮 158
Timaru, New Zealand 🕮 163
Timmins, Canada 🕮 55
Tionesta, U.S.A. 🕮 333
Tipperary, Ireland 🕮 138
Titusville, U.S.A. 🕮 293
Tokyo, Japan 🕮 147
Toledo, U.S.A. 🕮 322
Toms River, U.S.A. 🕮 293
Tønsberg, Norway 🕮 167
Toowooba, Australia 🕮 29
Topanga, U.S.A. 🕮 223
Topeka, U.S.A. 🕮 258
Torino, Italy 🕮 144
Toronto, Canada 🕮 55
Torquay, England 🕮 73
Torrington, U.S.A. 🕮 232
Toscana, Italy 🕮 145
Toulon, France 🕮 106
Toulouse, France 🕮 106
Tours, France 🕮 106
Townsville, Australia 🕮 29
Trandheim, Norway 🕮 166
Transvaal, South Africa 🕮 171
Traverse City, U.S.A. 🕮 278
Travis, U.S.A. 🕮 223
Trellech, Wales 🕮 359
Trentino, Italy 🕮 146
Trento, Italy 🕮 146
Trenton, U.S.A. 🕮 293
Treviso, Italy 🕮 147
Trier, Germany 🕮 134
Trieste, Italy 🕮 141
Troisdorf, Germany 🕮 134
Trois-Rivières, Canada 🕮 63
Trollhättan, Sweden 🕮 176
Tromdheim, Norway 🕮 166
Troms, Norway 🕮 166
Tromsø, Norway 🕮 166
Trondheim, Norway 🕮 166
Troy, U.S.A. 🕮 312
Trumbull, U.S.A. 🕮 232
Truro, England 🕮 72
Tübingen, Germany 🕮 134
Tucson, U.S.A. 🕮 194, 223
Tujunga, U.S.A. 🕮 223
Tulare, U.S.A. 🕮 223
Tulsa, U.S.A. 🕮 323
Turkey 🕮 180
Turku, Finland 🕮 96
Turunporin Lääni, Finland 🕮 96
Tuscaloosa, U.S.A. 🕮 192
Tustin, U.S.A. 🕮 223
Tuttlingen, Germany 🕮 134
Tweed Heads, Australia 🕮 27
Twickenham, England 🕮 87
Tyler, U.S.A. 🕮 344
Tyne & Wear, England 🕮 92
Tysons Corner, U.S.A. 🕮 349
U.S.A. 🕮 180
Uden, The Netherlands 🕮 158
Udine, Italy 🕮 141
Uelzen, Germany 🕮 134
Uithoorn, The Netherlands 🕮 158
Ukiah, U.S.A. 🕮 223
Ulm, Germany 🕮 134
Umbria, Italy 🕮 146
Umeå, Sweden 🕮 176
Union City, U.S.A. 🕮 293
Unionville, U.S.A. 🕮 232
Universal City, U.S.A. 🕮 223
University Park, U.S.A. 🕮 295
Unna, Germany 🕮 134
Upland, U.S.A. 🕮 224
Uppland, Sweden 🕮 176
Uppsala, Sweden 🕮 176
Utah, U.S.A. 🕮 345
Utica, U.S.A. 🕮 312
Utrecht, The Netherlands 🕮 158
Uudenmaan Lääni, Finland 🕮 96
Uxbridge, England 🕮 87
Vaasa, Finland 🕮 97
Vaasan Lääni, Finland 🕮 97
Valdosta, U.S.A. 🕮 246
Valencia, U.S.A. 🕮 224
Valkenswaard, The Netherlands 🕮 158
Valle D'Aosta, Italy 🕮 146
Vallejo, U.S.A. 🕮 224
Valley Village, U.S.A. 🕮 224
Van Nuys, U.S.A. 🕮 224
Vancouver, Canada 🕮 45
Vancouver, U.S.A. 🕮 354
Varese, Italy 🕮 143
Värmland, Sweden 🕮 176
Västerås, Sweden 🕮 176
Västerbotten, Sweden 🕮 176
Västergötland, Sweden 🕮 176
Västmanlands län, Sweden 🕮 176
Växjö, Sweden 🕮 175
Veerle-Laakdal, Belgium 🕮 39
Veghel, The Netherlands 🕮 158
Veneto, Italy 🕮 146
Venezia, Italy 🕮 147
Venlo, The Netherlands 🕮 158
Venray, The Netherlands 🕮 158
Ventura, U.S.A. 🕮 224
Vermont, U.S.A. 🕮 345
Verona, Italy 🕮 147
Vest-Agder, Norway 🕮 166
Vestal, U.S.A. 🕮 312
Vestfold, Norway 🕮 166
Viborg, Denmark 🕮 67
Vicenza, Italy 🕮 147
Victoria Park, Australia 🕮 34
Victoria, Australia 🕮 31
Victoria, Canada 🕮 46
Victoriaville, Canada 🕮 63
Victorville, U.S.A. 🕮 224
Viersen, Germany 🕮 134
Viganello, Switzerland 🕮 179
Villa Park, U.S.A. 🕮 253
Villingen-Schwenningen, Germany 🕮 134
Vineyard Haven, U.S.A. 🕮 272
Virginia Beach, U.S.A. 🕮 349
Virginia, U.S.A. 🕮 346
Visalia, U.S.A. 🕮 224
Visby, Sweden 🕮 173
Visp, Switzerland 🕮 179
Vlissingen, The Netherlands 🕮 159
Voorburg, The Netherlands 🕮 159
Waco, U.S.A. 🕮 345
Wageningen, The Netherlands 🕮 159
Wagga Wagga, Australia 🕮 27
Wakefield, England 🕮 94
Wales 🕮 358
Walkersville, U.S.A. 🕮 266
Walla Walla, U.S.A. 🕮 354
Walnut Creek, U.S.A. 🕮 224
Walnut, U.S.A. 🕮 224
Walsall, England 🕮 93
Waltham, U.S.A. 🕮 273
Warren, U.S.A. 🕮 278
Warrington, England 🕮 72
Warwick, England 🕮 92
Warwickshire, England 🕮 92
Waseca, U.S.A. 🕮 282
Washington Township, U.S.A. 🕮 293
Washington, U.S.A. 🕮 233, 253, 350
Waterbury, U.S.A. 🕮 232
Waterford, Ireland 🕮 138
Waterloo, Canada 🕮 60

Waterloo, U.S.A. 257
Watertown, U.S.A. 273
Waterville, U.S.A. 263
Waukesha, U.S.A. 358
Wausau, U.S.A. 358
Wayland, U.S.A. 273
Wayne, U.S.A. 293, 333
Webster, U.S.A. 312
Weert, The Netherlands 159
Weimar, Germany 134
Weirs Beach, U.S.A. 288
Wellington, New Zealand 163
Welshpool, Wales 359
Wenatchee, U.S.A. 354
Wentzville, U.S.A. 285
Wesel, Germany 135
West Allis, U.S.A. 358
West Chester, U.S.A. 333
West Columbia, U.S.A. 335
West Franklin, U.S.A. 288
West Haddon, England 89
West Hollywood, U.S.A. 224
West Medford, U.S.A. 273
West Midlands, England 92
West Newton, U.S.A. 273
West Palm Beach, U.S.A. 243
West Point, U.S.A. 333
West Virginia, U.S.A. 354
West Yorkshire, England 94
Westcliff On Sea, England 75
Westerland, Germany 135
Western Australia, Australia 33
Westford, U.S.A. 273
Westmount, U.S.A. 293
Weston, U.S.A. 232
Weston-Super-Mare, England 70
Weymouth, U.S.A. 273
Whangarei, New Zealand 163
Wheaton, U.S.A. 253, 266
Wheeling, U.S.A. 355
Whitby, Canada 61
White Cross, England 79
Whitehorse, Canada 64
Whitewater, U.S.A. 358
Whittier, U.S.A. 225
Wichita Falls, U.S.A. 345
Wichita, U.S.A. 258
Wick, Scotland 168
Wien, Austria 35
Wiesbaden, Germany 135
Wigan, England 76
Wildwood, U.S.A. 293
Wilhelmshaven, Germany 135
Wilkes-Barre, U.S.A. 333
Williamsburg, U.S.A. 349
Williamsport, U.S.A. 333
Williamstown, U.S.A. 273
Williamsville, U.S.A. 312
Willimantic, U.S.A. 232
Willmington, U.S.A. 233
Willow Grove, U.S.A. 333
Wilmington, U.S.A. 233, 316
Wilnsdorf, Germany 135
Wilrijk, Belgium 39
Wilton, Ireland 137
Wiltshire, England 94
Windhoek, Namibia 149
Windsford, England 72
Windsor, Canada 61
Windsor, U.S.A. 232
Winfield, U.S.A. 253
Winnetka, U.S.A. 253
Winnipeg, Canada 47
Winona, U.S.A. 282
Winston-Salem, U.S.A. 316
Winter Park, U.S.A. 243
Winterthur, Switzerland 179
Wisconsin, U.S.A. 355
Witten, Germany 135
Wivenhoe, Australia 31
Woburn, U.S.A. 273
Woerden, The Netherlands 159
Wokingham, England 71
Wolfsburg, Germany 135
Wollongong, Australia 27
Wolverhampton, England 94
Wondelgem, Belgium 39
Wood Dale, U.S.A. 253
Woodbridge, England 91
Woodbridge, U.S.A. 293, 350
Woodcliff Lake, U.S.A. 293
Woodland Hills, U.S.A. 225
Woodlawn, U.S.A. 338
Woodridge, U.S.A. 253
Woodside, U.S.A. 312
Woodstock, U.S.A. 312, 350
Worcester, U.S.A. 273, 346
Worms, Germany 135
Worthing, England 92
Wrexham, Wales 359
Wupperthal, Germany 135
Würzburg, Germany 135
Wyoming, U.S.A. 358
Yakima, U.S.A. 354
Yellow Springs, U.S.A. 322
Yellowknife, Canada 48
Yorba Linda, U.S.A. 226
York, England 88
York, U.S.A. 333
Youngstown, U.S.A. 322
Ypsilanti, U.S.A. 278
Yukon, Canada 64
Zaragoza, Spain 172
Zephyrs Hills, U.S.A. 243
Zoetermeer, The Netherlands 159
Zug, Switzerland 179
Zürich, Switzerland 179
Zwickau, Germany 136
Zwolle, The Netherlands 159

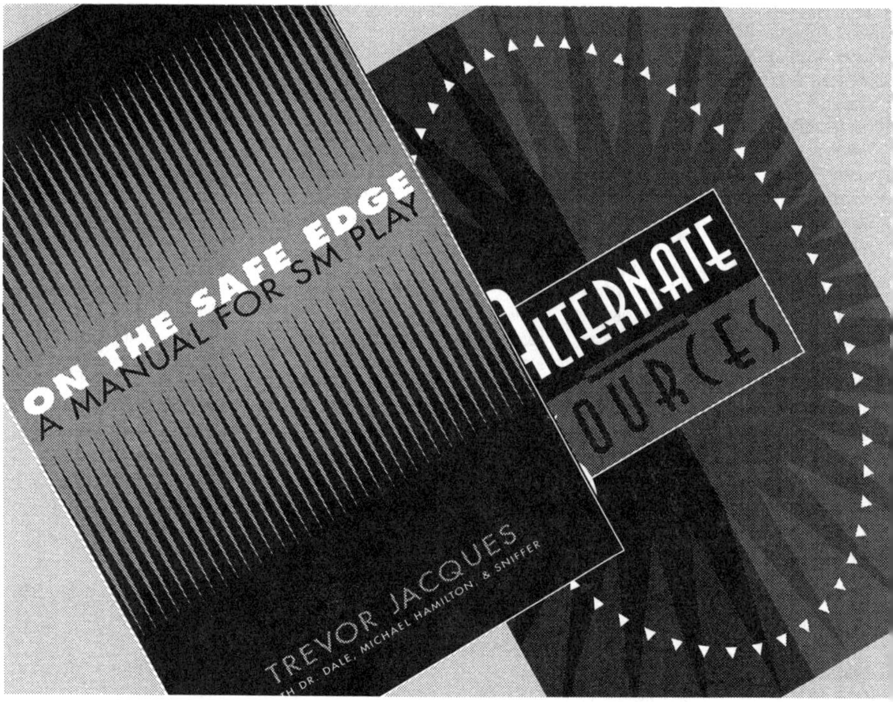

International Resources

Accommodation: BDSM

☺▼ **Logden House**
4320 8th. Street North West, Washington, District of Columbia 20011. U.S.A.
☎ 202 726 5159 ✆ 202 726 6495
✉ lvalentine@aol.com
⏰ 24hrs.
♣ ✓ $
Bed & breakfast catering to people who enjoy BDSM. Age statement of 18 is required.

Archives: BDSM

☺ **Leather Archives & Museum**
5015 North Clark Street, Chicago, Illinois 60640. U.S.A.
☎ 312 878 6360 ✆ 312 878 5184

☺ ☐ **Tom of Finland Foundation**
P.O. Box 26658, 1421 Laveta Terrace, Los Angeles, California 90026. U.S.A.
☎ 213 250 1685 ✆ 213 481 2092
⏰ 09:00 - 17:00
♣ ✓ $ 💳
Erotic art archive & resource centre for artists, curators, collectors, & educators. Publishes *Dispatch* quarterly. Yearly subscription is a $35, $100, or $250 donation.

Archives: Sexuality

⚥▽ **International Gay & Lesbian Archives**
P. O. Box 38100, Los Angeles, California 90038. U.S.A.
☎ 213 662 9444
⏰ Mon - Fri 10:00 - 22:00
Publishes *ILGA Bulletin*.

Artists: Erotic

⚥▼ **Galerie Leon**
P. O. Box 16825, Phœnix, Arizona 85011-6825. U.S.A.

☎ 602 263 0463
♣ ✓ $ 💳
Custom erotic portraits & fantasies. Notecards, prints. Catalogue, $2U.S.. Age statement of 18 is required.

BBSs: BDSM

⚥▼ **Hot Pockets BBS**
P. O. Box 3921, Portland, Oregon 97208. U.S.A.
☎ 503 232 2803 ✆ 503 232 9657
✆ 503 232 2803. 19800 baud maximum.
✉ daniel@hotpckts.rain.com
⏰ 24hrs.
♣ ✓ $ 💳
Spanish also spoken.

⚥▼ **Metropolitan Slave Online**
Selective Publishing, P. O. Box 4597, Oakbrook, Illinois 60522-4597. U.S.A.
☎ 708 986 8550 ✆ 708 323 3190
✆ 708 986 0294. 28800 baud maximum.
✉ jeb@metroslave.com
🌐 http://metroslave.com or telnet://metroslave.com
⏰ 24hrs.
♣ ✓ $ 💳
On-line edition of Metropolitan Slave magazine. Revelling in the slave lifestyle & honouring our masters. All masters / slaves interested are invited, regardless of gender / orientation. 2 hours free on sign-up. 30 min. a day subscriptions available. Free internet e-mail to all! Age statement of 21 is required.

☺▼ **SM Board**
P. O. Box 354, Wyoming, Pennsylvania 18644-0354.
☎ 717 655 2880 ✆ 717 655 7191
✆ 213 623 4732. 14400 baud maximum.
🌐 telnet://telcen.com
♣ ✓ 💳
System password: ALTERNATE. Age statement of 18 is required.

BBSs: Sexuality

⚥▼ **Back Door Computing Services**
P. O. Box 282720, San Francisco, California 94128-2720. U.S.A.
☎ 415 756 2906
✆ 415 756 6238. 28800 baud maximum.
✉ sysop@backdoor.com
⏰ 24hr. BBS. Voice 09:00 - 22:00
♣ ✓ $ 💳
Adult 98-line BBS for the gay or bisexual male. Full internet & web server. Chat, messages, online doctor, games, files. Age statement of 18 is required.

☺ **Lifestyle Online**
U.S.A.
✆ 516 698 5390. 14400 baud maximum.
✉ syslife@unet.net
🌐 http://www.unet.net/lifestyle or telnet://lifestyle.com or 166.82.150.22
♣ ✓ $ 💳
The largest adult (swingers, BDSM, bi, TV/TS, fetish) system in the world! It's an award winning system with 97 lines. Please see our display advertisement.

☺ ☐ **The Village**
c/o International Sexual Minorities Information Resource (ISMIR), P. O. Box 81869, Pittsburgh, Pennsylvania 15217-0869. U.S.A.
☎ 412 422 3060 ✆ 412 359 3878
✆ 412 422 1529. 14400 baud maximum.
✉ ismir@aol.com
♣
Public BBS free to everyone. ISMIR Events Calendar is available to members through BBS.

Competitions & Conventions: BDSM

⚥ **International Mr. Leather, Inc.**
5015 North Clark Street, Chicago, Illinois 60640. U.S.A.
☎ 800 545 6753 (in U.S.A.) ✆ 312 878 5184
☎ 312 878 6360

⚥ ▽ **International Ms Leather**
4332 Browne Street, Omaha, Nebraska 68111-1829. U.S.A.
☎ 402 451 7987 ✆ 402 457 5350
✉ imsl@synergy.net
⏰ Held in various cities every July
Competition is produced by Bare Images Productions, Ltd. from this address. Age statement of 21 is required.

⚥ ▽ **Mr. Deaf International Leather**
P. O. Box 226963, Dallas, Texas 75222-6963. U.S.A.
☎ 214 540 6439 TDD

Counsellors

☺ ■ **PMC Transgender Counseling & Consultation**
P. O. Box 5265, Coralville, Iowa 52241. U.S.A.

☎ 319 354 3189 📱 319 377 2045
🕐 By appointment
🚫 💳 ＭＣ 💳 📧
All types of gender counselling, legal financial, & psychological. All the romance languages also spoken.

Distributors: Books: Erotic

☺ ■ **Prestige Periodical Distributors**
P. O. Box 470, Port Chester, New York 10573. U.S.A.
☎ 914 939 2362 📱 914 939 5138
🚫 ✓ $ ⚡ ℓ
Free catalogue published once a year. Age statement of 18 is required.

Distributors: Erotica: General

⚧ **Paragon**
Postbus 23347, 1100 DV Amsterdam. The Netherlands
🚫 $ ⚡ ℓ
Distributes books, erotic videos, & magazines. Free catalogue. English & German also spoken.

Distributors: Magazines: General

☺ **Desert Moon Periodicals**
♿ 1226A Calle De Commercio, Santa Fe, New Mexico 87505. U.S.A.
☎ 505 474 6311 📱 505 474 6317
📧 xines@nets.com
🌐 http://www.swcp.com/xines/homepage.htm
🕐 Mon - Fri 08:30 - 17:00
🚫 ✓ $ 💳 ＭＣ
128-page catalogue published once a year, $4. Age statement of 18 is required.

Film Festivals: Sexuality

⚧▽ **Question de Genre**
c/o Cahiers Gai-Kitsch-Camp (CKC), Boîte Postale 36, 59009 Lille Cedex. France
☎ 20 06 3391 📱 20 78 1876
🕐 Held in Nov - Dec
🚫 ✓ $ ⚡ ℓ
English, French, & Arabic also spoken.

Health Services

⚧ ▽ **Concord Feminist Health Center**
♿ 38 South Main Street, Concord, New Hampshire 03301. U.S.A.
☎ 603 224 1737 📱 603 228 6255
Women-centred health provider, abortion services, feminist issues in general. Publishes *WomanWise* quarterly. Yearly subscription is $10 suggested donation, $20 suggested for businesses.

Helplines: Miscellaneous

⚧ ▽ **Discipline Support-Line for Women**
B. M. Elegance, London WC1N 3XX. England
☎ 181 989 0281
🕐 09:00 - 21:00
Women may telephone to discuss feelings / thoughts about discipline. Visits to household using corporal punishment as part of daily life possible. Age statement of 18 is required.

Helplines: Sexuality

⚧▽ **Pan Information**
♿ Postboks 1023, Teglgaardsstraede 13, 1452 København K. Denmark
☎ 33 13 0112
📧 hanschr@cybernet.dk
🕐 Mon Thu Fri Sun 20:00 - 23:00
Information about events & places in Denmark & other countries. We are always available for a talk. The service is anonymous.

Internet Mailing Lists: Academic

☺ ☐ **ACESGLBI**
📧 acesglbi@tasmvm1.tamu.edu
Gay, Lesbian, & Bisexual Interests in Counselor Education.

⚧▽ **EURO-QUEER-STUDIES**
📧 majordomo@queernet.org
European Gay & Lesbian Studies Discussion List.

⚧▽ **LGBPSYCH**
Canada
📧 listserv@vm1.mcgill.ca
Lesbian, Gay, & Bisexual Psychology Discussion List.

⚧▽ **MEDGAY-L**
📧 medgay-l@ksuvm.bitnet
Gay-Lesbian Medieval Studies Discussion Group. Gay & lesbian medieval studies.

⚧▽ **QSA**
New Zealand
📧 majordomo@massey.ac.nz
🌐 http://cc-server9.massey.ac.nz/~wwwms
Queer Studies Aotearoa Discussion List. Discussion of issues relating to lesbian, gay, bisexual & transgendered people in New Zealand. To

subscribe, send e-mail to: majordomo@massey.ac.nz with body text of: subscribe qsa.

⚧▽ **QSTUDY-L**
New Zealand
📧 listserv@ubvm.cc.buffalo.edu
Queer Studies Discussion List.

Internet Mailing Lists: AIDS

☺ ☐ **4ACURE-L**
📧 4acure-l@albnydh2.bitnet
AIDS Cure.

⚧☐ **ACT-UP AIDS-L**
📧 act-up-request@world.std.com
Discussion of HIV/AIDS issues & politics.

☺ ☐ **AIDS**
📧 aids-moderator@wubios.wustl.edu
AIDS Mailing list. A mirror of the newsgroup sci.med.aids. To subscribe, send e-mail to majordomo@wubios.wustl.edu with body text of: subscribe aids.

☺ ☐ **AIDS-STAT-L**
📧 AIDS-stat-request@wubios.wust1.edu

☺ ☐ **AIDSBKRV**
📧 aidsbkrv@uicvm.bitnet
AIDS Book Review Journal.

☺ ☐ **RETHINKING AIDS**
📧 Rethinking_AIDS@family.hampshire.edu
Rethinking AIDS. Discussion of issues relating to the reappraisal of the HIV/AIDS hypotheses.

Internet Mailing Lists: BDSM

☺ ☐ **AUSBDSM**
📧 listserv@cltr.uq.oz.au
Australian BDSM Discussion List. Australians & others interested in BDSM. To subscribe send e-mail to listserv@cltr.uq.oz.au with body text of: subscribe ausbdsm-1 <name>.

☺ ☐ **BAST**
U.S.A.
📧 bast-request@node.com
🌐 bast-announce@node.com
Mailing list for BDSM-minded people in the San Francisco Bay area. For information send e-mail to the e-mail address.

🏃 ☐ **FEMDOM-L**
📧 listserv@netcom.com
Feminine Domination Discussion List.

🏃 ☐ **FEMSUPREM**
📧 femsuprem-request@renaissoft.com
Feminine Supremacy Discussion List. To subscribe, send e-mail to: femsuprem-request@renaissoft.com with subject of: subscribe.

⚧▽ **GL-ASB**
📧 majordomo@queernet.org
Gay & Lesbian BDSM Discussion List.

☺ ☐ **MASTER-SLAVE**
📧 MSRList@aol.com
Master/Slave Discussion List. Discussion of master & slave relationships & related topics. To subscribe, send e-mail to: MSRList@aol.com with body text of: subscribe master-slave <your e-mail address>.

☺ ☐ **NLA-FRIENDS**
📧 nla-friends@tpe.com
Members Friends of the National Leather Association. Unofficial Internet mailing list for NLA members & friends of NLA.

Internet Mailing Lists: Bears

⚧▽ **BEARS**
📧 majordomo@queernet.org
Bears Discussion List. To subscribe, send e-mail to: majordomo@queernet.org with a text body of: subscribe bears-digest.

⚧▽ **BEARS-L**
📧 bears-request@spdcc.com
Bears Discussion List.

Internet Mailing Lists: Family

☺ ▽ **PFLAG-TALK**
U.S.A.
📧 pflag-talk@vector.casti.com
Parents & Friends of Gays, Lesbians, Bisexuals, & Transgendered Discussion List.

Internet Mailing Lists: Fetish: Cigars

⚧ **CS**
U.S.A.
📧 cs-owner@Queernet.ORG
Cigar &/or pipe smokers, & those sexually turned to them. Members often travel & meet each other. E-mail only.

Internet Mailing Lists: Library

GAYLIB-N
listproc@usc.edu
Gay, Lesbian, & Bisexual Librarians Network. To subscribe, send e-mail to: listproc@usc.edu with a body text of: sub gaylib-n <your first name> <your last name>.

Internet Mailing Lists: Sexual Politics

ACT-UP
act-up-request@world.std.com
Discussion of the activities of the world-wide chapters of ACT UP. Also to discuss HIV/AIDS issues & poiktics.

BIACT-L
biact-l@brownvm.bitnet
Bisexual Activist's Discussion List. To subscribe, send e-mail to: listserv@brownvm.brown.edu with body text of subscribe biact-l <your full name>.

QN
qn-request@queernet.org
Queer Nation. Discussion of issues relating to Queer Nation. To subscribe, send e-mail to: majordomo@queernet.org with body text of: subscribe qn.

STOPRAPE
stoprape@brownvm.bitnet
Sexaul Assault Activist List.

Internet Mailing Lists: Sexuality

ADDICT-L
listserv@kentvm.kent.edu
Sex Addiction Discussion List.

ALTERNATES
alternates-request@ns1.rutgers.edu
Open Sexual Lifestyle Discussion List.

AMAZONS
amazons-request@ifi.uio.no
Amazons International. Digest newsletter about amazons (physically & psychologically strong women). List owner: thomas@ifi.uio.no.

ARENAL
P. O. Box 6065, Bloomington, Indiana 47407. U.S.A.
listserv@lut.fi
To subscribe, send e-mail to listserve@lut.fi, with body text of: subscribe Arenal <Your Name>. Send articles to arenal@lut.fi.

ARENAL-L
arenal-l@brownvm.bitnet
Bisexuality Discussion List.

AUGLBC-L
auglbc@auvm.bitnet

AUSGBLF
ausgblf-request@minyos.xx.rmit.oz.au
Australian Gay, Lesbian, & Bisexual Discussion List.

BA-SAPPHO
ba-sappho-request@labrys.mti.sgi.com
Bay Area Lesbian Discussion List.

BGALA-L
listserv@brownvm.browm.edu
Brown Gay, Lesbian, & Bisexual Alumni Discussion List.

BIFEM-L
bifem-l@brownvm.bitnet
Bisexual Women's Discussion List. To subscribe, send e-mail to: listserv@brownvm.brown.edu with body text of subscribe bifem-l <your full name>.

BISEXU-L
bisexu-l@brownvm.bitnet
Bisexuality Discussion List. Discussion of issues relating to bisexuality. Everyone welcome to this list. To subscribe, send e-mail to: listserv@brownvm.brown.edu with body text of subscribe bisexu-l <your full name>.

BITHRY-L
bisexu-l@brownvm.bitnet
Bisexuality Theory Discussion List. Theoretical discussion of bisexuality. Not a social, support, anouncement, or news group. Cross postings from other groups are discouraged. To subscribe, send e-mail to: listserv@brownvm.brown.edu with body text of subscribe bithry-l <your full name>.

CD-FORUM
cd-request@therev.losalamos.nm.us
Cross Dressing Discussion List.

DC-MOTSS
dc-motss-request@vector.intercon.com
Abuse Victims Discussion List.

DDMM-L
ddmm-l@surplus.demos.su
Lesbigay list primarily in Russian. To subscribe, send e-mail to gala@surplus.demos.su.

DIGNITY
dignity@listserv.american.edu
LesBiGay Catholic List.

EURO-QUEER
majordomo@queernet.org
For all the messages, send e-mail to majordomo@queernet.org with body of: subscribe euro-queer. For a digest of the messages send body text of: subscribe euro-queer-digest.

EURO-SAPPHO
Finland
majordomo@seta.fi
http://www.helsinki.fi/~kris_ntk/esappho.html
To subscribe, send e-mail to majordomo@seta.fi with body of: subscribe euro-sappho <Name@Address>. If you have problems, send e-mail to euro-sappho-request@seta.fi.

FL-MOTSS
fl-motss-request@pts.mot.com
Florida Lesbian, Gay, & Bisexual DiscussionList.

GAY NETWORKS MAILING LIST
gaynet@athena.mit.com

GENDER
majordomo@indiana.edu
Gender Discussion List. Discussion of all aspects of gender. To subscribe, send e-mail to: majordomo@indiana.edu with a body text of: subscribe gender.

GLB-NEWS
listserv@brownvm.brown.edu
Gay, Lesbian & Bisexual News List.

GLBPOC
glbpoc-request@geri.pa.dec.com
Gay, Lesbian & Bisexual People of Colour Discussion List.

GLQSOC-L
glqsoc-l@binvmb.bitnet
Gay, Lesbian, Queer Social Sciences.

GRANITE
granite@nic.surfnet.nl
Gender Research Discussion List.

LA-MOTSS
U.S.A.
majordomo@langevin.usc.edu
Los Angeles MOTSS Discussion List. Discussion of all social & political lesbian, gay, & bisexual issues in the LA & southern California areas.

LA-MOTSS-ANNOUNCE
U.S.A.
majordomo@langevin.usc.edu
Los Angeles MOTSS Announcements List. Announcements of social & political lesbian, gay, & bisexual events in the LA & southern California areas.

LIS
lis-request@kenyon.edu
Lesbians In Science. Discussion of lesbian issues for women only. To subscribe, send e-mail to: lis-request@kenyon.edu with body text of: subscribe <your e-mail address> <your name>.

NE-SOCIAL-MOTSS
majordomo@plts.org
North East U.S.A. Discussion List. Discussion of lesbian, gay, bisexual & transgendered issues in the North East United States. To subscribe, send e-mail to: majordomo@plts.org with body text of: subscribe ne-social-motss.

NZGBLF
New Zealand
proffitt@iconz.co.nz
New Zealand Lesbian, Gay, & Bisexual Discussion List. Discussion of lesbian, gay, bisexual & transgendered issues in New Zealand. To subscribe, send e-mail to: proffitt@iconz.co.nz with body text of: subscribe nzgblf <your e-mail address>.

OH-MOTSS
U.S.A.
oh-motss-request@cps.udayton.edu
Ohio Gay, Lesbian, Bisexual, & Transgendered Discussion List.

PARTNERS
request-partners@starwars.com
Discussion between women whose partners are transsexual, transgendered, or cross dressers. To subscribe, send e-mail to: request-partners@starwars.com.

PDX-MOTSS
U.S.A.
pdx-motss-request@agora.rdrop.com
Portland Gay, Lesbian, Bisexual, & Transgendered Discussion List.

PLAYBOY MAILING LIST
U.S.A.

✉ playboy-request@lovesexy.com
Playboy Magazine Discussion List.

⚢⚤☐ **POLY**
✉ majordomo@hal.com
Non-Monogamous Relationships Discussion List. Discussion of non-monogamy, polyfidelty, & group marriage. To subscribe, send e-mail to: majordomo@hal.com with body text of: subscribe poly.

⚢⚤☐ **POLYFIDELITY**
✉ polyfi@cats.ucsc.edu
Non-Monogamous Relationships Discussion List. To subscribe, send e-mail to: polyfi@cats.ucsc.edu with body text of: subscribe polyfidelity.

⚥▽ **QNA**
New Zealand
✉ proffitt@iconz.co.nz
🌐 http://nz.com/NZ/Queer.qna.html & http://nz.com/glb/
Queer News Aotearoa. Weekly news service describing events & other items of interest to lesbian, gay, bisexual & transgendered people in New Zealand. To subscribe, send e-mail to: proffitt@iconz.co.nz with body text of: subscribe qna <your e-mail address>.

⚥▽ **QUEERCAMPUS**
✉ majordomo@vecto.casti.com
To subscribe, send e-mail to majordomo@vecto.casti.com with body of: subscribe QUEERCAMPUS.

⚢▽ **SAPPHO**
✉ sappho-request@apocalypse.org
Sappho. Discussion & support for all women. List is limited to female members.

☺▽ **SEX-L**
✉ sex-l@tamvm1.tamu.edu
General Sexual Topics Discussion List.

☺▽ **SEXTALK**
✉ sextalk@tamvm1.tamu.edu
Intellectual Sexuality Discussion List.

⚧▽ **TRANSGEN**
✉ transgen@brownvm.bitnet
TS/TV/TG Discussion List.

⚥▽ **UK-MOTSS**
England
✉ uk-motss-request@dircon.co.uk
U.K. MOTSS Discussion List. Discussion of lesbian, gay, bisexual & transgendered issues in the U.K.. For additional information, send e-mail to: uk-motss-request@dircon.co.uk with subject line of: send misc/info.

⚥▽ **UK-MOTSS-WOMEN**
England
✉ uk-motss-request@dircon.co.uk
U.K. MOTSS Women's Discussion List. Discussion of lesbian issues in the U.K.. This list is limited to female members. For additional information, send e-mail to: uk-motss-request@dircon.co.uk with subject line of: send misc/info.

Internet Mailing Lists: Spanking
⚥▽ **SPANK-L**
✉ craftman@iglou.com
Spanking Discussion List. For information, send e-mail to the e-mail address.

Internet Mailing Lists: Student
⚥▽ **CLGSG-L**
✉ listserv@ricevm1.bitnet
Coalition of Lesbian & Gay Students Discussion List.

⚥▽ **DSA-LGB**
✉ dc-motss-request@vector.intercon.com
Midway University Lesbian, Gay, & Bisexual Student Discussion List.

⚥▽ **GAYNET**
✉ gaynet-request@queernet.org
Discussions of gay, lesbian, & bisexual issues. To subscribe, send e-mail to: majordomo@queernet.org with body text of: subscribe gaynet.

⚥▽ **GGALA-L**
✉ ggala-l@ubcm.bitnet
Lesbian, Gay, Bisexual, Transgender, & Queer Graduate Students.

⚥▽ **LAMBDA**
U.S.A.
✉ listserv@ukcc.uky.edu
University of Kentucky Discussion Gay, Lesbian, & Bisexual List. Discussion of lesbian, gay, & bisexual issues, with a focus on the university. To subscribe, send e-mail to: listserv@ukcc.uky.edu with body text of: sub lambda <your first name> <your last name>.

⚥▽ **TAMUGLB**
✉ tamuglb@tamvm1.tamu.edu
Lesbian, Gay, & Bisexual Issues Discussion List.

Internet Mailing Lists: Support
☺☐ **COURAGE**
✉ majordomo@asarian.org

Abuse Victims Discussion List.

⚥☐ **EJINTVIO**
✉ listserv@uriacc.uri.edu
The Journal of Intimate Violence.

☺▽ **RECOVERY**
✉ recovery@wvnvm.wvnet.edu
Childhood Sexual Abuse Discussion List.

Internet Newsgroups: Academic: Anthropology
☺☐ **sci.anthropology**

Internet Newsgroups: Academic: Psychiatry
☺☐ **fj.sci.medical**
☺☐ **fj.sci.psychology**
☺☐ **francom.medical**
☺☐ **sci.psychology**
☺☐ **sci.psychology.journals.psyche**
☺☐ **sci.psychology.research**
☺☐ **sci.psychology.research.psychotherapy**
☺☐ **sfnet.keskustelu.psykologia**
☺☐ **tw.bbs.sci.psychology**
☺☐ **zer.z-netz.wissenschaft.psychologie**

Internet Newsgroups: Academic: Sexuality
☺☐ **tw.bbs.sci.sex**

Internet Newsgroups: AIDS
⚥▽ **gay-net.aids**

Internet Newsgroups: BDSM
☺☐ **alt.sex.bondage**
☺☐ **alt.sex.femdom**
☺☐ **alt.sex.sm.fig**
☺☐ **aus.sex.bondage**
⚥▽ **gay-net.lederecke**
☺☐ **sm-org**
✉ majordomo@vector.casti.com
SM Organizations.
☺☐ **uw.alt.sex.bondage**

Internet Newsgroups: Bears
⚥▽ **alt.sex.bears**

Internet Newsgroups: Body Size
☺☐ **alt.sex.fat**
☺☐ **alt.sex.fetish.fa**
☺☐ **alt.sex.fetish.size**
☺☐ **alt.sex.fetish.waifs**

Internet Newsgroups: Body Type
⚦☐ **alt.amazon-women.admirers**
☺☐ **alt.sex.furry**

Internet Newsgroups: Bondage
☺☐ **alt.fax.bondage**

Internet Newsgroups: Erotica
☺☐ **alt.magazine.playboy**
☺☐ **alt.magazines.pornographic**
☺☐ **alt.sex.erotica.marketplace**
☺☐ **alt.sex.magazines**
☺☐ **rec.arts.erotica**
This list is moderated.

Internet Newsgroups: Fetish: Adult Baby
☺☐ **alt.sex.fetish.diapers**

Internet Newsgroups: Fetish: Age
☺☐ **alt.sex.boys**
☺☐ **alt.sex.girls**

☺ ☐ alt.sex.pedophilia
☺ ☐ alt.sex.pedophilia.boys
☺ ☐ alt.sex.pedophilia.girls
☺ ☐ alt.sex.preteens
☺ ☐ alt.sex.young
☺ ☐ alt.support.boy-lovers

Internet Newsgroups: Fetish: Amputee
☺ ☐ alt.sex.fetish.amputee

Internet Newsgroups: Fetish: Animal
☺ ☐ alt.sex.animals
☺ ☐ alt.sex.bestiality
☺ ☐ alt.sex.hello-kitty
☺ ☐ alt.sex.reptiles
☺ ☐ alt.sex.zoophile
☺ ☐ alt.sex.zoophilia

Internet Newsgroups: Fetish: Balls
☺ ☐ alt.sex.balls

Internet Newsgroups: Fetish: Breasts
☺ ☐ alt.sex.breast

Internet Newsgroups: Fetish: Breathing
☺ ☐ alt.sex.asphyx
☺ ☐ alt.sex.breathless

Internet Newsgroups: Fetish: Clothing
☺ ☐ alt.clothing.lingerie
☺ ☐ alt.lycra
☺ ☐ alt.pantyhose
☺ ☐ alt.sex.fetish.fashion
☺ ☐ alt.sex.fetish.sportswear

Internet Newsgroups: Fetish: Enemas
☺ ☐ alt.sex.enemas

Internet Newsgroups: Fetish: Exhibitionism
☺ ☐ alt.sex.exhibitionism

Internet Newsgroups: Fetish: Foot
☺ ☐ alt.sex.fetish.feet
☺ ☐ alt.sex.fetish.feet.toes

Internet Newsgroups: Fetish: Foreskin
⚥▽ alt.sex.uncut

Internet Newsgroups: Fetish: Hair
☺ ☐ alt.sex.fetish.hair

Internet Newsgroups: Fetish: Mess
☺ ☐ alt.mud.sex
☺ ☐ alt.sex.fetish.wet-and-messy
☺ ☐ alt.sex.jello

Internet Newsgroups: Fetish: Miscellaneous
☺ ☐ alt.sex.fetish.orientals
▷▽ alt.sex.fetish.robots
☺ ☐ alt.sex.nasal-hair

Internet Newsgroups: Fetish: Motorcycle
☺ ☐ alt.sex.fetish.motorcycles

Internet Newsgroups: Fetish: Necrophilia
☺ ☐ alt.sex.necrophilia

Internet Newsgroups: Fetish: Smoking
☺ ☐ alt.sex.fetish.smoking

Internet Newsgroups: Fetish: Tickling
☺ ☐ alt.sex.fetish.tickling

Internet Newsgroups: Fetish: Voyeurism
☺ ☐ alt.sex.voyeurism

Internet Newsgroups: Library
☺ ☐ relcom.sci.libraries
☺ ☐ rpi.libraries
☺ ☐ soc.libraries.talk

Internet Newsgroups: Literature
☺ ☐ alt.censorship
▽ alt.lesbian.feminist.poetry

Internet Newsgroups: Masturbation
☺ ☐ alt.sex.masturbation

Internet Newsgroups: Medical: AIDS
☺ ☐ clari.tw.health.aids
☺ ☐ misc.health.aids
☺ ☐ sci.med.aids

Internet Newsgroups: Medical: Drugs
☺ ☐ zer.z-netz.gesundheit.drogen

Internet Newsgroups: Medical: General
☺ ☐ alt.support.herpes
☺ ☐ bit.listserv.medforum
☺ ☐ bit.listserv.medlib-l
☺ ☐ bit.listserv.mednews
☺ ☐ bit.med
☺ ☐ clari.tw.health
☺ ☐ misc.education.medical
☺ ☐ sci.med.diseases.hepatitis
☺ ☐ tw.bbs.sci.medicine
☺ ☐ zer.z-netz.gesundheit.diskussion
☺ ☐ zer.z-netz.gesundheit.krankheiten

Internet Newsgroups: Miscellaneous
☺ ☐ alt.nudism

Internet Newsgroups: Motorcycle
☺ ☐ tw.bbs.rec.motorcycle

Internet Newsgroups: Piercing
☺ ☐ rec.arts.bodyart

Internet Newsgroups: Polyfidelity
⚤ ☐ alt.polyamory

Internet Newsgroups: Sexual Politics
☺ ☐ alt.privacy
☺ ☐ alt.sex.advocacy

Internet Newsgroups: Sexuality: Youth
⚥▽ soc.support.youth.gay-lesbian-bi

Internet Newsgroups: Sexuality
☺ ☐ alt.books.anne-rice
☺ ☐ alt.christnet.nudism
☺ ☐ alt.foreplay
⚥▽ alt.homosexual
⚥▽ alt.journalism.gay-press
☺ ☐ alt.magick.sex
☺ ☐ alt.safe.sex
☺ ☐ alt.sex
☺ ☐ alt.sex.anal

☺ □ alt.sex.cd-rom
☺ □ alt.sex.historical
⚥▽ alt.sex.homosexual
☺ □ alt.sex.incest
☺ □ alt.sex.intergen
☺ □ alt.sex.jp
⚥▽ alt.sex.motss
☺ □ alt.sex.orgy
☺ □ alt.sex.safe
⚊▽ alt.sex.trans
♀▽ alt.shoe.lesbians
⚤▽ alt.support.transgendered
⚤▽ alt.transgendered
⚥▽ aus.culture.lesbigay
☺ □ aus.sex
⚥▽ can.motss
☺ □ cl.freie_liebe.hetero
⚥▽ cl.freie_liebe.schwule
☺ □ clari.news.crime.sex
⚥▽ clari.news.gays
☺ □ clari.news.law.crime.sex
☺ □ clari.news.sex
☺ □ es.alt.sex
　　⚒ http://latoso.cheme.cornell.edu:80/Spain/News/es.alt.sexo/
　　Spanish version of alt.sex. Not a normal newsgroup, but a set of web
　　pages.
⚥▽ fido.ger.gay
☺ □ fido.ger.sex
☺ □ fido7.sex
☺ □ finet.sex
⚥▽ gay-net.diskussionen
⚥▽ gay-net.general
⚥▽ gay-net.gesundheitsecke
⚥▽ gay-net.guide.bundesweit
⚥▽ gay-net.heteros
⚥▽ gay-net.international
♀▽ gay-net.lesben
⚥▽ ne.motss
♂▽ nv.bi
⚥▽ nv.motss
⚥▽ pa.motss
⚥▽ pgh.motss
⚥▽ pnw.motss
⚥▽ sdnet.motss
☺ □ slo.sex
♂▽ soc.bi
⚥▽ soc.gender.issues
⚥▽ soc.motss
⚤▽ soc.support.transgendered
⚥▽ su.gay
⚥▽ triangle.motss
⚥▽ uc.motss
♂▽ uiuc.soc.bisexuals
⚥▽ uiuc.soc.gay-men
⚥▽ uk.gay-lesbian-bi

☺ □ uw.alt.sex.beastiality
♂▽ vegas.bi
⚥▽ vegas.motss
☺ □ zer.t-netz.sex

Internet Newsgroups: Spanking
☺ □ alt.sex.spanking

Internet Newsgroups: Spirituality
☺ □ alt.christnet.sex
☺ □ alt.pagan
☺ ▽ alt.religion.sexuality
☺ □ alt.sex.cthulhu
☺ □ alt.sex.wizards

Internet Newsgroups: Support
☺ □ alt.recovery.addiction.sexual
☺ □ alt.recovery.sexual-addiction
☺ □ alt.sexual.abuse.recovery
☺ □ alt.sexual.abuse.recovery.d
☺ □ alt.support.abuse-partners
⚹ □ alt.support.cant.urinate.in-public
⚥▽ gay-net.coming-out
☺ □ talk.rape

Internet Newsgroups: Swingers
⚥⚹□ alt.sex.swingers

Internet Newsgroups: Watersports
☺ □ alt.sex.fetish.watersports
☺ □ alt.sex.watersports

Internet Newsgroups: Wrestling
☺ □ alt.sex.fetish.wrestling

Internet Organizations: Sexuality
♀▽ **Daughters of Aphrodite**
　　B.M. Elegance, London WC1N 3XX. England
　　☎ 181 989 0281
　　✉ embassy@pronews.pro-net.co.uk
　　⚒ http://www.zynet.net/elektra/aphrodite or
　　http://www.zynet.net/elektra/femmeworld
　　We exist to promote delicate ideals of female to female subtle
　　sensuality. '50s style glamour photos on the web. Age statement of 18
　　is required.

Internet Relay Chat (IRC) Channels
☺ □ #AIDS/HIV
☺ □ #analsex
☺ □ #anne-rice
☺ □ #bdsm
☺ □ #bdsmlounge
⚥▽ #bearcave
⚥▽ #bearlake
⚥▽ #bearlake2
⚤ ▽ #BiFEM!!!!
⚤ ▽ #bifemteens
♂▽ #bisex
☺ □ #bondage
☺ □ #breasts
⚊□ #crossdres
☺ □ #d&s
☺ □ #desade
☺ □ #Dom/Sub
☺ □ #erotic

☺ ☐ #erotica
☺ ☐ #eroticsex
☺ ☐ #exhibitionists
☺ ☐ #familysex
☺ ☐ #femdom
☺ ☐ #femuscle
☺ ☐ #FistFuck
☺ ☐ #fuck
⚥▽ #Gay
⚥▽ #gayboysex
⚥▽ #gaycouples
⚥▽ #gayhelp
⚥▽ #gayjackoff
⚥▽ #gaynz
　　New Zealand
⚥▽ #gaynz1
　　New Zealand
♀▽ #gaynzgirls
　　New Zealand
⚥▽ #gaysex
⚥▽ #gaySM
⚥▽ #gaysm
⚥▽ #gayteenchat
⚥▽ #gaytexas
⚥▽ #gayuncut
⚥▽ #GayWI
⚥▽ #gayworld
⚥▼ #gayyouth
　　🌐 http://www.bawue.de/~vba
☺ ☐ #goddess
☺ ☐ #HighHeels
☺ ☐ #intergen
⚥▽ #jack-off
⚥▽ #Jacks
⚥▽ #jerk-off
☺ ☐ #kinkysex
☺ ☐ #LeChambre
♀▽ #lesbian
♀▽ #lesbians
♀▽ #lesbos
♀▽ #lezsex
♀▽ #lezsex2
☺ ☐ #pagan
☺ ☐ #pantyhose
☺ ☐ #peesex
☺ ☐ #pervert
👫 ☐ #polyamory
☺ ☐ #pornshop
☺ ☐ #sex
☺ ☐ #sex&stuff
☺ ☐ #spanking
☺ ☐ #submission
👫 ☐ #Swing
☺ ☐ #teensex
🗯▽ #transgen
☺ ☐ #vampire

☺ ☐ #vampires
☺ ☐ #voyeurs
☺ ☐ #Weirdsex
☺ ☐ #wetstuff
☺ ☐ #wildsex
☺ ☐ #youngsex

Internet Search Engines: General

☺ ■ **DejaNews Partners**
U.S.A.
✉ help@dejanews.com
🌐 http://www.dejanews.com/
Largest collection of indexed archived Usenet news. Searches through mountains of Usenet archives in seconds to find the information you need.

☺ ■ **Excite**
U.S.A.
🌐 http://www.excite.com/

☺ ▽ **Lycos Incorporated**
293 Boston Post Road West, Marlborough, Massachusetts 01752. U.S.A.
☎ 508 229 0717　　　　　✆ 508 229 2866
✉ webmaster@lycos.com
🌐 http://www.lycos.com/

☺ □ **Yahoo Corporation**
Suite F, 10 Pioneer Way, Mountain View, California 94041. U.S.A.
☎ 415 934 3230　　　　　✆ 415 934 3248
✉ info@yahoo.com
🌐 http://www.yahoo.com/
🕐 Mon - Fri 08:30 - 17:00

Mailorder: Books: BDSM

☺ ▼ **QSM**
P.O. Box 880154, San Francisco, California 94188-0154. U.S.A.
☎ 800 537 5815　　　　　✆ 415 550 7117
☎ 415 550 7776
✉ Info@qualitysm.com
🕐 Mon - Fri 11:00 - 17:00
💰 ✓ $ ⚞ 💳 ⬤
Over 600 books, magazines, & adult comics. Also educational classes on BDSM in San Francisco. Free 24-page catalogue published quarterly. Age statement of 21 is required.

Mailorder: Books: BDSM

☺ ■ **WPC**
P. O. Box 19591-885, 55 Bloor Street West, Toronto, Ontario M4W 3T9.
☎ 416 962 1040　　　　　✆ 416 962 1044
✉ wpc@inforamp.net
🌐 http://www.inforamp.net/~wpc
🕐 Mon - Fri 09:00 - 17:00, voice mail at other times
💰 ✓ 💳
Publishers of the best seller "On The Safe Edge: A Manual for SM Play." Paperback edition $24.95Cdn. (plus G.S.T.) in Canada, £14.99 in U.K., $19.95U.S. in U.S. & elsewhere. Hardcover & signed limited edition black leather library binding also available. Shipping to U.S. & Canada (plus G.S.T. in Canada) $5 for the first book, $2 for each additional book; to U.K. £4 for the first book, £1.50 for each additional book; elsewhere $8U.S. for the first book, $2.50U.S. for each addional book. Please see our display advertisement.

Mailorder: Books: Erotic

☺ **Daisy Publications Ltd.**
P. O. Box 49, Bexhill-on-Sea, East Sussex TN39 3BZ. England
☎ 142 845 018　　　　　✆ 142 845 018
💰 ✓ $
Mail order books & erotic magazines. Catalogue available, published monthly. Age statement of 18 is required.

☺ ■ **Delectus Books**
27 Old Gloucester Street, South Kensington, London WC1N 3XX. England
☎ 181 963 0979　　　　　✆ 181 963 0502
🕐 Mon - Fri 10:00 - 18:00, Sat 10:00 - 12:30
💰 💳 ⬤
Catalogue published every two months, $2. Age statement of 18 is required.

Mailorder: Books: General

☺ **Body Art, Publications Ltd.**
P.O. Box 32, Great Yarmouth, Norfolk NR29 5RD. England
💰 ✓ $ ⚞ 💳 ⬤ ⚢
Publisher & distributor of body decoration magazines & books. Free catalogue published twice a year.

Mailorder: Books: Sexuality

⚥▼ **Books Bohemian**
P.O. Box 17218, Los Angeles, California 90017-0218. U.S.A.
☎ 213 385 6761
🕐 Mon - Sat 08:00 - 20:00
🚗 ✓ $ 💳
Free catalogue. Some Spanish also spoken.

☺▼ **Circlet Press Bookshop**
Suite 278, 1770 Massachusetts Avenue, Cambridge, Massachusetts 02140. U.S.A.
☎ 617 864 0492 ✆ 617 864 0492
📧 catalog@circlet.com
🌐 http://www.circlet.com/circlet/home.html
🚗 ✓ $ 💳
Hundreds of BDSM-related books & magazines, how-to erotica, graphic novels, & more. Catalogue, free with SASE or IRC. Age statement of 18 is required.

♀ **Fat Girl**
& Box 193, 2215 Market Street, San Francisco, California 94114. U.S.A.
☎ 714 550 7202
📧 airborne@advanced.com
🌐 http://www.icsi.berkeley.edu/~polack/fg/
🚗 ✓
The 'zine for fat dykes & the women who want them. Publishes *FaT GiRL* 3 times a year. Yearly subscription is $20U.S.. Age statement of 18 is required.

⚥▼ **Intermale**
Spuistraat 251, 1012 VR Amsterdam. The Netherlands
☎ 20 625 0009 ✆ 20 620 3163
🕐 Mon 12:00 - 18:00, Tue - Sat 10:00 -18:00, Thu - 19:00
🚗 $ ⚥ ✆
The largest bookstore in Amsterdam devoted entirely to books of interest to the gay male.

⚥■ **Lambda Rising Online**
1625 Connecticut Avenue North West, Washington, District of Columbia 20009-1013. U.S.A.
☎ 800 621 6969 ✆ 202 462 7257
☎ 202 462 6969
📧 lambdarising@his.com
🕐 Mon - Fri 10:00 - 24:00

✓ $ 💳
Gay & lesbian book & gift mail order service. On America Online, use keyword GAYBOOKS to reach full online service. Free catalogue published quarterly.

⚥▼ **Lambda Rising**
& 1625 Connecticut Avenue North West, Washington, District of Columbia 20009-1013. U.S.A.
☎ 800 621 6969 ✆ 202 462 7257
☎ 202 462 6969
📧 lambdarising@his.com
🕐 Mon - Fri 10:00 - 18:00
✓ $ 💳
Gay & lesbian book & gift catalogue & mail order service. Also videos, music, rainbow flags, & gifts. Publishes *Lambda Rising News* quarterly. Yearly subscription is free.

⚥ **Paragon**
Postbus 23347, 1100 DV Amsterdam. The Netherlands
🚗 $ ⚥ ✆
Free catalogue. English & German also spoken.

Mailorder: Clothing: Fetish

☺ **Demask**
Zeedijk 64, 1012 BA Amsterdam. The Netherlands
☎ 20 620 5603 ✆ 20 492 0393
☎ 20 620 7215 (2nd. facs.)
🕐 10:00 - 19:00
🚗 ✓ $ 💳 📺 ✆
Has shops & perhaps the largest manufacturing facility & production of fetish clothing, both rubber & leather in the world. Catalogue, FL30 ($20U.S.). English, German, Italian, Spanish, & Yugoslavian also spoken.

☺■ **The Fetish Factory Ltd.**
5 Flensburger Straße 5, 42655 Solingen. Germany
☎ 21 258 6151 ✆ 21 258 6156
🕐 09:00 - 13:00
🚗 ✓ $ 💳 ✆
Complete rubber fashion collection. Age statement of 18 is required. French & English also spoken.

⚥▼ **International Male Mail**
Postfach 10, 6170 Schüpfheim. Switzerland
☎ 41 485 0081 ✆ 41 485 0090

100136,3433@CompuServe.com
Mon - Sat 08:00 - 18:00
✓ $
Leather, rubber, uniforms, toys, etc.. Also immigration & legal services consulting. Catalogue published twice a year, $10U.S.. Age statement of 18 is required. French, English, & Russian also spoken.

Zipper Mail Order
283 Camden High Street, London NW1 7BX. England
171 267 0021 — 171 284 0329
171 267 7665
mailorder@gaytimes.co.uk
✓
Catalogue, £2. Age statement of 18 is required.

Mailorder: Clothing: Leather

Black Eagle Leather Co.
P. O. Box 950865, Mission Hills, California 91395-0865. U.S.A.
818 361 4674 — 213 426 4093
leather@painet.com
http://www.painet.com/~leather/
Mon - Fri 10:00 - 19:00
✓ $
On the cutting edge leather chaps, jackets, shorts. Also works in plastic, vinyl thigh-high custom boots. World acclaimed leather masks. Catalogue, $10U.S.. Age statement of 18 is required.

Saint Michael's Emporium
Suite 1, 156 East 2nd. Street, New York 10009. U.S.A.
212 995 8359
stmichemp@aol.com
Tue - Sat 13:00 - 19:00, Sun 13:00 - 17:00
✓ $
Specialist in fantasy medieval leather clothing & jewelry. Catalogue, $4.

Mailorder: Clothing: Rubber

Herta Gummi
BCM Box 6998, London WC1N 3XX. England
181 287 3839
09:00 - 18:00
Division of rubber manufacturer. Mail order only. Catalogue, £5. French also spoken.

Mailorder: Erotica: Adult Baby

Diaper Pail Friends (DPF)
Suite 127, 38 Miller Avenue, Mill Valley, California 94941. U.S.A.
08:00 - 20:00
✓ $
World's largest organization devoted to adult babies & diaper lovers. Huge selection. Publishes newsletter to help people meet, correspond & share their interests. Free 60-page catalogue. Publishes *DPF Newsletter* every two months. Yearly subscription is $30U.S.. Age statement of 18 is required. Please see our display advertisement.

Mummy Hazel High Heels - H. B. Enterprises
c/o 43 South Hill Road, Gravesend, Kent DA12 IJX. England
163 457 1396 — 163 485 2737
Mon - Fri 14:00 - 18:00
✓ $
Also runs the "Hush-A-Bye Baby Club" for contacts & parties. Has 2 fully equipped nurseries for hire. Publishes a newsletter every two months. Yearly subscription is £45. Age statement of 18 is required. French also spoken.

Mailorder: Erotica: BDSM

The Academy Club
P. O. Box 135, Hereford, Hereford & Worcester HR2 7PE. England
143 234 3241 — 143 234 3241 (manual)
guy@acopclub.demon.co.uk
$
Books, booklets, magazines, tapes, implements, uniform, etc., for the "Adult School" or corporal punishment fan. Must join to attend Muir Academy. Age statement of 21 is required.

Boutique Minuit
60 Galerie du Centre, 1000 Bruxelles 1. Belgium
2 223 0914 — 2 223 1009
Mon - Sat 10:30 - 18:30
✓
Over 4,000 different styles & 20 different catalogues available. Leather, lingerie, rubber, high heels, TV/TS, steelwear. In existence over 15 years. Catalogue available. Age statement of 18 is required. English & Dutch also spoken.

Hard Love Leather
Suite 485, 7620 East Mckellips, Scottsdale, Arizona 85257-4600. U.S.A.
602 947 3520
602 946 2375
Mon - Fri 12:00 - 20:00

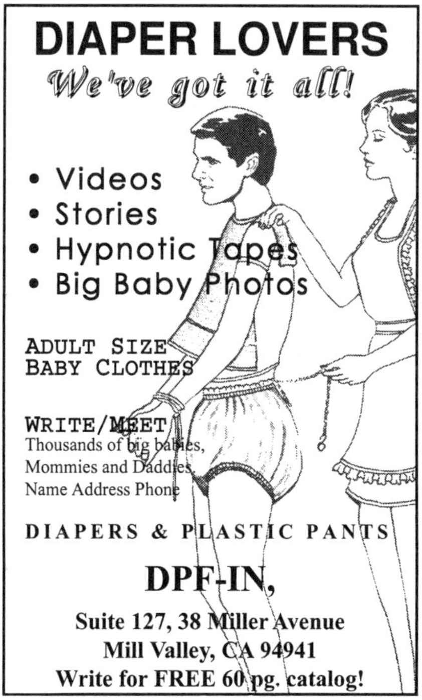

✓ $
Single-tail whips, floggers, cats, restraints, & harnesses made for the lifestyle by lifestylers. Cheques payable to Bob Clark or Roger Patterson. Age statement of 18 is required.

Hidebound
P.O. Box 10, Liverpool, Merseyside L36 6LD. England
151 252 2272 — 151 252 2273
✓
Chain mail leather, PVC, latex clothing, BDSM furniture, restraints, bondage. Also custom made. Catalogue, £7 airmail outside of U.K., p&p incl.. Age statement of 18 is required.

Leather Underground, Inc.
1170 North East 34th. Court, Fort Lauderdale, Florida 33334. U.S.A.
305 561 3977 — 305 561 4204
Mon - Sat 09:00 - 18:00
$
Also mail order. Catalogue, $20. Age statement of 21 is required.

Massad Mailorder
Postbus 3061, Zaagmolendrift 33, 3003 AK Rotterdam. The Netherlands
10 466 4368 — 10 465 9977
Tue - Sat 09:00 - 17:00
$
Leather manufacturer, bookshop, mail order. Also Massad magazine. Catalogue, $25U.S. incl. s&h. English & German also spoken.

The Other Pony Club
P. O. Box 135, Hereford, Herefordshire HR2 7PH. England
143 234 3241 — 143 234 3241 (manual)
guy@acopclub.demon.co.uk
09:00 - 20:00
✓ $
Books, harnesses, videos, etc.. Yearly subscription is £1 U.K., $5 U.S.. Age statement of 18 is required.

RGL Designs
Glenfield Park, Lomeshaye Industrial Estate, Nelson, Lancashire BB9 7DR. England
1282 697866 — 1282 697866
08:30 - 17:00
$
Manufacturer & supplier of leather bondage & discipline equipment direct to the public via catalogue, & to traders. Catalogue, £5. Age statement of 18 is required.

Strictly Stories
P. O. Box 15, Station A, Etobicoke, Ontario M9C 2V3. Canada
416 622 2485
09:00 - 21:00
$

Tom of Finland Company Inc.
P. O. Box 26716, Dept. AS, Los Angeles, California 90026. U.S.A.
800 334 6526 — Fax 213 666 2105
213 666 1052
tomfinland@earthlink.net
http://www.earthlink.net/~tomfinlandco/
Mon - Fri 09:00 - 17:00
✓ $ VISA MC
Sole resource for legendary Tom of Finland works in print, as well as an international source for erotic books, videos, prints, rubberwear, & more. Catalogue, $10. Age statement of 21 is required.

Mailorder: Erotica: Bondage

JuRonCo
P.O. Box 5992, Peoria, Illinois 61601. U.S.A.
309 673 8724
jlaredo@heartland.bradley.edu
✓ $
Mailoder supplier of institutional-type restraints. Catalogue, $3U.S.. Age statement of 21 is required.

KW Enterprises
Suite 803, 89 Fifth Avenue, New York 10003. U.S.A.
212 727 1973 — Fax 212 243 1630
Mon - Fri 10:00 - 18:00
✓ $ VISA MC AMERICAN EXPRESS
Subsidiary of The Outbound Press, specializing in male bondage. Videos, publications, books, equipment, toys, etc.. Also makes videos. Catalogue, $5. Age statement of 21 is required.

Mailorder: Erotica: Enemas

Arthur Hamilton, Inc.
P. O. Box 180145, Richmond Hill, New York 11418. U.S.A.
718 441 6066
Mon - Fri 10:00 - 17:00
✓ $ VISA MC AMERICAN EXPRESS
Furnishmedical quality enema equipment, including bags, nozzles, tubes, & bardexes. Mail order only. Catalogue, $2. Age statement of 21 is required. Please see our display advertisement.

Mailorder: Erotica: General

Blowfish
#284, 2261 Market Street, San Francisco, California 94114. U.S.A.
415 864 0880 — Fax 415 864 1858
blowfish@blowfish.com
http://www.blowfish.com
✓ $ VISA MC AMERICAN EXPRESS
Mail-order erotica source for all interests. Carries arts & crafts, books, videos, toys, & many other products, all with a sex-positive theme. Catalogue published 3 times a year, $3. Age statement of 18 required.

Q Things
P. O. Box 2230, London W14 9WD. England
171 384 2129 — Fax 171 610 6163
171 384 2130
10:00 - 18:00
✓ $ VISA MC ₡
Independent mail-order company specialising in quality lesbian & gay products, including music & clothing merchandise, as well as the exotic. Free catalogue published quarterly. German also spoken.

The Xandria Collection
The Lawrence Research Group, P. O. Box 31039, Dept. AS, San Francisco, California 94131. U.S.A.
415 468 3812 — Fax 415 468 3912
✓ $ VISA MC
Over twenty years marketing erotica to all people. Products with three guarantees in mind: 100% privacy, customer satisfaction, & product assurance. Catalogue published every two months, $4 U.S., $5 Cdn., £3 U.K.. Age statement of 21 is required. Spanish also spoken.

Mailorder: Erotica: Leather

Pleasure Place
1063 Wisconsin Avenue, Washington, District of Columbia 20007. U.S.A.
800 386 2386 — Fax 202 333 3997
202 333 8570
Mon Tue 10:00 - 22:00, Wed - Sat 10:00 - 24:00, Sun 12:00 - 19:00
$ VISA MC AMERICAN EXPRESS
Open for 16 years. Leather & latex clothes & toys, lingerie, stockings, patent thigh-high boots, 6'' heels, engineer boots, etc.. Catalogue, $3. Age statement of 18 is required. Spanish also spoken.

Remedy Versand
Gurlittstraße 47, 20099 Hamburg. Germany
40 24 5979 — Fax 40 24 6097
Mon - Wed Fri 10:30 -18:30, Thu 10:30 - 20:30, Sat 10:30 - 14:00
Catalogue, DM20.

Mailorder: Erotica

Bodyshot
P. O. Box 22051, Port Elizabeth, Cape Province 6000. South Africa
41 308016 — Fax 41 308017
Mon -Fri 09:00 - 16:00
$ VISA MC ₡
Catalogue, R10. Age statement of 18 is required.

Fantasy Erotique
P. O. Box 6412, London E7 9SB. England
181 555 2996 — Fax 181 503 0968
Mon - Sat 10:00 - 20:00
✓ $ VISA MC
Leather, rubber, toys, & clothing. Retail by appointment only. Catalogue, free upon written request. Age statement of 18 is required. German also spoken.

Good Vibrations
Suite 101, 938 Howard Street, San Francisco, California 94103. U.S.A.
800 289 8423 — Fax 415 974 8989
415 974 8990
goodvibe@well.sf.ca
Mon - Sat 07:00 - 19:00
✓ VISA MC
Mail order sex toys, books, videos, & catalogues. Free catalogue published quarterly. Age statement of 18 is required. Spanish spoken.

S. H. H. Services
291 Adsum Drive, Winnipeg, Manitoba R2P 0V9. Canada
204 694 3164 — Fax 204 697 1849
Mon - Fri 10:00 - 22:00
✓ $ VISA MC AMERICAN EXPRESS
Love shop supplies by mail order or appointment only. Catalogue, $4. Age statement of 21 is required.

Mailorder: Videos: Sexuality

Bluemoon Films
Bluemoon House, 89 London Lane, Bromley, Kent BR1 4HF. England

☎ 181 466 8296 ✆ 181 466 8295
🕐 7 days per week
🏧 ✓ $
Videos, books, sex aids. Promote Dr. Betty Dodson, Ph.D. - her video "Self Loving," & book "Sex For One" in the U.K.. Age statement of 18 is required.

Mailorder: Videos: Watersports
☺ ▼ **Michael Schein**
Suite 201, 76 Cranbrook Road, Cockeysville, Maryland 21030. U.S.A.
☎ 617 567 2000
🏧 ✓ $ ⚎ 💳 💳
Mail & facs. order watersports videos (VHS, Beta, 8mm). Mainly gay male, some hetero. Safe delivery of videos to Canada guaranteed. Free catalogue. Age statement of 18 is required.

Manufacturers: Adult Toys: Percussion
☺ ▼ **Hanson Percussion Instruments**
P.O. Box 085239, Racine, Wisconsin 53408-5239. U.S.A.
☎ 414 632 7330 ✆ 414 632 7101
✉ Rabj@mail.coretech.com
🕐 08:00 - 22:00 every day
🏧 ✓ $ ⚎ 💳 💳 ✉ ℓ
High quality original design paddles, straps, & our own version of the old-fashioned razor strap. We'll customize your fantasy percussion instrument. 6-page catalogue, $2, refundable with first purchase. Age statement of 21 is required. French, German, & Spanish also spoken.

Manufacturers: Clothing: Corsets
☺ ■ **Dark Garden Corsets**
Box 242A, 2215-R Market Street, San Francisco, California 94114. U.S.A.
☎ 415 522 9651
☎ 415 626 6264 (for appointments)
🕐 Tue - Fri 09:30 - 17:30, or by appointment
🏧 ✓ $ 💳
Custom corsets that fit! Beautifully crafted in leather, satin, silks, & brocade. Catalogue, $10U.S., redeemable on purchase, $12U.S. overseas.

☺ **Talana Gamah & leish**
BCM Blindfold, London WC1N 3XX. England
☎ 181 979 2429 ✆ 181 941 6909
 ☎ 585 760514
🏧 ✓ $ ⚎ 💳 💳
Dedicated to providing the finest fetish couture clothing in all materials (except rubber): corsets to the most elaborate fantasy garments.

Manufacturers: Clothing: Leather
☺ **Liz Lewitt - Wholesale**
6 Perry Road, Bristol, Avon BS1 5BQ. England
☎ 117 929 3754 ✆ 117 929 3754
🕐 11:00 - 18:00
🏧 ✓ $ ℓ
Designer inspired fetish clothing for dressers of all sexes - Leather, powernet mesh, spandex, transparent silk organza, & PVC. Commissions undertaken.

Manufacturers: Clothing: Rubber
☺ ■ **The Fetish Factory Ltd.**
5 Flensburger Straße 5, 42655 Solingen. Germany
☎ 21 258 6151 ✆ 21 258 6156
🕐 09:00 - 13:00
🏧 ✓ $ ⚎ 💳 💳 ℓ
Complete rubber fashion collection. Age statement of 18 is required. French & English also spoken.

☺ **Ripplesmooth**
Unit 6, 100 Spencer Street, Birmingham, West Midlands B18 6DB. England
☎ 121 515 1994
🕐 Mon - Fri 10:00 - 18:00
🏧 ✓ $ ⚎ ℓ
Specializing in bodysuits & restrictive rubberwear. Mail order & open to visitors. Free catalogue. Age statement of 18 is required.

☺ **Tentacle**
P.O. Box 20, Grantham, Lincolnshire NG33 5RB. England
☎ 1572 768440 ✆ 1572 768156
🕐 Flexible opening hours. Call first
🏧 ✓ $ 💳 ℓ
Friendly company designing & manufacturing unusual rubber clothing for both sexes. Trained tailor incorporates sculpted rubber with surreal & erotic style. Catalogue published once a year, £7. Age statement of 18 is required.

Manufacturers: Enema Equipment
☺ ■ **Mediquip**
⚤ Folly Gate, Okehampton, Devon EX20 3AQ. England
☎ 1837 53710 ✆ 1837 54972

✉ booth@mediquip.zynet.co.uk
🌐 http://www.zynet.co.uk/mediquip/
🕐 Mon - Fri 09:00 - 17:00
🏧 ✓ $ 💳 💳
Established 12 years for the mail order sales of medical equipment, including rubber sheeting & enema equipment, also ballon catheters. Catalogue, $5 cash or equivalent.

Manufacturers: Erotica: Leather
☺ ■ **Klix Leather Products**
P.O. Box 5, Bury, Lancashire BL8 2UQ. England
☎ 161 763 7488 ✆ 161 763 7488
 ☎ 378 314 902
✉ ako@klixgb.win-net.uk
🕐 09:00 - 18:00
🏧 ✓ $ ⚎ ℓ
Run by enthusiasts for enthusiasts. Designs in leather, rubber, metal, & wood, made to your ideas or from our vast range. Catalogue, £6. Age statement of 18 is required. Polish also spoken.

Manufacturers: Furniture: BDSM
☺ ■ **TFM Co.**
88 Chaple Street, Tiverton, Devon EX16 6BU. England
☎ 1884 34958 ✆ 1884 255330
☎ 1884 255330
🏧 $ ⚎
Erotic & BDSM furniture, from a rack with a 2-way pull, that will fit into a car, to convertible dining tables. Catalogue, £5, $10U.S.. Age statement of 21 is required.

Manufacturers: Piercing Jewelry
☺ ■ **Asgard International**
P. O. Box 69, Southampton, Hampshire SO9 7EQ. England
☎ 170 332 5059
Surgical steel solid ball closure rings, labret studs, nipple shields, nipple spreaders, & body piercing kits.

☺ **Chaotic Creations**
155 Britannia Street, Meriden, Connecticut 06450. U.S.A.
☎ 203 639 6105
🏧 ✓

☺ **The Wildcat Collection**
16 Preston Street, Brighton, East Sussex BN1 2HN. England
☎ 1273 323758 ✆ 1273 323758
🕐 Mon - Sat 10:00 - 18:00
🏧 ✓ $ ⚎ ℓ
Purveyors of sophisticated body adornment products & paraphernalia, jewelry, postcards, books, posters, toys, gadgets, video documentaries, & more. Free catalogue. Age statement of 18 is required. French & German also spoken.

Organizations: AIDS: Support
⚥ ▼ **Positive Image**
P.O. Box 1501, Pomona, California 91769. U.S.A.
☎ 909 622 6312 ✆ 909 623 1810
🕐 Erratic Mon - Fri 09:00 - 17:00
🏧 ✓ $
Contact: Mr. Kenneth Schein
A social & sexual communication network for men who are HIV+ or have AIDS. Publishes *Positive Image* quarterly. Yearly subscription is $25 (higher outside U.S. & Canada). Age statement of 18 is required.

Organizations: Balls
⚥ ▼ **Ball Club**
⚤ P.O. Box 1501, Pomona, California 91769. U.S.A.
☎ 909 622 6312 ✆ 909 623 1810
🕐 Erratic Mon - Fri 09:00 - 17:00
🏧 ✓ $
Contact: Mr. Kenneth Schein
A communications network set up in 1985 for men who have 'em & men who want 'em. Publishes *Ball Club Quarterly* quarterly. Yearly subscription is $45 (higher outside U.S. & Canada). Age statement of 18 is required.

Organizations: BDSM: Pony
☺ ■ **The Other Pony Club**
P. O. Box 135, Hereford, Herefordshire HR2 7PH. England
☎ 143 234 3241 ✆ 143 234 3241 (manual)
✉ guy@acapclub.demon.co.uk
🕐 09:00 - 20:00
🏧 ✓ $ ℓ
Contact: Sir Guy Masterleigh, B.Sc., Director
Club for would-be human "ponies," "puppies", etc., trainers, owners, & fans. Events & 1:1 training. Publishes *The Other Pony Express* 3 times a year. Yearly subscription is £25 for U.K., £30 for Europe, $60U.S. for U.S./Canada etc.. Age statement of 18 is required.

Organizations: BDSM
☺ **The Backdrop Club**

P.O. Box 390486, Mountain View, California 94039-0486. U.S.A.
415 965 4499 — 415 964 3879
415 964 3100. 28800 baud maximum.
info@backdrop.com
http://www.fantasies.com
✓ $ ¢
Contact: Mr. Robin Roberts
Publishes *Partylines* every month. Yearly subscription is $25. Age statement of 21 is required. French, Spanish, & Japanese also spoken.

Boots
P. O. Box 46001, RPO Quadra, Victoria, British Columbia V8T 5G7. Canada
604 744 5881

Contact Centre (S/M)
BCM Cuddle, London WC1V 6XX. England
✓ $
Contact: Ms. Irene Arsha Subiela, Adj. Secretary
Friendship for adults interested in any form of BDSM. Ladies seeking (among others) single males are enrolled free. Support & advice. Age statement of 18 is required.

Delta International
P. O. Box 825, Wilkes-Barre, Pennsylvania 18703-0825. U.S.A.

The International Dungeon & Playroom Association (IDPA)
P. O. Box 5979, Pasadena, California 91117. U.S.A.
213 627 8373
idpaclub@aol.com

Leather Scribes
Box 482, 7985 Santa Monica Boulevard, Los Angeles, California 90046. U.S.A.
213 665 5343
cuirhomme@aol.com
Leather writers.

Leather / SM / Fetish Community Outreach
Suite 806, 874 Broadway, New York 10003. U.S.A.
ixion@dorsai.org
gopher://unix.tpe.com.:70/11/outreach
Contact: Mr. Leonard Dworkin

Leathermasters International
P. O. Box 291532, Los Angeles, California 90027. U.S.A.
213 664 6422
✓ $ ¢
Contact: Mr. Jerome Stevens
Members in many countries. Training & counselling is available in many cities. Also mail order. Publishes *Leathermasters Guide*. Age statement of 21 is required.

Masters & Slaves Together
Box 482, 7985 Santa Monica Boulevard, West Hollywood, California 90046. U.S.A.
cuirhomme@aol.com
Women welcome.

Masters & Slaves Together
P.O. Box 410261, San Francisco, California 94141-0261. U.S.A.

The National Leather Association (NLA)—Deaf International
P. O. Box 30286, Columbus, Ohio 43230. U.S.A.
Publishes *NLA Deaf Leather Reporter* every two months.

The National Leather Association (NLA)—International Headquarters
Box 444, 584 Castro Street, San Francisco, California 94114-2500. U.S.A.
614 899 4406 (information/message line)
NLAi@aol.com
Mail box only. Publishes *The Link*. Age statement of 21 is required.

SM / Leather / Fetish Community Outreach Project (SM-COP)
U.S.A.
ixion@ dorsai.org
gopher://unix.tpe.com.:70/11/outreach

Vagevuur
Hemelrijken 18, 5612 LD Eindhoven. The Netherlands
40 244 2744
Fri 22:00 - 02:00, Sat - ?
Leather, rubber, uniform only. Specials: golden shower, fisting, BDSM, spanking, scat, mud, oil, etc. Check first for strict dress code. Publishes *Itch* twice a year. Yearly subscription is $20. Age statement of 21 is required. English & German also spoken.

Organizations: Bears

Bear History Project
P. O. Box 1427, Brookline Station, Boston, Massachusetts 02146. U.S.A.
617 262 4472 — 617 262 4472
codybear@delphi.com
By appointment only
Contact: Mr. Les Wright, Ph.D., Curator
Archive & periodicals collection, preserving the history of bears as it happens. Actively seeks videos & other materials for archive. Publishes *BHP Newsletter* once a year. Yearly subscription is free. Age statement of 21 is required. French, German, Dutch, & Russian also spoken.

Bears International
Box F4, 332 Bleeker Street, New York 10014-2818. U.S.A.
212 367 7484
Age statement of 21 is required.

Girth & Mirth—Belgium
Boîte Postale 1514, 6000 Charleroi 1. Belgium
71 56 0580 — 71 51 8401
phil-s3@pophost.eunet.be
http://www.eunet.be/rent-a-page/bigmen
08:00 - 20:00
✓ $
Social club for bears & big men. Hosts activities including dinners & jack-offs. Publishes *The Fat Angel Times* quarterly. Yearly subscription is 1400FB. Age statement of 18 is required. English & Dutch also spoken.

South Florida Bears
13520 North West 11th. Avenue, Miami, Florida 33168-6722. U.S.A.
305 685 1841
mredbear@aol.com
Meets twice a month
✓ $
Contact: Mr. Ed Morgan
For hairy men & their admirers. Our motto is "Congregate, not hibernate." Come join the bears & rub fur. Spanish also spoken.

Organizations: Fetish: Clothing: Rubber

Mecs En Caoutchouc (M. E. C.)
Boîte Postale 19, 77191 Dammarie Les Lys Cedex. France
✓ $
Approximately 200 members. Publishes *Plan K* 3 times a year. Age statement of 18 is required.

New World Rubber Men
1602 Lincoln Street, Port Townsend, Washington 98368-8031. U.S.A.
206 385 3811
Contact: Mr. Bill Bailey
Publishes *Rubber Sheets*.

Organizations: Fetish: Enema

The Fraternity of Enema Buddies
Suite 1116, 2421 West Pratt Boulevard, Chicago, Illinois 60645. U.S.A.
312 561 7188
Until 22:00
✓ $
Contact: Mr. Frank Ball, Founder
Specializes in the social & information needs of all enema oriented men, whether gay, bi, or straight. Established in 1983. Publishes a newsletter 3 times a year. Age statement of 21 is required. Please address envelopes to Mr. Frank Ball, do NOT address them to The Fraternity of Enema Buddies.

Organizations: Fetish: Hair

BROS
P. O. Box 17931, Rochester, New York 14617. U.S.A.
716 323 2419
$
Membership club for long-haired men & their admirers. Magazine has updates on club gatherings, stories, homoerotic art, personals, etc.. Yearly subscription is $29. Age statement of 21 is required.

Organizations: Fetish: Smoking

Hot Ash
P.O. Box 20147, London Terrace Station, New York 10011. U.S.A.
718 789 6147 — 717 789 6147
20:00 - 24:00
✓
Contact: Mr. Tony Shenton
All cigar fetishists & smokers welcome. Most NY events men only; most SF events open to all. Contacts throughout North America. Publishes *Hot Tips*. Yearly subscription is $25U.S. for U.S., $30U.S. overseas. Age statement of 18 is required.

The Smoke Exchange
Suite 265, 1562 First Avenue, New York 10028. U.S.A.
✓ $
Contact: Smokin' Jack, Editor
For gay men who are turned on by masculine cigarette-smoking men. Newsletter has erotic smoking stories, free personals, & more. Publishes *The Smoke Exchange*. Age statement of 21 is required.

Organizations: Fetish: Uniforms

☺▽ **The American Uniform Association (AUA)—New York**
P. O. Box 1074, Franklin D. Roosevelt Station, New York 10150. U.S.A.

☺▽ **Fits Like A Glove (FLAG)**
P. O. Box 79243, North Dartmouth, Massachusetts 02747-0993. U.S.A.
☎ 508 996 1394
Contact: Mr. Jim Maciel
Glove, leather, & uniform fetish. Publishes *Flagship*.

☺▽ **Military & Police Club International**
Suite 142, 1043 University, San Diego, California 92103-3392. U.S.A.
✉ mpcted@aol.com

Organizations: Motorcycle

☺▽ **Inter-Bike Denmark**
Postboks 2037, 1012 København K. Denmark
📞 33 116335
✉ eurolin2@inet.uni-c.dk
🕐 09:00 - 16:00
🍴 ✓ $
Contact: Tim
Members-only contact club for all bisexual / gay bikers & MC-lovers wordwide. Newsletter with articles of interest to members. Publishes a newsletter quarterly. Yearly subscription is 150DK. Age statement of 18 is required. English, Spanish, German, & French also spoken.

Organizations: Piercing

☺ **The Stainless Steel Ball**
c/o Wildcat International, 16 Preston Street, Brighton, East Sussex BN1 2HN. England
☎ 1273 323758 📞 1273 323758
🕐 An infrequent event. Call Mon - Sat 10:00 - 18:00 for info
🍴 ✓ $ ♂
The only pure event for pierced poeple. Dress-code: you must have a piercing. Sometimes held out of the U.K.. Please send SAE or IRC for reply. Age statement of 18 is required.

Organizations: Scat

☺▽ **Martifoto**
Postbus 669, 2501 CR Den Haag. The Netherlands
☎ 70 368 1865 📞 70 368 1865
🕐 Bi-monthly parties
Also sells videos (not to U.K., U.S., or Canada) for profit. Please include $1 or an IRC for information. Publishes a newsletter 3 times a year. Yearly subscription is $60U.S.. English, German, & some French also spoken.

Organizations: Sexual Politics

☺ ☐ **The Spanner Trust**
BM Box 99, London WC1 3XX. England
🕐 Meets quarterly
🍴 ✓ $ ♂ ♂̶
Contact: Mr. Rob Grover, Secretary
Supports the Spanner appeal to the European Court of Human Rights, defend BDSM in the U.K., & support BDSM rights internationally.

Organizations: Sexuality: Disabilities

☺ ☐ **Outsiders**
P. O. Box 4ZB, London W1A 4ZB. England
☎ 171 739 0388 📞 171 739 0355
🕐 Call Mon - Sat 12:00 - 18:30
🍴 ✓ $ ⚓ 🍴 VISA ⬜ ⬜ ⬜ ⬜ ℯ
Contact: Ms. Tuppy Owens, Dip.H.S.
Self-help group for people isolated because of social or physical disability & who want to find partners. Age statement of 18 is required.

Organizations: Sexuality

☺▽ **Gay Naturists International (GNI)**
Suite 201, 324 Main Avenue, Norwalk, Connecticut 06851. U.S.A.
Holds Mr. GNI Leather contest at its annual gathering.

☺ ☐ **International Sexual Minorities Information Resource (ISMIR)**
P. O. Box 81869, Pittsburgh, Pennsylvania 15217-0869. U.S.A.
☎ 412 422 3060 📞 412 359 3878
📠 412 422 1529. 14400 baud maximum.
✉ ismir@aol.com
🍴 ✓
Contact: Mr. Lee Kikuchi, President & Editor
Newsletter describes the activities of ISMIR. Publishes *ISMIR Chronicle* twice a year. Yearly subscription is free. Spanish, German, & Russian also spoken.

☞▽ **The Outreach Institute of Gender Studies**
K Suite 246, 126 Western Avenue, Augusta, Maine 04330. U.S.A.
☎ 207 621 0858 📞 207 621 0858

🕐 Mon - Fri 09:00 - 17:00
🍴 ✓ VISA MC
Contact: Mr. Ari Kane, Director
Programs & services to health care professionals who work with gender conflict issues. Call for more details. Publishes *The Journal of Gender Studies*. French, German, Spanish, Italian, & Greek also spoken.

Organizations: Spanking

☺▼ **C. L. E. F.**
Boîte Postale 73, 75922 Paris Cedex 19. France
☎ 142 70 3132
🍴 ✓ $
Publishes *Fessée Magazine*.

Organizations: Tattoo

☺▽ **Friends of the Tattoo Archive**
2804 San Pablo, Berkeley, California 94702. U.S.A.

☺▽ **T & P Men**
Im Brunnen, 9467 Fruemsen. Switzerland
☎ 81 757 1144 📞 81 757 1185
🍴 ✓ $
Contact: Herr Rudy Inhelder
Fraternity of tattooed &/or pierced men who are into permanent body art & other modifications. Publishes a newsletter quarterly. Yearly subscription is free. Age statement of 16 is required. English & French also spoken.

Organizations: Watersports

☺ **NYPT**
P. O. Box 783, New York 10025-0783. U.S.A.
🕐 Weekly events
Private watersports club. Memberships & guests.

Organizations: Wrestling

☺▽ **Alternative Sports**
P. O. Box 437, Glasgow, Strathclyde G42 8HU. Scotland
☎ 141 423 4175 📞 141 423 4175
✉ altspor@coloquium.co.uk
🍴 ✓ $
Alternative wrestling organization, organizes events, provides training & contacts for gay/bi guys/women into wrestling. Sponsors similar clubs. Publishes *Alternative Wrestlers*. Yearly subscription is £24.

☺ ☐ **Global Wrestling Alliance**
P. O. Box 352, Farmington, Connecticut 06034. U.S.A.
☎ 203 524 4288 📞 203 278 9898
Contact: Mr. Gary Crouch

Photographers: Erotic

☺ **Victoria Musson**
c/o Midian Books, 69 Park Lane, Bonehill, Staffordshire B78 3HZ. England
☎ 1827 281391 📞 1827 281391
Fetish photographer & artist, helping turn fantasies into reality. Commissions welcome. Age statement of 18 is required.

Piercers

☺ ■ **Asgard Body Piercing**
P. O. Box 69, Southampton, Hampshire SO9 7EQ. England
☎ 170 332 5059

Public Speakers: Sexuality

☺ **Barbara Carellas**
Suite C2, 420 West 46th. Street, New York 10036. U.S.A.
☎ 212 247 2354 📞 212 581 0299
✉ 103270,2134@compuserve.com
🍴 ✓ $ ♂
A Sex Positivist, metaphysical counsellor, teacher, & artist, lecturing & leading workshops internationally on Sexual Evolution, Sex & Healing, & Sex & Spirituality. Age statement of 18 is required.

☺ ■ **Trevor Jacques**
P. O. Box 19591-886, 55 Bloor Street West, Toronto, Ontario M4W 3T9. U.S.A.
☎ 416 962 1040 📞 416 962 1044
✉ Editor@Alternate.com
🕐 Mon - Fri 09:00 - 17:00, voice mail at other times
🍴 ✓ $ ♂
Speaker & best-selling author on BDSM & other alternate sexualities. Also workshops, & radio & television interviews. French, & some German also spoken.

Publishers: Books: BDSM

☺▼ **GLB Publishers**
♿ P.O. Box 78212, San Francisco, California 94107. U.S.A.
☎ 415 621 8307 📞 415 621 8307
🕐 09:00 - 17:00
🍴 ✓ $ ♂

Coöperative publisher of books by & for gay men, lesbians, & bisexuals. Fiction, non-fiction, & poetry. Free catalogue.

👫 ■ **Marquis Magazine**
The Fetish Factory Ltd., 5 Flensburger Straße 5, 42655 Solingen. Germany
☎ 21 258 6151 📞 21 258 6156
🕐 09:00 - 13:00
🐾 ✓ $ ✉ ▬ *VISA* 💳 ℓ
Publisher & distributor of fetish erotica: magazines, books, comics, videos, calendars, & photo archives. Published quarterly. Yearly subscription is DM100. Age statement of 18 is required. French & English also spoken.

☺ **Virtjack Studios**
♿ 7 Route de Saint Loup, 1200 Genève. Switzerland
📧 virtjack@iprolink.ch
🕐 09:00 - 12:00 15:00 - 20:00
ℓ
Video, audio, computer-based products, from CD-ROM to reference works about femdom, sexuality, psychology, & entertainment. Age statement of 21 is required. English & Spanish also spoken.

Publishers: Books: Erotic

☺ ■ **Tease!**
Pure Imagination, P. O. Box 669902, Marietta, Georgia 30066. U.S.A.
☎ 770 424 5151
📧 75451,3472@compuserve.com
🕐 13:00 - 23:00
✓ $
Tease! magazine is devoted to the timeless allure of classic pin-up art & dazzling feminine beauty. Published quarterly. Yearly subscription is $28. Age statement of 18 is required.

Publishers: Books: General

☺ ■ **Body Art**
Body Art, Publications Ltd., P. O. Box 32, Great Yarmouth, Norfolk NR29 5RD. U.S.A.
🐾 ✓ $ ✉ ▬ *VISA* 💳 ℓ
Publisher & distributor of body decoration magazines & books. SAE or IRC for free illustrated catalogue. Published twice a year. Yearly subscription is £30 for U.K. residents, £34 ($70U.S.) overseas surface mail.

☺ ■ **The Crossing Press**
P. O Box 1048, Freedom, California 95019. U.S.A.
☎ 800 777 1048 📞 408 722 2749
☎ 408 722 0711
📧 crossing@aol.com
🕐 Mon - Fri 08:00 - 12:00 12:30 - 16:00
✓ $ ▬ *VISA* 💳
Publish leather, fetish, & BDSM books, as well as gay, lesbian, bisexual, & transgendered titles. Catalogue available, published twice a year. Spanish also spoken.

Publishers: Books: Sexuality

☺ ■ **Artemis Creations Publishing**
#2J, 3395 Nostrand Avenue, Brooklyn, New York 11229-4053. U.S.A.
☎ 718 648 8215
📧 msgartemis@aol.com
🕐 24hrs.
🐾 ✓ $ ▬ *VISA* 💳
Age statement of 21 is required.

☺ ■ **Down There Press**
✍ Box 101, 938 Howard Street, San Francisco, California 94117. U.S.A.
☎ 415 974 8985 📞 415 974 8989
📧 goodvibe@well.com
🖥 http://www.bookfair.com/publishers/downther/asrc
🕐 Mon - Fri 09:00 - 17:00
✓ $ ▬ *VISA* 💳 ▬ 🐾 ✉ ℓ
Sexual health books for children & adults, & erotica. Titles include: Herotica, Femalia, Anal Pleasure & Health. Publishing arm of Good Vibrations. Free catalogue.

♂▽ **Gai-Kitsch-Camp (CKC)**
Cahiers Gai-Kitsch-Camp, Boîte Postale 36, 59009 Lille Cedex. France
☎ 20 06 3391 📞 20 78 1876
🐾 ✓ $ ✉ ℓ
Publishers of modern studies & "oldies." Erotics, literature, history, & social sciences (gender, & gay & lesbian studies). Published quarterly. English, French, & Arabic also spoken.

♂ ▼ **Kitchen Table, Women of Color Press**
✍ P. O. Box 40-4920, Brooklyn, New York 11240-4920. U.S.A.
☎ 718 935 1082 📞 718 935 1107
🕐 10:00 - 18:00
✓ $ ✉

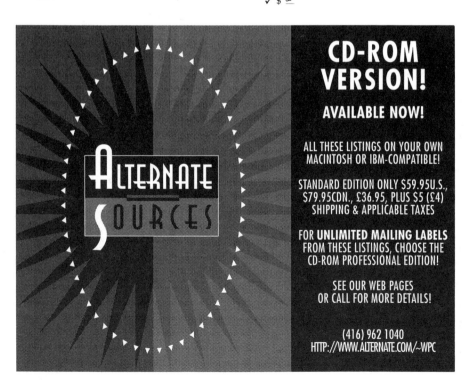

The only publisher for lesbians & feminists of colour in the U.S.. Publishes books, pamphlets, & magazines. Free catalogue.

☺ **Re/Search Publications**
Suite B, 20 Remolo Street, San Francisco, California 94133. U.S.A.
☎ 415 362 1465
🕐 Mon - Fri 10:00 - 18:00
🛍 ✓ $ ⚊ 💳 💿
Publishes many books about the margins of society & alternate sexual expression. Age statement of 21 is required.

Publishers: Books: Spanking

☺▼ **Imperia Press**
B. M. Empress, London WC1N 3XX. England
☎ 181 989 0281
🕐 09:00 - 21:00
🛍 ✓ ⚊ £
Publishers of all-female disciplinary fiction & non-fiction, including The Corporal Punishment of Schoolgirls, A Documentary Survey. Age statement of 18 is required.

☺▼ **The Wildfire Club**
B. M. Elegance, London WC1N 3XX. England
☎ 181 989 0281
📧 embassy@pronews.pro-net.co.uk
🌐 http://www.zynet.net/wildfire
🕐 09:00 - 21:00
🛍 ✓ ⚊ £
Publishers of high-quality fiction & non-fiction about females disciplining females. Suppliers of genuine school straps, canes & other implements. Yearly subscription is $1 cash, one U. K. stamp, or one IRC. Age statement of 18 is required.

Publishers: Directories: BDSM

☺ ■ **Alternate Sources**
♿ Kink, Ink, P. O. Box 19591-884, 55 Bloor Street West, Toronto, Ontario M4W 3T9. Canada
☎ 416 962 1040 📞 416 962 1044
📧 Editor@Alternate.com
🌐 http://Alternate.com/~wpc/Books/ASInfo.html
🕐 Mon - Fri 09:00 - 17:00, voice mail at other times
🛍 ✓ $
The world's most complete directory of resources for people of alternate sexualities. Each entry is exhaustive, listing all the information that your

Checkmate
INCORPORATING
DungeonMaster

The practical "how to" manual of S/M. Equipment reviews, dungeon construction projects, technique. $14.00 US, $16.00 Canada, $23.00 elsewhere for 4 issues per year mailed first class. $4.95 sample issue. Send check, money order or credit card order to:
Telecentral dept AS
PO Box 354
Wyoming, PA 18644-0354.
State that you are over 21. Include phone number with Visa, MasterCard, American Express or Discover orders

users might want. Published once a year. Yearly subscription is $34Cdn., $24.95U.S., plus s&h & applicable taxes. Age statement of 18 is required. French, & some German also spoken.

☺▼ **The Black Book**
Amador Communications, P.O. Box 31155, San Francisco, California 94131-0155. U.S.A.
☎ 415 431 0171 📞 415 431 0172
📠 415 431 0173 (orders)
📧 BlackB@ios.com
🕐 Mon - Fri 10:00 - 18:00 Pacific
🛍 ✓ $ ⚊ 💳 💿 ⚊
Amador publishes & distributes pansexual books & magazines that encourage a healthy, informed outlook on sexuality. Published every two years. Yearly subscription is $18 U.S., $20 Cdn/Mex, $24 elsewhere (in Calif. $19.25, due to sales tax). Age statement of 21 is required. Spanish also spoken.

☺▼■ **Black Pages International**
Blackline Press & Services, Meinekestraße 24, 10719 Berlin. Germany
☎ 30 883 3922 📞 30 229 4114

☺▼ **Womanlink**
Womanlink, #257, 2124 Kittridge, Berkeley, California 94704. U.S.A.
✓ $ ⚊
Roster & newsletter for women who do BDSM with other women. Resource list. SASE or IRC for information. Mail order only. Published quarterly. Yearly subscription is $25 - $30U.S.. Age statement of 21 is required.

Publishers: Directories: Fetish

☺ ■ **The Fetasy Guide**
Gear, Inc., P. O. Box 66306, Los Angeles, California 90066. U.S.A.
☎ 213 683 8313

Publishers: Directories: Sexuality

☺ **Alternative Lifestyles Directory**
Winter Publishing, Inc., P. O. Box 80667, South Dartmouth, Massachusetts 02748-0667. U.S.A.
☎ 508 999 0078 📞 508 984 4040
🛍 ✓ $ ⚊ 💳 💿 ⚊
Comprehensive directory of alternative lifestyles magazines. Includes review of over 375 publications, from mainstream to taboo, mild to wild. Published once a year. Yearly subscription is $10U.S., plus $3 s&h. Age statement of 21 is required.

☺▼ **The Gay & Lesbian Periodicals Directory**
New Vista Publishing, #J-437, 770 Sycamore Avenue, Vista, California 92083. U.S.A.
☎ 619 727 8718

☺ ▢ **Planet Sex The Handbook**
♿ The Leydig Trust, P.O. Box 4ZB, London W1A 4ZB. England
☎ 171 739 0388 📞 171 739 0355
🕐 Call Mon - Sat 12:00 - 18:30
🛍 ✓ $ ⚊ 💳 💿 ⚊ 🅳 ⚊ £
Age statement of 18 is required.

Publishers: Documentaries: Sexuality

☺ ▢ **Cambridge Documentary Films, Inc.**
P. O. Box 385, Cambridge, Massachusetts 02139. U.S.A.
☎ 617 354 3677 📞 617 492 7653
📧 cdf@shore.net
🌐 http://www.shore.net/~cdf/
🕐 09:00 - 17:00, voice mail at other times
🛍 ✓
Documentary Pink Triangles, a historical look at prejudice against lesbians & gay men, 35 minutes, educational, colour 16mm video. Free catalogue published once a year.

Publishers: Guides: Sexuality

☺ ■ **Complete Guide to Internet Sex Resources**
📧 Phillip@kingdom.win.net
🌐 http://www.win.net/~kingdom/2244zz.html

☺ ▢ **ISMIR Events Calendar**
International Sexual Minorities Information Resource, P. O. Box 81869, Pittsburgh, Pennsylvania 15217-0869. U.S.A.
☎ 412 422 3060 📞 412 359 3878
📞 412 422 1529. 14400 baud maximum.
📧 ismir@aol.com
🛍 ✓
Lists events up to year 2000 for gay, lesbian, bisexual, & other sexual minorities. Also available on Mac or IBM disk (specify which). Published every month. Yearly subscription is $35U.S. for U.S., $45U.S. for Canada & Mexico, $60U.S. elsewhere. German, Spanish & Russian also spoken.

☺ ▢ **Pointer to Sex Information on the Net (PtSIotN)**
📧 viaverde@netcom.com
Updated & posted to alt.sex on the 1st of every month.

Publishers: Magazines: Arts

Women's Review of Books
Center for Research on Women, Wellesley College, Wellesley, Massachusetts 02181. U.S.A.
617 283 2087 — 617 283 3645
✓ $
Monthly review of books by & about women. Published 11 times a year. Yearly subscription is $20U.S.. French, Spanish & Italian also spoken.

Publishers: Magazines: BDSM

Checkmate & DungeonMaster
Telecentral Electronics, P.O. Box 354, Wyoming, Pennsylvania 18644-0354.
717 655 2880 — 717 655 7191
hcox@microserve.com or bobr@microserve.com
✓
Incorporates DungeonMaster. Published quarterly. Yearly subscription is $14 U.S., $16 for Cdn., $23 foreign. Age statement of 21 is required. Please see our display advertisement.

Le Fer Rouge
RM Distribution, Ltd., Suite 271, 3539 Boulevard Saint Charles, Kirkland, Québec H9H 5B9. Canada
514 851 0264
princess.sheeba@linq.com
Mon - Fri 09:00 - 17:00
✓ $
Covering the scene of consensual domination & submission in its many, various facets, with informative articles, photography & art work. Published quarterly.

Katharsis
Katharsis, P. O. Drawer 98, Bunnell, Florida 32110-0098. U.S.A.
904 437 2642 — By prior arrangement
12:00 - 24:00
✓ $
Since 1987. All male. Beyond BDSM. Male victim fantasies. Torture, genitorture, castration, amputation, pillow conversions, gladiators, serial killers, vigilantes, military executions. Core (60+ pages) $35/month, $350/year. Full magazine (core plus more experimental drawings & stories) $95/month. Curious but cautious? Sampler $20. Outside North America, add 20%.. Published every month. Yearly subscription is $1,000. Age statement of 21 is required. Please see our display advertisement.

The Leather Journal
The Leather Journal, Box 109-368, 7985 Santa Monica Boulevard, West Hollywood, California 90046. U.S.A.
213 656 5073 — 213 656 3120
tljandcuir@aol.com
http://users.aol.com/tljandcuir
Mon - Fri 09:30 - 17:00
✓ $
International pan-sexual leather community magazine of record. Interviews, politics, humour, & pan-sexual personals. Extensive photo coverage of events. Published every month. Yearly subscription is $63. Age statement of 21 is required. Please see our display advertisement.

Manifest Reader
Alternate Publishing Company, 15 Harriet Street, San Francisco, California 94103. U.S.A.
415 864 3456 — 415 826 2736
09:00 - 18:00
✓ $
Also has direct mail division. Published every two months. Yearly subscription is $30.

Metropolitan Slave
Selective Publishing, Inc., P. O. Box 4597, Oakbrook, Illinois 60522-4597. U.S.A.
708 986 8550 — 708 323 3190
708 986 0294. 28800 baud maximum.
jeb@metroslave.com
http://metroslave.com or telnet://metroslave.com
24hrs.
✓ $
Dedicated to the celebration of slavery. Masters welcome! We seek to teach slaves to serve, & to match masters with slaves. Subscription includes free ad for master or slave. Primarily gay male, but all welcome. Published quarterly. Yearly subscription is $32 U.S.. Age statement of 18 is required. Korean also spoken.

Mistress
Olympia Publishing (UK) Ltd., 36 Union Street, Ryde, Isle of Wight PO33 2LE. England
1983 811783 — 1983 811785
09:00 - 17:00
✓ $ ¢

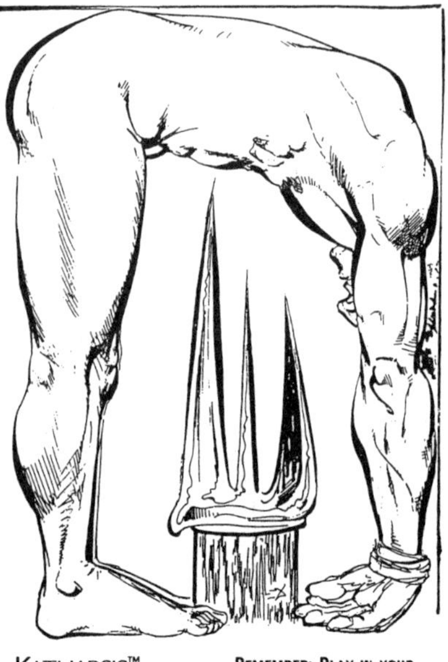

Fem/Dom magazine. Age statement of 18 is required.

Olympia Publishing (UK) Ltd.
36 Union Street, Ryde, Isle of Wight PO33 2LE. England
1983 811783 | 1983 811785
09:00 - 17:00
✓ $
Publishers of BDSM literature & bondage & corporal punishment books. Sells secondhand books in the genre. Also sells by mail order. Free catalogue. Age statement of 18 is required.

Projet X
Editions du Triangle Rose, Rue Sedaine 45, 75557 Paris Cedex 11. France
143 57 5205 | 143 57 8040
143 38 1221
Mon - Fri 09:00 - 18:00
✓ $
French leather & BDSM magazine: information, reports about European events, calendar, & personal ads. Published every month. Yearly subscription is FF60. Age statement of 18 is required. English & German also spoken. Please see our display advertisement.

Pussywhipped!
Six of the Best Publishing, Box 11724, Berkeley, California 94712. U.S.A.
510 208 2835
bearpaws@sirius.com
http://www.sirius.com/~bearpaws
10:00 - 18:00
✓ $
A leatherdyke BDSM 'zine that celebrates our sexualities. We welcome submissions. Published 3 times a year. Yearly subscription is $14U.S.. Age statement of 21 is required. German also spoken.

The Sadean
Katharsis, P. O. Drawer 98, Bunnell, Florida 32110-0098. U.S.A.
904 437 2642 | By prior arrangement
12:00 - 24:00
✓ $
Encore presentation of Katharsis™ & Disciples of Semiramis™. Fantasies plus bulletin board & reviews. $25/issue, $69/3. Published every month. Yearly subscription is $269. Age statement of 21 is required. Please see our display advertisement.

The Servant's Quarters
Six of the Best Publishing, Box 11724, Berkeley, California 94712. U.S.A.
510 208 2835
bearpaws@sirius.com
http://www.sirius.com/~bearpaws
10:00 - 18:00
✓ $
A BDSM 'zine that celebrates our sexualities; by & for submissives of all flavours. We welcome submissions. Published 3 times a year. Yearly subscription is $14U.S.. Age statement of 21 is required. German also spoken.

Subculture
Strictly Stories, P. O. Box 15, Station A, Etobicoke, Ontario M9C 2V3. Canada
416 622 2485
clare@the-wire.com
09:00 - 21:00
$
Stories, articles, & artwork for leather, latex, & fetish people. Published quarterly. Yearly subscription is $50. Age statement of 21 is required.

Wanda
N. S. P., 38 rue Servan, 75544 Paris Cedex 11. France
140 09 6969 | 140 09 6971
nsp10@calcucom.fr
$
Also mail order of BDSM erotica. Published every two months. Yearly subscription is FF250. Age statement of 18 is required.

Women who Administer Punishment (WhAP)
Retro Systems, Suite 1261, 1850 Union Street, San Francisco, California 94123. U.S.A.
✓ $
Women's guide to maternal discipline: Women spank, diaper, & humiliate their men. Published quarterly. Yearly subscription is $40. Age statement of 18 is required.

Publishers: Magazines: Bondage

Bondage Life
Harmony Concepts, Inc., P.O. Box 69976, Los Angeles, California 90069. U.S.A.
818 766 1448 | 818 766 9679
24hr. facs. & order lines
✓ $
Age statement of 21 is required. Please see our display advertisement.

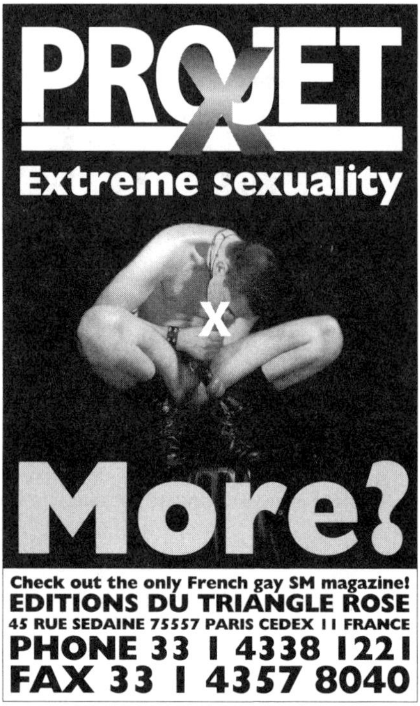

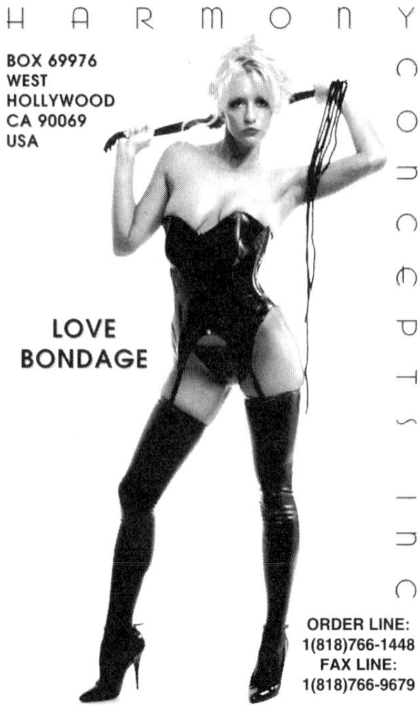

Bound & Gagged
The Outbound Press, Suite 803, 89 Fifth Avenue, New York 10003. U.S.A.
212 727 2751 — fax 212 243 1630
bobbg@aol.com
Mon - Fri 10:00 - 18:00
Also produces the Fleetwood/Academy & the Bound & Gagged videos. Published every two months. Yearly subscription is $30U.S. for U.S., $36U.S. for Cdn.. Age statement of 21 is required. French & Spanish also spoken. Please see our display advertisement.

Pleasure Bound
Olympia Publishing (UK) Ltd., 36 Union Street, Ryde, Isle of Wight PO33 2LE. England
1983 811783 — fax 1983 811785
09:00 - 17:00
✓ $
Bondage magazine by enthusiasts for enthusiasts. Age statement of 18 is required.

Publishers: Magazines: Erotic

Beau Magazine
Sportomatic, Ltd., P. O. Box 470, Port Chester, New York 10573. U.S.A.
914 939 2362 — fax 914 939 5138
✓ $
Beau is now America's #1 selling erotic gay digest. Available on newstands across the U.S. & Canada or by subscription. Published 8 times a year. Yearly subscription is $18.69U.S.. Age statement of 18 is required.

Libido
Libido, Inc., P. O. Box 146721, Chicago, Illinois 60614. U.S.A.
312 275 0842 — fax 312 275 0752
312 728 5957
rune@mcs.com
http://www.indra.com/libido/
✓ $
The literary answer to the horizontal urge. Published quarterly. Yearly subscription is $30. Age statement of 21 is required.

Magayzine
Bodyshot, P. O. Box 22051, Port Elizabeth, Cape Province 6000. South Africa
41 308016 — fax 41 308017
Mon -Fri 09:00 - 16:00
$ ₵
Published every two months. Yearly subscription is R120. Age statement of 18 is required.

Penthouse Variations
General Media Inc., 277 Park Avenue, New York 10172. U.S.A.
212 702 6000
09:00 - 17:00
✓
Lifestyle exposés within a wide range of sexual pleasure categories, accompanied by complementary explicit reader letters. Published 13 times a year. Yearly subscription is $29.97. Age statement of 18 is required.

TopHat's Calendar of Erotica
Champagne Productions, Suite 5C, 315 East 5th. Street, New York 10003-8823. U.S.A.
212 982 0384
tophat@bway.net
10:00 - 20:00
Detailed event calendar for the various fetish communities; available via e-mail or discrete paper mail; parties, lectures, seminars, demo's, etc.. Published every month. Age statement of 21 is required.

Publishers: Magazines: Fetish

Boot Lovers' Digest
Strictly Speaking Publishing Co., P. O. Box 8006, Palm Springs, California 92263. U.S.A.
fax 619 363 6030
✓ $
Published twice a year. Some French & German also spoken.

Disciples of Semiramis
Katharsis, P. O. Drawer 98, Bunnell, Florida 32110-0098. U.S.A.
904 437 2642 — fax By prior arrangement
12:00 - 24:00
✓ $
Males as absolute property of women. Humiliation, punishment, torture, castration, gladiators, skinning, butchering, cannibalism, execution. Fantasy. Sample $20, otherwise $45/issue. Published every month. Yearly subscription is $425. Age statement of 21 is required. Please see our display advertisement.

Fetish Times
Mang Publishing, BCM Box 9253, London WC1N 3XX. England
171 436 0385 — fax 171 436 0767
✓
Celebrates sexual diversity. Covers all sorts of sexual difference from a scene rather than fashion perspective. Articles on everything from Spanner to tickling fetishism. French, German, & Spanish also spoken.

Hair to Stay
Winter Publishing, Inc., P. O. Box 80667, South Dartmouth, Massachusetts 02748-0667. U.S.A.
508 999 0078 — fax 508 984 4040
✓ $
The world's only magazine for lovers of natural, hairy women, featuring high-quality photos, video reviews, & more. Published quarterly. Yearly subscription is $30U.S. for U.S., $45U.S. elsewhere. Age statement of 21 is required.

Marquis Magazine
The Fetish Factory Ltd., 5 Flensburger Straße 5, 42655 Solingen. Germany
21 258 6151 — fax 21 258 6156
09:00 - 13:00
✓ $ ₵
Publisher & distributor of fetish erotica: magazines, books, comics, videos, calendars, & photo archives. Published quarterly. Yearly subscription is DM100. Age statement of 18 is required. French & English also spoken.

The Noose Letter
Winter Publishing, Inc., P. O. Box 80667, South Dartmouth, Massachusetts 02748-0667. U.S.A.
508 999 0078 — fax 508 984 4040
✓ $
Publication of The Hangman's Noose Club. For gay men turned on by stories of hangings, breath control, ultimate BDSM, & edge play. Published quarterly. Yearly subscription is $50U.S. for U.S., $75U.S. elsewhere. Age statement of 21 is required.

«O» Magazine
P. O. Box 3075, Venice, California 90212.
310 289 1412
Mon - Fri 09:00 - 17:00
✓ $
A bold, wide-ranging spectrum of talented creators & their extraordinary works, challenging the conventions of the fetish genre. The boldest broadest panorama of the fetish world available anywhere. Published quarterly. Yearly subscription is $38, including s&h. Age statement of 21

is required. French, German, & Japanese also spoken.

Offrande
A. P. M. C., Boîte Postale 6, 75462 Paris Cedex 10. France
24hrs.
✓ $
Magazine of erotic culture. Also publishes newspaper on modern eroticsm. Available by mail order. Send IRC for catalogue. Published 10 times a year. Yearly subscription is $50U.S.. English & Italian spoken.

A Taste of Latex
DM International, P. O. Box 16188, Seattle, Washington 98116-0188. U.S.A.
Mon - Fri 09:30 - 18:00
✓ $
Fetish & erotica for people who test their limits. Insights on fashion, music, trends, clubs, events, body modifications, experiments, & experiences. Published 3 times a year. Yearly subscription is $24U.S. for North America, $32U.S. overseas. Age statement of 21 is required. Please address envelopes to DM International, do NOT address them to A Taste of Latex. Please see our display advertisement.

Publishers: Magazines: Literary

Porno Pen
Amador Communications, P. O. Box 31155, San Francisco, California 94131. U.S.A.
415 431 0171 — Fax 415 431 0172
415 431 0173 (orders)
BlackB@ios.com
Mon - Fri 10:00 - 18:00 Pacific
✓ $
Amador publishes & distributes pansexual books & magazines that encourage a healthy, informed outlook on sexuality. Published every two months. Yearly subscription is $14, $18 Cdn/Mex, $22 elsewhere. Age statement of 21 is required. Spanish also spoken.

Publishers: Magazines: Piercing

Body Modification Ezine
Canada
bme@io.org
http://www.io.org/~bme

Piercing Fans International Quarterly (PFIQ)
Gauntlet, Inc., Box 801, 2155-R Market Street, San Francisco, California 94114. U.S.A.
415 252 1404 — Fax 415 252 1407
kane@gauntlet.com
http://www.gauntlet.com/
08:30 - 16:30
✓ $
World's premier quarterly devoted to piercing... the art & the people. Published quarterly. Yearly subscription is Call for exchange. Age statement of 21 is required.

Publishers: Magazines: Scat

The Scat Times
Winter Publishing, Inc., P. O. Box 80667, South Dartmouth, Massachusetts 02748-0667. U.S.A.
508 999 0078 — Fax 508 984 4040
✓ $
Publication of BROWN HANKY MEN, for gay men into scat. Published quarterly. Yearly subscription is $35U.S. to U.S., $50 elsewhere. Age statement of 21 is required.

Publishers: Magazines: Sexuality

The Black Sheets
Amador Communications, P. O. Box 31155, San Francisco, California 94131. U.S.A.
415 431 0171 — Fax 415 431 0172
415 431 0173 (orders)
BlackB@ios.com
Mon - Fri 10:00 - 18:00 Pacific
✓ $
Amador publishes & distributes pansexual books & magazines that encourage a healthy, informed outlook on sexuality. Published quarterly. Yearly subscription is $20 U.S., $24 Cdn/Mex, $32 elsewhere. Age statement of 21 is required. Spanish also spoken.

The Journal of Gay & Lesbian Psychotherapy
Haworth Press, 10 Alice Street, Binghamton, New York 13904-1580. U.S.A.
607 722 5857 — Fax 607 722 6362
subscribe@haworth.com
✓
Published quarterly.

The Journal of Gay & Lesbian Social Services
Haworth Press, 10 Alice Street, Binghamton, New York 13904-1580.

Bitches with Whips

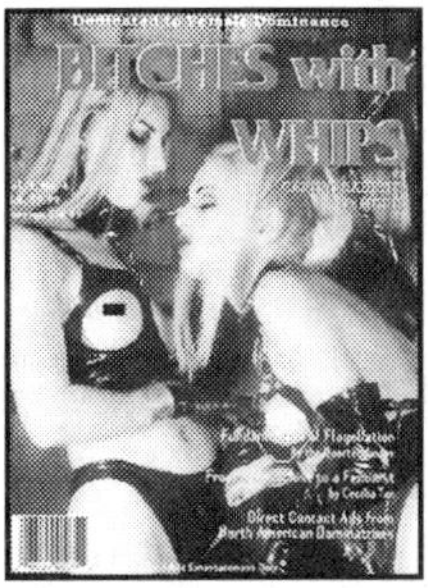

The power of female domination

Professional dominatrix ads, how-to articles, stories featuring dominants' lust and slaves' servitude.

SAMPLE ISSUE $10

Taste of Latex

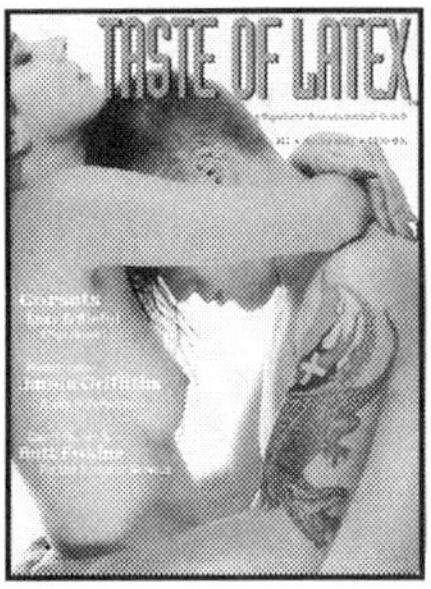

All sexual flavors with no apologies

Corsets, leather, rubber, club scenes, Practicing Pervert, famous & upcoming fetish photographers, sexy prose and poetry.

SAMPLE ISSUE $9

KPPT

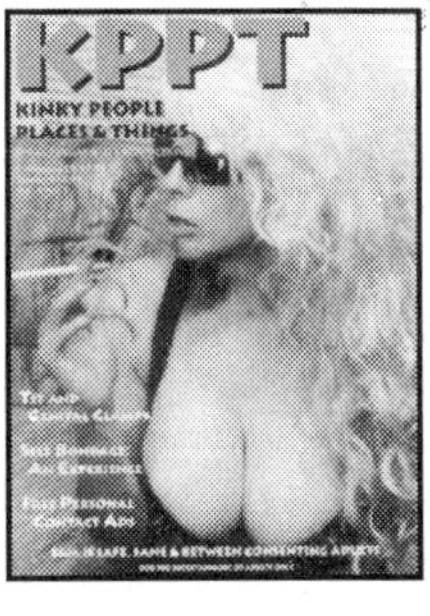

Where fantasy meets nonfiction

Stories featuring SM, B&D, and kinky hijinx. How-to articles, large contact ad section, kinky fiction for pervs of all persuasions.

SAMPLE ISSUE $8

TV Connection

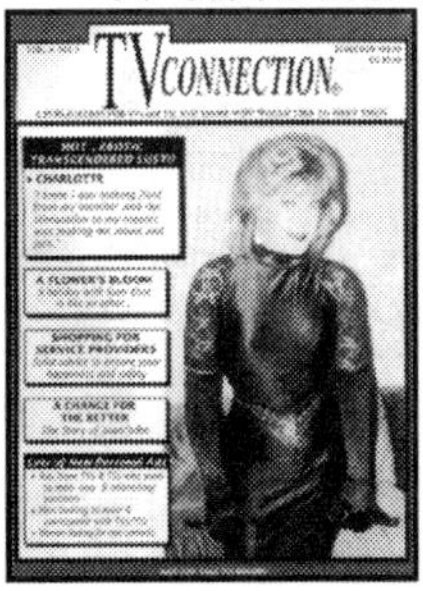

Lusty TV's and TS's & those who love'em

Beautiful transvestites and transgendered ladies. Beauty tips, educational support, hot fiction, and a contact ad section.

SAMPLE ISSUE $8

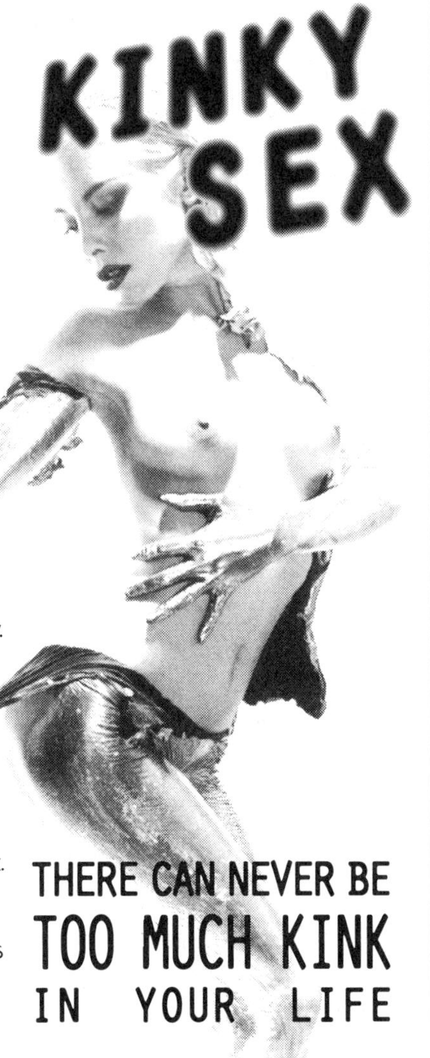

Photo ©Justice Howard

TO ORDER THESE FINE PUBLICATIONS: *For sample issues or subscriptions, please send check or money order made out to:* ***DM International, PO Box 16188, Seattle, WA 98116-0188.*** *All prices are US funds. Signed age 21 statement required for all purchases. Sample overseas must add $4 per magazine for 1st class mail. Personal checks held 2-8 weeks. Prices subject to change. Sorry, no credit cards.*

U.S.A.
☎ 607 722 5857 📞 607 722 6362
📧 subscribe@haworth.com
🛒 ✓ 💳 💳 💳
Published quarterly.

☺ *The Journal of Homosexuality*
Haworth Press, 10 Alice Street, Binghamton, New York 13904-1580.
U.S.A.
☎ 607 722 5857 📞 607 722 6362
📧 subscribe@haworth.com
🛒 ✓ 💳 💳 💳
Published quarterly.

⚧▼ *Lesbian & Gay Pride*
🌐 http://www.dircon.co.uk/flavour/pride/index.html

⚧▼ *The LGB Guide to Great Britain*
🌐 http://phymat.bham.ac.uk/LGB

⚧▽ *OMPO*
Via Einaudi 33, 00040 Frattochie RM, Lazio. Italy
☎ 6 93 54 7567 📞 6 93 54 7483
🛒 ✓ $
OMPO is the oldest gay publication in Italy. Published 10 times a year.
Yearly subscription is a voluntary donation.

⚧▼ *The Oral Majority*
Winter Publishing, Inc., P. O. Box 80667, South Dartmouth,
Massachusetts 02748-0667. U.S.A.
☎ 508 999 0078 📞 508 984 4040
🛒 ✓ $ 〜 💳 💳 💳
Publication of LIGHT-BLUE HANKY MEn, for gay men heavily into oral sex.
Published quarterly. Yearly subscription is $35U.S., $50U.S. foreign. Age
statement of 21 is required.

⚧▼ *Queer-e*
U.S.A.
📧 Queer-e-owner@vector.casti.com
🌐 http://www.qrd.org/QRD/media/journals/queer-e-v1.n1
Electronic lesbigay magazine. For information send e-mail to
majordomo@vector.casti.com with contents reading: info queer-e-text.

⚥ *Radiance, The Magazine For Large Women*
P. O. Box 30246, Oakland, California 94604. U.S.A.
☎ 510 482 0680 📞 510 482 0680
📧 radmag@aol.com
🕐 Mon - Fri 09:00 - 17:00, answering machine at other times
🛒 ✓ $
A unique magazine that provides inspiration, information, & support to
women all sizes of large. Leader in size acceptance. Published quarterly.
Yearly subscription is $20U.S., $26U.S. for Canada, $34U.S. elsewhere.

☺ *Redemption*
Borxan Publications, P. O. Box 54063, Vancouver, British Columbia V7Y
1B0. Canada
☎
 604 264 8666
🛒 ✓ $
A fanzine dedicated to those individuals who wish to explore the
extremities of sexuality, irrespective of orientation or extremity.
Published quarterly. Yearly subscription is $10U.S. for U.S., $10Cdn for
Cdn.. Age statement of 21 is required. German also spoken.

☺▽ *Rome Gay News*
RGN, Via Einaudi 33, 00040 Frattochie RM, Lazio. Italy
☎ 6 93 54 7567 📞 6 93 54 7483
RGN is a press agency which sends gay & AIDS related information by
facs. to its subscribers (especially the mainstream press). Published
every week. Yearly subscription is 4,000,000L.

☺▽ *Sabazio*
Via Einaudi 33, 00040 Frattochie RM, Lazio. Italy
☎ 6 93 54 7567 📞 6 93 54 7483
🛒 ✓ $
Periodical about spirituality (gay oriented). Published every week. Yearly
subscription is 4,000,000L.

⚥▽ *Shamakami*
Shamakami, Incorporated, P. O. Box 460456, San Francisco, California
94146-0456. U.S.A.
☎ 415 442 7958 📞 301 681 0115
📧 mretina@capaccess.org
Lesbian & bisexual literary magazine. Published quarterly. Yearly
subscription is $12U.S.. many other languages also spoken.

⚥▽ *Transsisters, The Journal of Transsexual Feminism*
Skyclad Publishing, 4004 Troost Avenue, Kansas City, Missouri 64110.
U.S.A.
☎ 816 753 7816 📞 816 753 7816
📧 davinaanne@aol.com
🛒 ✓ $
Published quarterly. Yearly subscription is $30.

⚥ *TransVamp*

TransVamp Publications, Ltd., Suite 405, 2300 Walnut Street,
Philadelphia, Pennsylvania 19103. U.S.A.
☎ 215 898 4714
📧 isato@a.chem.upenn.edu
🕐 10:00 - 18:00
🛒 ✓ $
Books & magazines of well-known Internet trans-vixen Kalina Isato, the
Sexy Vampire. Published quarterly. Age statement of 18 is required.

⚧▽ *Wicked Women*
⚤ Wicked Women, P. O. Box 1349, Strawberry Hills, New South Wales
2012. Australia
☎ 2 517 2163 📞 2 517 2163
🕐 09:00 - 17:00
🛒 ✓ $
Lesbian magazine of sex & sexuality, with national & international
news, sex radical journalism, feature articles, photo spreads, interviews,
& reviews. Published quarterly. Yearly subscription is $A38 for AUS,
$A48 overseas. Age statement of 18 is required.

⚧▽ *Young Gays Club (YGC)*
📧 ygc@lava.net
Newsletter about young men over 18 years of age. Network-wide ID is
YGC. To subscribe, send e-mail to: ygc@lava.net with subject line of:
subscribe ygc & a body text of: I am over age 18 subscribe ygc. Age
statement of 18 is required.

☺ □ *Zoomorph*
🌐 http://www.zoom.com/personal/aberno/zoomorph/

Publishers: Magazines: Spirituality

⚥ *The Crucible*
🖊 P. O. Box 951, Stevens Point, Wisconsin 54481-0951. U.S.A.
🛒 ✓ $
Newsletter for gay Wiccans or neo-pagans, focussing on BDSM & pain
aspects of spirituality. Published every two months. Yearly subscription is
$20 U.S. for U.S. & Cdn., $30 U.S. elsewhere. Age statement of 21 is
required.

Publishers: Magazines: Watersports

⚥▼ *Gold'n Stream*
Winter Publishing, Inc., P. O. Box 80667, South Dartmouth,
Massachusetts 02748-0667. U.S.A.
☎ 508 999 0078 📞 508 984 4040
🛒 ✓ $ 💳 💳 💳
Publication of YELLOW HANKY MEN, for gay men into watersports.
Published quarterly. Yearly subscription is $35U.S. to U.S., $50U.S.
elsewhere. Age statement of 21 is required.

Publishers: Miscellaneous

☺ □ *93 S/M Designs*
P. O. Box 10, Derby, Derbyshire DE1 9SN. England
🛒 ✓ $
Small independent company specializing in the magickal aspects of
BDSM. All products, including world's first magickal tarot deck, are
limited editions.

Publishers: Newspapers: Sexuality

♂ ▽ *Mail2Male*
FFT Publishing, P. O. Box 7407, Cairns, Queensland 4870. Australia
📞 15 964852
🛒 ✓ $
Male-to-male contacts, erotic fiction, issues / information on same-sex
(male) issues, encourages organization of same-sex (male) social /
sexual groups. Published every month. Yearly subscription is A$25 plus
p&p.

Publishers: Videos: BDSM

⚧□ *AVI Productions*
26 rue des Rigoles, 75020 Paris. France
☎ 143 66 6194 📞 143 66 6424
🕐 09:00 - 18:30
🛒 ✓ 〜 ℮
BDSM videos. Also put on fetish & domination nights, private nights for
members only, & information for couples exploring BDSM pleasures. Age
statement of 18 is required.

⚥▼ *Marathon Films*
P. O. Box 2194, Toluca Lake, California 91610-0194. U.S.A.
☎ 800 426 4207 📞 818 769 9751
✓ $ 💳
Manufacture tapes for the gay male BDSM community. Catalogue,
$3U.S.. Age statement of 21 is required.

Publishers: Videos: Bears

♂ ▼ *Girth & Mirth—Belgium*
Boîte Postale 1514, 6000 Charleroi 1. Belgium
☎ 71 56 0580 📞 71 51 8401
📧 phil-s3@pophost.eunet.be
🌐 http://www.eunet.be/rent-a-page/bigmen
🕐 08:00 - 20:00

✓ $
Catalogue, $10. Age statement of 18 is required. English & Dutch also spoken.

Publishers: Videos: Sexuality

Avalon Video International
P. O. Box 91257, Los Angeles, California 90009. U.S.A.
800 222 9622
Also distributes videos.

Publishers: Videos: Spanking

Camera Art
Suite 348, 217755 Ventura Boulevard, Woodland Hills, California 91367. U.S.A.
818 766 1448 — 818 766 9679
24hr. facs. & order lines
✓ $
Produces 2 girlie girl spanking videos a month, & they are real. Age statement of 21 is required. Please see our display advertisement.

Radio: Sexuality

Outwaves
Christchurch Lesbian Gay Radio Collective, c/o Plains-FM 96.9, P. O. Box 25-165, Christchurch. New Zealand
3 3657 999
w.abell@lincoln.ac.nz
Mon 20:00 - 21:00
Radio program for lesbian, gay, bisexual, & transgendered people. News, views, interviews, music from Christchurch, New Zealand & the world. Age statement of 18 is required.

Sculptor: Erotic

Anthony Wojnowski's Artworks
218 Weber Street, Kitchener, Ontario N2H 1E8. Canada
519 576 0381 — 519 576 0381
Mon - Fri 07:00 - 14:00
✓ $
Self-taught scultor, with 14 years of private & institutional training.

Gary Van Velsor
Suite 110, 555 Fulton Street, San Francisco, California 94102. U.S.A.
415 558 9977 — 415 558 9977
By appointment

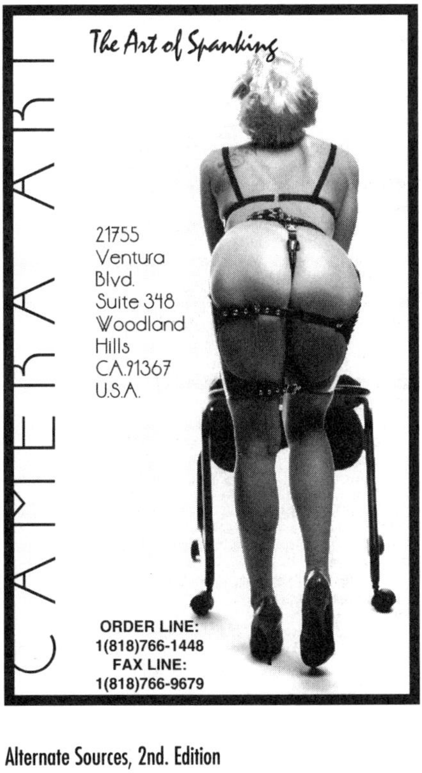

✓ $
Deep carved glass male torsos. Age statement of 21 is required.

Stores: Books: General

Big & Tall
15 Harriet Street, San Francisco, California 94103. U.S.A.
415 864 3456 — 415 826 2736
09:00 - 18:00
✓ $
Books, videos, & other merchandise.

Frontline Books
1 Newton Street, Manchester, Greater Manchester M1 1HW. England
161 236 1101 — 161 236 1103
161 236 1102
frontline-books@mcr1.geonet.de
http://www.poptel.org.uk/Bookfinder/
Mon - Sat 10:00 - 18:00, Sun 11:00 - 16:00
✓
Radical bookshop specializing in lesbian & gay books, magazines, cards, jewelry, t-shirts. Also kids, politics, & women's studies books. Urdu also spoken.

Stores: Clothing: Leather

Hide & Sleek
14 Saint Leonard's Place, Kinghorn, Fife KY3 9UL. Scotland
1592 891344 — 1592 891344
✓ $ ₵
Manufacture made-to-measure leather clothing. Also mail order.

Stores: Clothing: Lingerie

Agent Provocateur
6 Broadwick Street, London W1V 1FH. England
171 439 0229 — 171 494 1102
Mon - Sat 11:00 - 19:00
Very sexy provocative high-end exclusive lingerie shop selling mostly good french lingerie, hosiery, & shoes. Also mail order.

Stores: Clothing: Sexuality

Kentucky Woman
P. O. Box 2732, Brighton, East Sussex BN2 1LX. England
1273 674631
09:00 - 18:00
✓ $ ₵
Set in an exclusive Regency building overlooking the English Channel, the new Kentucky Woman studio now has the most extensive & exciting range of handmade Regency & Victorian gowns, dresses, maid uniforms, corsets, silk & satin lingerie, stockings, & stilettos, all made to measure by our expert seamstresses in the finest threads & materials. Everything in one complete studio for the 'new woman' in your life. For full details, & newsletter, send £10 to above address. Publishes *Kentucky Woman Newsletter*. Age statement of 18 is required.

Stores: Erotica: BDSM

Mister B
Postbus 789, 1000 AT Amsterdam. The Netherlands
20 422 0003 — 20 627 6868
mrb@euronet.nl
http://neturl.nl/mrb/
10:00 - 18:30, Sat 11:00 - 18:00
✓ $ ₵
Well-designed, open shop with highest quality leather & rubber clothing & toys, art exhibitions, magazines, piercing, etc.. Also mail order. English, German, French, & Italian also spoken.

Stores: Erotica: Corsets

Romantasy
199 Moulton Street, San Francisco, California 94123. U.S.A.
415 673 3137 Ext.: 03 — 415 567 2466
info@romantasy.com
http://www.romantasy.com
Mon - Sat 12:00 - 20:00, Sun 12:00 - 18:00
✓
Erotic boutique specializing in Victorian corsets, women-produced videos, pheromone perfume, washable massage oils, & non-piercing jewelry. Also mail order. Publishes *Touché* quarterly. Yearly subscription is free. Spanish also spoken.

Suppliers: Photoprinting

Magic Color Photo Lab
312 Mission Avenue, Oceanside, California 92054-2553. U.S.A.
619 967 6014 — 619 967 1706
magiccolor@aol.com
Mon - Sat 10:00 - 17:00
✓ $
Discreet, uncensorded photoprocessing by mail. Send for free price list & mailer. Age statement of 18 is required.

Suppliers: Travel Arrangements: BDSM

☺ ▼ **SunMaster**
Suite 312, 66 Oakmount Road, Toronto, Ontario M6P 2M8. Canada
☎ 416 763 5830
🕐 24hrs. voice mail
🔷 ✓ $ 💳 🚗 VISA MC 🚚 D 📧 ℓ
Empathic, reliable travel consultant, for those planning their next trip to a more-than-mainstream destination. Underground interests understood.

Training: BDSM

☺ ■ **Miss Prim's Muir Reform Academy**
🖐 P. O. Box 135, Hereford, Hereford & Worcester HR2 7PE. England
☎ 143 234 3241 📞 143 234 3241 (manual)
📧 prim@acopclub.demon.co.uk
🔷 ✓ $ ℓ
School for naughty (adult) boys, girls, & "boys who would be girls." To come, you must join The Academy Club . Publishes *The Muir Journal* 3 times a year. Yearly subscription is £30 for U.K., £35 for Europe, S60U.S. for overseas. Age statement of 21 is required.

☺ ■ **Miss Tresse's Finishing Academy**
🖐 Strictly Stories, P. O. Box 15, Station A, Etobicoke, Ontario M9C 2V3. Canada
☎ 416 622 2485
📧 clare@the-wire.com
🕐 09:00 - 21:00
🔷 $ 📧
Correspondence courses of instruction for adults interested in various forms of "age play," cross-dressing, maid, & slave training. Age statement of 21 is required.

Australia

Area: Approximately 7.6 million square kilometres
Population: Approximately 17,350,000
Capital City: Canberra
Currency: Australian Dollar
Official Language: English
Major Religions: 26% Protestant, 24% Roman Catholic
National Holiday: Australia Day, 26th. January
Time zone: GMT plus 8 - 10 hours
Country Initials: AUS
Electricity: 220-240 volts
Country Dialing Code (from elsewhere): 61
Intl. Dialing Prefix (out of the country): 0011
Long Distance Dialing Prefix: 0
Climate: Summer is in January. Inland, temperatures often surpass 35°C, with frequent heat waves above 40°C. Winter temperatures from 30°C inland to 5°C in the south east of the country.
Age of consent & homosexuality legislation: Age of consent for sexual activity is 18 in the Australian Capital Territory, 16 in Victoria, & 17 in South Australia. In New South Wales the age is 16 for heterosexual sex and 18 for homosexual sex. In Western Australia the age is 16 for heterosexual and lesbian sex, but 16 for gay male sex. Since 1991, there has been legal recognition of homosexual relationships. There is no longer a ban on homosexual people in the military (ban lifted in 1992). Also in 1992, the government made it illegal to discriminate against people with HIV/AIDS.
Legal drinking age: 18 in all states.

NATIONAL RESOURCES

Archives: Sexuality

⚥▽ **Australian Lesbian & Gay Archives**
P. O. Box 124, Parkville, Victoria 3052.
☎ 39 499 6334

Mailorder: Clothing: Footwear

☺ ■ **Shoecraft**
P. O. Box 389, Prahran, Victoria 3181.
☎ 5 221 4802

Mailorder: Erotica: BDSM

☺ ■ **Feelings**
P. O. Box 7059, Lismore Heights, New South Wales 2480.
Catalogue, S2.50AUS.

Mailorder: Erotica

⚥▼ **The Beat**
P. O. Box 168, Prahran, Victoria 3181.
☎ 39 827 8748

Mailorder: Erotica: Leather

☺ **Sax Leather**
P. O. Box 1193, Darlinghurst, New South Wales 2010.
☎ 1800 674 340 (order line)

Mailorder: Erotica

④ **The Pleasure Spot**
P. O. Box 213, Woolahra, New South Wales 2025.
☎ 2 361 0433 📞 2 331 6120

Mailorder: Videos: BDSM

☺ **Kayser Novelty Co.**
P. O. Box 6, Austal, New South Wales 2171.
☎ 2 606 0002 📞 2 606 0609
🔷 $ VISA MC
Catalogue, £5 to £12, depending on catalogue.

Organizations: AIDS: Education

☺ ☐ **AIDS Trust of Australia**
P. O. Box 1272, Darlinghurst, New South Wales 2010.
☎ 2 211 2044
Fundraising for HIV/AIDS research, care, & education.

☺ ☐ **Australian Foundation of AIDS Organizations (AFAO)**
Level 8, Kindersley House, 33 Bligh Street, Sydney, New South Wales 2000.
☎ 6 231 2111
Represents local AIDS organizations at national & international levels.

☺ **Australian National Council on AIDS**
P. O. Box 9849, Canberra, Australian Capital Territory 2601.
☎ 6 289 7186

Organizations: AIDS: Support

☺ **Bobby Goldsmith Foundation—South Australia**
P. O. Box 247, Norwood, South Australia 5067.
☎ 8 362 3106
☎ 8 212 2382
Financial assistance for those infected with HIV/AIDS & in financial difficulty.

Organizations: Sexuality

▷⚥☐ **The Gender Centre, Inc.**
P. O. Box 266, Petersham, New South Wales 2049.
☎ 2 569 2366 📞 2 569 1176
🕐 Mon - Fri 10:00 - 21:00
Counselling, information, accomodation, & emergency housing.

▷⚥▽ **Les Girls CD Group**
c/o P. O. Box 504, Burnwood, New South Wales 2134.

Piercers

☺ **The Piercing Urge**
🖐 P. O. Box 2145, Prahran MDC, Victoria 3181.
☎ 3 9530 2244 📞 3 9530 2427
☐ Check with store
🔷 ✓ 💳 📧 VISA MC 🚚 D
Body piercing of all kinds. Jewelry sales & custom made jewelry. Store on 1st. Floor, 206 Commercial Road. Age statement of 18 is required.

Publishers: Guides: Sexuality

⚥▼ **G'Day Guide**
4 Baker Street, Saint Kilda, Victoria 3182.
☎ 3 525 4040
Travel guide listing accomodations, beaches, etc.. Published twice a year.

Publishers: Magazines: BDSM

⚥▼ **Australian Leather Men (ALM)**
P. O. Box N124, Bexley North, New South Wales 2207.
Published quarterly. Yearly subscription is AS22.

Publishers: Magazines: Sexuality

⚥▼ **Burn**
P. O. Box 130, Brooklyn, New South Wales 2083.
Articles on culture & politics. Published every month.

⚥▼ **Campaign**
Worlander Pty. Ltd., P. O. Box A228, Sydney South, New South Wales 2000.
☎ 2 332 3620 📞 2 361 5962
☎ 2 332 3666
Australia's oldest national gay publication. Published every month.

⚥▼ **Gayzette**
P. O. Box 108, Carlton North, Victoria 5054.
Published 10 times a year.

⚥▼ **Outrage**
P. O. Box 121, Carlton South, Victoria 3053.
☎ 39 419 9877 📞 39 419 0827
Events, news, & reviews. Published every month.

Stores: Erotica: BDSM

☺ **Eagle Leather**
P. O. Box 202, Abbotsford, Victoria 3067.
☎ 39 417 2100 ℻ 39 416 4235
🕐 Wed - Sun 14:00 - 22:00
VISA MC
Black leather & related goods - clothing, BDSM gear, video bookings, repairs, cleaning, piercing jewelry, latex clothing; fetish eagles & skulls. Age statement of 18 is required.

AUSTRALIAN CAPITAL TERRITORY

Population: Approximately 250,000
Capital City: Canberra
Official Language: English
Time zone: GMT plus 10 hours
Age of consent & homosexuality legislation: Age of consent for heterosexual activity is 16, 18 for homosexual. No sodomy legislation.
Legal drinking age: 18

Canberra

Helplines: Sexuality

⚤▽ **Gayline**
P. O. Box 229, Canberra, Australian Capital Territory 2601.
☎ 6 247 2726
🕐 18:00 - 22:00

Organizations: Motorcycle

⚤▽ **Griffins Motor Club**
P. O. Box 1048, Canberra, Australian Capital Territory 2601.
🕐 Meets twice each month

Organizations: AIDS: Education

⚤□ **AIDS Action Council of the Australian Capital Territory**
P. O. Box 229, Braddon, Australian Capital Territory 2601.
☎ 6 257 2855 ℻ 6 257 4839
🕐 Mon - Fri 09:00 17:00

Radio: Sexuality

⚤▽ ***Gay Wave Length***
🕐 Wed 21:30 - 22:30

Stores: Erotica: General

☺ ■ **Adam & Eve**
125 Gladstone Street, Fyshwick, Australian Capital Territory.
☎ 6 239 1121

Coffs Harbour

Organizations: AIDS: Education

☺ □ **AIDS Council of New South Wales**
P. O. Box 990, Coffs Harbour, Australian Capital Territory 2450.
☎ 6 651 4056

NEW SOUTH WALES

Population: Approximately 5,200,000
Capital City: Sydney
Major Festival: Gay Mardi Gras celebration in Sydney in the Spring
Time zone: GMT plus 10 hours
Age of consent & homosexuality legislation: Age of consent for heterosexual activity is 16, 18 for homosexual male activity. No sodomy legislation. There is no mention in law for lesbian activity.
Legal drinking age: 18

Albury

Organizations: AIDS: Support

☺ □ **AIDS Task Group**
P. O. Box 1076, Albury, New South Wales 2640.
☎ 6 023 0340
Information, support, & education for those infected with & affected by HIC/AIDS.

Armidale

Organizations: Sexuality

⚤▽ **Armidale Gay Society**
P. O. Box 581, Armidale, New South Wales.
Counselling & social activities.

Publishers: Magazines: Literary

☺ ■ ***The Independent Review***
P. O. Box 492, Armidale, New South Wales 2350.
☎ 67 711724 ℻ 67 711724
✉ rledwidge@metz.une.edu.au

Callaghan

Organizations: Sexuality: Student

⚤▽ **Lesbian & Gay Convenors**
University of Newcastle, University Drive, Callaghan, New South Wales 2308.
☎ 49 68 1281 ℻ 68 3559
Position on student council to deal with non-heterosexual issues on campus. Also provides social group for staff & students.

Castle Hill

Organizations: Family

☺ □ **Parents & Friends of Lesbians & Gays (PFLAG)—Castle Hill**
P. O. Box 1152, Castle Hill, New South Wales 2154.

Lismore

Organizations: AIDS: Education

☺ □ **AIDS Council of New South Wales**
P. O. Box 6063, Lismore, New South Wales 2480.
☎ 6 622 1555 ℻ 6 622 3978

Radio: Sexuality

⚤▽ ***Gaywaves***
2NCR-FM 92.9, P. O. Box 157, Lismore, New South Wales 2480.
☎ 66 20 3929 ℻ 66 22 1266
✉ fm-2ncr@scu.edu.au
🕸 http://www.scu.edu.au:80/cbaa/2ncr/
🕐 Mon 22:00 - 24:00
Programme for the gays & lesbians on community radio station owned by Southern Cross University.

Milsons Point

Publishers: Magazines: Spanking

☺ ***Paddles***
P. O. Box 524, Milsons Point, New South Wales 2061.
For consenting adults with an interest in spanking & related activities. Published every month. Yearly subscription is $99AUS.

Newcastle

Helplines: AIDS

☺ □ **Newcastle AIDS Hotline**
c/o Royal Newcastle Hospital, Pacific Street, Newcastle, New South Wales.
☎ 4 926 6866
HIV testing & information for those infected with or affected by HIV/AIDS.

Helplines: Sexuality

⚤▽ **Newcastle Gay & Lesbian Information Service**
P. O. Box 425, Newcastle, New South Wales 2300.
☎ 4 929 6733
🕐 18:00 - 22:00

Organizations: AIDS: Education

☺ □ **AIDS Council of New South Wales**
P. O. Box 1081, Newcastle, New South Wales 2300.
☎ 4 929 3464 ℻ 4 929 4469

Penrith

Stores: Books: General

☺ ■ **Way Out West Bookshop**
Shop 2, Carmina Arcade, Penrith, New South Wales 2750.
☎ 4 731 3094
Gay & lesbian section.

Petersham

Organizations: BDSM

⚤▽ **Marked Men**
P. O. Box 252, Petersham, New South Wales 2049.

Rozelle

Organizations: BDSM

⚤▽ **Ringed Men**
P. O. Box 712, Rozelle, New South Wales 2039.
✉ lexw@sue.econ.su.oz.au

Publishers: Magazines: Sexuality

⚢▼ ***Lesbian Network***
P. O. Box 215, Rozelle, New South Wales 2039.
Published quarterly. Yearly subscription is $18.

Sydney
Bars: BDSM
♂▼ **The Stronghold at the Clock Hotel**
Crown Street / Collins Street, Surry Hills, New South Wales 2010.
☎ 2 360 4373
🕐 17:00 - 03:00
Enter from Collins Street.

BBSs: Sexuality
♂▼ **Pinkboard**
P. O. Box 1252, Darlinghurst, New South Wales 2010.
✆ 2 331 6370. 14400 baud maximum.

Distributors: Books: General
☺ **Bulldog Books**
P. O. Box 155, Broadway, New South Wales 2007.
☎ 2 699 3507 ✆ 2 699 3527
☺ ■ **Edition Habit Press Ltd.**
112 Bronte Road, Bondi Junction, New South Wales 2022.
☎ 2 387 4339 ✆ 2 389 2966

Distributors: Magazines: General
☺ **Wrapaway**
36A 1/34 Fizroy Street, Marrickville, New South Wales 2204.
☎ 2 550 1622

Helplines: AIDS
☺ ☐ **AIDS/HIV Info Line**
☎ 2 332 4268 ✆ 008 45 16 00

Helplines: Sexuality
♂▽ **Gay & Lesbian Line**
☎ 2 360 2211
🕐 16:00 - 24:00
Information & counselling.
♂▽ **Gay & Lesbian WotsOn**
☎ 2 361 0655
🕐 24hrs.
Recorded information.

Manufacturers: Clothing: Fetish
☺ **The Wild One**
20 Enmore Road, Newtown, New South Wales 2042.
☎ 2 557 1550

Manufacturers: Piercing Jewelry
☺ ■ **Bowerbird Designs**
2nd. Floor, 472 George Street, Sydney, New South Wales.
☎ 2 267 5471
Custom pieces available.

Organizations: AIDS: Education
☺ ☐ **AIDS Council of New South Wales**
P. O. Box 350, Darlinghurst, New South Wales 2010.
☎ 2 206 2000 ✆ 2 206 2069
☎ 2 283 2088 (TTY)
🕐 Mon -Fri 10:00 - 18:00

Organizations: AIDS: Support
☺ ☐ **Albion Street (AIDS) Centre**
150 Albion Street, Surry Hills, New South Wales 2010.
☎ 2 332 1090
🕐 08:00 - 19:00
Full medical clinic providing support for those infected with or affected by HIV/AIDS.
☺ ☐ **Bobby Goldsmith Foundation**
P. O. Box 97, Darlinghurst, New South Wales 2010.
☎ 2 360 9755
Financial support & accommodation in two locations for people with AIDS & AIDS related complex.
☺ ☐ **Community Support Network of New South Wales, Inc.**
P. O. Box 415, Darlinghurst, New South Wales 2010.
☎ 2 283 3234
🕐 10:00 -18:00
Physical care for people with AIDS.

Organizations: BDSM
♂▽ **The Club Australia**
P. O. Box 416, Darlinghurst, New South Wales 2010.
☺ ▽ **The National Leather Association (NLA)—New South Wales**

8/102 Burton, Darlinghurst, New South Wales 2010.
☺ ☐ **Sydney Leather Pride Association**
P. O. Box 1524, Darlinghurst, New South Wales 2010.
Organizes events throughout the year, including Leather Pride Week.

Organizations: Bears
♂▽ **Bears Down Under**
P. O. Box 108, Newton, New South Wales 2042.
☎ 2 550 1331
📧 bobh@triode.apana.org.au
🌐 http://www.skepsis.com/.gblo/bears/CLUBS/Bears_Down_Under/
♂▽ **Harbour City Bears**
P. O. Box 252, Petersham, New South Wales 2049.
☎ 2 9904 1603
☎ 2 568 3029
📧 s.hyslop@student.anu.edu.au
🌐 http://douglass.magna.com.au/html/hcb.htm
♂▽ **Ozbears Australia Inc.**
P. O. Box 108, Newtown, New South Wales 2042.
☎ 2 550 1331
☎ 2 690 1730
📧 bobh@triode.apana.org.au
Contact: Mr. Bob Hay

Organizations: Bondage
♂▽ **Sydney Bondage Club**
P. O. Box 293, Sydney, New South Wales 2007.

Organizations: Motorcycle
♂▽ **Australian Club Run Association (ACRA)**
P. O. Box A882, Sydney South, New South Wales 2000.
♂▽ **Dolphins Motor Club**
P. O. Box E362, Saint James, New South Wales 2000.
☎ 2 699 6588
🕐 Meets Thu 21:30
♂▽ **South Pacific MC**
P. O. Box 823, Sydney, New South Wales 2001.
🕐 Meets Fri Sat

Organizations: Sexual Politics
⚥▽ **Transgender Liberation Coalition (TLC)**
P. O. Box 208, Kings Cross, New South Wales 2011.
☎ 2 358 5664

Organizations: Sexuality
⚥▽ **Boys Will Be Boys**
P. O. Box 1349, Strawberry Hills, New South Wales 2012.
☎ 2 319 2034
Female-to-male support network, counselling. Publishes a newsletter every month.
♂▽ **Coming Out Group**
197 Albion Street, Sydney, New South Wales.
☎ 2 360 2211
🕐 Sun 15:00 - 17:30
♂▽ **Cronulla Gay Group**
P. O. Box 195, Cronulla, New South Wales 2230.
☎ 2 660 4615
🕐 20:00 each 2nd. Wed
Support group.
♂▽ **Gay & Lesbian Counselling Service of New South Wales**
P. O. Box 5074, Surry Hills, New South Wales 2001.
☎ 2 360 3063 (office)
☎ 008 80 53 79
🕐 Mon - Fri 09:00 - 16:00
Support & counselling. Office number not for counselling.
♂▽ **Gay Fathers**
#103, 412 Oxford Street, Paddington, New South Wales 2021.
☎ 2 360 3063
Telephone is provided by the Gay & Lesbian Counselling Service.
⚥▽ **The Seahorse Society—New South Wales**
P. O. Box 168, Westgate, New South Wales 2048.
☎ 2 569 6239
🕐 Call Thu evening
♂ ☐ **Sydney Bisexual Support Network (SBSN)**
66 Albion Street, Surry Hills, New South Wales.
☎ 2 310 2798
☎ 2 698 1207
🕐 Meets 2nd. & 4th. Mon of month

Organizations: Sexuality: Student

Gay & Lesbian Teachers & Students Association, Inc. (GaLTaS)
P. O. Box 399, Darlinghurst, New South Wales 2010.
☎ 2 350 9544
☎ 008 636 693
Support & education group.

Macquarie University Gay & Lesbian Association
Union Box 96, Students' Council, Macquarie University, Sydney, New South Wales 2109.

University of New South Wales Gay & Lesbian Department
☎ 2 663 0461
Information, support, needle exchange.

Photographers: Erotic

Chris Ireland
☎ 2 331 2689
Erotic & fantasy portraits a speciality.

Christian L'Hermite
Krystan Photo, 7th. Floor, 74 Reservoir Street, Surry Hills, New South Wales 2010.
☎ 2 212 2088
Mr. L'Hermite's agent is Joanne Milne, Captive Liberation, P. O. Box 87, Five Docks, New South Wales 2046, Telephone / facsimile 2 747 3148.

Piercers

The Bee's Knees
399 Liverpool Street, Darlinghurst, New South Wales 2010.
☎ 2 361 4888

The Body Piercer
1st. Floor, 143a Oxford Street, Darlinghurst, New South Wales 2010.
☎ 2 360 4823
Also manufactures body jewelry in surgical steel, Titanium, gold, & silver. Custom service & mail order also available.

David
P. O. Box 95, Westgate, New South Wales 2048.
☎ 2 550 9448
By appointment only

The Piercing Urge
P. O. Box 180, Darlinghurst, New South Wales 2010.
☎ 2 360 3179 Fax 2 332 3845
Check with store
✓
Body piercing of all kinds. Jewelry sales & custom made jewelry. Store at 332 Bourke Street. Age statement of 18 is required.

Polymorph Body Art Gallery
82 Enmore Road, Newtown, New South Wales 2042.
☎ 2 519 8923

Publishers: Newspapers: Sexuality

Capital Q
15-19 Boundary Street, Rushcutters Bay, New South Wales 20011.
☎ 2 332 4988 Fax 2 380 5104
Free at gay & lesbian locations. Published every week.

Sydney Star Observer
P. O. Box 179, Darlinghurst, New South Wales 2010.
☎ 2 380 5577
Free at gay & lesbian locations. Published every two weeks.

Radio: Sexuality

Gay Radio Information News Service (Grins)
P. O. Box 380, Broadway, New South Wales 2007.

Gaywaves
2SER FM 107.3, P. O. Box 473, Broadway, New South Wales 2007.
☎ 2 330 3000 (during program)
Thu 20:00 - 22:30

Out & Out
2SER FM 107.3, P. O. Box 123, Broadway, New South Wales 2007.
☎ 2 330 3000 (during program)
Tue 21:30

Wild G.A.L.S.
2RSR FM 88.9, P. O. Box 16, Paddington, New South Wales 2021.
☎ 2 550 9552
Sat 19:00 - 20:00

Stores: Books: General

The Bookshop—Darlinghurst
207 Oxford Street, Darlinghurst, New South Wales 2010.
☎ 2 331 1103 Fax 2 331 7021
☎ 2 331 4140
Sun - Wed 10:00 - 22:00, Thu - Sat 10:00 - 24:00
$
Australia's oldest & largest specialist gay / lesbian bookshop. Comprehensive range of titles. Friendly staff. Happy to advise visitors to Sydney.

The Bookshop—Newtown
186 King Street, Newtown, New South Wales 2010.
☎ 2 557 4244 Fax 2 331 7021
Mon - Wed 10:00 - 21:00, Thu - Fri 10:00 - 22:00, Sat 10:00 - 20:00, Sun 12:00 - 19:00
$
Australia's oldest & largest specialist gay / lesbian bookshop. Comprehensive range of titles. Friendly staff. Happy to advise visitors to Sydney.

Gleebooks
49 Glebe Point Road, Glebe, New South Wales 2037.
☎ 2 660 2578
Gay & lesbian section.

Stores: Clothing: Fetish

Purr...effect
62 Oxford Street, Paddington, New South Wales 2021.
☎ 2 332 1370 Fax 2 332 1370

Stores: Erotica: BDSM

Mephisto Leather
1st. Floor, 112 Oxford Street, Darlinghurst, New South Wales 2010.
☎ 2 332 3218
Mon - Sat 10:00 - ?

Radical Leather
P. O. Box 617, Darlinghurst, New South Wales 2010.
☎ 2 331 7544
Wed - Fri 14:00 -18:00, Sat 10:30 - 17:00

Sax Leather
110A Oxford Street, Darlinghurst, New South Wales 2010.
☎ 1800 674 340 (order line)

Stores: Erotica: General

The Land Beyond
583 George Street, Sydney, New South Wales 2001.

Numbers
95 Oxford Street, Darlinghurst, New South Wales 2010.
☎ 2 361 6099
24hrs.

The Tool Shed
P. O. Box 534, Newton, New South Wales 2010.
☎ 2 565 1599
11:00 - 01:30, Fri 11:00 - ?, Sat Sun 12:00 - ?
Toys, books, magazines, leatherwear, etc.. Three stores in Darlinghurst & Newtown.

Tattooists

Mischief Moon
1st. Floor, 143a Oxford Street, Darlinghurst, New South Wales 2010.
☎ 2 361 3332

Television: Sexuality

Queer TV
P. O. Box 636, Newtown, New South Wales 2042.
Community access television.

Tweed Heads

Stores: Books: General

Borderline Books
28 Bay Street, Tweed Heads, New South Wales 2485.
☎ 7 536 4275

Keyhole Bookshop
9 Bay Street, Tweed Heads, New South Wales 2485.
☎ 7 536 3197

Wagga Wagga

Organizations: AIDS: Education

Wagga Wagga AIDS Task Force
P. O. Box 159, Wagga Wagga, New South Wales 2650.
☎ 6 923 4811
Counselling & support for people infected with or affected by HIV/AIDS.

Wollongong

Organizations: AIDS: Education

AIDS Council of New South Wales
P. O. Box 1073, Port Kembla, New South Wales 2505.
☎ 4 276 2399 Fax 4 226 9838

Organizations: Sexuality
⚥▽ **Men's Gay & Bisexual Coming Out Group**
P. O. Box 1144, Wollongong, New South Wales 2500.
☎ 4 221 4012

Organizations: Sexuality: Student
⚥▽ **Alliance of Lesbian, Bi, & Gay Students**
P. O. Box 1144, Wollongong, New South Wales 2500.
☎ 4 221 4012

Stores: Erotica: General
☺ ■ **Venus Adult Book Shop**
121 Wentworth Road, Port Kembla, New South Wales 2505.
☎ 4 275 2121

NORTHERN TERRITORY
Population: Approximately 140,000
Capital City: Darwin
Official Language: English
Time zone: GMT plus 9 hours
Age of consent & homosexuality legislation: Age of consent for heterosexual activity is 16, 18 for homosexual. No sodomy legislation. Anti-gay discrimination laws are in force.
Legal drinking age: 18

Alice Springs
Health Services
☺ □ **Alice Springs Hospital**
STD Unit, Gap Road / Steward Terrace, Alice Springs, Northern Territory.
☎ 8 950 2638
⏱ Mon - Fri 08:00 16:00

Helplines: Sexuality
⚥▽ **Crisis Line**
☎ 8 981 9227
⏱ 24hrs.

Organizations: AIDS: Education
☺ □ **AIDS Council of Central Australia**
P. O. Box 910, Alice Springs, Northern Territory 0871.
☎ 8 953 1118 ✆ 8 953 4584
⏱ Mon - Fri 09:00 - 17:00
Community-based information, support, education for HIV/AIDS issues. Licensed, confidential needle exchange.

Darwin
Health Services
☺ □ **Royal Darwin Hospital**
Communicable Diseases Centre, Block 4, Rocklands Drive, Darwin, Northern Territory 0800.
☎ 8 720 8007
HIV testing.

Organizations: AIDS: Education
☺ □ **Northern Territory AIDS Council, Inc.**
P. O. Box 2826, Darwin, Northern Territory 0800.
☎ 8 41 3288 ✆ 8 412 590
☎ 008 011 180

Organizations: Sexuality: Student
⚥▽ **Territory University Gay Society (TUGS)**
P. O. Box 2849, Darwin, Northern Territory 0801.
☎ 8 941 1711

Radio: Sexuality
⚥▽ **Sexual Reality**
☎ 8 941 1711
⏱ Wed 22:00 - 24:00

QUEENSLAND
Population: Approximately 3,000,000
Capital City: Brisbane
Official Language: English
Time zone: GMT plus 10 hours
Age of consent & homosexuality legislation: There is no longer any mention of homosexual activity in law. Homosexual acts were decriminalized in 1982.
Legal drinking age: 18

Annerley
Organizations: Sexuality
▽▽ **The Seahorse Society—Queensland**

P. O. Box 574, Annerley, Queensland 4103.

Brisbane
Bars: BDSM
⚥▼ **Sportsman Hotel**
130 Leichardt Street, Brisbane, Queensland 4004.
☎ 7 831 2892
⏱ 13:00 - 01:00

Bars: Sexuality
⚤▼ **The Beat**
677 Ann Street, Fortitude Valley, Queensland 4006.
☎ 7 252 2543
Live shows.

⚤▼ **Empire Hotel**
Veranda Bar, 339 Brunswick Street, Fortitude Valley, Queensland 4006.
Shows Fri & Sat.

⚤▼ **Options Nightclub**
18 Little Edward Street, Brisbane, Queensland.
☎ 7 831 4214
Live shows Wed - Sun.

Counsellors
▽▼ **The Gender Clinic**
484 Adelaide Street, Brisbane, Queensland 4000.
☎ 7 639 8262 ✆ 1 819 7699
⏱ Wed 13:00 - 17:30

Health Services
⚥▽ **Gay & Lesbian Health Service**
38 Gladstone Road, Highgate Hill, Queensland 4101.
☎ 7 844 6806 ✆ 7 844 4206
⏱ Mon - Thu 08:00 - 20:00, Fri 08:00 - 18:00, Sat 09:00 - 12:00

Helplines: Sexuality
♂▽ **Bi-Line**
☎ 7 846 2770
⏱ 24hrs Mon - Fri
Operated by the Queensland AIDS Council.

⚥▽ **Gay Line—Brisbane**
☎ 7 839 3277

♀▽ **Lesbian Line—Brisbane**
☎ 7 839 3288
⏱ 19:00 - 22:00
Information & counselling.

Organizations: AIDS: Support
☺ □ **Queensland AIDS Committee—Townsville**
P. O. Box 1103, Fortitude Valley, Queensland 4006.
☎ 7 721 1384

☺ □ **Queensland AIDS Council**
522 Stanley Street, Mater Hill, Queensland 4101.
☎ 7 844 1990 ✆ 7 844 4206
☎ 008 17 7434
⏱ 24hrs.
Counselling, education, & welfare service for those infected with HIV/AIDS.

☺ □ **Queensland Positive People**
P. O. Box 3142, South Brisbane, Queensland 4101.
☎ 7 846 3939
Support & information. Publishes a newsletter.

Organizations: BDSM
⚥▽ **The Boot Co.**
P. O. Box 187, Red Hill, Brisbane, Queensland 4170.

Organizations: Motorcycle
⚥▽ **Rangers MC**
P. O. Box 449, Spring Hill, Brisbane, Queensland 4004.

Organizations: Sexuality
♂▽ **Australian Bisexual Network**
c/o Brisbane Bisexual Centre, P. O. Box 490, Lutwyche, Queensland 4030.
☎ 7 254 0692
✉ robertw@planet.mh.dpi.qld.gov.au
Publishes *National Biways* every month. Yearly subscription is $20AUS.

▽▽ **Boys Will Be Boys**
P. O. Box 212, West End, Queensland 4005.
☎ 7 846 3787

♂▽ **Brisbane Bisexual Centre**
P. O. Box 490, Lutwyche, Queensland 4030.
☎ 7 391 6025
Contact: Wayne, Coördinator

⚢▽ **Gay & Lesbian Counselling & Information Service**
P. O. Box 1078, Fortitude Valley, Queensland 4006.
☎ 7 3839 3277 (gayline)
☎ 7 3839 3288 (lesbianline)
⏲ 19:00 - 22:00
Contact: Mr. David McKelvey, Secretary
Opertated by Gay & Lesbian Welfare Association, Inc..

⚢ **Queensland Bisexual Network**
c/o Brisbane Bisexual Centre, P. O. Box 490, Lutwyche, Queensland 4030.

Organizations: Sexuality: Student

⚢▽ **QUT Campus Queers**
P. O. Box 5196, West End, Queensland 4101.

Publishers: Magazines: Sexuality

⚢▼ *Queensland Pride*
P. O. Box 591, Mount Gravatt, Queensland 4122.
☎ 7 349 1613 ☏ 7 849 7184
Free. Published every month.

Radio: Sexuality

⚢▽ *Gaywaves*
☎ 7 252 1555
⏲ Wed 18:00 -21:00

Bundaberg

Organizations: Sexuality

⚢▽ **Bundaberg Gay & Lesbian Support**
P. O. Box 2695, Bundaberg, Queensland 4670.
☎ 7 152 9999

Cairns

Organizations: AIDS: Support

☺☐ **Queensland AIDS Council**
P. O. Box 1284, Cairns, Queensland 4870.
☎ 7 051 1028 ☏ 7 031 2016
⏲ 10:00 - 16:00

Organizations: Sexuality

⚢▽ **Gayline—Cairns**
☎ 7 051 9083
☎ 7 051 0279
⏲ Wed - Sun 19:00 - 23:00

Radio: Sexuality

⚢▽ *Gay FM*
☎ 7 053 5866
⏲ Sun 22:00

New Farm

Organizations: Sexuality

⚧▽ **Australia TransGenerist Support Association, Inc.**
P. O. Box 212, New Farm, Queensland 4005.
☎ 7 236 2400 ☏ 2 236 2398
☎ 7 846 3787 (hotline)
⏲ Meets monthly
Publishes a newsletter.

Noosa

Organizations: AIDS: Education

☺☐ **Queensland AIDS Council**
P. O. Box 1191, Noosa, Queensland 4558.
☎ 7 443 7702 ☏ 7 443 3743

Nundah

Organizations: Bears

⚢▽ **Brisbears**
P. O. Box 6, Nundah, Queensland 4012.
☎ 7 3226 8847
✉ jasonk@eis.net.au
🌐 http://www2.eis.net.au/~jasonk/bb.html

Rockhampton

Organizations: Sexuality: Student

⚢▽ **Galileo**
Student Union CQU Box 5316, Rockhampton Mail Centre, Rockhampton, Queensland 4702.
Support for lesbian, gay, bisexual, & transgender students at Central Queensland University.

Surfer's Paradise

Organizations: AIDS: Education

☺☐ **Queensland AIDS Committee—Gold Coast**
P. O. Box 1330, Surfer's Paradise, Queensland 4217.
☎ 7 538 4611
⏲ Wed 19:00 - 22:00

☺☐ **Queensland AIDS Council**
P. O. Box 826, Runaway Bay, Queensland 4216.
☎ 7 532 2673 ☏ 7 591 1471

Toowooba

Organizations: AIDS: Education

☺☐ **Queensland AIDS Council**
P. O. Box 2469, Toowooba, Queensland 4350.
☎ 7 639 1820

Townsville

Health Services

☺☐ **Townsville General Hospital**
Clinic, Block A, Eyre Street, Townsville, Queensland 4810.
☎ 7 781 9369
⏲ Mon - Fri 09:00 17:00

Helplines: Sexuality

⚢▽ **Townsville Gayline**
P. O. Box 6247, Townsville, Queensland 4810.
☎ 7 772 6622
⏲ Sun 15:00 - 18:00
Counselling & information.

Organizations: AIDS: Education

☺☐ **Queensland AIDS Council**
P. O. Box 2106, Townsville, Queensland 4810.
☎ 7 721 1384
Community-based counselling, information, & education.

Organizations: Sexuality

⚢▽ **Townsville Gay & Lesbian Resource & Information Network**
P. O. Box 6247, Townsville, Queensland 4810.
☎ 7 772 6446
⏲ Meets every 2nd. Mon 19:00. Office hrs. 09:00 - 17:00. Telephones Tue Thu 19:00 - 20:00.
Counselling & information.

Radio: AIDS

⚢▼ *QuAC Voice*
4TTT FM 103.9, P. O. Box 2106, Townsville, Queensland 4810.
☎ 7 721 1384
⏲ Sat 18:30 - 19:30

Stores: Erotica: General

☺■ **Dreams Adult Shop**
461b Finders Street, Townsville, Queensland 4810.
☎ 7 771 4300

☺■ **Sweethearts Adult Bookshop**
206a Charters Towers Road, Townsville, Queensland 4810.
☎ 7 251 1431

SOUTH AUSTRALIA

Population: Approximately 1,400,000
Capital City: Adelaide
Official Language: English
Time zone: GMT plus 9 hours
Age of consent & homosexuality legislation: There is no longer any mention of homosexual activity in law. Anti-gay discrimination laws are in force. Homosexual acts were decriminalized in 1984.
Legal drinking age: 18

State Resources

Organizations: Family

☺☐ **Parents & Friends of Lesbians & Gays (PFLAG)—South Australia**
☎ 8 837 7108
☎ 8 241 0616

Organizations: Sexuality

⚧▽ **Carrousel Club, Inc.**
P. O. Box 721, Marleston, South Australia 5033.
☎ 8 281 6190

☎ 8 388 3644
⏱ Call until 21:30 nightly
Contact: Ms. Carol Seely, Secretary
For the transgendered & those with an interest in same. Publishes a
newsletter every two months. Yearly subscription is free to members.

Publishers: Newspapers: Sexuality
⊕ *Liberation*
c/o W. S. R. C., 64 Pennington Terrace, North Adelaide, South Australia
5006.
⚘ ✓ $
Local information for women put together by volunteers. Published every
month. Yearly subscription is $24AUS.

Adelaide
Archives: Sexuality
⚥▽ **Lesbian & Gay Community Library**
Darling House, 64 Fullarton Road, Norwood, South Australia 5067.
☎ 8 362 3106
⏱ Mon - Fri 09:30 - 17:30, Sat 14:00 - 17:00
Free membership library with one of the largest collections in Australia.

Bars: BDSM
⚥▼ **The Edinburgh Castle Hotel**
Gray Street / Currie Street, Adelaide, South Australia.
⏱ Leather Wed 21:00 - 24:00

Health Services
☺ ☐ **Clinic 275**
1st. Floor, 275 North Terrace, Adelaide, South Australia.
☎ 8 226 6025
⏱ Mon Thu Fri 10:00 - 16:30, Tue Wed 12:00 - 19:30
HIV testing.

☺ ☐ **Flinders Medical Centre**
Flinders Drive, Bedford Park, South Australia 5042.
☎ 8 204 5192
⏱ By appointment only Wed mornings
HIV testing & clinic.

Helplines: Sexuality
⚥▽ **Gayline**
P. O. Box 459, North Adelaide, South Australia 5006.
☎ 008 11 22 33
☎ 8 362 3223
⏱ 19:00 - 22:00, Sat Sun 14:00 - 17:00
Information, counselling, & support. Calls free from outside metropolitan
area (1st. number).

Organizations: AIDS: Support
☺ ☐ **AIDS Council of South Australia**
P. O. Box 907, Kent Town, South Australia 5071.
☎ 8 362 1611
☎ 8 362 3208
Support services for those infected with or affected by HIV/AIDS.
Recorded message.

☺ ☐ **CARA - Carers for People Living with AIDS**
64 Fullarton Road, Norwood, South Australia 5067.
☎ 8 362 3208

☺ ☐ **People Living With AIDS (PLWA)—South
Australia**
P. O. Box 2603, Kent Town, South Australia 5071.
☎ 8 362 2799
⏱ Call between 13:00 - 17:30

Organizations: Family
⚥▽ **Bisexual & Married Homosexual Men's Support
Group (BAMH)**
☎ 8 362 7931
⏱ Call Wed Sat 10:00 - 12:00. Meets Wed afternoon monthly, Thu
eve weekly

☺ ☐ **Parents of Lesbian & Gay Children**
☎ 8 267 5366

Organizations: Fetish: Clothing
☺ ☐ **South Australia Fetish / Fantasy Enthusiasts
(SAFE)**
P. O. Box 139, North Adelaide, South Australia 5006.

Organizations: Motorcycle
⚥▽ **Southern Region Motor Club (SRMC)**
P. O. Box 252, Adelaide, South Australia 5001.
☎ 8 266 3268
☎ 8 297 2468
⏱ Wed 21:00 - 24:00

Organizations: Sexuality
♂▽ **Adelaide Bisexual Collective**
P. O. Box 3391, Rundall Mall, Adelaide, South Australia 5000.
☎ 8 352 5715
Education & support for bisexuals & their friends.

✉▽ **Carousel Club of South Australia**
P. O. Box 721, Cowandilla, South Australia 5033.
☎ 8 388 3644
☎ 8 281 6190
Publishes a newsletter every month.

✉▽ **Chameleons**
P. O. Box 907, Kent Town, South Australia 5071.
☎ 8 362 3208
⏱ Meets 3rd. Fri of month. Call Tue & Fri 09:00 - 17:00
Group for transexuals, transvestites, & cross-dressers.

⚥▽ **Gay & Lesbian Counselling Service of South
Australia**
P. O. Box 2011, Kent Town, South Australia 5071.
☎ 8 362 3223

⚥▽ **Lesbian Network**
P. O. Box 3185, Adelaide, South Australia 5015.
☎ 8 341 6964
Contact: Seja

♂▽ **South Australia Bisexual Network**
P. O. Box 3391, Adelaide, South Australia 5000.
☎ 8 344 6146

✉☐ **South Australia Transexual Support**
☎ 1800 182 233
☎ 8 362 3223
⏱ Mon - Fri 19:00 - 22:00, Sat Sun 14:00 - 17:00

Organizations: Sexuality: Student
⚥▽ **Flinders University Gay Society**
☎ 8 201 2276
⏱ Meets every two Fri 12:00

⚥▽ **Gay & Lesbian Association of Adelaide University
(GALA)**
c/o Gayline, P. O. Box 459, Adelaide, South Australia 5006.
☎ 8 362 3223

Organizations: Sexuality: Youth
⚥▽ **Young Gays**
Second Storey Youth Centre, 57 Hyde Street, Adelaide, South Australia.
☎ 8 362 3223
⏱ 19:00 - 22:00
Support group for men 17 - 25.

Organizations: Uncircumcision
☾ ☐ **Uncirc South Australia**
P. O. Box 8106, Adelaide, South Australia 5000.
⏱ Meets 3rd. Tue of month 19:30
Information for men who want to reverse their circumsized state.

Publishers: Newspapers: Sexuality
⚥▼ **Adelaide GT**
Adelaide Gay Times, P. O. Box 101, 41 Grouger Street, Adelaide, South
Australia 5000.
☎ 8 232 1544 ✆ 8 232 1560
Free at gay locations. Published every two weeks. Yearly subscription is
A$25.

Radio: Sexuality
⚥▽ **Gay Radio**
☎ 8 410 0937
⏱ Sun 12:00 - 14:00

⚥▽ **Out Loud**
⏱ Sat 13:00 - 14:00

Stores: Books: General
☺ ■ **Imprints - Booksellers**
80 Hindley Street, Adelaide, South Australia.
☎ 8 231 4454
⏱ 09:00 - 18:00, Sun 12:00 - 18:00

Stores: Erotica: General
☺ ■ **Aphro Adult Products**
49 Morphett Street, Adelaide, South Australia.
☎ 8 231 3632
⏱ 10:00 - 24:00
Has gay section.

☺ ■ **Pink Pussy**
135b Goodwood Road, Adelaide, South Australia 5034.
☎ 8 271 5975
Adult books & toys.

⚧ ▼ **Femme Erotica**
73 Hindley Street, Adelaide, South Australia.
☎ 8 410 0636

Daw Park
Piercers
☺ ■ **Bodylink Body Piercing**
☎ 8 381 5093
⏲ After 17:00

Elizabeth Vale
Health Services
☺ ☐ **People In The North**
Lyell McEwin Community Centre, Haydown & Oldham Roads, Elizabeth Vale, South Australia.
☎ 8 282 1206
Free, confidential STD & HIV testing for men & women.

Ingle Farm
Organizations: Sexuality: Student
⚧▽ **University of South Australia Gay, Lesbian, & Bisexual Association**
c/o Out & About, Student Union, P. O. Box 1, Ingle Farm, South Australia 50095.
☎ 8 302 3212

Lobethal
Organizations: Bears
⚧▽ **Ozbears of South Australia**
P. O. Box 89, Lobethal, South Australia 5241.
☎ 8 389 4292

Plympton
Organizations: Sexuality: Student
☺ ▽ **Out & About**
♿ P. O. Box 553, Plympton, South Australia 5038.
☎ 8 302 3212 ✆ 8 303 4392
☎ 41 119 0553 ✆ 41 119 0553
⏲ 09:00 - 17:00 at 302 3212, 08:00 - 01:00 at 41 119 0553

Contact: Mr. Wayde Masters, Founder / Coördinator
The University of South Africa's social & support group for non-heterosexual students.

TASMANIA
Population: Approximately 480,000
Capital City: Hobart
Official Language: English
Time zone: GMT plus 10 hours
Age of consent & homosexuality legislation: Tasmania is the only Australian state where homosexual male acts are still illegal. There is no mention in law for lesbian activity. Anti-gay discrimination laws were approved in 1991
Legal drinking age: 18

Hobart
Health Services
☺ ☐ **AIDS Unit**
78 Hampden Road, Battery Point, Tasmania 7004.
☎ 0 230 2872

Helplines: Sexuality
⚧▽ **Gay Information Line**
☎ 0 234 8179
24hr. recorded message.

Organizations: AIDS: Support
☺ ☐ **AIDS Council of Tasmania**
P. O. Box 595F, Hobart, Tasmania 7001.
☎ 0 224 1034
☎ 008 00 5900 (24hrs.)
Information, education, & support for those infected with or affected by HIV/AIDS.

Radio: Sexuality
⚧▽ **Gaywaves**
⏲ Wed 19:00 - 20:00

Stores: Erotica: General
☺ ■ **The Black Rose**
108 Harrington Road, Hobart, Tasmania 7000.

Wivenhoe
Organizations: Sexuality
⚧▽ **North West Gay Support**
c/o Post Office, Wivenhoe, Tasmania 7320.
⏲ Meets monthly

VICTORIA
Population: Approximately 4,200,000
Capital City: Melbourne
Official Language: English
Time zone: GMT plus 10 hours
Age of consent & homosexuality legislation: Age of consent for sexual activity is 16. There is no longer any mention of homosexual activity in law.
Legal drinking age: 18

State Resources
Organizations: Sexuality
⚧▽ **Bendigo Gay Society, Inc.**
P. O. Box 1123, Bendigo, Victoria 3550.
☎ 54 270 312
Social activities, weekly drop-in nights, monthly functions. Age statement of 18 is required.

Publishers: Newspapers: Sexuality
⚧▽ **Melbourne Star Observer**
Bluestone Media, P. O. Box 205, Fitzroy, Victoria 3065.
☎ 39 419 9877 ✆ 39 419 0827
✉ mso@bluestone.com.au
⏲ 09:00 - 17:30
♿ ✓ $ 💳 VISA 🅫 💳
Victoria's gay & lesbian newspaper. Published every week.

Radio: Sexuality
⚧▽ **Gay Radio Programme**
3CR Community Radio, AM 855 kHz, P. O. Box 1277, Collingwood, Victoria 3066.
☎ 39 419 8377 ✆ 39 417 4472
♿ ✓ $ 💳 VISA 🅫 💳
Community radio station which provides access to minority & disadvantaged groups, including lesbian & gay, indigenous, womens', ethnic, etc. groups.

Bendigo
Organizations: Family
☺ ☐ **Parents & Friends of Lesbians & Gays (PFLAG)— Bendigo**
☎ 53 483 033

Melbourne
Accommodation: BDSM
⚧▼ **The Gatehouse**
c/o Club 80, 10 Peel Street, Collingwood, Victoria 3066.
☎ 39 417 2182 ✆ 39 416 9474
♿ ✓ $ 💳 VISA 🅫 💳
Australia's only guesthouse specifically designed to cater to male BDSMers. Four double rooms. Slings are standard equipment. Close to Nugget's Bar. Age statement of 18 is required.

Bars: BDSM
⚧▼ **Nugget's Bar**
149 Gipps Street, Collingwood, Victoria 3066.
☎ 39 417 2832 ✆ 39 416 0474
⏲ Tue, Thu - Sun 21:00 - 01:00
♿ ✓ $ 💳 VISA 🅫 💳
Melbourne Leather Men & Jackaroo's meet here. Melbourne's only true leather bar. In operation for 15 years. Part of Laird Hotel. Age statement of 18 is required.

BBSs: Sexuality
⚧▽ **Alternative Access BBS**
✆ 39 576 1507. 14,400 baud maximum.
⏲ 24hrs.
Alternative number: 3 576 1508.

Distributors: Erotica: General
☺ ■ **Studio Strak**
P. O. Box 4838, GPO, Melbourne, Victoria 3001.
☎ 3 809 2632

Health Services

☺ ☐ **Melbourne Sexual Health Centre**
580 Swanston Street, Carlton, Victoria 3053.
☎ 39 347 0244 (& TTY)
☎ 008 03 2017

Helplines: Sexuality

⚧▽ **Gay & Lesbian Switchboard**
P. O. Box 5197, Melbourne, Victoria 3001.
☎ 39 510 5488
☎ 055 12504 (24hr. recorded information)
🕐 18:00 - 22:00, Wed 14:00 - 22:00
Confidential counselling, information, & referral.

⚧▽ **Monash University Gayline**
☎ 39 565 4195

Organizations: AIDS: Education

☺ ☐ **Victorian AIDS Council**
Beats Outreach Project, 117 Johnston, Collingwood, Victoria 3066.
☎ 39 483 6700
☎ 39 416 1387

Organizations: AIDS: Support

☺ ☐ **AIDS Line**
☎ 39 347 6099
☎ 008 133 392
🕐 Mon - Fri 11:00 - 22:00, Sat Sun 11:00 - 14:00 19:00 - 22:00
Trained volunteers provide support, education, & counselling.

⚧▽ **Victorian AIDS Council**
Gay Men's Community Health Centre, 117 Johnston Street, Collingwood,
Victoria 3066.
☎ 39 483 6777 ✆ 39 419 9595
🕐 Mon Thu 09:30 - 21:30, Wed 14:00 - 17:00, Fri 09:30 - 17:30

⚧▽ **Victorian AIDS Council**
Gay Men's Community Health Centre, 46 Acland Street, Melbourne,
Victoria 3000.
☎ 39 483 6788
🕐 Mon Fri 10:00 - 18:00, Tue - Thu 10:00 - 22:00, Sat 10:00 -
15:00

⚧▽ **Positive Friends**
P. O. Box 2770, Saint Kilda, Victoria 3182.
☎ 39 481 3413

Organizations: BDSM

⚧▽ **Melbourne Leather Men, Inc.**
P. O. Box 252, Abbottsford, Victoria 3067.
☎ 39 645 3747
🕐 Meets Thu 21:30
Contact: Mr. Paul Brathwaite, Run Captain
For men who have an interest in leather & the leather lifestyle. Affiliated
with clubs in Melbourne & Sydney. Publishes a newsletter every month.

☺ **Melbourne Leather Pride Association**
P. O. Box 359, Abbottsford, Victoria 3067.
☎ 9 530 2244 ✆ 9 530 2427
☎ 9 531 2545
✉ mpla@polyester.com.au
🌐 http://union4.su.swin.edu.au/~skud/mlpa.html
Pan-sexual group of leather men & women interested in BDSM & fetish
sexual practices. Educational workshops, social events, & leather
competitions. Age statement of 18 is required.

⚧▽ **Vision SM Club**
P. O. Box 1615, Collingwood, Victoria 3066.

Organizations: Family

☺ ☐ **Parents & Friends of Lesbians & Gays (PFLAG)—
Melbourne**
☎ 39 700 7190
🕐 Meets 4th. Tue of month 19:30

Organizations: Masturbation

⚧▽ **Melbourne Wankers**
c/o Club Spa Caulfield, 482d Glenhuntly Road, Elsternwick, Victoria.
🕐 Meets 2nd. Mon of month

Organizations: Motorcycle

⚧▽ **Jackaroos MC**
P. O. Box 5064Y, Melbourne, Victoria 3001.
☎ 39 885 1612
🕐 Wed 21:30

Organizations: Sexuality

▽▽ **The Elaine Barrie Project**
P. O. Box 405, Altona, Victoria 3018.
☎ 3 69 2613
Publishes Nu-Scene International. Age statement of 18 is required.

⚧▽ **Gamma Line**
P. O. Box 41, Richmond, Victoria 3141.
☎ 39 899 0509
🕐 Tue 20:00 - 11:00. Meets last Mon at 20:00
Support for married gay men.

⚧▽ **Goulburn Valley Gay Group**
P. O. Box 2255, Shepparton, Victoria 3630.
☎ 58 299218
🕐 Monthly meetings

▽▽ **The Seahorse Society—Victoria**
P. O. Box 2337V, Melbourne, Victoria 3001.
🕐 Meets 2nd. Sat of month
Publishes Seahorse Victoria.

Organizations: Sexuality: Student

⚧▽ **Melbourne University Gay Society**
P. O. Box 54, Melbourne Union, Parkville, Victoria 3052.
🕐 Wed 13:00 - 14:00

⚧▽ **Monash University Gay Collective**
☎ 39 565 4195

Organizations: Sexuality: Youth

⚧▽ **Young & Gay**
☎ 39 865 6700
Support for youth under 26. A project of the Victorian AIDS Council.

Publishers: Newspapers: Sexuality

⚧▼ **Brother Sister**
57 Bevan Street, Albert Park, Victoria 3206.
☎ 39 690 9733 ✆ 39 696 7321
🕐 10:00 - 17:30
Free. Published every month.

Radio: Sexuality

⚧▽ **Joy Melbourne**
FM 90.7, P. O. Box 907, South Melbourne, Victoria 3205.
☎ 39 690 0907
🕐 Sat 00:00 - 24:00

Stores: Books: General

⚧▼ **Hares & Hyenas**
360 Brunswick Street, Fitzroy, Victoria 3065.
☎ 3 9419 4445

⚧▼ **Hares & Hyenas**
135 Commercial Road, Prahran, Victoria 3181.
☎ 3 9824 2839

☺ ▪ **Hartwigs Bookshop**
245 Brunswick Street, Fitzroy, Victoria 3065.
☎ 39 417 7147

Stores: Clothing: Fetish

☺ ▪ **Lucrezia & De Sade**
441 Brunswick Street, Fitzroy, Victoria 3065.
☎ 3 9416 3826 ✆ 3 9416 0947
✉ lucrezia@ozemail.com.au
🌐 http://www.ozemail.com.au/~lucrezia
Fetish clothing store with BDSM items.

Stores: Clothing: Rubber

☺ ▪ **Studio Strak**
P. O. Box 4838, GPO, Melbourne, Victoria 3001.
☎ 3 809 2632
Catalogue, £2 or AUS$5.

Stores: Erotica: BDSM

☺ ▪ **Hellfire Emporium**
305 Swanson Street, Melbourne, Victoria 3000.
☎ 39 639 4755 ✆ 39 639 4755

☺ ▪ **Laurie Lane's Leather World**
157a Commercial Road, South Yarra, Victoria.
☎ 3 9827 9974 ✆ 3 9885 5783
Leather clothing, toys, corsets, & accessories. Also custom work.

Stores: Erotica: General

⚧▼ **The Beat**
157 Commercial Road, Prahran, Victoria 3181.
☎ 39 827 8748
🕐 Mon - Wed 09:00 - 19:00, Thu Fri 09:00 - 21:00, Sun 14:00 -
20:00

♂ ▪ **City East Adult Bookstore**
147-149 Russell Street, Melbourne, Victoria 3000.
☎ 39 650 4763
🕐 07:00 - 21:00

⌕▼ **Gemini**
164 Acland Street, Saint Kilda, Victoria 3182.
☎ 39 534 6074
⏰ 10:00 - 03:00

⌕▼ **Gemini**
235a Smith Street, Fitzroy, Victoria 3065.
☎ 39 419 6270
⏰ 10:00 - 24:00, not Sun
Adult book shop with leather toys, sex aids, etc..

☺ ■ **Kill City**
126 Greville Street, Prahran, Victoria.

☺ ■ **Polyester Books**
P. O. Box 73, Fitzroy, Victoria 3065.
☎ 3 9419 5223 📱 3 9419 5451
✉ fools@polyester.com.au
🌐 http://www.polyester.com.au

Stores: Leatherwork Supplies: General
☺ ■ **Leffler's**
66 York Street, South Melbourne, Victoria 3205.
☎ 3 9690 3577
Not part of the scene or scene friendly, but they can supply items from whole hides to findings.

Northcote
Organizations: Sexuality
✉▽ **Boys Will Be Boys**
P. O. Box 328, Northcote, Victoria 3070.

Piercers
☺ ■ **Nomad**
95 High Street, Northcote, Victoria 3070.

WESTERN AUSTRALIA
Population: Approximately 1,420,000
Capital City: Perth
Time zone: GMT plus 8 hours
Age of consent & homosexuality legislation: Age of consent for heterosexual activity is 18, 21 for male homosexual activity. No sodomy legislation. Homosexual acts were decriminalized in 1990. It is still an offence to "promote & encourage" homosexual behaviour
Legal drinking age: 18

State Resources
Publishers: Newspapers: Sexuality
⌕▼ **WSO - Westside Observer**
Westside Publishing, P. O. Box 131, North Perth, Western Australia 6006.
☎ 9 242 2146 📱 9 242 2209
☎ 9 242 2210
⏰ 09:00 - 17:00
♠ ✓ $ [VISA] 💳
Publisher of the Western Australian gay & lesbian newspaper. News (local, national, international), features (health, lifestyle, etc.), entertainment, social, & classifieds. Published 25 times a year. Yearly subscription is $40AUS.

Stores: Books: General
⌕▼ **Arcane Bookshop**
212 William Street, North Bridge, Western Australia 6000.
☎ 9 328 5073 📱 9 228 0410
⏰ Mon - Fri 10:00 - 17:30, Sat 10:00 - 16:00, Sun 12:00 - 16:00
Specialises in gay / lesbian fiction / non-fiction, literature (fiction), art, literary studies, communications studies, womens' studies, history, philosophy, science, film, etc..

Bentley
Organizations: Sexuality: Student
⌕▽ **Curtin Stonewall Club**
Student Guild, Curtin University of Technology, Kent Street, Bentley, Western Australia 6102.
☎ 9 351 2907

Cloverdale
Organizations: Family
☺ ☐ **Parents & Friends of Lesbians & Gays (PFLAG)—Cloverdale**
P. O. Box 72, Cloverdale, Western Australia 6105.
Support for parents & friends of lesbians & gays.

Doublview
Organizations: Sexuality
✉▽ **WATS Support, Unity, & Pride (WATSUP)**
P. O. Box 771, Doublview, Western Australia 6018.

Gosnells
Organizations: Sexuality
✉▽ **The Gender Council of Australia (W. A.), Inc.**
P. O. Box 573, Gosnells, Western Australia 6110.
☎ 9 362 5447
✉ laura@cougar.multiline.com.au

Morley
Organizations: Polyfidelity
☺ ■ **Beyond Monogamy, Inc.**
P. O. Box 907, Morley, Western Australia 6062.

Murdoch
Organizations: Sexuality: Student
⌕▽ **Murdoch University Gay & Lesbian Society (MUGALS)**
Student Guild, Murdoch University, South Street, Murdoch, Western Australia 6105.
☎ 9 332 6335

Northbridge
Organizations: Sexuality: Student
⌕▽ **Stonewall Union of Students**
P. O. Box 158, Northbridge, Western Australia 6000.
Student support group.

Perth
Health Services
☺ ☐ **Mount Lawley Medical Centre**
689 Beaufort Street, Mount Lawley, Western Australia 6050.
☎ 9 227 2455
⏰ 09:00 - 18:00

☺ ☐ **Murray Street STD Clinic**
70 Murray Street, Perth, Western Australia 6000.
☎ 9 270 1122

Helplines: AIDS
☺ ■ **Western Australian AIDS Council**
107 Brisbane Street, Perth, Western Australia 6000.
☎ 9 227 8619
⏰ Mon - Fri 09:00 - 22:00

Helplines: Sexuality
⌕▽ **Gay & Lesbian Counselling Service**
P. O. Box 406, Perth, Western Australia 6000.
☎ 9 328 9044
⏰ Mon - Fri 10:00 - 16:00, 19:30 - 22:30, Sat Sun 14:00 - 17:00
Information & counselling.

⌕▽ **Gayline**
P. O. Box 406, Perth, Western Australia 6001.
☎ 9 328 9044
⏰ Mon - Fri 10:00 - 16:00, Mon - Sun 19:00 - 22:30, Sun 14:00 - 17:00
Information & counselling.

Organizations: AIDS: Education
☺ ☐ **Western Australian AIDS Council**
P. O. Box 1510, West Perth, Western Australia 6872.
☎ 9 429 9900 📱 9 429 9901
☎ 9 429 9933 (AIDS Youthline)
⏰ Mon - Fri 09:00 - 22:00

Organizations: AIDS: Support
☺ ☐ **People Living with AIDS**
P. O. Box 8440, Stirling Street, Perth, Western Australia 6849.
☎ 9 221 3002 📱 9 221 3035

Organizations: Bears
⌕▽ **West Oz Marsupial Bears And Their Supporters (Wombats)**
P. O. Box 242, Bassendean, Western Australia 6054.
☎ 9 279 7949 📱 9 446 5092
✉ rindos@perth.dialix.com.au
🌐 http://www.skepsis.com/.gblo/bears/CLUBS/wombats.html
Contact: Mr. Dave Rindos

Organizations: Sexuality: Student

Wilde Alliance
Box 28, Guild of Undergraduates, Stirling Highway, Nedlands, Western Australia 6009.
Support group.

Organizations: Sexuality: Youth

Breakaway - Gay Youth Group
P. O. Box 406, Perth, Western Australia 6001.
☎ 9 328 9044 ☏ 9 328 1345
Mon - Fri 10:00 - 16:00, Mon - Sun 19:00 - 22:30, Sun 14:00 - 17:00
Coming out support group for men up to 26. Fortnightly meetings for activities, guest speakers, education, friendship, & social support.

Publishers: Newspapers: Sexuality

Grapevine
P. O. Box K788, Perth, Western Australia 6001.

Radio: Sexuality

Ethos
6RTR FM 92.1, P. O. Box 949, Nedlands, Western Australia 6009.
Thu 24:00

Stores: Books: General

Hyde Park News
322 Bulwer Street, North Perth, Western Australia 6006.
☎ 9 328 5265

Stores: Erotica: General

Club X Shop 25
Dogswamp Shopping Centre, Yokina, Western Australia 6000.
☎ 9 444 5572

Vibration
354A Charles Street, North Perth, Western Australia 6000.
☎ 9 242 4501

Victoria Park

Organizations: Sexuality

Chamleon Society
P. O. Box 367, Victoria Park, Western Australia 6163.
☎ 15 771753
Call 20:00 - 22:00. Meets 1st. & 3rd. Thu of month 20:30 - 23:00

Austria

Area: Approximately 83,851 square kilometres
Population: Approximately 7, 510,000
Capital City: Wien (Vienna)
Currency: Schilling (Sch.)
Official Language: German
Major Religions: 81% Roman Catholic
National Holiday: 2nd. Republic Day, 27th. April
Time zone: GMT plus 1 hour.
Country Initials: A
Electricity: 220 volts
Country Dialing Code (from elsewhere): 43
Intl. Dialing Prefix (out of the country): 00
Long Distance Dialing Prefix (inside country): 0
Climate: Hot summers & cold winters.
Age of consent & homosexuality legislation: Age of consent for heterosexual activity is 14, 18 for male homosexual activity, & 14 for lesbian activity. Homosexual acts were decriminalized in 1971. Homosexual prostitution has been on the same legal basis as heterosexual prostitution since 1979. There are still sections of the penal code that discriminate against homosexual people: one cannot "advocate or approve of homosexuality (both male & female) or bestiality;" one cannot be a member of an organization the "favours homosexual lewdness." Some refugees have been granted asylum on grounds of their sexual orientation, however.

NATIONAL RESOURCES

Organizations: AIDS: Education

AIDS-Informationszentrale Austria
Lenaugasse 17, 1080 Wien.
☎ 222 402 2353
Mon - Fri 10:00 - 16:00
Central information office for Austrian AIDS organizations.

Bregenz

Organizations: AIDS: Support

AIDS-Hilfe—Voralberg
Neugasse 5, 6900 Bregenz.
☎ 5574 465 26
Tue Thu 16:00 - 19:00, Wed Fri 10:00 - 13:00. HIV testing Tue Thu 17:00 - 19:00

Dornberg

Organizations: Sexuality

Homosexuelle Initiative (HOSI)—Voralberg
Postfach 841, 6854 Dornberg.
☎ 557 436 8675

Dornbirn

Helplines: Sexuality

Rosa Telefon—Dornbirn
☎ 557 436 8675
Thu 18:00 - 20:00

Graz

Organizations: AIDS: Support

AIDS-Hilfe—Graz
Schmiedgasse 38, 8010 Graz.
☎ 316 81 5050
Mon - Wed 11:00 - 13:00, Tue Thu Fri 17:00 - 19:00

Organizations: Sexuality

Rosarote Panthe-Schwul-Lesbische Aktiongemeinschaft Steiermark
Postfach 34, 8010 Graz.
Meets Thu 19:00
Publishes *Rosa-Lila Buschtrommel.*

Innsbruck

Health Services

Landeskrankenhaus Innsbruck / Department of Dermatology & Venerology
Anichstraße 35, 6020 Innsbruck.
☎ 512 2 8711 Ext.: 448
Mon - Fri 09:00 - 11:00
STD testing.

Organizations: AIDS: Support

AIDS-Hilfe—Tirol
Ground Floor, Bruneckestraße 8, 6020 Innsbruck.
☎ 512 56 3621
Tue 16:00 -19:00, Wed Fri 12:00 - 15:00

Klagenfurt

Helplines: Sexuality

GayHotline
c/o ÖH Klagenfurt, Universitätstraße 65-67, 9020 Klagenfurt.
☎ 463 50 4690
Wed 18:00 - 20:00

Organizations: AIDS: Support

AIDS-Hilfe—Kärten
8.-Mai-Straße 19, 9020 Klagenfurt.
☎ 463 5 5128
Mon Tue Thu 17:00 - 19:00
HIV/AIDS counselling, information, & anonymous testing.

Linz

Organizations: AIDS: Support

AIDS-Hilfe—Oberösterreich
Langgasse 12, 4020 Linz.
Mon 15:00 - 18:00, Wed 17:0 - 20:00, Thu 10:00 - 13:00, Fri 14:00 -17:00
HIV/AIDS counselling, information, & anonymous testing.

Organizations: Sexuality

Lesbische & Schwule Aktiongemeinschaft
Postfach 160, 4010 Linz.
☎ 732 274 7382
Tue 19:00 - 21:00

Salzburg

Health Services

Landeskrankenhaus Salzburg, Dept. Dermatologie
Müllner Hauptstraße 48, 5020 Salzburg.
☎ 662 3 1581
Mon - Fri 08:00 - 19:00, Sat Sun 10:00 - 12:00
STD testing.

Helplines: Sexuality

Rosa Telefon—Salzburg
Müllner Hauptstraße 11, 5020 Salzburg.
☎ 662 43 5927
Fri 19:00 - 21:00

Organizations: AIDS: Support

AIDS-Hilfe—Salzburg
Saint-Julien-Straße 31, 5020 Salzburg.
☎ 662 88 1488
Mon Wed Thu 17:00 - 19:00
HIV/AIDS information & anonymous testing.

Organizations: Sexuality

Homosexuelle Initiative (HOSI)—Salzburg
Müllner Hauptstraße 11, 5020 Salzburg.
☎ 662 43 5927
Tue 20:00 - 22:00, Wed 18:00 - 24:00, Fri 21:00 - 24:00, Sat 20:00 - 01:00

Wien

Bars: BDSM

The Eagle
Blümelgasse 1, 1060 Wien.
☎ 1 587 2661
21:00 -04:00

Nightshift
Corneliusgasse 8, 1060 Wien.
☎ 1 586 2337
Sun - Fri 22:00 - 04:00, Sat 22:00 - 05:00
Entrance is not well marked.

Stiefelknecht
Wimmergasse 20, 1050 Wien.
☎ 1 545 2301
22:00 - 02:00, Fri Sat - 04:00
Enter from Stolberggasse.

Health Services

Allgemeines Krankenhaus
Alerstraße 4, 1060 Wien.
☎ 1 438 9510
STD testing & information.

Helplines: Sexuality

Rosa Telefon—Wien
☎ 1 26 6604
Fri 18:00 - 20:00

Organizations: AIDS: Education

Safe Way / Verien für Prävention für Schwule und Bisexuelle Männer
Linke Wienzeile 102, 1060 Wien.
Information about HIV/AIDS for gay & bisexual men.

Organizations: AIDS: Support

AIDS-Hilfe—Wien
Wickenburggasse 14, 1080 Wien.
☎ 1 408 6186
Tue 16:00 - 19:30, Thu 10:00 - 13:30, Fri 14:00 - 17:30

Organizations: Motorcycle

CFLM Austria
Khunngaße 18-26, 1030 Wien.
☎ 1 786 0835

LMC Vienna
Waaggaße 5-16, 1040 Wien.
☎ 1 798 5484 Fax 1 587 3630
Contact: Herr Sepp Engelmaier

Organizations: Sexuality

Homosexuelle Initiative (HOSI)—Wien
Novaragasse 40, 1020 Wien.
☎ 1 216 6604
Tue 20:00 - ?

TVS Verein Transvestitin & Arbeitsgruppe TS
Postfach 331, 1171 Wien.
Meets 1st. Mon & 3rd. Wed of month

Photographers: Erotic

Harald Jahn
Viennaslide, Seisgasse 2, 1040 Wien.
☎ 1 505 5490 Fax 1 505 5491

Helmut Wolech
Voltag 55 63/1/4/14, 1210 Wien.
☎ 222 30 6988

Piercers

Freizeitverein Priapos
Lehrbachgasse 4/1, 1120 Wien.
☎ 1 812 4716
Also make custom gold & platinum jewelry. Age statement of 18 is required.

Publishers: Magazines: Sexuality

Lambda-Nachrichten
Homosexuelle Initiative, Novaragasse 40, 1020 Wien.
Austria's oldest newsmagazine for gays & lesbians. Published quarterly.

Xtra!
Postfach 77, 1043 Wien.
Articles, local calendar, & listings. Free at gay & lesbian locations. Published every two weeks.

Radio: Sexuality

Radio Filzlaus
Wiener Warmenradio FM 107.3, 1A, Rembrandtstraße 32, 1020 Wien.
☎ 1 332 1096 Fax 1 332 1097
Wed Sun 18:00

Stores: Clothing: Fetish

Bizarr-Mode
Schopenhauer Straße 8, 1180 Wien.

Stores: Erotica: BDSM

Tailors Unlimited
Graf Starhemberg Gasse 9, 1040 Wien.
☎ 1 505 4941 Fax 1 505 4945
By appointment only
Made to measure leather.

Tiberius ASC
Arbeitgasse 10, 1050 Wien.
☎ 1 55 8319 Fax 1 587 2353
By appointment only
Custom leather clothing & toys.

Belgium

Area: Approximately 83,850 square kilometres
Population: Approximately 10,500,000.
Capital City: Bruxelles / Brussel / Brussels
Currency: Belgian Franc (FB)
Official Language: French / Flemish / German
Major Religions: 84% Roman Catholic.
National Holiday: Independence Day, 21st. July
Time Zone: GMT plus 1 hour.
Country Initials: B
Electricity: 220 volts
Country Dialing Code (from elsewhere): 32
Intl. Dialing Prefix (out of the country): 00
Long Distance Dialing Prefix (inside country): 0
Climate: Sea climate with warm-cool summers & mild winters.
Age of consent & homosexuality legislation: Age of consent for heterosexual activity is 16. Homosexual acts were decriminalized in 1985.
Legal drinking age: 18

NATIONAL RESOURCES

Helplines: AIDS

AIDS Telephone
Postbus 169, 2060 Antwerpen.
☎ 7 815 1515
☎ 3 236 6969

Helplines: Sexuality

Gay Info Line
☎ 9 223 9399 Fax 9 223 5821
☎ 9 223 5821
Main number 09:00 - 17:00, second number 16:00 - 24:00

Organizations: AIDS: Support

Het AIDS Team
Brugstraat 16, 2060 Antwerpen.
☎ 3 226 6969

De Witte Raven
Schifwerperstraat 145, 2020 Antwerpen.
☎ 3 828 6900
Mon - Fri 09:00 - 12:00 13:00 - 17:00
Support for people infected with HIV.

Organizations: Sexuality

English-Speaking Gay Group (EGG)
Boîte Postale 198, 1060 Bruxelles.
Meets once a month Sun 15:00 - 17:00
Very relaxed, casual atmosphere; no music or dancing. Alternative to bars & discos. Newsletter only for members. Publishes *The Group* every month. Age statement of 18 is required.

Organizations: Spanking

Spankclub
c/o Duquesnoy, Duquesnoystraat 12, 1000 Bruxelles.
2 523 6878 — 2 502 3883
Meets 3rd. Sun of month 15:00 - 16:00
Private spanking club with daily & yearly memberships.

Photographers: Fetish

Heïdi Kâa
c/o Secret Magazine, Boîte Postale 1400, 1000 Bruxelles 1.
2 223 0914 — 2 223 1009
Specialises in fetish & theatre pictures, virtual reality, & CD-ROM interactive programming. English also spoken.

Publishers: Magazines: BDSM

Secret Magazine
Boîte Postale 1400, 1000 Bruxelles 1.
2 223 0914 — 2 223 1009
Started in 1992, now circulation of 13,000 in 15 different countries. Entirely by fetish-minded people. Over 108 glossy pages, with very good articles & pictures. Probably one of the best European fetish/SM magazines in the world. (We are also very modest...) Catalogue $17.50U.S.. Published quarterly. Yearly subscription is $70. Age statement of 18 is required. English also spoken.

Publishers: Magazines: Sexuality

Amigo/CPC
Lambermontlaan 102, 1030 Bruxelles.
2 242 6740

Homo- und Lesbiennejongerenkrant
Lange Leemstraat 337, 2018 Antwerpen.
3 230 3764

Regard
Infor Homo, Boîte Postale 215, 1040 Bruxelles 4.
2 733 1024 — 2 733 1336
2 735 1599
✓ $
Principally for the francophone gay & lesbian community. Others welcome. Published every two months. Yearly subscription is 850FB. French, Dutch, English, & German also spoken.

Tels Quels
Rue du Marché au Charbon 81, 1000 Bruxelles.
Articles & listings. Published every month.

Zizo
Zizo, Vlanderenstraat 22, 9000 Gent.
9 223 6929
09:00 -17:00
✓
Covering news - local & international - culture, literature, fiction, lesbigay movement. Published every two months. Yearly subscription is 950FB. Dutch, French, & English also spoken.

Publishers: Newspapers: Sexuality

Uitkomst
Gesprecks- en Onthaalcentrum u. z. w., Dambruggestraat 204, 2060 Antwerpen.
3 233 1071 — 3 234 3339
14:00 - 24:00
✓
National gay rights organization with several subdivisions (youth, married, seniors, etc.). Several locations in Belgium. Published 10 times a year. Yearly subscription is $30, plus postage. French & English also spoken.

Aalst / Alost

Helplines: Sexuality

HAK - Advies Kontakt Centrum 't Koerken
St. Martinsplein 2, 9300 Aalst.
5 378 4279
10:30 - 13:30, 15:30 - 24:00

Stores: Erotica: General

Libidos-Erotheek
Gentsestraat 73, Aalst.
5 370 6428
12:00 - 22:00

Antwerpen / Anvers

Bars: BDSM

The Boots
Van Aerdtstraat 22, 2060 Antewerpen.
3 233 2136
3 233 2376
Fri Sat 22:00 - 05:00

Hanky Code
V. D. Wervestraat 69, 2060 Antwerpen.
3 226 8172 — 3 239 3025
19:00 - 02:00, Sat Sun 15:00 - ?
Small, intimate, & pleasant bar where "leatherboys" are free to do what they please. Already known for its warm welcome. English, Dutch, French, Spanish, & Italian also spoken.

Health Services

Konsultatieburo voor Relaties en Seksualiteit (DOK)
Osystraat 39, 2060 Antwerpen.
3 234 0848
Mon - Fri 09:00 12:30 13:30 - 17:00, Tue Thu also 19:00 - 21:30

Radio: Sexuality

Chocopot
Radio Centraal FM 101.6, Postbus 554, 2000 Antwerpen.
3 236 5076
Tue 21:00 - 22:00

Stores: Erotica: BDSM

Walhalla
St. Paulusstraat 21, 2000 Antwerpen.
3 233 6291

The Warehouse
c/o Boots, Van Aerdtstraat 22, 2060 Antwerpen.
3 225 2376
Fri Sat 22:30 - 05:00
Shop is inside Boots.

Stores: Erotica: General

Libidos-Erotheek
Carnotstraat 35, Antwerpen.
3 226 0245
12:00 - 22:00

Libidos-Erotheek
Gemeentestraat 11, Antwerpen.
3 233 1001
12:00 - 22:00

Bruxelles / Brussel

Bars: BDSM

Le Big Noise
44 Rue du Marché au Charbon, 1000 Bruxelles.
2 512 2525
Mon - Fri 18:00 - ?, Sat Sun 17:00 - ?

Moda Moda
343 Chaussée de Waterloo, 1060 Bruxelles.
2 537 6919

Le Sept
7 Rue Platesteen, 1000 Bruxelles.
2 513 1414
Fri - Wed 20:00 - 05:00

Le Why Not
7 Rue des Riches Claires, 1000 Bruxelles.
2 512 7587
22:00 - 06:00

Health Services

Asbl Aide Cliniques Universitaires Saint Luc
1200 Woluwe Saint Lambert, 1000 Bruxelles.
2 764 1582

Free Clinic
154a Chaussée de Wavre, 1050 Bruxelles.

Helplines: Sexuality

Infor Homo

Boîte Postale 215, 1040 Bruxelles 4.
☎ 2 733 1024 — Fax 2 733 1336
☎ 2 735 1599
100626.2434@compuserve.com
Mon Tue 18:00 - 20:00, Wed 19:00 - 23:00

Tels Quels Meeting Point
81 Rue du Marché au Charbon, 1000 Bruxelles.
☎ 2 512 4587
17:00 - 02:00, library/bookshop Mon Tue 17:00 - 19:00
Support, information, library, & bookshop.

Organizations: AIDS: Education

Association pour la Lutte Contre le SIDA
322 Rue Haut, 10000 Bruxelles.
☎ 2 538 9192
Mon - Fri 08:30 - 12:30 14:00 - 17:00

Groupe de Santé d'Antenne Rose
Boîte Postale 88, 1000 Bruxelles 1.

Organizations: AIDS: Support

Aide Info SIDA
45 Rue Duquesnoy, 1000 Bruxelles.
☎ 2 511 4529
☎ 2 514 2965
Mon - Fri 09:00 - 20:00, recording at other times

Centre Elisa Centrum
Oude Graanmarktstraat 48, 1000 Bruxelles.
☎ 2 513 2651
Mon Thu 17:00 - 21:00, Tue Wed Fri 10:00 - 14:00
De Médecins Sans Frontiers / van Artsen zonder grenzen.

The Foundation
49-51 Diksmuidelaan, 1000 Bruxelles.
☎ 2 219 3351
Mon - Thu 10:00 - 13:00 14:00 - 18:00, Fri 10:00 - 13:00 14:00 - 17:00
Counselling, information, & HIV testing.

Service aux Séro-Positifs
☎ 2 219 6795

Organizations: Fetish: Clothing

Nuit du Desir
Boîte Postale 443, 1000 Bruxelles.
Please write for more information.

Organizations: Motorcycle

MSC Belgium
Box 699, 1000 Bruxelles.
☎ 2 479 9692
Meets 1st. Fri of month

Organizations: Sexuality

De Andere Kant
Boîte Postale 389, 1000 Bruxelles 1.

Infor Homo
Boîte Postale 215, 1040 Bruxelles 4.
☎ 2 733 1024 — Fax 2 733 1336
☎ 2 735 1599
100626.2434@compuserve.com
Mon Tue 18:00 - 20:00, Wed 19:00 - 23:00

Organizations: Sexuality: Student

Cercle Homosexuel Etudiant de l'ULB (CHE)
38 Avenue Jeanne, 1050 Bruxelles.
☎ 2 650 2540
Thu 19:30 - ?

Photographers: Erotic

Jean-François Soyez
84 Avenue Panthéon, 1080 Bruxelles.
Fetish & gothic pictures.

Dany Willems
Adolph Max Laan 116, 1000 Bruxelles.
☎ 2 218 5126

Photographers: Fetish

L. Boeki
c/o Secret, Boîte Postale 1400, 1000 Bruxelles 1.
Specializes in fetish portraits.

Publishers: Books: BDSM

Editions Jaybird
Rue Scailquin 31, 1030 Bruxelles.
☎ 2 219 8007

Publishers: Magazines: BDSM

Contact S. M.
Chaud Business SPRL, 7 Rue de L'Eglise, 1060 Bruxelles.
☎ 2 537 8404 — Fax 2 537 5669
Published every two months. Yearly subscription is $40.

Rendez-Vous
Chaud Business SPRL, 7 Rue de L'Eglise, 1060 Bruxelles.
☎ 2 537 8404 — Fax 2 537 5669
Published every two months. Yearly subscription is $60.

Radio: Sexuality

Antenne Rose
Air Libre FM 107.6, Rue du Marché au Charbon 81, 1000 Bruxelles.
☎ 2 512 4587
Wed 20:00 23:00

Stores: Books: BDSM

Editions Jaybird
Rue Scailquin 31, 1030 Bruxelles.
☎ 2 219 8007
Specialises in rare BDSM & fetish photographs & drawings.

Stores: Books: General

Darakan
9 Rue du Midi, 1000 Bruxelles.
☎ 2 512 2076

Euro X
Boulevard Adolph Max 60, 1000 Bruxelles.

JP L'Agora
Rue de la Madelaine 21, 1000 Bruxelles.
☎ 2 511 1220 — Fax 2 511 1220
08:00 - 20:00, Sun 09:30 - 20:00

Librairie du Bon Secours
100A Rue du Marché au Charbon, 1000 Bruxelles.
☎ 2 512 2303
Mon - Fri 07:30 - 18:00

Lidéfix
Place de la Patrie, 1030 Bruxelles.
☎ 2 241 1804
Thu - Tue 17:00 - 03:00

Pepperland
47 Rue Namur, 1000 Bruxelles.
☎ 2 513 5751

Stores: Clothing: Fetish

Boutique Minuit
60 Galerie du Centre, 1000 Bruxelles 1.
☎ 2 223 0914 — Fax 2 223 1009
Mon - Sat 10:30 - 18:30
Probably the best & biggest fetish/SM store in Europe, with over 4,000 different styles & 20 different catalogues available. Leather, lingerie, rubber, high heels, TV/TS wear, & steelwear. In existence for 15 years, & has a very good reputation. Catalogue available. Age statement of 18 is required. English & Dutch also spoken.

Les Folies de Sade
Galerie Piccadilly 28b, Rue Fossé-aux-Loups, 1000 Bruxelles.
☎ 2 219 7997
Mon - Sat 10:00 - 18:00

Gwendoline
5 Passage Saint Honoré, Rue des Fripiers, 1000 Bruxelles.
☎ 2 523 3589

Stores: Clothing: Leather

Man To Man
9 Rue des Riches Claires, 1000 Bruxelles.
Imports items from RoB of Amsterdam.

Stores: Erotica: General

Hair Club
22 Boulevard Lemonnier, 1000 Bruxelles.
Costumes, wigs, high-heels for stage performances.

Stores: Safer Sex Products

Condomi
3 Rue Borgval, 1000 Bruxelles.

Training: Æsthetics

La Loge de Thalie
☎ 2 734 5705
Aesthetics for transvestites.

Charleroi
Organizations: AIDS: Education

Belgium

Charleroi
Organizations: AIDS: Education
☺ ☐ **SIDA MST Info**
Boîte Postale 1514, 6000 Charleroi.
☎ 7 156 0580 ✆ 7 151 8401
🕐 Mon - Fri 08:00 - 16:00

Publishers: Magazines: Fetish
☺ **The Delice Garden**
c/o Thierry Tillier, Boîte Postale 336, 6000 Charleroi.

Stores: Books: General
☺ ■ **Du Beffroi**
32 Rue du Beffroi, 6000 Charleroi.
☺ ■ **Nouvelle**
4-6 Passage de la Bourse, 6000 Charleroi.
☎ 7 131 8133

Deurne
Organizations: Sexuality
⚥▽ **Franjeppot**
Postbus 53, 2100 Deurne 1.

Gent / Gand
Bars: Sexuality
⚤▼ **Gold Club**
Rodelijvekenstraat 17, 9000 Gent.
☎ 9 225 0353
🕐 Thu - Tue 21:00 - ?

Organizations: AIDS: Support
☺ ☐ **De Witte Raven**
Elcker-Ik Gewad 13, 9000 Gent 12.
☎ 9 220 4197
🕐 Fri 20:00

Organizations: Sexuality
⚥▽ **Homo- en Lesbiennegroep Gehoor**
St. Niklaasstraat 7, 9000 Gent.
☎ 9 225 7599
🕐 Café 2nd. & 4th. Sat of month 21:00
♨ ✓ ℓ
Social gay & lesbian group. Cultural activities, sportsclub, badminton.
Dutch also spoken.

Organizations: Sexuality: Youth
⚥▽ **Verkeerd Geparkeerd Homojongeren**
Postbus 535, 9000 Gent 1.

Stores: Books: General
☺ ■ **Argos**
Kortrijksesteenweg 424, 9000 Gent.
☎ 9 222 5404
🕐 Mon - Sat 07:30 - 12:30 12:00 - 18:30
☺ ■ **De Brug**
Phœnixstraat 1, 9000 Gent.
☎ 9 226 3869
🕐 06:30 - 22:00, Sun 09:00 - 21:00

Stores: Erotica: General
☺ ■ **Libidos-Erotheek**
Kuiperstraat 4, Gent.
☎ 9 223 9388
🕐 12:00 - 22:00
♨ 💳 💳
Flemish also spoken.

Hainault
Helplines: Sexuality
⚥▽ **ASBL Gai Info**
☎ 6 828 0552
🕐 Tue - Sat 11:00 - 20:00

Herentals
Stores: Clothing: Leather
☺ ■ **Philippe Moda Pelle**
Bovenrij 25, 2200 Herentals.
☎ 1 421 9103 ✆ 1 422 3581
🕐 Mon - Fri 10:00 - 17:00

Kortrijk / Courtrai
Organizations: Sexuality
⚥▽ **Genderstichting (Belgian Gender Foundation)**
Pluimstraat 48, 8500 Kortrijk.
☎ 56 21 9541
🕐 Call Mon - Fri 09:00 - 11:30, 13:00 - 16:30, Mon Wed - 20:00
⚥■ **Leschemins de Trans**
c/o Belgische Gender Stichting, Plumstraat 48, 85000 Kortrijk B.

Stores: Erotica: General
☺ ■ **Libidos-Erotheek**
Zwevegemsestraat 28, 8500 Kortrijk.
☎ 5 625 7601
🕐 12:00 - 22:00
♨ 💳 💳
Flemish also spoken.

Leuven / Louvain
Helplines: Sexuality
⚥▽ **De Rose Drempel**
Maria Theresiastraat 114, 3000 Leuven.
☎ 1 620 0606

Organizations: AIDS: Support
☺ ☐ **De Witte Raven**
St. Michielcentrum, Naamsestraat 57a, 3000 Leuven.
☎ 1 620 0906
🕐 Fri 20:00

Liège / Luik / Luttich
Bars: BDSM
⚥▼ **Spartacus**
22 Rue Saint Jean-en-Ile, 4000 Liège.
☎ 4 123 1259
🕐 22:00 - 06:00
Some leather/fetish.

Organizations: Family
⚥▽ **Parents d'Enfants Homosexuels**
30 Monfort, 4050 Esneux.
☎ 4 180 3491

Organizations: Sexuality
⚥▽ **Association Gais & Lesbiennes à Liège**
Boîte Postale 15, 4000 Liège 1.
☎ 4 135 0968

Photographers: Erotic
☺ **Guy Lemaire**
Boîte Postale 441, 4020 Liège.

Stores: Books: General
☺ ■ **Hors Château**
33 Rue Château, 4000 Liège.
☎ 4 123 5588

Stores: Clothing: Fetish
☺ ▼ **Les Larmes D'Hollywood**
Galerie Cathédrale 82, 4000 Liège.
☎ 4 122 0472
🕐 Tue - Sat 11:00 - 18:00
Also clothing for transvestites.

Lovendegem
Organizations: Sexual Politics
☺ ☐ **V. V. S. M.**
Azaleastraat 58, 9920 Lovendegem.
Campaigns for legal acceptance of BDSM in Belgium. Send 3 IRCs for information.

Mechelen / Malines
Organizations: Sexuality
⚥▽ **Homo- Lesbiennewerking—Mechelen**
Hanswijkstraat 74, 2800 Mechelen.
☎ 1 543 2120
🕐 Fri 20:00 - 01:00

Stores: Erotica: General
☺ ■ **Libidos-Erotheek**
Nekkerspoelstraat 26, Mechelen.
☎ 1 555 6845
🕐 12:00 - 22:00

⚜ 💳 🅮,

Namur / Namen
Organizations: AIDS: Support
☺ ☐ **Entraide SIDA**
3bis Château des Balances, 5000 Namur.
☎ 8 122 2422

Organizations: Fetish: Clothing
☺ **Fantasmatic & Fetish Club**
Boîte Postale 184, 5000 Namur 1.
Contact: M. Jacques L.

Photographers: Erotic
☺ **Jacques Leurquin**
Boîte Postale 184, 5000 Namur 1.
☎ 81 22 7502
M. Leurquin's agent is Jürgen Boedt at Secret magazine.

Oostende / Ostende
Organizations: AIDS: Support
☺ ☐ **De Witte Raven**
Nieuwpoortsesteenweg 85, 8400 Oostende.
☎ 5 950 2882

Stores: Erotica: BDSM
☺ ■ **Walhalla**
Madridstraat, 8400 Oostende.

Stores: Erotica: General
⚥▼ **Paradise**
Madridstraat 15, 8400 Oostende.
☎ 5 951 3672
Leather, piercing jewelry, magazines, etc..

Schoten
Organizations: Fetish: Uniforms
⚥▽ **European Uniform Club**
Postbus 17, 2120 Schoten.

Sint Niklaas
Organizations: AIDS: Support
☺ ☐ **De Roze Waas**
Dalstraat 64, 9100 Sint Niklaas.
☎ 3 776 7270

Veerle-Laakdal
Organizations: Sexuality
⚥▽ **Homocentrum Laakdal en Omstreken**
Vortsebaan 38, 2431 Veerle-Laakdal.
☎ 1 484 0455
⊙ Fri 21:00 - 02:00, Sat Sun 21:00 - 24:00

Wilrijk
Organizations: BDSM
☺ **Club J & G**
Postbus 138, 2610 Wilrijk 1.
Private club in small farm with fully equipped playroom. Sponsorship may be required.

Wondelgem
Organizations: Sexuality
⚥▽ **Werkgroep Gehuwde Homo's Lesbiennes en Partners**
c/o Kalkoenlaan 3, 9032 Wondelgem.
☎ 9 153 8065

Brazil

Area: Approximately 8,510,000 square kilometres
Population: Approximately 146,000,000
Capital City: Brasilia
Currency: Cruzeiro (C)
Official Language: Portuguese
Major Religions: 89% Roman Catholic.
National Holiday: Independence Day, 7th. September
Time zone: GMT minus 3 hours
Country Initials: BR
Electricity: 220 volts
Country Dialing Code (from elsewhere): 55
Intl. Dialing Prefix (out of the country): 00

Long Distance Dialing Prefix (inside country): 0
Climate: Tropical weather in the north, sub-tropical in the south. Cooler temperatures at high altitudes. The east coast & the Amazon valley experience heavy rainfall, whereas the northeast of the country is much dryer, with regular periods of drought.
Age of consent & homosexuality legislation: There is no legislation against homosexuality. The age of consent for sexual activity is 18. There is a law that prevents discrimination on the basis of sexual orientation, but the police still use a law that allows them to "safeguard morality & public decency" to arrest homosexuals.

Rio de Janeiro
Helplines: AIDS
☺▽ **AIDS Hotline - AIDS Pela Vida**
☎ 21 221 2221
☎ 21 239 5171

Organizations: AIDS: Education
☺ ☐ **Associação Brasileira Interdisciplinar de AIDS**
Rua sete de Setembro 48/12, Rio de Janeiro.
☎ 21 224 1654 ☏ 21 224 3414
☎ 21 239 5171

Organizations: Sexuality
⚥▼ **Núdeo de Orientção em Saude Social (NOSS)**
☎ 21 262 6362
Publishes *Nós por Exemplo*.

São Paulo
Bars: Sexuality
⚲▼ **Bug House**
Rua Santa Antonio 1000, São Paulo.
☎ 11 257 3131
⊙ Thu - Sun 20:00 - 01:00

⚲▼ **Nostro Mondo**
Rua da Consolação 2554, São Paulo.
☎ 11 257 4481
⊙ Wed - Sat 23:00 - 04:00, Sun 19:00 - 01:00
Gay bar with many transvestites.

Health Services
☺ ☐ **Centro de Orientção e Aconselhamento em AIDS e Doeças Sexualmente Transmissiveis**
Galeria Prestes Maia, Terreo, São Paulo.
☎ 11 239 2224
⊙ Mon - Fri 08:00 - 14:00
Information about HIV/AIDS & free HIV testing.

☺ ☐ **Centro de Saude Santa Cecilia**
Rua Vitorino Camila 599, São Paulo.
☎ 11 826 7970
⊙ Mon - Fri 07:00 - 17:00
Free HIV tests & treatment.

☺ ☐ **Hospital das Clinicas da Faculdade de Medicina**
Liga de Combate a Sifilis e Outras Doenças Venereas, Rua Dr. Ovidio Pires de Campo, São Paulo.
☎ 11 282 2811
STD information & treatment.

☺ ☐ **Hospital Emilio Ribas**
165 Avenida Dr. Arnaldo, São Paulo.
☎ 11 881 2433
⊙ 24hrs.

☺ ☐ **Hospital São Paulo**
Rua Napoleão de Barras 715, São Paulo.
☎ 11 549 8777
☎ 11 544 0676

☺ ■ **Solidariedade, Apoio Moral e Psicologico Aplicados a AIDS (SAMPA)**
Rua Manuel de Paiva 218, São Paulo.
☎ 11 571 7396
Counselling by appointment only. Charges according to patient's means.

Organizations: AIDS: Education
☺ ☐ **AIDS Center of Reference**
122 Rua Antonio Carlos, São Paulo.
☎ 11 284 4206
☎ 11 284 9724
⊙ 07:00 - 21:00
Free HIV tests & treatment.

Organizations: AIDS: Support
☺▽ **Ambulatorio de Saude Mental SUD**
Rua Carlos Comenale 35, São Paulo.
☎ 11 283 0005
⊙ Mon Wed 09:00 - 11:30, Tue Thu 13:30 - 16:00

Organizations: AIDS: Support

Free counselling for people with AIDS.

☺ □ **Grupo de Apoio a Pacientes de AIDS (GAPA)**
Rua Barão de tatui 375, São Paulo.
Free counselling by appointment.

Bulgaria

Area: Approximately 110,900 square kilometres
Population: Approximately 9,000,000
Capital City: Sophia
Currency: Lev (BGL)
Official Language: Bulgarian
Major Religions: 88% Eastern Orthodox Christian
National Holiday: Liberation Day, 3rd. March.
Time zone: GMT plus 2-3 hours
Country Initials: BG
Electricity: 220 volts, 50Hz
Country Dialing Code (from elsewhere): 359
Intl. Dialing Prefix (out of the country): 00
Long Distance Dialing Prefix (inside country): 0
Climate: Continental climate, but milder on the coast of the Black Sea.
Age of consent & homosexuality legislation: Homosexual acts were decriminalized in 1968.

NATIONAL RESOURCES

Organizations: Sexuality

▽ **Bulgarian Lesbian & Gay Association (BULGA)**
P. O. Box 32, Sofia 1330.
☎ 2 58 5271 — Fax 44 3804
Please address envelopes to BULGA, do NOT address them to Bulgarian Lesbian & Gay Association.

Publishers: Magazines: Sexuality

▼ ***Flamingo***
Kiss Contact, P. O. Box 63, Sofia.
☎ 2 22 5607 — Fax 2 56 5856
🕘 09:00 - 17:00
Also helpline for gays, lesbians, & bisexuals. Published every month.

Byelorussia

Area: Approximately 208,000 square kilometres
Population: Approximately 10,270,000
Capital City: Minsk
Currency: Belarus Ruble (BRB)
Official Language: Byelorussian & Russian
Major Religions: Russian Orthodox
Country Initials: BEL
Country Dialing Code (from elsewhere): 810
Climate: Warm summers & cold winters.
Age of consent & homosexuality legislation: The legislation that barred homosexuality has been repealed. Society is still hostile toward homosexual activities.
Legal drinking age: 18

Minsk

Organizations: AIDS: Education

☺ □ **Stop AIDS Byelarus**
P. O. Box 398, Minsk 220090.

Canada

Area: Approximately 9,976,150 square kilometres
Population: Approximately 27,300,000
Capital City: Ottawa
Currency: Canadian Dollar ($Cdn.)
Official Language: English & French
Major Religions: 47% Roman Catholic, 41% Protestant
National Holiday: Canada Day, 1st. July
Time zone: GMT minus 5-8 hours
Country Initials: CDN
Electricity: 110 volts, 60Hz
Country Dialing Code (from elsewhere): 1
Intl. Dialing Prefix (out of the country): 011
Long Distance Dialing Prefix (inside country): 1
Climate: Dependent on province, but generally cold winters & hot summers. Coastal areas of British Columbia have mild winters & cool summers, due to the effects of the nearby Pacific ocean.
Age of consent & homosexuality legislation: Age of consent for sexual activity is 14. Homosexual acts were decriminalized in the 1960s. Anal intercourse has been legal for consenting adults of 18 years & older since 1988. A system of age and power between the partners has been adopted, also since 1988. In 1992, Canada abolished the restrictions of homosexuals in the military. Some refugees have been granted asylum on grounds of their sexual orientation. All provinces, except Alberta, Newfoundland, Prince Edward Island, and the Northwest Territories have passed legislation preventing discrimination based upon sexual orientation.
Legal drinking age: 18

NATIONAL RESOURCES

Archives: General

Canadian Women's Movement Archives
♿ Room 603, Marriset Library, 65 University, Ottawa, Ontario K1N 9A5.
☎ 613 562 5910
Material from contemporary Canadian Women's Movement (post-1960). Records from women's groups, events, periodicals, etc.. Substantial collection of lesbian material. French also spoken.

Mailorder: Books: General

☺ ■ **The Omega Centre Bookstore**
♿ 29 Yorkville Avenue, Toronto, Ontario M4W 1L1.
☎ 416 975 9086 — Fax 416 975 0731
✓ VISA MC

Mailorder: Books: Sexuality

▼ **Glad Day Books**
598A Yonge Street, Toronto, Ontario M4Y 1Z3.
☎ 416 961 4161 — Fax 416 961 1624
✓ $ VISA MC AMERICAN EXPRESS

▼ **Little Sister's Book & Art Emporium**
1221 Thurlow Street, Vancouver, British Columbia V6E 1X4.
☎ 800 567 1662 — Fax 604 685 0252
☎ 604 669 1753
🕘 10:00 - 23:00
VISA MC AMERICAN EXPRESS

Mailorder: Clothing: Fetish

☺ ▼ **B&B Leatherworks**
6802 Ogden Road South East, Calgary, Alberta T2C 1B4.
☎ 403 236 7072 — Fax 403 236 1304
http://www.cadvision.com/Home_Pages/accounts/bbent/
🕘 Tue - Fri 09:30 - 18:00, Sat 12:00 - 18:00
✓ $ VISA
Custom leather clothing, sub / dom equipment, latex wear, & made to order items. Virtually anything you can imagine in leather. Catalogue, $9.95.

☺ ■ **Classic Shoe Company**
P. O. Box 76081, Calgary, Alberta T2Y 2Z9.
☎ 403 938 6491 — Fax 403 938 6491
VISA AMERICAN EXPRESS
Catalogue, $7.

☺ ■ **Crossland Shoes**
P. O. Box 68147, Bonnie Doon Post Office #70, Edmonton, Alberta T6C 4N6.
☎ 403 448 0173 Ext.: 5665
🕘 Leave message on voice mail
Distributors of high-heel shoes & boots. Catalogue, $10.

☺ ■ **X-Treme Designs Ltd**
Box 34121, Suite 19, 1200 37th. Street South West, Calgary, Alberta T3C 3W0.
Catalogue, $15 for all 3 catalogues.

Mailorder: Clothing: Rubber

Dark Side Creations
4311 Dovercrest Drive South East, Calgary, Alberta T2B 1X6.
☎ 403 272 3134 — Fax 403 272 8781
darkside@canuck.com
http://www.canuck.com/Darkside/access.html
✓ $
North America's only manufacturer of moulded latex fashion wear.

☺ ■ **Rubbertree Rainwear**
P. O. Box 35135, Station E, Vancouver, British Columbia V6M 4G1.
☎ 604 885 1282
Rubber clothing & sheets. Catalogue available.

Mailorder: Erotica: Adult Baby

☺ ■ **Adult Baby World (ABW)**
Suite 697, 5468 Dundas Street West, Toronto, Ontario.

■ **Ashely's Boutique**
Suite 200, 2854 Dundas Street West, Toronto, Ontario M6P 1Y8.
☎ 416 767 3518
VISA MC
All items made to order. Also transvestite items. Also mail order. Catalogue, $10. Age statement of 19 is required.

■ **Babykins Products Ltd.**

8171 Seafair Drive, Richmond, British Columbia V7C 1X3.
☎ 604 275 2255 Ext.: 800 665 2229 ✆ 604 275 2255
♪♪ ■ **BBW**
Unit 11-239, 4040 Creditview Road, Mississauga, Ontario L5C 3Y8.
Catalogue available.
☺ ▼ **Cozy Time**
6802 Ogden Road South East, Calgary, Alberta T2C 1B4.
☎ 403 236 7072 ✆ 403 236 1304
🕐 Tue - Fri 09:30 - 18:00, Sat 12:00 - 18:00
🍴 ✓ $ 🌫 VISA
Custom manufacturer of adult baby wear. Several styles in stock, or made to order. Catalogue, $6.

Mailorder: Erotica: BDSM
⊘▼ **Aslan Leathers**
58, 363 Sorauren Avenue, Toronto, Ontario M6R 2G5.
☎ 416 538 9759
🕐 By appointment
🍴 $
Leather & rubber dildo harness, restraints, body harnesses, & custom orders. Made from heavy leather with women's bodies in mind. Catalogue published twice a year, $1U.S..
☺ ■ **Anne Esthesia**
P. O. Box 42014, Acadia Postal Outlet, Calgary, Alberta T2J 7A6.
✉ xpc@nucleus.com
🌐 http://www.nucleus.com/~xpc/xmag/fetfash.html
✓ $
Canadian cheques only, please.
☺ ■ **Northbound Leather Ltd.**
⚲ 7 Saint Nicholas Street, Toronto, Ontario M4Y 1W5.
☎ 416 972 1037 ✆ 416 975 1337
✉ leather@northbound.com
🌐 http://www.northbound.com/
🍴 ✓ 🌫 VISA MC 🌫 ♪
Canada's largest selection of fetish fashion & accessories, including corsetry, leather clothing, books, toys, & footwear. Also has large, inviting, & beautifully designed store. 116-page catalogue, $30Cdn. (taxes included). Shipping $5Cdn., to Cdn.$9.95Cdn. to U.S., $12.95Cdn. elswhere. Please see our display advertisements on the front & back covers.

Mailorder: Erotica
☺ ■ **Fantasyland Products**
P. O. Box 682, Owen Sound, Ontario N4K 5R4.
☎ 519 371 1215 ✆ 519 371 2975
🕐 10:00 - 17:30, Fri - 20:30, Sun by appointment
🍴 $ VISA MC 🌫
Corsetry, maids wear, sugar'n'spice creations (little girls wear), shoes, boots, wigs, silicone breasts, makeup, jewelry, & spanker, PVC, & Lycra clothing. 16 catalogues for $80; $25 sampler pack; New! Fantasy videos! Fashion $59.95, wedding $39.95, "Lil Girl Birthday" $29.95. For info only: SASE (or IRC) plus $1Cdn.. Catalogue, $5 for catalogue of catalogues. Age statement of 18 is required.

Mailorder: Erotica: General
⊘▼ **Caught In The Act**
P. O. Box 2512, Station D, Ottawa, Ontario K1P 5W6.
Catalogue available.
⊘▼ **Gayroute**
P. O. Box 1036, Station C, Montréal, Québec H2L 4V3.
Catalogue, $2U.S. cash or 3IRCs. Age statement of 21 is required. English, German, Spanish, & Italian also spoken.
⊘▼ **Priape**
1311 Sainte Catherine Est, Montréal, Québec H2L 2H4.
☎ 800 461 6969 ✆ 514 521 1309
☎ 514 521 8451
✉ ber_ber@cam.org
🍴 🌫 VISA MC 🌫
⊘▼ **Rubyfruit Erotica**
P. O. Box 386, Station P, Toronto, Ontario M5S 2S9.
☺ ■ **Séduction**
1315, Tellier, Laval, Québec H7C 2H1.
🍴 $
Also mail order. Catalogue, $5.

Mailorder: Erotica
☺ ■ **Groupe B. A. I., Inc.**
5169 Boulevard Métropolitain Est, Montréal, Québec H1R 1Z7.
☎ 514 852 2429 ✆ 514 852 3403
🕐 Mon - Fri 09:00 - 17:00
🍴 ✓ $ MC
Also showroom. C. O. D. available. Free catalogue. Age statement of 19 is required.

Mailorder: Erotica: Leather
⊘▼ **Mack's Leathers**
1043 Granville Street, Vancouver, British Columbia V6Z 1C4.
☎ 604 688 6225
🕐 Mon - Wed 11:00 - 19:00, Thu Fri 11:00 - 20:00, Sat 11:00 - 18:00, Sun 12:00 - 17:00
🍴 🌫 VISA MC
Catalogue is on video. Catalogue, $20.
☺ ■ **Sir Steve's Leather**
P. O. Box 1282, Guelph, Ontario N1H 6N6.

Mailorder: Erotica
⊘▽ **Malebox Warehouse**
⚲ P. O. Box 166, Station B, Ottawa, Ontario K1P 6C4.
☎ 613 237 7133 ✆ 613 237 6651
🕐 09:00 - 18:00
🍴 ✓ $ VISA MC
National mail order company offering discount prices on toys for bad boys: condoms, lubes, pumps, dildos, cock rings, etc.. Free catalogue. Age statement of 18 is required.

Mailorder: Erotica: Pony
☺ ■ **JG Leathers**
5325 10A Avenue, Delta, British Columbia.
✉ 75703.2412@compuserve.com
Boy/girl pony tack & dress, & other discipline & suspension harnesses. Also custom orders. Catalogue available.

Organizations: AIDS: Research
☺ ☐ **Canadian Foundation for AIDS Research (CANFAR)**
Suite 800, 165 University Avenue, Toronto, Ontario M5H 3B8.
☎ 416 361 6281 ✆ 416 361 5736
🕐 09:00 - 17:00, answering machine at other times
National charitable foundation to raise awarenes about & raise funds for all aspects of HIV & AIDS.

Organizations: AIDS: Support
☺ ☐ **Canadian AIDS Society / Société Canadienne du**
⚲ **SIDA**
Suite 400, 100 Sparks Street, Ottawa, Ontario K1P 5B7.
☎ 613 230 3580 ✆ 613 563 4998
🕐 08:30 - 17:30, answering machine at other times
National coalition of more than 100 community-based AIDS groups. Provides services to member groups & distributes publications.

Organizations: Health
☺ **Sex Information & Education Council (SIECCAN)**
850 Coxwell Avenue, East York, Ontario M4C 5R1.
☎ 416 466 5304 ✆ 416 778 0785

Organizations: Human Rights
☺ ☐ **Canadian Human Rights Commission**
⚲ 13th. Floor, Tower A, 320 Queen Street, Ottawa, Ontario K1A 1E1.
☎ 613 995 1151 ✆ 613 996 9661
☎ 613 996 5211 TTY
🕐 Weekdays 09:00 - 17:00, answering machine at other times
Government body that aims to prevent discrimination & to educate the public about human rights & the harm discrimination causes. Accepts complaints based on, amongst others, sex, sexual orientation, & national or ethnic origin.

Organizations: Piercing
☺ ☐ **The Canadian Association of Body Arts**
🌐 http://www.io.org/~bme/caba/caba.html

Organizations: Sexuality
⊘▽ **Fondation Nationale du Transsexualisme**
☎ 514 526 5892

Organizations: Tattoo
⊘▽ **The Canadian Tattoo Association**
P. O. Box 327, Qualicum Beach, British Columbia V0R 2T0.

Publishers: Directories: General
☺ ■ **The Connexions Annual**
Connexions Information Sharing Services, P. O. Box 158, Station D, Toronto, Ontario M6P 3J8.
☎ 416 537 3949
✆ 416 229 4465. 28800 baud maximum.
✉ Connex@Sources.com
🌐 http://www.sources./com
🕐 Mon - Fri 09:00 - 17:00
🍴 ✓ $ 🌫
A source book of social & environmental alternatives. Also has Internet version. Published once a year. Yearly subscription is $30. German also spoken.

☺ ■ *Sources*
 ♿ Suite 109, 4 Phipps Street, Toronto, Ontario M4Y 1J5.
 ☎ 416 964 7799 ✆ 416 964 8763
 ✆ 416 229 4465. 28800 baud maximum.
 ✉ Sources@Sources.com
 🌐 http://www.sources./com
 🕐 Mon - Fri 09:00 - 17:00
 ♿ ✓ $ ⚥
 The directory Canadian journalists use to find experts & spokespeople to
 interview & quote. Published twice a year. Yearly subscription is $45.
 German also spoken.

Publishers: Guides: Sexuality

⚥▼ *The Bent Guide to Gay/Lesbian Canada*
 ECW Press, 2120 Queen Street West, Toronto, Ontario M4E 1E2.

Publishers: Magazines: Sexuality

⚥▼ *Gazelle*
 ♿ Les Editions Nitram, 1212 Saint Hubert, Montréal, Québec H2L 3H7.
 ☎ 514 499 9994 ✆ 514 845 7645
 🕐 09:00 - 18:00
 ♿ ✓ $ ⚥ [VISA]
 Québec's French magazine for lesbians. Published every month. Yearly
 subscription is $22Cdn..

⚥▽ *Malebox*
 ♿ Pink Triangle Press, P. O. Box 166, Station B, Ottawa, Ontario K1P 6C4.
 ☎ 613 237 7133 ✆ 613 237 6651
 🕐 09:00 - 18:00
 ♿ ✓ $ [VISA] [MC]
 Canada's national erotica & contact magazine for gay men, featuring
 stories, photo-personal ads, centrefold, video reviews, & true life
 experiences. Published every two months. Yearly subscription is
 $20Cdn.. Age statement of 18 is required.

Publishers: Mailing Lists: Sexuality

⚥▽ **Malebox Direct Mail Service**
 P. O. Box 166, Station B, Ottawa, Ontario K1P 6C4.
 ☎ 613 237 7133 ✆ 613 237 6651
 🕐 09:00 - 18:00
 ♿ ✓ $ [VISA] [MC]
 National mailing list service targetting approximately 1,000 gay men
 across Canada. Free catalogue. Age statement of 18 is required.

ALBERTA

Population: Approximately 2,500,000
Capital City: Edmonton
Time zone: GMT minus 7 hours (Mountain Time)
Climate: Summers are pleasant, with average temperatures of approximately
 16°-20°C. Winters are cold with average temperatures of approximately
 -16°C. Calgary experiences winter thaws when temperatures can change
 by over 30°C within a few hours and jump back again just as quickly.
Age of consent & homosexuality legislation: One of only three
 provinces not to have laws preventing discrimination based upon sexual
 orientation.
Legal drinking age: 18

Provincial Resources

Publishers: Magazines: Sexuality

⚥▼ *qc Magazine*
 qc Magazine, P. O. Box 64292, 5512 Fourth Street North West,
 Calgary, Alberta T2K 6J1.
 ☎ 403 630 2061 ✆ 403 275 6443
 ✉ qcmag@nucleus.com
 🌐 http://mindlink.net/moworks/club_z.html
 🕐 Mon - Fri 09:00 - 18:00, answering machine at other times
 ♿ ✓ $ ⚥
 Lifestyle, non-political magazine for the lesbian, gay & bisexual
 communities (but not exclusively). Covers arts, fashion, community
 profiles, & entertainment. Published 11 times a year. Yearly subscription
 is $19, plus taxes. German also spoken.

Banff

Organizations: AIDS: Education

☺ ☐ **Banff Regional AIDS Committee**
 P. O. Box 520, Banff, Alberta T0L 0C0.
 ☎ 403 762 0690 ✆ 403 762 2602

Calgary

Bars: BDSM

⚥▼ **Boystown**
 213 10th. Avenue South West, Calgary, Alberta T2R 0A4.
 ☎ 403 265 2028
 🕐 21:00 - 03:00
 ♿ [VISA] [MC] ⚥
 Catalogue, $10, latex $2.

⚥▼ **Rekroom**
 Lower Level, 213 10th. Avenue South West, Calgary, Alberta T2R 0A4.
 ☎ 403 265 4749
 🕐 16:00 - 03:00
 ♿ [VISA] ⚥
 Catalogue, $10, latex $2.

⚥▼ **Trax**
 1130 10th. Avenue South West, Calgary, Alberta T2R 0B6.
 ☎ 403 265 8477
 🕐 Mon - Sat 16:00 03:00. Men only on Tue
 ♿ [VISA] [MC] ⚥
 Private club. Catalogue, $10, latex $2.

Counsellors

⚥▼ **Jane Oxenbury, M. Ed., C. Psyc.**
 K ♿ 3425 26th. Avenue South West, Calgary, Alberta T3E 0N3.
 ☎ 403 240 2501 ✆ 403 249 3428
 🕐 09:00 - 17:00
 ♿ ✓ $
 Psychotherapy for individuals, couples, & families. Specializes in sexual
 abuse, domestic & family violence, & depression. Age statement of 18
 is required.

Helplines: Sexuality

⚥▼ **Gay Lines Calgary**
 Suite 205, 223 12th. Avenue South West, Calgary, Alberta T2R 0G9.
 ☎ 403 234 8973 ✆ 403 234 8973

⚥▽ **Lesbian Information Line/Womyn's Collective of**
 ♿ **Calgary**
 Suite 210, 223 12th. Avenue South West, Calgary, Alberta T2R 0G9.
 ☎ 403 265 9458

Organizations: AIDS: Education

☺ ☐ **AIDS Calgary Awareness Association**
 ♿ Suite 300, 1021 10th. Avenue South West, Calgary, Alberta T2R 0B7.
 ☎ 800 590 8795 (information) ✆ 403 229 2077
 ☎ 403 228 0155

☺ ☐ **Feather of Hope Aboriginal AIDS Prevention**
 Society
 c/o AIDS Network of Edmonton Society, Suite 201, 11456 Jasper
 Avenue, Calgary, Alberta T5K 0M1.
 ☎ 403 488 5773 ✆ 403 488 3735

Organizations: BDSM

⚥▽ **CLUB Calgary**
 ♿ Suite 201, 223 12th. Avenue South West, Calgary, Alberta T2R 0G9.
 ☎ 403 234 8973

☺ ☐ **Southern Alberta Association for Fetish / Fantasy**
 Education / Exploration (SAAFE)
 Box 42014, Acadia Postal Outlet, Calgary, Alberta T2J 7A6.
 ✉ xpc@nucleus.com
 🌐 http://www.nucleus.com/~xpc/saafe/saafe.html
 Educational support group for open-minded discreet adults of ALL sexual
 orientations who share an interest in the fetishes.

☺ ☐ **Western Canada Leather / Fetish Clans Council**
 71 Applewood Drive South East, Calgary, Alberta T2A 7K8.
 ☎ 403 273 1765

Organizations: Family

☺ ☐ **Parents & Friends of Lesbians & Gays (PFLAG)—**
 Calgary
 20 Hendon Drive, Calgary, Alberta T2K 1Y5.
 ☎ 403 282 6592
 Contact: Mr. Thomas Rash

Organizations: Sexuality

⚥▽ **Illusions Social Club**
 6802 Ogden Road South East, Calgary, Alberta T2C 1B4.
 ☎ 403 236 7072 ✆ 403 236 1304
 🕐 Meets 2nd. Sat & last Thu of month 19:30
 ♿ ✓ $
 Contact: Christine or Barbie
 Social support group for TV/TS lifestyle. Yearly membership of $40
 includes magazine. Publishes *Illusions Magazine*. Yearly subscription is
 $9.95.

⚥▽ **The Society for the Second Self (Tri-Ess)—Phi**
 Sigma
 P. O. Box 8115, 755 Lake Bonavista Drive South East, Calgary, Alberta
 T2J 7C9.

Organizations: Sexuality: Student

⚥▽ **Gay, Lesbian, & Bisexual Academics, Students &**
 ♿ **Staff (GLASS)**
 Office #209E, Box 47, 321 MacEwan Hall, 2500 University Drive,

Calgary, Alberta T2N 1N4.
☎ 403 282 8998

♂♀▽ **Lesbian & Gay Collective of Mount Royal College**
⟁ Students Association, 4825 Richard Road South West, Calgary, Alberta T3E 6K6.

Organizations: Sexuality: Youth

♂♀▽ **Gay Youth Calgary**
Suite 317, 233 12th. Avenue South West, Calgary, Alberta.
☎ 403 234 9873
⏰ Sun 13:00 - 15:00
Information & counselling.

♂♀▽ **Lesbian & Gay Youth/Calgary**
♀⟁ Suite 200B, 223 12th. Avenue South West, Calgary, Alberta T2E 0G9.
☎ 403 262 1626
Publishes *Lesbian & Gay Youth News*.

Piercers

☺■ **Quintessential Transfigurations**
116 10th. Street North West, Calgary, Alberta T2N 0N2.
☎ 403 270 7550 ✆ 403 283 2505
⏰ Mon - Fri 10:00 - 21:00, Sat 10:00 - 18:00, Sun 12:00 - 17:00, Hol 12:00 - 17:00. Mon - Fri 10:00 - 20:00 in winter
🍴 VISA MC
Also wholesales piercing jewelry.

Stores: Books: General

☺■ **Books 'n' Books**
⟁ 738A 17th. Street South West, Calgary, Alberta T2S 0B7.
☎ 403 228 3337

☺■ **Mount Royal College Bookstore**
⟁ 4825 Richard Road South West, Calgary, Alberta T2E 6K6.
☎ 403 240 6300 ✆ 403 240 6628
🍴 ✓ ⚥ VISA MC ℓ

☺■ **With The Times**
⟁ 2212A 4th. Street South West, Calgary, Alberta T2S 1W9.
☎ 403 244 8020 ✆ 403 244 8019

⚥■ **A Woman's Place Bookstore**
⟁ 1412 Centre Street South, Calgary, Alberta T2G 2E4.
☎ 403 263 5256
🍴 ✓ VISA MC AMERICAN EXPRESS

Stores: Clothing: Adult Baby

☺▼ **Cozy Time Adult Baby Wear**
6802 Ogden Road South East, Calgary, Alberta T2C 1B4.
☎ 403 236 7072 ✆ 403 236 1304
⏰ Tue - Fri 09:30 - 18:00, Sat 12:00 - 18:00
🍴 ✓ $ ⚥ VISA
Custom manufacturer of adult baby wear. Several styles in stock, or made to order. Catalogue, $6.

Stores: Clothing: Sexuality

↪▼ **Lingerie by Barbie**
6802 Ogden Road South East, Calgary, Alberta T2C 1B4.
☎ 403 236 7072 ✆ 403 236 1304
⏰ Tue - Fri 09:30 - 18:00, Sat 12:00 - 18:00
🍴 ✓ $ ⚥ VISA
Manufacturer of fetish clothing. Also wigs, high heels, make-up, make overs, breast forms, etc.. For all walks of life, particularly TV/TS.

Stores: Erotica: BDSM

☺▼ **B&B Leatherworks**
6802 Ogden Road South East, Calgary, Alberta T2C 1B4.
☎ 403 236 7072 ✆ 403 236 1304
⏰ Tue - Fri 09:30 - 18:00, Sat 12:00 - 18:00
🍴 ✓ $ ⚥ VISA
Custom leather clothing, sub / dom equipment, latex wear, & made to order items. Virtually anything you can imagine in leather. Catalogue, $10, latex $2.

☺■ **Stairwell Leathers**
210 4th. Avenue North East, Calgary, Alberta T2E 0J1.
☎ 403 276 2471

Stores: Erotica: General

☺▼ **After Dark**
⟁ 1314 1st. Street South West, Calgary, Alberta T2R 0V7.
☎ 403 264 7399 ✆ 403 269 4251
🍴 ⚥ VISA MC AMERICAN EXPRESS

☺▼ **After Dark Adult Warehouse**
⟁ 7248 Ogden Road South East, Calgary, Alberta T2C 1B6.
☎ 403 264 7399 ✆ 403 269 4251
🍴 ⚥ VISA MC AMERICAN EXPRESS

☺■ **Daily Globe**
1004 17th. Avenue South West, Calgary, Alberta T2T 0A5.

✆ 403 246 2957

☺▼ **Tad's Total Adult Discount Store**
⟁🔑 1217-A 9th. Avenue South East, Calgary, Alberta T2G 0S9.
☎ 403 237 8237

☺▼ **Tad's Total Adult Discount Store**
⟁🔑 1506 14th. Street, Calgary, Alberta T3C 1C9.
☎ 403 244 8239

Edmonton

Helplines: Sexuality

⚥ ▽ **Womonspace / Lesbian Lifeline**
☎ 403 425 0511

Organizations: AIDS: Support

☺□ **AIDS Network of Edmonton Society**
⟁ Suite 201, 11456 Jasper Avenue, Edmonton, Alberta T5K 0M1.
☎ 403 488 5816 (information) ✆ 403 488 3735
☎ 403 488 5742 (office)
🍴 ⚥ MC

☺□ **Edmonton Persons Living with HIV Society**
c/o AIDS Network of Edmonton Society, Suite 201, 11456 Jasper Avenue, Edmonton, Alberta T5K 0M1.
☎ 403 488 5768 ✆ 403 488 3735

Organizations: Sexual Politics

♂♀▽ **Gays & Lesbians Awareness Civil Rights Committee**
P. O. Box 53, Edmonton, Alberta T5J 2G9.
☎ 403 469 4286

Organizations: Sexuality

♂♀▽ **Gay & Lesbian Community Centre of Edmonton**
⟁🔑 P. O. Box 1852, Edmonton, Alberta T5J 2P2.
☎ 403 488 3234 ✆ 403 988 4018
⏰ Mon - Fri 19:00 - 22:00, Wed 13:00 - 16:00
🍴
Drop-in centre offering peer support counselling, library, periodicals, calendar of events, & infoline. In basement of 10112 124th. Street North West. Publishes a newsletter 8 times a year. Yearly subscription is $10Cdn..

↪▽ **Illusions Social Club II**
P. O. Box 33002, Edmonton, Alberta T5P 4V8.
✓

Organizations: Sexuality: Student

♂♀▽ **Gays & Lesbians on Campus**
⟁ Box 75, Student Building, University of Alberta, Edmonton, Alberta T6G 2J7.
☎ 403 403 988 4166
🌐 http://gpu.srv.uablerta.ca/cbidwell/OUT/out.html
Publishes *OUTreach*.

Organizations: Sexuality: Youth

♂♀▽ **Pink Triangle Youth of Edmonton**
⟁🔑 P. O. Box 1852, Edmonton, Alberta T5J 2P2.
☎ 403 488 1754 ✆ 403 988 4018
⏰ Sat 20:00 - 22:00
🍴
Drop-in centre for Edmonton youth. Peer support counselling. In basement of 10112 124th. Street North West. Age statement of 16 is required.

Stores: Books: General

☺▼ **The Front Page**
⟁ 10846 Jasper Avenue, Edmonton, Alberta T5J 2B2.
☎ 403 426 1206
✓

☺ **Greenwood's Bookshoppe**
10355 Whyte Street, Edmonton, Alberta T6B 1Z9.
☎ 403 439 2005 ✆ 403 433 5774
☎ 800 661 2078 (orders only)

⚥▼ **Woman to Womon Books**
Suite 106, 12404 114th. Avenue, Edmonton, Alberta T5M 3M5.
☎ 403 454 8031

Stores: Erotica: General

♂♀▼ **Executive Express**
Suite 203, 11745 Jasper Avenue, Edmonton, Alberta T5K 2P2.
☎ 403 482 7480
⏰ Wed - Mon 13:00 - 21:00
🍴 VISA
Totally gay video outlet, with leather goods, toys, books, magazines, cards, etc.. Also mail order. Age statement of 18 is required.

Stores: Military Surplus

Stores: Military Surplus
☺ ■ **S O S Army Surplus Ltd.**
10247 97th. Street, Edmonton, Alberta.
☎ 403 422 3348

Grande Prairie
Organizations: AIDS: Education
☺ ☐ **South Peace AIDS Council**
P. O. Box 902, Grande Prairie, Alberta T8V 3Y1.
☎ 403 538 3388 ✆ 403 538 3368

Jasper
Organizations: AIDS: Education
☺ ☐ **AIDS, A Positive Coördinated Response Society of Jasper**
P. O. Box 1090, Jasper, Alberta T0E 1E0.
☎ 403 852 5274 ✆ 403 852 4019

Lethbridge
Organizations: AIDS: Support
☺ ☐ **Lethbridge AIDS Connection Society**
& Suite 421, 515 7th. Street South, Lethbridge, Alberta T1J 2G8.
☎ 403 328 8186 ✆ 403 328 5934 (call first)

Okotoks
Organizations: AIDS: Education
☺ ☐ **Foothills AIDS Awareness Association**
P. O. Box 758, Okotoks, Alberta T0L 1T0.
☎ 403 938 4911 ✆ 403 938 2783

Red Deer
Organizations: AIDS: Support
& **Central Alberta AIDS Network Society**
4935 51st. Street, Red Deer, Alberta T4N 2A8.
☎ 403 346 8858 ✆ 403 342 4154

Organizations: Motorcycle
♂ **Motorcycle Men of Alberta**
4141 40th. Street, Red Deer, Alberta T4N 1A5.
☎ 403 346 8927

Organizations: Sexuality
♂▽ **Gay & Lesbian Association of Central Alberta**
& P. O. Box 1078, Red Deer, Alberta T4N 6S5.
☎ 403 340 2198 (recorded message)

BRITISH COLUMBIA
Population: Approximately 3,400,000
Capital City: Victoria
Time zone: GMT minus 8 hours (PST)
Climate: Mild climate, with plenty or rain in the winter. Cool in the mountains in the north & east. Snow is rare in the Vancouver area. Average Vancouver summer temperatures are approximately
Age of consent & homosexuality legislation: All anal & oral sex is illegal in this state.
Legal drinking age: 19

Provincial Resources
Organizations: BDSM
☺ ☐ **The National Leather Association (NLA)—British Columbia**
Suite 151, 10090 152nd. Street, Surrey, British Columbia V6R 8X8.
☎ 604 945 3668
& ✓ $
Pansexual, alternative lifestyle, fetish-supportive. Bar nights & play parties. Publishes a newsletter. Age statement of 21 is required.

Burnaby
Organizations: Motorcycle
♂▽ **Highwaymen MC**
4673 Pender, North Burnaby, British Columbia V5C 2N2.
☎ 604 294 3559
Contact: Mr. John Sebastian

Organizations: Sexuality: Student
♂▽ **GALA TC**
321 Rotunda, Burnaby, British Columbia.
☎ 604 291 3182
Simon Fraser University students.

Stores: Erotica: General
☺ ■ **Imperial Books**
4924 Imperial Street, Burnaby, British Columbia.
☎ 604 432 9940

Coquitlam
Publishers: Magazines: BDSM
☺ ■ *Diversity Magazine*
P. O. Box 47558, Coquitlam, British Columbia V3K 6T3.
☎ 604 937 7447 ✆ 604 937 7555
☎ 604 650 6867 (pager)
Fiction, non-fiction, photographic essays, current events, reviews, etc.. Published quarterly.

Grand Forks
Organizations: AIDS: Support
☺ ☐ **West Kootenay-Boundry AIDS Network, Outreach & Support Society (ANKORS)**
P. O. Box 25, Grand Forks, British Columbia V0H 1H0.
☎ 800 421 2437 (information) ✆ 604 442 4305
☎ 403 365 2437 (office)

Kamloops
Organizations: Sexuality
▷◁▽ **Dream Girls**
P. O. Box 535, Kamloops, British Columbia V2C 5L7.
⊕ Meets every two weeks

Kelowna
Helplines: Sexuality
♂▽ **Gay Crisis Line**
☎ 604 860 8486
Lists local events.

Organizations: AIDS: Support
☺ ☐ **Kelowna & Area AIDS Resources, Education, & Support (KARES)**
Box 134, 435-2339 Highway 97 North, Kelowna, British Columbia V1X 4H9.
☎ 604 862 2437 ✆ 604 868 8662

Kootnays
Helplines: Sexuality
♂▽ **West Kootenays Gays & Lesbians**
☎ 604 325 3504
⊕ 24hrs.

Ladner
Counsellors
♂ **Virginia Walford, Ph.D.**
Suite 206, 4882 Delta Street, Ladner, British Columbia V4K 2T8.
☎ 604 940 2838

Langley
Organizations: Family
♂▽ **Langley Outreach**
5339 207th. Street, Langley, British Columbia.
☎ 604 534 7921

Nanaimo
Helplines: Sexuality
♂▽ **Gayline**
☎ 604 754 2585
⊕ Mon - Fri 18:00 - 21:00

New Westminster
Organizations: Sexuality: Student
♂▽ **Lesbian, Gay, & Bisexual Collective of Douglas College**
P. O. Box 2503, New Westminster, British Columbia.
☎ 604 527 5111

Prince George
Organizations: AIDS: Support
☺ ☐ **Prince George AIDS Society**
1371 4th. Avenue, Prince George, British Columbia V2L 3J6.
☎ 604 562 1172 ✆ 604 562 1172

Squamish

Publishers: Magazines: Sexuality

⊕ ▼ *Herspectives*
 ⅁ P. O. Box 2047, Squamish, British Columbia V0N 3G0.
 ☎ 604 892 5723

Terrace

Organizations: Sexuality

♂♀▽ **Terrace Gay Connection**
 ☎ 604 638 1632

Vancouver

Archives: Sexuality

♂♀▽ **Out On The Shelves**
 1170 Bute Street, Vancouver, British Columbia.
 ☎ 604 684 5307 ✆ 604 684 5309
 ⏰ Mon - Sun 19:30 - 21:30, Mon 11:00 - 14:00

Bars: BDSM

♂♀▽ **The Forge Tavern**
 900 Seymour Street, Vancouver, British Columbia.
 ☎ 604 683 2923

♂♀▼ **The Underground**
 1082 Granville Street , Vancouver, British Columbia.
 Some leather at weekends.

Counsellors

♂♀▼ **Lesbian & Gay Counselling & Consulting Services**
 ☎ 604 222 7807

Distributors: Books: General

☺ **MacNeill Library Service**
 1701 West 3rd. Avenue, Vancouver, British Columbia V6J 1K7.
 ☎ 604 732 1335 ✆ 604 732 3765

Health Services

▷□ **Centre for Sexuality**
 Gender Identity & Reproductive Health, Vancouver Hospital, Vancouver,
 British Columbia.

Organizations: AIDS: Education

☺ □ **AIDS Vancouver**
 c/o Pacific AIDS Resource Centre, 1107 Seymour Street, Vancouver,
 British Columbia V6B 5S8.
 ☎ 604 687 2437 (information) ✆ 604 893 2211
 ☎ 604 681 2122 (office)

Organizations: AIDS: Support

☺ □ **B. C. Coalition of People with Disabilities**
 Suite 204, 456 Broadway West, Vancouver, British Columbia V5Y 1R3.
 ☎ 604 875 0188 ✆ 604 875 9227

☺ □ **Healing Our Spirit**
 Suite 102, 1193 Kingsway Street, Vancouver, British Columbia V5V
 3C9.
 ☎ 604 879 0906 ✆ 604 879 1690
 First nations AIDS society.

☺ □ **Persons with AIDS Society of British Columbia**
 c/o Pacific AIDS Resource Centre, 1107 Seymour Street, Vancouver,
 British Columbia V6B 5S8.
 ☎ 604 681 2122 ✆ 604 893 2251

⊕ □ **Positive Women's Network**
 c/o Pacific AIDS Resource Centre, 1107 Seymour Street, Vancouver,
 British Columbia V6B 5S8.
 ☎ 604 681 2122 ✆ 604 893 2211

☺ □ **Victoria AIDS Respite Care Society**
 611 Superior Street, Vancouver, British Columbia V8V 1V1.
 ☎ 604 388 6220 ✆ 604 388 0711

Organizations: BDSM

☺ □ **A.S.B. Munch—Vancouver**
 ✉ dee@renaisoft.com
 ⏰ Meets Mon 19:00 - 21:00
 Contact: Mr. Peter Tupper

☺ ■ **The Betty Page Social Club**
 P. O. Box 28, 199 West Hastings Street, Vancouver, British Columbia
 V6B 1H4.
 ☎ 604 688 4458

♂♀▽ **The Post**
 5536 Knight, Vancouver, British Columbia V5P 2V2.

♂♀▽ **Vancouver Activists in SM (VASM)**
 P. O. Box 4579, Vancouver, British Columbia V6B 4A1.

 ☎ 604 434 1369
 ☎ 604 876 1914
 ✉ 70641.507@compuserve.com
 ⏰ Meets monthly
 ✓
 Publishes *Scene*.

☺ □ **Vancouver Leather Alliance**
 P. O. Box 2253, Vancouver, British Columbia V6B 3W2.
 ☎ 604 688 9378 Ext.: 2035

Organizations: Bears

♂♀▽ **BC Bears**
 Box 413, 1195 Davie Street, Vancouver, British Columbia V6E 1N2.

Organizations: Family

☺ □ **Parents & Friends of Lesbians & Gays (PFLAG)—Vancouver**
 ☎ 604 688 9378 Ext.: 2060

Organizations: Fetish: Smoking

♂♀▼ **Still Smokin'**
 P. O. Box 2253, Vancouver, British Columbia V6B 3W2.
 Contact: Northwind
 Publishes *On Wings of Leather* quarterly. Yearly subscription is 8 IRCs.

Organizations: Masturbation

♂♀▽ **Vancouver Jacks**
 P.O. Box 2682, Vancouver, British Columbia V6B 3W8.
 ☎ 604 688 9378 Ext.: 2034
 ⏰ Meets semi-regularly
 ♨
 Club for men who like safe jack-off with other men. Age statement of 21
 is required.

Organizations: Motorcycle

♂♀▽ **Border Riders MC**
 P. O. Box 21152, Seattle, Washington 98111.
 ☎ 503 256 0197
 ☎ 206 720 4774
 ✉ brmc95prez@aol.com

♂♀▽ **Knights of Malta MC—Dogwood**
 P. O. Box 3116, Vancouver, British Columbia V6B 3X6.

Organizations: Sexuality

♂▽ **Bi Face**
 ☎ 604 688 9378 Ext.: 2098

▷▽ **The Cornbury Society**
 P. O. Box 3745, Vancouver, British Columbia V6B 3Z1.
 For heterosexual crossdressers. Wives & girlfriends welcome.

▷▽ **Foundation for the Advancement of Transgendered People's Society (FATE)**
 Suite 1, 1727 William Street, Vancouver, British Columbia V5L 2R5.
 ☎ 604 254 9591

♂♀▽ **Gay & Lesbian Centre**
 Gay & Lesbian Centre, 1170 Bute Street, Vancouver, British Columbia.
 ☎ 604 684 6869

♀♀▽ **Lesbian Centre**
 876 Commercial Drive, Vancouver, British Columbia.
 ☎ 604 254 8458

♂▼ **Options Bisexual Group**
 ☎ 604 688 9378 Ext.: 2097

▷▽ **Vancouver General Hospital**
 Transsexual Support Group, 14905 32nd. Avenue, Vancouver, British
 Columbia V4P 1A4.
 ☎ 604 536 2053
 ☎ 604 875 4100
 ⏰ Meets Wed 19:00 - 22:00
 Contact: Dr. Angela Wensley, Director

▷▽ **Zenith Foundation**
 Box 46, 8415 Granville Street, Vancouver, British Columbia V6P 4Z9.

Organizations: Sexuality: Student

♂♀▽ **Gays, Lesbian, & Bisexuals of UBC**
 138 S. U. B. Boulevard, Vancouver, British Columbia.
 ☎ 604 228 4638

♂♀▽ **Lesbian, Gay, & Bisexual Students' Association**
 Student Union Building, Vancouver Community College, 100 West 49th.
 Avenue, Vancouver, British Columbia.
 ☎ 604 324 3881

♂♀▽ **Out On Campus**
 Simon Fraser University, Vancouver, British Columbia.
 ☎ 604 688 9378 Ext.: 2064

Organizations: Sexuality: Youth
⌕▽ **Lesbian, Gay, & Bi Youth**
Gay & Lesbian Centre, 1170 Bute Street, Vancouver, British Columbia.
☎ 604 688 9378 Ext.: 2067

Organizations: Shaving
⌕▽ **Men Shaving Men**
P. O. Box 381, 1215 Davie Street, Vancouver, British Columbia V6E 1N4.
Contact: Jim

Piercers
☺▼ **Next! Body Piercing**
1068 Granville Street, Vancouver, British Columbia.
☎ 604 684 6398

Printers: General
☺■ **Mitchell Press Ltd.**
Box 6000, 1706 West First Avenue, Vancouver, British Columbia V6B 4B9.
☎ 604 731 5211 ✆ 604 731 0312

Publishers: Magazines: Sexuality
⚲▼ **Kinesis**
⛶ Suite 301, 1720 Grant Street, Vancouver, British Columbia V5L 2Y6.
☎ 604 255 5499

Publishers: Magazines: BDSM
☺ **Kink**
Dominant Publications, Suite 601, 1755 Robson Street, Vancouver, British Columbia V6G 3B7.
A fetishist magazine for people with alternate styles of life: Dominant females, kinky cvouples, TVs, TSs, etc..
⌕▼ **Northwind**
P. O. Box 2253, Vancouver, British Columbia V6B 3W2.
☎ 604 253 1258
Also organizes yearly Spring rubber event called Rubbout.

Publishers: Magazines: Sexuality
⌕▼ **The Loop**
1141 Davie Street, Vancouver, British Columbia V6E 1N2.
☎ 604 689 5056 ✆ 604 689 5056
✉ loopzine@aol.com
Also distributed in the Los Angeles area. Published every month. Yearly subscription is $20.

Publishers: Newspapers: Sexuality
⌕▼ **Angles**
Lavendar Publishing, 1170 Bute Street, Vancouver, British Columbia V6E 1Z6.
☎ 604 688 0265 ✆ 604 688 5405
⊕ Mon - Fri 12:00 - 14:00, Wed 18:00 - 21:00
✓ $
The magazine of Vancouver's lesbigay community. Published every month. Yearly subscription is $30 Cdn., $35 U.S..
⌕▽ **Xtra! West**
⛶ Pink Triangle Press, P. O. Box 93642, Nelson Park Post Office, Vancouver, British Columbia V6E 4L7.
☎ 604 684 9696 ✆ 604 684 9697
✉ xtrawest@descon.minet.com
⊕ Mon - Fri 09:00 - 18:00
News, arts, & entertainment newspaper geared to the gay & lesbian community. Published every two weeks. Yearly subscription is $45.95 Cdn., $52.95 U.S., $85.95 U.S. elsewhere.
⌕ **Sodomite Invasion Review**
Suite 109, 1744 Barclay Street, Vancouver, British Columbia V6G 1K3.

Radio: Sexuality
⌕▽ **The Coming Out Show**
☎ 604 684 8494
☎ 604 688 9378 Ext. 2088
⊕ Thu 19:00
⌕▽ **Heather's Show**
☎ 604 685 2746
⊕ Sun 18:00
⌕▽ **The Lesbian Show**
☎ 604 684 8494
☎ 604 688 9378 Ext. 2010
⊕ Thu 20:00

Stores: Books: General
☺■ **Ariel Books**
1988 West 4th. Avenue, Vancouver, British Columbia V6J 1M5.

☎ 604 733 3511
☺■ **Book Mantle**
1002 Commercial Drive, Vancouver, British Columbia V5L 3W9.
☎ 604 253 1099
⊕ 11:00 - 19:00
No mail order.
☺ **Granville Book Company**
850 Granville Street, Vancouver, British Columbia V6Z 1K3.
☎ 604 687 2213
⌕▼ **Little Sister's Book & Art Emporium**
1221 Thurlow Street, Vancouver, British Columbia V6E 1X4.
☎ 800 567 1662 ✆ 604 685 0252
☎ 604 669 1753
⊕ 10:00 - 23:00
☺■ **Octopus Books**
♿ 1146 Commercial Drive, Vancouver, British Columbia V5L 3X2.
☎ 604 253 0013
☺■ **R2B2 Books**
2742 West 4th. Avenue, Vancouver, British Columbia V6K 1R1.
☎ 604 732 5087
⌕■ **Spartacus Books**
311 West Hastings Street, Vancouver, British Columbia V5L 2K9.
☎ 604 688 6138
⚲■ **Women In Print**
3566 West 4th. Street, Vancouver, British Columbia.
⚲■ **Women's Book Store**
315 Cambie Street, Vancouver, British Columbia V6B 2N4.
☎ 604 684 0523

Stores: Clothing: Fetish
☺▼ **Ms. Charade**
1263 Granville Street, Vancouver, British Columbia.
☎ 604 669 2195
⊕ Tue - Thu 10:00 - 18:00, Fri Sat 10:00 - 17:00, Sun 12:00 - 17:00
Entrance is through the Plus One Dollar store.

Stores: Erotica: BDSM
☺■ **Mack's Leathers**
♿ 1043 Granville Street, Vancouver, British Columbia V6Z 1C4.
☎ 604 688 6225
⊕ Mon - Wed 11:00 - 19:00, Thu Fri 11:00 - 20:00, Sat 11:00 - 18:00, Sun 12:00 - 17:00
Leather & rubber clothing & toys.
☺■ **Womyn's Ware**
896 Commercial Drive, Vancouver, British Columbia.
☎ 604 254 2543

Stores: Erotica: General
☺■ **Return to Sender**
1076 Davie Street, Vancouver, British Columbia V6E 1M3.
☎ 604 683 6363

Stores: Military Surplus
☺■ **Camouflage**
334 West Pender Street, Vancouver, British Columbia.
☺■ **West Lynn Military Surplus**
623 Front Street North West, Vancouver, British Columbia.

Tattooists
☺■ **Mum'sTattoo**
291 Pemberton Avenue, North Vancouver, British Columbia V7P 2R4.
☎ 614 984 7831 ✆ 614 980 0154
⊕ Mon - Sat 10:00 - 20:00, Sun Hol 12:00 - 18:00

Television: Sexuality
⌕▽ **Prism**
☎ 604 688 9378 Ext.: 2087

Victoria
Helplines: Sexuality
⌕▽ **Gay Help Line**
☎ 604 383 9124

⊙ Sat Sun 20:00 - 01:00, recording at other times

Organizations: AIDS: Education
☺ ☐ **AIDS Vanvouver Island**
Suite 304, 733 Johnson Street, Victoria, British Columbia V8W 3C7.
☎ 604 384 4554 (information) ✆ 604 380 9411
☎ 604 384 2366 (office)

Organizations: AIDS: Support
☺ ☐ **Victoria Persons with AIDS Society**
613 Superior Street, Victoria, British Columbia V8V 1V1.
☎ 604 383 7494 ✆ 604 383 1617

Organizations: Family
☺ ☐ **Parents & Friends of Lesbians & Gays (PFLAG)—Victoria**
☎ 604 688 9378 Ext.: 2091

Organizations: Sexuality
⚥▽ **Island Gay Community Centre**
140 Oswago Street, Victoria, British Columbia.
☎ 604 383 9124

Organizations: Sexuality: Student
⚥▽ **Lambda Club, University of Victoria**
P. O. Box 3035, Victoria, British Columbia V8W 3P3.

Radio: General
☺ ☐ *Offbeat*
♿ CFUV FM 101.9, P. O. Box 3035, University of Victoria, Victoria, British Columbia V8W 3P3.
☎ 604 721 8702 ✆ 604 721 7111
✉ cfuv@sol.uvic.ca
⊙ Mon - Fri 09:00 - 17:00
10 issues per year.

Stores: Books: General
⚥■ **Everywoman Books**
♿ 641 Johnson Street, Victoria, British Columbia V8W 1M7.
☎ 604 388 9411
♿ ✓ 💳 📷
☺ **Ivy's Bookshop**
2184 Oak Bay Avenue, Victoria, British Columbia V8R 1G3.
☎ 604 598 2713 ✆ 604 595 1552
☺ **Munro's Bookstore**
1108 Government Street, Victoria, British Columbia V8W 1Y2.
☎ 604 382 2464 ✆ 604 382 2832

MANITOBA
Provincial Resources
Mailorder: Books: Sexuality
☺ ▼ **Gaie Livraison**
♿ P. O. Box 1912, Winnipeg, Manitoba R3C 2R2.
☎ 204 474 0212 ✆ 204 478 1160
☎ 204 284 5208
⊙ Mon - Fri 13:30 - 16:00, 19:30 - 22:00
♿ ✓ $
Publish or reprint useful titles on homosexuality & AIDS.

Brandon
Organizations: AIDS: Support
☺ ☐ **Brandon AIDS Support, Inc.**
P. O. Box 32, Brandon, Manitoba R7A 6Y2.
☎ 204 726 4020

Organizations: Sexuality
⚥▽ **BU GLASS**
Brandon University Students' Union (BUSU), 270 18th. Street, Brandon, Manitoba R7A 6A9.
☎ 204 727 4279
☎ 204 727 9660 (BUSU office)
⊙ Call direct line only on Sat 19:00 - 21:00

Dugald
Organizations: Sexuality
◖▽ **Prairie Rose Gender Club**
Box 23 Group 4, RR1, Dugald, Manitoba R0E 0K0.
☎ 204 257 2759
⊙ Meets 1st & 2nd Thu of month

Winnipeg
Health Services
☺ ☐ **The Village Clinic**
668 Corydon Avenue, Winnipeg, Manitoba R3M 0X7.
☎ 204 453 2144 (information) ✆ 204 453 5214
☎ 204 452 0045 (office)
⊙ 08:30 - 17:00

Organizations: AIDS: Support
☺ ☐ **AIDS Information Line**
☎ 204 945 2437
☺ ☐ **Body Positive Coalition of Manitoba**
Suite 460, 22 Furby Street, Winnipeg, Manitoba R3C 2A9.
☎ 204 783 5848
☺ ☐ **Kali-Shiva Society**
366 Oakwood Avenue, Winnipeg, Manitoba R3L 1G1.
☎ 204 477 9506

Organizations: BDSM
⚥▽ **Club Winnipeg**
P. O. Box 1697, Winnipeg, Manitoba R3C 2Z6.
⚥▽ **Winnipeg Leather/Levi Club**
P. O. Box 3079, Winnipeg General, Winnipeg, Manitoba R3C 4E5.

Organizations: Family
☺ ☐ **Parents & Friends of Lesbians & Gays (PFLAG)—Winnipeg**
☎ 204 284 5208

Organizations: Sexuality
⚥▽ **AIDS Shelter Coalition of Manitoba**
Suite 202, 222 Furby Street, Winnipeg, Manitoba R3C 2A7.
☎ 204 775 9173 ✆ 204 774 8895
⚥▽ **Winnipeg Gay / Lesbian Resource Centre**
P. O. Box 1661, Winnipeg, Manitoba R3C 2Z6.
☎ 204 284 5208 ✆ 204 478 1160
☎ 204 474 0212 (office)
⊙ Mon - Fri 19:30 - 22:00. Office Mon - Fri 13:00 - 16:30
♿ ✓
Support, information, referrals, & library. Publishes *The Alternative*.

Organizations: Sexuality: Student
⚥▽ **Gay & Lesbian Association of Students & Staff (GLASS)**
Box 27, University Centre, University of Manitoba, Winnipeg, Manitoba R3T 2N2.
☎ 204 477 8184
☺ ☐ **The University of Manitoba**
AIDS & Sexuality Peer Education Project, University Health Project, 104 University Centre, 65 Chancellors Circle, Winnipeg, Manitoba R3T 2N2.
☎ 204 474 8411 ✆ 204 261 7446

Printers: General
☺ ■ **Hignell Printing Limited**
488 Burnell Street, Winnipeg, Manitoba R3G 2B4.
☎ 204 783 7237 ✆ 204 774 4053
☺ ■ **Kromar Printing**
725 Portage Avenue, Winnipeg, Manitoba R3G 0M8.
☎ 204 775 8721 ✆ 204 783 8985
⊙ Mon - Fri 09:00 - 17:00
Offices in Oakville & Ottawa.

Stores: Books: General
⚥■ **Dominion News**
263 Portage Avenue, Winnipeg, Manitoba R3B 3L4.
☎ 204 942 6563 ✆ 204 942 4646
☺ ■ **McNally Robinson Booksellers**
♿ 100 Osborne Street, Winnipeg, Manitoba R3L 1Y5.
☎ 204 452 2644 ✆ 204 452 4160
♿ ✓ 💳 📷

Stores: Erotica: General
☺ **Discreet Boutique**
♿ 317 Ellice Avenue, Winnipeg, Manitoba R3B 1X7.
☎ 204 947 1307 ✆ 204 924 6516
☎ 800 247 0454 (order desk, Canada only)
⊙ Mon - Fri 10:00 - 22:00, Sat 10:00 - 18:00, Sun 12:00 - 17:00
♿ $ 💳 📷 🖨 ✎
Also mail order. Age statement of 18 is required.
☺ ■ **The News Stand**
559 Portage Avenue, Winnipeg, Manitoba.

☎ 204 453 2644
🕐 Mon - Sat 08:00 - 24:00, Sun 09:00 - 24:00
Gay & lesbian section.

Television: Sexuality

Coming Out
🕐 Fri 22:30 on cable channel 11

NEW BRUNSWICK

Fredricton

Helplines: Sexuality

Gayline
☎ 506 457 2156
🕐 Meets every other Fri 19:00

Organizations: AIDS: Education

AIDS New Brunswick
65 Brunswick Street, Fredricton, New Brunswick E3B 1G5.
☎ 800 561 4009 (information) 506 459 5782
☎ 506 459 7518 (office)

Organizations: Family

Parents & Friends of Lesbians & Gays (PFLAG)—Fredericton
P. O. Box 1556, Station A, Fredricton, New Brunswick 506 457 1256.

Organizations: Sexuality: Student

Gay & Lesbian Alliance at UNB/STU
c/o Help Centre, P. O. Box 4400, Fredricton, New Brunswick.
🕐 Meets Fri 19:00

Stores: Books: General

Westminster Books
445 King Street, Fredricton, New Brunswick E3B 1E5.
☎ 506 454 1442 506 452 9330

Moncton

Organizations: AIDS: Education

SIDA-AIDS Moncton
368 Cameron Street, Moncton, New Brunswick E1C 5Z6.
☎ 506 859 9616 506 855 4726

Riverview

Organizations: Sexuality

Pride in Life, Gays & Lesbians of Southeastern New Brunswick
P. O. Box 7102, Riverview, New Brunswick E1B 1V0.
☎ 506 855 8064
dickbain@nbnet.nb.ca
The only "gay activist" group in southeastern New Brunswick. Devoted to improving the environment of gays & lesbians in New Brunswick. Publishes *Pride Guide* every month. Yearly subscription is free.

Saint John

Archives: Sexuality

Archives for the Protection of Gay History & Literature
P. O. Box 6368, Station A, Saint John, New Brunswick.

Helplines: Sexuality

The Group
☎ 709 652 2848

Organizations: AIDS: Education

AIDS Saint John
115 Hazen Street, Saint John, New Brunswick E2L 3L3.
☎ 506 652 2437 506 652 2438

NEWFOUNDLAND

Saint John's

Organizations: AIDS: Education

Newfoundland & Labrador AIDS Committee Inc.
P. O. Box 626, Station C, Saint John's, Newfoundland A1C 5K8.
☎ 709 579 8656 709 579 0559

Stores: Books: General

Wordplay
221 Duckworth Street, Saint John's, Newfoundland A1C 1G7.
☎ 709 726 9193

NORTH WEST TERRITORIES

Yellowknife

Organizations: AIDS: Education

AIDS Yellowknife
P. O. Box 864, Yellowknife, North West Territories X1A 2N6.
☎ 800 661 0795 (information) 403 873 2626
☎ 403 873 2626 (office)
Second information number: 800 873 7017.

NOVA SCOTIA

Halifax

Helplines: Sexuality

Gay Line
☎ 902 423 7129
🕐 19:30 - 22:00

Organizations: AIDS: Education

AIDS Nova Scotia
Suite 300, 5675 Spring Garden Road, Halifax, Nova Scotia B3J 1H1.
☎ 902 425 2437 (information) 902 422 6200
☎ 902 425 4882 (office)

Atlantic First Nations AIDS Task Force
P. O. Box 47049, Halifax, Nova Scotia B3K 2B0.
☎ 800 565 4255 (information) 902 492 0500
☎ 902 492 4255
Publishes *Atlantic Standard.*

Metro Area Committee on AIDS
P. O. Box 1013, Station M, Halifax, Nova Scotia.
☎ 902 425 4882

Organizations: AIDS: Support

Nova Scotia PWA Coalition
Suite 300, 5675 Spring Garden Road, Halifax, Nova Scotia B3J 1H1.
☎ 902 429 7922 902 422 6200

Organizations: Bondage

Tightropes
P. O. Box 33067, Halifax, Nova Scotia B3L 4T6.

Organizations: Sexuality

Community Outreach Program
P. O. Box 3611, South Station, Halifax, Nova Scotia.
☎ 902 424 6551
Outreach to contact gays lesbians throughout Nova Scotia.

Organizations: Sexuality: Student

Bisexual, Gays, & Lesbian Association at Dalhousie (BGLAD)
Room 307, Dalhousie Student Union Building, 6136 University Avenue, Halifax, Nova Scotia.
☎ 902 494 1415

Publishers: Newspapers: Sexuality

Wayves
P. O. Box 34090, Scotia Square, Halifax, Nova Scotia B3J 3S1.
☎ 902 423 6999
wayves@fox.nstn.ca
Regional lesbigay newspaper for Atlantic Canada. Published 10 times a year. Yearly subscription is $18.

Stores: Books: General

Atlantic News
5660 Morris Street, Halifax, Nova Scotia B3J 1C2.
☎ 902 429 5468 902 425 8593
🕐 Mon - Fri 08:00 - 22:00, Sat Sun 09:00 - 22:00

Entitlement—The Book Company
5675 Spring Garden Road, Halifax, Nova Scotia B3J 1H1.
☎ 902 420 0565 902 420 3201

Red Herring Coöp Books
1555 Granville Street, Halifax, Nova Scotia B3J 1W7.
☎ 902 422 5087

New Glasgow

Organizations: AIDS: Education

Pictou County AIDS Coalition
P. O. Box 964, New Glasgow, Nova Scotia B2H 5K7.
☎ 902 755 4647 902 755 6775 (call first)

Sydney
Organizations: AIDS: Education
☺ ☐ **AIDS Coalition of Cape Breton**
P. O. Box 177, Sydney, Nova Scotia B1P 6H1.
☎ 902 567 1766 📞 902 539 2526

ONTARIO
Population: Approximately 10,250,000
Capital City: Toronto
Time zone: GMT minus 5 hours (EST)
Climate: Hot humid summers with average temperatures of approximately 25°C. Winters are cold, with temperatures averaging -4°C to -16°C. Northern regions are considerably colder than the southern regions in the winter.
Legal drinking age: 18

Provincial Resources
Counsellors
⚥▼ **Nick Mulé, M.S.W.**
& Suite 820, 77 Maitland Place, Toronto, Ontario M4Y 2V6.
☎ 416 926 9135
🕐 Answering machine with information
🐾 ✓
Psychotherapy or counselling for individuals, couples, & families. Coming out into BDSM, expanding & respecting limits, BDSM relationships. Confidential. Age statement of 18 is required.

Organizations: AIDS: Education
☺ ☐ **Ontario AIDS Network**
Suite 400, 100 Sparks Street, Ottawa, Ontario K1P 5B7.
☎ 613 230 3580 📞 613 563 4998

Organizations: Daddy / Boy
⚥▽ **boys & Dads Association**
& P. O. Box 333, 253 College Street, Toronto, Ontario M5T 1R5.
☎ 416 925 9872 Ext.: 2174
☎ 416 534 5096
🕐 Meets 2nd. & 4th. Thu of month (except Dec) 20:00
Contact: Bashir, President
Men's social group that shares in the joys of a daddy / boy lifestyle between adult males. Publishes a newsletter quarterly. Age statement of 21 is required. French, Hindi, & Czech also spoken.

Organizations: Sexual Politics
⚥ **Coalition for Lesbian & Gay Rights in Ontario**
P. O. Box 822, Station A, Toronto, Ontario M5W 1G3.
☎ 416 553 6824
Update on progress of the CLGRO campaigns to advance lesbian, gay, & bisexual rights & liberation. Publishes a newsletter quarterly. Yearly subscription is $25.

Organizations: Sexuality
☺ ☐ **Transequal**
Suite 609, 165 Ontario Street, Saint Catharines, Ontario L2R 5K4.
☎ 905 688 0276
✉ laura@vaxxine.com
🌐 http://vaxxine.com/laura or ftp://vaxxine.com/laura
🕐 By appointment only
Consulting for professionals & advocacy of transexual & transgenderist issues.

Publishers: Directories: Sexuality
⚥▼ **The Pink Pages**
392 King Street East, Toronto, Ontario M5A 1K9.
☎ 416 864 9132 📞 416 861 0174
🕐 Mon - Fri 09:00 - 17:00
🐾 ✓ $
Published once a year. Yearly subscription is free.

Barrie
Mailorder: Clothing: Chainmail
⚥ **Chained Male**
7 Collette Crescent, Barrie, Ontario L4M 3X6.
☎ 705 737 9791
🌐 http://inforamp.net/~thom/chained.htm
🕐 By appointment only
Catalogue, $10.

Organizations: AIDS: Support
☺ ☐ **AIDS Committee of Simcoe County**
P. O. Box 744, Barrie, Ontario L4N 4YS.
☎ 705 722 6778 📞 705 722 6560
🕐 09:00 - 17:00 (emergency calls transferred after hours)
Provides information/support to those infected &/or affected by

HIV/AIDS.
Stores: Erotica: General
☺ ■ **609 Novelty**
37 Mary Street, Barrie, Ontario L4N 1S9.
☎ 705 722 3244
🐾 💳
Also mail order. Catalogue available.

Belleville
Organizations: Health
⚥☐ **Sexual Assault Centre for Quinte & District**
& P. O. Box 22010, Belleville, Ontario K8N 5V1.
☎ 800 909 7007 (24hrs.) 📞 613 967 6527
☎ 613 967 6000
🕐 Weekdays 09:00 - 17:00. Answering machine at other times
Counselling & information for survivors of sexual abuse.

Bonfield
Organizations: BDSM
⚥▽ **Leathermen Yearning for Northern eXcitement (LYNX)**
Box 83, RR #1, Bonfield, Ontario P0H 1E0.
☎ 705 776 2638
🕐 Call 21:00 - 23:00
Contact: Mr. C. Haskins
Annual western camping weekend & other events. Please address envelopes to Mr. Charles Haskins, do NOT address them to Leathermen Yearning for Northern eXcitement.

⚥▽ **Sons of Capone**
c/o R. J., Box 83, RR#1, Bonfield, Ontario P0H 1E0.
Guys innerested in underworld scenarios involvin' gangsters, mob goons, cops, bikers, & other toughs.

Burlington
Organizations: Health
☺ ☐ **Halton Regional Health Department**
& Sexual Health Program, 123 Maurice Drive, Burlington, Ontario L7K 2W6.
☎ 905 825 6065 📞 905 849 3602
☎ 905 825 6222 (AIDS program)
🕐 08:30 - 16:30
Information about health, relationships, normal growth & development, fertility, birth control, & the prevention of STDs.

Cooksville
Printers: General
☺ ■ **Globe Graphics Communications**
5485 Tomken Road, Cooksville, Ontario L4W 3Y3.
☎ 905 625 1010 📞 905 625 1011

Don Mills
Printers: General
☺ ■ **Matthews, Ingham, & Lake Inc.**
180 Bond Avenue, Don Mills, Ontario M3P 3P3.
☎ 416 445 8800 📞 416 445 2731

Erin
Printers: General
☺ ■ **Porcupine's Quill Inc.**
68 Main Street, Erin, Ontario N0B 1T0.
☎ 519 833 9158

Guelph
Helplines: Sexuality
⚥▽ **Guelph Gayline**
☎ 519 836 4550
🕐 September to April, Monday - Thursday 19:30 - 21:30. Answering machine at other times
Support for those struggling with their sexuality.

Organizations: AIDS: Support
☺ ☐ **AIDS Committee of Guelph & Wellington County**
265 Woolwich Street, Guelph, Ontario N1H 3V8.
☎ 519 763 2255 📞 519 763 8125
🕐 08:30 - 16:30. Answering machine at other times
Provides education & supportive programs in response to HIV/AIDS.

Organizations: Family
☺ ☐ **Parents & Friends of Lesbians & Gays (PFLAG)— Guelph & Kitchener / Waterloo**

Organizations: Family

> P. O. Box 773, Guelph, Ontario N1H 6L8.
> ☎ 519 623 0492 (Hotline)
> ☎ 519 822 6912
> ☺ Best to call evenings & weekends. Anzwering machine at other times
> Support for parents, families, & friends of lesbians gays, & for gays & lesbians coming out to their families.

Organizations: Sexuality

♂♀☐ **Guelph Gay, Lesbian, & Bisexual Equality**
> P. O. Box 773, Guelph, Ontario N1H 6L8.
> ☎ 519 824 4120 Ext.: 8575 📱 519 736 9603
> ☺ Meets Wed 20:00
> Information & support for those struggling with their sexuality.

Haliburton

Organizations: Sexuality

☺ ☐ **Intersex Society of North America (INSA)—**
 ♿ **Canada**
> P. O. Box 1076, Haliburton, Ontario K0M 1S0.
> ✉ info@insa.org
> Peer support & counselling for intersexuals (i.e. hermaphrodites, pseudo hermaphrodites), parents of intersexed children, & those who have (or not) been medicalized or have experienced mutilating genital surgery.

Hamilton

Archives: Sexuality

♂♀▽ **Hamilton-Wentworth Lesbian/Gay Archives**
> c/o 230 Caroline Street South, Hamilton, Ontario L8P 3L4.
> ☎ 905 528 0156
> Archives include printed material, newspaper clippings, photographs, & audio-visual material. Answering machine.

Helplines: Sexuality

♂♀▽ **Gayline—Hamilton**
> ☎ 905 523 7055
> ☺ Wd - Fri 19:00 - 22:00

♂♀▼ **Lesbian/Gay Phoneline**
> ☎ 905 523 7055

Organizations: AIDS: Support

☺ ☐ **Hamilton AIDS Network**
> ♿ Suite 900, 143 James Street South, Hamilton, Ontario L8N 3Y3.
> ☎ 800 563 6919 📱 905 528 6311
> ☎ 905 528 0854
> ☺ Best to 'phone Mon - Thurs 09:00 - 21:00, Fri 09:00 - 17:00. Answering machine at other times
> Community-based volunteer AIDS organization providing support & education to anyone affected by AIDS.

Organizations: Family

☺ ☐ **Parents & Friends of Lesbians & Gays (PFLAG)—**
 ♿ **Hamilton-Wentworth**
> c/o Education Departmment, Suite 900, 143 James Street South, Hamilton, Ontario L8P 3A1.
> ☎ 905 528 0854 📱 905 528 6311
> ☺ Best to call 09:00 - 17:00. Answering machine at other times
> Support & education about issues relating to parents of lesbians & gays. Monthly meetings.

Organizations: Health

☺ ☐ **Sexual Assault Centre - Hamilton & Area**
> ♿ P. O. Box 955, Station A, Hamilton, Ontario L8N 3P9.
> ☎ 905 525 4162 (24 hrs.) 📱 905 525 7085
> ☎ 905 525 4753
> ☺ Best to call 09:00 - 17:00. Answering machine at other times
> Crisis line, education, referals, & outreach programs.

Organizations: Sexuality

♂♀▽ **Hamilton Gay & Lesbian Alliance (GALA)**
> ♿ 255 West Avenue North, Hamilton, Ontario L8L 5C8.
> ☎ 905 523 7055
> ☺ Men's group meets Tues 19:30 in room 5
> Support for the lesbian & gay community. Telephone number has answering machine with information. Publishes *The Phœnix*.

Organizations: Sexuality: Student

♂ **Bisexual, Gay, & Lesbian Association, McMaster University**
> P.O. Box 313, Hamilton, Ontario L8S 1C0.
> ☎ 416 525 9140 Ext.: 2041

♂♀▽ **Gay, Lesbian, & Bisexual Association of Mc**
 ♿ **Master**
> P. O. Box 313, McMaster University, Hamilton, Ontario L8S 1C0.
> ☎ 905 525 9140 Ext.: 27397

> ☺ Support meetins Wednesdays 18:30
> University club working towards a positive space for lesbians, gays, & bisexuals, & their friends. Telephone number has answering machine with information.

Radio: Sexuality

♂♀☐ **A Different Voice**
> CFMU 93.3 FM, P. O. Box 33, McMaster University, Hamilton, Ontario L8S 1C0.
> ☎ 905 525 9140 Ext.: 27397
> ☺ On air Thursdays 17:00 & Mondays 12:30
> Community news for lesbian, gay, & bisexual communities in Hamilton-Wentworth. Telephone number has answering machine with information.

Stores: Books: General

♿ ■ **Women's Bookshop**
> 333 Main Street, Hamilton, Ontario L8P 1K1.
> ☎ 905 525 2970

Kingston

Helplines: AIDS

☺ ☐ **AIDS Infoline**
> P. O. Box 120, Kingston, Ontario K7L 4V6.
> ☎ 800 565 2209 (from Kingston area)
> ☺ Best to call weekdays 08:30 - 16:30
> Information about HIV & AIDS.

Organizations: AIDS: Support

☺ ☐ **Kingston AIDS Project**
> ♿ P. O. Box 120, Kingston, Ontario K7L 4V6.
> ☎ 800 565 2209 (information) 📱 613 545 9809
> ☎ 613 545 3698 (office)
> ☺ Best to call weekdays 08:30 - 16:30
> Support & education for people infected with or affected by AIDS.

Organizations: Motorcycle

♂♀▽ **Trident—Kingston**
> #117, 75 Notch Hill Road, Kingston, Ontario K7M 2W9.

Organizations: Sexuality

♂♀▽ **Kingston Lesbian, Gay, & Bisexual Association**
> 51 Queen's Crescent, Kingston, Ontario K7L 2S7.
> ☎ 613 545 2960
> ☺ Best to call weekdays 19:00 - 21:00. Answering machine at other times
> Library, social activities, & a phone line staffed by trained volunteers who can give information, counselling, & referals.

Organizations: Sexuality: Student

♂♀▽ **Lesbian, Gay, & Bisexual Issues Committee (LGBIC)**
> Alma Mater Society, JDUC, Queen's University, Kingston, Ontario K7L 3N6.
> ☎ 613 545 4816
> ✉ LGBIC@qucdn.queensu.ca
> ☺ Meets Tue 17:30

Organizations: Sexuality: Youth

♂♀▽ **Outright Youth in Kingston (OYINK)**
> The Grey House, c/o 51 Queen's Crescent, Kingston, Ontario K7L 3N6.
> ☎ 613 545 2960
> ☺ Meets Wed 19:00. Telephone 19:00 - 22:00, Answering machine at other times
> Peer support for youth 26 years & under.

Kitchener

Organizations: AIDS: Support

☺ ☐ **AIDS Committee of Cambridge-Kitchener /**
 ♿ **Waterloo**
> 123 Duke Street East, Kitchener, Ontario N2H 1A4.
> ☎ 519 570 3687 📱 519 570 4034
> ☺ Weekdays 09:00 - 12:00, 13:00 - 17:00. Answering machine at other times
> Support, education, & health promotion to people infected with or affected by HIV & AIDS.

Organizations: Health

♿ ☐ **Kitchener / Waterloo Sexual Assault Support**
 ♿ **Centre**
> P. O. Box 2003, Kitchener, Ontario N2H 6K8.
> ☎ 519 741 8633 (Hotline) 📱 519 571 0522
> ☎ 519 571 0121
> ☺ Hotline 24 hours. Other line has answering machine with information
> Contact: Ms. Laurie Ann Roddick
> Support, education, & referrals for women 16 years & over.

Lindsay

Manufacturers: Erotica: Leather
⌀■ **L. C. Fantasia**
109 Kent Street, Lindsay, Ontario K9V 2Y5.
☎ 705 328 3998

London

Counsellors
⌀▼ **Kirk Bates**
1105 Richmond Street, London, Ontario N6A 3K4.
☎ 519 679 6197
Psychotherapy & counselling. Special interests include trauma survivors, sexual orientation issues, & HIV/AIDS. For lesbians, gays, bisexuals, & transgenderists, 16 & over.

Helplines: Sexuality
⌀▽ **Homophile Association of London Ontario Inc. (HALO)**
Gayline, 649 Colburne Street, London, Ontario N6A 3Z2.
☎ 519 433 3511
⏱ Mon - Thurs 19:00 - 22:00, answering machine at other times
Volunteer peer counselling. Provides information, resources, & referrals.

Organizations: AIDS: Education
☺□ **AIDS Committee of London**
&. Suite 301, 343 Richmond Street, London, Ontario N6A 3C2.
☎ 519 434 8160 (information) ✆ 519 434 1843
☎ 519 434 1601 (office)
⏱ 09:00 - 17:00, answering machine at other times. Hotline Mon - Thurs 09:00 21:00, Fri 09:00 - 17:00
Education & support to meet the challenges of HIV/AIDS.

Organizations: Health
☺□ **Options Clinic**
&. 659 Dundas Street East, London, Ontario N5W 2Z1.
☎ 519 673 4427 ✆ 519 642 4532
⏱ Mon, Tues, Fri 10:00 - 16:00, Wed 15:00 - 21:00, Thurs 13:00 - 17:00
Anonymous HIV testing with pre- & post-test counselling.

Organizations: Sexuality
⌀▽ **Homophile Association of London Ontario Inc. (HALO)**
&. 649 Colbourne Street, London, Ontario N6A 3Z2.
☎ 519 433 3762
⏱ Weekdays 09:00 - 12:00
Publishes *HALO Newsletter* 10 times a year.

Organizations: Sexuality: Student
⌀▽ **Gay & Lesbian Peer Counselling Group**
&. Student Centre, University of Western Ontario, London, Ontario N6A 3K7.
☎ 519 661 3031 ✆ 519 661 3949
⏱ 08:30 - 17:00, answering machine at other times
Support & counselling for students, & their friends, roommates, & families.

⌀▽ **University Students' Council - GLBi Commissioner**
&. Room 340 University Community Centre, University of Western Ontario, London, Ontario N6A 3K7.
☎ 519 661 3574 ✆ 519 661 2094
⏱ Weekdays 08:30 - 16:30
Support & information for the student body.

⌀▽ **UWOUT**
&. Room 340, University Community Centre, University of Western Ontario, London, Ontario N6A 3K7.
☎ 519 432 3078
Answering machine with information.

Organizations: Sexuality: Youth
⌀▽ **Positivity About Youth Sexual Orientation (PAYSO)**
c/o AIDS Committee of London, 343 Richmond Street, London, Ontario N6A 3C2.
☎ 519 434 1604
⏱ Meets 19:30 - 21:00. Telephone weekdays 09:00 - 17:00
Support group for gay, lesbian, & bisexual youth 21 & under.

Radio: Sexuality
⌀▽ **Rainbow Radio Network**
CHRW 94.7 FM, Room 250, University Community Centre, University of Western Ontario, London, Ontario N6A 3K7.
☎ 519 661 3601
⏱ Broadcasts Tues 22:00 - 00:00
Telephone is CHRW office administration that has answering machine with information.

Stores: Books: General
☺■ **Mystic Bookshop**
&. 616 Dundas Street, London, Ontario N5W 2Z1.
☎ 519 673 5440
☺▽ **Womansline Books**
711 Richmond Street, London, Ontario N6A 3H1.
☎ 519 679 3416
&. ✓ ✆ 💳 ◧

MacTier

Organizations: AIDS: Support
☺□ **Parry Sound - Muskoka AIDS Committee**
P. O. Box 173, MacTier, Ontario P0C 1H0.
☎ 800 267 2437 (Hotline) ✆ 705 375 0529
☎ 705 375 1080
⏱ 09:00 - 17:00, answering machine at other times
Support & education for people infected with or affected by HIV/AIDS.

Mississauga

Organizations: AIDS: Support
☺□ **Peel HIV/AIDS Network (PHAN)**
Suite 402, 10 Kingsbridge Garden Circle, Mississauga, Ontario L5R 3K6.
☎ 905 890 8770 ✆ 905 890 8505
⏱ 09:00 - 17:00, answering machine at other times
A group of people & organizations committed to serving people infected with & affected by HIV/AIDS, service providers, & the community of Peel through support, education, & advocacy.

Organizations: Health
♿□ **Sexual Assault/Rape Crisis Centre of Peel**
&. P. O. Box 2311, Square One Post Office, Mississauga, Ontario L5B 3C8.
☎ 905 273 3337
⏱ 09:00 - 17:00, answering machine at other times
24 hour crisis & support telephone service, counselling, public education for women.

Organizations: Sexuality
⌀▽ **Gay Information Mississauga**
&. ☎ 905 891 1716
⏱ Meets Tue 19:00. Answering machine has information
Provides up-to-date materials & pamphlets on gay issues, referral services, & support groups.

⚎■ **Monarch Social Club**
P. O. Box 386, Station A, Mississauga, Ontario L5A 3A1.
☎ 416 949 6602
Publishes a newsletter.

Organizations: Sexuality: Youth
⌀▽ **Coalition for Bisexual, Gay, & Lesbian Youth in Peel**
c/o Jean Clipsham, 3038 Hurontatio Street, Mississauga, Ontario L5B 3B9.
☎ 416 925 XTRA Ext.: 2142
Support, education, & advocacy for youth. Meets Tues 19:00 - 21:00. Call for details.

Photographers: Erotic
☺ **Ted Samotowka**
Darkside Studios, 941 Lakeshore Road East, Mississauga, Ontario L5E 1E3.
☎ 905 760 3390

Printers: General
☺■ **McLaren Morris & Todd Ltd.**
3270 American Drive, Mississauga, Ontario L4V 1B5.
☎ 905 677 3592 ✆ 905 677 3675
☺■ **RBW Graphics**
Suite 800, 5925 Airport Road, Mississauga, Ontario L4V 1W1.
☎ 905 677 7468 ✆ 905 677 7911

Stores: Erotica: General
☺■ **Lovecraft**
2200 Dundas Street East, Mississauga, Ontario L4X 2V3.
☎ 416 276 5772

Niagara Falls

Distributors: Books: General
☺ **John Coutts Library Services, Ltd.**
P. O. Box 1000, Niagara Falls, Ontario L2E 7E7.
☎ 905 356 6382 ✆ 905 356 5064
Wholesales books to libraries.

Helplines: Sexuality

North Bay
Helplines: Sexuality
☿▽ **Gays, Lesbian, & Bisexuals of North Bay Area (GLB NBA)**
P. O. Box 1362, North Bay, Ontario P1B 8K5.
☎ 705 495 4545
🕐 19:00 - 21:00, answering machine with recorded message at other times
🕯 ✓ $
Social & support group for gays, lesbians, & bisexuals. Recorded message has information about planned events. Age statement of 18 is required. French also spoken.

Organizations: AIDS: Education
☺☐ **AIDS Committee of North Bay & Area**
Suite 202, 240 Algonquin Avenue, North Bay, Ontario P1B 8J1.
☎ 705 497 3560 ✆ 705 497 7850
🕐 09:00 - 17:00, answering machine at other times
Support, education, & anonymous phoneline.

Organizations: Sexuality
☿▽ **Gays, Lesbian, & Bisexuals of North Bay Area (GLB NBA)**
P. O. Box 1362, North Bay, Ontario P1B 8K5.
☎ 705 495 4545
🕐 19:00 - 21:00, answering machine with recorded message at other times
🕯 ✓ $
Social & support group for gays, lesbians, & bisexuals. Recorded message has information about planned events. Age statement of 18 is required. French also spoken.

North York
Organizations: Sexuality: Student
☿▽ **Bisexual, Lesbian, & Gay Alliance at York (BLGAY)**
♿ Room 449C, Student Centre, York University, 4700 Keele Street, North York, Ontario M3J 1P3.
☎ 416 736 2100 Ext.: 20494
☎ 416 925 9872 #2116
Peer counselling, education, & meetings. Answering machine at main number, recorded information at 2nd. number.

Orillia
Organizations: Sexuality
☿▽ **Gay & Lesbian Association of Simcoe County**
P. O. Box 2224, Orillia, Ontario L3Z 6S1.
☎ 613 325 0033
Publishes *The Umbrella*.

Oshawa
Manufacturers: Whips
☺▼ **Sunnypatch Works**
341 Jarvis Street, Oshawa, Ontario L1G 5L1.
☎ 905 571 3896
🕐 Open every day, by appoinment only
Whips & floggers. Also, leather, skin, wood, & papier-maâché custom art.

Organizations: BDSM
☿▽ **Durham Alliance Association**
7-717 Wilson Road South, Oshawa, Ontario L1H 6E9.
☎ 905 434 4297

Printers: General
☺ **Maracle Press**
1156 King Street East, Oshawa, Ontario L1H 7N4.
☎ 905 723 3438 ✆ 905 428 6024

Stores: Erotica: General
☺■ **Naughty But Nice**
205 King Street, Oshawa, Ontario L1J 2J5.
☎ 416 576 5826
Also mail order. Catalogue available.

Ottawa
Archives: Sexuality
☿▽ **Pink Triangle Services Library**
♿ P. O. Box 3034, Station D, Ottawa, Ontario K1P 6H6.
☎ 613 563 4818
🌐 http://www.ncf.carleton.ca/freenet/rootdir/menus/sigs/life/gay/events/library
🕐 Mon Wed Thu 18:30 - 20:00, Sat 13:00 - 16:00

Over 3,000 items, both fiction & non-fiction, all on LGB issues. No-fee lending library. Located on 2nd. Floor, 78 Bank Street.

Bars: BDSM
☿▼ **The Cellblock**
340 Somerset Street West, Ottawa, Ontario K2P 0J9.
☎ 613 594 0233
🕐 21:00 - 01:30

BBSs: BDSM
☺■ **The Pig Pen**
✆ 613 723 3143

Counsellors
☿■ **Christianne Racine**
302 Saint Patrick, Ottawa, Ontario K1N 5K5.
☎ 613. 562 0523
Counselling for addiction, sexual abuse, & couple counselling.

Health Services
☺☐ **STD Clinic**
250 Besserer Street, Ottawa, Ontario.
☎ 613 234 0747
Free information & confidential testing for STDs.

Helplines: Sexuality
☿▽ **Lambda Line**
☎ 613 233 8212
☿▽ **Ottawa Gayline / Télégai Ottawa**
♿ P. O. Box 3043, Station D, Ottawa, Ontario K1P 6H6.
☎ 613 238 1717
☎ 613 237 XTRA #2017
🕐 19:00 - 22:00, answering machine at other times
Bilingual phoneline providing information, referrals, counselling, & AIDS information.

Organizations: AIDS: Education
☺☐ **AIDS Committee of Ottawa**
♿ 4th. Floor, 207 Queen Street, Ottawa, Ontario K1P 6E5.
☎ 613 238 5014 ✆ 613 238 3425
🕐 09:00 - 17:00, answering machine at other times
Individual & group counselling, education, legal clinic, & drop-in centre for those infected with/ or affected by HIV/AIDS.

Organizations: BDSM
☿▽ **Ottawa Knights**
P.O. Box 9174, Ottawa, Ontario K1G 3T9.
☎ 613 237 9872 Ext.: 2038 ✆ 613 237 9833
☎ 613 237 9833
🕐 Meets 2nd. Sat of month
✓
Organizes the Mr. Leather contest each November. French also spoken.

Organizations: Health
☿▽ **Ottawa Physicians for Lesbian & Gay Health**
Suite 207, 267 O'Connor Street, Ottawa, Ontario K2P 1V3.
☎ 613 563 3331
🕐 08:30 - 16:30, answering machine at other times
Support for lesbian & gay physicians, residents, interns, & medical students in the Ottawa region.
☺☐ **Sexual Assault Support Centre - Ottawa**
P. O. Box 4441, Station E, Ottawa, Ontario K1S 5B4.
☎ 613 234 2266 (24 hrs.) ✆ 613 725 9259
☎ 613 725 1657
🕐 09:00 - 16:00, answering machine at other times
24 hour crisis line, support, & counselling for women, referrals for men. Information also from 613 237 XTRA #2078.

Organizations: Sexuality
☿▽ **Association of Lesbians & Gays of Ottawa**
P. O. Box 2919, Station D, Ottawa, Ontario K1P 5W9.
☎ 613 233 0152 ✆ 613 237 8727
☎ 613 238 9872 #2047 (English), 613 238 9872 #2056 (Français)
🕐 Meets 4th. Tue of each month 18:30. Telephone number has answering machine with information
🕯 ✓ $ 💳
Bilingual, non-profit volunteer organization.
▽▽ **FACT—Ottawa**
P. O. Box 7421, Ottawa, Ontario K1L 8E4.
☎ 819 770 1945
▽▽ **Gender Mosaic**
P. O. Box 7421, Ottawa, Ontario K1L 8E4.
☎ 819 770 1945
☎ 613 749 5203
Publishes *Notes From the Underground*.

Organizations: Sexuality: Student

☿▽ **Algonquin College Lesbigays**
 ☎ 613 238 1717
 ➽ http://www.ncf.carleton.ca/freeport/sigs/life/gay/algonquin/menu
 ⏱ Telephone Gayline / Télégai 19:00 - 22:00

☿▽ **Carleton University Gay, Lesbian, & Bisexual**
 ♿ **Centre**
 401 Unicentre Building, Carleton University, Ottawa, Ontario K1S 5B6.
 ☎ 613 788 2600 Ext.: 1860 ✆ 613 788 3704
 ☎ 613 237 9872 Ext. 2022
 ➽ http://www.ncf.carleton.ca/freenet/rootdir/menus/sigs/life/gay/car
 leton/about
 ⏱ Meets Thu eve.. 2nd. number 09:00 - 17:00, answering machine
 at other times
 A safe place for gay, lesbian, & bisexual students. Resource centre &
 weekly coming out groups.

☿▽ **Cégep de l'Outaouais**
 ☎ 613 771 4344
 ☎ 613 237 9872 Ext. 2014
 ➽ http://www.ncf.carleton.ca/freeport/sigs/life/gay/cegep/menu

☿▽ **Lesbigays Cité Collégiale**
 ➽ http://www.ncf.carleton.ca/freeport/sigs/life/gay/colleg/menu

☿▽ **University of Ottawa Lesbigays**
 c/o OPIRG, University of Ottawa, Ottawa, Ontario.
 ☎ 613 230 3076
 ☎ 613 237 9872 Ext. 2027
 ✉ be167@freenet.carleton.ca
 ➽ http://www.ncf.carleton.ca/freeport/sigs/life/gay/uottawa/menu
 ⏱ Meets weekly during term time

Organizations: Sexuality: Youth

☿▽ **Lesbian & Gay Youth Ottawa Hull**
 P. O. Box 2919, Station D, Ottawa, Ontario K1P 5W9.
 ☎ 613 729 1000
 ☎ 613 237 9872 Ext. 2014
 ➽ http://www.ncf.carleton.ca/freenet/rootdir/menus/sigs/life/gay/org
 s/youth.res
 ⏱ Wed 19:30

Piercers

☺ ■ **Denise Robinson Body Art (DEXTRA)**
 P. O. Box 53063, Ottawa, Ontario K1N 1C5.
 ☎ 613 567 9033
 ✆ 613 567 6534
 ⏱ By appointment only
 Use BBS line to book appointments online. Custom orders available.

☺ ■ **Living Colour Tattoo**
 2nd. Floor, 70 George Street, Ottawa, Ontario K1N 8W5.
 ☎ 613 789 7187 ✆ 613 833 1596
 ✉ blckstar@magi.com
 ➽ http://infoweb.magi.com/~blckstar

Printers: General

☺ ■ **Tri-Graphic Printing (Ottawa) Ltd.**
 485 Industrial Drive, Ottawa, Ontario K1G 0Z1.
 ☎ 613 731 7441 ✆ 613 731 3741

Publishers: Directories: Libraries

☺ ■ **Canadian Library Association**
 Suite 602, 200 Elgin Street, Ottawa, Ontario K2P 1L5.
 ☎ 613 232 9626 Ext.: 301 ✆ 613 563 9895

Publishers: Directories: Sexuality

☿▼ **Lambda Press**
 P. O. Box 1445, Station B, Ottawa, Ontario K1P 5P6.

Publishers: Magazines: Sexuality

☿▽ **Go Info**
 P. O. Box 2919, Station A, Ottawa, Ontario K1P 5W9.
 ☎ 613 238 8990 ✆ 613 748 0076
 ♿ ✓ 𝗩𝗜𝗦𝗔
 The monthly revue of lesbians, gays, & bisexuals of Ottawa. Published
 10 times a year. Yearly subscription is $24.

☿▽ **OUTawa Magazine**
 111 Albert Street, Ottawa, Ontario K1P 1A5.
 ☎ 613 241 3432

⚢ ▼ **The Womanist**
 ♿ 3rd. Floor, 41 York Street, Ottawa, Ontario K1N 5S7.
 ☎ 613 562 4081
 ✓

Publishers: Newspapers: Sexuality

☿▽ **Capital Xtra!**
 ♿ Pink Triangle Press, P. O. Box 544, Station B, Ottawa, Ontario K1P 5P6.

 ☎ 613 237 7133 ✆ 613 237 6651
 ✉ ao993@freenet.carleton.ca
 ⏱ 09:00 - 18:00
 ♿ ✓ $ 𝗩𝗜𝗦𝗔 𝗠𝗖
 Professionally produced newspaper, covering the national capital region's
 lesbian & gay community. News, arts, culture, & politics. Published
 every month. Yearly subscription is $21.95.

☺ ▼ **Hot & Bothered**
 USECA Communications Inc., 3rd. Floor, 31 York Street, Ottawa, Ontario
 K1N 5S7.
 ☎ 613 241 9499 ✆ 613 241 9493
 Monthly newspaper on positive erotica that combines fun sexuality with
 sexual health information. Published every month. Yearly subscription is
 $24.95 Cdn.

⚲▼ **Lite & Lively**
 P. O. Box 56120, Minto Place Postal Outlet, Laurier Avenue West,
 Ottawa, Ontario.

Radio: Sexuality

☿▽ **People Like You**
 ⏱ Tue 18:00

Stores: Books: General

☿▼ **After Stonewall**
 2nd. Floor, 105 4th. Street, Ottawa, Ontario K1S 2L1.
 ☎ 613 567 2221 ✆ 613 567 0752
 ♿ ✓ 𝗩𝗜𝗦𝗔 𝗠𝗖

☺ **Food For Thought Books**
 11 William Street, Ottawa, Ontario.
 ☎ 613 236 3361

☺ ■ **Octopus Books**
 732 Bank Street, Ottawa, Ontario K1S 3V8.
 ☎ 613 236 2589

☿▼ **Ottawa Women's Bookstore**
 ♿ 272 Elgin Street, Ottawa, Ontario K2P 1M2.
 ☎ 613 230 1156 𝗠𝗖

Stores: Clothing: Fetish

☺ ■ **Skin Tight**
 1750 Boulevard Saint Laurent, Ottawa, Ontario.
 ☎ 613 523 2708

Stores: Erotica: General

☺ ■ **Marc's Smokeshop**
 420 Rideau Street, Ottawa, Ontario K1N 5Z1.
 ☎ 613 789 8886

☿▼ **Wilde's**
 631 Somerset Street West, Ottawa, Ontario K1R 5K3.
 ☎ 613 567 4858

Owen Sound

Manufacturers: Clothing: Fetish

☺ ■ **Fantasyland Products**
 ♿ P. O. Box 682, Owen Sound, Ontario N4K 5R4.
 ☎ 519 371 1215 ✆ 519 371 2975
 ⏱ 10:00 - 17:30, Fri - 20:30, Sun by appointment, Dec 15-23 10:00
 - 20:30. 24hr. answering machine
 ♿ $ 𝗩𝗜𝗦𝗔 𝗠𝗖 𝗔𝗠𝗘𝗫
 PVC, Lycra, & fantasy clothing. Custom cuts, private fashion consultation
 & designs for everyone's needs. Also little girl fashions for adults.
 Catalogue, $5 for catalogue of catalogues. Age statement of 18 is
 required.

Organizations: AIDS: Support

☺ ☐ **AIDS Committe of Grey-Bruce**
 P. O. Box 710, Owen Sound, Ontario N4K 5W9.
 ☎ 800 331 6831 (within 519 area)
 ☎ 519 372 9362
 ⏱ Tues & Thurs 19:00 - 21:00, answering machine at other times
 Up-to-date information on all aspects of HIV/AIDS. Support services for
 those infected with or affected by HIV/AIDS.

Organizations: Sexuality

☿▽ **People of Alternate Lifestyles (PALS)**
 ☎ 519 371 8707
 Support group for lesbian, gay, & bisexuals in Grey-Bruce counties.

Stores: Erotica: General

⚲ ■ **Fantasyland Products**
 ♿ P. O. Box 682, Owen Sound, Ontario N4K 5R4.
 ☎ 519 371 1215 ✆ 519 371 2975
 ⏱ 10:00 - 17:30, Fri - 20:30, Sun by appointment. 24hr. answering
 machine
 ♿ $ 𝗩𝗜𝗦𝗔 𝗠𝗖 𝗔𝗠𝗘𝗫

Store front (sex shoppe plus four private rooms catering to TVs). 16 catalogues for $80; $25 sampler pack; New! Fantasy videos! Fashion $59.95, wedding $39.95, "Lil Girl Birthday" $29.95. For info only: SASE (or IRC) plus $1Cdn.. Catalogue, $5 for catalogue of catalogues. Age statement of 18 is required.

Peterborough

Distributors: Books: General

☺ ■ **Marginal Distribution**
Unit 102, 277 George Street, Peterborough, Ontario K9J 3G9.
☎ 705 745 2326 ✆ 705 745 2326
marginal@ptbo.igs.net
http://ptbo.igs.net/~marginal/index.htm
Also mail order.

Organizations: AIDS: Support

☺ □ **Peterborough AIDS Resource Network**
♿ P. O. Box 1582, Peterborough, Ontario K9J 7H7.
☎ 800 361 2895 (information) ✆ 705 749 6310
☎ 705 749 9110 (office)
🕘 Mon - Wed & Fri 09:00 - 17:00, Thurs 09:00 - 19:00, answering machine
Support & information on HIV/AIDS issues.

Saint Catharines

Organizations: AIDS: Support

☺ □ **AIDS Niagara**
♿ Suite 200, 50 William Street, Saint Catharines, Ontario L2R 5G2.
☎ 905 984 8684 ✆ 905 988 1921
🕘 Weekdays 08:30 - 16:30, answering machine at other times
Education & support to improve the lives of those infected with or affected by HIV/AIDS, & to prevent the spread of HIV.

Organizations: Family

☺ □ **Parents & Friends of Lesbians & Gays (PFLAG)—Saint Catharines**
☎ 905 934 9933
🕘 09:00 - 23:00
Support group for parents, families, & friends of lesbians & gays.

Publishers: Magazines: Sexuality

☺ ■ ***It's Okay!***
Phœnix Counsel, Inc., 1 Springbank Drive, Saint Catharines, Ontario L2S 2K1.
☎ 905 685 0496
🕘 Mon - Thu 10:00 - 17:00
About sexuality for the disabled. Published quarterly. Yearly subscription is $23.95 Cdn. in Cdn., $23.95 U.S. elsewhere.

Saint Thomas

Publishers: Guides: Sexuality

⚢▼ ***London Pink Pathways***
P. O. Box 20072, Saint Thomas, Ontario N5P 1B9.

Sault Saint Marie

Organizations: AIDS: Support

☺ □ **Algoma AIDS Network**
789 Queen Street East, Sault Saint Marie, Ontario P6A 2A8.
☎ 800 361 2497 (information) ✆ 705 256 1182
☎ 705 256 2437 (office)
🕘 Weekdays 10:00 - 18:00, Sat 12:00 - 18:00, answering machine at other times
Support for People Living with HIV/AIDS (PHAs) & their friends & families.

Scarborough

Manufacturers: Regalia

☺ ■ **Muir Cap & Regalia**
1550 O'Connor Drive, Scarborough, Ontario.
☎ 416 757 2815
Makers of the Muir cap.

Printers: General

☺ ■ **Aprinco Book Manufacturers**
30 Casebridge Court, Scarborough, Ontario M1B 3M5.
☎ 416 286 6688 Ext.: 22

Stratford

Organizations: AIDS: Support

☺ □ **AIDS Action Committee of Perth County**
♿ 86 Saint John Street South, Stratford, Ontario N5A 2Y8.
☎ 519 272 2437 ✆ 519 272 2437
🕘 08:00 - 16:00, answering machine at other times
Support, counselling, & direct financial support for people infected with or affected by HIV/AIDS. Library & educational services. Meets 3rd. Wed of each month.

Stores: Books: General

☺ ■ **Fanfare Books**
30 Waterloo Street South, Stratford, Ontario N5A 6T1.
☎ 519 273 1010

Sudbury

Organizations: AIDS: Education

☺ □ **AIDS Committee of Sudbury ACCESS**
♿ Unit 203, 111 Elm Street, Sudbury, Ontario P3C 1T3.
☎ 800 465 2437 (information) ✆ 705 688 0423
☎ 705 688 0505 (office)
🕘 Weekdays 09:00 - 17:00, answering machine at other times
Education & support for people infected with or affected by HIV/AIDS. 800 number from 705 area only.

Organizations: Health

♀ □ **Sudbury Sexual Assault Crisis Centre**
3rd. Floor, 156 Durham Street, Sudbury, Ontario P3E 3M7.
☎ 705 675 1323 (24 hrs.) ✆ 705 675 2641
☎ 705 675 3032 TTY
🕘 09:00 - 17:00
Information, counselling, education, & outreach for women 16 & over.

Organizations: Sexuality

⚢▽ **Sudbury All Gay Alliance (SAGA)**
P. O. Box 1092, Station B, Sudbury, Ontario P3E 4S6.
☎ 705 670 2262
🕘 Answering machine with information
Peer counselling, support groups, & referrals. Also hosts P-FLAG (Parents & Friends of Lesbians & Gays).

Radio: Sexuality

⚢▽ ***Speaking Out***
c/o CFLR Radio, Cable 106.7 FM, 935 Ramsey Lake Road, Sudbury, Ontario P3E 2C6.
☎ 705 673 8152
🕘 Broadcast last Fri of the month 18:30
Monthly half-hour broadcasts containing issues relevant to local lesbians, bisexuals, & gays.

Thornhill

BBSs: Sexuality

⚢▼ **Gay Blade**
✆ 905 882 4800

Thunder Bay

Organizations: AIDS: Support

☺ □ **AIDS Committee of Thunder Bay (ACT-B)**
P. O. Box 24025, Downtown N Postal Outlet, Thunder Bay, Ontario P7A 4T0.
☎ 807 345 7233 (information) ✆ 807 345 2505
☎ 807 345 1516 (office)
🕘 Weekdays 09:30 - 17:00, answering machine with information at other times
Support, education, & prevention for anyone in the Thunder Bay & North-Western Ontario region infected with or affected by HIV/AIDS.

Organizations: Family

☺ □ **Parents & Friends of Lesbians & Gays (PFLAG)—Thunder Bay**
☎ 807 345 1516
🕘 09:30 - 17:00, answering machine
Supportive environment for parent, friends, & family to talk about issues relating to lesbian, gay, & bisexual relationships.

Organizations: Health

☺ □ **Thunder Bay District Health Unit**
♿ 999 Balmoral Street, Thunder Bay, Ontario P1B 5J5.
☎ 807 625 5981 ✆ 807 623 2369
🕘 Weekdays 08:30 - 16:30, answering machine at other times
HIV counselling & anonymous testing.

☺ □ **Thunder Bay Physical & Sexual Assault Centre**
♿ 385 Mooney Street, Thunder Bay, Ontario P7B 5L5.
☎ 807 344 4502 (24 Hrs.) ✆ 807 344 1981
☎ 807 345 0894
Counselling, referrals, & information services for men & women over 14 years of age.

Organizations: Sexuality: Student

☺ □ **Gender Issues Centre**
♿ Lakehead University Student Union, 955 Oliver Road, Thunder Bay,

Ontario P7B 5E1.
☎ 807 343 8897
🕾 807 343 8598
🕐 08:30 - 16:30

Stores: Books: General

☿▼ **Rainbow Books**
264 Bay Street, Thunder Bay, Ontario P7B 1R5.
☎ 807 345 6272

Timmins

Stores: Books: General

☺■ **Grapevine Books**
249 Third Avenue, Timmins, Ontario P4N 1E2.
☎ 705 268 0181

Toronto

Accommodation: BDSM

☿▼ **Muther's**
508 Eastern Avenue, Toronto, Ontario M4M 1C5.
☎ 416 466 8616

Archives: Sexuality

☿▽ **Canadian Lesbian & Gay Archives**
⚲ P. O. Box 639, Station A, Toronto, Ontario M5W 1G2.
☎ 416 777 2755
🕾 416 251 8285
☎ 416 925 XTRA #2033
🕐 Tues - Thurs 19:30 - 22:00
🕮 ✓ 📷 VISA
Repository, library, & research centre for all relevant, recordable information by & about lesbians & gays, their histories, ideas, lifestyles, cultures, politics, etc.. Open to the public for research or browsing. Answering machine with information.

Artists: BDSM

☺▼ **Dan Bowers**
Suite 333, 253 College Street, Toronto, Ontario M5T 1R5
☎ 416 962 6969
📧 danbowers@inforamp.net
🕐 09:00 - 17:00, answering machine at other times
Graphics designer, credited with over 100 leather / BDSM posters, magazine / book covers, & printed illustrations. Other services, include magazine & advertising design. Specializes in gay marketing & gay publications.

Bars: BDSM

☿▼ **The Barn**
2nd. Floor, 418 Church Street, Toronto, Ontario M5B 2A3.
☎ 416 977 4702

☺▼ **Black Eagle**
2nd. Floor, 459 Church Street, Toronto, Ontario M4Y 1C5.
☎ 800 387 1420
☎ 416 413 1219
📧 eagle@io.org
🌐 http://www.io.org/~eagle
🕐 Mon - Fri 16:00 - 01:00, Sat 14:00 - 01:00, Sun 12:00 - 01:00

☿▼ **Kurbash**
592 Sherbourne Street, Toronto, Ontario M4X 1L4.
☎ 416 921 0665
🕾 416 923 3177
🕐 21:00 - 01:00
🕮 ✓ $ ⚲ VISA 💳
Also hotel rooms.

☿▼ **The Toolbox**
Å⚲ 508 Eastern Avenue, Toronto, Ontario M4M 1C5.
☎ 416 466 8616

BBSs: BDSM

☺■ **Port Kar BBS**
☏ 416 975 4068. 28800 baud maximum.
📧 thom@inforamp.net
🌐 http://www.inforamp.net/~thom/index.html
🕐 24hrs.
Pan-sexual, fetish-oriented BBS, devoted to the BDSM, fetish lifestyle. In operation for over three years.

BBSs: General

☺▼ **POWERarts Presence Provider**
P. O. Box 19578-255, Manulife Centre, 55 Bloor Street West, Toronto, Ontario M4W 3T9.
☎ 416 962 9696
📧 inforequest@powerarts.com
🌐 http://www.powerarts.com
🕐 09:00 - 17:00, answering machine at other times
BDSM-friendly Internet presence provider & graphics studio with our own private & secure web servers. We also offer other types of services, including magazine & advertising design. We specialize in gay

marketing & gay publications.

Counsellors

☿■ **Paul Armstrong**
⚲ P. O. Box 65133, Toronto, Ontario M4K 3Z2.
☎ 416 351 9430
Individual, couple, & family consultations for relationships, coming out, HIV/AIDS issues, & sexual abuse & trauma. Answering machine.

☿▼ **Joyce Barnett**
☎ 416 698 5183
🕐 Weekdays 09:00 - 17:00, answering machine at other times
Counselling & psychotherapy for women & gay men from a feminist perspective. Background in clinical psychology & theology.

☺■ **Bob Burgoyne, M.S.W.**
661 Carlaw Avenue, Toronto, Ontario M4K 3K6.
☎ 416 463 0950
Over 15 years of experience in personal, relationship, & family counselling services. Advanced training in sexuality & sex therapy.

☿▼ **Michael Hazelton**
P. O. Box 65133, Toronto, Ontario M4K 3Z2.
☎ 416 604 3958
🕐 Call anytime, answering machine
Individual, couple, & family therapy & counselling. Specializes in coming out, men's issues, relationships, sexual orientation, & HIV/AIDS.

☿▼ **Donna MacAuley**
⚲ Suite 408, 550 Ontario Street, Toronto, Ontario M4X 1X3.
☎ 416 925 9497
🕐 Mon - Sat 09:00 - 20:00, answering machine
Psychotherapy & counselling for issues including coming out & partner abuse.

☿▼ **John Montague**
Suite 2103, 980 Broadview Avenue, Toronto, Ontario M4K 3Y1.
☎ 416 463 6097
Private practice counselling gay men with issues such as coming out, marriage, HIV/AIDS, relationships, & sexual abuse & addiction. Answering machine.

☿■ **Psychotherapy Institute**
Suite 312, 120 Carlton Street, Toronto, Ontario M5A 4K2.
☎ 416 968 0640
🕐 Mon & Wed 09:00 - 18:00, Tues & Thurs 09:00 - 16:00, Fri 09:00 - 13:00, call for appointment
Therapy provided by co-therapists; one medical practitioner & one non-medical practitioner. Individuals, couples, or groups.

☿▼ **Janet Richards**
☎ 416 588 2030
🕐 08:00 - 22:00, answering machine
Private practice offering psychotherapy & counselling from a feminist perspective.

☿■ **Peter Scargall**
⚲ Suite 212, 111 Davisville Avenue, Toronto, Ontario M4S 1G5.
☎ 416 486 0014
☎ 416 486 0014 TTY
Counselling groups, couples, & individuals with sexual orientation &/or coming out concerns. Answering machine.

Health Services

☺□ **AIDS Prevention & Sexual Health Program**
⚲ 6th. Floor, 277 Victoria Street, Toronto, Ontario M5B 1W1.
☎ 416 392 2437
🕐 Weekdays 10:00 - 21:00, weekends & holidays 11:00 - 17:00
City of Toronto Public Health Department program offering HIV/AIDS & sexuality information, counselling, & referrals for all Toronto residents, workers, & visitors.

☺□ **Bay Centre for Birth Control**
⚲ 8th. Floor, 790 Bay Street, Toronto, Ontario M5G 1N9.
☎ 416 351 3700
🕾 416 351 3727
☎ 416 351 3724 TTY
Counselling & information on family planning, sexuality, pregnancy testing, & STDs, & anonymous HIV testing & counselling.

☺■ **John Goodhew, M.D.**
Ⓚ 416 461 2200
BDSM, fetish, & body art/modification friendly doctor.

♂□ **Hassle Free Clinic - Men**
2nd. Floor, 556 Church Street, Toronto, Ontario M4Y 2E3.
☎ 416 922 0603
🕐 Mon & Wed 16:00 - 21:00, Tues & Thurs 10:00 - 15:00, Fri 16:00 - 19:00, Sat 10:00 - 14:00. Answering machine at other times
STD & anonymous HIV testing. Free condoms, bleach kits, & needle exchange. HIV/AIDS support & counselling by appointment.

♀□ **Hassle Free Clinic - Women**
2nd. Floor, 556 Church Street, Toronto, Ontario M4Y 2E3.
☎ 416 922 0556
🕐 Drop-in STD testing Tues & Thurs 16:00 - 18:00, appointments

required for oter times. Appointment required for anonymous HIV testing
STD, pregnancy, & anonymous HIV testing. Birth control information & counselling available. Sexuality counselling. Needle exchange.

Helplines: AIDS

Minstry of Health AIDS Hotline
800 668 AIDS (English)
800 267 SIDA (French)
Weekdays 10:00 - 21:00, weekends & holidays 11:00 - 17:00
Information & referrals for AIDS issues.

Helplines: Sexuality

Lesbian & Gay Bashing Reporting & Information Line
Community Centre, 519 Church Street, Toronto, Ontario M4Y 2C9.
416 392 6877 (Hotline)
416 392 6874 TDD
Support & information for those who have been assaulted (verbally or physically). Reports can be made anonymously. Witnesses are encouraged to report incidents of violence.

Lesbian Gay Bi Youth Line
P. O. Box 62, Station F, Toronto, Ontario M6G 3V6.
800 268 9688
416 962 9688
15:00 - 23:00 (all lines)
Peer support & information to youth of all cultures who identify as lesbian, gay, bisexual, queer, two-spirited, &/or transgendered. TDD on all line. For further information, call 416 925 XTRA #2179.

Toronto Area Gay/Lesbian Phoneline & Crisis Counselling (TAGL)
P. O. Box 632, Station F, Toronto, Ontario M4Y 2N6.
416 964 6600
416 925 XTRA #2119
Mon - Sat 19:00 - 22:00, answering machine at other times
Volunteer group providing information (from AIDS to bar locations), peer counselling, & support.

Manufacturers: Erotica: Leather

Mac Leather
416 469 3459 (Brian)
416 966 1851
By appointment only
Custom leather clothing.

Northbound Leather Ltd.
7 Saint Nicholas Street, Toronto, Ontario M4Y 1W5.
416 972 1037 — Fax 416 975 1337
leather@northbound.com
http://www.northbound.com/
Mon - Wed Sat 10:00 - 18:00, Fri Sat 10:00 - 19:30, Sun 12:00 - 17:00
Canada's largest selection of fetish fashion & accessories, including corsetry, leather clothing, books, toys, & footwear. Also has large, inviting, & beautifully designed store. Catalogue, $30Cdn. (taxes included). Shipping $5Cdn., to Cdn.$9.95Cdn. to U.S., $12.95Cdn. elswhere. Please see our display advertisements on the front & back covers.

Manufacturers: Whips

Roy Montgomery
228 Shuter Street, Toronto, Ontario M5A 4M9.

Organizations: Academic: Sexuality

Toronto Centre for Lesbian & Gay Studies
Suite 100-129, 2 Bloor Street West, Toronto, Ontario M4W 2E3.
Community-based organization to connect academic studies & community development. Provides limited grants.

Organizations: AIDS: Education

AIDS Committee of Toronto
4th. Floor, 399 Church Street, Toronto, Ontario M5B 2J6.
416 340 8844 (information) — Fax 416 340 8224
416 340 8122 (TTY)
act@hookup.net
Mon -Thurs 10:00 - 21:00, Fri 10:00 - 17:00, answering machine at other times
Support, education, counselling, & other services. Large library of HIV/AIDS information. Office number: 416 340 2437.

Community AIDS Treatment Information Exchange
Suite 420, 517 College Street, Toronto, Ontario M6G 4A2.
800 263 1638 (information) — Fax 416 928 2185
416 944 1916

Positive Youth Outreach
2nd. Floor, 399 Church Street, Toronto, Ontario M5B 2J6.
416 506 1400 — Fax 416 506 1404

Prostitutes for Safer Sex Project
P. O. Box 1143, Station F, Toronto, Ontario M4Y 2TB.
416 964 0150 — Fax 416 964 9653 (call first)

Organizations: AIDS: Research

Community Research Initiative of Toronto
Suite 1, 196 Carlton Street, Toronto, Ontario M5A 2K8.
416 324 9505 — Fax 416 324 9921

Organizations: AIDS: Support

AIDS Action Now!
suite 321, 517 College Street, Toronto, Ontario M6G 1A8.
416 928 2206 — Fax 416 928 2185

AIDS Committee of Etobicoke
399 The West Mall, Etobicoke, Ontario M9C 2Y2.
416 394 8833 (Hotline)
416 394 8893
08:30 - 17:00, answering machine at other times
Information & HIV/AIDS related services.

Positive Straight Men
Suite 232, 517 College Street, Toronto, Ontario M6G 4A2.
416 923 3253 — Fax 416 944 1803

Toronto People With AIDS Foundation
2nd. Floor, 99 Church Street, Toronto, Ontario M5B 2J6.
416 506 1400 — Fax 416 506 1404
Free support to people living with HIV/AIDS, treatment information, emergency financial assistance, etc..

Two-Spirited People of the First Nations Native Awareness Project
Suite 1006, 2 Carlton Street, Toronto, Ontario M5B 1J3.
416 944 9300 — Fax 416 944 8381

Voices of Positive Women
P. O. Box 471, Station C, Toronto, Ontario M6J 3P5.
416 324 8703 — Fax 416 324 9701

Organizations: BDSM

The Betty Page Social Club
c/o Northbound Leather, 7 Saint Nicholas Street, Toronto, Ontario M4Y 1W5.
416 972 1037
leather@northbound.com
http://www.northbound.com/bpinfo.htm

The Edge
Suite 508, 1025 Scarlet Road, Etobicoke, Ontario M9P 3V3.
416 244 9117
Meets last Fri of month
Contact: Mr. Marvin Gordon
Publishes *The Edge* quarterly. Age statement of 21 is required.

Leather Caucus of Toronto
P. O. Box 19591-882, 55 Bloor Street West, Toronto, Ontario M4W 3T9.
416 962 1040 — Fax 416 962 1044
wpc@inforamp.net
http://www.inforamp.net/~wpc/Caucus
Meets 3rd. Sun of month

The National Leather Association (NLA)—Toronto
P. O. Box 98, 268 Parliament Street, Toronto, Ontario M5A 3A4.
416 925 9872 Ext.: 2089 — Fax 416 604 3599
Local chapter of NLA International. Publishes *The Flogger*.

Spearhead
P. O. Box 1000, Station F, Toronto, Ontario M4Y 2N9.

X-Corrigia
109 Vaughan Road, Toronto, Ontario M5W 1B2.
thom@inforamp.net
http://www.inforamp.net/~thom/index.html
Meets 2nd. & 4th. Sat of the month 21:00
Contact: Mr. Thom Bowen
Age statement of 21 is required.

Organizations: Bears

Bear Buddies Toronto
P. O. Box 926, Station F, Toronto, Ontario M4Y 2N9.
cbela@hookup.net
http://www.skepsis.com/.gblo/bears/CLUBS/Bear_Buddies/

Southern Ontario Bears
P. O. Box 5542, Station A, Toronto, Ontario M5W 1N7.
SOBears@aol.com
http://www.skepsis.com:80/.gblo/bears/CLUBS/Southern_Ontario_Bears/

Organizations: Family

Children of Lesbians & Gays Everywhere

(COLAGE)
P. O. Box 187, Station F, Toronto, Ontario M4Y 2L5.

OK To Be Us
Human Sexuality Program, Toronto Board of Education, 155 College Street, Toronto, Ontario M5T 1P6.
416 397 3755 — 416 397 3758
Weekdays 09:00 - 17:00
Peer support for adolescents with lesbian, gay, & bisexual parents.

Parents & Friends of Lesbians & Gays (PFLAG)—Brampton
905 457 4570
070:00 - 22:00. Answering machine at other times
Contact: Ms. Mary Jones
Support for families & friends of lesbians & gays, & to those coming out to their families.

Parents & Friends of Lesbians & Gays (PFLAG)—Toronto
P. O. Box 2020, 3266 Yonge Street, Toronto, Ontario M4N 3P6.
416 322 0600 — 416 322 4852
416 925 XTRA #2023
Call anytime
Support & education.

Organizations: Health

The LINK
East York Health Unit Sexual Health Clinic, 850 Coxwell Avenue, East York, Ontario M4C 5R1.
416 466 7198 — 416 461 8564
Walk-in sexual health clinic in a high school for youth under 19. Suitable for one-time visits. Information, free condoms, & free medication for STD treatment.

Peel Health Department - Sexual Health Info-Line
c/o Suite 200, 180B Sandalwood Parkway East, Brampton, Ontario L6Z 4N1.
905 840 1333 — 905 840 5720
Free, confidential counselling to anyone in the community.

Sexual Assault Centre of Brantford
11 Nelson Street, Brantford, Ontario N3T 2M6.
519 751 3471 (24 hrs.) — 519 7511 4187
519 751 1164
Best to call between 09:00 & 17:00 on weekdays. Answering machine at other times

Organizations: Human Rights

Canadian Human Rights Commission—Toronto Office
10th. Floor, 175 Bloor Street East, Toronto, Ontario M4W 2R8.
416 973 5527 — 416 973 6184
416 973 8912 TTY
Weekdays 09:00 - 17:00, answering machine at other times
Government body that aims to prevent discrimination & to educate the public about human rights & the harm discrimination causes. Accepts complaints based on, amongst others, sex, sexual orientation, & national or ethnic origin.

Organizations: Publishing

Canadian Book Marketing Centre
Suite 301, 2 Gloucester Street, Toronto, Ontario.
416 413 4930
Marketing services in Canada for book publishers, includes distribution of radio interviews to Canadian radio stations.

Organizations: Sexuality

The 519 Church Street Community Centre
519 Church Street, Toronto, Ontario M4Y 2C9.
416 392 6874 — 416 392 6874
Weekdays 09:00 - 22:00, weekends 12:00 - 17:00
Amongst other services, provides support, information, & counselling for the lesbians, gay, bisexuals, & transexual community. Publishes *The Rainbow Book* once a year.

Canadian Crossdressers Club
161 Gerrard Street East, Toronto, Ontario M5A 2E4.
416 921 6112
Tues - Fri 10:00 - 19:00, Sat 11:00 - 20:00, answering machine with information
A safe, comfortable atmosphere for men to explore their feminine sides. Book & video library for education purposes. Publishes *The Canadian Crossdresser.*

The Clarke Institute of Psychiatry
Gender Identity Clinic, 250 College Street, Toronto, Ontario M5T 1R8.
416 979 2221 Ext.: 2339
Counselling, referrals, & treatment of all gender dysphoria issues. Staff also teach & are available for public speaking.

Toronto Bisexual Network
c/o The 519 Church Street Community Centre, 519 Church Street, Toronto, Ontario M4 2C9.
416 925 XTRA Ext.: 2015
Meets first Thurs of the month 18:00 - 20:00, third Thurs 20:00 - 22:00
Support, education, & information for & about bisexual men & women. Telephone has answering machine.

Transition Support
c/o The 519 Church Street Community Centre, 519 Church Street, Toronto, Ontario M4Y 2C9.
Meets 2nd. Fri of month 19:30
Publishes *Trans News*.

Xpressions
P. O. Box 223, Station A, Toronto, Ontario M5W 1B2.
416 812 6879

Organizations: Sexuality: Student

Bisexuals, Gays, & Lesbians of Ryerson (BGALOR)
c/o Ryerson Student Union, Room A62, 380 Victoria Street, Toronto, Ontario M5B 1W7.
416 979 5000 Ext.: 7527
bgalor@acs.ryerson.ca
During term time: weekdays 11:00 - 15:00, answering machine at other times
Resources centre & referrals.

Committee on Homophobia
Room 158, University College, Toronto, Ontario.
416 978 8087

Gays & Lesbians at U of T
University of Toronto, 12 Hart House Circle, Toronto, Ontario M5S 1A1.
416 971 7880

Gays & Lesbians of Humber (GLOH)
c/o SAC, 205 Humber College Boulevard, Etobicoke, Ontario M9W 5L7.
416 675 5051
09:00 - 17:00

Gays, Lesbians, & Bisexuals International
42A Saint George Street, Toronto, Ontario M5S 2E4.
416 591 7949
416 925 XTRA #2187
Weekdays 09:00 - 21:00, Sat 12:00 - 15:00, answering machine at other times
Support for gay, lesbian, & bisexual international students, visible minorites, & people for whom English is not their first language.

George Brown College Lesbian, Gay, & Bisexual Students
c/o George Brown College Student Association, 200 King Street East, Toronto, Ontario M5 3W7.
416 925 9872 Ext.: 2178
416 867 2373
dgalbrai@gbc.gbrownc.on.ca
Support for lesbian, gay, & bisexual students at the college. Telephone number has an answering machine.

Glendon Gay, Lesbian, & Bisexual Alliance (GLABA)
2275 Bayview Avenue, Toronto, Ontario M4N 3M6.
416 736 2100 Ext.: 88197
Weekdays 10:00 - 17:00, answering machine at other times

Lesbian & Gay Students of the Toronto Board of Education
c/o Human Sexuality Program, TBED, 155 College Street, Toronto, Ontario M5T 1P6.
416 397 3755 — 416 397 3758
09:00 - 17:00
Support for students in a gay/lesbian positive atmosphere.

University of Toronto Sexual Education & Peer Counselling Centre
42A Saint George Street, Toronto, Ontario M5S 2E4.
416 591 7949
416 925 XTRA #2159
Mon- Sat 09:00 - 21:00, answering machine at other times
Short term counselling, sex education, & information & referrals to the University of Toronto & surrounding community. Large resources on all aspects of sexuality.

Organizations: Sexuality: Youth

Lesbian, Gay, & Bisexual Youth of Toronto
c/o The 519 Church Street Community Centre, 519 Church Street, Toronto, Ontario M4Y 2C9.
416 925 XTRA Ext.: 2880
Meets Tues 19:30 - 22:00, Sat 13:00 - 16:00
Social, educational, peer support group for people under 25. Group is 17 years old.

☺ ☐ **Youthlink - Inner City**
149 Gerrard Street East, Toronto, Ontario M5A 2E4.
☎ 416 922 3335 📞 416 922 1282
🕐 Weekdays 09:00 - 16:00, answering machine at other times
Outreach program for street youth & youth living in the downtown core.
HIV/AIDS support, education, & prevention. Sexual abuse support &
counselling.

Organizations: Spanking

♂♀▽ **Society of Spankers**
☎ 416 925 9872 Ext.: 2102
Age statement of 18 is required.

Photographers: BDSM

☺ **Optic Verve**
☎ 416 515 7260
📧 verve@epas.utoronto.ca

Photographers: Erotic

☺ **Dan Couto**
Suite 6, 457 Richmond Street West, Toronto, Ontario M5V 1X9.
☎ 171 499 9493

Piercers

☺ ■ **Auroboros**
Suite 3, 580 Yonge Street, Toronto, Ontario M4Y 1Z3.
☎ 416 962 7499
🕐 Tue - Sat 12:00- 20:00
☺ **Body Piercing by Tee**
Suite 2, 473 Church Street, Toronto, Ontario M4Y 2C3.
☎ 416 929 7330
☺ ■ **Stainless Steel Body Art**
394A Queen Street West, Toronto, Ontario.
☎ 416 504 1433
📧 bodyart@io.org
🌐 http://www.io.org/~bodyart

Printers: General

☺ ■ **Best Book Manufacturers**
150 Front Street West, Toronto, Ontario M5A 1E5.

☎ 416 362 1872 📞 416 362 6081
☺ ■ **Metropole Lithographers**
25 Atlantic Avenue, Toronto, Ontario M6K 3E7.
☎ 416 538 4511 📞 416 530 0379

Publishers: Books: BDSM

☺ ▼ **WholeSM Publishing Corporation**
♿ P. O. Box 19591-883, 50 Bloor Street West, Toronto, Ontario M4W
3T9.
☎ 416 962 1040 📞 416 962 1044
📧 wpc@inforamp.net
🌐 http://www.inforamp.net/~wpc
🕐 Mon - Fri 09:00 - 17:00, voice mail at other times
💰 ✓ VISA
Publishers of the best seller "*On The Safe Edge: A Manual for SM Play.*"
Paperback edition $24.95Cdn. (plus G.S.T.) in Canada, £14.99 in U.K.,
$19.95U.S. in U.S. & elsewhere. Hardcover & signed, limited edition
black leather library bindings also available. Shipping $5 to U.S. &
Canada (plus G.S.T. in Canada), £7 to U.K., $8U.S. elsewhere.

Publishers: Books: Sexuality

♂♀▼ **Queer Press**
P. O. Box 485, Station P, Toronto, Ontario M5S 2T1.
☎ 416 978 8201 📞 416 978 1078
Volunteer-run community-based desktop publisher dedicated to providing
opportunities for queer self-expression.
⚤ ■ **Women's Press**
♿ Suite 233, 517 College Street, Toronto, Ontario M6G 4A2.
☎ 416 921 2425 📞 416 921 4428
💰 ✓ VISA ⬤

Publishers: Directories: Libraries

☺ ■ **McIntyre Media**
30 Kelfield, Toronto, Ontario.
☎ 416 245 7800
☎ 416 249 5907
Publishes lists of Canadian libraries.

Publishers: Guides: Sexuality

♂♀▼ **Larry's Guide to the Ghetto**

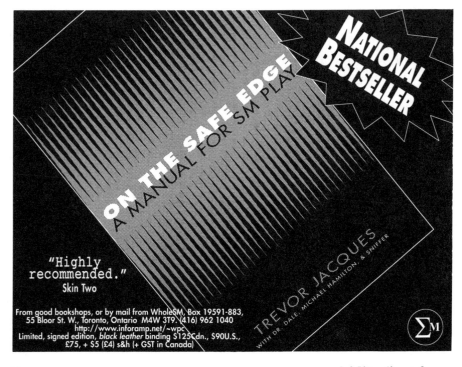

Suite 201, 219 Dufferin Street, Toronto, Ontario M6K 1Y9.
☎ 416 588 7339 ✆ 416 588 4519

Publishers: Magazines: BDSM

☺ ■ **The Boudoir Noir**
P. O. Box 5, Station F, Toronto, Ontario M4Y 2L4.
☎ 416 591 2387 ✆ 416 591 1572
✉ boudoir@the-wire.com
⌘ http://www.the-wire.com/boudoir.noir
Published quarterly. Yearly subscription is $30. Age statement of 21 is required.

♀▼ **Brazen Bitch Quarterly (BBQ)**
P. O. Box 57, 1172 Bay Street, Toronto, Ontario M5S 2B4.
✆ 416 944 3133
✉ brazenbq@aol.com
$
Lesbian SM sex magazine. Published quarterly. Yearly subscription is $24.95.

Publishers: Magazines: Fetish

☺ ■ **The Chatt**
Chatterly's, P. O. Box 128, Station A, Toronto, Ontario L5A 2Z7.
Fetish magazine for the sexually adventurous: dominants, submissives, TV, leather, rubber, BDSM, etc.. Send $12 for sample copy.

Publishers: Magazines: Literary

☺ ■ **Books In Canada**
♿ The Canadian Review of Books Ltd., Suite 603, 130 Spadina Avenue, Toronto, Ontario M5V 2L4.
☎ 416 601 9880

Publishers: Magazines: Sexuality

⚥▼ **Fab Magazine**
Suite 104, 25 Wood Street, Toronto, Ontario M4Y 2P9.
☎ 416 599 9273 ✆ 416 599 0964
Published every month. Yearly subscription is $24.

⚤ ■ **Fireweed**
P. O. Box 279, Station B, Toronto, Ontario M5T 2W2.
☎ 416 504 1339 ✆ 416 516 8869
✦ ✓

A 96 page
quarterly
lifestyle
magazine
published by,
for & about
gay women!

Photo: Wendy Jill York

Back Issues $ 6.95 One year subscription $ 25

PO Box 57 ▲ 1172 Bay Street,
Toronto, Ontario ▲ Canada M5S 2B4

⚥▼ **Icon**
P. O. Box 758, Station F, Toronto, Ontario M4Y 2N6.
☎ 416 461 6295 ✆ 416 461 0358
Monthly gay, lesbian, & bisexual newspaper. Published every month.

⚥▽ **PRIDENET**
PRIDENET, Incorporated, Suite 437, Communications Place, 366 Adelaide Street East, Toronto, Ontario M5A 3X9.
☎ 416 955 9050 ✆ 416 777 1169
✉ admin@pridenet.com
⌘ http://www.pridenet.com
🕐 09:00 - 17:00 Mon - Fri
✦ ✓ ℓ

⚤ ☐ **Resources for Feminist Research**
♿ OISE, 250 Bloor Street West, Toronto, Ontario M5S 1V6.

♀▼ **Sorority Magazine**
P. O. Box 57, 1172 Bay Street, Toronto, Ontario M5S 2B4.
✆ 416 944 3133
✉ soromat@aol.com
$
Magazine for gay women. Fiction, profiles, feature articles, & reports from the worlds of art, entertainment, & literature. Published quarterly. Yearly subscription is $24.95. Please see our display advertisement.

Publishers: Newspapers: Sexuality

☺ **Tab International**
Mailshoppe Inc., Suite 1801, 1 Yonge Street, Toronto, Ontario M5E 1E5.
☎ 416 921 6960 ✆ 416 921 1150
✓ $
Yearly subscription is $59.95.

⚥▽ **Xtra!**
♿ Pink Triangle Press, Suite 200, 491 Church Street, Toronto, Ontario M4Y 2C6.
☎ 800 268 9872 ✆ 416 925 6674
☎ 416 925 6665
🕐 09:00 - 24:00
✦ ✓ $ 💳 💳 ℓ
News, arts, & analysis for Toronto lesbians, gay men, & bisexuals. Published every two weeks. Yearly subscription is $62.60 Cdn.. Age statement of 18 is required.

Radio: Sexuality

▽ **Gaywire**
☎ 416 595 0909 ✆ 416 595 5604

⚥■ **Pink Antenna**
♿ c/o CKLN FM 88.1, 380 Victoria Street, Toronto, Ontario M5B 1W7.
☎ 416 595 5068 ✆ 416 595 0226
🕐 10:00 - 19:00, answering machine at other times
Covers local, national, & international lesbian & gay issues. First Tues of each month is dedicated to HIV/AIDS issues. Broadcasts Tues 19:00 - 20:00.

Stores: Art Galleries

☺ ▼ **O'Connor, A Gallery**
Suite 2, 473A Church Street, Toronto, Ontario.
☎ 416 921 7149

Stores: Books: General

☺ ■ **100th. Monkey Books**
2nd. Floor, 66 Wellesley Street East, Toronto, Ontario M4Y 1G2.
☎ 416 925 7633
🕐 Mon - Fri 10:00 - 18:30, Sat 10:00 - 18:00

☺ ■ **Bob Miller Bookroom**
Lower Concourse, 180 Bloor Street West, Toronto, Ontario M5S 2V6.
☎ 416 922 3557

☺ ■ **Common Knowledge Books**
♿ 602 Markham Street, Toronto, Ontario M6G 2L8.
☎ 416 539 8550 ✆ 416 539 8587
✦ ✓ $ 💳 💳 💳

⚥▽ **Glad Day Bookshop**
598A Yonge Street, Toronto, Ontario M4Y 1Z3.
☎ 416 961 4161 ✆ 416 961 1624
✦ ✓ $ 💳 💳 💳

☺ ■ **Pages**
256 Queen Street West, Toronto, Ontario M5V 1Z8.
☎ 416 598 1447 ✆ 416 598 2042

☺ ▼ **This Ain't The Rosedale Library**
483 Church Street, Toronto, Ontario M4Y 2C6.
☎ 416 929 9912

⚤ ☐ **Toronto Women's Bookstore**
73 Harbord Street, Toronto, Ontario M5S 1G4.
☎ 416 922 8744 ✆ 416 922 1417
✦ ✓ 💳 💳 💳

☺ ☐ **University of Toronto Bookstore**

⚹ 214 College Street, Toronto, Ontario M5T 3A1.
 ☎ 416 978 7918

☺ ■ **Volumes**
 Market Square, 74 Front Street East, Toronto, Ontario M5E 1T4.
 ☎ 416 366 9522

☺ ■ **World's Biggest Bookstore**
 20 Edward Street, Toronto, Ontario M5G 1C9.
 ☎ 416 977 7009

Stores: Clothing: Fetish

☺ ■ **He & She**
 ⚹ 263 Queen Street East, Toronto, Ontario M5A 2S6.
 ☎ 416 594 0171

Stores: Clothing: Leather

☺ ■ **Leathercraft**
 ⚹ 586 Yonge Street, Toronto, Ontario M4Y 1Z3.
 ☎ 416 924 5018 ✆ 416 975 1337
 ⚘ ✓ ⚲ 💳 🆔 ⬛

Stores: Clothing: Uniforms

☺ ■ **Frankel's**
 123 Church Street, Toronto, Ontario M5C 2G5.
 ☎ 416 366 4221
 ⏰ Mon - Sat 10:00 - 18:00
 Used military & commercial uniforms & other paraphernalia. Not part of
 the BDSM-fetish scene.

Stores: Erotica: BDSM

⚥▼ **Doc's Leathers & Harley Davidson Gear**
 2nd. Floor, 562 Parliament Street, Toronto, Ontario M4X 1P8.
 ☎ 416 324 8686 ✆ 416 929 1849
 ✉ docs@asgo.net
 ⚘ http://www.asgo.net/Docs
 ⬛

☺ ■ **Northbound Leather Ltd.**
 ⚹ 7 Saint Nicholas Street, Toronto, Ontario M4Y 1W5.
 ☎ 416 972 1037 ✆ 416 975 1337
 ✉ leather@northbound.com
 ⚘ http://www.northbound.com/
 ⏰ Mon - Wed Sat 10:00 - 18:00, Fri Sat 10:00 - 19:30, Sun 12:00 -
 17:00
 ⚘ ✓ ⚲ 💳 🆔 ⬛ ✆
 Canada's largest selection of fetish fashion & accessories, including
 corsetry, leather clothing, books, toys, & footwear. Large, inviting, &
 beautifully designed store. Catalogue, $30Cdn. (taxes included).
 Shipping $5Cdn., to Cdn.$9.95Cdn. to U.S., $12.95Cdn. elswhere.

☺ ■ **odd isn't. it?**
 P. O. Box 425, Station C, Toronto, Ontario M6J 3PS.
 ☎ 416 515 0009 ✆ 416 533 5790
 ☎ 416 533 5790
 Custom work in leather, wood, & metal. Art sculpture, jewelry, etc..

Stores: Erotica: General

⚹ ▼ **Cinéma Bleu Inc.**
 ⚹ 12 Roy's Square, Toronto, Ontario M4Y 2W2.
 ☎ 416 922 9112 ✆ 416 944 8612
 ⚘ 💳 🆔

☺ ■ **Lovecraft**
 63 Yorkville Avenue, Toronto, Ontario M5R 1B7.
 ☎ 416 923 7331 ✆ 416 923 4610

⚥▼ **Priape**
 465 Church Street, Toronto, Ontario M4Y 2C5.
 ☎ 800 461 6969 ✆ 416 586 0150
 ☎ 416 586 9914
 ✉ ber_ber@cam.org
 ⚘ ⚲ 💳 🆔 ⬛

☺ ■ **Private Pleasures**
 5114 Dundas Street West, Toronto, Ontario M9A 1C2.
 ☎ 416 237 0626 ✆ 416 455 4348
 Catalogue available.

Stores: Leatherwork Supplies: General

☺ ■ **Capital Findings & Leather**
 580 King Street West, Toronto, Ontario M5V 1M3.
 ☎ 416 363 8563
 Wholesalers of leather crafts goods open to general public.

Stores: Military Surplus

☺ ■ **Drolet's Army Surplus**
 2967 Dundas West, Etobicoke, Ontario M6P 1Z2.
 ☎ 416 762 6486

☺ **Hercules Outfitters**
 ⚹ 577 Yonge Street, Toronto, Ontario M4Y 1Z2.

 ☎ 416 924 7764

☺ ■ **M & J Army Surplus**
 2735 Lake Shore Boulevard West, Etobicoke, Ontario M8V 1S9.
 ☎ 416 253 0827

☺ ■ **Mr Surplus Army Navy Stores**
 371 Yonge Street, Toronto, Ontario M5B 1S1.
 ☎ 416 977 2769

☺ ■ **Save-More Sport Store**
 114 Queen Street East, Toronto, Ontario M5C 1S6.
 ☎ 416 368 3536
 ⏰ Mon - Wed Sat 09:00 -18:00, Thu Fri 09:00 - 20:00

Tattooists

☺ ▼ **Urban Primitive**
 Suite 2, 473 Church Street, Toronto, Ontario M4Y 2C3.
 ☎ 416 966 9155 ✆ 416 967 5373
 ✉ urbprim@io.org
 ⚘ http://www.io.org/~urbprim
 ⏰ 12:00 -19:00 every day
 Please see our display advertisement.

Training: BDSM

☺ ■ **Labyrinth**
 P. O. Box 41011, 2795 Bathurst Street, Toronto, Ontario M6B 4J6.
 ☎ 416 417 6583
 ✉ diva@inforamp.net
 ⚘ http://www.inforamp.net/~diva
 ⏰ Call between 11:00 - 19:00. By appointment only
 ⚘ ✓ $ ⚲

Waterloo

Organizations: Sexuality: Student

⚥▽ **Gay & Lesbian Liberation of Waterloo (GLLOW)**
 Room 110, Campus Centre, University of Waterloo, Waterloo, Ontario
 N2L 3G1.
 ☎ 519 884 4569
 ⚘ gopher://watserv2.uwaterloo.ca:70/11/departments/gllow
 ⏰ Mon - Fri 19:00 - 22:00

Radio: Sexuality

⚤▽ ***Nowhere To Hide***
Wed 20:00 - 21:00

⚤▽ ***Out & About - The Gay Radio Show***
CKWR FM 98.7, 56 Regina Street North, Waterloo, Ontario N2J 3A3.
☎ 519 886 9870 — 519 886 0090
09:00 - 22:00, answering machine at other times
News & information for the local gay, lesbian, & bisexual community. Broadcasts Tues 20:30 - 22:00.

⚤▽ ***We Are Everywhere***
Wed 12:20 & 15:15

Whitby

Organizations: AIDS: Education

☺ □ **AIDS Committee of Durham**
Suite 305, 209 Dundas Street East, Whitby, Ontario L1N 7H8.
☎ 905 665 0051 — 905665 0056
☎ 416 925 XTRA #2147
09:00 - 17:00, answering machine at other times
Community-based HIV/AIDS education & peer support to individuals, families, & groups infected with or affected by HIV/AIDS.

Windsor

Helplines: Sexuality

⚤▽ **Gay Phoneline of Windsor**
☎ 519 973 4951 — 519 977 5809
Thurs & Fri 20:00 - 22:00, answering machine with information at other times
Peer support for adult men who are gay or who have questions about homosexuality.

Organizations: AIDS: Support

☺ □ **AIDS Committee of Windsor**
♿ P. O. Box 2233, Windsor, Ontario N8Y 4R8.
☎ 519 256 2437 (information) — 519 973 7389
☎ 519 973 0222 (office)
Weekdays 09:00 - 17:00, answering machine with information at other times
Support & education for issues relating HIV/AIDS.

Organizations: Sexuality: Student

⚤▽ **Out on Campus**
Student Administrative Council, 2nd. Floor, 401 Sunset Street, Windsor, Ontario N9B 3P4.
☎ 519 971 7617
☎ 519 254 5067
Meets bi-monthly.
For lesbian, gay, & bisexuals in the University of Windsor community. Answering machine.

Stores: Erotica: BDSM

☺ ■ **Noir**
101 University Avenue, Windsor, Ontario N9A 5P3.
☎ 519 252 3653

PRINCE EDWARD ISLAND

Charlottetown

Helplines: Sexuality

⚤▽ **PEI Gay Phoneline**
☎ 902 566 9733

Organizations: AIDS: Support

☺ ■ **AIDS P. E. I.**
♿ P. O. Box 2762, Charlottetown, Prince Edward Island C1A 8C4.
☎ 902 566 2437 — 902 566 2437 (call first)

Stores: Books: General

☺ ■ **Bookmark**
172 Queen Street, Charlottetown, Prince Edward Island C1A 4B5.
☎ 902 566 4888 — 902 368 3651

QUÉBEC

Population: Approximately 7,000,000
Capital City: Québec
Time zone: GMT minus 5 hours (EST)
Climate: 22°C. Winters are cold and snowy, with temperatures averaging approximately -8°C. Considerably colder in the north during the winter.
Legal drinking age: 18

Provincial Resources

Archives: Sexuality

⚤▽ **Archives Gaies du Québec**
C. P. 395, Succursale Place du Parc, Montréal, Québec H2W 2N9.
☎ 514 287 4664

Organizations: AIDS: Education

☺ □ **Coalition des Organismes Communautaires Québecoise de Lutte Contre le SIDA**
4332A Rue Saint-Denis, Montréal, Québec H2J 2K8.
☎ 5114 844 2477 — 514 844 2498

☺ □ **Comité SIDA Québec**
101 rue Saint Denis, Montréal, Québec.
☎ 514 285 6471
Official government AIDS agency under the auspices of the Saint Luc hospital / Organisme officiel du Gouvernement du Québec sur le SIDA, sous la résponsabilité de l'hôpital Saint-Luc de Montréal.

Athelstan

Organizations: AIDS: Education

☺ □ **AIDS/AIDS Information & Ressources Québec Sud-Ouest**
2044 3e Consession, Athelstan, Québec J0S 1A0.
☎ 514 264 3379

Beaconsfield

Artists: BDSM

☺ **Princess Sheeba**
P. O. Box 664, Beaconsfield, Québec H9W 5V3.

Chicoutimi

Organizations: AIDS: Support

☺ □ **Mouvement d'Information, d'Education, & d'Entraide dans la Lutte Contre Le SIDA (MIENS)**
P. O. Box 723, Chicoutimi, Québec G7H 5E1.
☎ 418 693 8983 — 418 693 0409

Gatineau

Organizations: AIDS: Support

☺ □ **Bureau Régional d'Action SIDA**
Suite 103, 110 Rue de la Savane, Gatineau, Québec J8T 5B9.
☎ 819 568 2727 — 819 568 8765

Hull

Organizations: Sexuality

⚥ ▽ **Bi's R Us**
Suite 2, 11 Ettiene Brulé, Hull, Québec J8Z 1E4.
paula@proton.com

Organizations: Sexuality: Student

⚤▽ **Lesbigais de l'Université de Québec à Hull**
http://www.ncf.carleton.ca/freeport/sigs/life/gay/uqahul/menu

Stores: Erotica: General

☺ ■ **Erotica Plus**
22 Eddy, Hull, Québec.
☎ 613 777 4069
☎ 613 770 4442

Joliette

Helplines: AIDS

☺ □ **SISA Intervention Prévention Ecoute**
331 Rue Saint-Viateur, Joliette, Québec J6E 3A8.
☎ 514 752 4004

Laval

Organizations: AIDS: Support

☺ □ **Service Spécialisé SIDA Québec**
Suite 220, 226 Rue des Alpes, Pont-Vau, Québec H7G 3W2.
☎ 514 668 1230 — 514 668 6860 (call first)

Stores: Erotica: General

☺ ■ **Boutique Carrefour du Sexe Inc.**
1735 Boulevard Labelle, Laval, Québec H7T 1L1.
☎ 514 688 6969

Montréal

Bars: BDSM

⚤▼ **L'Aigle Noir**
1315 Rue Sainte Catherine Est, Montréal, Québec.
☎ 514 529 0040

⚤▼ **K. O. X.**

1450 Rue Sainte Catherine Est, Montréal, Québec.
☎ 514 523 0064
⌖▼ **Katacombes**
1450 Rue Sainte Catherine Est, Montréal, Québec.
☎ 514 523 0064
⌖▼ **Le Track**
1584 Rue Sainte Catherine Est, Montréal, Québec.
☎ 514 521 1419

BBSs: BDSM
☺■ **Montreal's Electronic Dungeon**
✆ 514 522 3866

BBSs: Sexuality
⌖▼ **S-TEK**
✆ 514 597 2409
⏲ 24hrs.
Must be over 18.

Competitions & Conventions: BDSM
⌖ **Concours M. Cuir Montréal**
2491, rue Centre, Montréal, Québec H3K 1J9.
☎ 514 933 3307 ✇ 514 933 3307

Health Services
☺☐ **Clinique Medicale de la Cité**
300 rue Léo Pariseau, Montréal, Québec.
☎ 514 281 1722
⏲ Mon - Fri 08:30 - 22:00, Sat 09:00 - 16:30, Sun 10:30 - 16:30
General clinic, with or without appointment.

Helplines: AIDS
☺☐ **Info SIDA**
☎ 514 521 7432 (SIDA)
Counselling information about HIV/AIDS / Ligne d'écoute et d'information consacré au SIDA.

Helplines: Sexuality
⌖▽ **Gai-Ecoute**
☎ 514 521 1508
⏲ 19:00 - 23:00
Ecoute confidentielle en Français. De l'aide quand vous en avez besoin.
⌖▽ **Gay Info**
☎ 514 768 0199
⏲ Fri Sat 19:30 - 22:30
Counselling & information in English.
⌖▽ **Gayline**
☎ 514 990 1414
⏲ 18:30 - 22:00
Information & counselling in English.

Organizations: AIDS: Education
☺☐ **Séro-Zéro**
☎ 514 286 0439
Information about HIV/AIDS.

Organizations: AIDS: Support
☺☐ **AIDS Community Care Montréal (ACCM)**
Suite 500, 231 Rue St. Jacques, Montréal, Québec H2Y 1M6.
☎ 5114 939 0075 (hotline) ✇ 514 287 9475
☎ 514 287 3551 (office)
Information, counselling, & support for people infected with or affected by HIV/AIDS.
♁☐ **Centre d'Action SIDA Montréal (Femmes)**
1831 Boulevard René Lévesque Ouest, Montréal, Québec H3H 1R4.
☎ 514 989 7997 ✇ 514 989 7811
Information, counselling, & support for women infected with or affected by HIV/AIDS.
☺☐ **Comité des Personnes Atteintes du VIH**
3600 Hôtel de Ville, Montréal, Québec H2X 3B6.
☎ 514 282 6673 ✇ 514 281 8004
☺☐ **Comité SIDA Aide Montréal**
P. O. Box 98, Succursale N, Montréal, Québec.
☎ 514 282 9888
☺☐ **L'Essentiel / HIV Anonyme**
CLSC Plateau Mont-Royal, 4689 rue Papineau, Montréal, Québec.
☎ 514 598 8402
⏲ Tue 19:30

Organizations: BDSM
☺■ **Megalesia**
P. O. Box 61043, 43399 Notre Dame Ouest, Montréal, Québec H4C 3N9.
Mainly couples.

Organizations: Motorcycle
⌖▽ **Iron Cross MC**
771 rue Versailles, Montréal, Québec H3C 1Z5.
☎ 514 931 2202
⌖▽ **MC Faucon, Inc.**
C. P. 5089, Station C, Montréal, Québec H2X 3M2.

Organizations: Sexuality
☒▽ **Club MET**
4113 Dorion Street, Montréal, Québec H2K 3B8.
☎ 514 528 8874
Publishes *Gender Press*.
☒▽ **FACT—Québec**
Succursale 293 Côte-des-Neiges, 5858 Boulevard Côte-des-Neiges, Montréal, Québec H3S 2S5.
Contact: Ms. Patricia Fisher
⌖▽ **The Gay & Lesbian Centre**
Marché St. Jacques, 2035 Rue Amherst, Montréal, Québec.
☎ 514 528 8424 ✇ 514 528 9708
⏲ Mon - Fri 10:00 - 22:00
☒▽ **Trans Post-Op Recovery Residence (TransPORRS)**
2006 Sherbrooke Est, Montréal, Québec H2K 1B9.
☒■ **Transsexuals In Prison**
Succursale 293 Côte-des-Neiges, 5858 Boulevard Côte-des-Neiges, Montréal, Québec H3S 2S5.
Contact: Ms. Patricia Fisher
Publishes a newsletter quarterly.

Organizations: Sexuality: Student
⌖▽ **L'Association des Lesbiennes & Gaies de l'Université de Québec à Montréal (ALGUQAM)**
Boîte Postale 8888, Succursale Centre-Ville, Montréal, Québec H3C 3P8.
☎ 514 987 3039
Publishes *Homo Sapiens* every month.
⌖▽ **Centre Gai & Lesbien de l'UQAM**
Bureau 9210, 1259 Rue Berri, Montréal, Québec.
☎ 514 987 3039
⌖▽ **Concordia Queer Collective**
2020 Mackay Street, Montréal, Québec H3G 2J1.
☎ 514 848 7414
⌖▽ **Lesbians, Bisexuals, & Gays of McGill**
Room 432, 3480 Rue McTavish, Montréal, Québec H3A 1X9.
☎ 514 398 6822
🖳 http://polestar.facl.mcgill.ca/vub/clubs/lbgm/

Organizations: Sexuality: Youth
⌖▽ **Project 10**
☎ 514 989 4585
⏲ Mon - Fri afternoons. Ask for Project 10
Information, counselling, & support for young gays, lesbians, & bisexuals.

Piercers
☺ **Black Sun Studio**
P. O. Box 1523, Place Bonaventure, Montréal, Québec H5A 1H6.
☎ 514 345 5701
⏲ As client requires
⚒ $
Private piercing studio open since 1990. Top quality piercing jewelry in steel, gold, niobium, acrylic, nylon, precious stones, exotic woods, etc.. Age statement of 18 is required. English also spoken.

Printers: General
☺■ **Lidec**
Boîte Postale 5000, Succursale C, Montréal, Québec H2X 3M1.
☎ 514 843 5991 ✇ 514 843 5252

Publishers: Guides: Sexuality
⌖▽ **Le Guide Gai du Québec**
C. P. 5245, Montréal, Québec H2X 3M4.
☎ 514 523 4992 ✇ 514 523 2214
Gay guide to the province of Québec. Published once a year. Yearly subscription is $15.

Publishers: Magazines: Sexuality
⌖▽ **Lesbian Information Line**
P. O. Box 509, Succursale Desjardins, Montréal, Québec H5B 1B6.
☎ 514 282 0100 ✇ 514 879 9722
⚒ ✓ 🆅🆈🆂🅰
⌖▼ **Magazine Fugues**
1212 Saint Hubert, Montréal, Québec H2L 3H7.

☎ 514 848 1854 📱 514 845 7645
🕐 09:00 - 18:00
The gay guide to Montréal & the province of Québec. Published every month. Yearly subscription is $30Cdn.. English also spoken.

⚥▼ *Magazine RG*
P. O. Box 5245, Station C, Montréal, Québec H2K 3M4.
☎ 514 523 9463 📱 514 523 2214
♣ $
Gay information in French. Personals section, etc.. Published every month. Yearly subscription is $50.

Radio: Sexuality

⚥▽ *Bulletin Lambda*
☎ 514 843 4564
🕐 Sun 23:00 - 24:00

Stores: Books: General

☺▼ **L'Androgyne**
 ♿ 3636 Boulevard Saint Laurent, Montréal, Québec H2X 2V4.
☎ 514 842 4765
♣ 🖊 💳 💳
Free catalogue.

Stores: Erotica: BDSM

⚥▼ **Cuir Plus**
 ♿ 1321 Sainte Catherine Est, Montréal, Québec H2L 2H4.
☎ 514 521 7587

☺■ **Il Bolero**
6842 rue Saint Hubert, Montréal, Québec.
☎ 514 270 6065

Stores: Erotica: General

☺■ **Boutique Carrefour du Sexe Inc.**
2067 Sainte-Catherine Ouest, Montréal, Québec H3H 1M6.
☎ 514 932 1311

⚥ **Choc Monsieur**
1881, avenue Mont-Royal Est, Montréal, Québec.
☎ 514 521 7558

⚥▼ **Priape**
1311 Sainte Catherine Est, Montréal, Québec H2L 2H4.
☎ 800 461 6969 📱 514 521 1309
☎ 514 521 8451
📧 ber_ber@cam.org
♣ 🖊 💳 💳

☺■ **Séduction**
38, Sainte-Catherine Ouest, Montréal, Québec H2X 3V4.
☎ 514 876 3636
♣ $
Also mail order. Catalogue, $5.

☺▼ **Videomag Plus**
 ♿ 1243 Bleury, Montréal, Québec H3B 3H9.
☎ 514 871 1653

Stores: Piercing Jewelry

☺■ **Shiny Things**
339 Terrace Saint-Denis, Montréal, Québec.
☎ 514 284 0868

Noranda

Organizations: AIDS: Support

☺☐ **Centre des R. O. S. É. S. de l'Abitibi-Témiscamingue**
C. P. 581, Rouyn, Québec J9C 5C6.
☎ 819 764 9111

Outremont

Organizations: BDSM

⚥▽ **Club de Cuir Predateurs**
Suite 5, 48 Joyce, Outremont, Québec H2V 1S6.
☎ 514 272 8638

Québec

Bars: BDSM

⚥▽ **Bar Mâle**
770 Côte Sainte Geneviève, Québec G1R 3L4.
☎ 418 523 8279
🕐 11:00 - 03:00
Some leather.

⚥▼ **Le Drague**
 ♿ 815 Rue Sainte Augustine, Québec.
☎ 418 649 7212 📱 418 649 0882
🕐 09:00 - 24:00

Some leather.

Helplines: Sexuality

⚥▽ **Relais d'Espérance**
617 rue Montmatre, Québec.
☎ 418 522 3301
Information & support.

Organizations: AIDS: Education

☺☐ **Mouvement d'Information & d'Entraide dans la Lutte Contre Le SIDA à Québec (MIELS)**
Suite 200, 175 Rue Saint-Jean, Québec G1R 1N4.
☎ 418 649 0788 (information) 📱 418 649 1256
☎ 418 649 1720 (office)

☺☐ **Mouvement SIDA Québec**
Bureau 200, 175 rue Saint-Jean, Québec G1R 1N4.
☎ 418 649 1720

Organizations: BDSM

⚥ **Club des Cuirassés de Québec**
C. P. 52064, Succursale Saint-Fidèle, Québec G1L 5A4.
☎ 418 525 8868
🕐 Meets monthly
♣ $
Social group devoted to wear & promote leather. Social activities to help AIDS organizations. Age statementof 18 is required. English also spoken.

Organizations: Sexuality: Student

⚥▽ **Groupe Gai de l'Université de Laval**
P. O. Box 2500, Pavillon Lemieux, Université Laval, Sainte Foy, Québec G1K 7P4.
☎ 418 649 9478
📧 stephane_couture@enap.uquebec.ca
Information, support, & library.

Stores: Erotica: General

⚥▼ **Delta**
875 rue Saint-Jean, Québec.
☎ 418 647 6808
🕐 Mon 12:00 - 19:00, Tue 10:00 - 19:00, Wed - Sat 10:00 - 21:00, Sun 12:00 - 17:00, less in the winter
Also mail order.

Saint Antoine des Laurentides

Organizations: AIDS: Support

☺☐ **Centre SIDA Amitié**
705 Boulevard des Laurentides, Saint Antoine des Laurentides, Québec J7Z 4M6.
☎ 514 431 7432

Sherbrooke

Organizations: AIDS: Education

☺☐ **Intervention Régionale & Information sur le SIDA (IRIS)**
Suite 204, 6 Rue Wellington, Sherbrooke, Québec J1H 5C6.
☎ 800 567 391 (information) 📱 819 823 5537
☎ 819 823 6704 (office)

Organizations: Sexuality: Student

⚥▽ **L'Association des Gais & Lesbiennes de l'Université de Sherbrooke**
Centre Social, 2500 Université, Sherbrooke, Québec.
☎ 819 564 5013

Trois-Rivières

Organizations: AIDS: Education

☺☐ **Sidaction Trois-Rivières**
C. P. 1142, Trois-Rivières, Québec G9A 5K8.
☎ 819 374 5740 📱 819 374 5932

Victoriaville

Organizations: AIDS: Support

☺☐ **Bureau Local d'Intervention Traitant du SIDA**
Suite 110, 59 Rue Monfette, Victoriaville, Québec G6P 1J8.
☎ 819 758 2662 📱 819 758 8270

SASKATCHEWAN

Population: Approximately 1,000,000
Capital City: Regina
Time zone: GMT minus 7 hours (CST)
Climate: Pleasant summers, with temperatures averaging approximately 24°C. Winters are cold & snowy, with temperatures averaging -16°C.
Legal drinking age: 18

Regina

Helplines: Sexuality

⌀♥▽ **Regina Gayline**
P. O. Box 3414, Regina, Saskatchewan.
☎ 306 569 0125
🕐 Mon Fri 20:00

Organizations: AIDS: Education

⌀♥□ **AIDS Regina**
1852 Angus Street, Regina, Saskatchewan S4T 1Z4.
☎ 306 924 8420 📠 306 525 0904
🖂 📠

Organizations: Sexuality: Student

⌀♥▽ **Regina Students Homophile Society, Inc.**
P. O. Box 3382, Regina, Saskatchewan.
☎ 306 522 7343
🕐 Meets Tue 19:30
Support, information, & library.

Stores: Books: General

☺ **Sutherland's Books**
1833 Hamilton Street, Regina, Saskatchewan S4P 4B4.
☎ 306 565 2808 📠 306 565 3188

Saskatoon

Health Services

⌀♥▽ **Gay & Lesbian Health Services of Saskatoon**
P. O. Box 8581, Saskatoon, Saskatchewan S7K 6K7.
☎ 306 665 1224 📠 306 244 2134

Helplines: Sexuality

⌀♥▽ **Saskatoon Gayline**
☎ 306 665 1224

Organizations: AIDS: Support

☺ □ **AIDS Saskatoon**
P. O. Box 4062, Saskatoon, Saskatchewan S7K 4E3.
☎ 306 667 6876 📠 306 665 9976
☎ 306 242 5005 (office)

Organizations: BDSM

⌀♥▽ **Levi/Leather Plainsmen**
P. O. Box 3043, Saskatoon, Saskatchewan S7K 3S9.

Organizations: Sexuality: Student

⌀♥▽ **Gays & Lesbians at the University of Saskatoon (GLUS)**
P. O. Box 369, Sub P. O. No. 6, Saskatoon, Saskatchewan S7N 4J8.
☎ 306 244 4782
🖂 Darrell.Broughton@usask.ca

Publishers: Newspapers: Sexuality

⌀♥▼ *Perceptions*
P. O. Box 8581, Saskatoon, Saskatchewan S7K 6K7.
☎ 306 244 1930
Published quarterly.

Stores: Erotica: General

☺ **Discreet Boutique**
⌖ 133 Third Avenue North, Saskatoon, Saskatchewan S7K 2H4.
☎ 306 665 6681 📠 306 665 6692
🕐 Mon - Wed, Sat 10:00 - 18:00, Thu Fri 10:00 - 22:00
🖂 $ 📠 💳 💳 📠 ℓ
Also mail order. Age statement of 18 is required.

YUKON

Whitehorse

Organizations: AIDS: Support

☺ □ **AIDS Yukon Alliance**
7221 7th. Avenue, Whitehorse, Yukon Y1A 1R8.
☎ 403 633 2437 📠 403 633 2447

The Channel Islands

The islands belong to the United Kingdom.
Area: Approximately 244,490 square kilometres for whole of U.K.
Population: Approximately 57,650,000 for whole of U.K.
Capital City: London
Currency: Pound Sterling (£)
Official Language: English & French
Major Religions: 57% Protestant, 13% Roman Catholic

National Holiday: Queen's Birthday, early June
Time zone: GMT
Country Initials: GB
Electricity: 240 volts, 50Hz
Country Dialing Code (from elsewhere): 44
Intl. Dialing Prefix (out of the country): 0101
Long Distance Dialing Prefix (inside country): 0
Climate: Warm, dry summers, cool, wet winters.
Age of consent & homosexuality legislation: Age of consent for sexual activity is 16, but 18 for homosexual activities. Homosexual acts were decriminalized in 1967. In 1992, Homosexual acts are not permitted for the members of the military.
Legal drinking age: 18
The is no gay scene to speak of. The only gay organization known to have existed disbanded "due to the age of the members."

GUERNSEY

County Resources

Helplines: Sexuality

⌀♥▽ **Solent Gay Switchboard & AIDSline**
☎ 1703 637363
☎ 1703 655077
🕐 1st. line: Tue Thu Sat 19:30 - 22:00, 2nd. line: Wed 19:30 - 22:00
Advice & information about HIV/AIDS & other sexual health & sexuality issues.

⌀○▽ **Solent Lesbian Line**
☎ 1703 405111
🕐 Tue Thu 19:30 - 22:00
Advice & information about HIV/AIDS & other sexual health & sexuality issues.

JERSEY

⌀♥▽ **Solent Gay Switchboard & AIDSline**
☎ 1703 637363
☎ 1703 655077
🕐 1st. line: Tue Thu Sat 19:30 - 22:00, 2nd. line: Wed 19:30 - 22:00
Advice & information about HIV/AIDS & other sexual health & sexuality issues.

⌀○▽ **Solent Lesbian Line**
☎ 1703 405111
🕐 Tue Thu 19:30 - 22:00
Advice & information about HIV/AIDS & other sexual health & sexuality issues.

Saint Helier

Organizations: AIDS: Support

☺ □ **Jersey AIDS Relief Group (JARG)**
☎ 1534 58886
🕐 Fri evening, Sat Sun daytime
Advice & information about HIV/AIDS & other sexual health issues.

Chile

Area: Approximately 760,000 square kilometres
Population: Approximately 13,240,000
Capital City: Santiago de Chile
Currency: Chilean Peso
Official Language: Spanish
Major Religions: 89% Roman Catholic
National Holiday: Independence Day, 19th. September
Time zone: GMT minus 4 hours
Country Initials: RCH
Electricity: 220 volts, 50Hz
Country Dialing Code (from elsewhere): 56
Intl. Dialing Prefix (out of the country): 00
Climate: Due to the north-south lenth of the country, it has three distinct climates. In the north, the weather is exptremely dry, with foggy coastal regions. In the centre, the weather is sub-tropical. In the south, the there is plenty of rain & the temperatures are lower.
Age of consent & homosexuality legislation: Homosexual activity is punishable with up to 1½-3 years imprisonment. The law has been enforced less & less in recent years, & the gay community is tolerated in large urban centres.

Santiago

Organizations: AIDS: Support

☺ □ **AIDS Committee**
Porvenir 464, Santiago.

Costa Rica

Area: Approximately 51,000 square kilometres
Population: Approximately 3,100,000
Capital City: San José
Currency: Costa Rica Colón
Official Language: Spanish
Major Religions: 89% Roman Catholic
National Holiday: Independence Day, 15th. September
Time zone: GMT minus 6 hours
Country Initials: CR
Electricity: 120/220 volts, 60Hz
Country Dialing Code (from elsewhere): 506
Intl. Dialing Prefix (out of the country): 00
Climate: May & june are mild. The dry season is from December until April.
Age of consent & homosexuality legislation: There is broad tolerance for hoomosexual activity. The age of consent for homosexual activity is 18.

San José

Organizations: AIDS: Support

☺ □ **Asociacion de Lucha Contra el SIDA**
P. O. Box 561-1002, San José 1000.

The Czech Republic

Area: Approximately 79,000 square kilometres
Population: Approximately 10,500,000
Capital City: Praha
Currency: Koruna
Official Language: Czech
Major Religions: 30% Roman Catholic, 8% Protestant
National Holiday: Independence Day, 28th. October
Time zone: GMT plus 1/2 hours
Country Initials: CS
Electricity: 220 volts
Country Dialing Code (from elsewhere): 42
Intl. Dialing Prefix (out of the country): 00
Climate: Temperate, continental climate. Warm summers, with temperatures averaging approximately 21°C. Winters are cold & snowy, with an average temperature of approximately -2°C.
Age of consent & homosexuality legislation: The age of consent for sexual activity is 15. Homosexual activity is frowned upon in the countryside, but the capital is tolerant of the gay community.

Praha

Bars: BDSM

⚣ **Lederklub SAM**
Cajkovskeho 34, Praha 3.
🕐 15:00 - 24:00

Denmark

Area: Approximately 43,070 square kilometres
Population: Approximately 5,125,000
Capital City: København (Copenhagen)
Currency: Krone (DK)
Official Language: Danish
Major Religions: 88% Protestant
National Holiday: Liberation Day, 5th. May
Time zone: GMT plus 1 hour
Country Initials: DK
Electricity: 220 volts
Country Dialing Code (from elsewhere): 45
Intl. Dialing Prefix (out of the country): 009
Climate: Mild & wet all year. Summer ranges from 15-16°C, winter hovers around 0°C.
Age of consent & homosexuality legislation: Age of consent for sexual activity has been 15 since 1976. In 1979, Denmark abolished the restrictions on homosexuals in the military. In 1976, Denmark permitted homosexual partners to register their union, but did not grant marriage licences to these couples.

NATIONAL RESOURCES

Mailorder: Clothing: Fetish

☺ ■ **Latexa**
Postboks 28, 4720 Praestoe.

☺ ■ **Passion**
Postboks 936, 8600 Silkeborg.
☎ 86 81 3370

Mailorder: Erotica: Adult Baby

⚤ ■ **Voksne Babyers Verden**
Postboks 27A, 5550 Langeskov.
☎ 65 38 3413
✉ babylai@vbv.ping.dk

Mailorder: Erotica

⚣ ▼ **Danske Bjørne ApS**
Postboks 1100, 6330 Padborg.
☎ 74 67 4727

Organizations: Sexuality

⚣ ▽ **Landsforeningen for Bøsser og Lesbiske (LBL)—Head Office**
Postboks 1023, 1007 København K.
☎ 33 13 1948
Founded in 1948. Pan lists LBL & non-LBL addresses & is free to members, libraries, etc.. Publishes *Pan* every month. Yearly subscription is DK150.

Ålborg

Health Services

☺ ▽ **Klinikken for Kønssygdomme**
Ladegaardsgase 10, 9000 Ålborg.
🕐 Mon 14:45 - 17:15, Tue - Fri 14:45 - 16:00

Organizations: Sexuality

⚣ ▽ **Landsforeningen for Bøsser og Lesbiske (LBL)—Rådgivning**
Anders Borksveij 18, 9000 Ålborg.
☎ 98 16 4507
🕐 Thu 18:00 - 20:00
Counselling & support in person or by 'phone.

Århus

Archives: Sexuality

⚣ ▼ **Biblioteket**
Postboks 362, 8000 Århus.
☎ 86 13 1948
Lends to members.

Organizations: AIDS: Support

☺ □ **AIDS Info**
Vestergade 48, 8000 Århus.
☎ 86 13 6513
🕐 19:00 - 23:00. Counselling Wed 16:00 - 18:00

⚣ ▽ **Body Positive Groups**
Vestergade 48, 8000 Århus.
☎ 86 18 1646

⚣ ▼ **HIV Groups**
☎ 86 12 4313
🕐 Members Mon 09:00 - 13:00, Tue 19:00 - 22:00; anyone Wed 19:00 - 22:00

Organizations: BDSM

⚣ ▽ **A-Men's Club**
Postboks 370, 8110 Århus C.
☎ 86 19 1089
🕐 Fri 23:00 - 02:00

Organizations: Family

☺ □ **Relatives Group**
Akt HIV-huset, Vestergade 48, 8000 Århus.
🕐 1st Thu of month 19:30 - 22:00

Organizations: Sexuality

⚣ ▽ **Landsforeningen for Bøsser og Lesbiske (LBL)—Århus**
Postboks 362, 8000 Århus.
☎ 86 12 1948
Support & counselling by 'phone or in person (Thu 18:00 - 19:00). Library.

Radio: Sexuality

⚣ ▽ ***Radio Rosa***
FM 106.7, 92.2, 89.5, & 98.7, Postboks 362, 8000 Århus.
☎ 86 19 3222
🕐 Mon 19:00 - 20:00, Fri 15:00 - 16:00

Broenshoej

Stores: Clothing: Fetish

☺ ■ **Ulf Dormann**
Islevhusvej 3, 2700 Broenshoej.
☎ 31 60 4818

Frederiksberg

Organizations: AIDS: Support

⚥ ▼ **Positivgruppen**
Postboks 159, 2000 Frederiksberg.
☎ 38 33 3244

Stores: Erotica: BDSM

☺ ■ **Conflicto**
Johnstrup Alle 1, 1923 Frederiksberg C.
☎ 31 35 0380

☺ ■ **Paradis**
95 Gl. Kongevej, 1850 Frederiksberg C.
☎ 31 12 6017

Greve

Organizations: Sexuality

⚢▽ **Freedom of Personality Expression (FPE)—
Northern Europe: Denmark**
Postboks 170, 2670 Greve.
☎ 42 13 9032
🕐 Call Mon Tue 18:00 - 21:00
Publishes *Feminform & Intermezzo.*

Holbæck

Publishers: Magazines: BDSM

⚥▼ *Mr. SM*
Orange Press ApS, Postboks 319, 4300 Holbæck.
📱 53 47 1268
🕐 Fri 23:00 - 02:00

København

Archives: Sexuality

⚥▽ **Arkiv for Bøsser & Lesbiske**
Postboks 1023, 1023 København.
☎ 33 11 1961
🕐 Tue 17:00 - 19:00
The only gay, lesbian, & bisexual archive in Denmark.

⚥▽ **Pan Biblioteket**
Knabrostræde 3, 1210 København K.
☎ 33 11 1961
🕐 Mon - Fri 17:00 - 19:00
Lends to members of LBL. Also sells books & magazines.

Bars: BDSM

⚥▼ **Men's Bar**
Teglgardstræde 3, 1452 København K.
☎ 33 12 7303
🕐 15:30 - 02:00, Sat 22:00 - 02:00

⚥▼ **Metro Place de Clichy**
Studiestræde 31B, 1455 København K.
🕐 Fri Sat 22:00 - 05:00

Helplines: AIDS

☺ ☐ **AIDS-linien (AIDS Hotline)**
Skindergade 27 2, 1159 København K.
☎ 33 91 1119
📱 33 91 3414
🕐 09:00 - 23:00
Counselling, support, & information about HIV/AIDS.

Helplines: Sexuality

⚥▽ **Gay Youth Switchboard / Ungdomstelefonen**
LBL - Teglgaardsstraede 13, 1452 København K.
☎ 33 13 0628
🕐 Tue 19:00 - 21:00
Counselling & support for young gays & lesbians.

⚥▽ **Landsforeningen for Bøsser og Lesbiske (LBL)—
Kobenhavn**
Postboks 1023, 1007 København K.
☎ 33 13 1948
Information, support, & counselling.

Organizations: AIDS: Support

⚥ ▼ **HIV-Hjælpen**
1st. Floor, Knabrostræde 3, 1210 København K.
Counselling, information, & support about HIV/AIDS.

Organizations: BDSM

⚥▽ **Scandinavian Leather Men (SLM)—Kobenhavn**
Studiestræde 14, 1455 København K.
☎ 33 32 0601
🕐 Fri 22:00 - ?

☺▽ **SMiL Denmark**
Sorgenfrigade 8B2, 2200 København.
☎ 1 81 05 50
🕐 Thu 18:00 - 20:00

Organizations: Sexuality

⚣▽ **Transvision**
Postboks 280, 1502 København.

Piercers

☺ ■ **The Black Universe**
Studiestræde 15, 1445 København K.
☎ 33 32 3113
☎ 31 57 8247

Radio: Sexuality

⚥▽ *Radio Rosa*
FM 98.9, Knabrostræde 3, 1210 København K.
☎ 33 33 0404
🕐 21:30 - 23:30, repeats next day 15:00 - 17:00. May - Sept English broadcast 2nd. & 4th. Wed of the month

Stores: Clothing: Fetish

☺ ■ **Subwave Design**
21 Studiestræde, 1455 København K.
☎ 33 12 1452

Stores: Clothing: Uniforms

☺ ■ **Hyssna**
Blegdamsvej 62, 2100 København E.
☎ 35 37 7700
📱 35 37 1642
Uniforms & other occupational clothing. Not part of the fetish scene.

Stores: Erotica: BDSM

⚥▼ **Cruz Leather Works**
Studiestræde 29, 1455 København K.
☎ 33 14 9017
🕐 11:00 - 17:30, Sat 11:00 - 14:00
Appointments available outside opeing hours (call for details).

☺ ■ **Renate Buccone**
Vesterbros Torv, 51 Vesterbrogade, 1620 København K.
☎ 31 22 1041

☺ ▼ **SM Bladet / SM Shop**
Studiestræde 12, 1455 København K.
☎ 33 32 3303
🕐 Mon - Thu 10:00 - 18:00, Fri 10:00 - 19:00
English, German, & Italian also spoken.

Kolding

Helplines: AIDS

☺ ☐ **AIDS Help Line**
☎ 75 50 5711
🕐 Wed 17:00 - 19:00

Organizations: Sexuality

⚥▽ **Landsforeningen for Bøsser og Lesbiske (LBL)—
Afdeling Sudjylland**
Dyrehavegårdsvej 38, 6000 Kolding.
☎ 75 54 1948
🕐 Help by 'phone Wed 19:00 - 21:00

Odense

Organizations: AIDS: Support

☺ ☐ **AIDS-Info**
Sankt Anne Plads 2, 5000 Odense.
☎ 65 91 1119
🕐 24hrs.
Information, counselling, & support.

Organizations: Sexuality

⚥▽ **Landsforeningen for Bøsser og Lesbiske (LBL)—
Odense**
Postboks 1192, 5000 Odense.
☎ 66 17 7692
🕐 Wed 18:00 - 20:00

Silkeborg

Piercers

☺ ■ **DK Profashion**
Virklundsvej 5, 8600 Silkeborg.
☎ 86 83 6470
📱 86 83 6489
🕐 24hr. ordering

Sønderborg

Organizations: Sexuality: Youth

☿▽ **Ungdomsgruppen for Bøsser og Lesbiske i Sønderjylland**
Postboks 51, 6400 Sønderborg.
☎ 74 62 1148
🕐 Fri 20:00 - 22:00
For youth under 28.

Viborg

Printers: General

☺ **Nørhaven A/S**

England

Area: Approximately 244,490 square kilometres for whole of U.K.
Population: Approximately 57,650,000 for whole of U.K.
Capital City: London
Currency: Pound Sterling (£)
Official Language: English & French
Major Religions: 57% Protestant, 13% Roman Catholic
National Holiday: Queen's Birthday, early June
Time zone: GMT
Country Initials: GB
Electricity: 240 volts, 50Hz
Country Dialing Code (from elsewhere): 44
Intl. Dialing Prefix (out of the country): 0101
Long Distance Dialing Prefix (inside country): 0
Climate: Warm, dry summers, cool, wet winters.
Age of consent & homosexuality legislation: Age of consent for sexual activity is 16, but 18 for homosexual activities. Homosexual acts were decriminalized in 1967. In 1992, Homosexual acts are not permitted for the members of the military.
Legal drinking age: 18

NATIONAL RESOURCES

Accommodation: BDSM

☺ ■ **Westward Bound**
P. O. Box 15, Launceston, Cornwall PL15 7YG.
☎ 1566 776907 ✆ 1566 774736
Bed & breakfast with dungeon. Catalogue available.

Counsellors

☺ □ **Red Admiral Project**
51A Philbeach Gardens, London.
Counselling for people with or affected by HIV/AIDS.

Helplines: AIDS

☺ □ **Blackliners**
☎ 171 738 5274
🕐 Mon - Fri 10:00 - 20:30, Sat 13:00 - 18:00
Advice & information about HIV/AIDS & other sexual health issues.

☺ □ **Body Positive**
51B Philbeach Gardens, London.
☎ 171 373 9124
Advice & information about HIV/AIDS & other sexual health issues.

☺ □ **Jewish AIDS Trust**
c/o HIV Education Unit, Colindale Hospital, Colindale Avenue, London NW9 5GH.
☎ 181 200 0369
🕐 Mon 19:30 - 22:00, except Jewish holidays
Advice & information about HIV/AIDS & other sexual health issues.

☺ □ **Mainliners**
☎ 171 737 3141
🕐 Mon - Fri 10:00 - 17:00
Advice & information about HIV/AIDS & other sexual health issues.

☺ □ **National AIDS Hotline**
☎ 800 567 123
☎ 800 521 3611 (Minicom)
🕐 24hrs.. Minicom 10:00 - 22:00
Advice & information about HIV/AIDS & other sexual health issues. In Bengali, Gujerati, Punjabi, Urdu, & English: 800 282 445. In Cantonese & English: 800 282 446. In Arabic & English: 800 282 447.

☺ □ **The NAZ Project**
☎ 181 563 0205
🕐 In Turkish, Mon 18:30 - 22:30; Punjabi, Tue 18:30 - 22:30; Urdu, Wed 18: 30 - 22:30; Bengali, Thu 18:30 - 22:30
Advice & information about HIV/AIDS & other sexual health issues.

☺ □ **The NAZ Project**
☎ 181 536 0208
🕐 In Farsi: Mon 18:30 - 22:30; Hindi, Tue 18:30 - 22:30; Gujerati,
Wed 18:30 - 22:30; Arabic, Thu 18:30 - 22:30
Advice & information about HIV/AIDS & other sexual health issues.

☻ □ **Positively Women**
☎ 171 490 2327
🕐 Mon - Fri 12:00 - 14:00
Advice & information about HIV/AIDS & other sexual health issues.

☺ □ **The Terrence Higgins Trust**
52-54 Grays Inn Road, London WC1X 8JU.
☎ 171 242 1010
🕐 12:00 - 22:00
Advice & information about HIV/AIDS & other sexual health issues.

Helplines: Sexuality

☺▽ **Jewish Lesbian & Gay Helpline**
☎ 171 706 3123
🕐 Mon Thu 19:00 - 22:00
Advice & information about HIV/AIDS & other sexual health issues.

☺▽ **London Lesbian & Gay Switchboard**
P. O. Box 7324, London N1 9QS.
☎ 171 837 7324
☎ 171 837 7606 (to volunteer)
🕐 24hrs.
Advice & information about HIV/AIDS & other sexual health issues.

Mailorder: Adult Toys: Miscellaneous

☺ ■ **Motail**
P.O. Box 19, Pangbourne, Berkshire RG8 8LW.
Catalogue, £1 each (or 4 IRCs), 3 for £2.5, all four for £3.

☺ **New Age**
BM 220, London WC1N 3XX.
☎ 181 809 6119

Mailorder: Books: BDSM

☺ ■ **Ryder Publishing**
BCM Box 3406, London WC1N 3XX.
Original & exclusive BDSM fiction.

Mailorder: Books: Erotic

☺ **Midian Books**
69 Park Lane, Bonehill, Staffordshire B78 3HZ.
☎ 1827 281391 ✆ 1827 281391
🕐 Mon - Sat 09:00 - 21:00
Specialises in erotic art, fiction, & studies in sexuality. Catalogue, £1. Age statement of 18 is required.

Mailorder: Books: General

☺ ■ **Books Direct**
Freepost, Nightingale House, 1 Fulham High Street, Fulham, London SW6 3YZ.
☎ 171 371 7004

☺ ■ **The Private Case**
P. O. Box 23, Royston, Hertfordshire SG8 8DT.
Books & magazines selected by women & couples.

☺ ■ **Prowler Press Ltd.**
33 Highgate Street, London N6 5JT.
☎ 181 348 9963 ✆ 181 347 7667

Mailorder: Books: Sexuality

☿▼ **Male Image**
P. O. Box 3821, London N5 1UY.
☎ 181 885 5488
[VISA] [MC] [AMEX]
Mail order arm of Gay Men's Press. Free catalogue.

☿▼ **Male Xpress Ltd.**
33 Highgate Street, London N6 5JT.
☎ 181 340 8644
Mail order arm of Prowler Press. Free catalogue.

☿▼ **Millivres Ltd.**
The Gay Times Book Service, 283 Camden High Street, London NW1 7BX.
☎ 171 267 0021

Mailorder: Catalogues: General

☺ ■ **Catalog Connection**
Freepost, Nightingale House, 7 Fulham High Street, Fulham, London SW6 3YZ.
☎ 171 371 7004
Clothing & catalogues from all the major manufacturers.

Mailorder: Clothing: Corsets

☺ ■ **Axfords**
82 Centurion Road, Brighton, East Sussex BN1 3LN.
☎ 127 332 7944 ✆ 127 322 0680
Catalogue available.

Mailorder: Clothing: Fetish

Alter Ego
P. O. Box 10, Bramhall, Cheshire SK7 2QF.
PVC skirts, capes, jackets, belts, etc.. Also newsletter. Catalogue, £5.

Après Noir
Unit 1, Erskine House, Union Street, Trowbridge, Wiltshire BA14 8RY.
1225 774164 — Fax 1225 774452
Services@bdyaware.demon.co.uk
Fetish underwear for men. Catalogue, £2 or $3U.S..

Cathouse Design Studio
2nd. Floor, Bennet Millbridge, Liversedge, West Yorkshire.
1924 412662
Custom work also available3.

D. B. Leisurewear
P. O. Box 2016, London NW6 4SD.
Schoolboy uniforms. Publishes *Devotee*.

Honour
5 Riverside, 28 Park Street, Waterloo, London SE1 9EQ.
171 378 8565 — Fax 171 378 8101
Mon - Fri 10:30 - 19:00, Sat 11:30 - 17:00
Catalogue, £5 in U.K. (refundable), £7 overseas.

The House of Harlot
171 706 2315
By appointment only
Made to measure leather & rubber for men & women.

Jay Fashions
P.O. Box 606, Stanford-Le-Hope, Essex SS17 9BE.

Lanem Fashions
4 Hillside, Chesham, Buckinghamshire HP5 2PQ.
PVC clothing & boots, magazines, & videos.

Lifestyle
P.O. Box 4, Holsworthy, Devon EX22 7YL.
Catalogue, £5.

Sh!
P. O. Box 3651, London N1 6HD.
171 613 5458
Mon Tue - Sat 11:30-18:30
✓
Mail order department of Sh! The U.K.'s only women's erotic emporium.
Catalogue, £5.

Showgrade Ltd.
P.O. Box 10, Bramhall, Stockport, Cheshire SK7 2QF.
Catalogue, £ 2.

Skint
P. O. Box 136, Norwich, Norfolk NR3 3LJ.

Tight Situation
P.O. Box 860, London SE12 0LL.
181 857 7146 — Fax 181 857 4251

Victoria Regine
P. O. Box 192, Wolverhampton, West Midlands WV4 5TS.
1902 336191
Also custom work. Catalogue, £1.50 each.

Yago Holdings Ltd.
Samantha Spade Division, Roman Way, Coleshill, West Midlands B46 1RL.
1675 464834
Catalogue available.

Mailorder: Clothing: Footwear

Roger Adams
31 North Road, Brighton, East Sussex BN1 1YB.
High heel shoes & boots.

Lady Elizabeth
P.O. Box 2, Ellesmere Port, Wirral L65 3EA.
151 353 0126 — Fax 151 353 0128

The Magic Shoe Company
Unit 6, 88 Mile End Road, London E1 4UN.
171 791 3331 — Fax 171 791 3331
171 791 3352
High-heeled boots & shoes.

Zenana
P. O. Box 192, Wolverhampton, West Midlands WV4 5TS.
✓
Source for erotic shoes & boots.

Mailorder: Clothing: General

Midnight Lady
20-24 Cardigan Street, Luton, Bedfordshire LU1 1RR.
158 239 1854
Catalogue available.

Mailorder: Clothing: Industrial

Cover Up
P.O. Box 40, Nuneaton, Warwickshire CV10 0XB.
1203 398809

Mailorder: Clothing: Leather

Elle For Leather
P. O. Box 47, Manchester, Greater Manchester M21 8EJ.

JDL
P. O. Box 32, Biddulph, Staffordshire ST8 7DW.
1782 518564
Visits by appointment only
VISA MC
High quality gear at low prices. Full range of leather & rubber belts, harnesses, jackets, chaps, waistcoats, etc.. Free catalogue.

Mailorder: Clothing: Lingerie

Body Aware
Unit 1, Erskine House, Union Street, Trowbridge, Wiltshire BA14 8RY.
1225 774164 — Fax 1225 774452
Services@bdyaware.demon.co.uk
Maid's dresses, panties, stockings, camisoles, etc. made to fit men.
Catalogue, £1 or $2U.S..

Mailorder: Clothing: Rubber

Abra Creations & Designs
10 High Street, Southminster, Essex CM0 7AA.
Stocks Images Plus rubber clothing. Catalogue available.

Bob's Rubberwear
37 Tenby Close, Forest Gate, London E7 8AX.
181 470 6635
Personal callers welcome by appointment seven days a week
Also custom work. Catalogue, free with SAE or IRS.

Essential Image
P. O. Box 5, Brixham, South Devonshire TQ5 9XR.
Makes fahsion & fetish rubber clothing. Also custom work.

Invincible
Unit 19E, 2nd. Floor, Tower Workshops, Riley Road, London SE1 3DG.
171 237 4017 — Fax 171 231 5416
171 237 5062
Mon - Fri 10:00 - 18:00, Sat 12:00 - 16:00
✓ $ VISA MC
Specialist in rubber for men & women, made to measure. Catalogue, £5, overseas £8.

Libidex
BCM Libidex, London WC1N 3XX.
171 613 3329

Loco
20a The Broadway, Stoneleigh, Surrey KT19 0RP.
181 786 7347
Catalogue available.

Remawear
Sherwood House, Burnley Road, Todmorden, Lancashire OL13 7ET.

Rubber Lady
P. O. Box 192, Barnet, Hertfordshire EN4 9LZ.

South Bucks Rainwear
Unit 5, Station Road, Didcot, Oxfordshire OX1 7NA.
1235 811666
Catalogue, $3U.S..

Kim West
BCM Box 8875, London WC1N 3XX.
171 729 6960
Catalogue, £8.

Wild Designs
1 Chestnut Road, London SE27 9EZ.
181 766 7550 — Fax 181 766 6896
Catalogue, £3.

Mailorder: Erotica: Adult Baby

Tinkerbell's Treasures
P.O. Box 3765, London SE5 8RY.

Mailorder: Erotica: BDSM

Bound II
P. O. Box 4, Weston-Super-Mare, Avon BS24 9BB.
Bondage, rubber, & corporal punishment gear.

Eagle Leathers
P. O. Box 57, Northolt, Middlesex UB5 4SB.
181 426 8047
Catalogue available.

Just Leathers

19 Cambridge Street, Caldmore, Walsall WS1 4BZ.
☺ **Leatherline**
Centenary Business Centre, Littlemore Lane, Loughborough, Leicestershire LE11 2RG.
☺ ■ **Monique**
P. O. Box 351, Ferndown, Dorset BH22 8U.
☺ ■ **Ram Leathers**
☎ 127 350 8272
Leatherwork & chainmail to order.

Mailorder: Erotica
☺ **Between The Sheets**
18 Calne Business Centre, Harris Road, Calne, Wiltshire SN11 9PT.
☎ 1249 822052 ✆ 1249 821517
Erotic bedsheets & duvet covers in latex, hi-gloss PVC, satin, velvet, & pure silk.

Mailorder: Erotica: Dildos
☺ **Babes Silicone Dildoes**
BMC Babes, London WC1N 3XX.

Mailorder: Erotica: Gas Masks
☺ **Restrictive Practice**
P. O. Box 3124, Newport Pagnell, Buckinghamshire MK16 0QD.

Mailorder: Erotica: General
♂▼ **Clone Zone**
3rd. Floor, Pollard Street, East Ancoats P. O., Greater Manchester M40 7FS.
☎ 161 273 5246 ✆ 161 272 8410
Free catalogue.
☺ ■ **Superia Supplies**
P. O. Box 424, Hove, East Sussex BN3 1EU.
☎ 127 377 8816 ✆ 127 374 6867
🕐 24hr. telephone & facsimile
Also some leather & rubber items. Does not ship to North America.

Mailorder: Erotica
☺ **Get Wet**
BCM Box 3564, London WC1N 3XX.
☎ 171 627 0290
Toys, clothing, & equipment. Catalogue, £5.
☺ ■ **Patrick Gilson**
859A Fulham Road, London SW6 5HA.
☎ 171 371 9454

Mailorder: Erotica: Leather
☺ **Belt Up & Buckle Off**
P.O. Box 593, London SW4 0HT.
☎ 171 737 6161
Catalogue available.
♂▼ **Expectations**
75 Great Eastern Street, London EC2A 3HU.
☎ 171 739 0292
London's largest collection of rubber, leather, & toys. Also sells the Detainer rubber & waxed cotton lines. Catalogue available.
☺ **Skin To Skin**
35 Newington Road, Ramsgate, Kent CT12 6EQ.

Mailorder: Erotica: Rubber
☺ **Lakeland Elements**
23 Broadway, Morecombe, Lancashire LA4 5BQ.
☎ 152 441 3607
Catalogue available.
☺ ■ **Wetlook Unlimited**
P.O. Box HP50, Leeds, West Yorkshire LS6 1TR.
Catalogue, £5.

Mailorder: Erotica
☺▼ **Sin-A-Matique**
22 Preston Street, Brighton, East Sussex BN1 2HN.
☎ 1273 329154
🕐 10:00 - 18:30
☺ **Spellbound Limited**
P. O. Box 4506, London SW19 1XU.
☺ **Tabby**
P.O. Box 916, Westcliff On Sea, Essex SS0 8QD.
Fashion for Purr-vs. Well-made, distinctive sex clothes for women. Catalogue, £5.
☺ **Una Deva**

P. O. Box 1426, Shepton Mallet, Somerset BA4 6HH.
☎ 174 983 1397
☺ ■ **Stephen Wyle**
134 Manor Street, Fenton, Stoke-On-Trent, Staffordshire ST4 2JD.

Mailorder: Safer Sex Products
☺ **Starlight**
P. O. Box 10, Buckhurst Hill, Essex IG9 5EU.
☎ 181 559 2369

Mailorder: Videos: BDSM
☺ **GVNS**
P. O. Box 173, Folkestone, Kent CT19 5YT.

Organizations: BDSM
♂▼ **Blackline Interchain**
P. O. Box 4293, London SW11 1ZF.
☎ 171 978 4820 ✆ 171 924 6740
Contact: Mr. Alan Turner
Club for men who enjoy leather, uniform, rubber, & BDSM, & gay skinheads & bootboys.
♂ ▽ **SM Bisexuals**
c/o Central Station, 37 Wharfdale Road, Kings Cross, London N1 9SE.
☎ 171 278 3294
✉ smbi@andelain.demon.co.uk
🕐 Meets monthly
National network for bisexual BDSMers, friends, & supporters. Publishes Ungagged quarterly. Yearly subscription is free in the U.K..
♂▽ **SM Gays**
BM SM Gays, London WC1N 3XX.
✉ smgays@powerhouse.co.uk
🌐 http://www.powerhouse.co.uk/
🕐 Meets 3rd. Wed of month 20:00 - 02:00
Social & educational group for consensual sexual BDSM. Also organizes annual Dungeon In The Sky event. Publishes SM Resources Book once a year. Age statement of 18 is required.

Organizations: Fetish: Clothing: Rubber
♂▽ **Gummi**
BM 414, London WC1N 3XX.
✉ gummi@powerhouse.co.uk
🌐 http://www.powerhouse.co.uk/powerhouse/gummi
🕐 Meets Last Sat of month in London 22:00 - 02:00
Men only, rubber only club. Strict dress code. Publishes Rubber Sheet every two months. Yearly subscription is £10. Age statement of 18 is required.

Organizations: Fetish: Mess
♂▽ **The Society for Lovers Of Slapstick Happenings (SLOSH)**
P. O. Box 73, Harrogate, North Yorkshire HG1 4TS.
Contact: Mr. Don McLeod, Secretary
Play with food, water, mud, & messy things.

Organizations: Sexual Politics
☺ □ **Countdown on Spanner**
c/o Central Station, 37 Wharfdale Road, Kings Cross, London N1 9SE.
☎ 171 278 3294
✉ spanner@honour.demon.co.uk
🌐 http://www.csv.warwick.ac.uk/~esrhi/span1.html
🕐 Workshops last Sun of month 20:00
Group campaigning to legalise BDSM.

Organizations: Tattoo
☺ **Tattoo Club of Great Britain**
389 Cowley Road, Oxford, Oxfordshire OX4 2BS.
☎ 186 571 6877

Publishers: Books: Sexuality
♂▼ **éditions aubrey walter**
P. O. Box 247, London N6 4BW.
☎ 181 341 7818 ✆ 181 341 7467
Free catalogue.
♂▼ **Gay Men's Press**
P. O. Box 247, 50 South Ealing Road, London N6 4BW.
☎ 181 341 7818 ✆ 181 341 7467
Free catalogue.

Publishers: Magazines: AIDS
♂▼ **Positive Times**
Silveraim Ltd., 72 Holloway Road, London N7 8NZ.
☎ 171 296 6000 ✆ 171 296 0026
✉ bz72@Cityscape.Co.UK

Published every month.

Publishers: Magazines: BDSM

👫▼ *The Key*
Sussex Mailbox, P. O. Box 314, Haywards Heath, Sussex RH16 2FH.
☎ 1444 482443
Mail order only. Published quarterly.

Stores: Books: General

♂▽ **Gay's The Word**
♿ 66 Marchmont Street, London WC1N 1AB.
☎ 171 278 7654
🕐 Mon - Sat 10:00 - 18:00, Sat - 19:00, Sun 14:00 - 18:00
🚗 ✓ ▦ VISA MC AMEX 🌑
Bookshop selling as wide a range as space allows of lesbian & gay literature. Good range of BDSM literature. Irish also spoken.

Stores: Clothing: Rubber

☺ ■ **Wild Designs**
1 Chestnut Road, London SE27 9EZ.
☎ 181 766 7550 ✆ 181 766 6896
Catalogue, £3.

AVON

Bath

Helplines: Sexuality

♂▽ **Bath Gay & Lesbian Switchboard**
☎ 122 546 5793
🕐 Tue 18:00 - 19:30

Organizations: AIDS: Education

☺ □ **Aled Richards Trust**
Hetling House, 2 Hetling Court, Bath, Avon.
☎ 127 255 3355
Advice & information about HIV/AIDS & other sexual health issues.

Bristol

Bars: BDSM

☺ **The Inner Circle**
6 Perry Road, Bristol, Avon BS1 5BQ.
☎ 117 929 3754 ✆ 117 929 3754
🕐 Monthly
🚗 ▦ VISA ℮
Strict dress code event for serious scene members. Membership only. Good food Jazz & classical music. Market stalls, massage, furniture, etc..

☺ **Spank Promotions**
6 Perry Road, Bristol, Avon BS1 5BQ.
☎ 117 929 3754 ✆ 117 929 3754
🕐 Club is monthly 21:30 - 02:00. Call 11:00 - 18:00 for information
🚗 ✓ ▦ VISA ℮
Dress code club night with DJs, dancing, massage, grope box, fun, fantasy, & fetishism.

Helplines: Sexuality

☺▽ **Bristol Lesbian & Gay Switchboard**
☎ 117 942 0842
☎ 117 942 5927
🕐 19:30 - 22:30
Advice & information about HIV/AIDS & other sexual health & sexuality issues.

Manufacturers: Clothing: Rubber

☺ ■ **Maxitosh**
P. O. Box 1377, Long Ashton, Avon BS18 9JW.
Rubber-lined satin & nylon underwear. Custom work available.

Organizations: AIDS: Support

☺ □ **Aled Richards Trust**
Queen Anne House, 8-10 West Street, Bristol, Avon BS2 0BH.
☎ 117 955 3355
🕐 Tue Fri 13:00 - 16:00 19:00 - 21:00
Advice & information about HIV/AIDS & other sexual health issues.

Organizations: BDSM

☺ **ACS**
P. O. Box 1504, Bristol, Avon BS12 3BL.
For people interested in fetish & BDSM.

Organizations: Fetish: Clothing

☺ □ **Cruise Club**
The Lochiel, Bristol, Avon BS1 5UH.
☎ 117 929 2447
🕐 Every Sat.
The Lochiel is a boat.

Organizations: Motorcycle

♂▽ **Excess Motorcycle Club**
P.O. Box 685, Bristol, Avon BS99 1YY.

Piercers

☺ ■ **Body Art Studios**
201 Two Mile Hill Road, Kingswood, Avon.
☎ 127 260 3923

Publishers: Magazines: Fetish

☺ ■ *Dominique & Rubber Fun*
154 Bedminster Down Road, Bristol, Avon BS13 7AF.
Contact magazine for those who enjoy dominance & submission. Also contains stories.

☺ ■ *Knickers & Upskirts*
154 Bedminster Down Road, Bristol, Avon BS13 7AF.

Stores: Books: General

☺ **Greenleaf Bookshop**
82 Colston Street, Bristol, Avon.
☎ 117 921 1369

Stores: Clothing: Fetish

☺ ■ **Crazy World**
81 Ponsford Road, Bristol, Avon BS4 2UT.

☺ **Religion**
6 Perry Road, Bristol, Avon BS1 5BQ.
☎ 117 929 3754 ✆ 117 929 3754
🕐 11:00 - 18:00
🚗 ▦ VISA ℮
Designer fetish inspired clothing & club wear for males, females, & she-males. Also, wigs, shoes, boots, magazines, books, corsetry. Commissions undertaken.

Stores: Clothing: Sexuality

⚦■ **Abigail Louise**
50 Park Row, Bristol, Avon BS1 5LH.
☎ 117 976 0969
Clothing , wigs, & shoes for TVs. Also adult baby clothes.

⚦ **Transformation Ltd.**
273 Southmead Road, Southmead, Avon B21 9RH.
☎ 117 959 3413
🕐 Mon - Sat 09:00 - 20:00
The world's leading TV specialists.

Weston-Super-Mare

Bars: BDSM

☺ **De Sade**
P. O. Box 4, Weston-Super-Mare, Avon BS24 9BB.
🕐 Last Sat of month 20:30 - 02:00 (write for more info)

BEDFORDSHIRE

County Resources

Helplines: Sexuality

☺▽ **Bedfordshire Lesbian & Gay Helpline**
☎ 123 421 8990
🕐 Tue 19:30 - 22:00
Advice & information about HIV/AIDS & other sexual health & sexuality issues.

♂▽ **Luton Switchboard**
☎ 1234 218990

Bedford

Organizations: AIDS: Support

☺ □ **Body Positive—Bedfordshire**
☎ 1582 484499
🕐 Mon Tue Thu 10:00 - 14:00, Wed 10:00 - 14:00 19:30 - 22:30
Advice & information about HIV/AIDS & other sexual health issues.

Leighton Buzzard

Organizations: BDSM

☺ □ **Valkyrie**
P.O. Box 148, Leighton Buzzard, Bedfordshire LU7 8ZH.

Publishers: Magazines: Sexuality

⚦■ *Taffeta*
P. O. Box 65, Leighton Buzzard, Bedfordshire OU7 8TJ.

Luton

Piercers

☺ ■ **Gary Simpson**
☎ 1582 505839
EPPA & APTA member.

BERKSHIRE

County Resources

Helplines: Sexuality

⚢▽ **Berkshire Gay Switchboard**
☎ 1753 856521
Wed 20:00 - 22:00
Advice & information about HIV/AIDS & other sexual health & sexuality issues.

Maidenhead

Organizations: BDSM

Submissive Females
P.O. Box 1504, Maidenhead, Berkshire SL6 7PT.
Contact: Jane

Reading

Helplines: AIDS

☺ □ **AIDSLine**
P.O. Box 358, Reading, Berkshire RG6 3DJ.
☎ 173 450 3377

Helplines: Sexuality

⚢▽ **Reading Lesbian & Gay Helpline**
P. O. Box 75, Reading, Berkshire RG1 7DU.
☎ 1734 597269
Tue Fri 20:00 - 22:00, Sun 16:00 - 18:00
Advice & information about HIV/AIDS & other sexual health & sexuality issues.

Slough

Organizations: AIDS: Support

☺ □ **Thames Valley Positive Support (TVPS)**
P. O. Box 1433, Slough, Berkshire SL1 6YG.
☎ 1628 603 400 — Fax 1628 669 797
Tue - Thu 11:00 - 16:00
Advice & information about HIV/AIDS & other sexual health issues.

Stores: Books: General

☺ ■ **R B Books**
6 Fairview Road, Slough, Berkshire SL2 2JL.
☎ 175 353 9565

Thatcham

Stores: Safer Sex Products

⚢ **Condomania**
5 Rivermead, Pipers Way, Thatcham, Berkshire RG19 4EP.
☎ 1635 874393

Wokingham

Manufacturers: Clothing: Corsets

☺ ■ **C & S Constructions**
40 Whaley Road, Wokingham, Berkshire RG40 1QA.
hourglass@staylace.win-uk.net
High standards in the traditions of English custom corsetry. Mail order only. No catalogue, but ordering pack $3 to cover postage costs.

☺ □ **True Grace Corsets**
43 Emmbrook Road, Wokingham, Berkshire RG11 1HG.
☎ 1734 785577
Custom made corsets. Also sell the C&S Constructions corset catalogue for $3U.S..

BUCKINGHAMSHIRE

High Wycombe

Helplines: AIDS

☺ □ **ChilternAIDS**
☎ 1494 444818
Thu 20:00 - 22:00
Advice & information about HIV/AIDS & other sexual health issues.

Helplines: Sexuality

⚢▽ **Milton Keynes Lesbian & Gay Switchboard**
☎ 1908 666266
Men Mon 19:00 - 21:00, Women Thu 19:00 - 21:00
Advice & information about HIV/AIDS & other sexual health & sexuality issues.

Milton Keynes

Helplines: Sexuality

⚢▽ **Milton Keynes Lesbian & Gay Switchboard**
☎ 1908 666266
Men Mon 19:00 - 21:00, Women Thu 19:00 - 21:00
Advice & information about HIV/AIDS & other sexual health & sexuality issues.

CAMBRIDGESHIRE

Cambridge

Helplines: AIDS

☺ □ **AIDS Helpline**
P.O. Box 257, Cambridge, Cambridgeshire CB2 1XQ.
☎ 122 369 765
Mon - Sat 08:00 - 18:00

☺ □ **Cambridge AIDS Helpline**
☎ 800 697 697
Sat 12:00 -14:00
Advice & information about HIV/AIDS & other sexual health issues.

Helplines: Sexuality

⚢▽ **Cambridge Friend**
☎ 122 324 6013
Wed 18:30 - 21:30
Advice & information about HIV/AIDS & other sexual health & sexuality issues.

Peterborough

Helplines: AIDS

☺ □ **Peterborough AIDS Helpline**
☎ 1733 62334
Tue Thu 19:30 - 21:30
Advice & information about HIV/AIDS & other sexual health issues.

Helplines: Sexuality

⚢▽ **Peterborough Friend**
☎ 1733 61499
Tue Thu 19:30 - 21:30
Advice & information about HIV/AIDS & other sexual health & sexuality issues.

Publishers: Newspapers: Sexuality

⚢▼ ***Gay Anglia***
P. O. Box 161, Peterborough, Cambridgeshire PE3 8HL.
☎ 1733 267373

CHESHIRE

Chester

Organizations: AIDS: Support

☺ □ **Chester & District AIDS Relief (CADAR)**
☎ 1244 390300
Mon Fri 19:30 - 22:00
Advice & information about HIV/AIDS & other sexual health issues.

Crewe

Helplines: Sexuality

⚢▽ **Crewe L&G Switchboard**
c/o Volunteer Bureau, 1a Gatefield Street, Crewe, Cheshire CW1 2JP.
☎ 1270 250980

Organizations: AIDS: Education

☺ □ **Crewe Action for Sexual Health**
P.O. Box 47, Crewe, Cheshire CW1 1WT.
☎ 127 025 1135

Organizations: AIDS: Support

☺ □ **AIDS Relief**
P.O. Box 47, Crewe, Cheshire CW1 1WT.
☎ 127 062 8938

Liverpool

Stores: Military Surplus

☺ ■ **Army & Navy Stores**
19b Church Street, Frodsham, Cheshire.
☎ 1928 731925

Macclesfield
Stores: Military Surplus
☺ ■ **Army & Navy Stores**
21 Chestergate, Macclesfield, Cheshire.
☎ 1625 425164

Runcorn
Stores: Clothing: Fetish
☺ ■ **Nightstyle Designs**
10 Leaside, Holton Brook, Cheshire WA7 2NQ.

Sandbach
Helplines: Sexuality
⚥▽ **North Staffordshire Lesbian & Gay Switchboard**
☎ 1782 266998
🕘 Mon Wed Fri 20:00 - 22:00, Sun 13:00 - 15:00
Advice & information about HIV/AIDS & other sexual health & sexuality issues.

Manufacturers: Whips
☺ ■ **AE Services**
P. O. Box 941, Sandbach, Cheshire CW11 0ZD.
High quality disciplinary implements: canes, tawses, paddles, straps, whips, etc. Efficient & discreet mail order service. Free catalogue.

Stalybridge
Organizations: Bondage
☺ **Axis**
P. O. Box 27, Stalybridge, Cheshire SK15 2ED.
Publishes a newsletter every month.

Stockport
Publishers: Magazines: BDSM
☺ ***Divinity***
Divine Press, P.O. Box 108, Stockport, Cheshire SK1 4DD.
☎ 153 274 6319

☺ ***Headpress Magazine***
P.O. Box 160, Stockport, Cheshire SK1 4ET.
Published 5 times a year. Yearly subscription is $40.

Warrington
Helplines: AIDS
☺ □ **Warrington AIDSline**
☎ 1925 417134
🕘 Mon Wed 19:00 - 21:00
Advice & information about HIV/AIDS & other sexual health issues.

Helplines: Sexuality
⚥▽ **Warrington Switchboard**
☎ 1925 59572
☎ 1925 59557
🕘 Mon Wed 19:00 - 22:00

Windsford
Stores: Clothing: Fetish
☺ ■ **Clingline**
417 Station Road, Windsford, Cheshire CW7 3NE.

CORNWALL
Cambourne
Helplines: Sexuality
☺ ▽ **Gay & Lesbian Switchboard Cornwall**
☎ 120 931 4449
🕘 Mon Fri 20:00 - 23:00
Advice & information about HIV/AIDS & other sexual health & sexuality issues.

Stores: Books: General
⚥▼ **Red River Books**
25 Chapel Road, Tuckingmill, Cornwall TR14 8QY.
☎ 1209 714805

Launceston
Manufacturers: Furniture: BDSM
☺ **Mr. & Mrs. Beech**
Braeside, Tavistock Road, Launceston, Cornwall PL15 9LF.

Penryn
Distributors: Books: General
☺ ■ **J Barnicoat Ltd.**
Parkengue, Penryn, Cornwall TR10 9EN.
☎ 132 637 2628 — Fax 132 637 6 423

Penzance
Helplines: Sexuality
⚢▽ **Penzance Lesbian Line**
☎ 1736 62869
🕘 Thu 19:00 - 22:00
Advice & information about HIV/AIDS & other sexual health & sexuality issues.

Saint Austell
Helplines: Sexuality
⚥▽ **Saint Austell Switchboard**
☎ 1726 69111
🕘 Wed 18:00 - 22:00

Truro
Organizations: AIDS: Support
☺ □ **Cornwall AIDS Council (CAC)**
☎ 1872 225022
🕘 Mon - Fri 12:00 - 17:00
Advice & information about HIV/AIDS & other sexual health issues.

CUMBRIA
Carlisle
Helplines: AIDS
☺ □ **Carlisle Citizens Advice Bureau**
☎ 122 859 1986
🕘 19:30 - 23:00
Advice & information about HIV/AIDS & other sexual health issues.

Kendal
Helplines: Sexuality
⚥▽ **Lancaster Lesbian & Gay Switchboard**
☎ 1524 847437
🕘 Thu Fri 19:00 - 21:00
Advice & information about HIV/AIDS & other sexual health & sexuality issues.

Penrith
Helplines: Sexuality
⚥▽ **Lancaster Lesbian & Gay Switchboard**
☎ 1524 847437
🕘 Thu Fri 19:00 - 21:00
Advice & information about HIV/AIDS & other sexual health & sexuality issues.

Seascale
Organizations: Fetish: Mess
⚥▽ **Mud Maniacs**
P. O. Box 7, Seascale, Cumbria CA20 1JE.

DERBYSHIRE
Chesterfield
Organizations: AIDS: Education
☺ □ **HIV & AIDS in North Derbyshire (HAND)**
☎ 1246 550550
Advice & information about HIV/AIDS & other sexual health issues.

Organizations: Sexuality
⚧▽ **Trans-Net**
3 Saint Augustines Road, Chesterfield, Derbyshire S40 2SF.
☎ 1246 275799 — Fax 1246 275799
Contact: Mr. R. Floyd
Publishes a directory.

Derby
Helplines: AIDS
☺ □ **Derby AIDS Line**
☎ 800 622738
🕘 Mon 19:00 - 21:00, Thu 14:00 - 16:00 19:00 - 21:00
Advice & information about HIV/AIDS & other sexual health issues.

Helplines: Sexuality

☿▽ **Derby Friend**
☎ 1332 349333
🕐 Wed 19:00 - 22:00
Advice & information about HIV/AIDS & other sexual health & sexuality issues.

Publishers: Magazines: BDSM

☺ ■ *Cruella*
Rogue-Hagen Publications, P. O. Box 122, Derby, Derbyshire DE22 4XA. For dominant females. Also mail order fetish gear.

☺ ■ *Goddess*
Rogue-Hagen Publications, P. O. Box 122, Derby, Derbyshire DE22 4XA. For dominant females.

Stores: Books: General

☺ **Abbey Books**
45 Bank Road, Derby, Derbyshire.

☺ ■ **Bookworm**
16 Bishop Street, Derby, Derbyshire.
☎ 150 426 1616

Heanor

Manufacturers: Rubber Sheeting

☺ ■ **Four D Rubber Co. Ltd.**
Heanor Gate Industrial Estate, Heanor, Derbyshire DE75 7SJ.
☎ 1773 763134 📠 1773 763136
Manufacturers of sheet rubber used by the world's leading rubber fashion & fantasy clothing designers. Over thirty colours in nine thicknesses.

Middleton

Manufacturers: Furniture: BDSM

☺ **Woodworks**
Oakstone House, Middleton, Derbyshire DE45 1LS.
Makes furniture & other wooden items.

DEVON

County Resources

Helplines: Sexuality

☿▽ **North Devon Lesbian & Gay Switchboard**
P. O. Box 13, Barnstaple, Devon EX31 7YU.
☎ 1271 321111
🕐 Thu Sun 19:00 - 21:00

Barnstaple

Organizations: AIDS: Education

☺ □ **Action Against AIDS—North Devon**
Barum House, The Square, Barnstaple, Devon.
☎ 127 124 555
🕐 Mon, Wed, Fri 19:00 - 22:00

Exeter

Helplines: AIDS

☺ □ **Exeter AIDS Line**
☎ 1392 411600
🕐 Mon - Fri 19:00 - 22:00
Advice & information about HIV/AIDS & other sexual health issues.

Helplines: Sexuality

☿▽ **Gay & Lesbian Counselling South West**
☎ 1392 422 016
🕐 Moon 19:30 - 22:00
Advice & information about HIV/AIDS & other sexual health & sexuality issues.

Newton Abbot

Publishers: Magazines: Fetish

☺ *Necronomicon*
15 Jubilee Road, Newton Abbot, Devon TQ12 1LB.

Plymouth

Organizations: AIDS: Support

☺ □ **Plymouth Eddystone Group (PEG)**
☎ 1752 251666
🕐 24hrs.
Advice & information about HIV/AIDS & other sexual health issues.

Stores: Books: General

☺▼ **In Other Words, Ltd.**
♿ 72 Mutley Plain, Plymouth, Devon PL4 6LF.
☎ 1752 663 889 📞 1752 252 232
🕐 Mon - Sat 09:00 - 18:00
🛍 ✓ 💳 💳 ℮
Gay-friendly bookshop. Clientele generally "alternative." Lesbian owned, Wide range of gay & lesbian books, magazines, etc.. Advice on local scene.

Torquay

Organizations: AIDS: Support

☺ □ **Torbay AIDS Group Supporters**
Braddan Hill Road West, Torquay, Devon.
☎ 180 329 9266

☺ □ **Torquay AIDS Support Group (TAGS)**
☎ 1803 299266
🕐 Mon - Fri 16:00 - 22:00
Advice & information about HIV/AIDS & other sexual health issues.

DORSET

County Resources

Helplines: Sexuality

☿▽ **Dorset Gay & Lesbian Switchboard**
☎ 1202 318 822
🕐 Mon - Fri 19:30 - 22:30

☺ ▽ **Dorset Lesbian & Gay Helpline**
☎ 1202 318822
🕐 Mon - Fri 19:30 - 22:30
Advice & information about HIV/AIDS & other sexual health & sexuality issues.

Bournemouth

Manufacturers: Restraints: Leather

☺ ■ **Dean's of Bournemouth**
☎ 1202 314584
Leather restraints handmade using traditional methods.

Organizations: AIDS: Support

☺ □ **Body Positive—Bournemouth**
☎ 1202 297386
🕐 Mon -Wed Fri 20:00 - 22:00
Advice & information about HIV/AIDS & other sexual health issues.

Organizations: Motorcycle

☺▽ **Bournemouth Leather MSC (BLMSC)**
P. O. Box 932, Bournemouth, Dorset BH3 7YG.
🕐 Meets Fri 21:00

Stores: Clothing: Rubber

☺ **Sealwear**
Regent Chambers, 15 Westover Road, Bournemouth, Dorset BH1 2BY.
☎ 1202 290675
Also custom cat suits & masks. Catalogue, £10.

Stores: Erotica: General

☺ **Cerebus**
25 The Triangle, Bournemouth, Dorset BH2 5SE.
☎ 1202 290529
Catalogue, £4.

Ferndown

Publishers: Magazines: BDSM

⚲ ■ *Sapphire*
P. O. Box 1643, Stone Castle, Ferndown, Dorset BH22 0YP.

☺ ■ *Scorpion*
P. O. Box 1643, Stone Castle, Ferndown, Dorset BH22 0YP.

Stoke Abbot

Stores: Erotica: General

☺ ■ **Mac Mac**
Brimley Mill, Beaminster, Dorset.
☎ 1308 68227
Raincoats & mackintoshes in cotton-backed rubber.

DURHAM

Darlington

Stores: Books: General

☺ ■ **Book Exchange**

NMA, 43 Grange Road, Darlington, Durham DL1 5NB.

Stores: Erotica: General
☺ ■ **N. M. A.**
43 Grange Road, Darlington, Durham DL1 5NB.
☎ 132 548 1631
Clothes, toys, books, & magazines.

Durham
Stores: Books: General
☺ **Alternatives**
28b Sutton Street, Durham DH1 4BW.
☎ 1209 612234

EAST SUSSEX
Brighton
Bars: BDSM
♂▼ **Schwarz Bar**
New Europe Hotel, 31-32 Marine Parade, Brighton, East Sussex.
☎ 1273 624462
⏱ Fri Sat 22:00 - 02:00
Dress code leather, denim, rubber, & uniform.

♂▼ **The Village Club**
74 Saint James Street, Brighton, East Sussex.
☎ 127 367 4816
Age statement of 18 is required.

Helplines: AIDS
☺ ☐ **Sussex AIDS Helpline**
☎ 127 357 1660
⏱ Mon - Fri 10:00 - 17:00, Minicom 20:00 - 22:00
Advice & information about HIV/AIDS & other sexual health issues.

Organizations: AIDS: Support
☺ ☐ **AIDS Centre**
P.O. Box 17, Brighton, East Sussex BN2 5NQ.
☎ 127 357 1660

Organizations: Motorcycle
♂▽ **Sussex Lancers MSC**
P.O. Box 890, Brighton, East Sussex BN2 2DA.

Piercers
☺ ■ **Perforations**
16A Preston Street, Brighton, East Sussex BN1 2HN.
☎ 127 332 6577
⏱ Mon - Sat 12:00 - 17:30

☺ ■ **Rings & Things**
39a Beaconsfield Road, Brighton, East Sussex.
☎ 127 367 0619
Makes body jewellery.

Radio: Sexuality
♂▼ **Pride FM**
G-Spot Productions, 20 Great College Street, Brighton, East Sussex BN2 1HL.
☎ 1273 676435

Stores: Books: General
☺ ▼ **Cardome**
47A Saint James Street, Brighton, East Sussex BN2 1RG.
☎ 127 369 2916
⏱ Mon - Sat 09:30 - 17:30
👗 ✓
Caters to gay people. Sells adult cards, magazines, poppers, etc.. Age statement of 18 is required.

♂▼ **Out! Books**
4 & 7 Dorset Street, Brighton, East Sussex BN2 1WA.
☎ 1273 623356

☺ **Public House Bookshop**
21 Preston Street, Brighton, East Sussex BN1 2HN.
☎ 127 328 357

☺ **Read All About It**
69 East Street, Brighton, East Sussex.
☎ 127 320 5824

Stores: Clothing: Fetish
☺ ■ **E-Garbs**
9 Boyces Street, The Lanes, Brighton, East Sussex BN1 1AN.
☎ 1273 748887
Catalogue available.

Stores: Clothing: Sexuality
⚥■ **Another World**
40 Preston Road, Brighton, East Sussex BN1 4QF.
☎ 1273 675167 📱 1273 887553
Also mail order.

Stores: Erotica: BDSM
☺ **The Leather Workshop**
94a Gloucester Road, Brighton, East Sussex BN1 4AP.
☎ 1273 600427
Makes & sells leather toys, restraints. Also some fetish wear & leather underwear. 24 hour service available.

Stores: Erotica: General
☺ ■ **Kooky Shop**
5 Kensington Gardens, Brighton, East Sussex BN1 4AL.
♂▼ **Out! Looks**
4 & 7 Dorset Street, Brighton, East Sussex BN2 1WA.
☎ 1273 623356
☺ **Scene 22**
129 Saint James Street, Brighton, East Sussex BN1 3AA.
☎ 127 362 6682

Stores: Safer Sex Products
☺ **Sussex Safer Sex Supplies Ltd.**
3 Cavendish Street, Brighton, East Sussex BN2 5NQ.
☎ 1273 625222

Eastbourne
Manufacturers: Piercing Jewelry
☺ ■ **Merlins Ear & Body Piercing Jewelry**
23 Susans Road, Eastbourne, East Sussex.
☎ 132 343 0595 📱 132 343 0283

Organizations: BDSM
♂▽ **Boots & Breeches Club**
P.O. Box 1465, Eastbourne, East Sussex BN22 9QP.
Contact: The Secretary

Hailsham
Stores: Erotica: General
☺ ■ **Leisure Look**
P. O. Box 709, Hailsham, East Sussex BN27 3US.

Hastings
Publishers: Magazines: Fetish: Mess
♀ ■ **Splosh**
P. O. Box 70, Saint Leonards-on-Sea, East Sussex TN38 0PX.
📱 1424 433747
Published quarterly. Yearly subscription is $60. Age statement of 18 is required.

Stores: Erotica: General
☺ ■ **Magic Moments**
14 Rock Close, Hastings, East Sussex.
☎ 1424 853366
Free catalogue.

Hove
Publishers: Directories: Sexuality
♂▼ **Queer Guide - Brighton**
Goldsmid Mews, 15a Farm Road, Hove, East Sussex BN3 1FB.
☎ 1273 773547

Publishers: Magazines: General
☺ **Caress Magazine**
The Write Solution, c/o Flat 1, 11 Holland Avenue, Hove, East Sussex BN3 1JF.
☎ 1273 726281
Newsletter for writers of erotica. Published 10 times a year. Yearly subscription is £10.

ESSEX
Basildon
Organizations: Sexuality
⚥ **TransEssex**
P. O. Box 3, Basildon, Essex SS14 1PT.
☎ 1268 583761
⏱ Meets 4th, Fri of month. Call Wed Sun 19:00 - 22:00
Support group for TVs & TSs. Holds regular parties. Publishes *Reflections*

quarterly. Yearly subscription is £15.

Braintree

Piercers

☺ ■ **Blake House Studios**
Blake End, Rayne, Essex CM7 8SH.
Catalogue, £4.50, overseas ₵5 or $15U.S..

Buckhurst Hill

Stores: Clothing: Fetish

☺ ■ **Michelle Fashions**
105 Epping New Road, Buckhurst Hill, Essex IG9 5TQ.
☎ 181 504 0418

Chelmsford

Helplines: Sexuality

⚢▽ **Chelmsford Lesbian & Gay Switchboard**
☎ 124 542358
🕘 Wed Fri 18:00 - 22:00

Stores: Books: General

☺ **The Paper Shop**
11 High Street, Chelmsford, Essex.

Chigwell

Photographers: Erotic

☺ **Jeanette Jones**
120 Hainault Road, Chigwell, Essex IG7 5DL.

Colchester

Helplines: AIDS

☺ □ **Colchester HIV/AIDS Helpline**
☎ 1206 767043
🕘 Mon - Fri 19:00 - 22:00
Advice & information about HIV/AIDS & other sexual health issues.

Helplines: Sexuality

☺ ▽ **Colchester Gay Switchboard**
☎ 1206 767043
🕘 Mon - Fri 19:00 - 22:00
Advice & information about HIV/AIDS & other sexual health & sexuality issues.

Publishers: Magazines: Sexuality

⚢▼ ***Broad Magazine***
The Pink House, Maldon Road, Colchester, Essex CO2 0NU.
☎ 1206 330549

Hadleigh

Stores: Erotica: BDSM

☺ ■ **Essex Intim**
393 London Road, Hadleigh, Essex S7 2BY.
☎ 1702 555407

Harlow

Helplines: Sexuality

⚢▽ **Harlow Switchboard**
☎ 1279 639637
🕘 Sun Wed Thu 20:00 - 23:00, Fri 20:00 - 24:00

Leytonstone

Publishers: Magazines: Bears

⚣▼ ***Big Boys & Buddies***
18 Cookes Close, Leytonstone, Essex E11 3EF.

Romford

Publishers: Magazines: Fetish

☺ ***Shiny***
G & M Fashions Ltd., P. O. Box 42, Romford, Essex RM4 1QT.

Stores: Erotica: General

☺ ■ **Mebray Ltd**
Century House, 100 George Street, Romford, Essex RM1 2EB.

Southend

Helplines: Sexuality

⚢▽ **Southend Lesbian & Gay Switchboard**
☎ 1702 480344

Stanford-Le-Hope

Publishers: Magazines: Fetish

☺ ■ ***Footsy***
FLAS, P.O. Box 867, Stanford-Le-Hope, Essex SS17 7JJ.

Thornton Heath

Organizations: BDSM

⚢▽ **SM Group**
c/o PJs Bar, Brigstock Road, Thornton Heath, Essex.

Westcliff On Sea

Organizations: BDSM

⚣ **Essex Leather**
P.O. Box 184, Westcliff On Sea, Essex SS0 3SN.

GLOUCESTERSHIRE

Gloucester

Helplines: Sexuality

⚢▽ **Gloucester Friend**
☎ 1452 306800
🕘 Wed 12:00 - 15:00
Advice & information about HIV/AIDS & other sexual health & sexuality issues.

Nailsworth

Manufacturers: Piercing Jewelry

☺ ■ **Barbary Products**
Uplands, Watledge, Gloucestershire GL6 0AP.
☎ 145 383 4426
🕘 Visits by appointment
Catalogue available.

GREATER MANCHESTER

County Resources

Helplines: Sexuality

⚢▽ **Manchester Lesbian & Gay Switchboard**
P. O. Box 153, Manchester, Greater Manchester M60 1LP.
☎ 161 274 3999
🕘 16:00 - 22:00
Advice & information about HIV/AIDS & other sexual health & sexuality issues.

Organizations: Family

☺ □ **Manchester Gay Parents Group**
P. O. Box 153, Manchester, Greater Manchester M60 1LP.

Beswick

Organizations: BDSM

⚣▽ **Bear Club U.K.**
56 Albert Street, Beswick, Greater Manchester M11 3SU.
✉ JLD1@cus.cam.ac.uk
🕸 http://www.skepsis.com/.gblo/bears/CLUBS/Bears_Club_UK/
🕘 Monthly meetings held in Bournemouth, Bristol, Edinburgh, Manchester, Newcastle, Norwich, St. Albans, Sheffield, Warwick, & Wolverhampton, & weekly meetings in London
Contact: Mr. John Dawson
Also area contacts in Birmingham, Blackpool, Brighton, Cardiff, Hastings, Gateshead, Great Yarmouth, Knutsford, Leeds, Nottingham, & Stourbridge. Publishes a newsletter every two months.

Manchester

Bars: BDSM

⚣▼ **Cellar Leather Club**
Napoleon's, Sackville Street at Bloom Street, Manchester, Greater Manchester.
☎ 161 236 8800

⚣▼ **Mineshaft**
4-6 Whitworth Street, Manchester, Greater Manchester.
☎ 161 237 9937
Four nights a week (Thurs., Fri., Sat., & Mon.) fetish club.

Helplines: Sexuality

⚧▽ **Manchester Transvestite / Transgender Hotline**
☎ 161 274 3705

Manufacturers: Clothing: Rubber

☺ ▼ **Murray & Vern**

63 Whitworth Street, Manchester, Greater Manchester M1 3NY.
☎ 161 236 7440 📞 161 228 1776

Organizations: AIDS: Support

☺ □ **Body Positive—North West**
P.O. Box 185, Manchester, Greater Manchester M60 2DD.
☎ 161 237 9717
Advice & information about HIV/AIDS & other sexual health issues.

Organizations: Family

☺ □ **Families & Friends of Lesbians & Gays (FFLAG)**
P. O. Box 153, Manchester, Greater Manchester M60 1LP.

Organizations: Motorcycle

♂▽ **Manchester Superchain MSC**
P.O. Box 18, Chorlton District Office, Manchester, Greater Manchester M21 1QQ.

Organizations: Sexuality

▷◁▽ **FTM Network—Manchester**
367 Upper Brook Street, Victoria Park, Greater Manchester M13 0EP.

▷◁▽ **Northern Concord**
P. O. Box 258, Manchester, Greater Manchester M60 1LN.
☎ 161 274 3705
✉ francsca@nconcord.u-net.com
🌐 http://www.u-net.com/~nconcord/
🕐 Wed 19:30 - 21:00
Publishes *Cross Talk*.

Publishers: Newspapers: Sexuality

♂▼ **All Points North**
Silveraim Ltd., 330-331 IMEX House, 40 Princes Street, Manchester, Greater Manchester M1 6DE.
☎ 161 236 4999 📞 161 237 5333

Radio: Sexuality

♂▼ **Outspoken Productions**
111 Ducie House, 37 Ducie Street, Manchester, Greater Manchester M1 2JW.
☎ 161 228 6228

Stores: Books: General

☺ ■ **Cornerhouse Books**
6-8 Oxford Road, Manchester, Greater Manchester.
☎ 161 228 7621

☺ ■ **Golden Dawn Books**
2 Palatine Mews, 6 Palatine Mews, Manchester, Greater Manchester M20 9JH.

♂▼ **Village Bookshop**
105/107 Princess Street, Manchester, Greater Manchester M1 6DD.
☎ 161 236 6441

☺ ■ **Waterstones**
Deansgate, Manchester, Greater Manchester.

Stores: Clothing: Sexuality

⚥ **Ethos**
1102 Stockport Road, Manchester, Greater Manchester M19 2SU.
☎ 161 442 3030

Stores: Clothing: Rubber

☺ ■ **Studio 2**
Market Buildings, 17 Thomas Street, Manchester, Greater Manchester M3 1EU.
☎ 1475 837930

Stores: Erotica: General

☺ ■ **Aphrodite/Elle**
P. O. Box 47, Manchester, Greater Manchester M21 8EJ.

♂▼ **Clone Zone**
37-39 Bloom Street, Manchester, Greater Manchester M1 3LY.
☎ 161 236 1398 📞 161 236 5178
💳 VISA MC
Free catalogue.

☺ **Harmony**
41 Cross Street, Manchester, Greater Manchester M2 4JE.
Clothes, books, & magazines.

☺ ■ **Savoy**
279 Deansgate, Manchester, Greater Manchester M3 4EW.

☺ **Stallion Book & Video Centre**
43 Bloom Street, Manchester, Greater Manchester.
☎ 161 237 3401

Stores: Military Surplus

☺ ■ **New Cross Army Surplus**

31A Tib Street, Manchester, Greater Manchester.
☎ 161 832 9683

Stores: Safer Sex Products

☺ **Rubber Plantation**
Unit 24, Afflecks Arcade, Oldham Street, Manchester, Greater Manchester.
☎ 161 839 5920

Oldham

Stores: Military Surplus

☺ ■ **New Cross Army Surplus**
100 Yorkshire Street, Oldham, Greater Manchester.
☎ 161 633 6967

Prestwich

Stores: Clothing: Sexuality

⚥ **Transformation Ltd.**
413 Bury Old Road, Prestwich, Greater Manchester M25 1PS.
☎ 161 773 4477 📞 161 773 6358
🕐 Mon - Sat 09:00 - 20:00
The world's leading TV specialists.

⚥ **Transformation Ltd.**
428 Bury Old Road, Prestwich, Greater Manchester M25 1PS.
☎ 161 773 2572 📞 161 773 6358
🕐 Mon - Sat 09:00 - 20:00
The world's leading TV specialists.

Rochdale

Helplines: Sexuality

♂▽ **Rochdale Lesbian & Gay Switchboard**
c/o Rochdale Law Centre, Smith Street, Rochdale, Greater Manchester OL16 1HE.
☎ 1706 59964
🕐 Tue 19:00 - 21:00
Advice & information about HIV/AIDS & other sexual health & sexuality issues.

Wigan

Stores: Books: General

☺ **Lamp Bookshop**
91 Bradshawgate, Wigan, Greater Manchester.

HAMPSHIRE

Andover

Publishers: Books: Sexuality

♂▼ **Routledge Press**
Freepost, Andover, Hampshire SP10 5BR.
☎ 1264 342923

Northam

Bars: BDSM

♂▽ **Gaol House**
Northam Road, Northam, Hampshire.
☎ 170 333 2830

Portsmouth

Helplines: Sexuality

♂▽ **Portsmouth Lesbian & Gay Switchboard**
☎ 1705 655 077
🕐 Wed 19:30 - 22:00

Manufacturers: Clothing: Corsets

☺ ■ **Voller's**
112 Kingston Road, North End, Portsmouth, Hampshire PO2 7PB.
☎ 1705 660 740 📞 1705 652 070

Organizations: AIDS: Support

☺ □ **Positive People Portsmouth**
☎ 1705 816429
🕐 Sun 19:00 - 21:00
Advice & information about HIV/AIDS & other sexual health issues.

Stores: Clothing: Fetish

☺ ■ **Forbidden**
58 Charlotte Street, Portsmouth, Hampshire PO1 4AW.
☎ 1705 826655
Fags, perverts, TVs, & everyone else are always warmly welcomed. Catalogue, free with SAE.

Southampton
Helplines: AIDS
☺ ☐ **AIDSline Southampton**
☎ 1703 339467
🕐 Fri 19:30 - 22:00
Advice & information about HIV/AIDS & other sexual health issues.

Helplines: Sexuality
⚥▽ **Solent Gay Switchboard & AIDSline**
☎ 1703 637363
☎ 1703 655077
🕐 1st. line: Tue Thu Sat 19:30 - 22:00, 2nd. line: Wed 19:30 - 22:00
Advice & information about HIV/AIDS & other sexual health & sexuality issues.

⚥▽ **Solent Lesbian Line**
☎ 1703 405111
🕐 Tue Thu 19:30 - 22:00
Advice & information about HIV/AIDS & other sexual health & sexuality issues.

Publishers: Magazines: Spanking
☺ ■ *Cul D'Or*
Omega Marketing, P.O. Box 81, Southampton, Hampshire SO18 5BP.
Spanking magazine with fiction, letters, & contact ads.

Stores: Books: General
☺ **October Books**
4 Onslow Road, Southampton, Hampshire SO2 0JB.
☎ 1703 224489

HEREFORD & WORCESTER
County Resources
Helplines: Sexuality
⚥▽ **Hereford & Worcester Lesbian & Gay Switchboard**
☎ 1905 723097
🕐 Tue - Fri 19:30 - 22:00
Advice & information about HIV/AIDS & other sexual health & sexuality issues.

Hereford
Helplines: AIDS
☺ ☐ **Herefordshire HIV/AIDS Advice Helpline**
☎ 1432 278787
🕐 Wed 19:30 - 21:30
Advice & information about HIV/AIDS & other sexual health issues.

Kidderminster
Stores: Erotica: General
☺ ■ **Cocoon**
Mackintosh House, Green Street, Kidderminster, Hereford & Worcester DY10 1JF.
☎ 156 282 9419

HERTFORDSHIRE
Letchworth
Stores: Clothing: Rubber
☺ ■ **Modern Armour**
Unit 82, Spirella Buildings, Bridge Road, Letchworth, Hertfordshire SG6 4HD.
☎ 1462 483458

Saint Albans
Organizations: Shaving
⚥▽ **Clippers**
9A Fishpool Street, Saint Albans, Hertfordshire AL3 4RS.
☎ 181 940 3084

HUMBERSIDE
Bridlington
Organizations: AIDS: Education
☺ ☐ **AIDS Action**
☎ 126 240 0440
Advice & information about HIV/AIDS & other sexual health issues.

Grimsby
Helplines: AIDS
☺ ☐ **Grimsby & District AIDS Line**
☎ 1472 240840
🕐 Mon Thu 19:30 - 21:30, Tue 11:00 - 15:00
Advice & information about HIV/AIDS & other sexual health issues.

Hull
Bars: Fetish
☺ **Stimulation**
The Tower Nightclub, Anlaby Road, Hull, Humberside.
☎ 1482 218068
🕐 Monthly event
Relaxed atmosphere with opened-minded dress code. A chance to meet local fetishists. Voyeurs are not welcome. Call for details.

Helplines: Sexuality
⚥▽ **Hull Lesbian Line**
☎ 1482 214331
🕐 Mon 19:00 - 21:00
Advice & information about HIV/AIDS & other sexual health issues.

⚥▽ **Humberside Friend**
☎ 1482 443333
🕐 Mon - Thu 20:00 - 22:00, Sat 19:00 - 21:00
Advice & information about HIV/AIDS & other sexual health & sexuality issues.

Organizations: AIDS: Education
☺ ☐ **AIDS Action North Humberside**
Cornerhouse, 29 Percy Street, Hull, Humberside HU2 8HL.
☎ 1482 27060
🕐 Mon Thu 10:00 - 13:00, Wed 19:00 - 21:00, Sat 10:00 - 12:00

Stores: Books: General
☺ **Page One Books**
9 Princes Avenue, Hull, Humberside.
☎ 148 241 925

Scunthorpe
Health Services
☺ ☐ **Ebb & Flow**
Centre for HIV & Sexual Health, Scunthorpe, Humberside.
☎ 1724 289292
🕐 Mon - Fri 10:00 - 17:00
Advice & information about HIV/AIDS & other sexual health issues.

Helplines: Sexuality
⚥▽ **Scunthorpe Gay Helpline**
☎ 1724 271661
🕐 Wed Fri 19:00 - 21:00
Advice & information about HIV/AIDS & other sexual health & sexuality issues.

ISLE OF MAN
Douglas
Helplines: Sexuality
⚥▽ **Carrey Friend**
☎ 1624 611600
🕐 Thu 19:00 - 22:00
Advice & information about HIV/AIDS & other sexual health & sexuality issues.

ISLE OF WIGHT
County Resources
Helplines: Sexuality
⚥▽ **Isle of Wight Switchboard**
☎ 1983 525123

Freshwater
Organizations: Sexuality
✉▽ **International Gender Transient Affinity (IGTA)**
Box 2, 1 Banks Building, School Green Road, Freshwater, Isle of Wight PO40 9AJ.
Contact: Miss Phaedra Kelly, Director

Sandown
Organizations: AIDS: Education
⚥▽ **Gay Men's Health Project**
P.O. Box 16, Sandown, Isle of Wight PO36 9NH.

KENT
Ashford
Publishers: Newspapers: Sexuality
♂▼ *Our Times*
P. O. Box 92, Ashford, Kent TN23 7AZ.
☎ 1233 662813

Canterbury
Helplines: Sexuality
♂▽ **East Kent Friend**
☎ 184 358 8762
🕓 Tue 19:30 - 22:00
Advice & information about HIV/AIDS & other sexual health & sexuality issues.

Chatham
Helplines: Sexuality
☺▽ **Medway & Maidstone Lesbian & Gay Switchboard**
P. O. Box 53, Chatham, Kent ME4 5QQ.
☎ 1634 826925
🕓 Thu Fri 19:30 - 21:30
Advice & information about HIV/AIDS & other sexual health sexuality issues.

Chislehurst
Stores: Safer Sex Products
☺ **Brush Away**
Chislehurst Railway Station, Station Approach, Chislehurst, Kent BR7 5NN.
☎ 181 467 1998

Folkestone
Helplines: AIDS
☺☐ **Kent County Council**
☎ 1303 248 177
🕓 17:00 - 20:00 for emergencies
Advice & information about HIV/AIDS & other sexual health issues.

Organizations: Fetish: Clothing: Rubber
☺ **International Mackintosh Society**
P.O. Box 202, Folkestone, Kent CT20 3YE.
Contact: Mr. Jim Price

Gravesend
Helplines: Sexuality
♂▽ **Gravesend Switchboard**
☎ 163 482695
🕓 Thu Fri 19:30 - 21:30

Organizations: Sexuality
☺☐ **Hush-A-Bye Baby Club**
c/o 43 South Hill Road, Gravesend, Kent DA12 1JX.
☎ 163 457 1396 📞 163 485 2737
Adult baby club with clothing catalogues. Catalogue available.

Maidstone
Stores: Clothing: Fetish
☺ **Pillow Talk**
46 Sandling Road, Maidstone, Kent ME14 2RH.
☎ 1622 661504
🕓 Mon - Sat 10:00 - 18:00
🔥 ✓ $ ⚏ 💳 📇
Sells whole range of sex items: sex aids, lingerie, TV fetish shoes, leather, leather toys, magazines, novels, restraints, etc..

Margate
Stores: Clothing: Fetish
☺ **Pillow Talk**
12 & 13 Marine Drive, Margate, Kent CT9 1DH.
☎ 1843 294069
🕓 Mon - Sat 10:00 - 18:00
🔥 ✓ $ ⚏ 💳 📇
Sells whole range of sex items: sex aids, lingerie, TV fetish shoes, leather, leather toys, magazines, novels, restraints, etc..

Near Marden
Manufacturers: Furniture: Bondage
☺ ■ **Ian King Engineering Designs Ltd.**
The Studio, Moors Farm, Collier Street, Near Marden, Kent TN12 9PR.

Royal Tunbridge Wells
Helplines: Sexuality
♂▽ **Tunbridge Wells Switchboard**
☎ 1892 535876
🕓 Mon 20:00 - 22:00

LANCASHIRE
County Resources
Helplines: Sexuality
♂▽ **Bolton Lesbian & Gay Switchboard**
P. O. Box 153, Manchester, Greater Manchester M60 1LP.
☎ 161 274 3999
🕓 16:00 - 22:00
Advice & information about HIV/AIDS & other sexual health & sexuality issues.

☺▽ **East Lancashire Lesbian & Gay Switchboard**
P. O. Box 50, Burnley, Lancashire BB1 1RX.
☎ 128 245 4978
☎ 128 245 4404 (minicom)
🕓 Tue Thu 19:30 - 21:30
Advice & information about HIV/AIDS & other sexual health & sexuality issues.

♂▽ **Lancaster Lesbian & Gay Switchboard**
☎ 1524 847437
🕓 Thu Fri 19:00 - 21:00
Advice & information about HIV/AIDS & other sexual health & sexuality issues.

Blackpool
Organizations: AIDS: Education
☺☐ **Health Education AIDS Liaison (HEAL)**
☎ 123 532 9 0052
🕓 Thu 19:00 - 20:00
Advice & information about HIV/AIDS & other sexual health issues.

Stores: Erotica: General
♂▼ **Clone Zone**
3 The Strand, Blackpool, Lancashire FY1 1NX.
☎ 125 329 4850 📞 125 329 4850
🔥 💳 📇
Free catalogue.

Bolton
Bars: BDSM
♂ **Cell Bar**
174 Crook Street, Bolton, Lancashire.
☎ 120 421 856

Burnley
Helplines: AIDS
☺☐ **Burnley AIDS Line**
☎ 800 220 704
🕓 Mon - Fri 19:00 - 21:00
Advice & information about HIV/AIDS & other sexual health issues.

Helplines: Sexuality
☺☐ **Burnley Switchboard**
☎ 1772 51122
🕓 Tue Thu Fri 19:30 - 21:30
Advice & information about HIV/AIDS & other sexual health & sexuality issues.

Darwen
Manufacturers: Clothing: Rubber
☺ ■ **Kastley**
Unit 2, Darwen Enterprise Centre, Railway Road, Darwen, Lancashire BB3 3EH.
☎ 125 487 3247
Catalogue, £5.

Lancaster
Helplines: AIDS
☺☐ **Positive Action for HIV**
☎ 800 220704
🕓 Mon Fri 19:00 - 21:00. Also minicom
Advice & information about HIV/AIDS & other sexual health issues.

Stores: Books: General
☺ **Single Step Co-op**
78a Penny Street, Lancaster, Lancashire.

☎ 1524 63021
Leyland
Organizations: Family
☺□ **Lancashire Family & Partners Support**
　☎ 1772 621111
　🕐 Mon Thu 13:00 - 16:00, Thu also 19:00 - 22:00, Sun 19:00 - 22:00
　Advice & information about HIV/AIDS & other sexual health issues.
Preston
Helplines: Sexuality
⚥▽ **Preston Gay Information Service**
　☎ 1772 51122
　🕐 Men Tue Thu Fri 19:30 - 21:00, Sat 13:00 - 15:00
　Advice & information about HIV/AIDS & other sexual health & sexuality issues.
Organizations: AIDS: Education
☺□ **Health Education AIDS Liason (HEAL)**
　☎ 1772 555525
　🕐 Mon 19:30 - 21:30
　Advice & information about HIV/AIDS & other sexual health issues.
Organizations: AIDS: Support
☺□ **Community AIDS Support Team (CAST)**
　☎ 1772 200911
　🕐 Tue Thu 19:30 - 21:30
　Advice & information about HIV/AIDS & other sexual health issues.
Organizations: Sexuality
♂▽ **Preston Bisexual Group**
　P. O. Box 375, Preston, Lancashire PR2 2UP.
White Cross
Helplines: AIDS
☺□ **AIDSLine**
　Unit 10, Lancaster Enterprise Workshops, White Cross, Lancashire LA1 4XH.
　☎ 152 484 1011

LEICESTERSHIRE
County Resources
Helplines: Sexuality
⚥▽ **Leicester Lesbian & Gayline**
　☎ 116 255 0667
　🕐 Mon - Fri 19:30 - 22:00. Staffed by women on Tue
　Advice & information about HIV/AIDS & other sexual health & sexuality issues.
Leicester
Organizations: AIDS: Support
☺□ **Leicestershire AIDS Support Services (LASS)**
　c/o Leicester CVS, 29 New Walk, Leicester, Leicestershire LE1 6TE.
　☎ 116 255 9995
　✆ 116 255 9000
　🕐 Mon - Fri 09:30 - 16:00
　Advice & information about HIV/AIDS & other sexual health issues.
Organizations: Sexuality
⚥▽ **Leicester Lesbian & Gay Communities' Resource Centre**
　☎ 116 255 0667
　🕐 Mon - Fri 19:30 - 22:00. Staffed by women on Tue
　Advice & information about HIV/AIDS & other sexual health & sexuality issues.
Piercers
☺ **The House of David**
　📞 153 081 5 966
　📞 585 261 413
　Confidential piercing in Leicester & Loughborough.
Stores: Books: General
☺ **Blackthorn Books**
　70 High Street, Leicester, Leicestershire.
　☎ 116 221896

LINCOLNSHIRE
County Resources
Helplines: Sexuality
⚥▽ **Lincoln Gay & Lesbian Switchboard**
　☎ 152 253 5553
　🕐 Thu Sun 19:00 - 22:00
Boston
Helplines: AIDS
☺□ **Boston AIDS Helpline**
　☎ 120 535 4462
　🕐 09:00 - 10:30
　Advice & information about HIV/AIDS & other sexual health issues.
Grantham
Helplines: AIDS
☺□ **Grantham HIV/AIDS Helpline**
　☎ 1476 60192
　🕐 Mon - Fri 08:30 - 16:30
　Advice & information about HIV/AIDS & other sexual health issues.
Lincoln
Manufacturers: Clothing: Corsets
☺■ **Wilbro**
　490-410 High Street, Lincoln, Lincolnshire LN5 8HX.
　Both ready-to-wear & custom orders are available.
Organizations: AIDS: Support
☺□ **Lincolnshire AIDS Voluntary Group (LAVG)**
　☎ 1522 513999
　🕐 Mon Wed Fri 09:00 - 21:00, Tue Thu 09:00 - 17:30
　Advice & information about HIV/AIDS & other sexual health issues.
Organizations: Health
☺■ **Health Shop**
　Portland House, 3 Portland Street, Lincoln, Lincolnshire.
　☎ 152 252 9222

LONDON
County Resources
Helplines: Sexuality
♂▽ **Bisexual Helpline**
　☎ 181 569 7500
　🕐 Tue Wed 19:30 - 21:30
　Advice & information about HIV/AIDS & other sexual health issues.
⚥▽ **London Lesbian Line**
　P. O. Box 1514, London WC1N 3XX.
　☎ 171 251 6911
　☎ 171 253 0924 (minicom)
　🕐 Mon - Fri 14:00 - 22:00
　Advice & information about HIV/AIDS & other sexual health & sexuality issues.
⚥▽ **S. E. London's Lesbian, Gay, & Bisexual Helpline**
　☎ 181 316 5954
　🕐 Mon - Thu 17:00 - 20:00
⚥▽ **South Asian Lesbian & Gay Network (Shakti)**
　☎ 171 837 2782
　🕐 Daytime. Ask for Shakti
　Advice & information about HIV/AIDS & other sexual health & sexuality issues.
Organizations: Spanking
👫■ **Public Eye**
　P. O. Box 2529, Ealing, London W5 4NY.
　☎ 181 840 4027
　☎ 175 365 2199
　🕐 All hours
　✉ ✔
　Contact: Mr. Kent Boulton, B.A.Hons, Dip.Ed., M.A.
　Spanking club. Publishes *Slightly Sinful*. Age statement of 18 is required. French also spoken.
London
Archives: BDSM
☺ **Lives of the Secular Saints**
　BCM Judgement, London WC1N 3XX.
　BDSM sex-pain archive. Preserving your words (& your anonymity). SAE (or IRC) for information (including extracts from the archive).

Artists: Fetish

Chris
104 Birchanger Road, South Norwood, London SE25 5BG.
181 655 2332
Fetish drawings: leather, stilettos, etc..

Bars: BDSM

The Anvil
88 Tooley Street, London SE1 2TF.
171 407 0371
Mon - Wed 22:30 - 01:00, Thu - Sat - 02:00, Sun 14:00 - 23:00

Attitude
The Trafalgar, Trafalgar Avenue & Sumner Road, London SE15.
171 701 2175
Mon - Fri 07:00 - 23:00, Sat 12:00 - 23:00, Sun 12:00 - 22:30

The Backstreet
Wentworth Mews, London E3.
181 980 8557 (club hours)
181 980 7880 (other times)
Thu - Sat 22:00 - 03:00, Sun 21:00 - 01:00
Strict black leather & rubber dress code.

The Block
1-5 Parkfield Street, London N1.
171 226 7453

Brompton's
294 Old Brompton Road, Earl's Court, London.
171 370 1344

The Colherne
261 Brompton Road, London SW5.
181 373 9859
Mon - Fri 12:00 - 15:00 19:00 - 22:30

The Dungeon Club
Corner of Parry Street & South Lambeth Place, Vauxhall, London.
171 932 0755
Dress code: black rubber, black leather, black PVC, black collar, black lead, black fantasy....

The London Apprentice
333 Old Street, London EC1.
171 739 5949
Mon - Thu 21:00 - 03:00, Fri Sat 21:00 - 05:00, Sun - 04:00

The Market Tavern
Market Towers, 1 Nine Elms Lane, London SW8.
171 622 5655
Mon 22:00 - 05:00, Thu 22:00 - 03:00, Fri 22:00 - 04:00, Sat 22:00 - 05:00, Sun 14:00 - 20:00 21:00 - 02:00

Underground
c/o Central Station Underground, 37 Wharfdale Road, Kings Cross, London N1 9SE.
181 875 1607
Sun 21:00 - 24:00, Tue 02:00

Bars: Fetish

Submission
BCM Box 4542, London WC1N 3XX.
171 284 2180 — Fax: 171 284 2189
Fetish club. Call for locations & times.

Bars: Sexuality

The Black Cap
171 Camden High Street, London NW1.
171 485 1742
Mon - Thu 13:00 - 02:00, Fri Sat - 03:00, Sun pub hours

Wayout Club
143 Knightsbridge, London W1.
Sat 20:30 - 01:30
For boys, girls, & in-betweenies.

Wayout Wine Bar
11 Kingly Court, London W1.
181 363 0948
Wed 21:00 - 03:00

Competitions & Conventions: BDSM

Fetish/SM Market
10 Caxton Road, Wood Green, London N22.
Held 2nd. Sun of month

Competitions & Conventions: Fetish: Clothing

The Planet Sex Ball
The Leydig Trust, P. O. Box 4ZB, London W1A 4ZB.
171 739 0388 — Fax: 171 739 0355
Call Mon - Sat 12:00 - 18:30 for details
Annual ball.

Competitions & Conventions: Fetish: Clothing: Rubber

Rubber Ball
c/o Tim Woodward Publishing Ltd., 23 Grand Union Centre, Kensal Road, London W10 5AX.
181 968 0234 — Fax: 181 960 8404

Counsellors

The Albany Trust
24 Chester Square, London SW12 9HS.
181 675 6669

Ian Brown
84 Marylebone High Street, London W1M 3DE.
171 916 2834
Counsellor & psychotherapist.

Careline
181 514 1177
Mon - Fri 10:00 - 16:00 19:00 - 22:00

Mark Elmer, Dip. Couns.
171 249 1351

Nick Gundry
181 995 1590

Sarah Jack
181 509 9751
Psychotherapy.

Moira Lake
181 943 5507
Psychotherapy.

Robert Lawrence
40 Boleyn Road, London E7 9QE.
181 472 2430

Phil Parkinson
181 767 7464

Graham Perlman
171 274 2754
Psychotherapy.

The Pink Practice
BM Box Practice, London WC1N 3XX.
181 809 7218

Three Worlds
181 767 7464

Alan Weeks
171 284 2621
Psychotherapy.

Distributors: Books: General

Central Books
99 Wallis Road, London E9 5LN.
181 986 4854 — Fax: 181 533 5821

Pipeline Books
32 Paul Street, London EC2A 4LB.
171 729 3491 — Fax: 171 729 6149

Turnaround
27 Horsell Road, London N5 1XL.
171 609 7836 — Fax: 171 700 1205

Venue Services Limited
156-158 Grays Inn Road, Holborn, London WC1X 8ED.
171 916 0162 — Fax: 171 713 0899
956 855004

Health Services

The Audre Lorde Clinic
Ambrose King Centre, Royal London Hospital, London E1 1BB.
171 377 7311
HIV/AIDS clinic.

The Bernhard Clinic
GU Department, Charing Cross Hospital, Fulham Palace Road, London W6.
181 846 1576

Herpes Association
41 North Road, Islington, London N7 9DP.
171 607 9661

The Rainbow Clinic
The Caldecot Centre, King's College Hospital, 15-22 Caldecot Road, Camberwell, London SE5 9RS.
171 346 3488
Wed 16:00 - 19:00. By appointment only. Ask for the Rainbow Clinic

Helplines: AIDS

☺ ☐ **Lesbian & Gay Bereavement Project**
☎ 181 455 8894
⏱ 19:00 - 24:00
Advice & information about HIV/AIDS & other sexual health issues.

☺ ☐ **The Metro**
☎ 181 316 5954
⏱ Mon - Thu 14:00 - 19:00
Advice & information about HIV/AIDS & other sexual health issues.

Helplines: Sexuality

♂▽ **Haringey Lesbian & Gay Helpline**
☎ 181 802 0840

♂▽ **Lewisham Friend**
☎ 181 690 6195

♂▽ **London Friend**
86 Caledonian Road, London N1.
☎ 171 837 3337 (men)
☎ 171 837 2782 (women)
⏱ 19:30 - 22:00. Women's line Sun Mon Tue 19:30 - 22:00.
Minicom on both lines
Advice & information about HIV/AIDS & other sexual health & sexuality issues.

♂▽ **National Friend**
BM National Friend, London WC1N 3XX.
Over 25 years old with over 30 Friend helplines, befriending, & coming out groups around the British Isles. Write for details.

Manufacturers: Clothing: Fetish

☺ **Black Magic**
451 Roman Road, London E3 5LX.
☎ 181 980 1365 ✆ 181 981 0338
Leather warrior woman designs.

☺ ■ **Lush**
Unit 310, Clerkenwell Workshop, 310 Clerkenwell Close, London EC1R OAT.
☎ 171 253 2975
Hand made leather corsets, basques, jackets, & coats. Wholesale only.

☺ **Pure**
Unit 20A, Tower Workshops, 58 Riley Road, London SE1 3DG.
☎ 171 394 1717 ✆ 171 394 1809
⏱ Mon -Sat 11:00 - 18:00
💳 ✓ 💳 💳
Clothing by Murray & Vern. Wholesale & retail enquiries welcome. Catalogue, free, with large SAE or 2 IRCs.

☺ **Valhalla**
P. O. Box 6144, London SW2 2NB.
☎ 181 674 9002

Manufacturers: Clothing: Leather

☺ ■ **Vic Wilder**
Unit 6, 86-96 Garratt Lane, London SW18 4DJ.
☎ 181 871 2443 ✆ 181 877 9367
The ultimate leather original jeans & divine software.

Manufacturers: Clothing: Rubber

☺ **Clothes For Practitioners**
140c Kennington Lane, London SE11 4UZ.
☎ 171 820 9393
Custom PVC, spandex, & leather clothing.

☺ ■ **Ectomorph**
Unit 1, 3rd. Floor, 42-44 DeBeauvoir Crescent, London N1 5SB.
☎ 171 249 6311 ✆ 171 241 6047
💳 💳
Rubber & PU clothes. Wholesale & retail. Catalogue, £10 for U.K., £12 overseas.

☺ **Jensen & Morrow**
The Studio, 65 Leonard Street, London EC2.
☎ 171 729 1115 ✆ 171 729 1300

Manufacturers: Erotica: BDSM

♂ **Fantasy Erotique**
P. O. Box 6412, London E7 9SB.
☎ 181 555 2996 ✆ 181 503 0968
 ✆ 385 346976
⏱ Mon - Sat 10:00 - 20:00
💳 ✓ $ 💳 💳 💳
Leather, rubber, toys, & clothing. Retail by appointment only. Catalogue, free upon written request. Age statement of 18 is required. German also spoken.

Manufacturers: Erotica: Leather

☺ **Leatherworks Ltd.**
77-79 Southgate Road, London N1 3IS.

☎ 171 359 9778 ✆ 171 226 6745
Clothes, & fetish & theatrical footwear. Catalogue, £7.

☺▼ **The Smart Alternative**
20-21 Wilmot Place, London W7 3TZ.
☎ 181 840 6431

Manufacturers: Erotica: Pony

☺ **BBL Pony Girl Club**
BCM Judgement, London WC1N 3XX.
Made-to-measure clothes, riding harnesses, & toys.

Manufacturers: Erotica: Rubber

☺ ■ **Chris Anderson**
☎ 181 293 1947
Made to measure rubberwear & masks.

☺ **Craig Morrison**
P. O. Box 2975, London N1 0RZ.
☎ 171 278 5367 ✆ 171 708 4594
Spiky rubber clothing & furniture.

♂ **The Sentry Box**
P. O. Box 722, London SE17 3NT.
☎ 171 735 1116
Catalogue, £2.

Manufacturers: Furniture: BDSM

☺▼ **Abusive Furniture**
P. O. Box 2153, London E7 0JZ.
Mail order only.

☺ ■ **Adam Bottomley**
☎ 181 964 5058

Manufacturers: Piercing Jewelry

☺ ■ **PW Multitek Services**
4 Victor Road, London NW10 5XD.
☎ 181 960 5759
Piercing kits & rings. Catalogue, £1 in coins, U.K. stamps, or IRCs.

Manufacturers: Restraints: BDSM

♂▼ **Fetters**
Unit 2B, North Building, Westminster Business Centre, Vauxhall, London SE11 5JH.
☎ 171 820 7780 ✆ 171 820 7790
⏱ By appointment only
Catalogue, £7, plus £1 post to Europe.

Manufacturers: Restraints: Metal

☺ ■ **Luke Morgan**
☎ 171 790 1346
Makes steel sculpture & furniture.

Manufacturers: Rubber Sheeting

☺ **Pentonville Rubber Company**
50 Pentonville Road, London N1 9FG.
☎ 171 837 0283
☎ 171 837 4582

Manufacturers: Slings

☺ **Chardmore Services**
BCM Box 2071, London WC1N 3XX.
☎ 181 392 9052

Organizations: Academic: Psychiatry

☺ ☐ **The Institute of Psychiatry**
De Crespigny Park, Denmark Hill, London SE15 8AS.
☎ 171 703 5411
Contact: Dr. Stuart Checkley, Dean

☺ ☐ **The Institute of Psycho-Analysis**
63 New Cavendish Street, London W1.
☎ 171 580 4952

☺ ☐ **The Institute of Psycho-Synthesis**
The Barn, Nan Clarks Lane, London NW7.
☎ 181 959 2330

☺ ☐ **The Institute of Psychosexual Medicine**
11 Chandos Street, London W1.
☎ 171 580 0631
☎ 171 979 6922
Contact: Dr. Heather Montford

☺ ☐ **The Institute of Psychotherapy & Social Studies**
18 Laurier Road, London NW5.
☎ 171 284 4762

☺ ☐ **The Tavistock Centre**
Sexual Disorders, 120 Belsize Lane, London NW3 5BA.
☎ 171 435 7111
Contact: Mr. Caplan

☺ ■ **University College London**
Department of Psychology, Gower Street, London WC1E 6BT.
Contact: Mrs. June Rathbone

Organizations: AIDS: Chinese

☺ ☐ **Chinese HIV/AIDS Support**
43 Dean Street, London W1V 5AP.
☎ 171 287 0904

Organizations: AIDS: Education

☺ ☐ **Black HIV/AIDS Network**
111 Devonport Road, London W12 8PB.
☎ 181 792 9223

☺ ☐ **FACTS**
23/25 Weston Park, Crouch End, London N8 9SY.
☎ 181 348 9195　　　　　　📞 181 340 5864

☺ ☐ **Greenwich Health Project**
☎ 181 854 2966
🕐 Wed 13:00 - 16:30
Advice & information about HIV/AIDS & other sexual health issues.

☺ ☐ **HIV Education Unit**
Colindale Hospital, Colindale Avenue, London NW9 5HG.
☎ 181 200 0369

☺ ☐ **NW Thames HIV Project**
82-86 Seymour Place, London W1H 5BD.
☎ 171 724 7443

☺ ☐ **PACE**
34 Harthan Road, London N7 9JL.
☎ 171 700 1323

☺ ☐ **Positively East**
P.O. Box 2224, London E15 4SL.

☺ ☐ **Positively Irish Action on AIDS**
☎ 181 983 4293
🕐 Mon - Fri 11:00 - 13:00 14:00 - 16:00
Advice & information about HIV/AIDS & other sexual health issues.

☺ ☐ **Safe Afro-Arab Health & AIDS Respite Action (SAHARA)**
☎ 181 795 3317
🕐 Mon - Fri 09:30 - 17:30, Sat 10:30 - 15:30, Sun 12:00 - 14:30
Advice & information about HIV/AIDS & other sexual health issues.

☺ ☐ **The Terrence Higgins Trust**
52-54 Grays Inn Road, London WC1X 8JU.
☎ 171 831 0330
☎ 171 405 2381 (legal line)
🕐 Mon - Fri 09:30 - 17:30. Legal line Mon Wed 19:00 - 21:00
HIV support & advice.

Organizations: AIDS: Jewish

☺ ☐ **Jewish AIDS Trust**
c/o HIV Education Unit, Colindale Hospital, Colindale Avenue, London NW9 5GH.
☎ 181 200 0369

Organizations: AIDS: Support

☺ ☐ **Association Française d'Aide aux Séro-Positifs**
☎ 171 287 2363
🕐 Mon 13:30 - 16:30, Wed 15:00 - 18:00
Advice & information about HIV/AIDS & other sexual health issues.

☺ ☐ **Body Positive—London**
51B Philbeach Gardens, London.
☎ 171 373 9124

☺ ☐ **Catholic AIDS Link**
P.O. Box 646, London E9 6QP.
☎ 171 485 7298

☺ ☐ **Globe Centre**
148 Brick Lane, London E1.
☎ 171 377 2003

☺ ☐ **London East AIDS Network**
35 Romford Road, London E15 4LY.
☎ 181 519 9545

☺ ☐ **London Lighthouse**
111-117 Lancaster Road, London W11 1QT.
☎ 171 792 1200　　　　　　📞 171 229 1258
Contact: Ms. Lisa Power

☺ ☐ **Oasis AIDS Care Centre**
9 Ram Street, Wandsworth, London SW!8 1TJ.
☎ 181 874 3230

☺ ☐ **The Positive Place**
52 Deptford Broadway, London SE8 4PH.
☎ 181 694 9988
📞 181 695 6113

📧 info@posnet.co.uk
🌐 http://www.posmet.co.uk

☺ ☐ **Survivors**
☎ 171 833 3737
🕐 Tue - Thu 19:00 - 22:00
Advice & information about HIV/AIDS & other sexual health issues.

Organizations: BDSM

♂▽ **Blue Haze**
BM Box Blue Haze, London WC1N 3XX.
Contact: Mr. Jock Blakey

♂▽ **DSSM**
Box BCM DSSM, London WC1N 3XX.

♂ **Fantasy Youth**
P.O. Box 1440, London N22 5JRM.
☎ 171 229 5672

☺ ☐ **Feminine Disciplinary Society**
BM Perfect, London WC1N 3XX.

♀ ☐ **The Lady O Society**
BCM Box 3406, London WC1N 3XX.
Contact: Ms. Deborah Ryder
For submissive ladies & dominant men: recognizing that a sub/dom relationship is more fulfilling & stimulating than a "normal" sexual association. Intends to provide reassurance & reinforcement. Publishes a newsletter quarterly.

♂♀ ☐ **Moonglow Dining Club**
BCM 7889, London WC1N 3XX.
🕐 Meets every six weeks
Dining club for dominant gentlemen & submissive ladies. Meal & chat, followed by an afternoon of realistic scenarios.

♀ **Re-Enchantment for Women**
BM Perfect, London WC1N 3XX.

♂▽ **SNC London**
P.O. Box SNC 69, London WC1N 3XX.

☺ **The Thunderbolt Book Club**
BCM Thunderbolt, London WC1N 3XX.
Specialises in erotic spanking literature, by bottoms for bottoms. $5 membership. Books only available to members. Cheques to Thunderbolt Publishing.

☺ ☐ **The Torture Garden**
BM Torture Garden, London WC1N 3XX.
☎ 171 490 0379
🕐 Meets monthly. Write for details

♀ **Women's SM Group**
c/o New Recessions, Brunswick Centre, Russell Square, London WC1.
☎ 171 833 8554

Organizations: Bears

♂▽ **Bear Club U. K.**
30 Forest Street, Forest Gate, London E7 0HW.
📧 JLD1@cus.cam.ac.uk
🌐 http://www.skepsis.com/.gblo/bears/CLUBS/Bears_Club_UK/
Contact: Mr. B. Bucan

♂▽ **BearHug - U. K.**
P. O. Box 3147, London E5 9RX.

Organizations: Body Size

♂▽ **Bulk Club U.K.**
P. O. Box 1155, London E11 3EF.

Organizations: Counselling

☺ **Identity**
Marylebone Counselling Centre, 17 Marylebone Road, London NW1 5TT.
☎ 171 487 3797

Organizations: Family

☺ **Parent's Enquiry**
☎ 181 698 1815
Contact: Ms. Rose Robertson

Organizations: Fetish: Clothing

☺ ■ **Club Whiplash**
P.O. Box 2610, London W14 0TP.
☎ 171 603 9654
🕐 Party 2nd. Wed of month 21:00 - 03:00. Events 2nd. Sun of month 11:00 - 17:00

☺ **Felicity**
BM Box 5395, London WC1N 3XX.

☺ ■ **Repentence**
c/o The Intrepid Fox, 99 Wardour Street, Soho, London W1.

☺ **Severin's Kiss**
BCM Box 2578, London WC1N 3XX.
☎ 181 342 9136

Organizations: Fetish: Clothing: Corsets

☺ ■ **Fantastic!**
Vox, 9 Brighton Terrace, London SW9.
☎ 181 674 1076
Annual corset ball & fashion show held in the spring.

Organizations: Fetish: Clothing: Denim

♂ **The London Blues**
c/o 9A Fishpool Street, Saint Albans, Hertfordshire AL3 4RS.
☎ 181 940 3084
Contact: Tony

Organizations: Fetish: Clothing: Rubber

♂▽ **Rubber Men's Club**
BCM RMC, London WC1N 3XX.

☺ **The Rubber Nipple Club**
Chancery House, 319 City Road, London EC1V 1LJ.
Write for event details. Send £3 or equivalent IRCs for 1 year's mailings.

Organizations: Motorcycle

♂ **East Anglia Bikers**
P. O. Box 1865, London N7 8QQ.

♂ **MSC London**
BM Box 8370, London WC1N 3XX.
☎ 181 840 4041
Contact: Ted

Organizations: Piercing

♂▽ **Tyger Tyger**
P.O. Box 1155, London SW2 1EE.
☎ 171 622 5655
Body art.

Organizations: Publishing

♂▽ **The Book Marketing Council**
19 Bedford Square, London WC1B.
☎ 171 580 6321

Organizations: Research: Sexuality

♂▽ **Project Sigma**
64 Eurolink Business Centre, 49 Effra Road, London SW2 1BZ.

Organizations: Sexual Politics

⊕ **Feminists Against Censorship**
BM Box 207, London WC1N 3XX.
☎ 181 552 4405

♂▽ **Lesbian & Gay Freedom Movement**
BM Box 207, London WC1N 3XX.
☎ 181 552 4405 ✆ 171 407 5354
Publishes *Lesbian & Gay Freedom Movement Newsletter* quarterly.
Yearly subscription is $4.

☺ **Libertarian Alliance**
25 Chapel Chambers, London SW1P 4NN.
☎ 171 821 5502

☺ **Liberty**
21 Tabard Street, London SE1 4LA.
☎ 171 403 3888
Contact: Ms. Nettie Pollard

☺ □ **National Campaign for Reform of the Obscene Publications Acts**
15 Sloane Court West, London SW3 4TD.

Organizations: Sexuality

✉■ **The Beaumont Society**
27 Old Gloucester Street, London WC1N 3XX.
☎ 1582 412220
Advice & support for TVs/TSs & their partners. Publishes *Beaumont Magazine*.

✉□ **The Beaumont Trust**
BM Charity, London WC1N 3XX.
☎ 171 730 7453
⏰ Call 19:00 -23:00 Thu (transsexuals), 19:00 - 23:00 Tue (transvestites)

♂▽ **Black Lesbian & Gay Centre**
Arch 196, 230 Bellenden Road, London.
☎ 171 732 3885
⏰ Tue Thu 14:00 - 16:30

Advice & information about HIV/AIDS & other sexual health & sexuality issues.

⚥■ **Club Travestie Extraordinaire**
Tudor Lodge, 95 Bromley High Street, London E3.
☎ 181 788 4154
⏰ Meets monthly 20:30 - 02:00. Call for details

✉▽ **Fanny's**
c/o Ted's Place, 305A North End Road, London W14.
⏰ Thu & Sat
TV winebar.

✉▽ **The Gender Trust**
BM Gentrust, London WC1N 3XX.
☎ 1305 269222 (infoline)
⏰ Call before 22:00

♂▽ **Greenwich Lesbian & Gay Centre**
3rd. Floor, 17 Bowater Road, Woolwich, London.
☎ 181 316 5954

♂ ▽ **London Bisexual Group (LGB)**
P. O. Box 3325, London N1 9EQ.
⏰ Meets Fri 19:00

✉▽ **Phoenix Centre**
12 Barnbury Road, Islington, London N1 1NB.

✉▽ **The Seahorse Society**
Newsletter, BM Seahorse, London WC1N 3XX.
For heterosexual transvestites & transsexuals.

⚥▽ **TV Self Help Group**
BM Box 3281, London E1 6JG.
☎ 171 289 5240

☺ □ **Women of the Beaumont Society (WOBS)**
BM WOBS, London WC1N 3XX.
☎ 1223 441246 (South)
☎ 1203 717528 (Midlands & Wales)
Support group for partners & families of crossdressers.

Organizations: Sexuality: Youth

♂▽ **Peer Education Project**
Health First, 15 Saint Thomas' Street, London Bridge, London SE1 9RY.
☎ 181 955 4366 Ext.: 4383
Addresses sexual health needs of young men in south east London who have sex with men.

Photographers: Erotic

☺ **Bob Carlos Clarke**
c/o Hamiltons, 13 Carlos Place, Mayfair, London W1.
☎ 171 499 9493
Still life photographer, also well known for his fetish work. Hamiltons is his gallery.

☺ **Randall Housk**
Flat 2, 42 Baldry Gardens, London SW16 3DJ.
☎ 181 764 8248

☺ **David Leslie**
5 Pragnell Road, London SE12 0LF.
☎ 181 857 7146 ✆ 181 857 4251

☺ **Gordon Rondelle**
50A Haverstock Hill, London NW3 2BH.
☎ 171 485 0134 ✆ 171 485 0134

☺ **Trevor Watson**
53C Unbridge Road, London W12 8LA.
☎ 181 749 2881 ✆ 181 749 2881

Photographers: Sexuality

⚥▼ **Girls Like Us, Ltd.**
197 Upper Street, Islington, London N1 1QR.
☎ 171 359 2289
Transvestite make-up & photography. Lessons, shoots, clothing rental, & dressmaking. Also has large photo library.

Piercers

☺ **The Bodyworks**
Suite 008, The Chandlery, 50 Westminster Bridge Road, London SE25.
☎ 171 721 7466

☺ ■ **Denis Cockell**
5 Walkers Court, London W1.
☎ 171 437 0605

☺ ■ **Cold Steel**
228 Camden High Street, London NW1 8QS.
☎ 171 267 7970 ✆ 181 908 4670
Member of the European Professional Piercers Association.

☺ ■ **The London Piercing Clinic**
55 Portland Road, South Norwood, London SE25.
☎ 181 656 7180

🕐 7 days a week
♿ 💳 💳 💳
☺ ■ **Metal Morphosis**
10-11 Moor Street, Westminster, London W1.
☎ 171 434 4554 📞 171 434 3279
 📞 831 511844
🕐 Mon - Sat 11:00 - 19:30, Sun 13:00 - 18:00
♿ 🚗 💳 💳 💳
☺ ■ **Multitek Services**
☎ 181 960 5759
☺ ■ **Pagan Metal**
29 Brewer Street, Soho, London W1R 3FE.
☎ 171 287 3830

Promoters

☺ **Chain Gang Promotions**
BCM Box 4542, London WC1N 3XX.
☎ 171 284 2180 📞 171 284 2189
☎ 171 494 3701
Major fetish club organizers.

Publishers: Books: Erotic

☺ **Nexus**
332 Ladbrook Grove, London W10 5AH.

Publishers: Books: Fetish

⚦ **Quartet Books Limited**
27/29 Goodge Street, London W1P 1FD.
☺ ■ **Tim Woodward Publishing Ltd.**
23 Grand Union Centre, Kensal Road, London W10 5AX.
☎ 181 968 0234 📞 181 960 8404
📧 info@skintwo.co.uk
🌐 http://www.dungeon.com/~SkinTwo

Publishers: Books: General

☺ ■ **Picador, Div. of Pan Macmillan**
Cavaye Place, London SW10 9PG.
Have published books about BDSM & fetish.

Publishers: Books: Sexuality

⚥ **Bottomliners**
P. O. Box 3628, London NW1 8EL.
☎ 171 267 8882
⚥▼ **Lesbian & Gay Studies**
Wellington House, 125 The Strand, London WC2R 0BB.
☎ 171 420 5555 📞 171 240 7261
⚥▼ **The Other Way Press**
9 Sovereign Close, London W5 1DE.
☎ 181 998 1519

Publishers: Directories: AIDS

☺ **AIDS Directory**
The Nam Charitable Trust, 52 The Eurolink Centre, 49 Effra Road, London SW2 1BZ.
☎ 171 737 1846 📞 171 737 6190
Current information on all the HIV & AIDS services in the U.K.. Published once a year.

Publishers: Directories: Books

☺ ■ **J. Whitaker & Sons**
12 Dyott Road, London WC1A 1DS.
☎ 171 836 8911 📞 171 836 2909
Lists books published in U.K..

Publishers: Directories: Sexuality

⚥▼ **BJ Ventures**
6 Dean Street, Soho, London W1W 5RN.
☎ 171 734 4585
⚥▼ **Gay To Z Directory**
Gay To Z Publishing, Ltd., 24 Offley Road, Oval, London SW9 0LS.
☎ 171 793 7450 📞 171 820 1366
📧 s-coote@dircon.co.uk
🌐 http://freedom.co.uk/gaytoz/
🕐 Mon - Fri 09:00 - 17:00
The U.K.'s gay phonebook—contains over 3,000 businesses, services, & organizations that serve the lesbian, gay, & bisexual communities. Published twice a year. Yearly subscription is $10. French also spoken.
⚥▼ **Visitors Guide to Gay Britain**
Gay To Z Publishing, Ltd., 24 Offley Road, Oval, London SW9 0LS.
☎ 171 793 7450 📞 171 820 1366
📧 s-coote@dircon.co.uk
🌐 http://freedom.co.uk/gaytoz/
🕐 Mon - Fri 09:00 - 17:00
Gay to Z guide to the U.K.. Maps, travel information, hotels, & the most

up-to-date listings on pubs, clubs, & saunas. Published once a year. Yearly subscription is $20. French also spoken.

Publishers: Guides: Sexuality

⚥▼ **Freedom Editions**
Wellington House, 125 The Strand, London WC2R 0BB.
☎ 171 420 5555 📞 171 240 7261
☺ ■ **The Transvestite's Guide**
The WayOut Publishing Company, P. O. Box 941, London SW5 9UT.
160-page listing guide, with information about shops, services, & places to go all over the world for transvestites & fetishists. Published once a year. Yearly subscription is £10 for U.K., or $20U.S. (in bills) elsewhere.

Publishers: Magazines: Arts

☺ ■ **Time Out**
3 Stockwell Terrace, London SW9.
☎ 171 813 3000

Publishers: Magazines: BDSM

⚥▼ **Corporal Contacts**
BCM Corpco, London WC1N 3XX.
☺ ■ **Domina**
27 Old Gloucester Street, South Kensington, London WC1N 3XX.
Fetish magazine with two sections in colour. Stories, articles, photos, listings, & mail order. Also has U.S. office in New York. Published quarterly. Yearly subscription is $100.
⚦ ■ **Pussy Cat**
Black Box Productions Ltd., 52 Bermondsey Street, London Bridge, London SE1 3UD.
Magazine of female domination.
☺ ■ **QUIM**
BM 2182, London WC1N 3XX.
⚥▼ **Sir!**
ST Publishing, P.O. Box 2153, London E7 0JZ.
Mail order only.

Publishers: Magazines: Erotic

☺ ■ **Desire**
Red Sky Publishing, Limited, 192 Clapham High Street, Clapham, London SW4 7UD.
☎ 171 627 5155 📞 171 627 5808
Sex & sexuality for women & men.
⚥▼ **Mike Arlen's Guys**
Wetherby Studios, 23 Wetherby Mansions, Earl's Court Square, Earl's Court, London SW5 9BH.
☎ 171 373 1107
Volumes 8, 9, 10, 11, & 12 $10, Volume 13 $12, plus $10 each air mail p&p, or $5 each for surface.

Publishers: Magazines: Fetish

☺ ■ **Aggressive Women Magazine**
Swish Publications Ltd., 47 Great Guildford Street, London SE1 0ES.
⚥ ■ **Detonator**
132 Buckingham Palace Road, London SW1W 9SA.
☺ ■ **Pagan Metal**
29 Brewer Street, Soho, London W1R 3FE.
☎ 171 287 3830
☺ ■ **Redeemer**
Redemption Films, BCM P.O. Box 9235, London WC1N 3XX.
☺ ■ **Ritual Magazine**
Ritual World, 29 Brewer Street, London W1R 3FE.
☎ 171 287 1025 📞 171 287 1025
☎ 171 287 2096
🌐 http://www.ritualmag.co.uk/
☺ ■ **Skin Two**
Tim Woodward Publishing Ltd., 23 Grand Union Centre, Kensal Road, London W10 5AX.
☎ 181 968 0234 📞 181 960 8404
📧 info@skintwo.co.uk
🌐 http://www.dungeon.com/~SkinTwo
Published quarterly.
☺ ■ **Zeitgeist**
Zeitgeist International, 66 Holloway Road, London N7 8JC.
☎ 171 607 2977 📞 171 607 8144

Publishers: Magazines: General

⚥ **Arena**
Exmouth House, Pine Street, London EC1.
☎ 171 837 7270
⚤ **Everywoman**
34 Islington Green, London N1 8DU.
☺ **The Face**

Exmouth House, Pine Street, London EC1.
☎ 171 837 7270

⚲▼ *Rouge Magazine*
Breakaway Publications Ltd., BM Rouge, London WC1N 3XX.
☎ 171 377 9426 📞 171 377 9426
📧 jjohnson@cix.compulink.co.uk

Publishers: Magazines: Sexual Politics
☺ *Body Politic*
P.O. Box 2898, London NW1 5RL.
☎ 171 486 2188 📞 171 486 2217

Publishers: Magazines: Sexuality
⚲▼ *Attitude*
Northern & Shell, Northern & Shell Tower, City Harbour, London E14 9GL.
☎ 171 987 5090

⚲ *Bad Attitude*
121 Railton Road, Brixton, London.
☎ 171 978 9057

⚲▼ *Diva*
Millivres Ltd., Worldwide House, 116-134 Bayham Street, London NW1 0BA.

⚲▼ *Gay Times*
Millivres Ltd., Ground Floor, Worldwide House, 116-134 Bayham Street, London NW1 0BA.
☎ 171 482 2576 📞 171 284 0329
Published every month.

⚲▼ *IQ Magazine*
93a Balls Pond Road, London N1 4BL.
☎ 171 275 8359

⚲▼ *Phase*
Blasé Ltd., 8 Neal's Yard, Covent Garden, London WC2H 9DP.
☎ 171 240 6525 📞 171 240 6529

⚲▼ *Prime*
Virtual Universe Publications Ltd., 5 Langley Street, Covent Garden, London WC2H 9JA.
☎ 171 240 9156 📞 171 240 9157

⚲▼ *QX*
Unit 14, 132 Charing Cross Road, London WC2H 0LA.
☎ 171 379 7525

Publishers: Magazines: Spanking
⚲▼ *Report*
ST Publishing, P. O. Box 2153, London E7 0JZ.
Mail order only.

Publishers: Miscellaneous: BDSM
☺ ■ *Comba-Borel*
BCM 3714, London WC1N 3XX.
☎ 171 738 2085 📞 171 738 2085
BDSM postcards (with envelopes). Catalogue, free with SAE.

Publishers: Newspapers: General
☺ ■ *The Daily Mail*
2 Derry Road, London W8.
☎ 171 938 6000

☺ ■ *The Guardian*
199 Farringdon Road, London WC1.

☺ ■ *The Times*
1 Virginia Street, London E1.
☎ 171 782 5000

Publishers: Newspapers: Sexuality
⚲■ *Boy's Own*
FTM Network, BM Network, London WC1N 3XX.
☎ 161 432 1915
Newsletter for female-to-male transsexuals with information of treatment, social issues, etc.. Published quarterly. Yearly subscription is $20.

⚲▼ *Boyz*
Silveraim Ltd., 72 Holloway Road, London N7 8NZ.
☎ 171 296 6000 📞 171 296 0026
Published every week.

⚲▼ *The Gay Gazette*
Silveraim Ltd., 72 Holloway Road, London N7 8NZ.
☎ 171 296 6000 📞 171 296 0026

⚲▼ *MX*
Out of London Limited, 6 Palace Gate, London W8 5LY.
☎ 171 581 1521
Published every week.

⚲▼ *The Pink Paper*
Silveraim Ltd., 72 Holloway Road, London N7 8NZ.
☎ 171 296 6000 📞 171 296 0026

⚲▼ *She Bang*
13 Hercules Street, London N7 6AT.
☎ 171 607 2696

⚲▼ *Thud*
156-158 Grays Inn Road, Holborn, London WC1X 8ED.
☎ 171 837 7333

Radio: General
☺ ■ *G.A.Y, The Radio*
Spectrum Radio AM 558, Endeavour House, Brent Cross, London NW2 1JT.
☎ 181 905 5000
🕐 Mon - Fri 01:00 - 03:00

Radio: Sexuality
⚲▼ *Freedom FM*
156-158 Grays Inn Road, Holborn, London WC1X 8ED.
☎ 171 916 0162

☺ ■ *Gay & Lesbian London*
Greater London Radio, 35C Marylebone High Street, London W1A 4LG.
☎ 171 224 2424

⚲▽ *Out This Week*
All Out Productions, 49 Wellington Street, Covent Garden, London WC2E 7BN.
☎ 171 240 2070

Stores: Art Galleries
☺ *Akehurst Gallery*
345 Portobello Road, London W10 5SA.
☎ 181 969 0453 📞 181 960 0085
Also represents many of the most important English fetish photographers.

Stores: Books: General
☺ *Bookmarks*
265 Seven Sisters Road, London N4 2DE.
☎ 181 802 6145

☺ ■ *Books, Etc.*
122 Charing Cross Road, London WC2H 0JR.
☎ 171 379 7313 📞 171 836 0373

⚲▼ *Colt Bookstore*
2 Berwick Street, London W1.

☺ *Compendium*
234 Camden High Street, Camden, London NW1.
☎ 171 485 8944

☺ *Houseman's*
5 Caledonian Road, London N1.
☎ 171 837 4473

☺ ■ *Intabooks*
112 Norfolk Place, London W2.

☺ ■ *Janus*
40 Old Compton Street, London W1V 5PB.
☎ 171 437 1741
Books & magazines.

☺ *Lance Publications*
707, High Road, Finchley, London N12 0BT.

☺ *Lovejoys*
99 Charing Cross Road, London.
☎ 171 437 0811
Large erotic & fetish magazine section downstairs.

☺ *The Pink List*
26c Denholme Road, London W9 3HX.
☎ 181 964 4523

☺ *Pipeline Bookshop*
37 Neal Street, Covent Garden, London WC2.
☎ 171 240 3319

⚱ ■ *Silver Moon*
64-68 Charing Cross Road, London WC2H 0BB.
☎ 171 836 7906 📞 171 379 1018

☺ ■ *W. & G. Foyles*
113-119 Charing Cross Road, London WC2H 0DT.

☺ ■ *W. H. Smith*
Surrey Quays Shopping Court, Redriff Road, London SE.
☎ 171 237 5235

☺ ■ *W. H. Smith*
7 Holbein Place, London SW1W 8NR.

☎ 171 730 1200
☺ **Waterstones**
121-125 Charing Cross Road, London WC2.
☎ 171 434 4291
☺ **Waterstones**
128 Camden High Street, Camden, London NW1 0NB.
☎ 171 284 4948
☺ **The Women's Book Club**
45/46 Poland Street, London W1C 4AU.
☎ 171 437 1019

Stores: Clothing: Corsets
☺ **Banned**
2 Cross Street, London N1 2BL.
☎ 171 704 2766

Stores: Clothing: Fetish
☺ **Ad Hoc**
38a Camden high Street, Camden, London W8.
☎ 171 938 1664
☺ ■ **Atom Age**
Unit 3A, 98 Victoria Road, London NW10 6NB.
☺ ■ **Cocoon**
1st. Floor, 250 Kilburn High Road, London NW6 3JU.
☎ 171 624 1074
🕐 Mon - Fri 10:00 - 18:00, Sat 10:00 -16:00
Rubber fetish clothes. Catalogue, £7, £10 overseas.
☺ **East of Eden**
519/523 Cambridge Heath Road, London E2 9EU.
☎ 171 251 4960
Wetlook, PVC, & lycra clothing.
☺ **Fantasy Fayre**
43 Anerley Road, Crystal Palace, London SE19 2AS.
☺ **Fetish Fetish**
4A Peter Street, London W1 3RR.
☎ 171 734 8343
Catalogue available.
☺ ■ **Honour**
86 Lower Marsh, Waterloo, London SE1 7AB.
☎ 171 401 8219 📞 171 401 8220
🕐 Mon - Fri 10:30 - 19:00, Sat 11:30 - 17:00
Catalogue, £5 in U.K. (refundable), £7 overseas.
⚥ ■ **Libido**
1 The Parkway, London NW1 7PG.
☎ 171 916 0180 📞 171 916 1262
Dress to Express. Hot clothes for cool women.
☺ ■ **Pagan Metal**
29 Brewer Street, Soho, London W1R 3FE.
☎ 171 287 3830
Clothes from corsets to warrior.
☺ ■ **Paradiso Bodyworks**
🚻 41 Old Compton Street, Soho, London W1V 5PN.
☎ 171 287 2487 📞 171 348 9352
☺ ■ **Regulation**
17a Saint Albans Place, Islington, London N1 0NX.
☎ 171 226 0665
🕐 Mon - Sat 10:00 - 18:30, Sun 12:00 - 17:00
Wholesale enquiries welcome. Catalogue, £5.
⚥ ▼ **Sh!**
🚻 43 Coronet Street, London N1 6HD.
☎ 171 613 5458
🕐 Wed-Thurs 12-5, Fri-Sat 12-10
Women's erotic emporium selling toys, books, all manner of clothing,
body jewelry, lubes, bondages. Men welcome only if with a woman.
Coffee & advice offered. Catalogue, £5.
☺ ■ **She'an'Me Fun Fashions**
123 Hammersmith Road, West Kensington, London W14.
☎ 171 603 2402
☎ 1753 663479 (24hr. order line)
40-page catalogue, £5.
☺ ■ **Skin Two**
23 Grand Union Centre, Kensal Road, London W10 5AX.
☎ 181 968 0234 📞 181 960 8404
✉ info@skintwo.co.uk
🌐 http://www.dungeon.com/~SkinTwo
🕐 Mon - Sat 11:00 - 19:00
☾ **Zipper Store**
283 Camden High Street, London NW1 7BX.
☎ 171 284 0537 📞 171 284 0329
☎ 171 267 0021

✉ zipper@gaytimes.co.uk
🕐 Mon - Thu 10:00 - 18:30, Fri 10:00 - 19:00, Sat 10:00 - 18:30,
Sun 12:00 - 17:00
Also BDSM toys. Catalogue, £2.

Stores: Clothing: Footwear
⚳ **The Little Shoe Box**
89 Holloway Road, London N7 8LT.
☎ 171 607 1247
Shoe manufacturers welcoming TVs.

Stores: Clothing: Rubber
☺ **Doc Roc**
59 Camden High Street, London NW1 7JL.
☎ 171 916 9273
☺ ▼ **Invincible**
🚻 Unit 19E, 2nd. Floor, Tower Workshops, Riley Road, London SE1 3DG.
☎ 171 237 4017 📞 171 231 5416
☎ 171 237 5062
✉ Invin@latex.demon.co.uk
🕐 Mon - Fri 10:00 - 18:00, Sat 12:00 - 16:00
Specialist in rubber for men & women, made to measure. Catalogue,
£5, overseas £8.

Stores: Clothing: Sexuality
⚳ ■ **Cover Girl Shoes**
44 Cross Street, London N1.
☎ 171 354 2883
Clothing for TVs.
⚳ ■ **Transformation Ltd.**
50-52 Eversholt Street, Camden, London NW1 1DA.
☎ 171 388 0627
🕐 Mon - Sat 09:00 - 20:00
The world's leading TV specialists. Some adult baby items, also. Next to
Euston station.

Stores: Clothing: Sports
☾ **Sports Locker**
53 Pembridge Road, London W11.
☎ 171 221 9166

Stores: Erotica: BDSM
☾▼ **Expectations**
75 Great Eastern Street, London EC2A 3HU.
☎ 171 739 0292
London's largest collection of rubber, leather, & toys. Also sells the
Detainer rubber & waxed cotton lines. Catalogue available.
☺ **Key Largo**
2 Bow Street, London WC2.
☎ 171 ?49 7599
☾ **The London Leather Cave**
Units A233/4, 2nd. Floor, Riverdale Business Centre, Bendon Valley,
London SW18.
☎ 181 875 1607
♂ ▼ **RoB—London**
24 Wells Street, London W1P 3FG.
☎ 171 735 7893 📞 171 637 4510

Stores: Erotica: General
☺ ■ **Ann Summers**
155 Charing Cross Road, London W1.
☎ 171 437 1886
☾▼ **Clone Zone**
🚻 64 Old Compton Street, Soho, London W1.
☎ 171 287 3530 📞 171 287 3531
Free catalogue.
☾▼ **Clone Zone Head Office**
Units 8 & 10, Eurolink Business Centre, 49 Effra Road, Brixton, London
SW2 1BZ.
☎ 171 737 3636 📞 171 737 3571
Head office, not a store. Free catalogue.
☺ ■ **Lovecraft**
46 Cranbourn Street, London WC2H.
☺ ■ **Ritual Shoes**
29 Brewer Street, London W1R 3FE.
☎ 171 287 2096 📞 171 242 2887
Shoes, boots, & magazines (including Ritual magazine).
☺ **Sign of the Times**
1st. Floor, Kensington Market, Kensington High Street, London W8.

☎ 171 938 4744
☺ ■ **Smorgasmatron!**
 39 Cranleigh Road, London N15 3AB.
 🕐 Weekends only
 🔥 ✓
 Small bookshop, specializing in cult / underground literature, comics, &
 magazines. Also mail order.

Stores: Military Surplus
☺ ■ **Army Classics**
 47 Pembridge Road, London W11.
 ☎ 171 247 8452
☺ ■ **Fulham Army & Navy Store**
 375 North End Road, London SW6.
 ☎ 171 610 3577
☺ ■ **Islington Army & Navy Store**
 32 Chapel Market, Islington, London N1.
 ☎ 171 833 4805
☺ ■ **Lawrence Corner**
 62 Hampstead Road, London NW1.
☺ ■ **Lawrence Corner**
 145 Drummond Street, London NW1.
☺ ■ **Romeo Trading Co. Ltd.**
 81 Roman Way, London N7 8UP.
 ☎ 171 607 7212 📞 171 607 5458
☺ ■ **Silvermans Ltd.**
 2 Hartford Street, Mile End, London E1 4PS.
 ☎ 171 790 5257

Suppliers: Safer Sex Products
☺ **John Bell Croyden**
 50 Wigmore Street, London W1.
 ☎ 171 935 5555
 Supplies catheters.
⚥▽ **Rubberstuffers**
 P. O. Box 246, London WC1H 8HU.
 ☎ 171 278 0508
 Provides safer sex packs at local venues.

Tattooists
☺ ■ **Into You**
 144 Saint John Street, London EC1R 0AT.
 ☎ 171 253 5085

Television: General
☺ ■ *The James Whale Show*
 Mike Mansfield TV, 5-7 Carnaby Street, London W1 1PG.
 ☎ 171 494 3061

MERSEYSIDE
County Resources
Helplines: Sexuality
⚥▽ **Saint Helens Lesbian & Gay Helpline**
 ☎ 1744 454823
 🕐 Mon Wed 19:00 - 21:00
 Advice & information about HIV/AIDS & other sexual health & sexuality
 issues.

Birkenhead
Helplines: AIDS
☺ □ **AIDS Care & Support In Action (ACASIA)**
 ☎ 185 003 2925
 🕐 24hrs. emergency cellular contact number
 Advice & information about HIV/AIDS & other sexual health issues.

Liverpool
Bars: BDSM
⚥ **Fascination**
 P.O. Box 10, Liverpool, Merseyside L36 6LD. England
 ☎ 151 252 2272 📞 151 252 2273
 🕐 Held 2nd. Tue of month
 🔥 ✓ VISA 🔥
 Fetish club. Catalogue, £7 airmail outside of U.K., p&p incl.. Age
 statement of 18 is required.

Health Services
☺ □ **Healthwise**
 ☎ 800 665544
 🕐 09:00 - 21:00. Fri women only
 Advice & information about HIV/AIDS & other sexual health issues. Free
 phone from Cheshire & Merseyside only. Minicom available.

Helplines: AIDS
☺ □ **AIDS Helpline**
 P.O. Box 11, Liverpool, Merseyside L69 1SN.
 ☎ 151 709 9000

Helplines: Sexuality
☺ □ **Merseyside Friend**
 36 Bolton Street, Liverpool, Merseyside L3 5LX.
 ☎ 151 708 9552 (men)
 ☎ 151 708 0234 (women)

Organizations: AIDS: Support
☺ □ **Merseyside AIDS Support Group (MASG)**
 ☎ 151 709 9000 (also TTY)
 🕐 Mon Wed Fri 19:00 - 22:00
 Advice & information about HIV/AIDS & other sexual health issues.
☺ □ **Body Positive—Merseyside**
 ☎ 151 707 2324
 🕐 24hrs.
 Advice & information about HIV/AIDS & other sexual health issues.

Organizations: Sexuality
⚥▽ **Liverpool Bisexual & Married Gays Group**
 ☎ 161 708 9552
⚥▽ **Liverbirds**
 c/o Merseyside Friend, 36 Bolton Street, Liverpool, Merseyside L3 5LX.
 ☎ 151 709 3181
 🕐 Call Fri 19:30 - 21:00. Meets Fri 20:00 - 22:00

Stores: Books: General
☺ **News from Nowhere**
 112 Bold Street, Liverpool, Merseyside L1.
 ☎ 151 708 7270

Stores: Military Surplus
☺ ■ **Callan Military Surplus**
 51 Whitechapel, Liverpool, Merseyside L1.
 ☎ 151 236 8753

Saint Helens
Organizations: Fetish: Foot
⚥▽ **Footmen**
 P. O. Box 53, Saint Helens, Merseyside WA10 2HN.

MIDDLESEX
Feltham
Stores: Erotica: General
☺ ■ **Valentine Products**
 P. O. Box 63, Feltham, Middlesex TW13 7QN.

Teddington
Photographers: Erotic
☺ **John Marshall**
 P. O. Box 88, Teddington, Middlesex TW11 0JG.
 ☎ 181 977 6180 📞 181 943 2396

Twickenham
Manufacturers: Clothing: Rubber
☺ **I, I & E Group**
 P. O. Box 1, Twickenham, Middlesex TW2 6AP.
 ☎ 181 894 2835 📞 181 287 3839
 🕐 09:00 - 18:00
 Produces latex clothing, etc. for trade customers only. No retail sales.
 Established 1971. French also spoken.

Manufacturers: Safe Sex Products
☺ **Bodywise**
 The Arches, Richmond Bridge, Twickenham, Middlesex TW1 2EF.
 ☎ 181 891 1485
 Make the lubricant adotped by the Terence Higgins Trust, Red Ribbon, &
 other National Health Service trusts.

Uxbridge
Organizations: AIDS: Support
☺ □ **Hillingdon AIDS Response Trust**
 Sterling House, 276A High Street, Uxbridge, Middlesex UB8 1LQ.
 ☎ 189 581 3874

Stores: Clothing: Fetish
☺ **She'an'Me Fun Fashions**
 48 Windsor Street, Uxbridge, Middlesex UB8.

☎ 1895 271668
☎ 1753 663479 (24hr. order line)
Catalogue, £5.

NORFOLK

Great Yarmouth

Helplines: Sexuality

⚥▽ **Norwich Lesbian & Gayline**
☎ 1603 592505
🕘 Mon 20:00 - 22:00
Advice & information about HIV/AIDS & other sexual health & sexuality issues.

King's Lynn

Helplines: AIDS

☺ □ **Eastern AIDS Support Triangle**
☎ 1553 776655
🕘 Wed Sun 19:00 - 22:00
Advice & information about HIV/AIDS & other sexual health issues.

Helplines: Sexuality

⚥ **West Norfolk Gay & Lesbian Helpline**
P. O. Box 40, King's Lynn, Norfolk PE32 1HF.
☎ 1553 630012

Publishers: Magazines: BDSM

■ ***Halcyon***
16 Tuesday Market Place, King's Lynn, Norfolk PE30 1JN.

Norwich

Helplines: AIDS

☺ □ **AIDS Helpline**
36 Unthank Road, Norwich, Norfolk NR2 2RB.
☎ 160 361 5816

☺ □ **Norwich AIDS Helpline**
☎ 1603 615816
🕘 Sat 11:00 - 15:00
Advice & information about HIV/AIDS & other sexual health issues.

Helplines: Sexuality

⚥▽ **Norfolk Friend**
☎ 1603 628055
🕘 Men Fri 19:00 - 21:00, women Tue 19:00 - 21:00
Advice & information about HIV/AIDS & other sexual health & sexuality issues.

⚥▽ **Norwich Lesbian & Gayline**
☎ 1603 592505
🕘 Mon 20:00 - 22:00
Advice & information about HIV/AIDS & other sexual health & sexuality issues.

Organizations: AIDS: Education

⚥▽ **Gay Men's Health Project**
46 Bethel Street, Norwich, Norfolk NR2 1NR.
☎ 160 362 7514

Organizations: AIDS: Support

☺ □ **The Fightback Trust—East Anglia**
☎ 1603 762656
🕘 Mon - Thu Sat 10:00 - 18:00 Fri 10:00 - 21:00
Advice & information about HIV/AIDS & other sexual health issues.

Organizations: Sexuality

⚥▽ **Norwich Gay Men's Health Project**
☎ 1603 62514
🕘 Wed 15:00 - 19:00
Advice & information about HIV/AIDS & other sexual health issues.

Stores: Books: General

☺ **Bookmark Bookstore**
83 Unthank Road, Norwich, Norfolk NR2 2PE.
☎ 160 376 2855

NORTH YORKSHIRE

Harrogate

Helplines: AIDS

☺ □ **AIDS Concern North Yorkshire**
☎ 1423 505222
🕘 Mon Thu 10:00 - 15:30, 19:00 - 21:00, Tue Wed Fri 10:00 - 15:30
Advice & information about HIV/AIDS & other sexual health issues.

Helplines: Sexuality

⚥▽ **Harrogate Switchboard**
☎ 1423 524101
🕘 19:30 - 22:00

Stores: Military Surplus

☺ ■ **The Harrogate Army & Navy Store**
22 Commercial Street, Harrogate, North Yorkshire.
☎ 1423 504035

Stores: Safer Sex Products

☺ **Boys Own**
LTC, Stuart House, 15/17 North Park Road, Harrogate, North Yorkshire.
☎ 1423 526467

Middlesbrough

Helplines: Sexuality

⚢▽ **Cleveland Lesbian Line**
☎ 1642 217955
🕘 Mon 20:00 - 22:00
Advice & information about HIV/AIDS & other sexual health & sexuality issues.

⚥▽ **Teeside Friend**
☎ 1642 248888
🕘 Tue Fri 19:00 - 21:30
Advice & information about HIV/AIDS & other sexual health & sexuality issues.

Organizations: AIDS: Support

☺ □ **Cleveland AIDS Support**
☎ 1642 244588
🕘 Mon Thu 19:00 - 21:30
Advice & information about HIV/AIDS & other sexual health issues.

Organizations: Sexuality: Student

⚥▽ **University of Teeside LGB Group**
Students Union, Borough Road, Middlesbrough, North Yorkshire TS1 3BA.
☎ 164 234 2234
Contact: LGB Officer

Scarborough

Stores: Erotica: General

☺ ■ **Hobson De Nero**
P. O. Box 34, Scarborough, North Yorkshire YO11 1AA.
☎ 172 335 1515
Deerskin basques, gloves, jackets, & jeans for men & women.

York

Helplines: Sexuality

⚥▽ **York Gay Line**
P. O. Box 284, York, North Yorkshire YO1 1TX.
☎ 1904 612828
🕘 Tue 19:30 - 22:00, Thu 22:00 - 24:00

⚢▽ **York Lesbian Line**
P. O. Box 225, York, North Yorkshire YO1 1AA.
☎ 1904 646812
🕘 Fri 19:00 - 21:00
Advice & information about HIV/AIDS & other sexual health & sexuality issues.

Organizations: AIDS: Support

☺ □ **Positive Advocacy**
☎ 13774 229133
🕘 24-hour crisis line
Advice & information about HIV/AIDS & other sexual health issues.

☺ □ **York AIDS Action Ltd.**
☎ 1904 639595
🕘 Thu 15:00 - 19:00
Advice & information about HIV/AIDS & other sexual health issues.

Stores: Books: General

☺ **Blue Star Publications**
1 Victoria Street, York, North Yorkshire YO2 1LZ.
☎ 190 462 4901

NORTHAMPTONSHIRE

County Resources

Helplines: Sexuality

⚥▽ **Northampton Lesbian & Gayline**
☎ 1604 39722 (men)
☎ 1604 39723 (women)

🕐 Men Tue 15:00 - 21:30, women Tue 19:00 - 21:30
Advice & information about HIV/AIDS & other sexual health & sexuality issues.

☿▽ **Northamptonshire Gayline**
☎ 1933 223591
🕐 Thu 19:00 - 22:00
Advice & information about HIV/AIDS & other sexual health & sexuality issues.

Northampton
Helplines: AIDS
☺ ☐ **Northampton AIDS Information Line**
☎ 1604 28999
🕐 Mon - Fri 09:00 - 18:00
Advice & information about HIV/AIDS & other sexual health issues.

West Haddon
Organizations: Fetish: Clothing: Stockings
☺ **SSSH**
P. O. Box 122, West Haddon, Northamptonshire NN8 7DS.
Send $10U.S. cash or equivalent for information package & sample photo. Publishes *Seamed Stockings & Stiletto Heels Newsletter*.

NOTTINGHAMSHIRE
County Resources
Helplines: Sexuality
☿▽ **Nottingham Lesbian & Gay Switchboard**
☎ 115 941 1454
🕐 Mon - Fri 19:00 - 22:00
Advice & information about HIV/AIDS & other sexual health & sexuality issues.

Mansfield
Stores: Clothing: Rubber
☺ ■ **James Adult Centre**
2 Station Road, Mansfield, Nottinghamshire NG18 1DG.
☎ 1623 420425
Custom made latex & PVC clothes.

Nottingham
Helplines: Sexuality
☿▽ **Nottingham Friend**
☎ 115 947 4717
🕐 Tue 19:00 - 22:00
Advice & information about HIV/AIDS & other sexual health & sexuality issues.

Manufacturers: Erotica: Leather
☺ **The Federation**
20 Chaucer Court Workshops, Chaucer Street, Nottingham, Nottinghamshire NG1 5LP.
☎ 115 941 3435 ✆ 115 941 3435
☎ 115 950 0154
Only mail order, no retail shop.

Organizations: AIDS: Education
☺ ☐ **Nottingham AIDS Information Project**
8 Eldon Chambers, Nottingham, Nottinghamshire NG1 2NS.
☎ 115 941 1989

Organizations: AIDS: Support
☺ ☐ **Nottingham AIDS Bereavement Support (ABS)**
☎ 115 962 0920
🕐 24hrs.
Advice & information about HIV/AIDS & other sexual health issues.
☺ ☐ **Positive Support**
☎ 115 942 5133
🕐 24hrs.
Advice & information about HIV/AIDS & other sexual health issues.

Organizations: BDSM
☿▽ **East Mercia MSC**
c/o Glaramara Close, The Meadows, Nottingham, Nottinghamshire NG2 1LD.
☎ 133 236 1056 ✆ 115 986 2462
🕐 Meets 2nd. Fri & 4th. Sat of the month
Contact: Mr. Peter Yates, President & Editor
Motorcycle club with strict dress code, for men into leather, rubber, uniforms, etc.. Publishes *The Messenger* quarterly.

Organizations: Fetish: Clothing
☺ **Marquis Masquerade**

25 Monks Way, Silverdale, Nottinghamshire NG11 7FG.
☎ 115 981 9113 ✆ 115 920 9861
☎ 115 920 9861
🕐 Meets for fetish parties approximately every two months
Contact: Mr. Nick Coleman
A celebration of fetish & Gothic fantasy. Larger parties alternate between London & the Midlands. Live bands & performances. Age statement of 18 is required.

Organizations: Motorcycle
☿▽ **Gay Bikers (GBMCC)**
c/o Gay Switchboard, 31-A Mansfield Road, Nottingham, Nottinghamshire NG1 3FF.
☎ 115 941 1454

Organizations: Sexuality
♂▽ **Nottingham Women's Bi Group**
c/o Nottingham Women's Centre, 30 Chaucer Street, Nottingham, Nottinghamshire NG1 5LP.

Publishers: Directories: Sexuality
☿▼ *The Gai Guide*
The Gai Project, The Health Shop, Broad Street, Nottingham, Nottinghamshire.
☎ 115 947 5414

Publishers: Magazines: Fetish
☺ *Marquis Masquerade*
25 Monks Way, Silverdale, Nottinghamshire NG11 7FG.
☎ 115 981 9113 ✆ 115 920 9861
☎ 115 920 9861
🕐 Meets for fetish parties approximately every two months
Very visual with erotic art, sexual photography, stories, music reviews, club reviews, & special features on the erotic & obscure. Published quarterly. Yearly subscription is £20 plus £6 p&p (U.K.£ or IRCs). Age statement of 18 is required.

Publishers: Magazines: Sexuality
☿▼ *Outright!*
P. O. Box 4, West PDO, Nottingham, Nottinghamshire NG7 2DJ.
☎ 115 978 0124

Stores: Books: General
☺ ■ **Bookscene**
70 Alfreton Road, Nottingham, Nottinghamshire NG7 3MN.
☺ **Mushroom Bookshop**
10 Heathcote Road, Nottingham, Nottinghamshire NG1 3AA.
☎ 115 958 2506
☺ **Soho Books**
147 Radford Road, Nottingham, Nottinghamshire.
☎ 115 978 3567

Stores: Clothing: Fetish
☺ **Barbarella (Armoury)**
10 Greyhound Road, Nottingham, Nottinghamshire NG1 2DP.
☎ 115 950 0508 ✆ 115 950 0749
Catalogue, £6 for U.K., £7 for Europe, £9 overseas.

OXFORDSHIRE
County Resources
Helplines: Sexuality
☿▽ **Oxford Lesbian & Gay Switchboard**
☎ 1865 793 999
🕐 19:00 - 21:00

Oxford
Helplines: Sexuality
☿ **Oxford Friend**
☎ 1865 726 893
🕐 Tue Wed Fri 19:00 - 21:00
Advice & information about HIV/AIDS & other sexual health & sexuality issues.

Organizations: AIDS: Education
☺ ☐ **OxAIDS**
☎ 800 393999
🕐 Mon - Wed Fri 18:30 - 20:30
Advice & information about HIV/AIDS & other sexual health issues.

Organizations: AIDS: Support
☺ ☐ **Body Positive—Oxford**
Ebor House, 5 Blue Street, Oxford, Oxfordshire OX1 4E2.
☎ 186 520 4606

Organizations: Sexuality

⚥▽ **Bisexuals in Oxford**
c/o OLGC, North Gate Hall, Saint Michael's Street, Oxford, Oxfordshire OX1 2DU.
☎ 186 520 0030

▽ **Oxford Gay & Lesbian Centre**
North Gate Hall, Saint Michael's Street, Oxford, Oxfordshire OX1 2DU.
☎ 186 520 0030

Publishers: Magazines: Sexuality

▼ ***Pink Times***
P.O. Box 28, 34 Cowley Road, Oxford, Oxfordshire.

Stores: Books: General

☺ **Inner Bookshop**
111 Magdalen Road, Oxford, Oxfordshire OX4 1RQ.
☎ 186 524 5301

SHROPSHIRE

County Resources

Helplines: Sexuality

▽ **Shropshire Lesbian & Gay Switchboard**
☎ 1743 232393
🕘 Tue Fri 20:00 - 22:00
Advice & information about HIV/AIDS & other sexual health & sexuality issues.

Hollinswood

Manufacturers: Furniture: BDSM

☺ ■ **S&M Fabrications**
63 Dalford Court, Hollinswood, Shropshire TF3 2BP.
☎ 195 229 9978

Shrewsbury

Helplines: AIDS

☺ □ **Shrewsbury AIDS Helpline**
☎ 1743 261113
🕘 Mon 09:00 - 12:00 14:00 - 17:00, Wed 09:00 - 12:00, Thu 13:00 - 17:00
Advice & information about HIV/AIDS & other sexual health issues.

Organizations: AIDS: Support

☺ □ **Body Positive—Shropshire**
☎ 1743 350075
🕘 Mon 10:00 -16:00
Advice & information about HIV/AIDS & other sexual health issues.

Telford

Manufacturers: Clothing: Rubber

☺ ■ **The Rubber Mask & Costume Company**
Studio 1, Maws Craft Workshops, Ferry Road, Jackfield, Telford, Shropshire TF8 7LS.
☎ 1952 883994 📠 1952 884413

SOMERSET

Bridgwater

Stores: Books: General

☺ **Bookworm**
25 Saint John Street, Bridgwater, Somerset.
☎ 127 842 3512

Bristol

Organizations: Motorcycle

Severn Links
c/o Oasis Club, 14 Park Row, Bristol, Somerset.

Burnham-on-Sea

Suppliers: Photoprinting

☺ **Brent Photographics**
23 Abingdon Street, Burnham-on-Sea, Somerset TA18 1PL.
☎ 1278 784557
Confidential film processing & printing. Same day. Free catalogue.

Evercreech

Publishers: Magazines: Fetish

■ ***Marquis Magazine***
The Fetish Factory Ltd., 2 Sherston Terrace, High Street, Evercreech, Somerset BA 6HZ.
☎ 1749 831397 📠 1749 831380
🕘 09:00 - 13:00
Publisher & distributor of fetish erotica: magazines, books, comics, videos, calendars, & photo archives. Published quarterly. Yearly subscription is DM100. Age statement of 18 is required. French & German also spoken.

Taunton

Organizations: AIDS: Support

☺ □ **Body Positive—Somerset**
☎ 1823 324417
🕘 Mon Wed 19:00 - 21:0
Advice & information about HIV/AIDS & other sexual health issues.

☺ □ **Somerset AIDS Advice**
☎ 1823 332727
🕘 Tue Thu 10:00 - 16:00
Advice & information about HIV/AIDS & other sexual health issues.

SOUTH YORKSHIRE

County Resources

Helplines: Sexuality

☺ ▽ **South Yorkshire Connections**
☎ 122 673 0703
🕘 Thu 19:00 - 22:00, Sun 15:00 - 20:00
Advice & information about HIV/AIDS & other sexual health & sexuality issues.

Sheffield

Helplines: AIDS

☺ □ **South Yorkshire AIDSline**
☎ 800 844334
🕘 Tue - Thu 19:00 - 22:00
Advice & information about HIV/AIDS & other sexual health issues. Free call, but only available from South Yorkshire & North Derbyshire.

Helplines: Sexuality

▽ **Sheffield Friend**
☎ 114 275 8880
🕘 Helpline: Thu Fri 19:30 - 21:30
Advice & information about HIV/AIDS & other sexual health & sexuality issues.

▽ **Sheffield Gayphone**
☎ 114 258 8199
🕘 Mon Wed 19:30 - 21:30
Advice & information about HIV/AIDS & other sexual health issues.

⚢▽ **Sheffield Lesbian Line**
☎ 114 258 1238
🕘 Thu 19:00 - 22:00
Advice & information about HIV/AIDS & other sexual health issues.

Manufacturers: Chastity Belts

☺ ■ **Tollyboy Products**
P.O. Box 27, Dronfield, Sheffield, South Yorkshire S18 6DN.
☎ 1742 890575
Mail order only.

Organizations: Sexuality

■ **Rose's Club**
29 Roundel Street, Sheffield, South Yorkshire S9 3LE.
☎ 114 261 9444
Help, support, & social events for TVs. A4 sized magazine with features, stories, help & advice, reviews, letters, ads, etc.. Publishes *International TV Repartee* quarterly. Yearly subscription is $35U.S..

⚥▽ **Sheffield Bisexual Women's Group**
c/o General Office, Voluntary Action, 69 Division Street, Sheffield, South Yorkshire S1 4GE.

Stores: Books: General

☺ **Independent Bookshop**
69 Surrey Street, Sheffield, South Yorkshire S1 2LH.
☎ 114 273 7722

Stores: Clothing: Fetish

☺ ■ **Desire**
619 Attercliffe Road, Sheffield, South Yorkshire S9 3RD.
☎ 114 244 2626

STAFFORDSHIRE

County Resources

Helplines: Sexuality

⚤▽ **North Staffordshire Lesbian & Gay Switchboard**
☎ 1782 266998
🕘 Mon Wed Fri 20:00 - 22:00, Sun 13:00 - 15:00
Advice & information about HIV/AIDS & other sexual health & sexuality issues.

Hanley

Stores: Erotica: General

☺ ■ **Fantasy World**
10 Market Square, Hanley, Staffordshire ST1 1NU.

SUFFOLK

County Resources

Helplines: Sexuality

⚤▽ **Suffolk Lesbian & Gay Switchboard**
☎ 1473 232212
🕘 Tue Sat 19:30 - 21:30
Advice & information about HIV/AIDS & other sexual health & sexuality issues.

Bury Saint Edmund's

Organizations: AIDS: Support

☺ □ **The Fightback Trust—East Anglia**
☎ 1284 725600
🕘 Mon - Thu Sat 10:00 - 18:00 Fri 10:00 - 21:00
Advice & information about HIV/AIDS & other sexual health issues.

Organizations: BDSM

⚤ **The Cellar**
P.O. Box 17, Bury Saint Edmund's, Suffolk IP32 7AT.

Ipswich

Helplines: AIDS

☺ □ **Ipswich AIDS Helpline**
☎ 1473 232007
🕘 Tue Fri 19:30 - 22:00
Advice & information about HIV/AIDS & other sexual health issues.

Organizations: AIDS: Support

☺ □ **The Fightback Trust—East Anglia**
☎ 1473 289200
🕘 Mon - Thu Sat 10:00 - 18:00 Fri 10:00 - 21:00
Advice & information about HIV/AIDS & other sexual health issues.

Lowestoft

Manufacturers: Furniture: BDSM

☺ ■ **Eroteak**
Unit 3A, Norwich Road Industrial Estate, Lowestoft, Suffolk NR32 2BN.
☎ 1502 519222
Erotic furniture. By appointment only. Catalogue, £5.

Organizations: AIDS: Support

☺ □ **The Fightback Trust—East Anglia**
☎ 1502 501509
🕘 Mon - Thu Sat 10:00 - 18:00 Fri 10:00 - 21:00
Advice & information about HIV/AIDS & other sexual health issues.

Woodbridge

Photographers: Erotic

☺ **China Hamilton**
c/o Brooklyn Holdings, Badington, Suffolk IP13 8JJ.
☎ 1728 638415 📠 1728 638680

SURREY

Camberley

Organizations: AIDS: Education

☺ □ **Positive Action**
☎ 127 668 6377
🕘 Thu Fri 20:00 - 22:00
Advice & information about HIV/AIDS & other sexual health issues.

Croydon

Helplines: Sexuality

⚤▽ **Croydon Friend**
☎ 181 683 4239

Publishers: Magazines: Photography

☺ ***Scenario***
P. O. Box 900, Croydon, Surrey CR9 6AG.
☎ 181 681 7817
Art photography magazine with some fetish & bondage.

Stores: Clothing: Fetish

☺ **Pillow Talk**
48 Lower Addiscombe Road, Croydon, Surrey CR0 6AA.
☎ 181 688 8197
🕘 Mon - Sat 10:00 - 18:00
✓ $ VISA MC
Sells whole range of sex items: sex aids, lingerie, TV fetish shoes, leather, leather toys, magazines, novels, restraints, etc..

East Molesley

Organizations: Tattoo

☺ ■ **Flesh Canvas**
P. O. Box 139B, East Molesley, Surrey KT8 9YQ.

Egham

Distributors: Books: Fetish

☺ **Flywheel, Ltd.**
Brunel License Park, Egham, Surrey TW20 0JZ.

Godlaming

Organizations: AIDS: Support

☺ □ **Body Positive—West Surrey**
☎ 1483 418657
🕘 Wed Thu 20:00 - 22:00
Advice & information about HIV/AIDS & other sexual health issues.

Guildford

Helplines: AIDS

☺ □ **Surrey & East Hants AIDSlink Ltd.**
☎ 1483 300150
🕘 20:00 - 22:00
Advice & information about HIV/AIDS & other sexual health issues.

Organizations: BDSM

⚤ **GSN**
P.O. Box 234, Guildford, Surrey GU4 7TX.

Organizations: Sexuality

⚤▽ **Gay Skinhead Group**
P. O. Box 234, Guildford, Surrey GU4 7TX.

Kew Gardens

Stores: Clothing: Rubber

☺ ■ **Weathervain**
283 Sandycombe Road, Kew Gardens, Surrey TW9 3LU.
☎ 181 940 0156 📠 181 940 0156
Rubber & PVC clothes, & magazines.

SUSSEX

Chichester

Organizations: AIDS: Support

☺ □ **Community AIDS Network**
☎ 1243 538484
🕘 Tue - Fri 18:00 - 19:00
Advice & information about HIV/AIDS & other sexual health issues.

Hastings

Helplines: Sexuality

☺ □ **Hastings Befrienders**
☎ 1424 444777
🕘 Men Fri 20:00 - 22:00, women Mon 19:00 - 21:00
Advice & information about HIV/AIDS & other sexual health issues.

☺ □ **Hastings Switchboard**
☎ 1424 721394
🕘 Fri 20:00 - 22:00

Organizations: AIDS: Support

☺ □ **AIDS Support Society**
49 Cambridge Gardens, Hastings, Sussex.
☎ 142 442 9901

Organizations: BDSM

👫 **The Alice Kerr Sutherland Society**

Box 12, Hastings, Sussex.
Publishes *The Governess*.

Worthing

Organizations: Fetish: Hair

☺ **T. S. C.**
P. O. Box 1409, Worthing, West Sussex BN14 8PE.
For devotees of hair-free bodies.

TEESIDE

Stockton-on-Tees

Publishers: Magazines: BDSM

☺ ■ ***Some Bizarre***
SB Publishing, Ltd., P. O. Box 28, Stockton-on-Tees, Teeside TS21 1YR.
Published every two months. Yearly subscription is $35.

TYNE & WEAR

Gateshead

Organizations: Sexuality

⚥ ▽ **North East Bi Group**
c/o Gateshead Law Centre, Swinburne House, Swinburne Street, Gateshead, Tyne & Wear.
🕘 Meets 2nd. Thu of month

Newcastle upon Tyne

Helplines: Sexuality

⚣⚢ ▽ **Newcastle Friend**
☎ 191 261 8555
🕘 Minicom Mon - Thu 19:00 - 22:00
Advice & information about HIV/AIDS & other sexual health & sexuality issues.

⚣⚢ ▽ **Newcastle Gay Youthline**
☎ 191 233 1551
🕘 Thu 15:30 - 17:30
Advice & information about HIV/AIDS & other sexual health & sexuality issues.

⚢ ▽ **Newcastle Lesbian Line**
☎ 191 261 2277
🕘 Minicom Tue 19:00 - 22:00
Advice & information about HIV/AIDS & other sexual health & sexuality issues.

Manufacturers: Clothing: Rubber

☺ ■ **Westgate Industrial Rubber**
Bakers Hill Industrial Area, 345 Shields Road, Newcastle upon Tyne, Tyne & Wear NE6 2UD.
☎ 1632 654858
Heavy rubber boots & chest waders.

Organizations: AIDS: Education

☺ □ **AIDS Community Trust**
P.O. Box 1DL, Newcastle upon Tyne, Tyne & Wear NE99 1DL.
☎ 191 224 4848

Organizations: AIDS: Support

☺ □ **SIDA Centre**
☎ 191 232 2855
🕘 Sat 10:00 - 16:00
Advice & information about HIV/AIDS & other sexual health issues.

Stores: Books: General

☺ **Alleycat Books Coöp**
46 Low Friar Street, Taylors Court, Blackfriars, Newcastle upon Tyne, Tyne & Wear NE1 5XD.
☎ 191 232 5478
🕘 10:00 - 18:00 Mon - Sat
✓
Radical bookshop including lesbian, gay & bisexual section. Fiction, non-fiction, travel guides, sex guides, magazines, cards, & postcards.

Stores: Clothing: Sexuality

Transformation Ltd.
39/41 Low Friar Street, Newcastle upon Tyne, Tyne & Wear NE1 5UE.
☎ 191 230 1105
🕘 Mon - Sat 09:00 - 20:00
The world's leading TV specialists.

Sunderland

Helplines: Sexuality

⚣⚢ ▽ **Sunderland Lesbian & Gay Young Peoples Group**
☎ 191 565 7905
🕘 Mon 19:00 - 20:00
Advice & information about HIV/AIDS & other sexual health & sexuality issues.

Organizations: Sexuality: Student

⚣⚢ ▽ **University of Sunderland LGB Group**
Carlton Bar, Stockton Road, Sunderland, Tyne & Wear.
Contact: LGB Coördinators

Radio: Sexuality

⚣⚢ ▽ ***Gay II Gay***
Wear FM 103.4FM, Forster Building, Chester Road, Sunderland, Tyne & Wear SR1 3SD.
☎ 191 515 2103

WARWICKSHIRE

Kenilworth

Helplines: Sexuality

☺ ▽ **West Midlands Lesbian & Gay Switchboard**
☎ 121 622 6589
🕘 19:00 - 22:00
Advice & information about HIV/AIDS & other sexual health issues.

Nuneaton

Manufacturers: Piercing Jewelry

☺ **P. A. U. K.**
153 Tomkinson Road, Nuneaton, Warwickshire CV10 8DP.

Publishers: Magazines: Piercing

☺ ***Piercing World***
P. A. U. K., 153 Tomkinson Road, Nuneaton, Warwickshire CV10 8DP.
Published quarterly. Yearly subscription is £25.

Royal Leamington Spa

Accommodation: BDSM

☺ **The Lodge**
P.O. Box 168, Royal Leamington Spa, Warwickshire CV33 0AD.

Helplines: Sexuality

☺ ▽ **West Midlands Lesbian & Gay Switchboard**
☎ 121 622 6589
🕘 19:00 - 22:00
Advice & information about HIV/AIDS & other sexual health issues.

Stratford-upon-Avon

Helplines: Sexuality

☺ ▽ **West Midlands Lesbian & Gay Switchboard**
☎ 121 622 6589
🕘 19:00 - 22:00
Advice & information about HIV/AIDS & other sexual health issues.

Warwick

Accommodation: BDSM

☺ ■ **Domino**
P.O. Box 159, Warwick, Warwickshire CV35 8JG.
Bed & breakfast with dungeon.

Manufacturers: Furniture: BDSM

☺ ■ **Domino**
P.O. Box 159, Warwick, Warwickshire CV35 8JG.

WEST MIDLANDS

County Resources

Helplines: AIDS

☺ □ **AIDS Line West Midlands**
☎ 121 622 1511
🕘 Mon - Fri 19:30 - 22:00
Advice & information about HIV/AIDS & other sexual health issues.

Helplines: Sexuality

☺ ▽ **West Midlands Friend**
P. O. Box 2405, Birmingham, West Midlands B5 4AL.
☎ 121 622 7351

☺ ▽ **West Midlands Lesbian & Gay Switchboard**
☎ 121 622 6589
🕘 19:00 - 22:00
Advice & information about HIV/AIDS & other sexual health issues.

Organizations: Sexuality

⚥ ▽ **Birmingham Bi Women's Group**

c/o Friend, P. O. Box 2405, Birmingham, West Midlands B5 4AL.
☎ 121 622 7351
⏲ Meets monthly

Birmingham

Counsellors

☺ **In Distress**
Yewcroft Mental Health Resource Centre, Court Oak Road, Harbourne, West Midlands.
☎ 121 428 3192

☺ **Pinkpot**
1 Kingston Court, Abdon Avenue, Selly Oak, West Midlands B29 4NZ.
☎ 121 476 4627

Helplines: AIDS

☺ ☐ **AIDS Lifeline**
St. Patrick's Centre for Health Promotion, Highgate Street, Birmingham, West Midlands B12 0YA.
☎ 121 235 3535

☺ ☐ **AIDSLine**
4th. Floor, Smithfield House, Digbeth, West Midlands B5 6BS.
☎ 121 622 1511

Manufacturers: Whips

☺ **Quality Control**
P. O. Box 4127, Selly Oak, West Midlands B29 4LF.
Handmade whips & bondage equipment.

Organizations: AIDS: Support

☺ ☐ **Body Positive—Birmingham**
☎ 121 212 3636
⏲ Wed 20:00 - 22:00
Advice & information about HIV/AIDS & other sexual health issues.

Organizations: BDSM

⚥ **BSG**
Suite 116, Victor Tower, Birmingham, West Midlands B7 5BW.

Organizations: Fetish: Clothing

☺ ☐ **The Events**
P.O. Box 2292, Acocks Green, West Midlands B27 7UD.
Write for details of their regular Midlands meetings.

Organizations: Motorcycle

⚥▽ **Midland Link MSC**
P.O. Box 1509, Castle Bromwich, West Midlands B36 9UD.

Organizations: Sexuality

⚥▽ **Lesbewell**
P. O. Box 4048, Moseley, West Midlands B13 8DP.
☎ 121 442 4481

Organizations: Sexuality: Student

⚥▽ **Birmingham University LGB Association**
Guild of Student, Birmingham University, Birmingham, West Midlands.
☎ 121 472 1841 Ext.: 254

Piercers

☺ **Needleworks**
☎ 121 622 6602

Stores: Books: General

☺ ■ **Book Exchange**
1014 Coventry Road, Birmingham, West Midlands B25 8DP.

☺ ■ **Midland Book Centre**
510 Stratford Road, Birmingham, West Midlands B11 4AH.

Stores: Clothing: Fetish

☺ **Cocoon**
182 High Street, Digbeth, West Midlands B12 0LD.
☎ 121 772 2800 📞 121 772 2882
⏲ Mon - Fri 10:00 - 18:00, Sat 10:00 -16:00

Stores: Clothing: Rubber

☺ ■ **Rage Fashions**
The Oasis Centre, Corporation Street, Birmingham, West Midlands B4.
☎ 121 233 4488

Stores: Clothing: Sexuality

⚤ **Transformation Ltd.**
62-64 Oxhill Road, Handsworth Wood, West Midlands B21 9RH.
☎ 121 554 2429
⏲ Mon - Sat 09:00 - 20:00
The world's leading TV specialists.

Stores: Erotica: General

⚥▼ **Clone Zone**
42 Bristol Street, Birmingham, West Midlands.
☎ 121 666 6640 📞 121 666 6640
♿ 💳 💳
Free catalogue.

Stores: Military Surplus

☺ ■ **Army Navy Stores**
214 Stratford Road, Birmingham, West Midlands B90.
☎ 121 744 5135

☺ ■ **Bordesley Army & Navy Stores**
460 Bordesley Green, Bordesley Green, West Midlands B9 5NS.
☎ 121 772 5947

☺ ■ **Q & M Stores**
633 Stratford Road, Sparkhill, West Midlands B11.
☎ 121 771 3134

☺ ■ **Q & M Stores**
1498 Pershore Road, Stirchley, West Midlands.
☎ 121 458 4614

Television: General

☺ ■ **CS4 Media Today**
University of Birmingham, Dept of Cultural Studies, Birmingham, West Midlands B15 2TT.
☎ 121 414 6060

Coventry

Helplines: Sexuality

⚥▽ **Coventry Friend**
☎ 1203 714199
⏲ 19:30 - 21:30
Advice & information about HIV/AIDS & other sexual health & sexuality issues.

☺ ▽ **West Midlands Lesbian & Gay Switchboard**
☎ 121 622 6589
⏲ 19:00 - 22:00
Advice & information about HIV/AIDS & other sexual health issues.

Organizations: AIDS: Support

☺ ☐ **The HIV Network**
12 Park Road, Coventry, West Midlands CV1 2LD.
☎ 1203 555616
Advice & information about HIV/AIDS & other sexual health issues.

Stores: Books: General

☺ **Wedge Bookshop**
13 High Street, Coventry, West Midlands.

Hockley

Stores: Erotica: General

☺ ■ **Kraze**
33 Heathcote Street, Hockley, West Midlands NG1 3AG.

Solihull

Stores: Military Surplus

☺ ■ **Army Navy Stores**
Unit 93, Inshops Chelmsly Wood Market, Solihull, West Midlands B37.
☎ 121 788 3739

Stourbridge

Organizations: AIDS: Support

☺ ☐ **Dudley HIV & AIDS Support Group**
☎ 1384 444300
⏲ Tue 19:00 - 21:00
Advice & information about HIV/AIDS & other sexual health issues.

Stores: Military Surplus

☺ ■ **Army & Navy Stores**
57 Enville Street, Stourbridge, West Midlands.
☎ 1384 395166

Walsall

Stores: Military Surplus

☺ ■ **Army & Navy Stores**
27 Stafford Street, Walsall, West Midlands.
☎ 1922 725755

Wolverhampton
Counsellors
☺ **Alan Woodhouse**
☎ 1902 331413

Organizations: AIDS: Support
☺ □ **Reach HIV Support Group**
☎ 1902 25702
🕘 Mon Wed Thu 18:00 - 20:45
Advice & information about HIV/AIDS & other sexual health issues.

WEST YORKSHIRE
Bradford
Helplines: Sexuality
☺ ▽ **Bradford Friend**
☎ 1274 723802

☺ ▽ **Bradford Gay & Lesbian Switchboard**
☎ 1274 722206
🕘 Tue Thu - Sat 19:30 - 21:30
Advice & information about HIV/AIDS & other sexual health issues.

Organizations: AIDS: Education
☺ □ **Pennine AIDS Link**
4 Duke Street, Bradford, West Yorkshire BD1 3QR.
☎ 127 439 5815

☺ □ **Yorkshire Mesmac**
c/o PAL, 4 Duke Street, Bradford, West Yorkshire BD1 3QR.
☎ 127 439 5815

Stores: Erotica: BDSM
☺ ■ **Adult Scene Supplies**
334 Leeds Road, Bradford, West Yorkshire BD3 92X.
☎ 127 472 4726

Stores: Erotica: General
☺ ■ **Scene One**
145 Manningham Lane, Bradford, West Yorkshire BD8.

Halifax
Helplines: Sexuality
☺ ▽ **Bradford Gay & Lesbian Switchboard**
☎ 1274 722206
🕘 Tue Thu - Sat 19:30 - 21:30
Advice & information about HIV/AIDS & other sexual health issues.

⚣ ▽ **Men on Men Project**
☎ 1422 366298
🕘 Mon 18:00 - 20:00
Advice & information about HIV/AIDS & other sexual health & sexuality issues.

Hebden Bridge
Stores: Books: General
☺ **Bookcase**
29 Market Street, Hebden Bridge, West Yorkshire.
☎ 1422 845353

Huddersfield
Helplines: Sexuality
⚣ ▽ **Kirklees Lesbian & Gay Switchboard**
☎ 1484 538070
🕘 Tue 19:00 - 21:00, Sun 18:00 - 21:00
Advice & information about HIV/AIDS & other sexual health & sexuality issues.

Organizations: AIDS: Education
☺ □ **Kirklees AIDS Response**
1-2 Estate Buildings, 11 Railway Street, Huddersfield, West Yorkshire HD1 1JY.
☎ 1484 432433
☎ 1484 434825 (helpline)

Leeds
Helplines: Sexuality
⚣ ▽ **Leeds Gay Switchboard**
☎ 113 245 3588
🕘 Wed - Mon 19:00 - 22:00
Advice & information about HIV/AIDS & other sexual health & sexuality issues.

⚢ ▽ **Leeds Lesbian Line**
☎ 113 245 3588
🕘 Tue 19:00 - 21:30
Advice & information about HIV/AIDS & other sexual health & sexuality issues.

Organizations: AIDS: Support
☺ □ **AIDS Advice**
50 Call Lane, Leeds, West Yorkshire.
☎ 113 242 3204

Organizations: Family
☺ □ **Leeds Parent's Friend**
VA Leeds Stringer House, 34 Lupton Street, Leeds, West Yorkshire LS10 2QW.
☎ 113 267 4627
🕘 Mon - Fri 19:30 - 23:00
Contact: Ms. Joy Dickens
Advice & information about HIV/AIDS & other sexual health & sexuality issues.

👫 □ **PASTELS**
VA Leeds Stringer House, 34 Lupton Street, Leeds, West Yorkshire LS10 2QW.
☎ 113 267 4627
🕘 Mon - Fri 19:30 - 23:00
Contact: Ms. Joy Dickens
Counselling for hetersexual partners & spouses.

Organizations: Fetish: Clothing
☺ **Northern Association of Fantasy Fetishists**
P.O. Box HP50, Leeds, West Yorkshire LS6 1TR.

Organizations: Sexuality: Student
⚣ ▽ **Leeds University Lesbian, Gay, & Bisexual Society**
LUV P.O. Box 157, Leeds, West Yorkshire LS1 1UH.

Publishers: Magazines: BDSM
☺ □ ***Unleashed***
Unlimited, P. O. Box HP 50, Leeds, West Yorkshire LS6 1TR.
🕸 http://www.ccs.neu.edu/home/pallando/BDSM/unleashed/unleashed.html
✓
Published quarterly. Yearly subscription is $72. Age statement of 18 is required.

Stores: Books: General
☺ ■ **L.U.U. Bookshop**
University of Leeds Campus, Leeds, West Yorkshire.
☎ 113 244 4974

Stores: Erotica: General
⚣ ▼ **All Points North**
Walk 34, Middleton Road, Morley, Leeds, West Yorkshire LS27 8BB.
☎ 113 238 0999

⚣ ▼ **Annares**
The Piazza, Corn Exchange, Leeds, West Yorkshire LS1 7BR.

Wakefield
Health Services
☺ □ **Claydon Hospital**
☎ 192 436 4144

WILTSHIRE
Salisbury
Helplines: Sexuality
⚣ ▽ **Salisbury Lesbian & Gay Switchboard**
☎ 1722 415051
🕘 Wed 19:00 - 22:00

Stores: Clothing: Leather
☺ ■ **JS Leather**
16 Dews Road, Salisbury, Wiltshire SP2 7SN.
☎ 1722 328588

Swindon
Helplines: Sexuality
⚣ ▽ **Thamesdown Lesbian & Gay Line**
☎ 1793 644585
🕘 Wed Fri 20:00 - 22:00
Advice & information about HIV/AIDS & other sexual health & sexuality issues.

Organizations: AIDS: Education
☺ □ **Swindon Project for AIDS Counselling & Education (SPACE)**

P.O. Box 2004, Swindon, Wiltshire SN1 3TJ.
☎ 1793 420620
🕓 Tue Thu 19:00 -21:00
Advice & information about HIV/AIDS & other sexual health issues.

Finland

Area: Approximately 337,050 square kilometres
Population: Approximately 5,030,000
Capital City: Helsinki
Currency: Markka (FM)
Official Language: Finnish & Swedish
Major Religions: 98% Protestant.
National Holiday: Independence Day, 6th. December
Time zone: GMT plus 2 hours
Country Initials: SF
Electricity: 220 volts
Country Dialing Code (from elsewhere): 358
Intl. Dialing Prefix (out of the country): 990
Long Distance Dialing Prefix (inside country): 0
Climate: In northern parts, cold, snowy winters with temperatures approximately -16°C, but summers are mild, with temperatures around 16°C. In the south west temperatures can reach 16°C in summer, but summer in the north of the country only reaches approximately 12°C.
Age of consent & homosexuality legislation: Although not in the law, the penal code permits heterosexual activity from 16, but 18 for homosexual activity. Homosexual acts were decriminalized in the 1960s. Anal intercourse has been legal for consenting adults of 18 years & older since 1988. A system of age and power between the partners has been adopted, also since 1988. In 1992, Canada abolished the restrictions of homosexuals in the military. Some refugees have been granted asylum on grounds of their sexual orientation.

NATIONAL RESOURCES

Helplines: Sexuality

⚥▽ **SETA Information Service**
Postboks 55, 00531 Helsinki, Uudenmaan Lääni.
☎ 90 135 8302 📳 90 135 8306
📧 seta@seta.fi
🌐 gopher://seta.fi
🕓 Mon Tue 12:00 - 16:00, Wed 12:00 - 18:00, Thu 12:00 - 16:00, Fri 12:00 - 14:00

Mailorder: Clothing: Fetish

☺ ■ **Decadence**
Postboks 245, 00181 Helsinki, Uudenmaan Lääni.
☎ 90 694 8898

Organizations: AIDS: Education

☺ ☐ **Finnish AIDS Council**
Postboks 106, 00161 Helsinki, Uudenmaan Lääni.
☎ 90 17 5822 📳 90 65 6806
🕓 Mon - Fri 13:00 - 21:00

Organizations: BDSM

☺ ☐ **Kinky Club**
PL 296 9, 00151 Helsinki, Uudenmaan Lääni.
🔱 ℓ
Contact: Irma
For happy perverts of all kinds. Organizes parties & special events for members. Member contacts throughout the world. Publishes a newsletter 3 times a year.

Organizations: Motorcycle

⚥▽ **MSC Finland**
🔱 Postboks 48, 00531 Helsinki, Uudenmaan Lääni.
☎ 0 680 2948
📧 msc@seta.fi
🕓 Sat 22:00 - ?
Contact: Mr. Pekka Teräsalmi, International Secretary
Club for gay men & women who are interested in leather, latex, rubber, boots, uniforms, other fetishes, & BDSM. Member of ECMC.

Organizations: Sexuality

⚥▽ **Seksuaalinen Tasavertaisuus ry (SETA)—Head**
🔱 **Office**
Postboks 55, 00531 Helsinki, Uudenmaan Lääni.
☎ 3580 135 8302 📳 3580 135 8306
☎ 3580 135 8305
📧 seta@seta.fi
🌐 gopher://seta.fi
🕓 Mon Tue 12:00 - 16:00, Wed 12:00 - 18:00, Thu 12:00 - 16:00, Fri 12:00 - 14:00
🔱 ℓ
National gay & lesbian organization. Works for human rights. Social services for individuals & others. Has AIDS support centres &

transsexuals' centres all over the country. Publishes *Z* every two months. Swedish & English also spoken.

⚥▽ **Seksuaalinen Tasavertaisuus ry (SETA)—Helsingin**
Seudun
Postboks 55, 00531 Helsinki, Uudenmaan Lääni.
☎ 3580 135 8302 📳 3580 135 8306
☎ 3580 135 8305
📧 bureau@seta.fi
🌐 gopher://seta.fi
🕓 Mon Tue 12:00 - 16:00, Wed 12:00 - 18:00, Thu 12:00 - 16:00, Fri 12:00 - 14:00
🔱 ℓ
Local Helsinki office of the national organization. Publishes *Z* every two months. Swedish & English also spoken.

▷▽ **Trasek**
Postboks 135, 00251 Helsinki, Uudenmaan Lääni.
☎ 90 241 1135 📳 90 241 1137
🕓 Mon Tue 12:00 - 16:00, Wed 12:00 - 18:00, Thu 12:00 - 16:00, Fri 12:00 - 14:00
🔱 ℓ
Information, support, & counselling. Swedish & English also spoken.

HÄMEEN LÄÄNI

Lahti

Organizations: Sexuality

⚥▽ **Seksuaalinen Tasavertaisuus ry (SETA)—Lahti**
Postboks 164, 15101 Lahti, Hämeen Lääni.
☎ 918 781 8954

Oulu

Organizations: AIDS: Support

☺ ☐ **Oulu AIDS-Tukikeskes**
Kikkokatu, 90100 Oulu, Hämeen Lääni.
☎ 98 137 9398
☎ 98 137 9458 (AIDS counselling)
🕓 Mon - Fri 09:00 - 15:00. HIV/AIDS counselling Mon - Fri 09:00 - 15:00, Tue Thu 17:00 - 19:00

Tampere

Organizations: AIDS: Support

☺ ☐ **Tampere AIDS-Tukikeskus**
Postboks 19, 33100 Tampere, Hämeen Lääni.
☎ 93 113 3307 📳 93 113 3307
☎ 93 113 3134 (Helpline)
🕓 Mon - Fri 11:00 - 18:00. Helpline Mon - Wed 15:30 - 18:30
Information & anonymous counselling & HIV testing.

Organizations: Sexuality

⚥▽ **Seksuaalinen Tasavertaisuus ry (SETA)—Tampere**
Postboks 381, 33101 Tampere, Hämeen Lääni.
☎ 93 114 8721
☎ 93 113 2969 (counselling)
🕓 Anonymous counselling Tue Fri 20:00 - 22:00. Secretary Thu 14:00 - 18:00
Written information available in Finnish, Swedish, English, & German if you send an IRC.

Stores: Erotica: General

☺ ■ **Eros**
Satamakatu 5, 33100 Tampere, Hämeen Lääni.
🕓 Mon - Fri 10:00 - 19:00, Sat 10:00 - 15:00

☺ ■ **Red Lights Sex Center**
Routatienkatu 12, 33100 Tampere, Hämeen Lääni.
🕓 Mon - Fri 10:00 - 18:00, Sat 10:00 - 14:00
Also mail order.

☺ ■ **Sex Shop**
Hämeenpuisto 12, 33100 Tampere, Hämeen Lääni.
🕓 Mon - Fri 10:00 - 18:00, Sat 10:00 - 14:00

KESKISUOMEN LÄÄNI

Jyväskylä

Helplines: Sexuality

⚥▽ **Seksuaalinen Tasavertaisuus ry (SETA)—**
Jyrässendun
☎ 941 310 0660
🕓 Wed 19:00 - 21:00

Organizations: Sexuality

⚥▽ **Seksuaalinen Tasavertaisuus ry (SETA)—**
Jyrässendun

Organizations: Sexuality

Postboks 410, 40101 Jyväskylä, Keskisuomen Lääni.
☎ 941 310 0660
🕐 Wed 19:00 - 21:00

KUOPION LÄÄNI
Kuopio
Organizations: AIDS: Support

☺ ☐ **Kuopion AIDS-Tukikeskus**
Postboks 305, 70101 Kuopio, Kuopion Lääni.
☎ 971 281 1959 ✆ 971 281 1957
🕐 Mon - Fri 09:00 - 11:00 12:00 - 15:00. 'Phone Mon - Fri 09:00 - 11:00 12:00 - 15:00, Mon Tue 17:00 - 19:00

Organizations: Sexuality

♂♀▽ **Seksuaalinen Tasavertaisuus ry (SETA)—Kuopio**
Hile ry, Postboks 213, 70101 Kuopio, Kuopion Lääni.
☎ 971 261 9566
🕐 Wed 18:00 - 20:00, Sun 15:00 - 17:00

LAPPIN LÄÄNI
Rovaniemi
Organizations: Sexuality

♂♀▽ **Seksuaalinen Tasavertaisuus ry (SETA)— Rovaniemi**
Postboks 1216, 96100 Rovaniemi, Lappin Lääni.
☎ 96 031 0141
☎ 920 651 7005 (Info line)
🕐 Fri 20:00 - ?
Info line is in Finnish.

OULUN LÄÄNI
Oulu
Organizations: Sexuality

♂♀▽ **Seksuaalinen Tasavertaisuus ry (SETA)—Oulu**
Kirkkokatu 19A15, 90100 Oulu, Oulun Lääni.
☎ 98 137 6932
🕐 Tue 19:00 - 21:00

POHJOIKARJALAN LÄÄNI
Joenssun
Organizations: Sexuality

♂♀▽ **Seksuaalinen Tasavertaisuus ry (SETA)—Joenssun**
Postboks 188, 80101 Joenssun, Pohjoikarjalan Lääni.
☎ 9 732 6033 ✆ 9 766 1325 (after 17:00)

TURUNPORIN LÄÄNI
Turku
Organizations: AIDS: Support

☺ ☐ **Turun AIDS-Tukikeskus**
Humalistonkatu 1018, 20501 Turku, Turunporin Lääni.
☎ 921 253 4746 ✆ 921 233 7963
🕐 Mon Tur 13:00 - 19:00, Wed - Fri 09:00 - 15:00

Organizations: Sexuality

♂♀▽ **Seksuaalinen Tasavertaisuus ry (SETA)—Turku**
Postboks 288, 20101 Turku, Turunporin Lääni.
☎ 921 250 0695
☎ 921 231 0335 (Helpline)
✉ haski@seta.fi
🕐 Wed 18:00 -21:00

UUDENMAAN LÄÄNI
Helsinki
Archives: Sexuality

♂♀▽ **SETA Library**
Postboks 55, 00531 Helsinki, Uudenmaan Lääni.
☎ 90 135 8302
✉ seta@seta.fi
🖳 gopher://seta.fi
🕐 Mon Tue 12:00 - 16:00, Wed 12:00 - 18:00, Thu 12:00 - 16:00, Fri 12:00 - 14:00

Bars: BDSM

♂▼ **Company Bar**
Iso Roobertinkatu 3, Helsinki, Uudenmaan Lääni.

☎ 90 64 4391
🕐 Wed Thu Sun 17:00 - 24:00, Fri Sat 18:00 - 01:00

Helplines: AIDS

☺ ☐ **AIDS Info Line**
Linnankatu 2B, Helsinki, Uudenmaan Lääni.
☎ 90 66 5081 ✆ 90 65 6806
☎ 90 17 5822
🕐 Mon - Thu 13:00 - 21:00, Fri 13:00 - 17:00, Sat 18:00 - 21:00, Sun 14:00 - 16:00
Information, counselling, support, & HIV testing.

Organizations: AIDS: Support

☺ ☐ **AIDS Centre**
Linnankatu 2B, Helsinki, Uudenmaan Lääni.
☎ 90 66 5081 ✆ 90 65 6806
☎ 90 17 5822
🕐 Mon - Thu 13:00 - 21:00, Fri 13:00 - 17:00, Sat 18:00 - 21:00, Sun 14:00 - 16:00
Information, counselling, support, & HIV testing.

☺ ☐ **Positiivi-yhdistys**
☎ 90 685 1846
🕐 Tue Thu Sat

Organizations: Sexuality

♂♀▽ **Dreamwear Club**
Postboks 159, 00251 Joensuu, Uudenmaan Lääni.
☎ 73 891396 ✆ 73 891396

♂♀▽ **Trans-tukipiste**
Postboks 135, 00251 Helsinki, Uudenmaan Lääni.
☎ 90 41 1135
☎ 90 41 1136 (helpline)
✉ ekt@seta.fi
🕐 Tue Wed 12:00 - 16:00, Thu 12:00 - 18:00, Fri 12:00 - 14:00. Helpline Sun 12:00 - 18:00. Open doors Thu 19:00 - 21:00
Help for transsexual people.

Organizations: Sexuality: Student

♂♀▽ **OHO**
5th. Floor, Mannerheimintie 5A, 00100 Helsinki, Uudenmaan Lääni.
🕐 Tue 19:00 - 21:00
Organization for sexual minorities.

Publishers: Directories: Sexuality

♂♀▼ **Queer Biz Oy**
Postboks 340, 001121 Helsinki, Uudenmaan Lääni.
☎ 0 7002 8710
Free in gay & lesbian locations.

Publishers: Miscellaneous

♂♀ **Meikänainen**
Viides Linja 14 C 73, 00530 Helsinki, Uudenmaan Lääni.
Queer publisher.

Radio: Sexuality

♂♀▽ **Radio Toinen linja**
🕐 Sun 21:00 - 21:30

♂♀▽ **Radio SETA**
🕐 Thu 17:00 - 17:30, Sat 13:00 - 13:30

Stores: Books: General

♂♀▼ **Baffin Books**
Postboks 50, Eerikinkatu 15-17, 00241 Helsinki, Uudenmaan Lääni.
☎ 90 694 7078
✉ baffin@freenet.hut.fi
🕐 Mon - Fri 10:00 - 19:00, Sat 11:00 - 17:00
The only gay, lesbian, & bisexual bookshop in Finland. Also mail order to Finland. Please address envelopes to Managing Director, do NOT address them to Baffin Books.

Stores: Clothing: Footwear

☺ **Boot Factory**
Forum Shopping Centre, Helsinki, Uudenmaan Lääni.
☎ 90 148 1525
Hand-made boots. Gay friendly.

☺ **Boot Factory**
Mäkelänkatu 62, Helsinki, Uudenmaan Lääni.
☎ 90 148 1525
Hand-made boots. Gay friendly.

Stores: Erotica: BDSM

♂♀ **Harness - Sin City**
Kalevankatu 28, Helsinki, Uudenmaan Lääni.
☎ 90 612 1513
🕐 Mon - Fri 11:00 - 18:00, Sat 10:00 - 14:00

Stores: Erotica: General

☺ ■ **Hot Love**
5 Linja 8, Helsinki, Uudenmaan Lääni.
☎ 90 773 3004
Also mail order.

⚣▼ **Mister Mosse's Boy Shop**
Iso Robertinkatu 38, Helsinki, Uudenmaan Lääni.
⏲ Mon - Fri 09:00 - 20:00, Sat 09:00 - 18:00, Sun 09:00 - 16:00

☺ ■ **RVG-Import Oy**
Pengerkatu 24, 00500 Helsinki, Uudenmaan Lääni.
☎ 90 719781
⏲ 24hr. telephone
Catalogue, FIM29.

⚣▼ **Sex 10**
Eerikinkatu 10, 00010 Helsinki, Uudenmaan Lääni.
☎ 90 60 2368

☺ ■ **Sex 42**
Iso Robertinkatu 42, Helsinki, Uudenmaan Lääni.
⏲ 09:00 - 18:00, Sat 09:00 - 14:00

Hyvinkää

Organizations: Sexuality

⚤▽ **Amigo Kerho 56**
Postboks 7, 05821 Hyvinkää, Uudenmaan Lääni.
☎ 91 453 2201
⏲ Tue 19:00 - 21:00. Meets every other Fri

Oulu

Stores: Erotica: General

☺ ■ **Sex Market**
Asemakatu 29, 90100 Oulu, Uudenmaan Lääni.

VAASAN LÄÄNI

Kokkola

Organizations: Sexuality

⚤▽ **Seksuaalinen Tasavertaisuus ry (SETA)—Kokkola**
Club Sebastian ry, Postboks 242, 67101 Kokkola, Vaasan Lääni.
☎ 96 831 0469
⏲ Thu 19:00 - 21:00

Vaasa

Stores: Erotica: General

☺ ■ **LL&SS**
Taidekustannus, PL 361, 65101 Vaasa, Vaasan Lääni.
☎ 962 42123
⏲ 24hr. telephone
All kinds of underclothing for men & women.

France

Area: Approximately 544,000 square kilometres
Population: Approximately 57,400,000
Capital City: Paris
Currency: Franc (FF)
Official Language: French
Major Religions: 77% Roman Catholic
National Holiday: Bastille Day, 14th. July
Time zone: GMT plus 1 hour
Country Initials: F
Electricity: 220 volts
Country Dialing Code (from elsewhere): 33
Intl. Dialing Prefix (out of the country): 19
Long Distance Dialing Prefix (inside country): 0
Climate: Maritime (mild winters, cool summers) in the north. More continental with cooler winter & warmer, dryer summers. Mediterranean hot summer & mild winters in the south. The coastal Riviera is sunny most of the year.
Age of consent & homosexuality legislation: Age of consent for sexual activity is 15, but it is not advisable for foreigners to become involved with anyone under 18. Homosexual acts were removed from the criminal code in 1982.

NATIONAL RESOURCES

Mailorder: Clothing: Fetish

⚣▼ **International Estetic Men (IEM)**
208 Rue Saint-Maur, 75010 Paris.
☎ 142 41 2141 — Fax 142 41 8680
Catalogue, FF50.

Mailorder: Clothing: Rubber

☺ ■ **Latex Seduction**
c/o Mme. Guerig, Boîte Postale 651, 44018 Nantes Cedex 01.

Publishers: Magazines: AIDS

☺ ■ ***Alerte***
11 bis rue du Moscou, 70558 Paris.
Published every month.

Publishers: Magazines: Erotic

⚣▼ ***All Man***
Fraction Presse SARL, 108 Avenue Gen. Michel Bizot, 75012 Paris.
☎ 144 75 7979 — Fax 144 75 3720

⚣▼ ***Espace MAN***
Fraction Presse SARL, 108 Avenue Gen. Michel Bizot, 75012 Paris.
☎ 144 75 7979 — Fax 144 75 3720
Published every month.

⚣▼ ***Gay Obscessions***
Publications Nouvelles, 49 Rue du Faubourg Poissoniere, 75009 Paris.
☎ 148 24 3955
Published every two months.

⚣▼ ***Hommes***
Editions SAN, 35 Rue de Clignancourt, 75018 Paris.
☎ 146 06 1035

⚣▼ ***Honcho***
Fraction Presse SARL, 108 Avenue Gen. Michel Bizot, 75012 Paris.
☎ 144 75 7979 — Fax 144 75 3720
Published every two months.

⚣▼ ***Jean Paul***
Editions SAN, 35 Rue de Clignancourt, 75018 Paris.
☎ 146 06 1035

Publishers: Magazines: Sexuality

⚤▼ **Adonis Atlantic Presse Editions**
Boîte Postale 7110, 44030 Nantes Cedex 04.

⚤▼ ***Double Face***
64 Rue Rambuteau, 75003 Paris.
☎ 128 04 5800 — Fax 148 04 0592
Free at gay locations. Published every month.

⚤▼ ***Journal Gaie Presence***
Boîte Postale 181, 75564 Paris Cedex 12.

Publishers: Newspapers: Sexuality

⚤▼ ***Exit***
75 Rue des Archives, 75004 Paris.
☎ 140 05 9402 — Fax 140 05 9642
Free at gay locations. Published every month.

⚤▼ ***Illico***
64 Rue Rambuteau, 75003 Paris.
☎ 128 04 5800 — Fax 148 04 0592
Free at gay locations. Published every month.

Aix-en-Provence

Health Services

☺ □ **Centre de Santé**
3 Avenue Paul Cézanne, 13100 Aix-en-Provence.
☎ 42 23 3519

Alençon

Health Services

☺ □ **Centre Hospitalier d'Alençon**
25 Rue Fresnaiz, 61000 Alençon.
☎ 33 32 3049
HIV testing.

Radio: Sexuality

⚤▽ ***Gaiement Vôtre***
⏲ Sun 21:00

Amiens

Health Services

☺ ■ **Centre Hospitalier d'Amiens**
Service Dermato-Vénérologie, Boîte Postale 5707, 80480 Saleux.
☎ 22 89 0222
HIV testing.

☺ □ **Centre Médico-Social**
16bis Rue Fernel, 80000 Amiens.
☎ 22 91 0770

☺ □ **Services Départmental de Vénérologie**
3 Boulevard Guyencourt, 80000 Amiens.

☎ 22 89 4630

Radio: Sexuality

⚢▽ ***Homophonies***

Angers

Counsellors

☺ ■ **J. P. Chiron**
36 Rue Florent-Cornilleau, 49000 Angers.
☎ 41 60 3876

Health Services

☺ □ **Centre Hospitalier d'Angers**
Service Consultations Externe, 1 Avenue de l'Hôtel Dieu, 49033 Angers.
☎ 41 35 3419
HIV testing.

Organizations: AIDS: Support

☺ □ **AIDES Anjou**
Boîte Postale 2321, 49023 Angers Cedex 02.
☎ 41 87 1144
🕘 Mon - Fri 17:00 - 19:00, 2nd. & 4th. Sat of month 14:30 - 17:00

Radio: Sexuality

⚢▽ ***Radio Gribouille***
FM 99.7, 160 Avenue Pasteur, 49000 Angers.
🕘 Mon 22:00 - 24:00

Annecy

Health Services

☺ ■ **Centre Hospitalier**
Avenue du Trésum, 74000 Annecy.
☎ 50 45 1649

Antibes

Stores: Erotica: General

☺ ■ **Eroshop**
6 Rue Vaubon, 69480 Antibes.
☎ 93 34 09 04
🕘 Mon - Sat 09:00 - 23:00

Argenteuil

Health Services

☺ □ **Centre Hospitalier**
Consultations Externes, 69 rue du Lieutenant Prudhon, 95100 Argenteuil.
☎ 34 23 2620
Confidential, free HIV testing.

Auxerre

Health Services

☺ ■ **Centre Hospitalier d'Auxerre**
Boîte Postale 5164, Résidence Saint Germain, 89000 Auxerre.
☎ 86 48 4718
HIV testing.

Beauvais

Health Services

☺ ■ **Centre Hospitalier de Belfort**
28 Avenue Jean-Jaurès, 90000 Beauvais.
☎ 84 28 1712
HIV testing.

Radio: Sexuality

⚢▽ ***Croque Monsieur***
🕘 Mon 21:30

Besançon

Organizations: AIDS: Support

☺ ■ **AIDES France-Comté**
15 Rue Petit Battant, 25000 Besançon.
☎ 81 81 8000
🕘 14:00 - 18:00
HIV testing.

Organizations: Body Size

⚢▽ **Girth & Mirth—Alpes-Jura**
Boîte Postale 972, 25022 Besançon Cedex.
☎ 16 81 880618

Béziers

Health Services

☺ ■ **Dispensaire Anti-Vénérien**
2 Boulevard Pérréal, 34500 Béziers.
☎ 67 76 9080
STD information & treatment.

Radio: Sexuality

⚢▽ ***Tendences Gaies***

Biarritz

Radio: Sexuality

⚢▽ ***Triangle Rose***
🕘 Tue Sat 20:00

Blanquefort

Helplines: Sexuality

⚢▽ **Vivre Autrement en Aquitaine**
Boîte Postale 66, 33290 Blanquefort.
☎ 56 81 8062
🕘 Mon - Fri 19:00 - 20:00

Bordeaux

Health Services

☺ ■ **Centre Hospitalier**
☎ 56 98 4607
HIV & STD testing.

☺ ■ **Centre Hospitalier de Charleville**
☎ 24 56 7070
HIV testing.

☺ ■ **Hôpital Pellegrin**
Plave Amélie-Raba-Léon, 33000 Bordeaux.
☎ 56 98 4607
HIV testing.

☺ ■ **Hôpital Saint-André**
86 Cours d'Albret, 33000 Bordeaux.
☎ 56 91 4424
STD prevention information & services.

Helplines: Sexuality

⚢▽ **ALLOGAY**
☎ Minitel 3615 ALLOGAY

Organizations: AIDS: Support

☺ ■ **AIDES Aquitaine**
Boîte Postale 18, 33037 Bordeaux Cedex.
☎ 56 52 7761
🕘 Mon - Fri 15:00 - 19:00, Tue Thu 15:00 - 23:00
Information & counselling about HIV/AIDS.

Organizations: Sexuality

⚢▽ **For'Hommes**
♿ Boîte Postale 194, 33000 Bordeaux Cedex.
☎ 56 50 6300
🕘 17:00 - 19:30
✓
Group living out their homosexuality quietly in their city. Involved with HIV/AIDS prevention. Publishes *For'Hommes* every two months. Age statement of 18 is required. English & Spanish also spoken.

Radio: Sexuality

⚢▽ ***Emission Homophobie***
Fréquence 4 FM 99.6, Boîte Postale 36, 33015 Bordeaux Cedex.
🕘 Wed 21:00 - 23:30

Stores: Books: General

☺ ■ **Librairie d'Albret**
52 Cours d'Albret, 33000 Bordeaux.
☎ 56 52 2929
🕘 06:30 - 19:30, Sun 07:30 - 12:00

Stores: Erotica: General

⚢▼ **Boîte à Films**
26 Rue Rolland, 33000 Bordeaux.
☎ 56 44 8221
🕘 10:00 - 01:00

Boulogne-sur-Mer

Health Services

☺ ■ **Centre Médico-Social**
1 Place Navarin, 62200 Boulogne-sur-Mer.

☎ 21 31 5656
HIV testing.

Brest

Health Services

☺ ■ **Centre Hospitalier de Brest**
☎ 98 22 3333
HIV testing.

Organizations: AIDS: Support

☺ ■ **AIDES Armor**
1 Rue de l'Harteloire, 29200 Brest.
☎ 98 43 1872
🕒 Mon 19:30 - 22:30

Caen

Health Services

☺ ■ **Centre de Prophylaxie et MST**
3 Rue des Cultures, 14000 Caen.
☎ 31 94 8422
HIV testing.

Organizations: AIDS: Support

☺ ■ **AIDES Basse-Normandie**
2 Ruede Marais, 14000 Caen.
☎ 31 84 3663
🕒 Mon -Fri 14:00 - 17:00

Radio: Sexuality

⚦▽ ***Abus de Confiance***
🕒 1st Sun of month 16:00

Cahors

Health Services

☺ ■ **Centre Hospitalier de Cahors**
Service de Médcine Interne, Rue Président Wilson, 46000 Cahors.
☎ 65 20 5050
HIV testing.

Cannes

Health Services

☺ ■ **Centre Médical**
74 Avenue Clémenceau, 06400 Cannes.
☎ 93 39 0636

Carcassone

Health Services

☺ ■ **Hôpital**
57 Rue d'Alsace, 11000 Carcassone.
☎ 68 25 7976

Châlons

Organizations: AIDS: Support

☺ ■ **AIDES Champagne-Ardennes**
Boîte Postale 135, 51008 Châlons.
☎ 26 66 8434

Chambéry

Health Services

☺ ■ **Centre Hospitalier de Chambéry**
☎ 79 96 5050
HIV testing.

Organizations: AIDS: Support

☺ ■ **AIDES Dauphiné-Savoie**
300 Chemin des Moulins, 73000 Chambéry.
☎ 79 85 5034
🕒 Thu 19:00 - 22:30

Cherbourg

Health Services

☺ ■ **Centre Hospitalier Louis Pasteur**
Service de Dermatologie, 46 Rue du Val-de-Seine, 50100 Cherbourg.
☎ 33 20 7000
HIV testing.

Clermont-Ferrand

Organizations: AIDS: Support

☺ ■ **AIDES Auvergne**
Boîte Postale 502, 63000 Clermont-Ferrand Cedex.
☎ 73 31 3103
🕒 Mon - Fri 009:30 - 12:00
Support & information about HIV/AIDS.

Corse

Health Services

☺ ■ **Centre Hospitalier Général Faconaja**
Route Impériale, 20200 Bastia.
☎ 95 55 1111
HIV testing.

☺ ■ **Centre Hospitalier Notre Dame de la Misericorde**
27 Avenue de l'Impératrice Eugénie, Ajaccio.
Anonymous HIV testing.

Courcouronnes

Organizations: Fetish: Clothing: Stockings

👫 □ **Nylon Club**
Rue de la Boisée, 91080 Courcouronnes.
☎ 164 97 0506

Créteil

Health Services

☺ ■ **Centre Hospitalier Intercommunal**
Service Médecine Interne, 40 Avenue de Verdun, 94000 Créteil.
☎ 48 98 7758
HIV testing.

Organizations: AIDS: Support

☺ ■ **Hôpital Henri Mondor**
Maladies Infecieuses, 551 Avenue de Maréchal de Lattre de Tassigny, 94010 Créteil.
☎ 49 81 2295
Support, information, & counselling for people infected with or affected by HIV/AIDS.

Dammarie les Lys

Organizations: Fetish: Clothing: Rubber

⚦▽ **Mecs en Caoutchouc**
Boîte Postale 77191, Dammarie les Lys Cedex.

Didenheim

Organizations: Sexuality

🦋▽ **Association Beaumont Continental (ABC)**
Boîte Postale 3, 68350 Didenheim.

Stores: Clothing: Fetish

☺ ■ **SCL «O» Fashion**
5 Rue des Vosges, 68200 Didenheim.
☎ 89 06 1040

Dijon

Organizations: AIDS: Support

☺ □ **AIDES Bourgogne**
Boîte Postale 408, 21101 Dijon Cedex.
☎ 80 30 3777
🕒 Mon - Fri 09:00 - 11:30

Stores: Erotica: General

⚦▼ **Librairie Erotique**
64 Rue Berbisey, 21000 Dijon.
☎ 80 30 7409
🕒 Mon - Fri 10:00 - 24:00, Sat 10:00 - 20:00

Dunkerque

Health Services

☺ ■ **Centre de Prophylaxie des MST**
4 Rue Monseigneur Marquis, 59240 Dunkerque.
☎ 28 24 0400
STD & HIV testing.

Epinal

Health Services

☺ ■ **Centre Hospitalier d'Epinal**
Consultations de Médecine Interne, Boîte Postale 3353, 88000 Epinal.
☎ 29 31 3131
HIV testing.

Gap

Health Services

☺ ■ **AIDES Provence**

24 Rue Saint Arey, 05000 Gap.
☎ 92 53 4393
⌚ 1st. Tue of the month 14:00 - 16:00

☺ ■ **Centre Hospitalier de Gap**
Service de Médecine, Boîte Postale 6284, 05000 Gap.
☎ 92 40 6161
HIV testing.

Grenoble

Health Services

☺ ■ **Centre Hospitalier de Grenoble**
Département de Santé, 23 Avenue Albert 1er. de Belgique, 38000 Grenoble.
☎ 76 87 6240
HIV testing.

Helplines: Sexuality

⚦▽ **ALLOGAY**
☎ Minitel 3615 ALLOGAY

Organizations: AIDS: Support

☺ ■ **AIDES Dauphiné-Savoie**
Boîte Postale 381, 38015 Grenoble Cedex.
☎ 76 46 0758
⌚ Mon Wed 19:30 - 22:00
Support & HIV/AIDS information.

Stores: Clothing: Fetish

☺ ■ **Planet Alice**
4 Rue Diodore Raoult, 38000 Grenoble.
☎ 76 42 7032

Stores: Erotica: General

⚦▼ **Sexashop**
2 Rue de Miribel, 38000 Grenoble.
☎ 76 46 7086
⌚ 09:00 - 22:00

Guéret

Health Services

☺ ■ **Centre Hospitalier de Guéret**
Service de Médecine, 39 Avenue de la Sénatorerie, 23011 Guéret.
☎ 55 51 7000
HIV testing.

Issy Les Moulineaux

Health Services

☺ ■ **Hôpital Corantins-Celton**
37 Boulevard Gambetta, 92130 Issy Les Moulineaux.
☎ 45 54 9533

Publishers: Books: Fetish

Editions Vents d'Ouest
31/33 Rue Ernest Renan, 92130 Issy Les Moulineaux.

La Rochelle

Health Services

☺ ■ **Centre Hospitalier de la Rochelle**
Service Médecine Interne, Boîte Postale 3849, 17019 La Rochelle Cedex.
☎ 46 27 3333
HIV testing.

Laval

Health Services

☺ ■ **Centre Hospitalier de Laval**
Service de Médecine Interne, Boîte Postale 4280, 53024 Laval Cedex.
☎ 43 66 5000
HIV testing.

Le Mans

Stores: Erotica: General

☺ ■ **Sex Shop**
72 Rue Bourg Bélé, 72000 Le Mans.
☎ 43 28 5139
⌚ 10:00 - 22:00

☺ ■ **Vénus**
36 Rue des Ponts, 72000 Le Mans.
☎ 43 23 0615
⌚ Mon - Thu Sat 16:30 - 22:30, Fri 16:30 - 23:30
VISA MC

Lille

Health Services

☺ ■ **Centre de Prophylaxie**
26 Rue d'Inhermann, 59000 Lille.
☎ 20 54 5773
HIV testing.

Helplines: Sexuality

⚦▽ **ALLOGAY**
☎ Minitel 3615 ALLOGAY

Organizations: AIDS: Support

☺ ■ **AIDES Nord-Pas-de-Calais**
Boîte Postale 106, 59000 Lille Cedex.
☎ 20 06 5959

Organizations: Sexuality

⚦▽ **Les Flamands Roses**
1-2 Rue Denis-du-Péage, 59000 Lille.
☎ 20 47 6265
⌚ Meets Tue 20:00

⚦▽ **Groupe Homo pour l'Expression des Minorités (GHEM)**
Boîte Postale 1277, 59000 Lille.
☎ 20 52 1884
⌚ Wed - Sun 21:00 - 24:00

Radio: Sexuality

⚦▽ ***Radio Bigoudi***
⌚ Sun 21:00 - 22:00

Stores: Erotica: General

⚦▼ **Golden Boy**
33 Rue des Ponts-de-Comines, 59000 Lille.
☎ 20 06 3426
⌚ Mon - Sat 10:00 - 23:00
VISA MC

☺ ■ **Sex Center**
56 Rue Esquermoise, 59000 Lille.
☎ 20 51 0891
⌚ 10:00 - 24:00
VISA MC

Limoges

Health Services

☺ ■ **Centre Hospitalier R. U. Dupuytren**
☎ 55 06 6652
HIV testing.

Organizations: AIDS: Support

☺ ■ **AIDES Limousin**
Boîte Postale 118, 87003 Limoges Cedex.
☎ 55 06 1819

Lyon

Health Services

☺ ■ **Hôpital Edouard Herriot**
Pavillon P, 5 Place d'Arsonval, 690008 Lyon.
☎ 72 34 4689
Free HIV testing.

☺ ■ **Hôtel Dieu**
71 Quai Jules Courmont, 69002 Lyon.
☎ 78 42 2926
☎ 78 92 2016
Free HIV testing.

☺ ■ **Médecins du Monde**
10 Rue Sévigné, 69003 Lyon.
☎ 78 60 2384
Free HIV testing.

Helplines: Sexuality

⚦▽ **Acceuil Rencontre Information Service (ARIS)**
Boîte Postale , 69203 Lyon Cedex 01.
☎ 78 27 1010
⌚ Mon Tue Thu 19:00 - 21:00, Fri 19:00 - 22:00, Wed 17:00 - 19:00 (parents / gay children) 19:00 - 21:00 (women only)
✓
Regional helpline.

⚦▽ **ALLOGAY**
☎ Minitel 3615 ALLOGAY

Organizations: AIDS: Education

☺ ■ **Association de Lutte Contre le SIDA**
16 Rue Pizay, 69000 Lyon.
☎ 78 27 8080
⏲ Wed 20:30 - 22:30, otherwise 14:00 - 18:00

Organizations: BDSM

⚥▽ **MSC Rhône-Alpes (MCRA)**
Boîte Postale 3010, 69394 Lyon Cedex 03.
☎ 72 33 0339

Organizations: Sexuality

⚥▽ **Acceuil Rencontre Information Service (ARIS)**
Boîte Postale 1125, 69203 Lyon Cedex 01.
☎ 78 27 1010
⏲ Mon Tue Thu 19:00 - 21:00, Fri 19:00 - 22:00, Wed 17:00 - 19:00 (parents / gay children) 19:00 - 21:00 (women only), dance (all sexes) 1st. Sat of month (21:00 - 01:00)
✓
Contact: Mme. Béatrice Bouillaut
Regional organization. Age statement of 18 is required.

Stores: Clothing: Leather

☺ ▼ **Tom's Boutic**
♿ 1 Rue Terme, 69001 Lyon.
☎ 78 30 1984
⏲ 11:00 - 19:00
✓ $ VISA MC ¢
Handcrafted original leather creations. Handmade clothes. Gays welcome. English also spoken.

Marseille

Helplines: Sexuality

⚥▽ **ALLOGAY**
☎ Minitel 3615 ALLOGAY

Organizations: AIDS: Support

☺ ■ **AIDES Marseille**
61 Rue Saint Ferreol, 13000 Marseille.
☎ 93 33 5401

Organizations: BDSM

⚥▼ **Club Cuir ESMC**
28 Rue Mazagran, 13005 Marseille Cedex.
☎ 91 48 4934
⏲ Fri Sat 23:00 - ?
Attendance requires an introduction.

Organizations: Masturbation

⚥▽ **Santé & Plaisir Gai (SPG)—Marseille**
Boîte Postale 203, 75921 Paris Cedex 19.
☎ 142 72 7386
Write to the Paris location for information.

Organizations: Motorcycle

⚥▽ **FSMC**
1528 Rue Mazagran, 13001 Marseille.

Publishers: Magazines: Sexuality

⚥▼ ***Ibiza***
Association Ibiza, 22 Rue Léon Bourgeois, 13001 Marseille.
☎ 91 50 5012 — Fax 91 84 6493
Available at gay & lesbian locations. Published 8 times a year.

Stores: Erotica: BDSM

⚥▼ **Boy's Cuir Leather Shop**
Boîte Postale 33, 13005 Marseille Cedex .
⏲ Tue - Sat 15:00 - 20:00
Also mail order.

Stores: Erotica: General

⚥▼ **Sexashop**
6, Rue Corneille, 13001 Marseille.
☎ 91 33 7191
⏲ 09:30 - 24:00
Also mail order.

Meaux

Health Services

☺ □ **Centre Hospitalier**
68 rue Saint Fiacre, 77108 Meaux.
☎ 64 35 3838
Confidential, free HIV testing.

☺ ■ **Centre Hospitalier Général**
6/8 Rue Saint Pierre, 77100 Meaux.
☎ 64 33 4935
HIV testing.

Metz

Health Services

☺ ■ **Centre Hospitalier Beausecours**
Service de Dermatologie, 1 Place Philippe de Vigneulles, 57038 Metz.
☎ 87 63 1313
HIV testing.

Organizations: AIDS: Support

☺ ■ **AIDES Lorraine-Nord**
Boîte Postale 4126, 57040 Metz Cedex 01.
☎ 87 36 89 63
⏲ Tue 20:00 - 22:00

Mons

Photographers: Erotic

☺ **Robert Chouraqui**
5 Impasse Le Stradic, 91200 Athis.
☎ 16 048 0917 — Fax 14 678 0791
Fashion & nude photographer, famous for his "Betty Bleu" photographs.

Montpellier

Bars: BDSM

⚥▼ **Le Block**
32 Rue du Plan de l'Olivier, 34000 Montpellier.
⏲ 19:00 - 02:00

Health Services

☺ ■ **Centre Hospitalier de Montpellier**
555 Route de Ganges, 34059 Montpellier Cedex.
☎ 67 33 9302

☺ ■ **Hôpital Saint Charles**
Consultations des MST, Rue Auguste Broussonet, 34000 Montpellier.
☎ 67 33 6490
STD & HIV testing.

Helplines: Sexuality

⚥▽ **ALLOGAY**
☎ Minitel 3615 ALLOGAY

Organizations: AIDS: Support

☺ ■ **AIDES Monpellier Languedoc Mediterannée**
Boîte Postale 9213, 34043 Montpellier Cedex 01.
☎ 67 72 6303
⏲ Tue Fri 20:30 - 23:00

Publishers: Magazines: Sexuality

⚥▼ ***Midi Gai Loisirs***
8 Rue Levant, 34000 Montpellier.
☎ 67 58 6142
Irregular free publication.

Stores: Erotica: General

☺ ■ **L'Arc en Ciel**
6bis Rue Cope Cambes, 34000 Montpellier.
☎ 67 60 6461
⏲ 10:00 - 20:00

Montréal La Cluse

Piercers

☺ ■ **Olivier Rocquet**
5 Montée Du Grapillon, 01460 Montréal La Cluse.

Mulhouse

Health Services

☺ ■ **Centre de Dépistage**
Hôpital de Moenchsberg, Rue de Dr. R. Laennée, 68100 Mulhouse.
☎ 89 54 9033
⏲ Mon 10:00 - 13:00, Tue 16:00 - 19:00, Wed 15:00 - 18:00
Free anonymous HIV testing.

☺ ■ **Centre Hospitalier E. Muller**
☎ 89 64 6464
HIV testing.

Organizations: AIDS: Support

☺ ■ **AIDES Alsace**
44 Rue des Fabriques, 68100 Mulhouse.
☎ 89 60 0077

Nancy
Health Services
☺ ■ **AIDES Lorraine-Sud**
67 Avenue Foche, 54000 Nancy.
☎ 83 27 9171
🕘 Mon - Fri 09:00 - 12:00 14:00 - 17:00, Sat 17:00 - 19:00

☺ ■ **Centre Hospitalier de Nancy**
29 Rue du Maréchal de Lattre de Tassigny, 54037 Nancy.
☎ 83 57 6161

Helplines: Sexuality
⚢▽ **ALLOGAY**
☎ Minitel 3615 ALLOGAY

Organizations: Sexuality
⚢▽ **Gai Amitié Initiative (GAI)**
Boîte Postale 258, 54005 Nancy Cedex.
🕘 Fri 18:00 - 19:00

Nantes
Health Services
☺ ■ **AIDES Atlantique**
13 Rue de la Tchécoslovaquie, 44000 Nantes.
☎ 40 47 9956
🕘 Mon - Fri 09:00 - 12:00, Mon Tue Thu 14:00 - 18:00, Wed 14:00 - 23:00

☺ ■ **Centre Hospitalier de Nantes**
Place Alexie Ricardeau, 44035 Nantes Cedex 01.
☎ 40 48 3333
HIV testing.

Helplines: Sexuality
⚢▽ **ALLOGAY**
☎ Minitel 3615 ALLOGAY

Organizations: AIDS: Support
☺ ■ **Amitié SIDA**
21 Rue Dufour, 44000 Nantes.
☎ 40 29 1228
Support & information for people infected with or affected by HIV/AIDS.

Organizations: Sexuality
⚢▽ **Homosaïque**
Boîte Postale 358, 44012 Nantes Cedex.
🕘 Tue 18:00 - 19:00. Meets 1st Fri of month

Nice
Helplines: Sexuality
⚢▽ **ALLOGAY**
☎ Minitel 3615 ALLOGAY

Organizations: AIDS: Support
☺ ■ **AIDES Côte d'Azur**
Boîte Postale 24, 06021 Nice Cedex.
☎ 93 56 9338

Nîmes
Health Services
☺ ■ **Centre Hospitalier Regional**
Centre Gaston Doumergues, 30000 Nîmes.
☎ 66 27 4111
HIV testing.

Organizations: AIDS: Support
☺ ■ **AIDES Languedoc-Nord**
Boîte Postale 183, 30012 Nîmes Cedex.
☎ 66 76 2607
🕘 Mon 18:00 - 20:00, Wed 18:00 - 22:00

☺ ■ **CHRU de Nîmes**
☎ 66 27 3175
Information, support, & counselling about HIV/AIDS.

Orléans
Health Services
☺ ■ **Centre Hospitalier Orléans-la-Source**
Service Maladies Infectieuses, Avenue de l'Hôpital, 45100 Orléans.
☎ 38 51 4361
HIV testing.

Organizations: AIDS: Support
☺ ■ **AIDES Orléans Region Centre**
Boîte Postale 2147, 45011 Orléans Cedex 1.
☎ 38 53 3031

Organizations: Sexuality
⚢▽ **Groupe Action Gai**
46 Rue Sainte Catherine, 45000 Orléans.

Palaiseau
Organizations: AIDS: Support
☺ ■ **Paips Essonne**
7 Avenue du 8-Mai, 91120 Palaiseau.
☎ 42 61 1522
Information & support for people infected with & affected by HIV/AIDS.

Paris
Archives: Sexuality
⚢▽ **Archives Recherches & Cultures Lesbiennes**
Boîte Postale 362, 75526 Paris.
☎ 148 05 2589
🕘 Fri 19:00 - 22:00
Library, museum, & video & sound archive.

Bars: BDSM
⚣▼ **Café Moustache**
138 Rue du Faubourg-Saint-Martin, 75010 Paris.
☎ 146 07 7207
🕘 18:00 - 02:00

⚣▼ **Docks**
150 Rue Saint-Maur, 75011 Paris.
☎ 143 57 3382

⚣▼ **Keller's**
14 Rue Keller, 75011 Paris.
☎ 143 55 1152
🕘 22:00 - 02:00
VISA MC
Strict leather & levi dress code.

⚣ **Le Manhattan**
8 Rue des Anglais, 75005 Paris.
☎ 143 54 9886
🕘 Wed - Sun 23:00 - ?
VISA MC AMERICAN EXPRESS
Cover charge on Fri & Sat.

⚣▼ **Mec Zone**
27 Rue Turgot, 75009 Paris.
☎ 140 82 9418
🕘 18:00 - 02:00
VISA MC
Strict dress code of leather & Levis.

⚣▼ **Le Mic-Man**
24 Rue Geoffrey-L'Angeuin, 75004 Paris.
☎ 142 74 3980
🕘 14:00 - 02:00, Sat Sun Holidays - 04:00
VISA MC

⚣▼ **One Way**
28 Rue Charlot, 75003 Paris.
☎ 148 87 4610
🕘 17:00 - 02:00

⚣▼ **QG**
12 Rue Simon Le Franc, 75004 Paris.
☎ 148 87 7418
🕘 12:00 - 02:00

⚣▼ **Stratègie**
170 Rue de la Convention, 75015 Paris.
☎ 145 32 1820
🕘 Tue - Sat 10:00 - 13:00 14:00 - 19:00

⚣▼ **Le Transfert**
3 Rue de laSourdière, 75001 Paris.
☎ 142 60 4842
🕘 23:00 - 05:00
VISA MC

⚣▼ **Le Trap**
10 Rue Jacob, 75006 Paris.
☎ 143 54 5353
🕘 23:00 - 04:00

Health Services
☺ □ **Centre Figuier**
2 Rue du Figuier, 75004 Paris.
☎ 142 78 5573
Confidential, free HIV testing.

☺ ■ **Centre Médico-Social**

Centre de Dépistage, 218 Rue de Belleville, 75020 Paris.
☎ 147 97 4049
🕘 Mon -Thu 17:00 - 20:00, 10:00 - 13:00
Confidential, free HIV & STD testing & treatment.

☺ □ **Centre Médico-Social**
3-5 rue Ridder, 75014 Paris.
☎ 145 43 8378
Confidential, free HIV testing.

☺ □ **Hôpital Antoine Beclere**
SOS SIDA, 157 Rue de la Porte de Triveaux, 92410 Paris.
☎ 145 37 4444 — Fax 145 37 4840
HIV testing.

☺ ■ **Hôpital Boucicaut**
78 Rue de la Convention, 75015 Paris.
☎ 145 54 9292

☺ □ **Hôpital de la Fontaine**
2 Rue de la Fontaine, 93200 Paris.
☎ 142 35 6808

☺ □ **Hôpital Lariboisère**
2 Rue Ambroise-Paré, 75010 Paris.
☎ 149 95 6565 Ext.: 2120
Confidential, free HIV testing.

☺ ■ **Hôpital Saint Antoine**
184 Rue du Faubourg Saint Antoine, 75012 Paris.
☎ 143 44 3333

☺ ■ **Hôpital Saint Louis**
40 Rue Bichot, 75010 Paris.
☎ 142 49 9924

☺ ■ **Hôpital Tarnier**
89 Rue d'Assas, 75006 Paris.
☎ 143 29 1289

☺ ■ **Institut Prophylactique**
36 Rue d'Assas, 75007 Paris.
☎ 145 55 3894

☺ □ **Pitié-Salpêtrière**
Médecine Interne, 47 boulevard de l'Hôpital, 75013 Paris.
☎ 145 70 2172
☎ 145 70 2173
Confidential, free HIV testing.

Helplines: AIDS

☺ ■ **AIDES Paris & Ile de France**
☎ Minitel 3615 AIDES

⚢▽ **Ecoute Gai**
190 Boulevard de Charonne, 75020 Paris.
☎ 144 93 0102
🕘 Mon - Fri 18:00 - 22:00
Confidential support.

Helplines: Sexuality

⚢▽ **ALLOGAY**
☎ Minitel 3615 ALLOGAY

⚢▽ **Infoline**
☎ 136 65 5678
Information recording.

Organizations: AIDS: Education

☺ ■ **Association des Artistes Contre le SIDA**
5 Rue du Bois de Boulogne, 75116 Paris.
☎ 145 00 5353

☺ □ **Association pour la Recherche Clinique sur le SIDA & sa Thérapie (ARCAT)**
13 boulevard Rochechuart, 75009 Paris.
☎ 149 70 8590
Fundraising for HIV/AIDS research & support. Publishes *SIDA*.

☺ ■ **Combattre le SIDA**
11 Rue du Général Cordonnuer, 92200 Neuilly sur Seine.
☎ 146 40 0303
🕘 Mon - Fri 09:00 - 19:00

☺ ■ **Vaincre le SIDA (VLS)**
41 rue Volta, 75003 Paris.
☎ 144 78 7550
☎ 144 78 7552
🕘 Wed - Sun 20:00 - 22:00

Organizations: AIDS: Information

☺ ■ **Centre Regional d'Information & de Prévention du SIDA (CRIPS)**
192 rue Lecourbe, 75015 Paris.
☎ 53 68 8888 — Fax 53 68 8889
🕘 Tue - Fri 13:00 - 20:00, Sat 10:00 - 17:00
Information, counselling, support for people infected with or affected by HIV/AIDS.

Organizations: AIDS: Support

☺ ■ **Actions Prévention SIDA & Aide aux Malades (APSAM - GPL)**
Boîte Postale 451, 75840 Paris Cedex 17.

☺ ■ **AIDES Pairs & Ile de France**
247 Rue de Belleville, 75019 Paris.
☎ 144 52 0000 — Fax 144 52 0201

☺ ■ **Banque de Sang Cochin**
☎ 143 29 8385
🕘 Tue Fri 17:00 - 19:00
Counselling & information about HIV/AIDS.

☺ ■ **Hôpital Antoine Beclere**
SOS SIDA, 157 Rue de la Porte de Triveaux, 92410 Clamart.
☎ 145 37 4444 — Fax 145 37 4840

Organizations: BDSM

⚢▽ **ASMF Paris**
Boîte Postale 2, 75965 Paris Cedex 20.

☺ ■ **Les Chandelles**
1 Rue Thérèse, 75001 Paris.
Swingers club that puts on periodc BDSM events.

⚢▽ **Clan Masters**
CM Boîte Postale 58, 75622 Paris Cedex 13.

Organizations: Bears

⚢▽ **Les Gais Nounours**
Boîte Postale 275-16, 75766 Paris Cedex 16.
Contact: M. Vincent de LaCroix

Organizations: Body Size

⚢▽ **Girth & Mirth—France**
Boîte Postale 275-16, 75766 Paris Cedex 16.
☎ 19 47 2745
Contact: M. V. de Lacroix

Organizations: Family

⚢▽ **Association des Parents & Futures Parents Gais (APG)**
Boîte Postale 253, 75866 Paris.
☎ 147 36 0487
🕘 Call Sat 16:00 - 19:00

☺ ▽ **Contact**
☎ 64 03 9794
☎ 38 85 6052
🕘 1st. number: Mon Thu 20:00 - 22:00; 2nd. number Fri 21:00 - 23:00
For parents of gays & lesbians.

Organizations: Motorcycle

⚢▽ **Gai Moto Club**
Boîte Postale 203, 75927 Paris Cedex 19.

Organizations: Sexuality

⚢▽ **Centre Gai & Lesbien (CGL)**
3 Rue Keller, 75011 Paris.
☎ 143 57 2147
🕘 14:00 - 20:00

⚢▽ **Partages**
Boîte Postale 122, 75023 Paris Cedex 01.
Support & information.

⚢▽ **Point Gai**
33 Rue Jules Charpentier, 37000 Paris.
☎ 47 20 5530
🕘 Thu 18:00 - 20:00

Organizations: Sexuality: Student

⚢▽ **Gage**
c/o Les Mots à la Bouche, 6 Rue Sainte Croix de la Bretonnerie, 75004 Paris.
☎ 146 03 2012

Organizations: Sexuality: Youth

⚢▽ **Jeunes & Etudiant(e)s Homosexuel(le)s de Tour (JEHT)**
Boîte Postale , 33 Rue Jules Charpentier, 37000 Paris.
☎ 47 20 5530
🕘 Tue 20:00 - 22:00

⚢▽ **MAG Jeunes Gais**
Boîte Postale 48, 75521 Paris Cedex 11.
☎ 143 70 5009 — Fax 148 07 8018

Organizations: Sexuality: Youth

🌐 http://fglb.qrd.org:8080/fqrd/assocs/mag/mag1.mtml
Contact: M. François Vauglin, Président

☺▽ **Maison des Homosexualités**
25 Rue Michel le Comte, 75003 Paris.
☎ 142 77 7277

Photographers: Erotic

☺ **Claude Alexandre**
24 Boulevard Beaumarchais, 75011 Paris.
☎ 143 38 7482

☺ **Gilles Berquet**
c/o Alexandre Dupouy, 58 Rue Amelot, 75011 Paris.
☎ 143 38 3343 📠 143 38 0995
M. Dupouy is M. Berquet's agent.

☺ **J. L. Del Valle**
69 rue der la Tombe-Issoire, 75014 Paris.
☎ 143 21 8487

☺ **Kelvin Kert**
77 Avenue Simon Bolivar, 75019 Paris.
☎ 148 03 2885
Mr. Kelvin's agent is Jean -François Krettly at the same address.

☺ **Christophe Mourthé**
8 Rue Frochot, 75009 Paris.
☎ 142 82 1054 📠 142 85 3904

☺ **Gerard Musy**
110 Rue Veille du Temple, 75003 Paris.

Piercers

☺▽ **Gauntlet, Inc.**
23 rue Keller, 75011 Paris.
☎ 147 007360 📠 145 806362
🌐 http://www.gauntlet.com/

Publishers: Books: Fetish

👥 **Editions Astarté**
58 rue Amelot, 75011 Paris.
☎ 143 38 3343 📠 143 38 0995

👥 **Editions Dominique Leroy**
61 Rue Monsieur Le Prince, 75006 Paris.
☎ 146 34 6361
☎ 143 54 8913

Publishers: Magazines: BDSM

☺■ *Demonia*
Société Comedit, 15 Cité Joly, 75011 Paris.
☎ 143 57 09 93 📠 148 06 6942
Also have a shop. Published 11 times a year.

👥■ *La Scene*
F. A., 102 Avenue des Champs Elysés, 75008 Paris.

☺■ *Sortilège*
C. P. 91, 189 rue d'Aubervilliers, 75886 Paris.

Publishers: Magazines: Fetish

👥 *Maniac*
Editions Astarté, 58 rue Amelot, 75011 Paris.
☎ 143 38 3343 📠 143 38 0995

Radio: Sexuality

☺▽ *Frequence Gaie*
FG FM 98.2, 45 Rue Rébéval, 75019 Paris.
☎ 140 13 8800
🕐 24hrs.

♀♀▽ *LMT 94.4 FM*
🕐 Wed 22:00 - 24:00

Stores: Art Galleries

☺ **Galerie Michel Vidal**
56 Rue du Faubourg Saint Antoine, 75011 Paris.
☎ 143 42 2271

☺■ **Les Larmes D'Eros**
58 Rue Amelot, 75011 Paris.
☎ 143 38 3343 📠 143 38 0995
🕐 Tue - Sat 14:30 - 19:30
Fetish & BDSM photographs, erotic drawings, paintings, vintage works, & old books.

Stores: Books: General

⚤ **La Fourmi Ailée**
8 Rue de Fouarre, 75005 Paris.
☎ 143 29 4099
🕐 Wed - Mon 12:00 - 19:00

⚤ **La Librairie des Femmes**

74 Rue de Seine, 75006 Paris.

☺■ **Librarie La Scarabée D'or**
61 Rue Monsieur Le Prince, 75006 Paris.
☎ 146 34 6361
☎ 143 54 8913
🕐 Mon - Sat 10:00 - 19:00
Catalogue, 2 IRCs.

☺▽ **Les Mots à la Bouche**
6 Rue Sainte Croix de la Bretonnerie, 75004 Paris.
☎ 142 78 8830
🕐 Mon - Sat 11:00 - 20:00

☺▽ **Neuens Co-Op**
33 Rue Des Rosiers, 75004 Paris.

Stores: Clothing: Fetish

☺■ **Les Artistes**
19 Boulevard de Clichy, 75009 Paris.
☎ 142 82 1190

☺■ **Galactica**
31 Boulevard de Clichy, 75009 Paris.
☎ 148 74 5671

☺▽ **International Estetic Men (IEM)**
4 Rue de Bailleul, 75001 Paris.
☎ 142 96 0574
🕐 Mon - Sat 13:00 -20:00

☺▽ **International Estetic Men (IEM)**
33 Rue de Liège, 75008 Paris.
☎ 145 22 6901
🕐 Mon - Sat 12:00 - 19:00

☺▽ **International Estetic Men (IEM)**
208 Rue Saint-Maur, 75010 Paris.
☎ 142 41 2141 📠 142 41 8680
🕐 Mon - Sat 12:00 -19:30

☺■ **Leader Ship**
20 Rue Saint Denis, 75001 Paris.
Uniforms, toys, etc..

☺■ **MGL Sexy Lingerie**
144 Rue Saint Denis, 75002 Paris.
☎ 142 21 3334

Stores: Erotica: BDSM

☺▽ **TTBM**
16 Rue Saint Croix de la Bretonnerie, 75004 Paris.
☎ 148 04 8088
🕐 Mon - Thu 13:00 - 21:00, Fri Sat 13:00 - 24:00, Sun 15:00 - 23:00

Stores: Erotica: General

☺■ **Boutique Demonia**
10 Cité Joly, 75011 Paris.

☺■ **Ets Cochon**
2 Rue les Lombards, 75004 Paris.
🕐 10:00 - 02:00

☺ **Hardclub 88**
88 Rue Saint-Denis, 75001 Paris.
🕐 Every day - 02:00

☺■ **Ligne 2**
2 impasse de la Gaîté, 75014 Paris.
☎ 143 20 9132
🕐 09:00 - 02:00

☺■ **Phylea**
61 Rue Quaincampoix, 75004 Paris.
☎ 142 76 0190
🕐 Mon - Sat 10:30 - 20:00

☺▽ **Yanko**
54 Rue de l'Arbre Sec, 75009 Paris.
☎ 142 60 5528
🕐 12:00 -20:00, Sun 14:00 - 20:00

☺▽ **Yanko**
10 Place de Clichy, 75001 Paris.
☎ 145 26 1841
🕐 12:00 -20:00, Sun 14:00 - 20:00

Pau

Health Services

☺■ **Centre Hospitalier de Pau**
17bis Rue E. Guichenne, 64000 Pau.

☎ 59 84 1350
Stores: Erotica: General
⌀▼ **Kitsch**
13 Cours Bosquet, 6400 Pau.
☎ 59 27 6867
🕐 Mon - Sat 14:00 - 20:00

Perpignan
Stores: Erotica: General
⌀▼ **Défi**
10 Avenue Leclerc, 66000 Perpignan.
☎ 68 52 4425
🕐 09:00 - 24:00
Mail order through Boîte Postale 4051, Perpignan, 66000 Cedex.

Poitiers
Health Services
☺ ■ **AIDES Poiteau-Charentes**
Boîte Postale 467, 86000 Poitiers.
☎ 49 42 4545
☺ ■ **Centre Hospitalier**
☎ 49 44 3905
HIV testing.

Poussan
Health Services
☺ ■ **Centre Hospitalier de Privas**
Service de Médecine, Boîte Postale 1623, Avenue Pasteur, 34560 Poussan.
☎ 75 64 1177
HIV testing.

Quimper
Health Services
☺ ■ **Centre Hospitalier Laennec**
Avenue Y. Theapot, 29000 Quimper.
☎ 98 90 3030
Stores: Erotica: General
☺ ■ **Duo Shop**
14 Rue de Concarneau, 29000 Quimper.
☎ 98 90 7357
🕐 14:00 - 01:00

Rennes
Health Services
☺ ■ **Centre Hospitalier R. Pontchaillou**
Bloc d'Urgences, 2 Rue Henri le Guilloux, 35000 Rennes.
☎ 99 28 4302
HIV testing.
Helplines: Sexuality
⌀▽ **ALLOGAY**
☎ Minitel 3615 ALLOGAY
Organizations: AIDS: Support
☺ ■ **AIDES Bretagne**
Boîte Postale 3757, 35037 Rennes Cedex.
☎ 99 79 0604
🕐 Mon - Fri 09:00 - 12:30 13:30 - 18:00
Support, counselling, & information for people infected with or affected by HIV/AIDS.
☺ ■ **SID'Aventure**
3 Place Saint Germain, 35000 Rennes.
☎ 99 78 2132
🕐 18:00 - 22:00

Riems
Organizations: AIDS: Support
☺ ■ **AIDES Champagne-Ardennes**
Boîte Postale 2180, 51081 Riems Cedex 10.
☎ 26 49 9610
🕐 19:00 - 22:00
Support & information about HIV/AIDS.

Rochefort
Stores: Erotica: General
☺ ■ **Sex Shop**
13 Rue Cochon Duvivier, 17300 Rochefort.
☎ 46 99 9363

Roissy
Stores: Erotica: General
☺ ■ **Enigma**
11 Avenue Charles De Gaulle, 95700 Roissy.

Rosny sous Bois
Photographers: Erotic
☺ **Philippe Serieys**
18 Avenue Kennedy, 93110 Rosny sous Bois.
☎ 145 28 2157 ✆ 148 94 0267

Rouen
Health Services
☺ ■ **AIDES Haute-Normandie**
Boîte Postale 8, 76120 Le Grand-Quevilly.
☎ 35 69 3232
☺ ■ **Hôpital Charles-Nicole**
☎ 35 008 8040
HIV testing.

Saint Denis
Health Services
☺ ■ **Centre Hospitalier de Saint Denis**
☎ 42 35 6067
HIV testing.
☺ ■ **Hôpital de la Fontaine**
2 rue de la Fontaine, 93200 Saint Denis.
☎ 42 35 6808
Confidential, free HIV testing.

Saint Etienne
Health Services
☺ ■ **Hôpital de Bellevue**
Service Maladies Infectieuses, 1bis Boulevard Pasteur, 42000 Saint Etienne.
☎ 77 42 7722
HIV testing.
Organizations: AIDS: Support
☺ ■ **AIDES Loire & Haute-Loire**
65 Rue des Docteurs Charcot, 42000 Saint Etienne.
☎ 777 80 7571
🕐 Mon Fri 15:00 - 19:00

Saint Lô
Organizations: AIDS: Support
☺ ■ **Syndicat PTT de la Manche CFDT**
75 Rue Torteron, 50001 Saint Lô.
☎ 33 57 0697
Support for people with HIV/AIDS.

Saint Louis
Radio: Sexuality
⌀▽ *Radio Dreyekland*
FM 104.6, Boîte Postale 198, 68300 Saint Louis.
☎ 89 67 6566
🕐 Sun 19:00 - 21:00

Saint Malo
Health Services
☺ ■ **Centre Médico-Social**
9 Boulevard Villebois Mareuil, 35400 Saint Malo.
☎ 99 56 1156
Stores: Erotica: General
☺ ■ **Boutique X**
4 Rue du Puits aux Braies, 35400 Saint Malo.
☎ 99 56 0151
🕐 10:00 - 12:30 13:30 - 19:30

Saint Michel
Health Services
☺ ■ **Centre Hospitalier de Saint Michel**
☎ 45 24 4040
HIV testing.

Saintes
Stores: Erotica: General
☺ ■ **Sex Shop**
10 Quai de la République, 17100 Saintes.
☎ 46 74 5172
🕘 Mon - Sat 10:00 - 12:00 14:00 - 19:00

Soissons
Health Services
☺ ■ **Centre Hospitalier de Soissons**
Consultations de Médecine, Boîte Postale 404, 46 Avenue Général de Gaulle, 02209 Soissons.
☎ 23 59 1102
HIV testing.

Strasbourg
Health Services
☺ ■ **Hospices Civils de Strasbourg**
1 Place de l'Hôpital, 67000 Strasbourg.
☎ 88 16 1718
STD & HIV testing.

Helplines: Sexuality
⚣▽ **ALLOGAY**
☎ Minitel 3615 ALLOGAY

Organizations: AIDS: Support
☺ ■ **AIDES Alsace**
6 Rue de Bischwiller, 67000 Strasbourg.
☎ 88 75 7363
🕘 Mon - Fri 18:00 - 20:00

Thionville
Health Services
☺ ■ **Hôpital Beauregard**
Service de Dermatologie, 21 Rue des Frères, 57100 Thionville.
☎ 82 55 8899
HIV testing.

Toulon
Health Services
☺ ■ **Cité Sanitaire**
132 Avenue Lazare Carnot, 83076 Toulon.
☎ 94 89 9020

Stores: Erotica: General
☺ ■ **Sexy Shop**
26 Rue Anatole France, 83000 Toulon.
☎ 94 62 6393
🕘 Closed Sun

Toulouse
Bars: BDSM
⚣▼ **N. Y. C.**
83 Allé Charles-de-Fitte, 31100 Toulouse.
☎ 61 59 4645
🕘 Tue - Sun 22:00 - ?

Health Services
☺ ■ **Centre Hospitalier de Toulouse Hôtel Dieu**
Rue Viguerie, 31052 Toulouse Cedex.
☎ 61 77 8133

☺ ■ **Centre Hospitalier la Grave**
Dispensaire Antivénérien, Place Lange, 31100 Toulouse.
☎ 61 77 7859
HIV testing.

Organizations: AIDS: Support
☺ ■ **AIDES Toulouse-Midi-Pyrénées**
Boîte Postale 77, 31013 Toulouse Cedex.
☎ 61 25 2571
🕘 Mon - Fri 09:00 - 17:00
Infomation, support, & counselling.

Stores: Erotica: BDSM
☺ ■ **Aphrodite**
13 Rue Denfert-Rochereau, 31100 Toulouse.
☎ 61 62 4882
🕘 Mon - Sat 11:00 - 02:00

Stores: Erotica: General
☺ ■ **Autan X**
23 Rue Denfert-Rochereau, 31100 Toulouse.
☎ 61 63 8790
🕘 12:00 - 24:00

☺ ■ **Eros**
22 Rue Denfert-Rochereau, 31100 Toulouse.
☎ 61 63 4472
🕘 13:00 - 02:00

⚣▼ **Spartacus**
29 Rue Héliot, 31100 Toulouse.
☎ 61 62 6145
🕘 Mon - Sat 12:00 - 01:00

Tours
Health Services
☺ ■ **Centre Hospitalier de Tours**
2 Boulevard Tonnelé, 37044 Tours.
☎ 47 34 8111

Helplines: AIDS
☺ ■ **Allo SIDA**
🕘 Tue 18:00 - 20:00, Thu 20:00 - 22:00, Sat 10:00 - 12:00
Counselling & support for HIV/AIDS & STD issues.

Organizations: AIDS: Support
☺ ■ **Tours Elisa 2000**
22B Avenue Grammont, 37000 Tours.
☎ 47 20 000899

Stores: Erotica: General
⚣▼ **Miroir des Hommes**
34 Rue Michelet, 37000 Tours.
☎ 47 37 4646

French Guiana

Area: Approximately 91,000 square kilometres
Population: Approximately 120,000
Capital City: Cayenne
Currency: French Franc (FF)
Official Language: French & Créole
Major Religions: Roman Catholic
Time zone: GMT minus 3 hours
Country Initials: FG
Country Dialing Code (from elsewhere): 594
Intl. Dialing Prefix (out of the country): 19
Climate: Warm weather. Plenty of rain in the tropical rainforests, direr savannah-like conditions further inland.
Age of consent & homosexuality legislation: Age of consent for sexual activity is 15, but it is not advisable for foreigners to become involved with anyone under 18. Homosexual acts were removed from the criminal code in 1982. Although the laws are French, the local customs are Latin-American.

Cayenne
Health Services
☺ ■ **Hôpital Jean Martial**
☎ 885
🕘 07:30 - 12:00, Mon Thu 17:00 - ?

Organizations: Sexuality
⚣▼ **Group Gai Guyanais (GGG)**
Boîte Postale 347, 97302 Cayenne.

Radio: Sexuality
⚣▽ ***Emission Gaie Cayenne***
🕘 Wed 22:00 - 24:00

Germany

Area: Approximately 356,950 square kilometres
Population: Approximately 80,990,000
Capital City: Berlin
Currency: Mark (DM)
Official Language: German
Major Religions: 41% Roman Catholic, 41% Protestant
National Holiday: Unification Day, 3rd. October
Time zone: GMT plus 1 hour
Country Initials: D
Electricity: 220 volts, 60Hz
Country Dialing Code (from elsewhere): 49
Intl. Dialing Prefix (out of the country): 00

Long Distance Dialing Prefix (inside country): 0
Climate: Maritime climate in the west, continental climate in the east.
Age of consent & homosexuality legislation: In West Germany, the age of consent for sexual activity is 14 for heterosexual & lesbian activity, but 18 for gay males. In East Germany, the age of consent for sexual activity is 14. The GDR has announced that it will unify the age of consent to 14 in the near future. Since 1992, homosexual activity has been permitted in the military, but these people are not considered suitable for higher ranks.

NATIONAL RESOURCES

Archives: Sexuality

&⋄▽ **Schwule Pressearchiv Bonn**
c/o Joachim Witt, Klufterstraße 99, 53175 Bonn.
☎ 228 21 6587

BBSs: Sexuality

&⋄■ **Arcisbox**
✆ 40 524 3510
Linked with GayNet, HIV-NET, LCH-NET, & den Niederlanden.

&⋄■ **SGBB Mailbox**
✆ 40 690 7117
🕐 24hrs.
Second BBS number 40 61 2794. Linked with GayNet, GNI, HIV-NET, & LCH-NET.

Distributors: Clothing: Fetish

☺▼ **Basta**
Gurlittstraße 47, 20099 Hamburg.
☎ 40 24 5979 ✆ 40 24 6097
Distributes Invincible rubberwear in Germany.

Helplines: Sexuality

&⋄▽ **Freies Tagungshaus Waldschlößhen**
☎ 559 2 2382

&⋄▽ **Mann-O-Meter e. V.**
♿ Motzstraße 5, 10777 Berlin.
☎ 30 216 8008 ✆ 30 215 7078
🕐 Mon - Sat 15:00 - 23:00, Sun 15:00 - 21:00
Information about gay life. Education & information on problems with HIV/AIDS. Help with coming out. Anti-gay-violence hotline.

Mailorder: Books: Sexuality

&⋄▼ **Bruno Gmünder Versand**
Postfach 110729, 10837 Berlin.
☎ 30 615 00342 ✆ 30 615 9134
🕐 24hr. answering machine
Free catalogue.

Mailorder: Clothing: Fetish

&⋄▼ **Apollo Contakt Versand**
Postfach 401960, 80719 München.

☺ **BMA**
Postfach 1114, 83484 Ramsau.
18 different sizes of false breasts in the form of bras, to be worn to give someone breasts or increase the size of existing breasts.

☺■ **Fairy Tales**
Postfach 103009, 44030 Dortmund.
 ✆ 231 128240

☺■ **Samanta**
Postfach 8035, 59035 Hamm.
☎ 2381 402586 ✆ 2381 404288
Catalogue, DM25.

☺■ **Schau Mode**
Paul-Hindemith-Ring 18, 63110 Rodgau.
☎ 610 61 8379
🕐 Visitors by appointment
Also custom orders.

☺■ **Schwarze Mode**
Grunewaldstraße 91, 10823 Berlin.
☎ 30 784 5922 (shop) ✆ 30 694 1297
☎ 30 694 5475 (mail order)
Supplies customers with books & goods from more than 10 catalogues.

Mailorder: Clothing: Rubber

☺▼ **Basta Boots**
Gurlittstraße 47, 20099 Hamburg.
☎ 40 24 5979 ✆ 40 24 6097

&⋄▼ **Fa. Dawi**
Peter Anders Straße 4B, 81245 München.
Catalogue, DM20.

⊕■ **Full Moon Fashions**
Postfach 520430, 22594 Hamburg.

Catalogue, DM20 for Europe, £8 for U.K., $15U.S. for North America.

☺■ **Lampe**
Postfach 500942, 22709 Hamburg.
Catalogue available.

Mailorder: Erotica: Adult Baby

♯♯■ **Hygia-Versand**
Postfach 140163, 7530 Pforzheim.
Only German spoken. Catalogue available.

Mailorder: Erotica: BDSM

☺ **Domination**
Postfach 810243, 81902 München.
☎ 89 930 6980
[VISA] [MC]
PVC, leather, latex, high heels, bondage toys, corsets. Catalogue, DM25.

☺■ **Dream & Fantasy Fashions**
Postfach 410309, 1000 Berlin 41.
☎ 30 792 7760
Catalogue available.

☺■ **Hard Line**
Müllerstraße 33, 80469 München.
☎ 89 260 6017 ✆ 89 260 8076
☎ 80 260 6018
🕐 Mon - Fri 12:30 - 18:00, Sat 11:00 - 13:30
♿ [VISA] [MC]
Manufacturers, wholesalers, & retailers of rubber & leather clothes, & BDSM toys.

&⋄▼ **K. A. B. Kühn / Clabes Versandhandel GbR**
Postfach 100840, 47008 Duisberg.
☎ 203 33 4482 ✆ 203 33 4482
Catalogue, DM5.

☺■ **Kastley GmbH**
Erwin Bälz Straße 73, 70597 Stuttgart.
☎ 711 76 9074 ✆ 711 765 1945
🕐 Mon - Fri 09:30 - 17:30, Sat 10:00 - 14:00
♿ $ [MC]
Mail order by catalogues: toys & clothes in leather, rubber, & steel, high heels (including large sizes). Age statement of 18 is required. English also spoken.

☺ **Moonlight Fashion**
Postfach 180128, 33691 Bielefeld.
Catalogue available.

☺ **SM Toy Hamburg**
Postfach 602568, 22768 Hamburg.

☺ **SM Versand**
Postfach 4024, 26030 Oldenburg.
☎ 441 72340 ✆ 441 777 5744
Catalogue, DM8.

☺ **Venus Versand**
Postfach 2723, 33057 Paderborn.

Mailorder: Erotica

☺■ **Ernst Fischer**
Postfach 251160, 69079 Heidelberg.

Mailorder: Erotica: General

☺ **Erosart**
Postfach 1132, 25557 Hanerau.
Catalogue available.

&⋄▼ **Pro-Fun**
Reifenburger Straße 57, 60489 Frankfurt.
☎ 69 59 3590 ✆ 69 789 6813
Catalogue, DM19.

Mailorder: Erotica

&⋄▼ **Keile Henkel**
Lindemunnstraße 75, 44137 Dortmund.

Mailorder: Erotica: Leather

&⋄▼ **Blackline Press & Services**
Postfach 150230, 10664 Berlin.
☎ 30 883 7013 ✆ 30 229 4114

&⋄▼ **Hot Leather Versand**
Postfach 2141, 30021 Hannover.
☎ 511 57 4251 ✆ 511 57 4251

&⋄▼ **PI Versand**
Brammer Hauptstraße, 27308 Kirchlinteln.
☎ 42 36 1058
🕐 Mon - Wed 10:00 - 13:00 17:00 - 18:30

&⋄▼ **Vimpex GmbH**
Postfach 1372, 24576 Bad Bramstedt.

☎ 419 25 0010

Mailorder: Erotica: Rubber
⚥▼ **Black Light**
Postfach 350208, 50793 Köln.
Catalogue, DM4.

Mailorder: Safer Sex Products
☺▼ **The Hot Rubber Company**
Postfach 610149, 10921 Berlin.

Organizations: AIDS: Education
☺■ **Deutsche AIDS-Hilfe e. V.**
Dieffenbachstraße 33, 10967 Berlin.
☎ 30 690 0870
Publishes *Aktuell* 5 times a year.

☺■ **Dignity-Dokumentationsstelle der Diskriminierung von Menschen mit HIV/AIDS**
c/o AIDS Archiv, Brönnestraße 9, 60313 Frankfurt.
☎ 69 29 6797 ✆ 69 28 9181

Organizations: Sexuality
⚥▽ **BVH - Bundesverband Homosexualität e. V.**
Boxhagener Straße 76/78, 10245 Berlin.
☎ 30 581 8306 ✆ 30 581 8307
🕐 Mon - Fri 10:00 - 12:00, Mon Tue Thu 14:00 - 18:00, Wed 14:00 - 20:00
Publishes *Schwule Zeiten*.

⚥▽ **Hannchen Mehrzweck Stiftung für Homosexuelle Selbsthilfe**
Postfach 126710, 10595 Berlin.
☎ 30 391 2651 ✆ 30 391 2651

⚥▼ **Homosexuelle Selbsthilfe e. V.**
Löwengasse 27, 60385 Frankfurt.
 ✆ 69 46 5068

⚥▽ **International Gay & Lesbian Association (ILGA)**
c/o Schultz, Bismarckstraße 17, 50672 Köln.
☎ 221 52 0206

⚥▽ **Zentrale Erfassung Homosexuellendiskriminierung (ZEH)**
c/o HSH, Postfach 4722, 30047 Hannover.
Registry of cases of discrimination based on sexual orientation.

Publishers: Books: Sexuality
⚥▼ **Albino Verlag**
Postfach 110729, 10837 Berlin.
☎ 30 615 0030 ✆ 30 615 9007
🕐 24hr. answering machine
Yearly subscription is free.

⚥■ **Verlag Rosa Winkel**
Postfach 620604, 10796 Berlin.
☎ 30 853 4042 ✆ 30 853 9995
Bibliophile reprints of gay writings.

Publishers: Directories: Sexuality
⚥■ **Der Stiefel**
c/o Venker, Palmstraße 39, 50672 Köln.
Club listings. Published quarterly.

Publishers: Guides: Sexuality
⚥▼ **Berlin & Brandenburg, Sachsen, Sachsen-Anhalt von Hinten**
Bruno Gmünder Verlag, Postfach 110729, 10837 Berlin.
☎ 30 615 00342 ✆ 30 615 9134
Published every month.

⚥▼ **Schwule Männer**
Bruno Gmünder Verlag, Postfach 110729, 10837 Berlin.
☎ 30 615 00342 ✆ 30 615 9134
Covers Austria, Germany, & Switzerland. Published once a year.

⚥▼ **Spartacus**
Bruno Gmünder Verlag, Postfach 110729, 10837 Berlin.
☎ 30 615 00342 ✆ 30 615 9134

Publishers: Magazines: Arts
⚥■ **Euros**
Bruno Gmünder Verlag, Postfach 110729, 10837 Berlin.
☎ 30 615 00342 ✆ 30 615 9134
Published every two months.

Publishers: Magazines: Sexual Politics
⚥■ **Box**
Postfach 290341, 50525 Köln.
☎ 221 54 2516

Published every month.

Publishers: Magazines: Sexuality
⚥■ **Die Andere Welt**
Postfach 24, 10371 Berlin.
☎ 30 588 0833
Published every month.

⚥■ **Don & Adonis**
Foerster Verlag, Redaction Darmstadt, Reidstraße 8, 64295 Darmstadt.
☎ 61 513 3468
Published every two months.

⚥■ **Du & Ich**
Leine Verlag, Postfach 3745, 30057 Hannover.
☎ 511 31 1619
Published every month.

⚥■ **Foerster Verlag**
Postfach 700362, 60533 Frankfurt.
☎ 69 297 8681

⚥▼ **Forum Homosexualität und Literatur**
Postfach 101240, 57012 Siegen.
☎ 271 740 4444

⚥■ **Lambda Edition**
Postfach 304171, 20324 Hamburg.
☎ 40 319 2836 ✆ 40 319 2096

⚥■ **Magnus**
Magnus Verlag, Postfach 620560, 10795 Berlin.
☎ 30 787 93431 ✆ 30 782 0453
☎ 30 787 93434
🕐 10:00 - 17:00
♠ ✓ 💳 MC AMERICAN 🔑
National gay magazine: politics, culture, news, trends, lifestyle, & more. Also book publisher & mail order. Published every month. Yearly subscription is 150DM. English & French also spoken.

⚥■ **Männer Aktuell**
Bruno Gmünder Verlag, Postfach 110729, 10837 Berlin.
☎ 30 615 00342 ✆ 30 615 9134
Published every month.

Publishers: Newspapers: Sexuality
⚥■ **Down Town**
Michael Sürth Verlag, In Der Bohnenbitze 68, 51143 Köln.
☎ 220 38 5767 ✆ 220 38 6818

⚥■ **First**
Breniger Straße 5, 50969 Köln.
☎ 221 36 4821
Free in gay & lesbian locations. Published every month.

⚥■ **Gay Express**
Verlag W.-D. Fritsch, Zimmerstraße 38a, 22085 Hamburg.
☎ 40 220 4001
Free at gay & lesbian location. Published every month.

⚥■ **Gay Life**
Schrötteringsweg 11, 22085 Hamburg.
☎ 40 229 6603 ✆ 40 229 6962
Free in gay & lesbian locations. Published every month.

Stores: Erotica: BDSM
⚥▼ **H•M - Lederwerk**
Neukrikstraße 18, 28215 Bremen.
☎ 421 37 1430 ✆ 421 37 4953
🕐 Mon - Fri 16:00 - 18:30, Sun - 20:30, 1st. Sat of month 10:00 - 16:00
♠ ✓ $ ⚡ VISA 🔑
Store, distibutor, & mail order. Also organization BDSM events. Catalogue, DM10. English also spoken.

Aachen
Helplines: Sexuality
⚥▽ **Rosa Telefon—Aachen**
☎ 241 3 4633
🕐 Tue 19:00 - 21:00

Organizations: AIDS: Support
☺□ **AIDS-Beratung im Gesundheitsamt Aachen**
Vereinsstraße 25, 52063 Aachen.
☎ 241 432 5326

☺□ **AIDS-Hilfe—Aachen**
Zollernstraße 1, 52070 Aachen.
☎ 241 1 9411
🕐 Mon 19:00 - 21:00 Thu 10:00 - 12:00

Organizations: Motorcycle
⚥▽ **MSC Black Angels Köln**

Postfach 1503, 52016 Aachen.
Contact: Herr Ferdi Wetzels

Organizations: Sexuality
⚥■ **Schwule in der AIDS-Hilfe (SidAH)**
Zollernstraße 1, 52070 Aachen.
☎ 241 52 2558

Organizations: Sexuality: Student
⚥■ **Schwulenreferat an den Aachener Hochschulen**
Königstraße 14-16, 52064 Aachen.
☎ 241 3 4633
🕐 Mon 20:00 coming out group, Thu 19:00 - 21:00 support
Also has a library of gay/lesbian literature.

Aalen
Organizations: Sexuality
⚥▽ **Homosexuelle Initiative Aalen (HIA)**
Postfach 1362, 73403 Aalen.
☎ 07361
🕐 Every 2nd. Mon 20:00

Ahaus
Organizations: AIDS: Support
☺ ☐ **AIDS-Hilfe—Westmünsterland**
Postfach 1120, 48661 Ahaus.
☎ 256 1 19411
🕐 Tue 10:00 - 16:00, Wed 20:00 - 22:00

Ahlen
Organizations: AIDS: Support
☺ ☐ **AIDS-Hilfe—Ahlen**
Königstraße 9, 59227 Ahlen.
☎ 238 2 4650 ✆ 238 28 1179
🕐 Mon 09:00 - 12:00 17:00 - 19:00, Tue Thu 09:00 - 12:00 15:00 -
17:00, Fri 15:00 - 17:00

Allmendingen
Stores: Books: General
☺ ■ **BMCF Antiquariat**
Postfach 5, 89602 Allmendingen.

Altenkirchen
Organizations: Sexuality
⚥▽ **Schwule im Westerwald (SIW)**
c/o Huas Felsenkeller, Heimstraße4, 57610 Altenkirchen.
🕐 Last Wed of month 19:30

Arnsberg
Organizations: Sexuality
⚥▽ **Rosa Gruppe Arnsberg**
Grotte, Hallenstraße 19, Arnsberg.
☎ 293 1 3670
🕐 1st. & 3rd. Wed of the month 19:00 - 21:30

Arnstadt
Organizations: AIDS: Support
☺ ☐ **AIDS-Hilfe—Arnstadt**
c/o Dieter Schettlock, Magerstraße 4a 11, 99310 Arnstadt.

Aschaffenberg
Stores: Erotica: General
☺ ■ **Shiwa**
Rossmarkt 24-26, 63739 Aschaffenberg.

Augsburg
Helplines: Sexuality
⚥▽ **Rosa Telefon—Augsburg**
☎ 821 15 9242
🕐 Fri 20:00 - 22:00

Organizations: AIDS: Support
☺ ☐ **AIDS-Hilfe—Augsburg**
Postfach 110125, 86026 Augsburg.
☎ 821 1 9411
🕐 Mon Wed 18:30 - 20:00, Fri 13:00 - 14:30

Bamberg
Helplines: Sexuality
⚥▽ **Rosa Telefon—Bamberg**
☎ 951 2 4729
🕐 Thu 19:30 - 21:00

Organizations: AIDS: Support
☺ ☐ **AIDS-Beratungstelle**
Kunigundenruhstraße 24, 96050 Bamberg.
☎ 951 2 7998
🕐 Mon Tue Thu 09:00 - 12:00 14:00 - 17:00, Fri 09:00 - 12:00
☺ ☐ **AIDS-Hilfe—Bamberg**
Eisgrube 18, 96049 Bamberg.
☎ 9551 1 9411
🕐 Sun 16:00 - 18:00, Mon 18:00 - 20:00

Organizations: Sexuality
⚥▽ **ASTA - Schwulen & Lesbenferat**
Fachschaftsbüro G/Geo, Austraße 37, 96047 Bamberg.
☎ 951 86 3347
🕐 Mon 16:00 - 18:00
⚥▽ **Initiative Homosexualität Bamberg (IHBa)**
Postfach 1742, 96008 Bamberg.
☎ 951 2 4729
🕐 Meets Thu 19:30 - 21:00

Bayreuth
Helplines: Sexuality
⚥▽ **Rosa Telefon—Bayreuth**
Postfach 101245, 95412 Bayreuth.
☎ 921 85 2928
🕐 Mon 18:30 - 20:00

Organizations: AIDS: Support
☺ ☐ **AIDS-Beratungstelle**
Schulstraße 15/III, 95444 Bayreuth.
☎ 921 8 2500
🕐 Mon - Fri 08:30 - 12:30 Thu 14:00 - 17:00

Organizations: Sexuality
⚥▽ **Vereinigung Homosexualität & Gesellschaft e. V.
(VHG)**
Postfach 101245, 95412 Bayreuth.
☎ 921 85 2928
🕐 Meet Mon 20:00

Bergkirchen
Manufacturers: Furniture: BDSM
☺ ■ **X-zess**
Postfach 32, 85232 Bergkirchen.
☎ 8131 78941 ✆ 8131 78941

Berlin
Accommodation: BDSM
⚥▼ **Le Moustache**
Gartenstraße 4, 10115 Berlin.
☎ 30 281 7277
🕐 21:00 - 03:00
⚥▼ **Tom's House**
Eisenacher Straße 10, 10777 Berlin.
☎ 30 218 5544 ✆ 30 213 4464
🕐 No check-in 15:00 - 18:00
Primarily leather/fetish/SM clients.

Archives: Sexuality
⚥■ **Lila Archiv e. V.**
Choriner Straße 9, 10119 Berlin.
☎ 30 448 5713 ✆ 30 448 5713
⚥▽ **Schwules Pressearchiv Berlin**
c/o SchwuZ, Hasenheide 54, 10967 Berlin.
☎ 30 694 1077

Bars: BDSM
⚥▼ **Adam**
Jungstraße 31, 10247 Berlin.
☎ 30 292 3089
🕐 Mon - Fri 10:00 - 21:00, Sat - 16:00
🍴 ✓
⚥▼ **Andreas Kneipe**
Ansbacher Straße 29, 10789 Berlin.
☎ 30 218 3257

Bars: BDSM

🕐 11:00 - 04:00
♂▼ **Knast**
Fuggerstraße 34, 10777 Berlin.
☎ 30 219 1026
🕐 21:00 - 05:00

♂▼ **Le Moustache**
Gartenstraße 4, 10115 Berlin.
☎ 30 281 7277
🕐 21:00 - 03:00

♂▼ **New Action**
Kleiststraße 35, 10787 Berlin.
☎ 30 211 8256 ✆ 30 213 4981
🕐 Mon - Sat 20:30 - ?, Sun 13:00 - ?

♂■ **Phönix**
Motzstraße 25, 10777 Berlin.
☎ 30 213 8580
🕐 Sun - Thu 21:00 - 07:00, Fri Sat 20:00 - ?

♂ **Snax Club**
c/o Bunker, Albrechtstraße 24/25, Berlin.
Holds occasional gay fetish parties for those into rubber, leather, piercing, & sweaty, kinky sex. Local press has times.

♂■ **Tom's Bar**
Motzstraße 19, 10777 Berlin.
☎ 30 213 4570
🕐 22:00 - ?

♂▼ **Twilight Zone**
Welserstraße 24, 10777 Berlin.
☎ 30 218 1432 ✆ 30 217 7686
🕐 Wed Thu Sun 23:00 - 05:00 (dress code), Fri Sat 23:00 - ?

Counsellors

☺□ **Centrum Für Sexualwissenschaft e. V.**
Joachim Friedrich Straße 3, 10711 Berlin.
☎ 30 891 6046
🕐 Mon Wed 10:00 - 12:00, Tue Thu 17:00 - 19:00
Counselling, information, & support for people with sexual & relationship difficulties.

Distributors: Videos: Erotic

♂▼ **Edition Manfred Salzgeber Berlin**
Motzstraße 9, 10777 Berlin.
☎ 30 215 3209 ✆ 30 215 4348

Helplines: AIDS

♂♀▽ **Allgemeine Homosexuelle Arbeitsgemeinschaft e. V. (AHA)**
Mehringdamm 61, 10961 Berlin.
☎ 30 692 3600

Manufacturers: Clothing: Fetish

☺■ **Schwarze Mode**
Grunewaldstraße 91, 10823 Berlin.
☎ 30 784 5922 (shop) ✆ 30 694 1297
☎ 30 694 5475 (mail order)
Makes latex & leather clothes, & corsets.

Manufacturers: Clothing: Rubber

☺■ **Atelier für Extravagante Mode**
Marienburger Straße 47, 10405 Berlin.
☎ 30 442 2740

Organizations: Academic: Sexuality

♂□ **Arbeitsgemeinschaft Humane Sexualität**
Ohlauer Straße 30, 10999 Berlin.
☎ 30 618 9039

Organizations: AIDS: Education

☺□ **Stop AIDS Projekt Berlin**
Kalckreuthstraße 7, 10777 Berlin.
☎ 30 218 2011
🕐 Mon - Thu 10:00 - 17:00, Fri 10:00 - 14:00

Organizations: AIDS: Support

☺□ **AIDS Forum**
Bredowstraße 14, 10551 Berlin.
☎ 30 395 7505

☺□ **AIDS-Hilfe—Berlin**
Meineckestraße 12, 10719 Berlin.
☎ 30 1 9411 ✆ 30 882 5194
🕐 Mon Tue Thu Fri 10:00 - 18:00, Wed 15:00 - 19:00
Publishes *Helferzelle*.

☺□ **HIV-Arbeitlung der Charité**
Luisenstraße, Berlin.
☎ 30 286 4596

Germany

☎ 30 286 2294
🕐 Mon - Fri 08:00 - 12:00, Wed also 14:00 - 18:00
Anonymous, free HIV testing, counselling, & support.

☺□ **Prenzelberger AIDS Projekt "JederMann" e. V.**
Greifenhagener Straße 6, 10437 Berlin.
☎ 30 448 1170
🕐 Mon - Fri 15:00 - 20:00

Organizations: BDSM

♂▽ **FSC**
Postfach 15 11 45, 1000 Berlin.

♂▼ **Quälgeister - FSG Berlin e.V.**
Hasenheide 54, 10967 Berlin.
☎ 30 694 7829
🕐 2nd. Fri of month. 1st. Fri social, 4th Fri beginners. Door open 22:00 -23:00
Sex parties & discussion groups for fans of BDSM, leather, rubber, fetish, fisting, & other alternate activities.

♂▽ **SKVdC Sekretariat**
c/o Herr christian Brückmann, Ebersstraße 35, 10827 Berlin.

Organizations: Bears

♂▽ **Berliner Bären Bartmänner**
Postfach 128, PA2, 1142 Berlin.
☎ 30 931 6173
🕐 Meets 1st. Fri of each month 21:00, 3rd. Fri of month 21:00, & 2nd. Sun 16:00
Contact: Herr Reiner Lachs

Organizations: Body Size

♂▽ **Girth & Mirth—Deutschland: Berlin**
☎ 30 325 5990

Organizations: Masturbation

♂▽ **Berlin Jacks**
c/o Mann-O-Meter, Motzstraße 5, 10777 Berlin.
🕐 Last Fri of month. Doors open 20:00 - 21:00

Organizations: Motorcycle

♂▽ **Motorradclub LederBären Berlin (MCLB)**
c/o Mann-O-Meter, Motzstraße 5, 10777 Berlin.
☎ 30 215 1458
🕐 Meets 1st. Sun of month
Club requires members to own a motorbike.

♂▽ **MSC Berlin e.V.**
Postfach 303969, 10725 Berlin.
☎ 30 861 8847
🕐 Meets 1st. Thu & 3rd. Sun of every month

Organizations: Sexuality

♂▽ **Schwule Internationale Berlin e. V.**
c/o Selman Arikboga, Schillerstraße 54, 10625 Berlin.
☎ 30 315 2615 ✆ 30 705 1462
🕐 Meets Sat 19:30

Organizations: Sexuality: Youth

♂▽ **Antarius**
Kulturhaus Spandau, Mauerstraße 6, 13597 Berlin.
☎ 30 432 8928 ✆ 30 432 9828
🕐 Sun 18:00

♂♀▽ **Jungendnetwerk Lambda e. V.**
Ackerstraße 12, 10115 Berlin.
🕐 18:00 - 21:00

Photographers: BDSM

☺ **Andreas Fux**
Marienburger Straße 18, 10405 Berlin.
☎ 30 442 5501 ✆ 30 442 6598

Piercers

☺■ **Tatau Obscur**
Leonhardstraße 19, 14057 Berlin.

Publishers: Books: Sexuality

♂▼ **Janssen Verlag**
Postfach 150701, 10669 Berlin.

Publishers: Magazines: BDSM

♂▼ *Disziplin*
Vogel Verlag, Postfach 151403, 10837 Berlin.

♂▼ *Kumpel*
Vogel Verlag, Postfach 151403, 10837 Berlin.

☺■ *Twilight*
Katzbachstraße 17, 10965 Berlin.

The information magazine for the new BDSM-erotic culture. Scene news, stories, photography, psychology & BDSM, & much more. Published every two months.

Z&O
Vogel Verlag, Postfach 151403, 10837 Berlin.

Publishers: Magazines: Sexuality

Pink Power
Erkstraße 5, 12043 Berlin.
☎ 30 688 09052 — Fax 30 688 09053
☎ 30 688 09051
pinkpower1@aol.com
http://users.aol.com/pinkpower1/homepage.htm
Mon - Fri 10:00 -17:00. Not published in Aug
✓ $
Published every month. English also spoken.

Siegessäule
Magnus Verlag, Postfach 620570, 10795 Berlin.
☎ 30 787 93431 — Fax 30 782 0453
☎ 30 787 93434
10:00 - 17:00
✓ VISA MC AMERICAN EXPRESS ₵
Gay programme magazine for Berlin. Published every month. English & French also spoken.

Stores: Art Galleries

Galerie Janssen
Pariser Straße 45, 10719 Berlin.

PPS. Gallery
Hirtenstraße 19, 10178 Berlin.

Stores: Books: General

Adam
Jungstraße 31, 10247 Berlin.
☎ 30 292 3089
Mon - Fri 10:00 - 21:00, Sat - 16:00
✓

Bruno's
1st. Floor, Kufürstendamm 227, 10719 Berlin.
☎ 30 882 4290
Mon - Sat 10:00 - 22:00

Prinz Eisenherz Buchladen
Bleibtreustraße 52, 10623 Berlin.
☎ 30 313 9936 — Fax 30 313 1795
10:00 - 18:30, Sat 10:00 - 14:00, 1st Sat of month - 18:00
✓ VISA MC
Gay men's community book shop with an international collection of books, magazines, postcards, etc.. Also worldwide mail order. Thematic catalogues available. English, Dutch, & French also spoken.

Stores: Clothing: Fetish

Black Stratsch
Lepsiusstraße 47, 12163 Berlin.
☎ 30 793 3692 — Fax 30 793 3692

Blackstyle
Malmoerstraße 25, 10439 Berlin.

Hautnah
Uhlandstraße 170, 10719 Berlin.
☎ 30 882 3434 — Fax 30 883 2401
On three levels.

Jeans Mode Trends
Uhlandstraße 33, 10719 Berlin.
☎ 30 881 4157
10:00 -18:30, Sat 09:00 - 14:00

Schwarze Mode
Grunewaldstraße 91, 10823 Berlin.
☎ 30 784 5922 (shop) — Fax 30 694 1297
☎ 30 694 5475 (mail order)
Clothes in latex & leather, corsets, lingerie, high heels, bondage equipment & other toys, & erotic literature, magazines, & videos.

Stores: Clothing: Leather

Tschul's
Oranienstraße 199, 10999 Berlin.
☎ 30 612 5143

Stores: Clothing: Rubber

Jox
Winnstraße 69, 10405 Berlin.
Mon - Fri 10:00 - 18:00, Sat 10:00 - 14:00

Zweite Haut
Wilhemstraße 16, 12161 Berlin.
☎ 30 821 8603
Custom work also available. Catalogue, DM30 or $18U.S..

Stores: Erotica: BDSM

Horsts Laden
Rankestraße 14, 10789 Berlin.
☎ 30 881 3929 — Fax 30 881 9767
Mon - Fri 11:00 - 18:00, Sat 11:00 - 14:00

Leder Boutique bei Günther
Fredericiastraße 7, 14050 Berlin.
☎ 30 302 8494
Mon - Fri 10:00 18:30, Sat - 14:00
Tailored leather & rubber clothing. Also bondage & piercing items.

Walter's Leder Boutique
Martin Luther Straße 45, 10779 Berlin.
☎ 30 211 1897
Mon - Fri 11:00 - 18:00, Sat 11:00 - 13:00
Separate catalogues for leather, "leather-bizzare," rubber, & toys. Also provides mail order. Catalogue, DM10.

Stores: Erotica: General

City Men Shop & Video
Fuggerstraße 26, 10777 Berlin.
☎ 30 218 2959
Mon - Thu 11:00 - 01:00, Fri Sat 11:00 - 02:00, Sun 14:00 - 01:00

Connection Garage
Fuggerstraße 33, 10777 Berlin.
☎ 30 218 1432 — Fax 30 217 7686
Mon - Thu 10:00 - 01:00, Fri Sat - ?, Sun 14:00 - 01:00

Ero Box
Leitzenburger Straße 54, 10719 Berlin.
☎ 30 882 1331
Mon - Sat 10:00 - 22:00

Go Up
Kantstraße 117, 10627 Berlin.
☎ 30 312 3045
10:00 - 01:00, Sun 14:00 - 01:00

Man's Pleasurechest
Kalckreuthstraße 15, 10777 Berlin.
10:00 - 01:00, Sun Hol 13:00 - 01:00

Sex Pool
Schaperstraße 11, 10719 Berlin.
☎ 30 214 1989
Mon - Sat 10:00 - 22:00

Sexbox
Frankfurter Allee 243, 10365 Berlin.
☎ 30 233 3953
Mon - Fri 09:00 - 18:00, Sat - 14:00

Tattooists

Tattoo Connection
Belziger Straße 53, 10823 Berlin.
Body piercing also available.

Bernberg

Organizations: Sexuality

Fürsorger für Homosexuelle im Caritas Verband
z. Hd. H.-P. Schulze, Altstäster Kirchhof 10, 03471 Bernberg.
Support meetings 2nd. & 4th. Mon of each month 15:00 - 19:00

Biberach

Organizations: Sexuality

Homosexuelle Emanzipationsgruppe (HELB)
Ehinger Straße 19, 88388 Biberach.
☎ 735 1 8384
Meets Thu 19:00

Biedenkopf

Helplines: Sexuality

Rosa Telefon Hinterland—Biederkopf
☎ 735 1 5055
Tue 19:00 - 21:00

Organizations: Sexuality

Schwulengruppen Biedenkopf
Bahnhofstraße 38, 35037 Biedenkopf.
Meets 2nd. & 4th. Wed 19:00

Bielefeld

Counsellors

Psychotherapeutische Beratungsstelle
☎ 521 12 3216

🕐 Mon - Fri 09:00 - 18:00

Helplines: Sexuality

⚥▽ **Homophon**
c/o AStA, Postfach 100131, 33501 Bielefeld.
☎ 521 106 3424
🕐 Tue 18:00 - 20:00

⚥▽ **HomoPhon**
☎ 521 106 3424
🕐 Tue 18:00 - 20:00

Organizations: AIDS: Support

☺ □ **AIDS Beratung im Gesundheitsamt**
☎ 521 51 3890

☺ □ **AIDS-Hilfe—Bielefeld**
Stapenhorststraße 5, 33615 Bielefeld.
☎ 521 1 9411
🕐 Counselling Thu 19:00 - 21:00

☺ □ **HIV-Positiven Treff**
☎ 521 79 1571

Organizations: Sexuality: Student

⚥▽ **Autonomes Schwulenreferat der Uni Bielefeld**
Postfach 100131, 33501 Bielefeld.
☎ 521 106 3424 📠 521 106 3032
🕐 Coming out group Wed 18:00 - 20:00

Bitterfeld

Organizations: AIDS: Support

☺ □ **AIDS-Hilfe—Halle**
☎ 349 32 1018

Bocholt

Organizations: Sexuality

⚥▽ **Homosexuelle Inititivgruppe & Freunde**
c/o Ewald Boekhorst, Moselstraße 10, 46395 Bocholt.
🕐 Meets 2nd. & 4th. Fri of the month 20:00

Bochum

Organizations: AIDS: Support

☺ □ **AIDS-Hilfe—Bochum**
Bergstraße 115, 44791 Bochum.
☎ 232 71 9411
🕐 Mon Tue 10:00 - 12:00, Thu 18:00 - 20:00

Organizations: Sexuality

⚥▽ **BoSchwul**
c/o Oase, Buschyplatz 3, 44801 Bochum.
☎ 232 36 8374
🕐 Sun 15:00

⚥▽ **Rosa Strippe e. V.**
☎ 232 71 9411
🕐 Mon 19:00 - 21:00, Fri 14:00 - 16:00
Support for people coming out & families of gays & lesbians.

⚥▽ **Schwulenzentrum Bochum**
c/o AIDS-Hilfe, Bergstraße 115, 44791 Bochum.
☎ 232 758 3858
🕐 Thu 15:00 - 17:00, Fri 10:00 - 13:00

Organizations: Sexuality: Student

⚥▽ **Schwulenreferat der Bochumer Ruhr-Universität**
AStA der Universität, Universitätstraße 150, 44801 Bochum.
☎ 232 700 2226
🕐 Mon - Wed 14:00, Thu 12:00 - 17:00, Fri 12:00 - 14:00

Publishers: Newspapers: Sexuality

⚥▼ *Rosa Zone*
Postfach 102168, 44721 Bochum.
☎ 232 362 0241
Free at gay locations.

Stores: Erotica: General

☺ ■ **Sexyland**
Humboldtstraße 34, 44787 Bochum.
🕐 Mon - Fri 09:00 - 18:00, Sat -14:00

Bonn

Helplines: Sexuality

⚥▽ **Rosa Telefon—Bonn**
c/o Schwulen & Lesben Zentrum, Endenicher Straße 51, 53113 Bonn.
☎ 228 63 00339
🕐 Wed 19:00 - 21:00

Organizations: AIDS: Education

⚥□ **AK Schwule**
c/o AIDS-Hilfe, Weberstraße 52, 53113 Bonn.
☎ 228 21 9021
🕐 Thu 20:00 - 22:00
Gay AIDS prevention.

Organizations: AIDS: Support

☺ ■ **AIDS-Hilfe—Bonn**
Weberstraße 52, 53113 Bonn.
☎ 228 1 9411 📞 228 21 9024
☎ 228 21 9021 (office)
Information & counselling about HIV/AIDS. 2nd. & 4th. Fri of month meeting for bisexuals.

Organizations: Sexuality

⚥▽ **Schwulen & Lesben Zentrum**
Endenicher Straße 51, 53115 Bonn.
☎ 228 63 0029
🕐 Mon 20:00 - 24:00, Sun 16:00 - 20:00
Counselling & support for gays, lesbians of all ages.

Stores: Books: General

⚥▼ **Buchladen 46**
Kaiserstraße 46, 53113 Bonn.
☎ 228 22 3608

Stores: Erotica: General

☺ ■ **Erotic Shop**
Berliner Freiheit 18, 53111 Bonn.
☎ 228 65 5041
🕐 Mon - Fri 10:00 - 20:00, Sat - 14:00

Bottrop

Organizations: AIDS: Support

☺ □ **AIDS-Hilfe—Bottrop**
Gerichtsstraße 3, 46236 Bottrop.
☎ 204 11 9411
🕐 Mon - Fri 09:00 - 12:00, Mon Thu 19:00 - 21:00

Brandenburg

Organizations: AIDS: Support

☺ □ **AIDS-Hilfe—Brandenburg**
Geschwister Scholl Straße 20, 14776 Brandenburg.
☎ 338 12 3917
🕐 Wed Fri 08:00 - 12:00

Organizations: Sexuality

⚥▽ **Homosexuelle Selbsthilfe**
c/o Gemeindehaus, Domlinden 23, 14776 Brandenburg.

Braunschweig

BBSs: Sexuality

⚥▼ **GayBox**
☎ 531 79 6054
📞 531 7 2054
Login: gast (return). Password: (return).

Helplines: Sexuality

⚥▽ **Rosa Telefon—Braunschweig**
☎ 531 1 9411
🕐 Thu 20:00 - 22:00

Organizations: AIDS: Support

☺ □ **AIDS-Hilfe—Braunschweig**
Echternstraße 15, 38100 Braunschweig.
☎ 531 1 9411
🕐 Mon Thu 18:00 - 20:00

Organizations: Sexuality

⚥▽ **Jungendnetzwerk Lambda Niedersachsen e. V.**
c/o Schwartz, Karlstraße 97, 38106 Braunschweig.

⚥▽ **Schwulenreferat beim AStA der TU**
Katharinstraße 1, 38106 Braunschweig.
☎ 531 391 4555

⚥▽ **Verein für Sexuelle Emanzipation e. V. (VSE)**
Echternstraße 15, 38100 Braunschweig.
☎ 531 33 2423 📞 531 34 1105

Organizations: Sexuality: Youth

⚥▽ **Come Out Jungengruppe**
c/o AStA-TU, Katharinstraße 1, 38106 Braunschweig.
☎ 531 391 4556

🕐 2nd. & 4th. Thu of the month 20:00

Stores: Books: General

☺ ■ **Magni**
Ölschlägern 9, 38100 Braunschweig.
☎ 531 4 2429

Stores: Erotica: General

☺ ■ **Boutique Intim**
Freidrich Wilhelm Straße 31, 38100 Braunschweig.
☎ 531 4 4922

☺ ■ **Orion**
Ägidinmarkt 9, 38100 Braunschweig.
☎ 531 4 3283

☺ ■ **Sex Bazar**
Wendenstraße 51, 38100 Braunschweig.
☎ 531 4 0440

☺ ■ **Sex Imtim**
Malertwete 3, 38100 Braunschweig.
☎ 531 4 3541

Bremen

Bars: BDSM

♂▽ **Bronx**
Bohnenstraße 1b, 28203 Bremen.
☎ 421 70 2404
🕐 Sun - Thu 20:00 - ?, Fri Sat 12:30 - ?

Organizations: AIDS: Support

☺ ☐ **AIDS-Hilfe—Bremen**
Am Dobben 66, 28203 Bremen.
☎ 421 1 9411
🕐 Wed 15:00 - 17:00

Organizations: BDSM

♂▽ **LC Nordwest**
c/o Joachim Driefmeier, Friesenstraße 88, 28209 Bremen.
Contact: Herr Kai Lohmüller

Organizations: Family

♂▽ **Eltern Schwuler Söhne & Lesbischwe Töchter**
Rat & Tat Zentrum, Theodor Körner Straße 1, 28203 Bremen.
☎ 421 70 4170
🕐 Call Mon Tue 20:00 - 22:00 for information. 3rd. Fri of month 20:00

♂▽ **Schwule Väter & Ehemänner**
Rat & Tat Zentrum, Theodor Körner Straße 1, 28203 Bremen.
☎ 421 70 4170
🕐 Call Mon Tue 20:00 - 22:00 for information. 1st. Tue of month 20:00

Organizations: Sexuality

♂▼ **Bisexuellengruppe**
Rat & Tat Zentrum, Theodor Körner Straße 1, 28203 Bremen.
☎ 421 70 4170
🕐 Call Mon Tue 20:00 - 22:00 for information. 1st. Thu of month 20:00

♂▽ **Rat & Tat Zentrum**
Theodor Körner Straße 1, 28203 Bremen.
☎ 421 70 4170
🕐 Call Mon Tue 20:00 - 22:00 for information

Organizations: Sexuality: Youth

♂▽ **Sappho & Apoll Schwulen & Lesben-Jungengruppe**
Rat & Tat Zentrum, Theodor Körner Straße 1, 28203 Bremen.
☎ 421 70 4170
🕐 Call Mon Tue 20:00 - 22:00 for information. Sat 17:00 - 19:00

Stores: Books: General

☺ ■ **Humboldt Buchhandlung**
Östertortsteinweg 76, 28203 Bremen.
☎ 421 7 7721
🕐 10:00 - 18:30, 1st. Sat of Month 10:00 - 18:00, else - 14:00

☺ ■ **Montanus Aktuell**
Sägestraße 46, 28195 Bremen.
☎ 421 17 1077

☺ ■ **Wohlthat'sche Buchhandlung**
Wenkenstraße 2, 28195 Bremen.
☎ 421 1 4320

Stores: Clothing: Fetish

☺ ■ **Fashion & Tools**
Herdentorsteinweg 6, 28195 Bremen.
☎ 421 339 8270 📞 421 3398271
🕐 Mon - Sat 09:00 - 18:00
📠 💳 💳
Leather, rubber, & wetlook.

Bremerhaven

Helplines: Sexuality

♂▽ **Rosa Telefon—Bremerhaven**
☎ 471 4 4010
🕐 Wed 20:00 - 22:00, Sun 18:00 - 20:00

♂▽ **Schwule Aktion Bremerhaven**
c/o Kulturcentrum Roter Sand, Karlsburg 7, 27568 Bremerhaven.
☎ 471 4 4010
🕐 Wed 20:00 - 22:00

Stores: Books: General

☺ ■ **Montanus Aktuell**
Columbus Center 55, 27568 Bremerhaven.

Stores: Erotica: General

♂▼ **Channel Six**
Rickmersstraße 77, 27568 Bremerhaven.
☎ 471 5 6595
🕐 Mon - Fri 14:00 - 23:00, Sat 16:00 - 23:00

Celle

Organizations: AIDS: Support

☺ ☐ **AIDS-Hilfe—Celle**
Großer Plan 12, 29221 Celle.
☎ 514 11 9411
🕐 Mon Thu 19:00 - 21:30

Stores: Erotica: General

☺ ■ **Buchfink**
Westcellertorstraße 12, 29221 Celle.
☎ 514 121 7420

☺ ■ **MMV Erotic Shop**
Hannoversche Straße 41, 29221 Celle.

Chemnitz

Health Services

☺ ☐ **Gesundheitsamt Chemnitz**
Rathausstraße 1112 , 09111 Chemnitz.
☎ 371 65 4347

☺ ☐ **Klinikum an Küchwald Infectktionsklinik**
Bürgerstraße 2, 09111 Chemnitz.
☎ 371 33 2644

Helplines: AIDS

♂☐ **Helpline**
☎ 371 1 9411
🕐 Mon Wed 18:00 - 21:00, Sun 15:00 - 18:00

Helplines: Sexuality

♂▽ **CheLSI e. V.**
Rößlerstraße 9, 09120 Chemnitz.
☎ 371 50094 📞 371 55867
🕐 Mon Tue Thu Fri 17:00 - ?, Sat 20:00 - ?, Sun 15:00 - ?

Organizations: AIDS: Support

☺ ☐ **AIDS-Hilfe—Chemnitz**
Hauboldstraße 6, 09111 Chemnitz. 📞 371 41 5223
☎ 371 41 5223
🕐 Tue Thu 15:00 - 20:00, Fri 09:00 14:00

Organizations: BDSM

♂▽ **CLSMC Eagle**
c/o CheLSI e.V., Rößlerstraße 9, 09120 Chemnitz.

Organizations: Sexuality

▷▽ **CheLSI e. V.**
TV/TS Treff Sachsen, Rößlerstraße 9, 09120 Chemnitz. 📞 371 55867
☎ 371 50094
🕐 Call Fri only. Meets 1st Wed of month 19:00

Clausthal-Zellerfeld

Organizations: Sexuality

♂☐ **Schwule Initiative**
c/o AStA, Silberstraße 1, 38678 Clausthal-Zellerfeld.
☎ 532 3 4794

Cottbus
Organizations: AIDS: Education
☺ □ **Mobiles Team AIDS des Landes Brandenburg**
Thiemstraße 104, 03050 Cottbus.
☎ 355 48 8156 ✆ 355 48 8156
🕘 Wed 14:00 - 18:00

Organizations: Sexuality
⚤▽ **Lebensart e. V.**
Thiemstraße 105, 03050 Cottbus.
☎ 355 48 8156 ✆ 355 48 8156

Darmstadt
Helplines: Sexuality
⚤▽ **Ratgeber Schwul Darmstadt**
Hindenburgstraße 35, 64295 Darmstadt.
☎ 615 16 5384
🕘 Mon Tue Fri 19:00 - 22:00
Counselling & information.

Organizations: Sexuality
⚤▽ **Schwulengruppe Darmstadt**
c/o Günter Koch, Mathildenstraße 54, 64285 Darmstadt.
☎ 615 14 5691
🕘 Meets Wed 21:00

Organizations: Sexuality: Student
⚤▽ **Pink & Purple**
Hochschulstraße 1, 64289 Darmstadt.
🕘 Tue 19:00

Dillenburg
Organizations: AIDS: Support
☺ □ **AIDS-Hilfe—Dillenburg**
☎ 277 11 9411
🕘 Wed 17:00 - 19:00

Dinslaken
Organizations: AIDS: Support
☺ □ **AIDS-Hilfe—Duisburg**
☎ 213 41 9411
🕘 Mon - Fri 09:00 - 17:00

Dollnstein
Organizations: AIDS: Support
☺ □ **AIDS-Hilfe—Eichstätt**
c/o Annett Schroer, Obere Dorfstraße 3, 91795 Dollnstein.
🕘 Tue 19:00 - 21:30

Donaueschingen
Stores: Erotica: General
☺ ■ **Intim Shop**
Bahnhofstraße 27, 78166 Donaueschingen.
🕘 Mon - Fri 09:00 - 12:30, 15:30 - 18:30, Sat 09:00 - 19:00

Dortmund
Bars: BDSM
⚤▼ **Don-Club**
Johannisborn Straße 6, 44135 Dortmund.
☎ 231 55 3221
🕘 21:00 - ?

Helplines: Sexuality
⚤▽ **Café Stonewall**
c/o Ché Coolala, Heyden Rynch Straße 2, 44149 Dortmund.
☎ 231 17 8145
🕘 Tue 20:00 - ?

⚤▽ **Rosa Hilfe**
c/o KCR, Braunschweiger Straße 22, 44145 Dortmund.
☎ 231 83 1919
🕘 Wed 19:00 - 22:00

Organizations: AIDS: Support
☺ □ **AIDS-Hilfe—Dortmund**
Klosterstraße 14, 44135 Dortmund.
☎ 231 52 7637
🕘 Mon Tue Thu 08:30 - 17:00, Wed 10:30 - 19:00, Fri 08:00 - 15:30

☺ □ **Klinik HIV Station**
Westfalendamm 403-307, 44143 Dortmund.
☎ 231 4 5090

Organizations: Motorcycle
⚤▽ **MSC Rote Erde Dortmund**
Postfach 102739, 44027 Dortmund.
🕘 Meets 1st. & 3rd. Fri of the month 21:00

Organizations: Sexuality
⚤▽ **BVH e. V. - Dortmund**
c/o Stephan Kleinschulte, Flemerskam 61, 44319 Dortmund.
☎ 231 28 3333
🕘 Mon 20:00

Organizations: Sexuality: Student
⚤▽ **Schwulen- & Lesben-Initiative der Universität Dortmund**
c/o AStA der Universität, Emil Figge Straße 50, 44227 Dortmund.
🕘 Thu 17:00 - ?

Radio: Sexuality
⚤▽ ***Homo laber***
FM 91.2, c/o KCR, Braunschweiger Straße 22, 44145 Dortmund.
🕘 2nd. & last Fri of the month 19:00 - 20:00

Stores: Books: General
⚤▼ **LITFASS Der Buchladen**
Münsterstraße 107, 44145 Dortmund.
☎ 231 83 4724 ✆ 231 83 0292
🕘 Mon - Fri 10:00 - 18:30, Sat 10:00 - 13:00
✓
English, French, & Dutch also spoken.

Stores: Erotica: General
⚤▼ **Adonis Center**
Bornstraße 14, 44135 Dortmund.
☎ 231 57 3619
🕘 12:00 - 18:30, Sat 10:00 - 14:00
Also mail order.

Dresden
Helplines: Sexuality
⚤▽ **Gerede-Dresdener Lesben, Schwule, & Alle Anderen**
1st. Floor, Haus der Jungend, Wiener Straße 41, 01219 Dresden.
☎ 351 464 0220 ✆ 351 464 0247
🕘 Mon - Fri 09:00 - 17:00

Organizations: AIDS: Support
☺ □ **AIDS-Beratung im Gesundheit Dresden**
Prellerstraße 5, 01309 Dresden.
☎ 351 3 0126
🕘 Tu Thu Fri 08:00 - 12:00 Tue 13:00 - 18:00, Thu 13:00 - 15:00
Information, counselling, & support for people infected with or affected by HIV/AIDS.

☺ ▽ **AIDS-Hilfe—Dresden**
2nd. Floor, Haus der Jungend, Wiener Straße 41, 01219 Dresden.
☎ 351 464 0213 ✆ 351 464 0247
🕘 Mon - Fri 09:00 - 12:00 13:00 - 14:00, Thu 18:00 - 21:00

Organizations: BDSM
⚤▽ **Lederclub Dresden**
Postfach 200118, 02291 Dresden.

⚤▽ **SMC Dresden**
Postfach 192402, 01282 Dresden.

Organizations: Sexuality: Youth
⚤▽ **Lambda-Junge Lesben & Schwule im Freistaat Sachsen e. V.**
Louisenstraße 56, 01099 Dresden.

Duisberg
Organizations: AIDS: Support
☺ ■ **AIDS-Hilfe—Duisburg**
Frieden Straße 100, 47053 Duisberg.
☎ 281 1 9411
☎ 203 1 9411
Office number: 203 66 6633.

Duisburg
Helplines: Sexuality
⚤▽ **Rosa Telefon—Duisburg**
☎ 203 66 3383
🕘 Tue 20:00 - 22:00

Organizations: Family

☺ □ **Pro Familia Homosexuellenberatung**
Oststraße 172, 47198 Duisburg.
☎ 203 35 0700
🕘 Tue 19:00 - 21:00

Organizations: Sexuality

⚥ ▽ **Homosexuelle Kultur Duisburg**
Postfach 100709, 47007 Duisburg.
🕘 3rd. Fri of month 20:00

⚥ ▽ **Lesch-Selbsthilfegruppe Lesben & Schwule**
Postfach 660226, 47131 Duisburg.
🕘 1st. & 3rd. Fri of month

⚥ ▽ **The Pink Homo**
c/o Beck, Friedrich Ebert Straße 115, 47119 Duisburg.
☎ 203 87 1083
🕘 Fri 18:00

Organizations: Sexuality: Student

⚥ ▽ **SchwBile Referat**
c/o AStA GH Duisburg, Lotharstraße 65, 47057 Duisburg.
☎ 203 37 0047

Stores: Erotica: General

⚦ ▼ **Man Shop**
Kasinostraße 4a, 47051 Duisburg.
☎ 203 2 3300
🕘 09:00 - 24:00, Sun 13:00 - 23:00

Düsseldorf

Bars: BDSM

⚥ ▼ **Musk**
Charlottenstraße 47, 40210 Düsseldorf.
☎ 211 35 2154
🕘 Thu - Sat 21:00 - 05:000, Sun - Wed 21:00 - 01:00

Helplines: Sexuality

⚥ ▽ **Gay Hotline**
c/o AStA-Schwulenreferat, Universitätstraße 1, 40225 Düsseldorf.
☎ 211 311 5283
🕘 Wed 18:00 - 21:00

Organizations: AIDS: Support

☺ ■ **AIDS-Hilfe—Düsseldorf**
Oberbilker Allee 310, 40227 Düsseldorf.
☎ 211 19411 — 📠 211 726 0536
☎ 211 726 0526

☺ □ **DGSS Institut**
Gerresheimer Straße 20, 40211 Düsseldorf.
☎ 211 35 4591 — 📠 211 36 0777
🕘 09:00 -22:00
Information, counselling, & support for people infected with or affected by HIV/AIDS.

☺ □ **Gesundheitsamt AIDS-Beratungstelle**
Kölner Straße 180, 40227 Düsseldorf.
☎ 211 899 2663
🕘 Mon - Fri 08:00 - 15:00

☺ □ **Treffpunkt Regenbogen**
BorsigStraße 34, 40227 Düsseldorf.
☎ 221 72 0186
🕘 Mon - Fri 11:00 - 17:00, Thu 19:00 - 22:00, Sun 16:00 - 20:00

Organizations: BDSM

⚥ ▽ **Black Hedgehogs Rheinland**
Adersstaße 80, 40000 Düsseldorf.
Contact: Herr Kai-Ralf Kunath

⚥ ▽ **Leather Men Düsseldorf**
Postfach 102005, 40011 Düsseldorf.
Contact: Herr Alf Dahlwitz

Organizations: Sexuality

⚥ ▽ **Schwulengruppe Düsseldorf**
c/o Luszd, Kronenstraße 72-74, 40217 Düsseldorf.
☎ 211 36 4260

Organizations: Sexuality: Student

⚥ ▽ **AStA-Schwulenreferat**
Universitätstraße 1, 40225 Düsseldorf.
☎ 211 311 5283
🕘 Mon - Thu 12:00, Tue 18:00 - ?

Organizations: Sexuality: Youth

⚥ ▽ **Jungendberatung Düsseldorf (JUB)**
Grafenberger Allee 115, 40237 Düsseldorf.
☎ 211 67 3058
🕘 Mon - Sat 11:00 - 21:00

Publishers: Newspapers: Sexuality

⚥ ▼ ***Facette***
c/o LuSzD, Postfach 320745, 40422 Düsseldorf.
☎ 211 34 4610 — 📠 211 28 4875
☎ 211 28 1404

Radio: Sexuality

⚥ ***Rosa Mickrowelle***
☎ 211 733 6540
🕘 1st Thu of the month 19:00

Stores: Books: General

⚥ ▼ **Gegen den Strich Buchcafé**
Bilker Straße23A, 40213 Düsseldorf.
☎ 211 323 7938 — 📠 211 323 7939
🕘 Tue - Fri 10:00 - 18:30, Sat 10:00 - 14:00

Stores: Clothing: Fetish

☺ ■ **Annette K Fashions**
Helmholtzstraße 28, 4000 Düsseldorf.
☎ 211 37 4476 — 📠 211 680 3826
Catalogue, £7 to U.K., $10U.S. to U.S., FF60 to France.

☺ ■ **Fashion Cats**
Vulkanstraße 33, 40277 Düsseldorf.
☎ 211 787276
🕘 Sun - Fri 10:00 - 18:30, Sat 09:00 - 14:00

☺ ■ **Sexy Cats**
Industriestraße 10, 40227 Düsseldorf.

Stores: Clothing: Footwear

☺ ■ **Buzios Mode**
Kronenstraße 48, 40217 Düsseldorf.
☎ 211 333736

Stores: Erotica: BDSM

⚥ ▼ **Schneiderei Ottokar Fischer**
Schützenstraße 71, 40211 Düsseldorf.
☎ 211 35 9486
🕘 Mon - Fri 09:00 - 13:00 15:00 - 18:30, Sat 10:00 - 14:00

Eckernförde

Health Services

☺ □ **Gesundheitsamt**
Schleswiger Straße 3, 24340 Eckernförde.
☎ 435 188 22567
🕘 Wed 16:00 - 18:00

Eichstätt

Organizations: AIDS: Support

☺ □ **AIDS-Hilfe—Eichstätt**
Postfach 1329, 850067 Eichstätt.
☎ 842 1 8488
🕘 Tue 19:30 - 21:30

Eisenach

Organizations: AIDS: Support

☺ □ **AIDS-Hilfe—Wartburgkreis**
Marienstraße 57, 99817 Eisenach.
☎ 369 121 4083
🕘 Tue 11:00 - 15:00, Thu 14:0 - 19:00, Fri 10:00 - 12:00

Organizations: Sexuality

⚥ ▽ **Schwul in Eisenach—Wartburgkreis**
c/o AIDS-Hilfe Eisenach, Marienstraße 57, 99817 Eisenach.
☎ 369 121 4083
🕘 Meets 2nd. & 4th. Thu of month 19:00

Elmshorn

Helplines: Sexuality

⚥ ▽ **Rosa Telefon—Elmshorn**
☎ 412 16 5058
🕘 Wed 19:00 - 20:00

Organizations: AIDS: Support

☺ □ **AIDS-Hilfe—Kreis Pinneberg / Steinfurt**
Postfach 422, 25304 Elmshorn.
☎ 412 11 9411
🕘 Thu 20:00

Organizations: Sexuality
⚦▽ **Schwulengruppe Elmshorn**
c/o AIDS-Hilfe, Vormstegen 25, 25336 Elmshorn.
☎ 412 18 8943
🕐 Thu 20:00

Emden
Organizations: Sexuality
⚦▽ **Lesben- & Schwuengruppe Emden**
c/o AIDS- & Drogenberatung Emden, Am Alten Binnenhafen 2, 26721 Emden.
☎ 49 212 6501
🕐 1st. Wed of the month 20:00
Contact: Ralf

Organizations: Sexuality: Youth
⚦▽ **Ostfreisische Schwulen- & Lesbeninitiative**
Früchteburgerweg 1, 26721 Emden.
☎ 492 12 9522
🕐 Every other Fri 20:00

Erfurt
Health Services
☺ □ **Gesundheitsamt Erfurt**
HIV-Antikörpertest, Turniergasse 17, Erfurt.
☎ 361 655 1744
HIV testing.

Helplines: Sexuality
⚦▽ **Gay Line**
☎ 361 66 6764
🕐 18:00 - 23:00
⚦▽ **Rosa Telefon—Erfurt**
☎ 361 731 2458
🕐 Wed 18:00 - 22:00

Organizations: AIDS: Support
☺ □ **AIDS-Hilfe—Thüringen**
Postfach 50, 99091 Erfurt.
☎ 361 731 2233
☎ 361 19411 (hotline)
📱 361 312458
🕐 Mon - Fri 10:00 - 15:00. Sun 14:00 - 18:00
Publishes *HIT Magazine.*

Organizations: BDSM
⚦▽ **Thüringer Lederclub (TLC)**
Postfach 124, 99003 Erfurt.
☎ 361 731 2233
🕐 Meets 2nd. Sun of month 17:00

Organizations: Family
⚦□ **Schwüle Väter**
c/o AIDS-Hilfe, Postfach 50, 99001 Erfurt.
☎ 361 731 2233
🕐 Meets 4th. Tue of month 18:00

Organizations: Sexuality
⚦▽ **Schwulengruppen**
c/o AIDS-Hilfe Thüringen, Postfach 50, 99091 Erfurt.
☎ 361 731 2233
📱 361 312458
🕐 Meets 2nd. & 4th. Fri of month 20:00
⚧▽ **TRANSITAS**
c/o AIDS-Hilfe Thüringen, Postfach 50, 99091 Erfurt.
☎ 361 731 2233
📱 361 312458
🕐 Meets 1st. & 3rd. Tue of month 18:00

Stores: Books: General
☺ ■ **Haus des Buches Carl Habel GmbH**
Juri Gagarin Ring 35, 99084 Erfurt.
☎ 361 2 3033
📱 351 2 6461

Erlangen
Organizations: Sexuality
⚦▽ **Magnus Hirschfeld Zentrum**
2nd. Floor, Hilpertstraße 23, 91052 Erlangen.
☎ 913 18 0050
🕐 14:00 - 01:00, Sun 14:00 - 20:00

Organizations: Sexuality: Student
⚦▽ **Schwulenreferat im SprecherInnenrat der Friedrich-Alexander Universität Erlangen Nürnberg**
Turnstraße 7, 91054 Erlangen.
☎ 913 185 6695

🕐 Meets Wed 18:00

Essen
Bars: BDSM
⚦▼ **Number One**
Lindenallee 71, 45127 Essen.
☎ 201 23 6682
🕐 Wed leather night

Competitions & Conventions: Fetish: Clothing
☺ **Feticon**
c/o Creative Business, Steeler Straße 137, 45138 Essen.

Helplines: Sexuality
⚦▽ **Gay Hotline**
c/o Schwulenreferat im AStA der GH Essen, Universitätsstraße 2, 45141 Essen.
☎ 201 183 3392
🕐 Thu 18:00 - 20:00

Organizations: AIDS: Support
☺ □ **AIDS-Hilfe—Essen**
Varnhorststraße 17, 45127 Essen.
☎ 201 1 9411
🕐 Tue Thu 16:00 - 22:00

Organizations: BDSM
⚦▽ **Lederfreunde Rhein-Ruhr Essen (LFRR)**
c/o Club Go-In, Steeler Straße 83, 45127 Essen.
☎ 201 236161
☎ 201 752023
🕐 Meets 1st. Mon of month

Organizations: Sexuality
⚦▽ **Homosexuelle Initiative Essen (HIE)**
Postfach 101530, 45015 Essen.
☎ 201 4 2924
🕐 Tue 19:30
⚦▽ **Rosa Aktionsgruppe Essen (RAGE)**
c/o AIDS-Hilfe Essen, Varnhorststraße 17, 45127 Essen.
☎ 201 23 6096
🕐 Sun 19:30
⚧▽ **TSH—Essen**
Caesar Straße 34, 45130 Essen.
☎ 201 78 6999
Contact: Fraulein Claudia Peppenhorst

Organizations: Sexuality: Student
⚦▽ **Schwulenreferat im AStA der GH Essen**
Universitätsstraße 2, 45141 Essen.
☎ 201 183 3392

Stores: Erotica: General
⚦▼ **Eros Boutique**
Klarastraße 19, 45130 Essen.
☎ 201 78 8321
🕐 Mon - Fri 10:00 - 18:00, Sat - 14:00

Esslingen
Piercers
☺ ■ **Suzie Q Pleasure & Pain**
c/o Tattoo You, Sirnauer Straße 23, 73728 Esslingen.

Finnentrop
Organizations: AIDS: Support
☺ □ **AIDS-Hilfe—Kreis Olpe**
Attendorner 45, 57413 Finnentrop.
☎ 276 11 9411
🕐 Mon 19:00 21:00

Flensburg
Helplines: Sexuality
⚦▽ **Rosa Telefon—Flensburg**
☎ 461 2 1347
🕐 Tue 18:00 - 19:00

Organizations: AIDS: Support
☺ □ **AIDS-Hilfe—Flensburg**
Postfach 1111, 24901 Flensburg.
☎ 461 1 9411
🕐 Wed 18:00 - 21:00, Thu 16:00 - 19:00

Organizations: Sexuality
⚥▽ **Flensburger Initiative & Treffpunkt für Schwule**
c/o AIDS-Hilfe, Postfach 1111, 24901 Flensburg.
☎ 461 2 5618

Frankfurt am Main
Archives: Sexuality
⚥▽ **Schwules Archiv**
c/o Archiv für Sexualpolitik, Brönnerstraße 9, 60313 Frankfurt.
☎ 69 29 6797 ✆ 69 28 9181

Bars: BDSM
⚥▽ **Construction Five**
Alte Gasse 5, 60313 Frankfurt.
☎ 69 29 1356
🕐 Fri Sat 22:00 - ?

⚥▽ **Stall**
Stiftstraße 20, 60313 Frankfurt.
☎ 69 29 1880
🕐 21:00 - 04:00

Helplines: AIDS
☺ ☐ **AIDS Telefon**
☎ 69 63 6036

Helplines: Sexuality
⚥▽ **Rosa Hilfe**
c/o V. S. B. N., Postfach 111903, 60019 Frankfurt.
☎ 69 28 8080
🕐 sun 18:00 - 22:00

⚥▽ **Switchboard**
☎ 69 28 3535
🕐 Tue - Sun 19:00 - 22:00

Organizations: AIDS: Support
☺ ☐ **AIDS-Beratung-Stelle der Stadt Frankfurt**
Mörfelder Landstraße 6, Frankfurt.

☺ ☐ **AIDS-Hilfe—Frankfurt**
Friedberger Anlage 24, 60316 Frankfurt.
☎ 69 1 9411
🕐 Mon Tue Thu Fri 17:00 - 19:00, Wed 17:00 - 21:00

Organizations: BDSM
⚥▽ **Frankfurter Lederclub e. V. (FLC)**
Große Friedbergerstraße 19, 60313 Frankfurt.
☎ 69 29 3904
🕐 Meets 1st. Wed of month
Contact: Herr Hans-J. Müller

Organizations: Bears
⚥▽ **AHF-Switchboard (CIC)**
Alte Gaße 36, 6000 Frankfurt.

Organizations: Sexuality
⚥▽ **Club für Gleichgeschlechtlich Liebende e. V. (GL)**
Franz Mehring Straße 20, 15230 Frankfurt (Oder).
☎ 335 32 1051
🕐 Mon - Fri 09:00 - 17:00

⚥▽ **Emanzipation e. V.**
Klingerstraße 6, 60313 Frankfurt.
☎ 69 297 7296

⋈▽ **Freedom of Personality Expression (FPE)—Frankfurt**
c/o Kröcher & Surhoff, Postfach 800442, 65904 Frankfurt.

⚥▽ **Informationszentrum für Männer**
Neuhofstraße 41, 60318 Frankfurt.
☎ 69 597 0959
🕐 Mon Thu 17:00 - 20:00
Information, counselling, & support.

Organizations: Sexuality: Student
⚥▽ **Frankfurter Schwule, Automones AStA-Schwulenreferat**
J. W. Goethe Universität, Mertonstraße 26-28, 60325 Frankfurt.
☎ 69 77 7575 ✆ 69 70 2039

Organizations: Sexuality: Youth
⚥▽ **Schwule Jungendclique Frankfurt**
c/o Switchboard, Alte Gasse 36, 60313 Frankfurt.
☎ 69 28 3535
🕐 Wed 21:00

Stores: Books: General
☺ ■ **Hugendubel**
Steinweg 12, 60313 Frankfurt.
☎ 69 29 9820

☺ ■ **Land in Sight**
Rotteckstraße 11-13, 60316 Frankfurt.
☎ 69 44 3095
🕐 Mon - Fri 10:00 - 18:30, Sat - 14:00

⚥▽ **Oscar Wilde Buchladen**
♿ Alte Gasse 51, 60313 Frankfurt.
☎ 69 28 1260 ✆ 69 129 77542
🕐 Mon - Fri 10:30 - 19:00, Sat 10:00 - 16:00
✓ ⤷ 🌐 💳 🅳
Books, videos, CDs, magazines, postcards, & accessories for gay guys & girls. Age statement of 18 is required. English & French also spoken.

Stores: Clothing: Fetish
☺ ■ **Fetische in Leder, Latex, & Lack**
Rotlinstraße 11, 60316 Frankfurt.
☎ 69 43 9187
🕐 Mon 14:00 - 17:00, Tue Wed Fri 10:00 - 18:00, Thu 10:00 - 17:30, Sat 10:00 - 13:00

Stores: Erotica: General
⚥▽ **Backdoor**
Schäffergasse 27, 60313 Frankfurt.
☎ 69 28 4311
🕐 Mon - Sat 10:00 - 20:00

☺ ■ **Beate Uhse**
Kaiserstraße 53, 60329 Frankfurt.
☎ 69 23 6280
🕐 09:00 - 18:30, Thu - 20:30, Sat - 14:00

☺ ■ **Beate Uhse**
Kaiserstraße 79, 60329 Frankfurt.
🕐 Mon - Wed Fri 11:30 - 18:30, Thu - 20:00, Sat 11:30 - 14:30, 1st. Sat of month - 18:00

☺ ■ **Kunomeiden GMBH**
Eckenheimer Landstraße 60b, 60318 Frankfurt.

Freiburg
Helplines: Sexuality
⚥▽ **Rosa Telefon—Freiburg**
☎ 761 2 5161
🕐 Thu 19:30 - 21:30

Organizations: AIDS: Support
☺ ☐ **AIDS-Hilfe—Freiburg**
1755, 79017 Freiburg.
☎ 761 1 9411 ✆ 761 28 8112
🕐 Mon - Fri 10:00 - 13:00, Mon Tue 15:00 - 17:00, Wed 17:00 - 19:00

Organizations: Motorcycle
⚥▽ **MSC Südwest**
Postfach 1105, 79010 Freiburg.

Organizations: Sexuality
⚥▽ **Rosa Hilfe**
Escholtzstraße 19, 79106 Freiburg.
☎ 761 2 5161
🕐 Meets Fri 19:00

Publishers: Newspapers: Sexuality
⚥▽ **Gay-Plus**
c/o Jos Fritz, Wilhelmstraße 15, 79098 Freiburg.
☎ 761 7 7188
Free at gay locations.

Fremdingen
Organizations: AIDS: Support
☺ ☐ **AIDS-Hilfe—Ansbach / Dinkelsbühl**
c/o Georg Großiebel, Rautstetten 9, 86742 Fremdingen.

Freudstadt
Organizations: Sexuality
⚥▽ **Schwulengruppe Freudstadt**
Postfach 902, 72239 Freudstadt.

Fulda
Helplines: Sexuality
⚥▽ **Schwule Beratung**

☎ 661 19446
Beratungsinititive & Schwulenorganization Fulda. Counselling, information, & support.

Organizations: AIDS: Support

☺ □ **AIDS-Hilfe—Fulda**
Friedrichstraße 4, 36037 Fulda.
☎ 661 77011
🕘 Walk-in Mon - Thu 19:00 - 21:00

Organizations: Sexuality

⚤▽ **BiSchoF e. V.**
Postfach 204, 36002 Fulda.
Beratungsinititive & Schwulenorganization Fulda. Counselling, information, & support. Publishes *GAYzette*.

Organizations: Sexuality: Student

⚤▽ **Schwulenreferat ASta in der FH Fulda**
Marquardstraße 35, 36039 Fulda.
☎ 661 60 2162 📠 661 6 6251
🕘 Mon - Fri 10:00 - 14:00
Counselling, information, & support.

Fürth

Stores: Clothing: Fetish

☺ ■ **Sin-A-Matic**
Glückstraße 13, 90763 Fürth.
☎ 911 709 017 📠 911 785 246
Leather, latex, PVC, magazines, high heels, & body jewelry & piercing. Mail order, retail, & wholesale.

Gaggenau

Organizations: Sexuality

⚤▽ **Gay Liberation Forum Baden-Baden**
Postfach 1471, 76554 Gaggenau.

Geldern

Organizations: Sexuality

⚤▽ **Schwül-lesbischer Stammtisch**
c/o Schwarzbrenner, Kapuzinerstraße 4, 47608 Geldern.
☎ 2831 89233
🕘 Wed 20:00
Gays & lesbians meeting for friendship & cultural & social intersts. Everybody is welcome.

Gelnhausen

Stores: Erotica: General

⚤■ **Rosa Blum**
c/o Mike Mathes, Carl Becker Straße 15, 63571 Gelnhausen.
☎ 605 11 2561
🕘 Fri 19:00

Gelsenkirchen

Organizations: AIDS: Support

☺ ▽ **AIDS-Hilfe—Gelsenkircher**
c/o Kontacktzentrum, Husemannstraße 39-41, 45879 Gelsenkirchen.
☎ 209 1 9411
🕘 Mon 20:00 - 22:00

Organizations: Sexuality

⚤▽ **Gelsenkirchen Lesben- & Schwulenintiative**
c/o Trotzalledam Intiativzentrum, Weberstraße 79, 45879 Gelsenkirchen.
☎ 209 20 1171
🕘 Fri 20:00

Photographers: Erotic

☺ **Wolfgang Eichler**
Beethovenstraße 17, 45884 Gelsenkirchen.
☎ 20 913 4794 📠 20 913 9888

Stores: Clothing: Rubber

☺ ■ **Leder-Gummistudio**
Bochumerstraße 76, 45886 Gelsenkirchen.
☎ 209 22214
🕘 Mon - Fri 09:00 - 18:30, 1st. Sat of month 09:00 - 18:00, else - 14:00
Also body piercing. Catalogue available.

Gera

Helplines: Sexuality

⚤▽ **Rosa Telefon—Gera**
☎ 365 710 6303
🕘 Wed 19:00 - 23:00

Organizations: Sexuality

⚤▽ **Schwule Akzeptanz Gera (SIAG)**
c/o HPA Postlagernd, 07845 Gera.

Stores: Art Galleries

☺ **Museum für Angewandte Kunst**
Im Ferbeschen Haus, Geizer Straße 37, 07545 Gera.

Germersheim

Organizations: Sexuality

⚤▽ **Schwule Gruppe Germersheim**
☎ 727 4 4089

Gießen

Helplines: Sexuality

⚤▽ **Rosa Telefon—Gießen**
☎ 641 38 9294
🕘 Fri 19:00 - 21:00

Organizations: AIDS: Support

☺ □ **AIDS-Hilfe—Gießen**
Diezstraße 8, 35390 Gießen.
☎ 641 1 9411
🕘 Thu 14:00 - 18:00

Organizations: Sexuality

⚤▽ **Selbsthilfegruppe Gießen**
Postfach 100401, 35334 Gießen.
☎ 641 38 9294
🕘 Fri 21:00 - ?. Telephone Fri 19:00 - 21:00

Gladbeck

Organizations: Sexuality

⚤▽ **Schwule Initiative Gladbeck**
Rosa Telephon, c/o Die Grünen, Friedenstraße 5, 45964 Gladbeck.
☎ 204 32 5412
🕘 'Phone Tue 19:00 - 22:00

Radio: Sexuality

⚤▽ ***Emscher-Lipper Andersrum***
FM 96.1 or FM 104.5, Freidenstraße 5, 45964 Gladbeck.
🕘 Last Fri of month 10:00 - 19:30

Görlitz

Organizations: Sexuality

⚤▽ **Görlitzer Homosexuelleninitiative**
c/o Laus Szczeszak, Schanze 13, 02826 Görlitz.

Göttingen

Helplines: Sexuality

⚤▽ **Telefonberatung Homosexualität**
☎ 551 4 3438
🕘 Mon 20:00 - 22:00

Organizations: AIDS: Support

☺ □ **AIDS-Hilfe—Göttingen**
Obere Karspüle 14, 37073 Göttingen.
☎ 551 1 9411
🕘 Tue 19:00 - 21:00, Wed 11:00 - 13:00, Thu 16:00 - 18:00

Organizations: Sexuality

⚤■ **Automones Schwulenreferat im AStA**
Goßler Straße 16a, 37073 Göttingen.
☎ 551 39 4571
🕘 Meets Tue 20:00. Call Tue 15:00 - 17:00, Thu 11:00 - 13:00

⚤▽ **Coming Our Gruppe**
c/o Pro Familia, Rote Straße 19, 37073 Göttingen.
🕘 Thu 20:00

⚤▽ **Schwule Hilfe Göttingen**
Postfach 1151, 37116 Göttingen.
☎ 551 8 3355

Stores: Books: General

☺ ■ **Montanus Aktuell**
Weender Straße 21, 37073 Göttingen.

Greifswald

Organizations: Sexuality

⚤▽ **Rosa Greif-Schwul-Lesbischer AK im Vorpommern e. V.**

Postfach 3, 17462 Greifswald.
☎ 383 4 3463
🕒 Thu 19:00

⚥▽ **Verein für Lesben & Schwule**
c/o Sozialkulturelles Zentrum St. Spiritus, Lange Straße 49, 17849 Greifswald.
🕒 Thu 18:00 - 22:00

Güdingen

Stores: Clothing: Leather

⚥▼ **Adler & Schmitt Lederwerkstatt**
Postfach 1306, Güdingen.
📠 681 85 2994

Gummersbach

Organizations: Sexuality

⚥▽ **Schwule Gruppe Oberberg**
Postfach 310123, 51616 Gummersbach.
☎ 226 59152
☎ 226 15 2477

Hagen

Helplines: Sexuality

⚥▽ **Gay Line Hagen**
c/o AIDS-Hilfe, Christian Rohlfs Straße 1, 58089 Hagen.
☎ 233 133 8833
🕒 Mon 20:00 - 22:00

Organizations: AIDS: Support

☺ □ **AIDS-Hilfe—Hagen**
Christian Rohlfs Straße 1, 58089 Hagen.
☎ 233 11 9411
🕒 Mon - 20:00 - 22:00, Tue 19:00 - 21:00, Wed 09:00 - 12:00, Fri 14:00 - 16:00

Organizations: Sexuality

⚥▽ **Homosexuelle Interessengruppe Hagen (HIGH)**
Lange Straße 30, 58089 Hinterhaus.
🕒 Fri 20:00

Stores: Books: General

☺ ■ **Montanus Aktuell**
Eberfelder Straße 31, 58095 Hagen.

Halberstadt

Organizations: AIDS: Support

☺ □ **AIDS-Hilfe—Halberstadt**
Finckestraße 7, 38820 Halberstadt.
🕒 Mon - Fri 10:00 - 14:00

Halle (Saale)

Film Festivals: Sexuality

⚥▽ **Schwul-lesbische Filmtage**
c/o BBZ "lebensart" e. V., Joliot-Curie Platz 29/30, 06108 Halle (Saale).
☎ 345 512 5103 📠 345 512 5103
🕒 Second half of October

Organizations: AIDS: Support

⚥▽ **AIDS-Hilfe—Halle**
Magdeburger Straße 34, 06112 Halle (Saale).
☎ 345 3 6419 📠 345 3 5419
☎ 345 1 9411
🕒 Office Mon - Fri 10:00 - 18:00. Health service Tue Thu 17:00 - 20:00

Organizations: Sexuality

⚥▽ **Begegnungs- & Beratungs-Zentrum lebensart e. V.**
Joliot Curie Platz 29/30, 06108 Halle (Saale).
☎ 345 512 5103 📠 345 512 5103
🕒 Mon Wed 14:00 - 18:00, Tue Thu - 20:00, Fri 14:00 - 22:00
Publishes *Homo Sum* every month.

♀ ▽ **Dornrosa - Frauenselbsthilfe e. V.**
Große Klausstraße 11, 06108 Halle (Saale).
☎ 345 202 4331 📠 345 202 4331

Stores: Books: General

☺ ■ **Litfass**
Rannische Straße 14-15, 06108 Halle (Saale).
☎ 345 2 4263

☺ ▼ **Proteus**
Thomas Müntzer Platz 2, 06114 Halle (Saale).
☎ 345 50 3649
🕒 Mon - Fri 09:00 - 18:00, Sat - 14:00

Hamburg

Accommodation: BDSM

⚥▼ **Hotel Adler**
Ernst Mercke Straße 10, 20099 Hamburg.
☎ 40 24 5640 📠 40 24 5619

Archives: Sexuality

⚥▽ **Verein Schwulenkultur e. V.**
c/o Café Tuc Tuc, Oelkersallee 5, 22769 Hamburg.
☎ 40 430 0695
🕒 Wed - Fri 20:30 - 23:00

Bars: BDSM

⚥▼ **Black**
Danziger Straße 21, 20099 Hamburg.
☎ 40 24 0804
🕒 Sun - Thu 22:00 - 03:00, Fri Sat 22:00 - ?

⚥▼ **Café Adler**
Ernst Mercke Straße 8, 20099 Hamburg.
🕒 09:00 - ?, Fri Sat 10:00 - ?

⚥▼ **Chaps**
Woltmanstraße 24, 20097 Hamburg.
☎ 40 23 0647
🕒 Fri Sat 22:00 - 04:00, Sun 15:00 - 02:00

⚥▼ **Tom's Saloon**
Pulverteich 17, 20099 Hamburg.
☎ 40 280 3056
🕒 22:00 - 04:00, Fri Sat - ?

Helplines: Sexuality

⚥ **Hein & Feite Switchboard**
♿ Kleiner Pulverteich 19, 20099 Hamburg.
☎ 40 24 0333 📠 40 24 0675
🕒 Mon - Fri 16:00 - 21:00, Sat - 19:00
Information on everything that's of interest to gay or bisexual men. Also streetwork & HIV prevention. English also spoken.

Manufacturers: Clothing: Fetish

⚥ **Karo Design**
Postfach 601303, 22213 Hamburg.
☎ 40 279 6121 📠 40 279 8910
Fetish clothes made from air-cushion film, plastic net, showercurtains, & other unusual materials. Catalogue available.

Manufacturers: Clothing: Rubber

☺ ▼ **Rik Production**
Gurlittstraße 47, 20099 Hamburg.
☎ 40 24 5979 📠 40 24 6097
🕒 Mon - Wed Fri 10:30 -18:30, Thu 10:30 - 20:30, Sat 10:30 - 14:00
VISA MC
Leather, rubber, & toys. Mail order service also available.

Organizations: AIDS: Support

☺ □ **AIDS-Hilfe—Hamburg**
Paul Roosen Straße 43, 22767 Hamburg.
☎ 40 1 9411 📠 40 319 6984
🕒 Telephone: Mon - Wed 18:00 - 21:00, Tue 16:00 - 21:00, Thu 18:00 - 21:00. In person: Tue 16:00 - 19:00, Wed 10:00 - 12:00

☺ □ **Ökumenischer Arbeitskreis AIDS**
Otzenstraße 19, 22767 Hamburg.
☎ 40 43 4696

☺ □ **Palette Hamburg e. V. im Schantezhof**
Bartelsstraße 12, 20357 Hamburg.
☎ 40 430 2777 📠 40 43 3096
Counselling for people infected with or affected by HIV/AIDS.

Organizations: BDSM

⚥▽ **Gruppe Leder SM (GLSM)**
Postfach 323448, 20119 Hamburg.
☎ 40 313540
🕒 Meets 2nd. Sat of month 23:45

⚥▽ **Lederclub Hamburg (LCH)**
Reineckstraße 16, 22761 Hamburg.
🕒 Meets Thu 22:00
Contact: Herr Reiner Hölscher

⚥▽ **Lederclub HH**
c/o Black, Danziger Straße 21, 20099 Hamburg.
☎ 40 24 0804

☺ □ **Molotov**

Spielbundenplatz 9, 20359 Hamburg.
☎ 40 319 2633
⏰ 1st. Fri of every 2nd month
BDSM parties.

Organizations: Bears
⚥▽ **Bären Hamburg**
Gurlittstraße 47, 2000 Hamburg.

Organizations: Body Size
⚥▽ **Girth & Mirth—Deutschland: Hamburg**
Postfach 302023, 20307 Hamburg.
☎ 40 28 0289

Organizations: Motorcycle
⚥▽ **MC Nordlicht Hamburg**
c/o Chaps, Woltmannstraße 24, 20097 Hamburg.
⚥▽ **MSC Hamburg e. V.**
Postfach 303683, 20312 Hamburg.

Organizations: Research: Sexuality
⚥□ **Sexuallberatungsstelle der Abteilung für Sexualforschung**
Universität Hamburg, Poppenhusenstraße 12, 22305 Hamburg.
⏰ Mon - Fri 09:00 - 12:00

Organizations: Sexuality
⚲▽ **Freie Transenstadt Hamburg**
Postfach 700767, 22007 Hamburg.
☎ 40 656 0585
⚥▽ **Homosexuellenberatung in Bartaungs- & Seelsorgenzentrum St. Petri**
Kreuslerstraße 6-8, 20095 Hamburg.
☎ 40 33 5845
⏰ Tue 18:00 - 20:00
Counselling for issues about homosexuality.
⚥▽ **Magnus Hirschfeld Centrum**
Borgweg 8, 22303 Hamburg.
☎ 40 279 0060
⏰ 15:00 -24:00, Sun 13:00 -24:00. Men's counselling Wed Fri 19:00 - 21:00, women's counselling Wed 17:00 - 19:00
Counselling & social centre for gays, lesbians, & bisexuals.
⚥▽ **Rosa Engel-SchwulLesbische Aktion Hamm**
c/o AIDS-Hilfe: Hamm, Werler Straße 105, 59063 Hamburg.
☎ 238 1 5575
⏰ Wed 20:00 - 22:00
⚲▽ **TS Gesellschaft Hamburg e.V.**
Kornweide 47, 21109 Hamburg.
☎ 40 7549 5910
Contact: Fraulein Iris Donaubauer

Organizations: Sexuality: Student
⚥▽ **AStA-Schwulenreferat der Uni Hamburg**
Von-Melle Park 5, 20146 Hamburg.
☎ 40 410 3064
⏰ Mon Tue Thu 16:00 - 18:00

Photographers: Erotic
☺ **Karo Design**
Postfach 601303, 22213 Hamburg.
☎ 40 279 6121 ✆ 40 279 8910
Catalogue available.
☺ **Peter Toko Koschnick**
Schulterblatt 58, 20357 Hamburg.
☎ 40 439 1847

Publishers: Guides: Sexuality
⚥▼ **Hinnerk**
Chemnitzstraße 78-80, 22767 Hamburg.
☎ 40 389 3446

Publishers: Magazines: BDSM
☺ **Schlagzeilen**
Postfach 304 199, 20324 Hamburg.
⚑ $
Published quarterly.

Publishers: Magazines: Literary
⚥▼ **Literatussi**
c/o Buchladen Männerschwarm GmbH, Neuer Pferdemarkt 32, 20359 Hamburg.
☎ 40 43 6093 ✆ 40 430 2932

Publishers: Newspapers: Sexuality
⚥▽ **Hamburger Gay Information**
Postfach 605420, 22249 Hamburg.
Free at gay & lesbian locations. Published every month.

Radio: Sexuality
⚥▽ **Pink Channel**
FM 96.0, Cable 95.4, c/o Hein & Feite, Gurlittstraße 47, 20099 Hamburg.
⏰ Sat 20:00
⚥▽ **Radio Lightfire**
FM 96.0, Cable 95.4, c/o Offener Kanal Hamburg, Hamburg.
☎ 40 43 6268
⏰ Every month

Stores: Art Galleries
☺ **Erotic Art Museum**
Bernhard-Nochtstraße 69, 20359 Hamburg.

Stores: Books: General
☺ ■ **Art of Fée**
Hallerplatz 15, 20146 Hamburg.
☎ 40 450 35353 ✆ 40 450 35355
[VISA] [MC]
Bookshop & gallery of erotic art owned by fetish-minded woman. Catalogue, £10, $15U.S., DM10.
☺ ■ **Bücherboom**
Bahrenfelder Straße 142, 22765 Hamburg.
☎ 40 390 5436
⏰ Mon - Fri 09:00 - 18:00, Sat - 14:00
⚥▼ **Männerschwarm Buchladen**
Neuer Pferdemarkt 32, 20359 Hamburg.
☎ 40 43 6093 ✆ 40 430 2932
⏰ Mon - Fri 10:00 - 18:30, Thu - 20:30, Sat 10:00 - 14:00
☺ ■ **Montanus Aktuell**
Mönkebergstraße 7, 20095 Hamburg.

Stores: Clothing: Fetish
☺ ■ **Boutique de Sade**
Erichstraße 41, 20359 Hamburg.
☎ 40 314 4119
☺ ■ **Fashion & Tools**
Reeperbahn 40, 20359 Hamburg.
☎ 40 319 2361 ✆ 40 319 2342
⏰ Mon - Sat 09:00 - 18:00
⚑ [VISA] [MC]
Leather, rubber, & wetlook.

Stores: Clothing: Leather
⚥▼ **Skarupe**
Cuxhaven Straße 266, 21149 Hamburg.
☎ 40 701 7048
Custom made leather clothing for men.

Stores: Clothing: Rubber
☺ ▼ **Basta Boots**
Gurlittstraße 47, 20099 Hamburg.
☎ 40 24 5979 ✆ 40 24 6097
☺ ▼ **Rik Production**
Gurlittstraße 47, 20099 Hamburg.
☎ 40 24 5979 ✆ 40 24 6097
⏰ Mon - Wed Fri 10:30 -18:30, Thu 10:30 - 20:30, Sat 10:30 - 14:00
⚑ [VISA] [MC]
Leather, rubber, & toys. Mail order service also available.

Stores: Erotica: BDSM
☺ ▼ **Mr. Chaps Leatherworks**
Gurlittstraße 47, 20099 Hamburg.
☎ 40 24 3109 ✆ 40 24 6097
⏰ Mon - Wed Fri 10:30 -18:30, Thu 10:30 - 20:30, Sat 10:30 - 14:00
⚑ [VISA] [MC]
Tailormade leather & latex clothing.
⚥▼ **Remedy Versand**
Gurlittstraße 47, 20099 Hamburg.
☎ 40 24 5979 ✆ 40 24 6097
⏰ Mon - Wed Fri 10:30 -18:30, Thu 10:30 - 20:30, Sat 10:30 - 14:00
Catalogue, DM20.

Stores: Erotica: General
☺ ■ **Eppendorfer**
Landstraße 95, 2247 Hamburg.

☺ ■ **Revolt Shop**
Clemens Schultz Straße 77, 20359 Hamburg 4.
☎ 40 31 2848 — Fax 40 319 2096
🕒 Mon - Sat 10:00 - 18:30
Leather, rubber, toys, books, magazines, etc..

Tattooists

☺ **Endless Pain Tattoo**
Am Grundwasserwerk 17, 22041 Hamburg.
Body piercing also available.

Hameln

Stores: Clothing: Fetish

☺ ■ **Love & Flash**
Zentralstraße 13-17, 31785 Hameln.
☎ 51 51 28769

Hamm

Organizations: AIDS: Support

☺ □ **AIDS-Hilfe—Hamm**
Werler Straße 105, 59063 Hamm.
☎ 238 1 5575
🕒 Mon - Fri 08:00 - 12:00 14:00 - 16:00

Stores: Erotica: General

☺ ■ **Sex & Gay Shop**
Gallbergerweg 37, 59063 Hamm.

Hannover

Archives: Sexuality

⚥▽ **Schwullesbisches Archiv Hannover (SARCH)**
c/o HSH, Postfach 4722, 30047 Hannover.
☎ 511 66 1055

Bars: BDSM

⚥▼ **Backstairs**
Lange Laube 24, 30159 Hannover.
☎ 511 1 3858
🕒 Wed Fri - Sat 22:00 - ?
Also uniforms. Entrance from Hausmannstraße above Vulcano.

⚥▼ **The Hole**
Franckesstraße 5, 30165 Hannover.
☎ 511 352 3895
🕒 Wed Fri Sat 21:00 - 03:00

Helplines: AIDS

☺ □ **Rosa Hilfe**
☎ 511 458 1624
☎ 511 39 1441
🕒 20:00 - 23:00
Extra number to call: 511 44 0253.

Helplines: Sexuality

⚥▽ **Beratungstelle für Homosexuelle**
c/o HOME Zentrum, Johannssenstraße 8, 30159 Hannover.
☎ 511 36 3344
🕒 Tue 18:00 -20:00, Wed 11:00 - 13:00, Thu 19:00 - 21:00

⚥▽ **Switchboard**
☎ 511 41 3932

Organizations: AIDS: Support

☺ □ **AIDS-Hilfe—Hannover**
c/o HOME Zentrum, Johannssenstraße 8, 30159 Hannover.
☎ 511 1 9411
🕒 Mon - Thu 10:00 - 16:00, also Mon -Fri 19:00 - 21:00, Fri 10:00 - 14:00. Personal counselling Mon - Fri 10:00 - 13:00 14:00 - 16:00

☺ □ **AIDS-Hilfe—Kreis Unna**
Markt 13, 59174 Hannover.
☎ 230 71 9411
🕒 Mon - Thu 09:00 - 17:00, Fri 09:00 - 14:00. Gayline Wed 19:00 - 22:00

Organizations: BDSM

⚥▽ **AG Leder**
c/o HOME Zentrum, Johannssenstraße 8, 30159 Hannover.
☎ 511 33 3636

⚥▽ **MSC Hannover**
Postfach 4149, 30041 Hannover.
☎ 511 66 8557

Organizations: Family

☺ □ **Pro Familia Homosexuellenberatung**
c/o Pro Familia, Am Hohen Ufer 3A, 30159 Hannover.
☎ 511 36 3606

Organizations: Research: Sexuality

⚥▽ **Verein zur Erforschung der Geschichte der Homosexuellen in Niedersachsen (VEHN)**
c/o Freizeit & Bildungszentrum Weiße Rose, Mühlenberger Markt 1, 30457 Hannover.
☎ 511 66 1055

Organizations: Sexuality

⚥▽ **Aktionsgruppe Homosexualität Hannover (HSH)**
Postfach 4722, 30047 Hannover.
☎ 511 66 1055
🕒 2nd. & 4th. Sun of month 17:00

⚥▽ **HOME Zentrum**
Johannssenstraße 8, 30159 Hannover.
☎ 511 36 3633
🕒 Thu Sun 20:00, Sep - May 15:00 - 18:00

⚥▽ **Homosexuelle Emanzitpation Gruppe (HOME)**
c/o HOME Zentrum, Johannssenstraße 8, 30159 Hannover.
☎ 511 36 3633
Publishes *Mimikry*.

Organizations: Sexuality: Student

⚥▽ **Schwule Hannöversche Studenten (SHS)**
AStA Gebäude, Welfengarten 1, 30167 Hannover.
☎ 511 49 4575
🕒 Wed 20:00 - 22:00

Organizations: Sexuality: Youth

⚥▽ **Outspace Schwul-Lesbische Jungendgruppe**
Postfach 5612, 30056 Hannover.
☎ 511 36 3633
🕒 Meets Fri 20:00

Piercers

☺ ■ **Bernhard Kellner**
Elsa-Brandstroimstraße 3, 30453 Hannover.

Publishers: Magazines: Sexuality

☺ ■ ***The Observer***
Allemannstraße 13, 30165 Hannover.
☎ 511 352 2962 — Fax 511 352 2962

Publishers: Newspapers: Sexuality

⚥▼ ***Down Town Redaktion Nord***
☎ 511 23 4141 — Fax 511 41 3939

Stores: Books: General

☺ ■ **Buchhandlung Decins**
Marktstraße 52, 30159 Hannover.
☎ 511 36 3663

Stores: Clothing: Fetish

☺ ■ **S. W. 3**
Herschelstraße 32, 30159 Hannover.
☎ 511 131 7279
Leather, rubber, & wetlook.

Stores: Erotica: BDSM

☺ ■ **Leder Art & Design**
Schulenburger Landstraße 48, 30165 Hannover.
☎ 511 350 5633
🕒 Mon - Fri 14:00 - 18:00
Also tailormade leather clothing.

Stores: Erotica: General

☺ ■ **Beate Uhse**
Kleine Packhofstraße 16, 30159 Hannover.
🕒 Mon - Fri 09:00 - 18:00, Sat 09:00 - 14:00

⚥▼ **Frankies Erotik Shop**
Fernroder Straße 8, 30161 Hannover.
☎ 511 262 1052
🕒 Mon - Fri 10:00 - 20:00, Sat 10:00 - 15:00

⚥▼ **Frontline**
Lilienstrasse 16, 3000 Hannover 1.

☺ ■ **Kools**
Scholvinstraße 2, 30159 Hannover.
☎ 511 262 1540
🕒 09:00 - 24:00, Sun 13:00 - 24:00

Pleasure
Kölnische Stra, Hannover.
Mon - Fri 10:00 - 21:00, Sat 09:30 - 18:00

Quasimode
Pavillionstraße 11, 30451 Hannover.

Zardoz
Fosse Straße10, 3000 Hannover 91.

Hattersheim

Organizations: Sexuality

TVV
Postfach 1148, 65780 Hattersheim.

Heide

Organizations: AIDS: Support

AIDS-Hilfe—Westküste
Große Westerstraße 30, 25746 Heide.
☎ 481 1 9411
Wed 20:00 - 22:00

Heidelberg

Helplines: Sexuality

Rosa Telefon—Heidelberg
☎ 622 118 3770
Fri 19:00 - 21:00

Organizations: AIDS: Support

AIDS-Hilfe—Heidelberg
Untere Neckarstraße 17, 69117 Heidelberg.
☎ 622 11 9411
Mon 15:00 - 17:00, 18:00 - 20:00

Stores: Art Galleries

Galerie Welker
Hauptstraße 126, 69120 Heidelberg.

Stores: Erotica: General

Sex Shop
Merianstraße 3, 69117 Heidelberg.
☎ 622 12 9899
Mon - Fri 09:00 - 23:00, 09:00 -14:00

Heilbronn

Organizations: AIDS: Support

AIDS-Hilfe—Unterland
Postfach 1146, 74001 Heilbronn.
☎ 713 11 9411
Tue 15:00 - 18:00, Thu 18:00 - 21:00

Organizations: Sexuality

Homosexuelle Emanzipationsgruppe (Heh!)
Postfach 2023, 74010 Heilbronn.
☎ 713 18 9064
Wed 19:30 - 21:30

Herne

Organizations: AIDS: Support

AIDS-Hilfe—Herne
Hauptstraße 94, 44651 Herne.
☎ 232 36 0990
Fri 17:00 - 22:00

Stores: Erotica: BDSM

MVS
Poststraße 46, 44629 Herne.
☎ 23 231 8028 Fax 23 235 1471
☎ 23 231 0493
Leather, latex, PVC, high heels, boots, & BDSM furniture. Catalogue, DM20.

Hildesheim

Organizations: AIDS: Support

AIDS-Hilfe—Hildesheim
Einumer Straße 74, 31135 Hildesheim.
☎ 512 11 9411 Fax 512 51 0051
Thu 19:00 - 21:00

Stores: Books: General

Montanus Aktuell
Almsstraße 19-20, 31134 Hildesheim.

Hirschhorn

Organizations: AIDS: Support

AIDS-Beratungsstelle Oberfranken
Wilhelmstraße 17, 95028 Hirschhorn.
☎ 627 28 7681
Wed 15:00 - 18:00

Hohenmölsen

Organizations: Sexuality

Ehe-Familien-Jungend & Schwulenberatung
Lindenstraße 12, 06679 Hohenmölsen.
Contact: Dr. Kurt Bach
Counselling for young gays & lesbians.

Holzminden

Organizations: Sexuality

Schwulengruppe HX/HOL
c/o Pro Familia, Wallstraße 2, 37603 Holzminden.
☎ 553 11 0807

Hoyerswerda

Organizations: Sexuality

Men Only Selbsthilfzentrum
Schulstraße 5, 02977 Hoyerswerda.

Ilmenau

Organizations: Sexuality

Homosexuelle Aktion Ilmenau (HAI)
c/o Uwe Schäfer, Naumannstraße 19, 98693 Ilmenau.
Meets Wed 1930

Ingolstadt

Helplines: Sexuality

Rosa Telefon—Ingolstadt
☎ 841 30 5608
Wed 20:00 - 22:00

Organizations: AIDS: Support

AIDS-Hilfe—Ingolstadt
c/o Thomas Thöne, Altenhofstraße 11, 85049 Ingolstadt.
☎ 841 8 5961

Organizations: Sexuality

Romeo & Julius
c/o Bürgertreff Alte Post, Kreutzstraße 12, 85049 Ingolstadt.
Thu 20:00 - 22:00

Insel

Organizations: Sexuality

Die Insel
Postfach 0216, 53569 Insel.
☎ 268 5 7612
☎ 264 4 4782

Ispringen

Stores: Clothing: Rubber

Kunzmann
Lanhaustraße 2, Ispringen.
Catalogue, DM30 or £7, refundable on first order.

Ittlingen

Stores: Clothing: Fetish

Shiny Fashion
Haptstraße 48, 74930 Ittlingen.
☎ 7266 3595 Fax 7266 3595
Mon - Fri 11:00 - 13:00 15:00 - 18:30, Thu - 20:00, Sat 10:00 - 13:00

Jena

Health Services

Universitätshautklinik
Erfurter Straße 35, 07743 Jena.
☎ 364 1 822 2048

Organizations: Sexuality

Gay's Innung—Jena
Eberstraße 7, 07743 Jena.
Meets Thu

Kaarst

Stores: Clothing: Rubber

☺ **Rubber Design Modevertriebsgesellschaft**
Industriestraße 8B, 41564 Kaarst.
Represents Craig Morrison on the continent of Europe.

Kaiserlautern

Organizations: AIDS: Support

☺ □ **AIDS-Hilfe—Kaiserlautern**
Pariser Straße 23, 67655 Kaiserlautern.
☎ 631 1 9411
🕘 Mon - Fri 19:00 - 21:00, Wed 18:00 - 20:00

Organizations: Sexuality: Student

⚤▽ **AStA-Schwulenreferat**
Erwin Schrödinger Straße, 67663 Kaiserlautern.
☎ 631 205 2228
🕘 Wed 11:00 - 12:00

Karlsruhe

Helplines: Sexuality

⚤▽ **Rosa Telefon—Karlsruhe**
☎ 721 37 9352
☎ 721 2 4744
🕘 Thu 20:00 - 21:30

Organizations: AIDS: Education

☺ □ **AIDS Initiative Karlsruhe e. V.**
Sophienstraße 59, 76133 Karlsruhe.
☎ 721 1 9411
🕘 Mon 16:00 - 18:00, Wed 14:00 - 16:00, Thu 20:00 - 22:00, Fri 10:00 - 12:00

Organizations: Sexuality

⚤▽ **SchwuZ-Schwules Zentrum**
Postfach 6001, 76133 Karlsruhe.
☎ 721 37 9352

Organizations: Sexuality: Student

⚤▽ **Schwule Uni Gruppe (SchWUnG)**
c/o AStA Universität Karlsruhe, Adenauerring 7, 76131 Karlsruhe.
☎ 721 69 1041
🕘 Tue 19:30

Stores: Books: General

☺ ■ **Montanus Aktuell**
Kaiserstraße 127, 76133 Karlsruhe.

Stores: Erotica: General

☺ ■ **Sex Shop**
Bürgerstraße 12, 76133 Karlsruhe.
☎ 721 2 9185
🕘 09:00 - 19:00

Kassel

Helplines: Sexuality

⚤▽ **Rosa Telefon—Kassel**
c/o Pro Familia, Frankfurter Straße 133a, 341221 Kassel.
☎ 561 2 7413
🕘 Fri 18:00 - 22:00

Organizations: AIDS: Support

☺ □ **AIDS-Hilfe—Kassel**
Frankfurter Straße 65, 34121 Kassel.
☎ 561 1 6801
🕘 Mon 16:00 - 18:00, Wed 18:00 - 20:00

Stores: Books: General

☺ ■ **ABC Buchladen**
Goethestraße 77, 34119 Kassel.
☎ 561 77 7704

Stores: Erotica: General

☺ ■ **City Sex Shop**
Grüner Weg 10, 34117 Kassel.
☎ 561 1 7587
🕘 Mon - Fri 10:00 - 18:30, Sat 10:00 - 13:00
VISA MC

☺ ■ **Pleasure**
Postfach , Kölnische Straße 7, 34117 Kassel.
☎ 561 77 4437
🕘 Mon - Fri 10:00 - 21:00, Sat 09:30 - 18:00

Kiel

Helplines: Sexuality

⚤▽ **Rosa Telefon—Kiel**
☎ 431 1 7099
🕘 Mon Wed Thu 18:00 - 20:00. Parents call Fri 18:00 - 20:00

Organizations: AIDS: Support

⚤▽ **AIDS-Hilfe—Kiel**
Goethestraße 23, 24116 Kiel.
☎ 431 1 9411
🕘 Wed Fri 18:00 - 20:00

Organizations: Sexuality

⚤▽ **Huch! Schwulen- & Lesben-Zentrum**
Westring 278, 24116 Kiel.
☎ 431 17090

⚤▽ **Schwule an der Christian Albrecht Universität**
c/o Café Kom, Max Eyth Straße 2, 24118 Kiel.
🕘 Thu 15:00

Organizations: Sexuality: Student

⚤▽ **Schwulenreferat im AStA der Christian Albrecht Universität**
Westring 385, 24118 Kiel.
☎ 431 880 2647
🕘 Mon - Fri 10:00 - 14:00

Stores: Books: General

☺ ■ **Zapata**
Jungfernstieg 27, 24103 Kiel.
☎ 431 9 3639

☺ ■ **Zapata**
Medusastraße 16, 24143 Kiel.
☎ 431 73 8323

Stores: Erotica: General

☺ ■ **Beate Uhse**
Wall 12, 24103 Kiel.
☎ 431 97 0833
🕘 09:00 - 23:30, Sun 14:00 - ?

☺ ■ **Wos Markt**
Eggerstraße 11, 24103 Kiel.
🕘 10:00 - 24:00

Kitzingen

Organizations: Sexuality

⚤▽ **Homosexuelle Interessengemeinschaft Unterfranken Warum**
Postfach 25, 97302 Kitzingen.
☎ 932 12 2666
🕘 19:00

⚤▽ **Neuer Freundeskreis Homosexueller**
Postfach 446, 97301 Kitzingen.
🕘 Every 2nd Thu 20:00

Kleve

Organizations: Sexuality

⚤▽ **Teestube Schwuler Treff**
c/o Familienbildungsstätte, Regenbogen 14, 47533 Kleve.
☎ 282 12 3157
🕘 Wed 20:00 - 22:00

Koblenz

Helplines: Sexuality

⚤▽ **Rosa Telefon—Koblenz**
c/o Huk, Postfach 1836, 56508 Koblenz.
☎ 261 6 3557
🕘 Tue 20:00 - 22:00

Organizations: AIDS: Support

☺ □ **AIDS-Hilfe—Koblenz**
Postfach 133, 56001 Koblenz.
☎ 261 1 9411
🕘 Wed 19:00 - 21:00

Organizations: Sexuality: Youth

⚤▽ **Schwule Jungendgruppe Koblenz (SJK)**
Rizzastraße 14, 56068 Koblenz.

Stores: Erotica: General

☺ ■ **Journal**

An der Liebfrauenkirche 12, 56068 Koblenz.
☎ 261 30 9768
🕐 Mon - Fri 09:30 - 22:00

Köln

Archives: Sexuality

⚥▽ **Schwulen-Archiv Köln**
Postfach 420625, 50900 Köln.
☎ 221 44 2757
🕐 Sun mornings
Also leather archives.

⚥▽ **Schwul-Lesbisches Presse-Archiv**
c/o Ralf Syben, Luisenstraße 8, 50679 Köln.
☎ 221 81 0451

Bars: BDSM

⚥▼ **Chains**
Stephanstraße 4, 50676 Köln.
☎ 221 23 8730
🕐 Mon - Thu 21:00 - 01:00, Fri Sat 21:00 - 03:00, Sun 19:00 - 01:00.
Minimum charge DM5 on Fri & Sat.

⚥▼ **Platzjabbeck**
Annostraße 96, 50678 Köln.
☎ 221 21 8173
🕐 Tue - Sat 20:00 - 01:00

⚥▼ **Stiefelknecht**
Pipinstraße 9, 50667 Köln.
☎ 221 21 3001
🕐 Sun - Fri 22:00 - 03:00, Sat 22:00 - 04:30

Helplines: Sexuality

⚥▽ **Rosa Telefon—Köln**
c/o Homosexuelle Initiative Konstanz, Freidrichstraße 21, 78464 Köln.
☎ 753 16 4535
🕐 Mon 20:00 - 22:00

⚥▽ **Schwules Überfalltelefon**
☎ 221 1 9228
Gay bashing helpline.

Organizations: AIDS: Education

☺ ☐ **Deutsche AIDS-Stiftung Positiv-Leben**
Pipinstraße 7, 50667 Köln.
☎ 221 24 3535

Organizations: AIDS: Support

☺ ☐ **AIDS-Beratungsstelle des Gesundheitsamt**
Neumarkt 15-21, 50667 Köln.
☎ 221 221 4602
🕐 Mon - Thu 08:00 - 12:30 14:00 - 16:30, Fri 09:00 - 12:00
HIV testin.

☺ ☐ **AIDS-Beratungsstelle für Kölner Studierende**
Zulpicher Straße 68, 50937 Köln. 📞 221 472 0101
🕐 Mon - Thu 09:00 - 15:00, Fri - 13:00. By appointment

☺ ■ **AIDS-Hilfe—Köln**
Beehovenstraße 1, 50674 Köln.
☎ 221 19411 📞 221 230325
☎ 221 20 2030 (office)
🕐 Helpline Mon Tue Thu Fri 19:00 - 21:00. Office Mon - Fri 09:00 - 17:00

☺ ☐ **AIDS-Hilfe—Nordrhein-Westfalen**
Hohenzollernring 48, 50672 Köln.
☎ 221 25 3596 📞 221 25 2495

Organizations: BDSM

⚥▽ **Gay Raiders**
Spinrad, Mauritiuswall 48, 5000 Köln.

☺ ▽ **LSMA Köln**
Postfach 290341, 50525 Köln.
☎ 221 54 2516
🕐 2nd. & 4th. Mon of the month 20:00
Events for people into BDSM.

Organizations: Bears

⚥▽ **Bartmäner Bären Köln**
Postfach 290341, 50525 Köln.
☎ 221 54 2516 📞 221 546 2235
🌐 http://www.skepsis.com:80/.gblo/bears/CLUBS/bears_cologne.html
🕐 1st. & 3rd. Mon of month

Organizations: Body Size

⚥▽ **Girth & Mirth—Deutschland: Köln**

☎ 234 925 55104

Organizations: Family

⚥☐ **Schwule Väter Köln**
c/o Lavendelschwert, Bayardsgase 5, 50676 Köln.
☎ 221 23 2626
🕐 Meets 1st. Fri of the month 20:00
Support & counselling for gay fathers.

Organizations: Fetish: Uniforms

⚥▽ **Köln Oliv**
c/o Hands, Mathiasstraße 22, 50676 Köln.
☎ 228 234451

Organizations: Masturbation

⚥▽ **Cologne Jacks**
Postfach 290341, 50525 Köln.
☎ 221 54 2516
🕐 17:00 - 20:00. Safer sex parties 3rd Thu of month 22:00

Organizations: Motorcycle

⚥▽ **MS Panther Köln e. V.**
Postfach 190325, 50500 Köln.
☎ 221 73 9483

⚥▽ **MSC Viking**
Postfach 60 05 23, 50685 Köln.

Organizations: Research: Sexuality

⚥▽ **Verein zur Förderung der Erforschung der Geschichte der Homosexuellen in Nordrhein-Westfalen**
Postfach 420625, 50900 Köln.

Organizations: Sexuality

⚥▽ **Checkpoint**
c/o Schwips e. V., Pipinstraße 7, 50667 Köln.
☎ 221 25 5009 📞 221 257 1471
🕐 17:00 - 21:00
Information & counselling for lesbians & gays.

⚥▽ **Schwulen- & Lesben-Zentrum (SchuLZ)**
Kaartäuserwall 18, 50678 Köln.
☎ 221 52 0206
🕐 18:00 - 00:30, Sat Sun 16:00 - 00:30

Organizations: Sexuality: Student

⚥▽ **Andere Fakultät / Schwulen- & Lesbenreferat**
Universitätsstraße 16, 50937 Köln.
🕐 Mon 17:00 - 18:00

Publishers: Books: Fetish

⚤ **Benedickt Taschen Verlag GmbH**
Hohenzollernring 53, 50672 Köln.
Specialises in high quality, cheap art books.

Radio: Sexuality

⚥▽ **Radio Tilla**
FM 107.1 & 97.8, c/o Bernd Winkelman, Ritterstraße 22, 50668 Köln.
☎ 221 13 3446
🕐 Every other Wed

Stores: Art Galleries

☺ **Galleria Erotica**
Heinsbergstraße 16, 50674 Köln.

☺ **Kunstbanett**
Kaesenstraße 19, 50677 Köln.

Stores: Books: General

⚥▼ **Lavendelschwert Buchladen**
Bayardsgasse 3-5, 50676 Köln.
☎ 221 23 2626
🕐 Mon- Wed Fri 10:00 - 18:30, Thu 12:00 - 20:00, Sat 10:00 - 14:00
Also provides mail order service.

Stores: Clothing: Fetish

☺ ■ **Cosmic Wear**
Mauritiuswall 30/32, 50676 Köln.
☎ 221 240 1201 📞 221 240 2094
🕐 Mon - Fri 12:00 - 18:30, Thu 12:00 - 20:30, Sat 11:00 - 14:00

☺ ■ **Modern Style**
Julicherstraße 10, 50674 Köln.
☎ 221 121 1080

Stores: Erotica: BDSM

☺ **Das Atelier**

Vogelsangstraße 286, 50825 Köln.
☎ 221 54 1972 📞 221 546 3367
🕐 - 18:30

⚥▼ **Man Leder Shop**
Mathiasstraße 9, 50676 Köln.
🕐 Tue - Fri 14:00 - 18:30, Sat 10:00 - 14:00

⚥▼ **Man's World**
Flanderische Straße 2, 50674 Köln.
☎ 221 25 2423
🕐 Mon - Wed 10:00 - 18:30, Sat 10:00 -14:00
Also tailormade leather clothing.

☺ ■ **Nima**
Wolfstraße 16, 5000 Köln 1.
☎ 22 123 6328
Catalogue available.

⚥▼ **Secrets Boutique**
Marienplatz 1, 50676 Köln.
☎ 221 24 4100
🕐 Tue Wed Fri 13:30 - 18:30, Thu - 20:30, Sat 10:00 - 14:00
Leather, rubber, wetlook, BDSM toys.

Stores: Erotica: General

⚥▼ **Hands**
Mathiasstraße 22, 50676 Köln.
☎ 221 24 3541
🕐 Mon - Thu 22:00 - 02:00, Fri Sat 22:00 - 03:00

☺ ■ **WIWA International**
Ehrenstraße 46, 50672 Köln.
☎ 221 25 3115 📞 221 25 6810

Konstanz

Organizations: AIDS: Support

☺▽ **AIDS-Hilfe—Konstanz**
Friedrichstraße 21, 87464 Konstanz.
☎ 753 11 9411
🕐 Wed 20:00 - 22:00

Organizations: Sexuality

⚥▽ **Homosexuelle Initiative Konstanz**
Friedrichstraße 21, 78464 Konstanz.
☎ 753 16 4535
🕐 Meets Tue 20:00

Stores: Erotica: General

☺ ■ **Sexy Shop**
Kreuzlinger Straße 5, 78462 Konstanz.
☎ 752 1220 2526
🕐 Mon - Fri 10:00 - 18:30, Sat 10:00 - 13:00

Krefeld

Helplines: Sexuality

⚥▽ **Rosa Telefon—Krefeld**
☎ 215 177 0643
🕐 Thu 19:00 - 21:00

Organizations: AIDS: Support

☺ □ **AIDS-Hilfe—Krefeld**
Postfach 108, 47701 Krefeld.
☎ 215 11 9411
🕐 Mon 12:00 - 14:00, Wed 18:00 - 21:30

Organizations: Sexuality: Student

⚥▽ **Schwulenreferat Fachhochschule Niederrhein**
Frankenring 20, 47798 Krefeld.
☎ 215 177 6878
🕐 Tue 12:00 - 14:00, Thu 15:00 - 17:00

Lahr

Organizations: Sexuality

⚥▽ **Homosexuelle Informationsgruppe Ortenau / Baden (HIOB)**
Kaiserstrase 80, 77933 Lahr.
☎ 782 13 8383

Landau

Helplines: Sexuality

⚥▽ **Rosa Telefon—Landau**
☎ 634 18 8688
🕐 Wed 20:00 - 22:00

Organizations: AIDS: Support

☺ □ **AIDS-Hilfe—Landau**

Weißenburger straße 2b, 76829 Landau.
☎ 634 11 9411
🕐 Tue 19:00 - 21:00

☺ □ **AIDS-Hilfe—Saar**
Im Bahnhof, 66822 Landau.
☎ 688 115 2222
🕐 Mon - Fri 10:00 - 12:00, Mon 19:00 - 21:00

Leipzig

Helplines: Sexuality

⚥□ **Beauftragte für Gleigeschlechtliche Lebensweisen**
Dezernat Soziales & Gesundheit, holzhäuserstraße 65, 04299 Leipzig.
☎ 341 882 1189 📞 341 882 1194
🕐 Tue 09:00 - 18:00

Organizations: AIDS: Support

☺ □ **AIDS Beratung & Betreuung**
c/o Gesundheitsamt Leipzig, Tschaikowskistraße 24, 04105 Leipzig.
☎ 341 29 5021
🕐 Mon Tue Thu 09:00 - 12:00, Mon Wed 13:00 - 16:00, Tue 13:00 - 18:00
HIV testing.

☺ □ **AIDS-Hilfe—Leipzig**
Ossietzkystraße 18, 04347 Leipzig.
☎ 341 232 3126
🕐 Tue Thu 15:00 - 21:00

Organizations: BDSM

⚥▽ **Hardcore**
c/o AIDS-Hilfe Leipzig e. V., Ossietzkystraße 18, 04347 Leipzig.
☎ 341 232126

⚥▽ **Lederclub Leipzig**
c/o Detlef Hüttig, Gießerstraße 56, 04229 Leipzig.

Organizations: Health

☺ □ **abc Leipzig e. V.**
Universitätstraße 5, 04109 Leipzig.
☎ 341 719 3565
🕐 Mon - Fri 14:00 - 18:00
Education, library, & condom programs.

Organizations: Sexuality

⚥▽ **Rosa Linse Leipzig**
c/o HdV, Lindenauer Markt 21, 04177 Leipzig.
🕐 Meets Mon 20:00

Organizations: Sexuality: Student

⚥▽ **Schwule an der Universität Leipzig (SchwUL)**
c/o Student Innenrat, Augustusplatz 9-11, 04109 Leipzig.
☎ 341 719 2261

Stores: Erotica: General

☺ ■ **Erotik Shop**
Universitätstraße 18, 04109 Leipzig.
☎ 341 28 41 44 📞 341 28 41 44
🕐 Mon - Fri 10:00 - 18:30, Sat 10:00 - 12:30

Leverhusen

Organizations: AIDS: Support

☺ □ **AIDS-Hilfe—Leverkusen**
c/o Volker Linhart, Okerstraße 30, 51371 Leverhusen.

Limburg

Helplines: Sexuality

⚥▽ **Rosa Telefon—Limburg**
☎ 643 12 3711
🕐 Thu 19:00 - 21:00

Organizations: AIDS: Support

☺ □ **AIDS-Hilfe—Limburg**
☎ 643 11 9411
🕐 Thu 17:00 - 19:00

Organizations: Sexuality

⚥▽ **Schwulengruppe Limburg / Weilburg**
☎ 643 12 3711
🕐 Thu 20:00
Telephone number is for the Rosa Telefon.

Lingen

Helplines: Sexuality

⚥▽ **Rosa Telefon—Lingen**
☎ 591 1 9411

Helplines: Sexuality
☺ 1st. & 3rd. Mon of month 19:00 - 21:00

Organizations: AIDS: Support
☺ ☐ **AIDS-Hilfe—Lingen**
Postfach 1165, 49871 Lingen.
☎ 591 1 9411
☺ Mon - Wed 14:00 - 17:00, FRI 17:00 - 21:00

Lübeck

Helplines: Sexuality
♂▽ **Rosa Telefon—Lübeck**
☎ 451 7 4619
☺ Wed 20:00 - 22:00

Organizations: AIDS: Support
☺ ☐ **AIDS-Hilfe—Lübeck**
Postfach 1931, 23507 Lübeck.
☎ 451 1 9411
☺ Thu 18:00 - 20:00

Organizations: Sexuality
♂▽ **Homosexuelle Initiative Lübeck (HIL)**
Postfach 1823, 23556 Lübeck.
☎ 451 7 4619
☺ Wed 20:00 - 22:00
♂▽ **Schwule Aktion Lübeck**
Postfach 1823, 23556 Lübeck.

Stores: Books: General
☺ ■ **Montanus Aktuell**
Briete Straße 58, 23522 Lübeck.

Stores: Erotica: General
☺ ■ **Sparta-Shop**
Hüxstraße 15, 23552 Lübeck.
☎ 451 7 2453
☺ 09:00 - 18:00

Lüdenscheid

Organizations: AIDS: Support
☺ ☐ **AIDS-Hilfe—Märkischen Kreis**
Duisbergweg 3, 58511 Lüdenscheid.
☎ 235 12 3202
☺ Mon 19:00 - 21:00

Organizations: Sexuality
♂▽ **Homosexuelle Initiative im Märkischen Sauerland (HIMS)**
c/o Die Grünen, Bahnhofstraße 44, 58507 Lüdenscheid.
☎ 235 13 9547
☺ Wed 19:00 - 21:00

Ludwigsburg

Stores: Erotica: General
☺ ■ **Beate Uhse**
Stuttgarter Straße 56, 71638 Ludwigsburg.
☎ 294 190 1821
☺ Mon - Sat 09:00 - 23:00, Sat 14:00 - 23:00

Ludwigshafen

Organizations: AIDS: Support
☺ ☐ **AIDS-Beratungstelle**
Falkenstraße 19, 67063 Ludwigshafen.
☎ 621 520 4440

Stores: Erotica: General
☺ ■ **Mike's**
Amtsstraße 1, 67059 Ludwigshafen.
☺ Mon - Sat 10:00 - 22:00, Sun 14:00 - 22:00
☺ ■ **Sexyland**
Ludwigstraße10, 67059 Ludwigshafen.
☺ Mon - Fri 09:00 - 18:30, Sat 09:00 - 14:00

Lüneburg

Organizations: AIDS: Support
☺ ☐ **AIDS-Hilfe—Lüneburg**
Katzenstraße 3, 21335 Lüneburg.
☎ 413 11 9411
☺ Mon Tue 09:00 - 13:00, Wed 09:00 - 13:00 14:00 - 18:00, Thu 09:00 - 14:00

Organizations: Sexuality
♂▽ **Lüneburger Schwulengruppe & Rosa Telefon— Lüneburg**
c/o AIDS-Hilfe, Katzenstraße 3, 21335 Lüneburg.
☎ 413 11 9411
☺ 2nd. & 4th. Wed of month 20:00, 1st Thu of month 20:00, 3rd Sun of month 15:00

Magdeburg

Helplines: Sexuality
♂▽ **Rosa Hilfe**
☎ 391 34 3364
☺ Mon 17:00 - 21:00, Fri 16:00 - 21:00

Organizations: AIDS: Support
☺ ☐ **AIDS-Hilfe—Magdeburg**
Schäfferstraße 28, 39112 Magdeburg.
☺ Mon - Fri 10:00 - 20:00

Organizations: Sexuality
♂▽ **Caritasverband Beratung Homosexueller Männer & AIDS Beratung**
Max-Josef Metzger Straße 3, 39104 Magdeburg.
☎ 391 3 8075
☺ Thu 14:00 - 18:00
♂▽ **Klub A-3 e. V. - Anders als Andere**
c/o AIDS-Hilfe, Schäfferstraße 28, 39112 Magdeburg.
☺ Sat 15:00

Mainz

Organizations: AIDS: Support
☺ ☐ **AIDS-Beratung des Gesundheitsamtes Mainz**
Große Langgasse 29, 55116 Mainz.
☎ 613 122 5353
☺ Mon - Thu 08:00 - 12:00, 14:00 - 16:00
☺ ☐ **AIDS-Hilfe—Mainz**
Postfach 1173, 55001 Mainz.
☎ 613 11 9411
☺ Mon - Fri 17:00 - 19:00, Wed Sun 19:00 - 21:00
☺ ☐ **Klinikum der Johan-Gutenburg Universit_at**
Langenbeckstraße 1, 55131 Mainz.
☎ 613 11 7197
☎ 613 117 2104

Organizations: Sexuality
♂▽ **Schwuguntia - Verein zur Förderung Sozialer & Kulturelle Interessen e. V.**
Marienborner Straße 15, 55128 Mainz.
✉ helmich@mzd.mza.zdv.uni-mainz.de
☺ Hosts large lesbigay festival at end of July
Serves cultural, social interests of the lesbigay community in the Mainz / Wiesbaden area. Connections to local AIDS & lesbigay organizations. English also spoken.

Organizations: Sexuality: Student
♂■ **Autonomes Schwulenreferat**
Staudingerweg21, 55128 Mainz.
☺ Tue 10:00 - 12:00, Wed 19:30 - 22:00, Thu 17:00 - 19:00

Stores: Books: General
☺ ■ **Wohlthat'sche Buchhandlung**
Große Bleiche 8, 55116 Mainz.
☎ 613 122 2353

Mannheim

Bars: BDSM
♂▼ **Jail**
Angelstraße 5-9, 68199 Mannheim.
☎ 621 85 9626
☺ Wed - Sun 21:00 - 01:00. Doors open 21:00 - 22:30

Helplines: Sexuality
♂▽ **Rosa Hilfe—Mannheim**
☎ 621 31 8594
☺ Tue 19:00 - 21:00

Organizations: AIDS: Support
☺ ☐ **AIDS-Hilfe—Mannheim**
Postfach 120113, 68052 Mannheim.
☎ 621 1 9411
☺ Mon Tue Thu Fri 10:00 - 13:00, Wed 15:00 - 18:00, Thu 19:00 - 21:00

Organizations: BDSM

⚥▼ **M & S Connexion**
Angelstraße 5-9, 68199 Mannheim.
☎ 621 85 8374 — Fax 621 86 1638
🕘 Thu - Sun 21:00 - 01:00

Organizations: Body Size

⚥▽ **Girth & Mirth—Deutschland: Mannheim / Stuttgart**
☎ 621 545 315

Organizations: Sexuality

⚥▽ **Schwule Aktion Mannheim e. V. (SchAM)**
Postfach 240117, 68069 Mannheim.
☎ 621 31 8594

Piercers

☺ ■ **Ars Subcutan**
AlphornStraße 41, 68169 Mannheim.
☎ 621 318 9183

Marburg

Helplines: Sexuality

⚥▽ **Rosa Telefon der Pro Familia—Marburg**
Universitätstraße 42, 35037 Marburg.
☎ 642 12 2800
🕘 Thu 18:00 - 20:00

Organizations: AIDS: Support

☺ □ **AIDS-Hilfe—Marburg**
Bahnhofstraße 38, 35037 Marburg.
☎ 642 11 9411
🕘 Mon 14:00 - 16: 00, Thu 19:00 - 21:00

Organizations: Sexuality

⚥▽ **Schwulengruppe Biedenkopf**
c/o AIDS-Hilfe, Bahnhofstraße 38, 35037 Marburg.
☎ 642 11 9411
🕘 Meets 2nd. & 4th. Wed 19:30

⚥▽ **Schwulengruppe Marburg**
c/o Automomes Schwulenreferat, Erlenring 5, 35037 Marburg.
☎ 642 12 6001
🕘 Mon - Fri 13:00 - 14:00

Menden

Organizations: Sexuality

⚥▽ **RosaLinde**
Hauptstraße 48, 58706 Menden.
☎ 237 390 3455
☎ 237 390 3457
🕘 Thu 20:00 - 22:00

Minden

Helplines: Sexuality

⚥▽ **Rosa Telefon—Minden**
c/o Schwulen Initiative Minden (SchwIM), Seidenbeutel 1, 32423 Minden.
☎ 571 88 0038
🕘 Tue Fri 17:00 - 19:00

Organizations: Sexuality

⚥▽ **Schwule Arbeitsgruppe Minden (SCHWARM)**
Postfach 1544, 32375 Minden.
🕘 Meets Thu 20:00
Also runs a group for youth.

⚥▽ **Schwule Initiative Minden (SchwIM)**
c/o BÜZ, Seidenbeutel 1, 32423 Minden.
☎ 571 88 0038
🕘 Meets Wed 20:00 - 22:00
Group for coming out, meeting point. Info line about all gay groups' activities in Minden, cinéma, TV, etc.. Age statement of 18 is required. English also spoken.

Moers

Organizations: AIDS: Support

☺ □ **AIDS-Hilfe—Duisburg**
☎ 284 11 9411
🕘 2nd. & 4th. Tue of month 20:00 - 22:00

Stores: Books: General

☺ ■ **Aragon Buchladen**
Homberger Straße 30, 47441 Moers.
☎ 284 12 9772

🕘 Mon - Sat 09:30 - 18:30

Mölln

Organizations: AIDS: Support

☺ □ **AIDS-Hilfe—Herzogtum Lauenburg**
Wasserkrüger Weg 14, 23879 Mölln.
☎ 454 21 9411
🕘 Wed 19:00 - 21:00

Mönchengladbach

Helplines: Sexuality

⚥▽ **Homophone**
c/o AIDS-Hilfe, Ertzberger Straße, 41061 Mönchengladbach.
☎ 216 14 5055
🕘 Sun 18:00 - 20:00

Organizations: AIDS: Support

☺ □ **AIDS-Hilfe—Mönchengladbach / Rheydt**
Ertzberger Straße 8, 41061 Mönchengladbach.
☎ 216 11 9411
🕘 Mon - Fri 08:00 - 12:00 14:00 - 16:00

Stores: Books: General

☺ ■ **Montanus Aktuell**
Hindenburgstraße 153, 41061 Mönchengladbach.
☎ 216 11 5527

Mülhausen

Organizations: AIDS: Support

☺ □ **AIDS-Hilfe—Mülhausen**
Postfach 415, 99964 Mülhausen.
☎ 360 144 6218 — Fax 360 144 8403
🕘 Mon 09:00 - 15:00, Tue 09:00 - 22:00, Wed - Fri 09:00 -15:00

Mülheim

Organizations: Sexuality

⚥▽ **Schwule Initiativ Gruppe Mülheim And der Ruhr (SIGMAR)**
c/o 3. Welt-Laden, Kaiserstraße 8, 45468 Mülheim.
☎ 208 806516
☎ 208 3 3624 (Information)
🕘 Thu 20:00 - 22:00. Meets Fri 20:00 - 22:00

Publishers: Magazines: Fetish

☺ ■ **Webeverlag**
Postfach 102140, 4330 Mülheim.
Rubber fetish magazines.

München

Bars: BDSM

⚥▼ **Bolt**
Blumenstraße 15, 80331 München.
☎ 89 26 4323
🕘 15:00 - 03:00

⚥▼ **Empire**
Thalkirchner Staße 2, 80337 München.
☎ 89 260 8403
🕘 Fri Sat 21:00 - 01:00, Fri Sat leather disco, Sun gay disco

⚥▼ **Löwengrube**
Reisingerstraße 15, 80337 München.
☎ 89 26 5750
🕘 Mon - Sat 20:00 - 01:00, Sun 18:00 - 01:00

⚥▼ **New York**
Sonnenstraße 25, 80331 München.
☎ 89 59 1056
🕘 23:00 - 04:00

⚥▼ **Ochsengarten**
Müllerstraße 47, 80469 München.
☎ 89 26 6446
🕘 20:00 - 01:00, Fri Sat - 03:00
Meeting place of Münchner-Löwen Club. Information for ECMC members.

⚥▼ **Pop As**
Thalkirchner Straße 12, 80337 München.
☎ 89 260 9191
🕘 20:00 - 01:00
Contact point & information for ECMC members.

Helplines: Sexuality

⚥▼ **Beratungsstelle**
☎ 89 1 9411
🕘 Mon - Fri 19:00 - 22:00

Helplines: Sexuality

Counselling for gays, lesbians, & bisexuals.

⚥▽ **Überfalltelefon**
☎ 89 1 9411
☎ 89 1 9226
🕐 Mon - Fri 19:00 - 22:00
Gay bashing line.

Manufacturers: Erotica: BDSM

☺ ■ **Hard Line**
Müllerstraße 33, 80469 München.
☎ 89 260 6017 ✆ 89 260 8076
☎ 80 260 6018
🕐 Mon - Fri 12:30 - 18:00, Sat 11:00 - 13:30
♿ [VISA] [MC]
Manufacturers, wholesalers, & retailers of rubber & leather clothes, & BDSM toys. Also mail order. .

Organizations: AIDS: Support

☺ □ **AIDS-Hilfe—München**
Postfach 140465, 80454 München.
☎ 89 1 9411 ✆ 89 26 3455
🕐 Mon - Fri 19:00 - 22:00

☺ □ **Anonyme AIDS-Beratungsstralle des Gesundheithauses**
Room 483, Dachauer Straße 90, 80335 München.
☎ 89 520 7387
☎ 89 520 7337
🕐 Mon - Fri 08:00 - 11:00, Tue 16:00 - 18:00
Counselling, information, & HIV testing.

Organizations: BDSM

⚥▽ **Münchner-Löwen Club e. V. (MLC)**
Postfach 330163, 80061 München.
Publishes *Löwenspiegel*.

Organizations: Body Size

⚥▽ **Girth & Mirth—Deutschland: München**
☎ 89 542 0407

Organizations: Sexuality

⚲▽ **Club Neues Leben Nova**
Postfach 710232, 81452 München.
☎ 89 311 3260
☎ 89 616808
🕐 Meets 1st. Fri of month 19:00. Call 18:00 - 18:300. German only

⚥▽ **Homosexuelle Alternative (HALT)**
c/o ESG, Friedrichstraße 25, 808801 München.
☎ 89 311 6172
🕐 Wed 20:30

⚥▽ **Verein für Sexuelle Gleichberechtigung e. V.**
Postfach 152208, 80052 München.
☎ 89 260 3056
🕐 Mon Fri 20:00 - 23:00

⚲▽ **Viva TS - Selbsthilfe München e. V.**
Hirschbergstraße 14, 80634 München.
☎ 89 13481 ✆ 89 162324
🕐 Call 18:00 - 18:30. German only. Regular meetings
Contact: Herr Peter Reidel

Organizations: Sexuality: Student

⚥▽ **Münchner Hochschwule - Schwulenreferat der LMU**
Leopoldstraße 15, 80802 München.
☎ 89 2180 2072
🕐 Thu 20:00 during term time

Photographers: Fetish

☺ **Nicolas Plakidas**
Mabliebchenstraße 17, 80935 München.
☎ 89 314 3540 ✆ 89 314 3540

Stores: Art Galleries

☺ **Gallerie Reygers**
Widmeyerstraße 49, 80538 München.

Stores: Books: General

⚥▽ **Max & Millian**
Gabelsbergerstrße 65, 80333 München 2.
☎ 89 52 7452 ✆ 89 523 1225
🕐 Mon - Fri 10:00 - 18:30, Thu - 20:20

☺ ■ **Montanus Aktuell**
Stachus Einkaufzentrum, Sonnenstraße, 80331 München.
☎ 89 59 4377

Stores: Clothing: Fetish

☺ ■ **Boutique Highlights**
Gabelsbergerstraße 68, 80333 München.
☎ 89 527475
🕐 10:30 - 18:30, Thu - 20:30, Sat - 14:00
Catalogue, DM20.

☺ **Kießling Handelsagentur**
Georgschwaigstraße 28, München.
☎ 89 35 65 1745

Stores: Clothing: Footwear

☺ ■ **Josef Hiegel**
Auguststraße 113, 80798 München.
☎ 89 527132
High-heeled shoes.

Stores: Erotica: BDSM

⚥▽ **Cornelius Men**
Corneliusstraße 19, 80469 München.
☎ 89 201 4753
🕐 Mon - Fri 10:00 - 18:30, Thi 10:00 - 20:30, Sat - 14:00

⚥▽ **Follow Me**
Corneliusstraße 32, 80469 München.
☎ 89 202 1208
🕐 10:00 18:30, Sat - 14:00
Leather, rubber, uniforms, BDSM toys.

☺ ■ **Hard Line**
Müllerstraße 33, 80469 München.
☎ 89 260 6017 ✆ 89 260 8076
☎ 80 260 6018
🕐 Mon - Fri 12:30 - 18:00, Sat 11:00 - 13:30
♿ [VISA] [MC]
Manufacturers, wholesalers, & retailers of rubber & leather clothes, & BDSM toys.

☺ ■ **Hot Shop**
Rosenhemer Straße 77, München.
☎ 89 487 214
🕐 Mon - Fri 10:00 - 18:00, Sat 10:00 - 13:00

Stores: Erotica: General

⚥▽ **Apollo**
Lindwurmstraße21, 80337 München.
☎ 89 26 7438
🕐 14:30 - 20:00, Sat 11:00 - 16:00

⚥▽ **Buddy**
Utzschneiderstraße 3, 80469 München.
☎ 89 26 8938 ✆ 89 26 8938
🕐 Mon - Fri 10:00 - 18:30, Sat 10:00 -14:00
♿ [VISA] [MC]

☺ ■ **Dr. Müller's Sex Shop**
Sonnenstraße 12, 80331 München.

⚥▽ **Erotic Shop**
Thalkircherstraße 10, 80337 München.
☎ 89 260 78709
🕐 Mon - Fri 09:00 - 20, Sat 09:00 - 14:00

Münster

Helplines: Sexuality

⚥▽ **Rosa Hilfe im KCM**
☎ 251 6 0440
🕐 Wed 20:00 - 22:00, Fri 18:00 - 20:00

Organizations: AIDS: Support

☺ □ **AIDS-Hilfe—Münster**
Herwarthstraße 2, 48143 Münster.
☎ 251 1 9411
🕐 Tue - Fri 14:00 - 19:00

Organizations: Sexuality

⚥▽ **Schwule Väter**
Herwarthstraße 2, 48143 Münster.
☎ 251 3 4969
🕐 Last Fri of month 20:00

⚥▽ **Schwulen- & Lesbenzentrum Münster (KCM)**
Postfach 4407, 48025 Münster.
☎ 251 66 56886
🕐 Wed Fri 20:00, Sun 15:00

⚲▽ **TSH—Münster**
☎ 251 43240
Contact: Fraulein Claudia Scholz

✉▽ **TV Selbsthilfegruppe—Münster**
Herwarthstraße 2, 48143 Münster.

Organizations: Sexuality: Student

⚥▽ **Schwulenreferat beim AStA der WW-Uni**
Schloßplatz1, 48249 Münster.
☎ 251 83 3057
🕐 Mon Tue 11:00 - 13:00, Thu 15:00 - 17:00

⚥▽ **Schwulenreferat im AStA der Fachhochschule**
Corrensstraße 25, 48149 Münster.
☎ 251 8 2001
☎ 251 8 2002
🕐 Tue 11:00 - 13:00, Thu 14:00 - 16:00

Publishers: Magazines: Sexuality

⚥▽ **Die Zauberflöte**
♿ Postfach 4407, 48025 Münster.
☎ 251 263545 📞 251 263555
🖎 ✓
Free local magazine with news, information, calendar, & contacts. Latest
issue can be ordered free. Published every month. English also spoken.

Stores: Books: General

☺ ■ **Hippopotame**
Ludgeristraße 55, 48143 Münster.
☎ 251 51 8011
🕐 Mon - Fri 09:00 - 18:30, Sat 10:00 - 14:00

Stores: Erotica: General

⚥■ **Erotic World**
Wolbecker Straße 1, 48155 Münster.
☎ 251 4 7833
🕐 10:00 - 24:00

⚥▼ **Gerotek**
Mauritzstraße 20, 48143 Münster.
☎ 251 51 1161
🕐 Mon - Sat 10:00 - 22:00, Sun 17:00 - 22:00
🖎 💳 💳

Neubrandenburg

Organizations: AIDS: Support

☺ □ **AIDS-Hilfe—Neubrandenburg**
Ziegelbergstraße 1, 17033 Neubrandenburg.
☎ 395 44 3083 📞 395 44 3083
🕐 Moon 18:00 - 20:00, Wed 09:00 - 11:00, Thu 14:00 - 17:00

Neumünster

Organizations: AIDS: Support

☺ □ **AIDS-Beratung**
Gesundheitsamt, Meßtorffweg 8, 24534 Neumünster.
☎ 432 1942 2837
🕐 Wed 09:00 - 11:00, Thu 14:00 - 17:00

☺ □ **AIDS-Hilfe—Neumünster**
Haart 15a, 24534 Neumünster.
☎ 432 11 9411
🕐 Mon 19:00 - 21:00

Organizations: BDSM

⚥▽ **Arbeits Gemeinschaft S/M & Offentlichkeit**
Holstenstraße 5, 2350 Neumünster.

Organizations: Sexuality

⚥▽ **Homosexuelle Initiative Neumünster (HIN)**
c/o AIDS-Hilfe, Haart 15a, 24534 Neumünster.
☎ 432 12 9097
☎ 432 15 4179(information)
🕐 Meets 1st. Tue 20:00 - ?
Contact: Herr Wolfgang Fehlberg

Neuss

Organizations: AIDS: Support

☺ □ **AIDS-Hilfe—Neuss**
Adolf Flecken Straße 10, 41460 Neuss.
☎ 210 122 2925
🕐 Mon - Fri 10:00 - 14:00, Tue 19:00 - 21:30

Neustadt

Organizations: Sexuality

⚥▽ **Andersrum**
Postfach 101051, 67410 Neustadt.
☎ 632 13 5208
🕐 Wed 20:00 - 22:00

Neustrelitz

Helplines: Sexuality

⚥▽ **Telefon des Vertrauens**
☎ 398 1 4995
🕐 Wed 19:00 - 22:00

Organizations: Sexual Politics

⚥▽ **Arbeitsgemeinschaft Homosexualität Magnus**
Postfach 40, 17221 Neustrelitz.

Nordhorn

Helplines: Sexuality

⚥▽ **Manphone-Schwulenberatung**
Postfach 1812, 48507 Nordhorn.
☎ 592 17 6590
🕐 Thu 19:00 - 20:00

Organizations: AIDS: Support

☺ □ **AIDS-Hilfe—Grafschaft Bentheim**
Postfach 1120, 48501 Nordhorn.
☎ 592 1 9411
🕐 Mon 17:00 - 19:00, Thu 19:00 - 21:00

Nürnberg

Bars: BDSM

⚥▼ **Backstage**
Lammsgasse 8, 90403 Nürnberg.
☎ 911 241 9383
🕐 Tue - Sun 21:00 - 03:00

Helplines: Sexuality

⚥▽ **Rosa Hilfe**
c/o Fliederlich e. V., Luitpoldstraße 15, 90402 Nürnberg.
☎ 911 1 9446
🕐 Wed 19:00 - 22:00

Organizations: AIDS: Support

☺ □ **AIDS-Hilfe—Nürnberg / Erlangen / Fürth**
Hessestraße 5-7, 90443 Nürnberg.
☎ 911 1 9411 📞 911 241 9988
🕐 Thu 19:00 - 21:00, Sun 17:00 - 19:00

Organizations: BDSM

⚥▽ **Leder Jeans Club Ost (LJC Ost)**
Zeltnerstraße 30, 90443 Nürnberg.
☎ 911 24 1471 📞 911 241 9238
📞 911 241 9238
Contact: Herr W. Schmidt

Organizations: Family

☺ □ **Eltern Telefon**
☎ 911 22 2377
🕐 1st Mon of month 19:00 - 22:00

Organizations: Sexuality

⚥▽ **Fliederlich e. V.**
Luitpoldstraße 15, 90402 Nürnberg.
☎ 911 22 2377
🕐 1st. & 3rd. Tue of the month 20:00

✉▼ **Trans Reality**
c/o Fliederlich, Luitpoldstraße 15, 90402 Nürnberg.
☎ 911 22 2377
🕐 2nd. Wed of month 20:00

Publishers: Newspapers: Sexuality

⚥▼ **Nürnberger Schwulenpost**
Luitpoldstraße 15, 90402 Nürnberg.
☎ 911 33 2010
Free at gay & lesbian locations or by subscription. Published every
month.

Radio: Sexuality

⚥▽ **Fliederfunk**
FM 95.8, c/o Radio Z, Hintere Ledergasse 10, 90403 Nürnberg.
☎ 911 20 4069
🕐 Thu 21:00 - 22:00

Stores: Books: General

☺ **Die Bücherkiste**
Schlehegasse 6, 90402 Nürnberg.
☎ 911 22 2423
🕐 Mon - Fri 10:00 - 18:00, Sat - 13:00

☺ **Männertreu**

Bauerngasse 14, 90443 Nürnberg.
☎ 911 26 2676 📠 911 26 9844
🕘 Mon 12:00 - 18:30, Tue Wed Fri 10:00 - 18:30, Thu 10:00 - 20:30, Sat 10:00 - 14:00, Sat - 18

☺▼ **Montanus Aktuell**
Briet Gasse 69, 90402 Nürnberg.
☎ 911 23 2803

☺■ **Regenbogen Buchhandlung**
Kirchenweg 25, 90419 Nürnberg.
☎ 911 33 7785
🕘 Mon - Fri 10:00 14:00 15:00 - 18:30, Sat 10:00 - 14:00

Stores: Clothing: Fetish

☺ **Crazy Fashion**
Schweiggerstraße 30, 90478 Nürnberg.
☎ 911 47 2769 📠 911 471 9350

Stores: Erotica: General

☺■ **Beate Uhse**
Königstraße 69, 90402 Nürnberg.
☎ 911 241 8915
🕘 Mon - Fri 09:00 - 18:30, Thu - 20:30, Sat - 14:00

⚤▼ **New Man im WOS**
Luitpoldstraße 11, 90402 Nürnberg.
☎ 911 20 3443
🕘 10:00 - 00:30, Sun 12:00 - 03:00

Oberhausen

Organizations: AIDS: Support

☺□ **AIDS-Hilfe—Oberhausen**
Langemarkstraße 12, 46045 Oberhausen.
☎ 208 80 6518
🕘 Mon 13:00 - 17:00, Wed 17:00 - 20:00

Radio: Sexuality

⚤▽ ***Blitz***
FM 92.2, Cable 106.2, c/o Förderverein Jungendring, Gerd-Rüdiger Wiechert, Oberhausen.
☎ 911 825 2662
🕘 Tue 10:00 - 18:45

Offenbach

Helplines: Sexuality

⚤▽ **Homosexuelle Selbsthilfe e. V. (HS)**
Postfach 101613, 63016 Offenbach.
☎ 69 84 1933

Organizations: AIDS: Support

☺□ **AIDS-Hilfe—Offenbach**
Frankfurter Straße 48, 63065 Offenbach.
☎ 69 99 3688
🕘 Tue 19:00 - 22:00

Organizations: Sexuality

▽ **Transidentitas**
Postfach 101046, 63010 Offenbach M.
☎ 69 800 1008
🕘 Frankfurt meets 3rd. Wed of month 20:00, Koblenz meets Mon 19:00 - 21:00
Support for transsexuals & transvestites. Groups in other German cities, also. Publishes a newsletter.

⚤▽ **Verein zur Verbesserung der Lebenssituation Homosexueller Frauen & Männer e. V.**
c/o DPVW, Frankfurter Straße 48, 63065 Offenbach.
☎ 69 87 2700

Stores: Books: General

☺■ **Buchladen am Markt**
Wilhelmsplatz 12, 63065 Offenbach.
☎ 69 88 3333
🕘 Mon - Fri 09:00 - 18:30, Sat 09:00 - 14:00

☺■ **Tucholsky Buchladen**
Mittelseestraße 14, 63065 Offenbach.
☎ 69 99 7090
🕘 09:00 - 14:00, 15:00 - 18:30, Sat 09:00 14:00, 1st. Sat of month - 16:00
Small gay lesbian section.

Offenburg

Stores: Erotica: General

☺■ **Erotic Shop**
Unionrampe 6, 77652 Offenburg.
☎ 781 2 3553
🕘 Mon - Fri 09:30 - 24:00, Sat 09:30 - 14:00

Oldenburg

Organizations: AIDS: Support

☺□ **AIDS-Hilfe—Oldenburg**
Nadorster Straße 24, 26123 Oldenburg.
☎ 441 1 9411
☎ 441 88 3010
🕘 Mon Wed 19:00 - 22:00

Organizations: Sexuality

⚤▽ **Na Und e. V.**
Postfach 3804, Ziegelhofstraße 83, 26028 Oldenburg.
☎ 441 777 5923 📠 441 76478
🕘 Wed 18:00 - 20:00. Rosa disco last Sat of month
Mixed gay & lesbian group with helpline, youth group, café, & other groups. Publishes *Rosige Zeiten* every two months.

Organizations: Sexuality: Student

⚤▽ **Schwulenreferat im AStA der Carl von Ossietsky Universität Oldenburg**
Uhlhornstraße 49-55, 26129 Oldenburg.
☎ 441 798 2578
🕘 Mon 12:00 - 16:00

Stores: Books: General

☺■ **Carl von Ossietsky Buchhandlung**
Acternstraße 16, 26122 Oldenburg.

☺■ **Montanus Aktuell**
Postfach , Lange Straße 74, 26122 Oldenburg.

Stores: Erotica: General

☺■ **Intimshop**
Kaiserstraße 11-14, 26122 Oldenburg.
☎ 441 2 7291
🕘 Mon - Sat 09:00 - 24:00

☺■ **Power of Passion**
Postfach 3905, 26029 Oldenburg.

☺■ **Shop 28**
Damm 28, 26135 Oldenburg.
🕘 Mon - Fri 14:30 - 23;00, Sat 15:00 - 23:00

Olpe

Organizations: AIDS: Support

☺□ **AIDS-Hilfe—Kreis Olpe**
Kampstraße 26, 57462 Olpe.
☎ 276 11 9411
🕘 Mon 19:00 - 21:00

Organizations: Sexuality

⚤▽ **Schwulen Selbsthilfegruppe**
Postfach 1549, 57445 Olpe.

Osnabrück

Organizations: AIDS: Support

☺□ **AIDS-Hilfe—Osnabrück**
Koksche Straße 4, 49080 Osnabrück.
☎ 541 1 9411
🕘 Mon - Fri 09:00 - 15:00

Organizations: Sexuality

⚤▽ **Aktionsgruppe Homosexualität Osnabrück e. V. (AHO)**
Postfach 1161, 49001 Osnabrück.
☎ 541 2 2722
🕘 Thu 20:30

⚤▽ **Schwule Coming Out Gruppe**
c/o Lagerhalle, Rolandsmauer / Heger Tor, 49074 Osnabrück.
☎ 541 2 2722
🕘 Tue 20:30

Stores: Books: General

☺■ **Montanus Aktuell**
Große Straße 15-16, 49074 Osnabrück.
☎ 541 2 2787

Paderborn

Organizations: AIDS: Support

☺□ **AIDS-Hilfe—Paderborn**
Postfach 1168, 33041 Paderborn.
☎ 525 11 9411
🕘 Thu Sun 19:00 - 21:00

Organizations: Sexuality

⚢▽ **Schwul in Paderborn**
c/o AIDS-Hilfe, Riemekestraße 15, 33102 Paderborn.
☎ 525 12 1959
🕘 Thu 19:00

Organizations: Sexuality: Student

⚢▽ **AStA-Referat Schwule & Lesben der Universität Paderborn**
Warburger Straße 100, 33098 Paderborn.
☎ 525 160 3174
☎ 525 160 3170
🕘 Mon Wed 16:00 -18:00

Passau

Helplines: Sexuality

⚢▽ **Rosa Telefon—Passau**
☎ 851 7 1973
🕘 Fri 20:00 - 22:00

Organizations: AIDS: Support

☺ □ **AIDS-Beratungsstelle Niederbayern**
Bahnhofstraße 16b, 94032 Passau.
☎ 851 7 1065
🕘 Mon - Fri 09:00 - 13:00

Organizations: Sexuality

⚢▽ **Homosexuelle Initiative Passau (HIP)**
Postfach 1611, 94006 Passau.
☎ 851 7 1973
🕘 Meets Fri 20:00 - 22:00

Pforzheim

Manufacturers: Clothing: Rubber

☺ ■ **Kunzmann**
Postfach 1047, 75110 Pforzheim.
☎ 7231 89774
Catalogue, DM30 or £7, refundable on first order.

Organizations: AIDS: Support

☺ □ **AIDS-Hilfe—Pforzheim**
Frankstraße 143, 75172 Pforzheim.
☎ 732 14 1110
🕘 Mon 18:00 - 20:00

Plauen

Organizations: Sexuality

⚢▽ **Schwul & Lesben in Plauen (SLiP)**
Postfach 712, 08525 Plauen.

Potsdam

Organizations: AIDS: Support

☺ □ **AIDS-Hilfe—Potsdam**
Berliner Straße 49, 14467 Potsdam.
🕘 Wed 19:00 - 20:00

Organizations: Sexuality

⚢▽ **Büro für Gleichgeschlectliche Lebensfragen in Land Brandenburg**
c/o Ministerium für Frauen, Arbeit, & Soziales, Heinrich Mann Allee 103, 14478 Potsdam.
☎ 331 866 5173 — Fax 331 866 5173
🕘 Tue 10:00 - 18:00

⚢▽ **Homosexuelles Integrationsprojekt Potsdam (HIP)**
c/o Haus der Jungend, Berliner Straße 49, 14467 Potsdam.
☎ 331 2 2065
☎ 331 48 2005
🕘 Mon Thu 20:00 - 24:00

Preetz

Organizations: Sexuality

⚢▽ **Schwul-Lesbische Initiative Preetz**
c/o Initiativbüro Der Laden, An der Mühlenau 10, 24211 Preetz.
☎ 434 2 4566
🕘 3rd. Sun of month 15:00

Putbus

Helplines: Sexuality

⚢▽ **Rosa Telefon—Putbus**
☎ 291 498
🕘 Thu 18:00 - 20:00

Recklinghausen

Stores: Clothing: Footwear

☺ ■ **Spezial Schuversand**
Bochumerstraße 100, 45661 Recklinghausen.
High-heeled shoes.

Regensburg

Organizations: AIDS: Support

☺ □ **AIDS-Hilfe—Regensburg**
Bruderwöhrdstraße 10, 93055 Regensburg.
☎ 941 1 9411
🕘 Mon Wed 18:00 - 20:00

Organizations: Sexuality

⚢▽ **Regensburger Schwulen & Lesben Initiative (RESI)**
Blaue-Lilien Gasse 1, 93047 Regensburg.
☎ 941 5 1441
🕘 Wed Fri Sat 20:00 - 01:00, Sun 15:00 - 20:00

Rendsburg

Stores: Erotica: General

☺ ■ **Intim Boutique**
Oberreiderstraße 16, 24768 Rendsburg.

Reutlingen

Photographers: Erotic

☺ **Stephan Richter Photography**
Herman Ehlerstraße 50 / 44, 72762 Reutlingen.
☎ 71 212 2525 — Fax 71 212 2124
Specialises in portraits of people with tattoos & piercings.

Rheine

Organizations: AIDS: Support

☺ □ **AIDS-Hilfe—Kries Steinfurt**
c/o Waltraud Rohlmann, Thiemauer 42, 48431 Rheine.
☎ 591 5 4023

Rosenheim

Stores: Clothing: Footwear

☺ ■ **First In Schumode**
Am Rossacker 13, 83022 Rosenheim.
☎ 803 11 3625
High-heel shoes.

Rostock

Helplines: Sexuality

⚢▽ **Telefon des Vertrauens**
☎ 381 45 3156
🕘 Thu 19:00 - 20:00

Organizations: AIDS: Support

☺ □ **AIDS-Hilfe—Rostock**
Gerberbruch 13-15, 18055 Rostock.
☎ 381 45 3156
🕘 Mon 10:00 - 13:00 16:00 - 18:00, Tue 14:00 - 16:30, Wed 18:00 - 20:00, Thu 14:00 - 18:00

Organizations: Sexuality

⚢▽ **Rat & Tat**
Gerbruch 13-15, 18055 Rostock.
🕘 Mon 10:00 - 13:00 16:00 - 18:00, Tue 15:00 16:30, Thu 14:00 - 16:00 19:00 22:00

⚢▽ **Referat für Schwule & Lesben**
August Bebel Straße 28, 18055 Rostock.
☎ 381 379 2481
🕘 Wed 18:00 - 20:00

Stores: Books: General

☺ ■ **Die Andere Buchhandlung**
Wismarsche Straße 18, 18057 Rostock.
🕘 Mon - Fri 08:00 - 18:00

Rottweil

Stores: Erotica: General

☺ ■ **Intim Boutique**
Königstraße 88, 78628 Rottweil.
☎ 741 1 2714
🕘 Mon - Fri 09:00 - 12:30, 14:00 - 18:30, Sat 09:00 - 13:00

Saarbrücken

Helplines: Sexuality

⚥▽ **Rat & Tat Rosa Telefon—Saarbrücken**
☎ 681 37 4650
🕐 Thu 18:00 - 20:00

Organizations: AIDS: Support

☺ □ **AIDS-Hilfe—Saar**
Nauwieser Straße 19, 66111 Saarbrücken.
☎ 681 1 9411
🕐 Mon - Fri 14:00 - 17:00

Organizations: BDSM

⚥▽ **LC Saar**
c/o Balbier, Mainzerstraße 28, 66111 Saarbrücken.
🕐 Sun - Thu 20:00 - 04:00, Fri Sat - 05:00

Organizations: Sexuality

⚥▽ **Lebensberatung Für Transsexuelle Menschem Im Saarland**
Schloss Straße 6, 66117 Saarbrücken.
☎ 681 583912
☎ 681 589 8449
Contact: Dr. Waltraud Schiffels
2nd. telephone contact is Herr Marc Elholz.

⚥▽ **Das Lesben & Schwulen Zentrum Saar (EZS)**
Bismarkstraße 6, 66111 Saarbrücken.
☎ 681 37 4055
🕐 Mon Wed Thu Fri 16:00 - 23:00, Sun 15:00 - 19:00

Stores: Books: General

☺ ■ **Buchhandlung Berliner Promenade**
Berliner Promenade 12, 66111 Saarbrücken.
☎ 681 3 2670

Stores: Erotica: BDSM

☺ ■ **Pourquoi Pas?**
Ludwigstraße 29, 66115 Saarbrücken.
☎ 681 417018
Catalogue, DM20, £7, $12U.S..

Salzwedel

Stores: Clothing: Fetish

☺ ■ **Shiny Fashion**
Reichstraße 21, 29410 Salzwedel.
☎ 3901 33927
☎ 172 715 9004
🕐 Mon - Fri 11:00 - 13:00 15:00 - 18:30, Thu - 20:00, Sat 10:00 - 13:00

Schatthausen

Photographers: Erotic

☺ **Günter Blum**
Hohenhardterstraße 15, Schatthausen.
Agent: Sylvie Neubauer, Brückenstraße 28, Heidelberg 69120, Germany. 161 164 5145 or 62 227 6378, Facs.: 62 227 6379.

Schwalmstadt

Organizations: Sexuality

⚥▽ **Rosa Hilfe Schwalm-Alsfed**
Jungendwerkstatt, Steingasse 54, 34613 Schwalmstadt.
☎ 669 2 7085 (helpline)
🕐 Meets Tue 20:00 - 22:0

Schwerin

Helplines: Sexuality

⚥▽ **Telefon des Vertrauens**
☎ 385 80 0618
🕐 Thu 17:00 - 22:00

Organizations: Sexuality

⚥▽ **Klub Einblick e. V.**
Dr. Külz Straße 3, 19053 Schwerin.
☎ 385 764 9720 📠 385 764 9720
🕐 Mon - Fri 14:00 - 20:00

Stores: Erotica: General

☺ ■ **Sex Shop Erotik Kaufhaus**
Goethestraße 62, 19053 Schwerin.

Siegen

Helplines: Sexuality

⚥▽ **Rosa Telefon—Siegen**
☎ 271 5 3297
🕐 Wed 19:30 - 21:30

Organizations: AIDS: Support

☺ □ **AIDS-Hilfe—Siegen-Wittgenstein**
Sandstraße 12, 57072 Siegen.
☎ 271 2 2222
🕐 Tue Thu 20:00 - 22:00

Organizations: Sexuality

⚥▽ **Schwule Initiative Siegen (SIS-ters)**
c/o ESG, Burgstraße 18, 57072 Siegen.
🕐 Sun 19:30

Soest

Organizations: AIDS: Support

☺ □ **AIDS-Hilfe—Soest**
Postfach 1101, 59471 Soest.
☎ 292 1 2888
🕐 Mon 18:00 - 20:00

Solingen

Organizations: AIDS: Support

☺ □ **AIDS-Hilfe—Solingen**
Postfach 190149, 42701 Solingen.
☎ 212 1 9411

Photographers: Erotic

☺ **Peter Czernich**
c/o Marquis Magazine, Flensburger Straße 5, 42655 Solingen.
☎ 21 258 6151 📠 21 258 6156

Stores: Books: General

☺ ■ **Montanus Aktuell**
Kölner Straße 99, 42651 Solingen.

Stuttgart

Bars: BDSM

⚥▼ **Boots**
Boperstraße 9, 70180 Stuttgart.
☎ 711 236 4764
🕐 20:00 - 01:00, Fri Sat - 02:00

⚥▼ **Eagle**
Mozartstraße 51, 70180 Stuttgart.
☎ 711 640 6183 📠 711 607 4436
🕐 Sun - Thu 19:00 - 01:00. 2nd. Sun of month dres code: leather, rubber, uniform

Health Services

☺ □ **Städtiches Gesundheitsamt-Beratungstelle für Geschlechtskrankheiten**
Mörikestraße14, 70178 Stuttgart.
🕐 Mon - Thu 09:00 - 11:00, Mon Wed also from 14:00 - 16:00
STD information, counselling, & testing.

Helplines: Sexuality

☺ □ **Leder Beratungstelefon**
☎ 711 61 7318
🕐 2nd. & 4th. Wed of month 19:00 - 21:00

⚥▽ **Rosa Telefon—Stuttgart**
c/o IHS, Postfach 102424, 70020 Stuttgart.
☎ 711 1 9446
🕐 Fri 19:00 - 21:00

Organizations: AIDS: Support

☺ □ **AIDS-Hilfe—Stuttgart**
Silberburgstraße 145B, 70176 Stuttgart.
☎ 711 19411 📠 711 61 6504
🕐 Mon - Thu 18:00 - 21:00

☺ □ **Städtisches Gesundheitsamt AIDS Beratungstelle**
Bismarkstraße 3, 70176 Stuttgart.
☎ 711 216 6292
🕐 Mon - Wed 12:00 - 15:00, Thu 12:00 - 19:00, Fri 09:00 - 13:00
Information, counselling, & anonymous HIV testing.

Organizations: BDSM

⚥▽ **LC Stuttgart e. V.**
Postfach 131216, 70069 Stuttgart.
☎ 711 640 6138 (Eagle bar)

For further information, call the Eagle bar.

Organizations: Bears

Bären Stuttgart
Bonnisheimerstraße 66, 7000 Stuttgart.
Contact: Herr Ralf Dieter Lenz

Organizations: Family

Schwule Väter
c/o AIDS Hilfe, Silberburgstraße 145B, 70176 Stuttgart.
Mon 20:00

Organizations: Sexuality

Initiativgruppe Homosexualität Stuttgart e. V. (IHS)
Postfach 102424, 70020 Stuttgart.
711 62 4870
Tue 20:00

Schwule Aktion Südwest (SAS)
Infotek, c/o Wolfgang Eckstein, Obere Waiblinger Straße 136, 70374 Stuttgart.
711 52 5341

Selbsthilfegruppe—Stuttgart
7143 33502
Contact: fraulein Minica Lusche

Verein für Sexuelle Emanzipation e. V. (VSE)
Postfach 105006, 70044 Stuttgart.

Organizations: Sexuality: Youth

Max & Moritz Jugendgruppe
c/o IHS, Postfach 102424, 70020 Stuttgart.
711 297936
Fri 19:30

Publishers: Magazines: Fetish

Club Caprice
Kastley GmbH, Postfach 700331, 70597 Stuttgart.
711 76 9074 — Fax 711 765 1945
Mon - Fri 09:30 - 17:30, Sat 10:00 - 14:00
$
Bizarre erotic magazine. Age statement of 18 is required. English also spoken. Please see our display advertisement.

Stores: Art Galleries

Kunsthaus Fischinger
Esslinger Straße 20, 70182 Stuttgart.

Stores: Books: General

Erlkœnig Buchladen
Bebelstraße 25, 70193 Stuttgart.
711 63 9139 — Fax 711 63 9139
Mon - Fri 10:00 - 18:30, Sat 10:00 - 14:00
Gay & lesbian bookshop with books, postcards, videos, CDs, etc.. Also mail order. Age statement of 18 is required.

Stores: Clothing: Fetish

Kastley GmbH
Erwin Bälz Straße 73, 70597 Stuttgart.
711 76 9074 — Fax 711 765 1945
Mon - Fri 09:30 - 17:30, Sat 10:00 - 14:00
$
Toys & clothes in leather, rubber, & steel, high heels (including large sizes). Also mail order by catalogues. Age statement of 18 is required. English also spoken.

Stores: Clothing: Footwear

High Heels
Hölderlinstraße 53, 70193 Stuttgart.
711 29 1676
Mon - Fri 15:00 - 18:00
Catalogue, DM20.

Stores: Erotica: General

Beate Uhse
Marienstraße 24, 70178 Stuttgart.
771 61 3748
09:00 18:30, Thu - 20:30, Sat 09:00 - 14:00, summer Sat 09:00 - 16:00

City Sex Boutique
Bärenstraße 5, 70173 Stuttgart.
711 24 4928
09:00 - 18:30, Thu - 20:30, Sat 09:00 - 14:00, summer Sat

09:00 - 16:00

☺ ■ **Dacapo Sexladen**
Blumenstraße 22, 70182 Stuttgart.
☎ 711 236 4734
⌚ 09:00 - 18:30, Thu - 20:30, Sat 09:00 - 14:00, summer Sat 09:00 - 16:00

☺ ■ **Dr. Müller's Sex Shop**
Alte Poststraße 2, 70173 Stuttgart.
☎ 711 29 5561
⌚ 09:00 - 18:30, Thu - 20:30, Sat - 14:00, summer Sat - 16:00

☺ ■ **Erotik Handlung Copenhagen**
Olgastraße 116, 70180 Stuttgart.
☎ 711 640 6778
⌚ 09:00 - 18:30, Thu - 20:30, Sat - 14:00, summer Sat - 16:00

☺ ■ **Sex Shop**
Rotebühlplatz 1, 70178 Stuttgart.
☎ 711 62 5340
⌚ 09:00 - 18:30, Thu - 20:30, Sat - 14:00, summer Sat - 16:00

Suhl

Organizations: AIDS: Support

☺ □ **AIDS-Hilfe—Suhl**
Am Bahnhof 15, 98523 Suhl.
☎ 368 12 0084 — Fax 368 12 0084
⌚ Tue Wed 10:00 - 15:00, Thu -19:00, Fri - 12:00

Organizations: Sexuality

⚥▽ **Schwulengruppe Suhl (Schwugs!)**
Postfach 264, 98529 Suhl.
⌚ Meets 2nd. & 4th. Fri 19:00

Thürmsdorf

Organizations: Sexuality

⚥▽ **Homogruppe Thürmsdorf**
Bärenklause 5, 01824 Thürmsdorf.
⌚ Wed 18:00 - 21:00

Trier

Helplines: Sexuality

⚥▽ **Rosa Telefon—Trier**
☎ 651 1 9411
⌚ Sun 20:00 - 22:00

Organizations: AIDS: Support

☺ □ **AIDS-Hilfe—Trier**
Postfach 2022, 54210 Trier.
☎ 651 1 9411 — Fax 651 2 5595
⌚ Tue 15:00 - 17:00, Wed 19:00 - 21:00

Organizations: Sexuality

⚥▽ **SchMIT-Z**
Postfach 4729, 54237 Trier.
☎ 561 14 1416
⌚ Office Thu 17:00 - 19:00, meetings Thu 20:00 - ?

⚥▽ **Schwulenforum Trier**
Postfach 4729, 54237 Trier.
☎ 651 14 1461
⌚ Meets Mon 20:00

Organizations: Sexuality: Student

⚥▽ **Schwulenreferat**
c/o AStA Universität Trier, Universitätsring 12b, 54290 Trier.
☎ 651 201 2117 — Fax 651 201 3902
⌚ Tue - Thu 12:00 - 14:00
Publishes *Anstoss*.

Piercers

☺ ■ **Baldo's Piercing Studio**
Postfach 2764, 54217 Trier.
☎ 651 2 8335 — Fax 651 2 8335
Fax 651 2 9434

Troisdorf

Organizations: AIDS: Support

☺ □ **AIDS-Hilfe—Rhein-Sieg-Kreis**
Postfach 1110, 53821 Troisdorf.
☎ 224 11 9411
⌚ Tue Wed 15:00 - 18:00, Fri 10:00 - 13:00

Tübingen

Helplines: Sexuality

⚥▽ **Rosa Telefon—Tübingen**
☎ 707 14 4843
⌚ Fri 20:00 - 22:00

Organizations: AIDS: Support

☺ □ **AIDS-Hilfe—Tübingen**
Postfach 1122, Herrenberger Straße 9, 07071 Tübingen.
☎ 707 11 9411
⌚ Counselling Mon 12:00 - 14:00, Tue 16:00 - 18:00 20:00 - 22:00, in person Wed 17:00 - 19:00

Organizations: Sexuality

⚥▽ **Innitiativgruppe Homosexualität Tübingen (IHT)**
Postfach 1772, 72007 Tübingen.
☎ 707 14 2763
⌚ Meets Thu 20:00

⚥▽ **Schwusos**
Postfach 1625, 72006 Tübingen.

Tuttlingen

Organizations: Sexuality

⚥▽ **Homosexuelle Selbsthilfe**
Postfach 4207, 78507 Tuttlingen.
☎ 746 17 6333
⌚ Meets Thu 20:00

Uelzen

Organizations: Sexuality

⚥▽ **Schwul-lesbische Jungendegruppe**
St. Viti Straße 22, 29525 Uelzen.
☎ 581 7007
⌚ Meets Wed 20:00

Ulm

Helplines: Sexuality

⚥▽ **Rosa Telefon—Ulm**
☎ 731 3 7332
⌚ Wed 20:00 - 22:00

Organizations: AIDS: Support

☺ □ **AIDS-Hilfe—Ulm**
Postfach 1670, 89006 Ulm.
☎ 731 3 3731
⌚ Mon - Fri 19:30 - 21:00

Organizations: Sexuality

⚥▽ **SchwUlm**
Furttenbachstraße 14, 89077 Ulm.
☎ 731 3 7332
⌚ Wed 20:00

Photographers: Fetish

☺ **Hard Art Design**
Rychartweg 40, 89075 Ulm.
☎ 731 5 6072 — Fax 731 55 2422

Unna

Organizations: AIDS: Support

☺ □ **AIDS-Hilfe—Kreis Unna**
Nordring 21, 59423 Unna.
☎ 230 31 9411

Viersen

Organizations: AIDS: Support

☺ □ **AIDS-Hilfe—Kreis Viersen**
Lambersartstraße 29, 41747 Viersen.
☎ 216 23 4987

Villingen-Schwenningen

Organizations: Sexuality

⚥▽ **Pink Panther**
c/o AWO Pro Familia, Benediktinerring 7, 78050 Villingen-Schwenningen.
☎ 772 05 9088
⌚ Meets Fri 20:30 - 22:30

Weimar

Health Services

☺ □ **HIV-Antikörpertest**
Postfach 510, Erfurter Straße 17, 99423 Weimar.
☎ 364 36 1451 (office) — Fax 364 35 9636
☎ 364 31 9411 (helpline)

🕐 Mon - Fri 11:00 - 15:00, Wed - 20:00
HIV testing.

Helplines: Sexuality
⚥▽ **Rosa Telefon—Weimar**
☎ 364 3 3407
🕐 Wed 16:00 - 23:00

Organizations: AIDS: Support
☺☐ **AIDS-Hilfe—Weimar**
Postfach 510, Erfurter Straße 17, 99423 Weimar.
☎ 364 36 1451 (office) ✆ 364 35 9636
☎ 364 31 9411 (helpline)
🕐 Mon - Fri 11:00 - 15:00, Wed - 20:00

Organizations: BDSM
⚥▽ **Café Schwarz**
c/o AIDS-Hilfe Weimar, Erfurter Straße 17, 99423 Weimar.
☎ 364 3 3407 ✆
🕐 1st Thu of month 19:00 - 24:00

Organizations: Family
☺☐ **Schwuler Väter—Weimar**
c/o AIDS-Hilfe, Weimar, Postfach 510, Erfurter Straße 17, 99423 Weimar.
☎ 364 36 1451 (office) ✆ 364 35 9636
🕐 Meets 4th. Thu of month 20:00

Organizations: Sexuality
⚥▽ **Felix Halle**
Postfach 107, 99402 Weimar.
☎ 364 342 0873
🕐 Helpline Mon Fri 18:00 - 20:00

Publishers: Newspapers: Sexuality
⚥▼ *GAYmeinsam*
Postfach 510, 99406 Weimar.
☎ 364 36 1451
Published every month.

Wesel
Organizations: AIDS: Support
☺☐ **AIDS-Hilfe—Duisberg / Zweigstelle Wesel**
Herzogenring 4, 46483 Wesel.
☎ 281 2 9980
🕐 Wed 19:00 - 21:00

Westerland
Organizations: AIDS: Support
☺☐ **AIDS-Beratung**
Gesundheitsamt, Hebbelweg 2, 25980 Westerland.
☎ 465 11 3784
🕐 Mon 15:00 - 18:00

Organizations: BDSM
⚥▽ **Sylter Männer Leder Club (SLMC)**
☎ 465 1 7849

Wiesbaden
Helplines: Sexuality
⚥▽ **Rosa Telefon—Wiesbaden**
Postfach 5406, 65044 Wiesbaden.
☎ 611 1 9446
🕐 Mon 18:00 - 21:00

Organizations: AIDS: Support
☺☐ **AIDS-Hilfe—Wiesbaden**
Karl Glässing Straße, 65183 Wiesbaden.
☎ 611 1 9411
🕐 Mon Wed Fri 20:00 - 22:00, Tue Thu 11:00 - 15:00

Organizations: Motorcycle
⚥▽ **MSC Rhein-Main, Frankfurt**
Eleonorenstraße 4, 65185 Wiesbaden.
Contact: Herr Jürgen Möller

Organizations: Sexuality
⚥▽ **Rosa Lüste**
Postfach 5406, 65044 Wiesbaden.
☎ 611 37 7765
🕐 Meets 2nd. Fri of month

⚥▽ **Schwule Initiative Rheingau (SIR)**
Postfach 5221, 65042 Wiesbaden.
☎ 611 7 5141
🕐 17:00

Publishers: Magazines: Sexual Politics
⚥▼ *Nummer*
Nummer Verlag, Postfach 5406, 65044 Wiesbaden.
☎ 611 37 7765
🕐 Mon 18:00 - 21:00

Publishers: Magazines: Sexuality
⚥▼ *Lust*
Nummer Verlag, Postfach 5406, 65044 Wiesbaden.
☎ 611 37 7765
🕐 Mon 18:00 - 21:00
Published every two months.

Wilhelmshaven
Organizations: AIDS: Support
☺☐ **AIDS-Hilfe—Wilhelmshaven**
Bremer Straße 139, 26382 Wilhelmshaven.
☎ 442 11 9411
☎ 442 12 1149 (office)
🕐 Tue Thu 19:00 - 21:00

Wilnsdorf
Organizations: AIDS: Support
☺☐ **AIDS-Hilfe—Kreis Siegen-Wittgenstein**
Wahbach 24, 57234 Wilnsdorf.
☎ 273 7 4253

Witten
Organizations: Sexuality
⚥▽ **Schwule Gruppe Witten**
c/o DPWV, Dortmunder Straße 13, 58455 Witten.
🕐 Meets Sun 16:30

Wolfsburg
Organizations: AIDS: Support
☺☐ **AIDS-Hilfe—Wolfsburg**
Schachtweg 5a, 38440 Wolfsburg.
☎ 536 1 9411
🕐 Mon - Fri 09:00 - 12:00, Mon Thu 19:30 - 21:00

Worms
Organizations: Sexuality
⚥▽ **Dinos**
Postfach 30, 67527 Worms.
☎ 635 98 5200

Wupperthal
Helplines: Sexuality
⚥▽ **Rosa Telefon—Wupperthal**
c/o AIDS-Hilfe Wupperthal, Hofaue 9, 42103 Wupperthal.
☎ 202 45 0004
🕐 Tue 20:00 - 22:00

Organizations: AIDS: Support
☺☐ **AIDS-Hilfe—Wupperthal**
Hofaue 9, 42103 Wupperthal.
☎ 202 1 9411
🕐 Mon - Fri 10:00 - 15:00, Mon 20:00 - 22:00

Organizations: Sexuality
⚥▽ **Schwule Gruppe Wupperthal**
c/o Die Börse, Viehofstraße 125, 42117 Wupperthal.
🕐 Meets Wed 20:00

Organizations: Sexuality: Student
⚥▽ **Die Bunte Tunte**
Max Horkheimer Straße 15, 42119 Wupperthal.
☎ 202 439 2874

Würzburg
Helplines: Sexuality
⚥▽ **Rosa Hilfe**
Postfach 6843, 97018 Würzburg.
☎ 931 1 9446
🕐 Wed 20:00 - 22:00

Organizations: AIDS: Support
☺☐ **AIDS-Beratungsstelle Unterfranken**
Sanderstraße 4a, 97070 Würzburg.
☎ 931 5 0599
🕐 Mon - Fri 09:00 - 12:00, 14:00 - 17:00

Organizations: AIDS: Support

Information, support, & counselling for people infected with or affected by HIV/AIDS.

☺ □ **AIDS-Hilfe—Würzburg**
Grombühlstraße 29, 97080 Würzburg.
☎ 931 1 9411
🕒 Tue Thu 19:00 - 21:00

Organizations: Sexuality

⚤▽ **Würzburger Schwulengruppe (WüHST)**
Postfach 6843, 97018 Würzburg.
☎ 931 41 2646
🕒 Thu 20:00 - 22:00

Stores: Books: General

☺ ■ **Neuer Weg**
Sanderstraße 23-25, 97070 Würzburg.
☎ 931 35 5910

Stores: Erotica: General

☺ ■ **Claudia Sexshop**
Bahnhofstraße 3, 97070 Würzburg.
☎ 931 1 4361
🕒 Mon - Fri 09:00 - 18:00, Sat 09:00 - 13:00

Zwickau

Organizations: AIDS: Support

☺ □ **AIDS-Hilfe (ZASA)—Zwickau**
Schlobigplatz 24, 08056 Zwickau.
☎ 375 78 1017 — Fax 375 85 5370
🕒 Tue 19:00 - 24:00

Hong Kong

Area: Approximately 1,071 square kilometres
Population: Approximately 5,700,000
Capital City: Victoria
Currency: Hong Kong Dollar (HK$)
Official Language: English, Chinese
Major Religions: Christian, Buddism, & Confucianism
National Holiday: Liberation Day, 30th. August
Time zone: GMT plus 8 hours
Country Initials: HK
Electricity: 220 volts, 50Hz
Country Dialing Code (from elsewhere): 852
Intl. Dialing Prefix (out of the country): 001
Climate: Warm in the spring, wet in the summer, cool in the winter, humid all year. Summer average temperature is approximately 28°C, winter average is approximately 15°C.
Age of consent & homosexuality legislation: Homosexual activity was illegal until 1991.

Hong Kong

Manufacturers: Clothing: Footwear

☺ ■ **Abelman Trading Company**
P. O. Box 4017, Hong Kong.
Makes fetish shoes & boots to order.

Iceland

Area: Approximately 103,000 square kilometres
Population: Approximately 258,000
Capital City: Reykjavik
Currency: Icelandic Crown (ikr)
Official Language: Icelandic
Major Religions: 93% Protestant
National Holiday: Independence Day, 1st. December
Time zone: GMT
Country Initials: IS
Electricity: 220 volts
Country Dialing Code (from elsewhere): 354
Intl. Dialing Prefix (out of the country): 90
Climate: Cool, wet ocean weather. Often foggy, with many storms.
Age of consent & homosexuality legislation: Age of consent for sexual activity is 14.

Reykjavik

Organizations: Motorcycle

⚤▽ **MSC Iceland**
Box 5321, Reykjavik 125.
☎ 1 17101
☎ 1 22072

Ireland

Area: Approximately 70,300 square kilometres
Population: Approximately 3,550,000
Capital City: Dublin
Currency: Irish Pound(Ir£)
Official Language: Gaellic & English
Major Religions: 88% Roman Catholic
National Holiday: Independence Day, 17th. April
Time zone: GMT
Country Initials: IRL
Electricity: 220 volts, 50Hz
Country Dialing Code (from elsewhere): 353
Intl. Dialing Prefix (out of the country): 16
Long Distance Dialing Prefix (inside country): 0
Climate: Very mild, particularly in winter. Ireland is wet throughout the year.
Age of consent & homosexuality legislation: Age of consent for sexual activity is 17. Homosexual acts were decriminalized in 1993. In 1992, homosexual acts are not permitted for the members of the military. In 1989, the Prohibition of Incitement to Hatred Act was passed, making it illegal to incite hatred on the basis of sexual orientation.
Legal drinking age: 18

NATIONAL RESOURCES

Helplines: Sexuality

⚨▽ **National Transvestite Line**
☎ 1 671 0939
🕒 Thu 20:00 - 22:00

☺ □ **Parent's Enquiry**
c/o Gay Switchboard, Dublin 7.
☎ 1 872 1055

Organizations: Sexuality

⚤▽ **Gaeilgeori Aerach Aontaithe**
c/o Roy O'Gealbhain, 10 Fownes Street, Dublin 2.
Irish speaking gay group.

⚤▽ **Gay & Lesbian Equality Network (GLEN)**
10 Fownes Street, Dublin 2.
☎ 1 872 1055
🕒 Mon - Fri 12;00 - 17:30

⚤▽ **National Lesbian & Gay Federation**
10 Fownes Street, Dublin 2.
☎ 1 671 0939
🕒 Mon - Fri 12:00 - 17:30

Publishers: Newspapers: Sexuality

⚤▼ ***Gay Community News (GCN)***
10 Fownes Street, Dublin 2.
Free at gay & lesbian locations. Published every month.

CAVAN

Cavan

Organizations: Sexuality

⚤▽ **Border Area Lesbian & Gay Group**
☎ 42 441 10
🕒 Evenings

CORK

County Resources

Film Festivals: Sexuality

⚤ **Lesbian & Gay Film Festival**
8 South Main Street, Cork.
☎ 21 27 8470 — Fax 21 96 5077
☎ 21 27 6582
🕒 Meets twice per month
♿ ✓
Held in conjunction with the annual Cork Film Festival. Organizes social events for the gay & lesbian community at film festival. Age statement of 17 is required.

Helplines: Sexuality

⚢ **Cork Lesbian Line**
8 South Main Street, Cork.
☎ 21 27 8470
🕒 Meets twice per month
Voluntary service run as a collective by women identifying as lesbians for women questioning their sexuality. Provides information on local events. Age statement of 17 is required.

⚣ **Gay Information Cork**

7/8 Augustine Street, Cork.
☎ 21 27 1087
🕐 Wed 19:00 - 21:00, Sat 15:00 - 17:00
Non-directive, non-judgemental listening, advice, & referrals on safer sex, family situations, discrimination, transvesticism, tourist information, etc. in Cork.

Organizations: AIDS: Education
⚥ Southern Gay Health Project
8 South Main Street, Cork.
☎ 21 27 8470 ✆ 21 96 5077
☎ 21 27 6582
🕐 Meets twice per month
Addresses the health issues of gay men in the region. Information on HIV & AIDS, as well as other issues. Age statement of 17 is required.

Organizations: Sexuality
⚥ The Other Place
Lesbian & Gay Resource Centre, 8 South Main Street, Cork.
☎ 21 27 8470 ✆ 21 96 5077
☎ 21 27 6582
🕐 Mon - Sat 10:00 - 17:30
♿ ✓ $
Provides a number of projects for the gay, lesbian, & bisexual community of Cork. Also runs bookshop, café, & weekend nightclub.

Organizations: Sexuality: Youth
⚥ The Other Place
Lesbian & Gay Youth Group, 8 South Main Street, Cork.
☎ 21 27 8470 ✆ 21 96 5077
☎ 21 27 6582
🕐 Meets twice per month
♿ ✓
Social group for lesbians, gay men, & bisexuals under 25 years. Though mainly a social group, we also do educational groupwork. Age statement of 17 is required.

Cork
Helplines: AIDS
⚥▽ AIDS Helpline Cork
☎ 21 27 6676
🕐 Mon - Fri 10:00 - 17:00

Organizations: AIDS: Education
☺ AIDS Alliance / Cairde
16 Saint Peter's Street, Cork.
☎ 21 27 5837 (office)
☎ 21 27 6676 (helpline)

Organizations: Sexuality: Student
⚥▽ University of County Cork Gay Society
c/o Students' Union, University of County Cork, Cork.
☎ 21 27 6871

Stores: Books: General
⚥ The Other Side Bookshop
♿ 8 South Main Street, Cork.
☎ 21 27 8470 ✆ 21 96 5077
☎ 21 27 6582
🕐 Mon - Sat 10:00 - 17:30
♿ ✓
Stocks new & secondhand books: lesbian, gay, women's, politics, & the environment. Also, cards, magazines, t-shirts, & jewelry. Information point.

☺ ■ Waterstones
69 Patrick Street, Cork.
☎ 21 27 6002

Wilton
Helplines: Sexuality
☺ ☐ Southern Health Board
☎ 21 96 6844
🕐 Mon 17:30 - 19:30, Wed 10:00 - 12:00

DUBLIN
County Resources
Helplines: Sexuality
⚥▽ Dublin Gay Switchboard
Carmichael House, North Brunswick Street, Dublin 7.
☎ 1 721 055
🕐 Sun - Fri 20:00 - 22:00, Sat 15:30 - 18:00

Dublin
Helplines: AIDS
☺ ■ AIDS Helpline
☎ 1 724277
🕐 Mon - Fri 19:00 - 21:00, Sat 15:00 - 18:00

Organizations: AIDS: Education
☺ AIDS Alliance
Avoca House, 189-193 Parnell Street, Dublin D1.
☎ 1 733799

Organizations: AIDS: Support
☺ ☐ Body Positive—Dublin
Dame House, 24-26 Dame Street, Dublin D2.
☎ 1 671 2363 ✆ 1 671 2404
☎ 1 671 2364
🕐 Phone for appointment

☺ ☐ CAIRDE
25 Saint Mary's Abbey, Dublin D7.
☎ 1 873 3799
🕐 Mon - Fri 10:00 - 13:00. 'Phone for appointment

⚥▽ Gay Men's Health Project
Baggot Street Clinic, 19 Haddington Road, Dublin D4.
☎ 1 602149
🕐 Tue Wed 20:00 - 21:30
Free HIV & STD testing, counselling, & information.

Organizations: Sexuality: Student
⚥▽ Gay College Societies
c/o Gay Switchboard Dublin, Carmichael House, North Brunswick Street, Dublin 7.
☎ 1 872 1055
Societies for University College Dublin, Trinity College. Call Gay Switchboard for details.

Organizations: Sexuality: Youth
⚥▽ Gay Switchboard Dublin
Carmichael House, North Brunswick Street, Dublin 7.
☎ 1 721 055
🕐 Sun - Fri 20:00 - 22:00, Sat 15:30 - 18:00

Stores: Books: General
☺ ■ Books Upstairs
36 College Green, Dublin.
☎ 1 796687
🕐 Mon - Fri 10:00 - 20:00, Sat - 18:00, Sun 14:00 - 18:00

☺ ■ Easons
340 Lower O'Connell Street, Dublin.
☎ 1 73 3811

☺ ■ Waterstones
7 Dawson Street, Dublin.
☎ 1 679 1415

GALWAY
County Resources
Helplines: Sexuality
⚥▽ Gay Help Line
☎ 91 661 34
🕐 Tue Thu 20:00 - 22:00

Galway
Health Services
☺ ☐ STD Clinic
☎ 91 460 00
🕐 By appointment only

Organizations: AIDS: Education
☺ Western AIDS Alliance/Cairde
Ozanam House, Saint Augustine Street, Galway.
☎ 91 66266

Organizations: AIDS: Support
☺ ☐ AIDS Help West
Oznam House, Galway.
☎ 91 252 00
🕐 Mon - Fri 10:00 - 12:00, Thu 20:00 - 22:00
Education, information, & support.

Stores: Books: General
☺ ■ Sheela-Na-Gig
Cornstore Mall, Middle Street, Galway.

☎ 91 668 49

KILDARE
Maynooth
Organizations: Sexuality: Student
⚥▽ **Maynooth Gay & Lesbian Society**
c/o Student Union, Saint Patrick's College, Maynooth, Kildare.
☎ 1 628 6035

LIMERICK
County Resources
Helplines: Sexuality
⚥▽ **Gay Switchboard Limerick**
P. O. Box 151, Henry Street, Limerick.
☎ 61 310101
🕐 Mon Tue 19:30 - 21:30

⚥▽ **Lesbian Line**
☎ 61 310101
🕐 Thu 19:30 - 21:30

Limerick
Helplines: Sexuality
☺☐ **Regional Hospital**
☎ 61 281 11
🕐 Fri 14:30 - 16:30

Organizations: AIDS: Support
☺☐ **AIDS Alliance**
103 Cecil Street, Limerick.
☎ 61 316661
🕐 Mon Thu 1930 - 21:30

MEATH
Drogheda
Organizations: Sexuality
⚥▽ **Outcomers**
c/o Resource Centre for the Unemployed, 8 North Quay, Drogheda, Meath.
☎ 1 872 1055
🕐 2nd. & 4th. Fri of month 19:00 - 21:00. Contact through the Gay Switchboard in Dublin

TIPPERARY
Clonmel
Organizations: Sexuality
⚥▽ **Clonmel Gay Group**
🕐 Meets twice per month. Contact Gay Switchboard in Dublin for details

Waterford
Stores: Books: General
☺■ **World Development Centre**
Saint John's Way, Waterford.
🕐 Mon - Fri 09:30 - 13:00 14:00 - 17:30

Israel

Area: Approximately 26,265 square kilometres
Population: Approximately 5,500,000
Capital City: Jerusalem
Currency: Shekel (IS)
Official Language: Hebrew & Arabic
Major Religions: 82% Jewish, 14% Moslem
National Holiday: Independence Day, 26th. April
Time zone: GMT plus 2 hours
Country Initials: IL
Electricity: 220 volts
Country Dialing Code (from elsewhere): 972
Intl. Dialing Prefix (out of the country): 00
Climate: Mediterranean to desert in the south. Winters are cool in the mountains & mild in the plains.
Age of consent & homosexuality legislation: Age of consent for homosexual activity is 18
Legal drinking age: 18

Tel-Aviv
Stores: Clothing: Fetish
☺■ **Air Transilvania**
Sheinkin 58, Tel-Aviv.
Latex & PVC clothing.

Italy

Area: Approximately 301,300 square kilometres
Population: Approximately 57,700,000.
Capital City: Roma (Rome)
Currency: Lira (Lit.)
Official Language: Italian
Major Religions: 90% Roman Catholic
National Holiday: Liberation Day, 25th. April
Time zone: GMT plus 1 hour
Country Initials: I
Electricity: 220 volts
Country Dialing Code (from elsewhere): 39
Intl. Dialing Prefix (out of the country): 00
Long Distance Dialing Prefix (inside country): 0
Climate: Mediterranean
Age of consent & homosexuality legislation: Age of consent for sexual activity is 14. Homosexual activity is still unacceptable in the military.
Legal drinking age: 18

NATIONAL RESOURCES
Archives: Sexuality
⚥▼ **Fondazione Sandro Penna**
Via S. Chiara 1, 10123 Torino, Piemonte.
☎ 11 43 4749
🕐 By appointment only
Student library.

⚥▽ **Libreria Gruppo Abele**
Via Melchiorre Gioia 8, 10100 Torino, Piemonte.
☎ 11 54 5420
🕐 09:00 - 13:00 16:00 - 20:00
Good library about homosexuality, transsexuality, & prostitution. Also large selection of press clippings.

Helplines: Sexuality
⚥▽ **Arci Gayline**
☎ 144 880988

Mailorder: Erotica
⚥▼ **Editrice Cassia**
Casella Postale 16089, 20160 Milano, Lombardia.
⚥■ **Frisco**
Via F. Veracini, 50144 Firenze, Toscana.
☎ 55 35 7351 ✆ 55 35 7351
Catalogue available.

Organizations: Bears
⚥▽ **Orsi Italiani Girth & Mirth**
Casella Postale 15028, 20148 Milano, Lombardia.
☎ 2 481 8685 ✆ 2 481 2381
☎ 2 610 2381
$
A club for big, hairy men. Publishes *Orsi Otaliani* every two months. Age statement of 18 is required. English & French also spoken.

Organizations: Body Size
⚥▽ **Magnum Club**
Casella Postale 17140, 20100 Milano, Lombardia.
☎ 2 536273
🕐 Call for more information

Organizations: Motorcycle
⚥▽ **Moto Leather Club Veneto (MLCV)**
Casella Postale 259, Str. Piancoli 13, 36100 Vicenza, Veneto.
☎ 444 32 1290 ✆ 444 32 1290
$
Contact: Mr. Tiziano Bedin.
Leather gay group. Members into uniform, BDSM, motorcycle, rubber. AIDS information. Member EFMC. Promotes international meeting (May), bikers camp (July). Publishes a newsletter every two months. Yearly subscription is 55,000Lira, $45U.S.. Age statement of 18 is required. English, French, & German also spoken.

Organizations: Sexuality
⚥▽ **Arci Gay—Genova**
🖊 Via S. Luca 11/4, 16123 Genova, Liguria.

☎ 10 247 0575
☎ 10 277 0739
🕐 Mon 17:30 - 19:30
English, French, German, & Spanish also spoken.

⚥▽ **Arci Gay—Nazionale**
Casella Postale 691, 40100 Bologna, Emilia Romagna.
☎ 51 644 7054 📞 51 644 6722
🕐 Mon - Fri 11:00 - 13:00
Italy's only national gay organization. Branches all over the country.
Publishes *Con-Tatto*.

Publishers: Books: Sexuality

⚥▼ **Edizione Gruppo Abele**
Via Giolitti 21, 10123 Torino, Piemonte.
☎ 11 839 5444
Publishes Italian gay bibliography & other books on gay subjects.

Publishers: Guides: Sexuality

⚥▼ *Guida Gay*
Babilonia Edizione, Via Ebro 11, 20141 Milano, Lombardia.
☎ 2 57 40 4788

Publishers: Information: Sexuality

☺▽ **ASPE**
Via Giolitti 21, 10123 Torino, Piemonte.
☎ 11 839 5444
Press agency that deals with gay, lesbian, & bisexual issues.

Publishers: Magazines: Erotic

⚥▼ *Babilonia*
Babilonia Edizione, Via Ebro 11, 20141 Milano, Lombardia.
☎ 2 569 6468 📞 2 552 13419
🕐 09:00 - 18:00
Published every month. Yearly subscription is L110,000 overseas
(surface), L130,000 (air).

⚥▼ *Gay Italia*
Casella Postale 16089, 20160 Milano, Lombardia.
Published every two weeks.

⚥▼ *Marco*
Via G. B. Sammartini 21, 20125 Milano, Lombardia.
☎ 2 29 551 7490
Also has a gay guide section.

Radio: Sexuality

⚥▽ **Radio Studio Aperto FM 88.25**
🕐 Tue 10:00 & 18:15

Stores: Books: General

⚥▼ **Libreria Babele**
🚻 Via Sammartini 23/25, 20125 Milano, Lombardia.
☎ 2 669 2986
🕐 Mon - Sat 09:30 - 19:30
💳 [VISA] [CD]
Milan's only completely gay & lesbian book & video shop. Near metro 2
stazione centrale. Catalogue available, published once a year.

Stores: Erotica: BDSM

☺▼ **Carpe Diem**
🚻 Via Marco Polo 32 bis, 10129 Torino, Piemonte.
☎ 11 50 0018 📞 11 59 0735
🕐 09:30 - 12:30 14:00 - 19:30
Specialized in magazines, videos of BDSM, fetish, wrestling, boxing,
spanking, fashion shoes, & boots. Exclusive Italian dealer for Festelle's
videos. Age statement of 18 is required. Spanish, English, & French also
spoken.

⚥▽ **Europa 92**
Via Stradella 12, 20100 Milano, Lombardia.
☎ 2 282 6356
🕐 Mon - Sat 09:30 - 19:30
Specializes in BDSM toys.

⚥▼ **Europa 92—Leather Shop**
Via G. B. Sammartini 21, 20125 Milano, Lombardia.
☎ 2 669 92448
🕐 Mon - Sat 09:30 - 19:30

Stores: Erotica: General

☺■ **Bushido**
Via Andrea Doria 48A, 20100 Milano, Lombardia.
☎ 2 670 6420
🕐 09:30 - 13:00 14:00 - 19:30, closed Sun Mon mornings
Leather & BDSM items, videos, magazines, etc..

☺■ **Europa 92**
Via Sirtori 24, 20100 Milano, Lombardia.
☎ 2 295 13708
🕐 Mon - Sat 09:30 - 19:30

⚥▽ **Europa 92**
Viale Umbria 80, 20100 Milano, Lombardia.
☎ 2 546 9582
🕐 Mon - Sat 09:30 - 19:30

ABRUZZO

Chieti

Health Services

☺□ **Ospedale S. Camillo de Lellis**
Via C. Forlanini, 66100 Chieti, Abruzzo.
☎ 871 64141

L'Aquila

Health Services

☺□ **Ospedale San Salvatore**
Viale Nizza, 67100 L'Aquila, Abruzzo.
☎ 862 7781
HIV testing.

Pescara

Health Services

☺□ **Ospedale Civile**
Via Paolini 45, 65100 Pescara, Abruzzo.
☎ 85 37 3111 Ext.: 406

Helplines: Sexuality

⚥▽ **Arci Gay—Helios**
Via C. Battisti 61, 65100 Pescara, Abruzzo.
☎ 85 294 2221

Rieti

Organizations: Sexuality

⚥▽ **Arci Gay—Rieti**
c/o Bartolucci, Via del Forno 14, 02100 Rieti, Abruzzo.

Teramo

Health Services

☺□ **Ospedale Civile**
☎ 861 4291

BASILICATA

Matera

Health Services

☺□ **Ospedale Provinciale**
☎ 835 2431
HIV information & testing.

Potenza

Health Services

☺□ **Ospedale Provinciale San Francesco di Paola (Pescopagano)**
Via San Pietro, 85100 Potenza, Basilicata.
☎ 971 26929

☺□ **Ospedale San Carlo**
Iazza dele Regione, 85100 Potenza, Basilicata.
☎ 971 3595
HIV testing.

CALABRIA

Catanzaro

Health Services

☺□ **Ospedale Civile**
Via Pio X, 88100 Catanzaro, Calabria.
☎ 961 42613
HIV testing.

☺□ **Ospedale Madonna dei Cieli**
Via Cortese, 88100 Catanzaro, Calabria.
☎ 961 41921
🕐 08:00 - 12:00

Cosenza

Health Services

☺□ **Ospedale Civile dell'Annunziata**
☎ 984 7291
HIV testing.

Stores: Books: General

☺ ■ **Domus**
Corsa d'Italia, 87100 Cosenza, Calabria.
Alternative bookshop. Gay & lesbian books upon request.

☺ ■ **Il Seme**
Via Nicola Serra, 87100 Cosenza, Calabria.
Alternative bookshop.

Crotone

Health Services

☺ □ **Ospedale Malacrino**
☎ 965 34711

CAMPANIA

Avellino

Health Services

☺ □ **Ospedale Civile**
HIV testing.

Capri

Stores: Books: General

☺ ■ **La Conchiglia**
Via le Bottaghe 12, 80073 Capri, Campania.
☎ 81 837 6577

Caserta

Health Services

☺ □ **Ospedale Civile**
☎ 81 23 1111

Napoli

Health Services

☺ □ **Clinica Malatte Infettive**
Via B. Cotugno 3, 80100 Napoli, Campania.
☎ 81 21095
HIV testing.

☺ □ **Ospedale Cotugno**
Via Quagliarello, 80100 Napoli, Campania.
☎ 81 25 7033

☺ □ **Ospedale Pascale**
Via Cappella Cangiani, 80100 Napoli, Campania.
☎ 81 25 7300
HIV testing.

☺ □ **Ospedale Pellegrini Nuovo**
Via Briganti 255, 80100 Napoli, Campania.
☎ 81 780 1122
HIV testing.

☺ □ **Policlinico**
Piazza Miraglia, 80100 Napoli, Campania.
☎ 81 45 5365
HIV/AIDS information & testing. Part of the Arci Gay centre.

Organizations: Sexuality

⚧▽ **Arci Gay—Antinoo**
Via S. Geroniom 17-20, 80100 Napoli, Campania.
☎ 81 552 8815
🕑 Mon - Fri 18:00 - 21:00

EMILIA ROMAGNA

Bologna

Archives: Sexuality

⚧▽ **Centro di Documentazione**
Piazza di Porta Saragozza 2, 40100 Bologna, Emilia Romagna.
☎ 51 644 6824
🕑 Every evening

⚥ □ **Centro per le Donne**
Via Gallera 8, 40100 Bologna, Emilia Romagna.
☎ 51 233863
🕑 Call for meeting times
Women's organization. Large women's & feminist library.

Artists: BDSM

☺ **Susi Medusa Gottardi**
C. P. 6024, 40138 Bologna, Emilia Romagna.
Images of the sophisticated states of libertinage, bizarre piercing, trans-sex, cerebral sadism, etc..

Distributors: Erotica: General

☺ ■ **Cybercore**
Via Lame 57/G, 40122 Bologna, Emilia Romagna.

Helplines: AIDS

☺ □ **Informazioni AIDS**
☎ 51 624 0644
🕑 Mon - Fri 16:00 - 19:00, Sat 09:00 - 12:00

Helplines: Sexuality

⚧▽ **Consultorio Gay**
☎ 51 644 6820
Also books HIV testing.

⚧▽ **Informazioni Gay**
☎ 51 624 7054
🕑 Mon - Fri 11:00 - 13:00

Organizations: Sexuality

⚥▽ **Visibilia**
Piazza di Porta Saragozza 2, 40100 Bologna, Emilia Romagna.
☎ 51 263592
🕑 Wed 21:00 - 23:00

Organizations: Sexuality: Student

⚧▽ **Gaya Mater Studiorum**
c/o Arci Gay, Piazza di Porta Saragozza 2, 40100 Bologna, Emilia Romagna.
☎ 51 644 6824
🕑 Mon 22:00 - 24:00

Stores: Erotica: General

☺ ■ **Andromeda**
Piazza San Simone 1/2, 40100 Bologna, Emilia Romagna.
☎ 51 225976
🕑 Closed Sun & Mon morning
Also sells leather & BDSM items.

⚧▼ **In Line Diffusion**
Via San Simone 1/2, 40100 Bologna, Emilia Romagna.
☎ 51 22 5976
🕑 Mon - Sat 09:30 - 13:00 14:30 - 19:30
Clothing & videos. Also mail order.

☺ ■ **Magic America**
Via Piella 2, 40100 Bologna, Emilia Romagna.
☎ 51 235882
🕑 Mon - Sat 09:00 - 12:30 15:00 - 19:30
In the basement.

Bolzano

Organizations: Sexuality

⚧▽ **Arci Gay—Bolzano**
Via Combattenti 7, 39100 Bolzano, Emilia Romagna.
☎ 471 27 2165

Ferrara

Organizations: Sexuality

⚧▽ **Arci Gay e Lesbica—Ferrara**
Via Cortevecchia, Ferrara, Emilia Romagna.
☎ 532 210597
🕑 Meets Wed

Forli

Health Services

☺ □ **Ospedale Morgagni**
☎ 545 73 1717
HIV information & testing.

Helplines: Sexuality

⚧▽ **Telephono Viola**
Via Fratelli Bandiera 3, 47100 Forli, Emilia Romagna.
☎ 543 34422
🕑 Tue Fri 21:00 - 23:00

Organizations: Sexuality

⚧▽ **Arci Gay—Forli**
Via Fratelli Bandiera 3, 47100 Forli, Emilia Romagna.
☎ 543 34422
🕑 Meetings Tue Fri 21:00 - 23:00

Modena

Stores: Erotica: General

☺ ■ **Magic America**
Via Rua Pioppa 42, 41100 Modena, Emilia Romagna.
☎ 59 21 6774

Parma

Health Services

☺ ☐ **Clinica Dermosifilopatica**
☎ 521 99 1630
HIV testing.

Stores: Erotica: General

☺ ■ **Magic America**
Borgo del Parmigianino 31D, 43100 Parma, Emilia Romagna.
☎ 521 20 6273
⏰ 09:00 - 12:30 15:00 - 19:30

Ravenna

Health Services

☺ ☐ **Lega Volontari Anti-HIV—Ravenna**
Via Roma 141, 48100 Ravenna, Emilia Romagna.
☎ 544 40 9625
⏰ Mon 21:00 - 23:00, Tue - Thu 17:30 - 19:00

Organizations: Sexuality

⚢▽ **Arci Gay—Ravenna**
Casella Postale 524, 48100 Ravenna, Emilia Romagna.
☎ 544 30151

Riccione

Distributors: Piercing Jewelry

☺ ■ **IMAX International**
Casella Postale 240, Via Emilia, 23, 47063 Riccione, Emilia Romagna.
☎ 541 642160 ✆ 541 64352
Distributes piercing jewelry, supplies, & Piercer Training Seminars, exclusively for Gauntlet.

Stores: Erotica: General

☺ ■ **Eros Center**
Via Dante 16, 47036 Riccione, Emilia Romagna.
☎ 541 64 8686
Also sells BDSM items.

Rimini

Organizations: Sexuality

⚢▽ **Eros Center**
Via le Vespucci 29A, 47037 Rimini, Emilia Romagna.
☎ 541 22465
Also sells BDSM items.

Stores: Erotica: General

☺ ■ **Magic America**
Viale Regina Elena 94, 47037 Rimini, Emilia Romagna.
☎ 541 39 1977

FRIULI-VENEZIA GIULIA

Gorizia

Health Services

☺ ☐ **Centro MTS**
Via Mazzini 7, 34170 Gorizia, Friuli-Venezia Giulia.

Pordenone

Health Services

☺ ☐ **Ospedale**
☎ 434 65 2512

Trieste

Health Services

☺ ☐ **Ospedale Di Cattinara**
☎ 40 79 5338
HIV testing.

Organizations: Sexuality

⚢▽ **Arci Gay—Arcobaleno**
Strada di Rozzol 79, 34100 Trieste, Friuli-Venezia Giulia.
☎ 40 94 1708

Stores: Books: General

☺ ■ **Serri di Piazza, Arcobaleno**
Via Felice Venezian 7, 34100 Trieste, Friuli-Venezia Giulia.
Sells gay magazines.

Udine

Helplines: Sexuality

⚢▽ **Arci Gay—Nuovi Passi**
Via Manzini 42, 33100 Udine, Friuli-Venezia Giulia.
☎ 432 51 3311
⏰ Wed 19:00 - 22:00

Organizations: Sexuality

⚢▽ **Arci Gay—Nuovi Passi**
Via Manzini 42, 33100 Udine, Friuli-Venezia Giulia.
☎ 432 51 3311
⏰ 19:00 - 21:00. Meetings Thu 21:00

Stores: Erotica: General

☺ ■ **Magic America**
Via Manzini 38/A, 33100 Udine, Friuli-Venezia Giulia.
☎ 432 29 7345

LAZIO

Roma

Archives: Sexuality

⚢▽ **Ompos's Gay House**
Via Ghiberti 8/B, Roma, Lazio.
☎ 6 93 54 7567 ✆ 6 93 54 7483
No entrance fee. English, French, & Spanish also spoken.

Bars: BDSM

⚢▼ **Hangar**
Via in Selci 69, 00184 Roma, Lazio.
☎ 6 488 1397
⏰ Wed - Sun 22:30 - 02:00
Leather welcome.

Health Services

☺ ☐ **Istituto Dermopatico dell'Immacolata**
Via del Monti di Creta 104, Roma, Lazio.
⏰ 08:00 - 12:00

☺ ☐ **Ospedale S. Gallicano**
Clinica Dermosifilopatica, Via delle Fratte di Travestevere, Roma, Lazio.

☺ ☐ **Ospedale Spallanzani**
Via Portuense 292, Roma, Lazio.
☎ 6 55 4021
⏰ 08:00 - 12:00

☺ ☐ **Policlinico Gemelli**
Clinica Dermosifilipatica, Largo Agostino Gemelli 8, 00100 Roma, Lazio.
☎ 6 330527
⏰ 08:00 - 12:00

Helplines: AIDS

☺ ☐ **Assistenza AIDS**
☎ 6 832 2315
⏰ Mon - Fri 18:00 - 20:00
Information, counselling, & support for people infected with or affected by HIV/AIDS.

Helplines: Sexuality

⚢▽ **Gay Counselling**
☎ 6 702 9037
☎ 6 702 2297

Organizations: AIDS: Support

☺ ☐ **Positif**
Via Ciancaleoni 6, 00100 Roma, Lazio.
☎ 6 488 1859

Organizations: Sexuality

⚢▽ **Arci Gay—Roma**
Via dei Mille 23, 00196 Roma, Lazio.
☎ 6 446 5839
⏰ Sat 18:00 - 20:00

⚢▽ **Cicolo Di Cultura Omosexxuale Mario Mieli**
♿ Via Ostiense 202, Roma, Lazio.
☎ 6 541 3985 ✆ 6 541 3971
⏰ Mon - Fri 18:00 - 20:00
Can arrange anonymous HIV tests.

⚢▽ **Coordinamento Lesbische Italiano**
Via San Francesco di Sales 1A, 0100 Roma, Lazio.
☎ 6 686 4201

Radio: Sexuality

⚢▽ *Effetto Diversita*
Radio Onda Rossa FM 93.3 & 93.45, Via dei Volsci 56, 00100 Roma,

Lazio.
☎ 6 491750
🕘 Fri 16:30

Stores: Books: General

☺ ■ **Grand Mello**
Via di Tor Millina 10/11, 00100 Roma, Lazio.
☎ 6 687 7309
🕘 Mon - Sat 09:30 - 1930

⚢▼ **Libreria Babele**
Via Paola 44, 00186 Roma, Lazio.
☎ 6 687 6628
🕘 Mon - Sat 09:30 - 1930

Stores: Erotica: General

☺ ■ **Cobra**
Via Barietta, Roma, Lazio.
☎ 6 38 5947

☺ ■ **Magic America**
Via Marco Valerio Corvo 118, 00100 Roma, Lazio.
☎ 6 769 02211

LIGURIA

Genova

Health Services

☺ □ **Ospedale San Martino**
Via Benedetto XV 10, 16100 Genova, Liguria.
☎ 10 35351
HIV testing.

Helplines: Sexuality

⚢▽ **Arci Gay—Genova**
Via S. Luca 11/4, 16100 Genova, Liguria.
☎ 10 247 0575
☎ 10 277 0739
🕘 Mon 17:30 - 19:30

Stores: Erotica: General

☺ ■ **Magic America**
Via Teodosia 7/R, 16100 Genova, Liguria.
☎ 10 31 6783
🕘 09:00 - 19:30

La Spezia

Health Services

☺ □ **Sezione Malattie Infettive dell'Ospedale**
Via Vittorio Veneto, 19100 La Spezia, Liguria.
☎ 187 53 5111

Stores: Erotica: General

☺ ■ **Privaty Shop**
Via San Ferarri 25, 19100 La Spezia, Liguria.
☎ 187 52 4268

LOMBARDIA

Bergamo

Health Services

☺ □ **Ospedali Riuniti**
Largo Barozzi 1, 24100 Bergamo, Lombardia.
☎ 35 26 9111
🕘 Mon 08:00 - 12:00 14:00 - 17:00

Organizations: Sexuality

⚢▽ **Arci Gay—Bergamo**
Via Baschenis 9, 24100 Bergamo, Lombardia.
☎ 35 23 0959
🕘 Meets Tue 18:00 - 19:00, Thu 21:00 - 22:30, Sat 15:00 - 18:00

Brescia

Health Services

☺ □ **Centro Democeltico**
Via Galilei 22, 25100 Brescia, Lombardia.
☎ 30 399 4615

☺ □ **Ospedale Santa Anna**
☎ 301 58 5329

Organizations: Sexuality

⚢▽ **Pianeta Viola**
c/o Arci, Via Cefalonia 41A, 25100 Brescia, Lombardia.
☎ 30 242 1840
🕘 Meets Mon Wed 20:30 - 22:30

Stores: Erotica: General

☺ ■ **Desiderio**
Viale Stazione 16A, 25100 Brescia, Lombardia.
☎ 30 41840

Cremona

Health Services

☺ □ **Gruppo C**
☎ 372 45 1755
Free anonymous HIV testing.

☺ □ **Istituti Ospedale**
Viale Concordia 1, 26100 Cremona, Lombardia.
☎ 372 40 5518

Organizations: Sexuality

⚢▽ **Arci Gay—Cremona**
Via Speciano 4, 26100 Cremona, Lombardia.
☎ 372 20484
🕘 Fri 21:00 - 23:00, except Aug

Milano

Archives: Sexuality

⚢▽ **Fondo Olivari**
c/o Centro d'Iniziativa Gay, Via Torricelli 19, 20100 Milano, Lombardia.
☎ 2 581 00299 — Fax 2 839 4604
🕘 15:00 - 20:00, also Wed - 24:00
Library of gay & lesbian publications.

Bars: BDSM

⚢▼ **Company Club**
Via Benadir 14, 20100 Milano, Lombardia.
☎ 2 282 9481
🕘 21:00 - 02:00, Fri Sat - 06:00
Some leather.

⚢▼ **Querelle**
Via de Castillia, 20100 Milano, Lombardia.
☎ 2 68 3900
🕘 Tue - Sun 20:00 - 02:00, closed Aug
Some leather.

Health Services

☺ □ **Centro Antivenereo (CAVE)**
Via Pace 9, 20100 Milano, Lombardia.
☎ 2 550 35226
☎ 2 551 16180
🕘 07:30 - 11:00
STD clinic for Italian residents only.

Helplines: Sexuality

⚢▽ **SOS Gay**
c/o L. I. L. A., Viale Tibaldi 41, 20100 Milano, Lombardia.
☎ 2 832 2762
☎ 2 832 3775
🕘 17:30 - 19:30
Also 2 835 7188.

⚢▽ **Telefono Amica**
c/o Centro d'Iniziativa Gay, Via Torricelli 19, 20100 Milano, Lombardia.
☎ 1678 27182
☎ 2 894 01749
🕘 Wed 20:00 - 24:00
Free from Lombardy.

⚢▽ **Telefono Amico Gay**
c/o Centro d'Iniziativa Gay, Via Torricelli 19, 20100 Milano, Lombardia.
☎ 1678 27182
☎ 2 894 01749
🕘 Mon Thu 21:00 - 24:00
Free from Lombardy.

⚢▽ **Telefono Gay**
c/o Centro d'Iniziativa Gay, Via Torricelli 19, 20100 Milano, Lombardia.
☎ 2 581 00299
🕘 Sun - Fri 11:00 - 20:00

Organizations: AIDS: Education

☺ □ **Associazione Solidarieta AIDS (ASA)**
Via Panzeri 11, 20100 Milano, Lombardia.
☎ 2 581 07084
🕘 10:00 - 19:00
Information, support, & counselling for people infected with or affected by HIV/AIDS.

Organizations: Body Size

⚢▽ **Girth & Mirth—Italia Magnum Club**

Casella Postale 17140, 20128 Precotto, Lombardia.
☎ 3 531 5998 📠 2 262 0000

Organizations: Family

☺ □ **Associazione Genitori di Omosessuali (AGEDO)**
c/o Centro d'Iniziativa Gay, Via Torricelli 19, 20100 Milano, Lombardia.
☎ 2 894 01749
🕒 Thu 14:00 -17:00
information & counselling for parents of gays.

Organizations: Motorcycle

⚥ ▽ **Italia Motor Club Milano (IMC)**
Via C. Battisti 13, 20090 Milano, Lombardia.
☎ 2 0250 4889
🕒 Meets Thu 22:00 - 24:00
Contact: Mr. Gabriel Molinari

Organizations: Sexuality

⚥ ▽ **Arci Gay—Milano**
c/o Centro d'Iniziativa Gay, Via Torricelli 19, 20100 Milano, Lombardia.
☎ 2 839 4604
🕒 11:00 - 20:00

⚢ ▽ **CDM**
Via Cicco Simonetta 15, 20100 San Agostino, Lombardia.
☎ 2 839 4604
🕒 Meets Sun 15:00 - 20:00

⚥ ▽ **Centro d'Iniziativa Gay**
Courtyard, Via Torricelli 19, 20100 Milano, Lombardia.
☎ 2 839 4604
🕒 Mon Thu Sun 15:00 - 20:00
Anti-AIDS programme, social, cultural, & political activities. Coördinates local university gay & lesbian groups.

Organizations: Sexuality: Student

⚥ ▽ **R. O. S. PO.**
Via Bonardi 3, 20100 Milano, Lombardia.

Photographers: Erotic

⚥ ▼ **Tony Patrioli**
Casella Postale 10273, 20110 Milano, Lombardia.

Radio: Sexuality

⚥ ▽ ***L'Altro Martedi***
Radio Popolare FM 105.5 & 107.6, Via Stradella 10, 20100 Milano, Lombardia.
☎ 2 80 8249
☎ 2 80 9100
🕒 Tue 22:00 - 23:00

Stores: Erotica: General

⚥ ▼ **In Line Diffusion**
Via Scarlatti 20, 20100 Milano, Lombardia.
☎ 2 20 1894
🕒 Mon - Sat 09:30 - 13:00 14:30 - 19:30

⚥ ▼ **Know How**
Piazza Duca d'Aosta 12, 20100 Milano, Lombardia.
☎ 2 66 98 7065
🕒 09:00 - 12:30 13:30 - 19:00

⚥ ▼ **Magic America**
Via Legnone 19, 20100 Milano, Lombardia.
☎ 2 688 1057
🕒 09:00 - 19:30, Sat - 17:00

☺ ■ **Magic America**
Via P. Castaldi 27, 20100 Milano, Lombardia.
☎ 2 29 52 4386
🕒 09:00 - 19:30, Sat - 17:00

☺ ■ **Magic America**
Via Bramate 20, 20100 Milano, Lombardia.
☎ 2 349 4118
🕒 09:00 - 19:30, Sat - 17:00

☺ ■ **Magic America**
Viale Umbria 50, 20100 Milano, Lombardia.
☎ 2 546 5679

☺ ■ **Magic America**
Via Inama 17, 20100 Milano, Lombardia.
☎ 2 761 0083

☺ ■ **Magic America**
Via Misurata 17, 20100 Milano, Lombardia.
☎ 2 423 9980

Pavia

Health Services

☺ □ **Ospedale San Matteo**
Piazzale Golgi 2, 27100 Pavia, Lombardia.
☎ 382 39 0660 Ext.: 3881
HIV testing & treatment.

Sondrio

Health Services

☺ □ **Ospedale Civile**
Via Stelvio 29, 23100 Sondrio, Lombardia.
☎ 342 81 3470

Varese

Health Services

⚥ ▽ **Arci Gay—Varese**
Via Piave 6, 21100 Varese, Lombardia.
☎ 332 23 4055 📠 332 23 0037
🕒 Wed 21:00 - 23:00

☺ □ **Ospedale Macchi—Varese**
Malattie Infettive, Viale Borri 57, 21100 Varese, Lombardia.
☎ 332 27 8234
🕒 11:00 - 12:00

MARCHE

Ancona

Health Services

☺ □ **Ospedale Umberto I**
Clinica Dermatologica, Largo Cappelli, 60100 Ancona, Marche.
☎ 71 5961 3270
🕒 08:00 - 12:00
HIV testing.

Organizations: Sexuality

⚥ ▽ **Arci Gay—Il Gabbiano**
Via Mazzini 64, 60100 Ancona, Marche.
☎ 71 203 0454 📠 71 203 3050
🕒 Wed 20:00 - 23:00

Radio: Sexuality

⚥ ▽ ***L'Altra Faccia della Luna***
Gay Radio Sibilla FM 103, c/o Arci Gay Il Gabbiano, Via Mazzini 64, 60100 Ancona, Marche.
☎ 71 203 0454 📠 71 203 3050
🕒 Mon every 2nd. week 21:00

Macerata

Health Services

⚥ ▽ **Ospedale Generale Provinciale**
☎ 733 2571

Pesaro

Health Services

☺ □ **Ospedale S. Salvatore di Muraglia**
Via Lombroso, 61100 Pesaro, Marche.
☎ 721 36 4052

Radio: Sexuality

⚥ ▽ **Radio Punto Stereo FM 88.5, 103.5**
🕒 Wed 23:00 - 03:00

MOLISE

Campobasso

Health Services

☺ □ **Ospedale A Cardanelli**
Via Petrella, 86100 Campobasso, Molise.
☎ 874 99791
HIV testing.

PIEMONTE

Regional Resources

Archives: Sexuality

⚥ ▽ **Arci Gay—Torino**
Centro di Documentazione, Via Basilica 5, 10122 Torino, Piemonte.
☎ 11 521 1116 📠 11 521 1132
🕒 Mon - Sat 15:00 - 19:00

Helplines: Sexuality

⚥ ▽ **Arci Gay—Torino**
Via Basilica 5, 10122 Torino, Piemonte.

Helplines: Sexuality

☎ 11 521 1116 📱 11 521 1132
🕐 Mon - Sat 15:00 - 19:00
⚓

Organizations: Family

☺ ☐ **Assoziazione Genitori di Omosessuali (AGEDO)**
c/o Arci Gay, Via Basilica 5, 10122 Torino, Piemonte.
☎ 11 521 1116 📱 11 521 1132
🕐 Fri 17:00 - 19:00
Support for parents of lesbians & gays.

Organizations: Sexuality

⚥♀▽ **Arci Gay e Lesbica—Torino**
Via Basilica 5, 10122 Torino, Piemonte.
☎ 11 521 1116 📱 11 521 1132
🕐 Mon - Sat 15:00 - 19:00
⚓
Contact: Mr. Maurice Circolo

Alessandria

Health Services

☺ ☐ **Ospedale San Antonio**
☎ 131 3061
HIV testing.

Asti

Health Services

☺ ☐ **Ospedale Civile**
☎ 141 3941
HIV testing & information.

Biella

Health Services

☺ ▽ **L'Araba Fenice**
Casella Postale 394, 13051 Biella, Piemonte.
🕐 Tue 18:00 - 20:00
HIV information & testing at Via Orfanotrofio 14.

☺ ☐ **Ospedale Civile**
☎ 15 35031
HIV information & testing.

Cuneo

Health Services

☺ ☐ **Ospedale Civile**
☎ 171 44182 Ext.: 441
HIV information & testing.

Torino

Counsellors

⚥▽ **Ospedale Mauriziano**
Consultorio di Sessuologia, Largo Turati 62, 10100 Torino, Piemonte.
☎ 11 50801
Information, counselling, & operations for transexuals.

Health Services

☺ ☐ **Ospedale Amedeo di Savoia**
Corso Svizzera 164, 10100 Torino, Piemonte.
☎ 11 771 0514 AIDS information
☎ 11 55421
🕐 08:00 - 12:00
HIV testing & treatment.

☺ ☐ **Ospedale Molinette**
Corso Bramante 89-90, 10100 Torino, Piemonte.
HIV testing.

☺ ☐ **Ospedale San Lazzaro**
Consultorio di Venereologia, Via Cherasco 23, 10100 Torino, Piemonte.
☎ 11 66251
No HIV testing available.

Helplines: Sexuality

⚥♀▽ **Informagay**
Via S. Chiara 1, 10100 Torino, Piemonte.
☎ 11 436 5000 📱 11 436 8638
🕐 Tue 17:00 - 20:00 21:00 - 23:00, Thu 21:00 - 23:00, Sat 17:00 - 20:00
Information, counselling, support for HIV/AIDS & sexuality issues.

Organizations: Motorcycle

⚥♀▽ **Leather Motor Club Torino**
Corso Marconi 9, 10125 Torino, Piemonte.
☎ 11 669 2599 📱 11 669 2599
🕐 Meets monthly
Contact: Franco Sobrito

Stores: Books: General

☺ ■ **Bottega di Monica e Patrick**
Via San Tommaso 27, 10100 Torino, Piemonte.
Gay literature available. Also mail order.

⚥♀▼ **Libreria Internazionale Luxemburg**
Via Battisti 7, 10100 Torino, Piemonte.
☎ 11 561 3896 📱 11 54 0370
🕐 Mon - Sat 09:00 - 12:30 15:00 - 19:30
International bookstore with gay & lesbian publications.

Stores: Erotica: BDSM

☺ ■ **L'Occhiolino**
Via Gioberti 40, 10128 Torino, Piemonte.
☎ 11 54 9440
🕐 Mon - Sat 09:00 - 19:30

Stores: Erotica: General

⚥♀▼ **In Line Diffusion**
Corso Racconigi 40, 10100 Torino, Piemonte.
☎ 11 38 6512
🕐 Mon - Sat 09:00 - 12:30 14:30 - 19:30
Leathers, toys, & videos.

☺ ■ **Magic America**
Via dell'Accademia Albertina 29, 10100 Torino, Piemonte.
☎ 11 817 7007
🕐 Mon - Sat 09:00 - 19:30
Large video shop.

PUGLIA

Bari

Health Services

☺ ☐ **Clinica Dermatologica**
Piazza G. Cesare 11, 70100 Bari, Puglia.
🕐 08:00 - 12:00
HIV testing.

☺ ☐ **Ospedale di Venere**
Centro Immunotrasfusionale, Via Amendola 207, 70100 Bari, Puglia.
☎ 80 35 0731
HIV testing.

☺ **Policlinico**
Malattie Infettive, Piazza G. Cesare 11, 70100 Bari, Puglia.
☎ 80 27 1111
☎ 80 36 9068
🕐 08:00 - 12:00
HIV testing.

Organizations: Sexuality

⚥♀▽ **Arci Gay—Bari**
Via Celentano 81, 70100 Bari, Puglia.
☎ 80 554 3474
🕐 Tue - Sun 20:30 - 22:30, Mon 16:00 - 20:00

Brindisi

Health Services

☺ ☐ **Ospedale di Summa**
☎ 831 2042
HIV testing & information.

Organizations: Sexuality

⚥♀▽ **Attika**
Via San Chiara, 72100 Brindisi, Puglia.
☎ 831 563051

Foggia

Organizations: Sexuality

⚥♀▽ **Arci Gay—Foggia**
Via Trieste 46, 71100 Foggia, Puglia.

Lecce

Health Services

☺ ☐ **Unita Sanitaria Locale (USL)**
☎ 832 6851
HIV information & testing.

Organizations: Sexuality

⚥♀▽ **Arci Gay—Arcobaleno**
Vico Conservatorio San Leonardo 20, 73100 Lecce, Puglia.
☎ 832 30 6138
🕐 Sat Sun 20:00 - 23:00

Taranto
Health Services
☺ ☐ **Ospedale SS. Annunziata**
Via Bruno, 74100 Taranto, Puglia.

SARDEGNA
Alghero
Health Services
☺ ☐ **Ospedale Civile**
☎ 79 95 0235
HIV testing & information about HIV/AIDS.

Cagliari
Health Services
☺ ☐ **Centro Epidemiologico Sardo**
Via Cadello 9B, 09100 Cagliari, Sardegna.

☺ ☐ **Ospedale SS. Trinita**
☎ 70 285 2294

Organizations: Sexuality: Youth
⚢▽ **Arci Gay—Cagliari**
Vicoprimo XX Settembre 6, 09100 Cagliari, Sardegna.
☎ 70 65 5998
🕘 19:00 - 22:00 every day
Counselling, support, information about sexuality & HIV/AIDS. Also has a library.

Sassari
Health Services
☺ ☐ **Istituto Malattie Infettive—Sassari**
Via Manno 54, 07100 Sassari, Sardegna.
☎ 79 231 1659

Organizations: Sexuality
⚢▽ **Arci Gay—Sassari**
Via dei Corsi 31, 07100 Sassari, Sardegna.
☎ 79 23 5366
🕘 Call Tue Thu for info. Meets Sun 20:00 - 22:00

SICILIA
Caltanissetta
Health Services
☺ ☐ **Ospedale V. Emanuele**
☎ 934 32611
HIV information & testing.

Catania
Health Services
☺ ☐ **Clinica Dermosifilopatica**
Piazza Sant' Agata le Vetere 5, 95100 Catania, Sicilia.
☎ 95 32 2720
🕘 08:00 - 12:00

☺ ☐ **Ospedale Maurizio Ascoli**
Via Passo Gravini, 95100 Catania, Sicilia.
☎ 95 759 1111
🕘 08:00 - 12:00

Organizations: Sexuality
⚢▽ **Arci Gay—Catania**
Via Canfora 11, 95100 Catania, Sicilia.
☎ 95 50 5830 — 📠 95 50 5830
🕘 Thu 21:00 - ?

⚢▽ **Arci Gay—Enna**
c/o Lega Ambiente, Via Bagni 39, 94100 Catania, Sicilia.
☎ 935 50 0021

Masalucia
Organizations: Bears
⚢▽ **Orsiciliani**
Casella Postale 16, 95030 Masalucia CT, Sicilia.

Messina
Health Services
☺ ☐ **Ospedale Regina Marherita**
Viale della Libertà, 98100 Messina, Sicilia.
☎ 90 292 6284
HIV testing.

Organizations: Sexuality
⚢▽ **Arci Gay—Messina**
Casella Postale 154, 98100 Messina, Sicilia.
☎ 90 69 3542
🕘 Fri 21:30 - 23:00

Palermo
Health Services
☺ ☐ **Ospedale Civico**
Via C. Lazzaro, 90100 Palermo, Sicilia.
☎ 91 48 9004
🕘 08:00 - 12:00
HIV testing.

☺ ☐ **Ospedale Guadagna**
Via Villa Grazia 46, 90100 Palermo, Sicilia.
☎ 91 39 7111
☎ 91 39 7270

Organizations: Sexuality
⚢▽ **Arci Gay e Lesbica—Palermo**
Via Genova 7, 90100 Palermo, Sicilia.
☎ 91 33 5688
🕘 Mon - Sat 11:00 - 13:00 17:00 - 20:00, closed Aug

Ragusa
Organizations: Sexuality
⚢▽ **Arci Gay—Coccioli**
Corso Italia 4, 97100 Ragusa, Sicilia.
☎ 932 20471

Radio: Sexuality
⚢▽ ***Gay Radio***
Arci Gay, Corso Italia 4, 97100 Ragusa, Sicilia.
☎ 932 20471
🕘 Tue 15:00 - 16:30

TOSCANA
Empoli
Organizations: Sexuality
⚢▽ **Arci Gay—Empoli**
Via Paladini 31, 50053 Empoli, Toscana.
☎ 571 71 0301
🕘 Mon - Thu 16:00 - 19:00 21:30 - 24:00, Tue Wed Fri 21:30 - 24:00
STD & HIV/AIDS information, counselling, & support..

Firenze
Health Services
☺ ☐ **Clinica Dermosifilopatica**
Via degli Alfani, 50100 Firenze, Toscana.
☎ 55 247 8351
🕘 Mon - Fri 08:00 - 12:00
HIV testing.

☺ ☐ **Policlinico di Careggi**
Viale Morgagni 85, 50100 Firenze, Toscana.
☎ 55 439 9620
🕘 Mon - Fri mornings
HIV testing.

Helplines: Sexuality
⚢▽ **Gay Line**
c/o Arci Gay, Via Paladini 31, 50053 Firenze, Toscana.
☎ 1678 69042 (free)
🕘 Mon 21:30 - 24:00

Organizations: Family
☺ ☐ **Associazione Genitori di Omosessuali (AGEDO)**
Via del Leone 5/11R, 50100 Firenze, Toscana.
☎ 55 28 8126 — 📠 55 239 8772
🕘 Thu 18:00 - 20:00
For parents of lesbians & gays.

Organizations: Motorcycle
⚢▽ **MCF Leather Motor Club Firenze**
Box 536, Via Galiano 29R, 50100 Firenze, Toscana.

Organizations: Sexuality
⚢▽ **Arci Gay—Firenze**
Via del Leone 5/11R, 50124 Firenze, Toscana.
☎ 55 28 8126

Organizations: Sexuality

 🕐 Mon Wed Fri 16:00 - 20:00. Men meet Mon, women meet Thu 21:00
Information, counselling, & support. Also has library/archive.

☿♀ **Tabasco**
Piazza S. Cecilia 3R, 50100 Firenze, Toscana.
 ☎ 55 21 3000
 🕐 Sun - Thu 21:00 - 03:00, Fri Sat - 06:00
Leather welcome.

Publishers: Books: Erotic

☺■ **Edizioni d'Essai**
Via Giovanni da Montorsoli, 37/39, 50142 Firenze, Toscana.
 ☎ 55 717 880
High quality books of prints from BDSM & fetish illustrators. Catalogue available.

Publishers: Books: Fetish

♟♟ **Glittering Images**
Via Giovanni da Montorsoli, 37/39, 50142 Firenze, Toscana.
 ☎ 55 717 880
Publishes an illustrated anthology about the Marquis de Sade.

Radio: Sexuality

☿♀ *Un Mercoledi da Leone*
 ☎ 55 30 8461
 🕐 Wed 22:00 - 24:00

Stores: Erotica: BDSM

☺□ **Studio Blu**
Via delle Panche 8R, 50100 Firenze, Toscana.
 ☎ 55 422 3767
 🕐 09:30 - 13:00 14:00 - 19:30, closed Sun Mon mornings

Stores: Erotica: General

☺■ **Magic America**
Via Guelfa 89-91, 50100 Firenze, Toscana.
 ☎ 55 21 2840

Pisa

Health Services

☺□ **Ospedale S. Chiara**
 ☎ 50 59 2111
 ☎ 50 59 2338

Organizations: Sexuality

☿♀ **Arci Gay—Pisa**
Vicolo della Croce Rossa 7, 56100 Pisa, Toscana.
 ☎ 50 54 4646
 🕐 Mon - Wed 17:00 - 19:30

Siena

Organizations: Sexuality

☿♀ **Logos**
Casella Postale 103, 53100 Siena, Toscana.

TRENTINO

Bolzano

Organizations: Sexuality

☿♀ **Arci Gay—Centaurus**
Casella Postale 64, 39100 Bolzano, Trentino.

Trento

Health Services

☺□ **Ospedale Civile S. Chiara**
Largo Medaglie d'Oro, 38100 Trento, Trentino.
 ☎ 461 92 5125
HIV testing.

Organizations: Sexuality

☿♀ **Arci Gay—Trento**
Casella Postale 226, 38100 Trento, Trentino.
 ☎ 461 41 0808

UMBRIA

Perugia

Health Services

☺□ **Ospedale Policlinico Monteluce**
Via Brunamonti, 06100 Perugia, Umbria.
 ☎ 75 66118
HIV testing.

Helplines: AIDS

☺□ **Telefono AIDS**
Via Antonio Fratti 18, 06100 Perugia, Umbria.
 ☎ 75 63942
 🕐 Mon Wed Fri 21:00 -23:00

Stores: Erotica: BDSM

☺■ **Paradise Sexy Shop**
Via Gerardo Dorotti 90, 06100 Perugia, Umbria.
 ☎ 75 527 0121 ✆ 75 840 0002
 🕐 Mon - Sat 09:30 - 13:00 15:30 - 20:00
Extensive range of leather & rubber.

Terni

Health Services

☺□ **Ospedale Generale Provinciale**
Viale Tristano di Ioannuccio, 05100 Terni, Umbria.
 ☎ 744 57141
HIV testing.

VALLE D'AOSTA

Aosta

Health Services

☺□ **Ospedale Civile**
Reparto Dermatologico, Via Ginevra, 11100 Aosta, Valle D'Aosta.
 ☎ 165 3041

☺□ **Unita Sanitaria Locale (USL)**
Centro Trasfusionale dell'Ospedale, Via St. Martin d'Orléans, 11100 Aosta, Valle D'Aosta.
 ☎ 165 55 2675
HIV testing.

VENETO

Belluno

Organizations: Sexuality

☿♀ **Arci Gay—Belluno**
Via Caffi 113, 32100 Belluno, Veneto.
 ☎ 437 94 0209

Legnano

Organizations: Sexuality

☿♀ **Arci Gay—Legnano**
Viale dei Caduti 28, 37045 Legnano, Veneto.
 ☎ 442 26053

Mestre

Health Services

☺□ **Centro Dermoceltico USL**
Via S. Maria dei Battuti, 30170 Mestre, Veneto.
HIV testing.

☺□ **Gruppo C**
c/o Ufficio d'Igiene, S. Maria dei Battuti, 30170 Mestre, Veneto.
 ☎ 41 98 7868
Free, anonymous HIV testing.

Organizations: Sexuality

☿♀ **Arci Gay—Mestre**
Via Olivi 2, 30170 Mestre, Veneto.
 ☎ 41 98 3653
 🕐 Thu 21:00 - ? Gay line Mon Wed Fri 19:00 - 23:00
Publishes a newsletter.

Radio: Sexuality

☿♀ *Onda Gay*
Radio Città Aperta FM 99.8 & 100.1, Via B. Marcello 10, 30170 Mestre, Veneto.
 🕐 23:15 - ?

Padova

Health Services

☺□ **Clinica Dermosifilopatica**
Via C. Battista 206, 35100 Padova, Veneto.
 ☎ 49 66 1011
 🕐 08:00 - 12:00
STD information & testing.

Helplines: Sexuality

☿♀ **Arci Gay—Padova**

Via Dante 41, 35100 Padova, Veneto.
☎ 49 875 6326
⏱ Tue 20:00 - 22:00

Organizations: Sexuality
☺▽ **Arci Gay—Padova**
Via Dante 41, 35100 Padova, Veneto.
☎ 49 875 6326
⏱ 20:30 - 23:00
HIV testing.

Stores: Erotica: General
☺■ **Magic Top Video Club**
Via Tommaseo 96C, 35100 Padova, Veneto.
☎ 49 807 2414
Leather & BDSM toys, videos, etc..

Rovigo
Organizations: Sexuality
☺▽ **Arci Gay—Rovigo**
Casella Postale 91, 45100 Rovigo, Veneto.

Treviso
Health Services
☺☐ **Ospedale Gen. Reg. S. M. Battuti**
☎ 422 58 2625
⏱ 08:00 - 12:00

Venezia
Health Services
☺☐ **Centro Dermoceltico**
Cannaregio, Fondamenta dell'Abbazia 3546, 30100 Venezia, Veneto.
☎ 41 522 1942
⏱ Tue 09:00 - 11:00
HIV testing.

☺☐ **Ospedale Civile Ruiniti**
Campo SS. Giovanni e Paolo, 30100 Venezia, Veneto.
☎ 41 78 4304
⏱ 08:00 - 12:00
HIV testing.

Helplines: Sexuality
☺▽ **Consultorio Gay—Venezia**
Via CAnnaregio 3546, 30100 Venezia, Veneto.
☎ 41 524 2121
⏱ Mon Wed Fri 18:00- 22:00
Counselling & onformation on HIV/AIDS & sexuality issues.

Organizations: Sexuality
☺▽ **Arci Gay—Venezia**
S. Croce 1507, 30100 Venezia, Veneto.
☎ 41 72 1842
⏱ Mon Wed Fri 18:00 - 24:00, Thu 21:00- 23:30

Verona
Health Services
☺☐ **Centro Ospedale di Borgo di Trento**
☎ 45 93 2647
⏱ 08:00 - 12:00

☺☐ **Gruppo C—Verona**
Via S. D'Acquisto, 37100 Verona, Veneto.
☎ 45 803 0843 📞 45 807 5043
Free, anonymous HIV testing.

Stores: Erotica: General
☺■ **Europa 92**
Via Scarsellini 30, 37100 Verona, Veneto.
☎ 45 800 9714
⏱ Mon - Sat 09:00 - 13:00 14:00- 19:30
Some leather & BDSM toys.

☺■ **Magic America**
Via Cantarene 27, 37100 Verona, Veneto.
☎ 45 800 5234
⏱ Mon - Sat 09:00 - 12:30 15:00- 19:30

Vicenza
Organizations: Sexuality
☺▽ **Arci Gay—Vicenza**
Via Fontanelle 5, 36100 Vicenza, Veneto.
☎ 444 50 7230
⏱ Tue 21:00 - 22:30

Stores: Books: General
☺■ **Emporio del Libro**
Via Beata Giovanna 34/36, 36100 Vicenza, Veneto.
☎ 444 22 8097
Lesbian & gay literature available.

Japan

Area: Approximately 378,000 square kilometres
Population: Approximately 124,600,000
Capital City: Tokyo
Currency: Yen (¥)
Official Language: Japanese
Major Religions: 80% Buddist or Shinto
National Holiday: Foundation Day, 11th. February
Time zone: GMT plus 9 hours
Country Initials: J
Electricity: 100 volts, 50-60Hz
Country Dialing Code (from elsewhere): 81
Intl. Dialing Prefix (out of the country): 001
Climate: The south of Japan is warm & sub-tropical, whereas the north tends to be cool, with plenty of snow in the mountains during winter.
Age of consent & homosexuality legislation: There is no mention of homosexuality in Japanese law. Age of consent for sexual activity is 13.
Call ahead for directions when visiting places. Streets are usually not marked with their names, nor are many buildings marked with street numbers. Companies are often located on high floors of office buildings. You can usually find someone able to explain the directions to you in English.

NAGOYA-SHI
Makamura-Ku
Stores: Clothing: Sexuality
▽ **Elizabeth**
1-13-15 Noritake, Makamura-Ku, Nagoya-shi 453.

Mizuho-Ku
Stores: Clothing: Fetish
☺■ **Dynasty**
♿ 3-2-4 Shioji-cho, Mizuho-Ku, Nagoya-shi.
☎ 52 853 1144

OSAKA
Nishi-Ku
Organizations: Sexuality
▽ **The Elizabeth Club**
1-1-9 Kujo, Nishi-Ku, Osaka 550.
Publishes *Queen*.

TOKYO
Adachi-Ku
Organizations: Sexuality
▽ **FTM Nippon**
Adachi-nishi Post Office, Adachi-Ku, Tokyo 123.
☎ 3 3683 6092
First Japanese FTM group. Publishes *FTM Nippon*.

Bunkyo-Ku
Publishers: Books: Fetish
♀♂ **Futami - Shobo Co., Ltd.**
1-21-11 Otowa, Bunkyo-Ku, Tokyo 112.
☎ 3 3942 2311

Kita-Ku
Photographers: BDSM
☺ **Masami Akita**
105 Parkside Corp., 7/32/14 Takinogawa, Kita-Ku, Tokyo.
Specializes in heavy bondage pictures.

Koto-Ku
Organizations: Sexuality
▽ **The Elizabeth Club**
5-32-18 Kameido, Koto-Ku, Tokyo 136.
☎ 3 3683 6092
Publishes *Queen*.

Minato-Ku
Organizations: Bears
♂♡▽ **Bear Club Japan**
c/o G-project Inc., 4-10-21-101, Akasaka, Minato-Ku, Tokyo 107.
✉ lonestar@st.rim.or.jp
🌐 http://www.skepsis.com/.gblo/bears/CLUBS/bear_club_japan.html
Contact: Mr. Akira Nakazawa

Shibuya-Ku
Publishers: Books: BDSM
⚥ **Treville Edition, Ltd.**
Suite 203, 2-11-17 Shoto, Shibuya-Ku, Tokyo 150.
☎ 3 3481 5611 📠 3 3481 5610

Shinjuku-Ku
Distributors: Erotica: General
☺ ■ **Tokyo Boeki Shokai Ltd.**
5-7 Shinjuku 1-chome, Shinjuku-Ku, Tokyo.

Photographers: Erotic
☺ ■ **Shinji Yamazaki**
21 Sakamachi, Shinjuku-Ku, Tokyo 160.
☎ 81 3 3225 4630 📠 81 3 3356 9810
✉ VYC00243@niftyserve.or.jp
$ VISA MC AMERICAN

Publishers: Books: BDSM
☺ ■ **AZZLO**
21 Sakamachi, Shinjuku-Ku, Tokyo 160.
☎ 81 3 3225 4630 📠 81 3 3356 9810
✉ VYC00243@niftyserve.or.jp
$ VISA MC AMERICAN

Stores: Clothing: Fetish
☺ ■ **AZZLO Discipline Co.**
21 Sakamachi, Shinjuku-Ku, Tokyo 160.
☎ 81 3 3225 4630 📠 81 3 3356 9810
✉ VYC00243@niftyserve.or.jp
$ VISA MC AMERICAN

Stores: Erotica: BDSM
☺ **Atomage**
8th. Floor, 2-15-26 Shinjuku, Shinjuku-Ku, Tokyo 160.

Liechtenstein

Area: Approximately 160 square kilometres
Population: Approximately 30,000
Capital City: Vaduz
Currency: Swiss Franc (Sfr.)
Official Language: German
Major Religions: 87% Roman Catholic, 481% Protestant
Time zone: GMT plus 1 hour
Country Initials: FL
Electricity: 220 volts
Country Dialing Code (from elsewhere): 41 75
Intl. Dialing Prefix (out of the country): 00
Long Distance Dialing Prefix (inside country): 0
Climate: Continental
Age of consent & homosexuality legislation: Homosexual acts are illegal.

NATIONAL RESOURCES
Helplines: AIDS
☺ □ **AIDS-Hilfe—Liechtenstein**
Postfach 207, Schaan 9494.
☎ 232 0520
⏰ Mon 18:00 - 20:00

Luxembourg

Area: Approximately 2,600 square kilometres
Population: Approximately 385,000
Capital City: Luxembourg
Currency: Luxemburg Franc (Flux)
Official Language: French, German, Letzebuergs
Major Religions: 95% Roman Catholic
National Holiday: Liberation Day, 9th. September
Time zone: GMT plus 1 hour
Country Initials: D
Electricity: 220 volts

Country Dialing Code (from elsewhere): 352
Intl. Dialing Prefix (out of the country): 00
Long Distance Dialing Prefix (inside country): There are no area codes here
Climate: Continental weather, with summers averaging approximately 24°C & winters approximately 6°C.
Age of consent & homosexuality legislation: Age of consent for sexual activity is 14 for heterosexual activity, but 18 for homosexual activity.

Crauthem
Photographers: Erotic
☺ **Etienne Braun**
4 rue Dr. Schumacher, Crauthem 3326.
☎ 35 236 5102
Fetish art photography.

Luxembourg
Helplines: Sexuality
☺ □ **Planning Familial**
18-20 Rue Glesener, Luxembourg.
☎ 48 5976

Organizations: AIDS: Support
☺ □ **AIDS-Beratung**
34 Boulevard Patton, Luxembourg 2316.
☎ 40 6251

Piercers
☺ ■ **Creative Art Collection**
Postbox 1317, Luxembourg 1013.
Catalogue, DM30, overseas $30U.S..

Stores: Erotica: General
☺ ■ **Boutique Amour**
4 Boulevard d'Avranches, Luxembourg 1160.

Malaysia

Area: Approximately 330,000 square kilometres
Population: Approximately 18,250,000
Capital City: Kuala Lumpur
Currency: Malayan Ringgit (M$)
Official Language: Maly, Chinese, & English
Major Religions: 53% Moslem, 17% Buddist, & some Confusciansim, tribal religions, & Christians
National Holiday: National Day, 31st. August
Time zone: GMT plus 8 hours
Country Initials: MAL
Electricity: 220 volts
Country Dialing Code (from elsewhere): 60
Intl. Dialing Prefix (out of the country): 007
Long Distance Dialing Prefix (inside country): 0
Climate: Warm all year, with temperatures between 21°C & 32°C. Rainy season is from May & September.
Age of consent & homosexuality legislation: Due to the proportion of Moslems in the country, homosexuality is generally considered to be taboo. Voluntary offences of "carnal intercourse against the order of nature with any man, woman, or animal" are punishable with a prison sentencce of up to 20 years.

Kuala Lumpur
Organizations: Sexuality
♂♡▽ **Pink Triangle Group**
P. O. Box 11859, Kuala Lumpur 50760.
☎ 3 981 2863 📠 3 981 2864
⏰ Office Mon - Fri 10:00 - 18:00, counselling Mon - Fri 19:30 - 21:30
Contact: Mr. Yee Khim Chong, Human Resources & Training Coördinator
Office moved in late 1995. Call directory enquiries for new telephone numbers.

Martinique

Population: Approximately 360,000
Capital City: Fort-de-France
Currency: Franc (FF)
Official Language: French & Créole
Major Religions: Mostly Roman Catholic
National Holiday: Bastille Day, 14th. July
Country Initials: F
Country Dialing Code (from elsewhere): 596
Intl. Dialing Prefix (out of the country): 19
Climate: Warm, tropical weather, with sea breezes.

Age of consent & homosexuality legislation: Age of consent for sexual activity is 15, but it is not advisable for foreigners to become involved with anyone under 18. Homosexual acts were removed from the criminal code in 1982.

Martinique is a French "Departement d'Outre-Mer" (D.O.M.) and is, therefore part of France, not an owned territory. Hence, the laws of France apply, here.

Fort-de-France

Helplines: Sexuality

☺ ☐ **Centre Hospitalier La Meynard**
 ☎ 50 1515
 HIV testing.

Organizations: AIDS: Support

☺ ☐ **AIDES—Martinique**
 Boîte Postale 1075, Fort-de-France 97209.
 ☎ 63 1236
 ⏲ Call Wed 15:00 - 18:00, Thu 19:00 - 21:00

Mexico

Area: Approximately 1,960,00 square kilometres
Population: Approximately 86,160,000
Capital City: Mexico City
Currency: Peso (mex$)
Official Language: Spanish
Major Religions: 92% Roman Catholic
National Holiday: Independence Day, 16th. September
Time zone: GMT -6-8 hours
Country Initials: MEX
Electricity: 110 volts, 60Hz
Country Dialing Code (from elsewhere): 52
Intl. Dialing Prefix (out of the country): 00
Long Distance Dialing Prefix (inside country): 0
Climate: Tropical to sub-tropical throughout the country. The average temperature is 27°C.
Age of consent & homosexuality legislation: Male prostitution is illegal. Public morality laws are often used against homosexual people.

NATIONAL RESOURCES

Organizations: AIDS: Education

☺ ☐ **Mexicanos Contre el SIDA**
 Calazada de Tlalpan 613, Mexico City, D. F. 03400.
 ☎ 5 530 2771
 ☎ 5 530 2549

Organizations: Sexuality

⚥▽ **Centro de Informacion y Documentacion de las Homosexualidades en Mexico Celectivo Sol, A. C. (CIDHOM)**
 P. O. Box 13-424, Mexico City, D. F. 3500.
 Centre for information & archives of the gay community in Mexico.
 Publishes *Soñar Fantasmas.*

Publishers: Magazines: Sexuality

⚥▼ *Apolo*
 P. O. Box 141-30, Mexico City, D. F. 15630.

⚥▼ *Del Otro Lado*
 Colectivo Sol, A.C., P. O. Box 13-4242, Mexico City, D. F. 03500.

⚥▼ *¡Y Que!*
 P. O. Box 904, Oficina Tijuana, Tijuana, Baja California Norte.
 ☎ 66 80 9963

BAJA CALIFORNIA NORTE

Tijuana

Helplines: Sexuality

⚥▽ **Gay & Lesbian Info Line**
 ☎ 66 88 0267

D. F.

Mexico City

Archives: Sexuality

⚥▽ **Colectivo Sol**
 P. O. Box 13-320, Mexico City, D. F. 03500.
 ☎ 5 658 3534

Organizations: AIDS: Education

☺ ☐ **Tijuana AIDS / SIDA Organization**
 P. O. Box 663, Oficini Central, Mexico City, D. F..

 ☎ 66 80 9963

Organizations: Sexuality

⚥▽ **Colectivo Masiorare**
 P. O. Box 5607, Mexico City, D. F..

⚥▽ **Serhume**
 P. O. Box 10-33, Mexico City, D. F. 06002.

Organizations: Sexuality: Youth

⚥▽ **POLEN**
 P. O. Box 3404, Oficina Central, Mexico City, D. F..
 Publishes *Asi Somos* twice a month.

Publishers: Magazines: Sexuality

⚥▼ *Hermes*
 Febo Editores, S. A. de C. V., P. O. Box 03311, Mexico City, D. F..

Stores: Erotica: General

☺ ■ **Multi Sexy Boutique**
 Insurgentes Sur 271, Mexico City, D. F..
 ☎ 5 264 4195
 ⏲ Mon - Sat 10:00 - 20:00

JALISCO

Guadalajara

Organizations: Sexuality

⚥▽ **Communidad Triangulo Rosa (CTR)**
 P. O. Box 9136, Guadalajara, Jalisco.

⚥▽ **Grupo Neuróticos Anónimos Gay**
 P. O. Box 14045, Guadalajara, Jalisco.
 Support group for gays.

⚥▽ **Grupo Nueva Generación**
 P. O. Box 36218, Guadalajara, Jalisco.
 Publishes *CRISALDA.*

⚥▽ **Grupo Orgullo Homosexual de Liberación (GOHL)**
 P. O. Box 11693, Guadalajara, Jalisco 44100.

Puebla

Counsellors

⌕■ **Morena & Orta Gender Issues Specialists**
 Instituto de Estudios Sobre Sexualidad y Pareja, A. C., C. P. 72590, Puebla.
 ☎ 22 44 3826 📞 22 44 3826

Namibia

Area: Approximately 823,000 square kilometres
Population: Approximately 1,550,000
Capital City: Windhoek
Currency: South African Rand (R)
Official Language: English, Afrikaans, & German
Major Religions: 90% Christian
Country Initials: NAM
Country Dialing Code (from elsewhere): 264
Intl. Dialing Prefix (out of the country): 09
Age of consent & homosexuality legislation: There is still legislation against homosexual activity.

Swakopmund

Organizations: BDSM

⚥▽ **Namibian Leather Corps**
 P. O. Box 525, Swakopmund.
 ☎ 641 4979 📞 641 4978
 Contact: Mr. Frank Passano

Windhoek

Organizations: Sexuality

⚥ **United Gay Organization of Namibia (UGON)**
 P. O. Box 21429, Windhoek.
 Contact: Ms. Yvonne Isaacs

The Netherlands

Area: Approximately 41,865 square kilometres
Population: Approximately 15,185,000
Capital City: Den Haag (The Hague)
Currency: Dutch Guilder/Florin (Dfl)
Official Language: Dutch
Major Religions: 36% Roman Catholic, 26% Protestant
National Holiday: Liberation Day, 5th. May

Time zone: GMT plus 1 hour
Country Initials: NL
Electricity: 220 volts
Country Dialing Code (from elsewhere): 31
Intl. Dialing Prefix (out of the country): 09
Long Distance Dialing Prefix (inside country): 0
Climate: Cool, wet, & windy winters. Summers are cool.
Age of consent & homosexuality legislation: Age of consent for sexual activity is 16, since 1971. The Dutch military has activity recruited homosexual people for several years.

NATIONAL RESOURCES

Archives: Sexuality

⚥▽ **Homodok**
Oudezijds Achterburgwal 185, 1012 DK Amsterdam.
☎ 20 525 2601 ✆ 20 525 3010
🕐 Wed - Fri 10:30 - 16:30
Archive with biographies, reference books, theses, research papers, & a comprehensive collection of gay & lesbian periodicals.

BBSs: Sexuality

♂▽ **Bi-Link**
✆ 10 413 7340. 28800 baud maximum.
✉ maurice@bi-link.tdcnet.nl

⚥▼ **GAYTEL**
Postbus 10, 5680 AA Best.
✆ 499 839 1000
🕐 24hrs.

Distributors: Videos: Political

⚥▽ **Gay Film Association Lambda**
Cabralstraat 51, Amsterdam.
☎ 20 618 5374
International distribution of gay & lesbian political films.

Helplines: Sexuality

⚥▽ **Infofoon Amsterdam**
☎ 20 675 3026
Non-stop recorded information.

Mailorder: Books: Sexuality

⚥▼ **Delta Boek**
Postbus 92, 2980 AB Ridderkerk.

Mailorder: Clothing: Fetish

☺■ **Rimba**
Postbus 33, 4840 AA Prinsenbeek.
☎ 76 541 4484
Catalogue, £5, $10U.S..

Mailorder: Erotica: BDSM

☺■ **Ben's Fashion**
Postbus 3184, 3101 ED Schiedam.
☎ 10 425 0785 ✆ 10 435 0785
Catalogue, £5 or €6U.S..

⚥■ **Mail & Female**
Postbus 16668, 1001 RD Amsterdam.
☎ 20 693 6074 ✆ 20 668 4990
Catalogue, DFl.15.

Mailorder: Erotica

⚥▽ **Europost**
Postbus 1019, 1000 BA Amsterdam.

Mailorder: Erotica: General

☺■ **Christine Le Duc**
Postbus 170, 1130 AD Volendam.
Mail order arm of a chain of shops with a lot of fetish & BDSM items.
Catalogue available.

Mailorder: Erotica: Leather

⚥▼ **Expectations**
Warmoesstraat 32, 1012 JE Amsterdam.
VISA 💳
Catalogue available.

⚥▼ **P+E**
Postbus 6102, Rotterdam.
☎ 10 474 8360

Mailorder: Videos: Erotic

⚥▼ **Euro Men**
Postbus 10923, 1001 EX Amsterdam.

Organizations: AIDS: Education

⚥▽ **Stuurgroep AIDS Preventie Homo's**

c/o Buro G. V. O., Prins Hendricklaan 12, 1075 BB Amsterdam.
☎ 20 671 2815
🕐 Mon - Fri 09:00 - 17:00

Organizations: BDSM

⚥□ **Vereniging Studiegroep Sado-Masochisme (VSSM)**
♿ Werkgroep Vrouwen en SM, Postbus 3570, 1001 AJ Amsterdam.
☎ 20 420 2117
✉ vssm@dds.nl
🖥 http://sparkie.riv.net/fetish/vssm
♨ ℰ
Aims to bring BDSM men & women together, no matter what their background, colour, or interests are. About 650 members. English & German also spoken.

Organizations: Fetish: Clothing

☺▼ **Fetish Street**
🖥 http://sparkie.riv.nl/fetish/

Organizations: Fetish: Clothing: Rubber

☺□ **Vereniging Studiegroep Sado-Masochisme (VSSM)**
♿ Rubbergroep, Postbus 3570, 1001 AJ Amsterdam.
☎ 20 420 2117
✉ vssm@dds.nl
🖥 http://sparkie.riv.net/fetish/vssm
🕐 Meets 4th. Fri of the month every two months
♨ ℰ
Aims to bring BDSM men & women together, no matter what their background, colour, or interests are. About 650 members. English & German also spoken.

Organizations: Sexuality

⚥▽ **COC—Head Office**
Nieuwezijds Vorburgwal 68 - 70, 1012 SE Amsterdam.
☎ 20 623 4596 ✆ 20 626 7795
COC is the main national gay & lesbian organization with offices all over the country. COC is short for Nederlandse Vereniging tot Integratie van Homosexualiteit COC. Publishes *XL* 11 times a year.

☺□ **Martijn**
Postbus 43548, 1009 NA Amsterdam.
☎ 20 693 4793
Pædophile organization.

☺□ **Nederlandse Vereniging voor Sexuele Hervorming (NVSH)**
Postbus 13117, 3507 LC Utrecht.
Society for sexual reform, with groups for tranvestites, transexuals, bisexuals, & pædophiles.

♂▽ **Vereniging Landelijk Netwerk voor Bisexualiteit (LNBi)**
Postbus 75087, 1070 AB Amsterdam.
☎ 77 354 9776 ✆ 10 476 6313
✉ lnbi@bi-link.tdcnet.nl
♨ ✓ ℰ
Contact: Mr. Maurice Snellen, Secretary
The LNBi (or Dutch National Bi Network) tries to organize bisexuals & publishes information about bisexuality & activities concerning bisexuality. Publishes *Bi-Nieuws* quarterly. Yearly subscription is FL30 in NL, FL40 elsewhere. English & German also spoken.

🗫▽ **Vereniging LKGT&T**
Postbus 11575, 1001 GN Amsterdam.
☎ 76 593 3901
🕐 Meets monthly in Alkmaar, Amsterdam, Eindhoven, Groningen, Leiden, Rotterdam, Utrecht, & Zwolle
Publishes *Transformatie*.

Organizations: Spanking

⚥▽ **Castigatio**
♿ Postbus 279, 2300 AG Leiden.
🕐 Meets twice a month in various cities
♨
Contact: Goedhals, Secretary
Publishes *Strafblad* every two months. Yearly subscription is FL45 (part of membership). Age statement of 18 is required. French, German, & English also spoken.

Publishers: Books: Sexuality

⚥▼ **The Acolyte Press**
Postbus 12731, 1100 AS Amsterdam.

Publishers: Guides: Sexuality

⚥▼ **Best Guide**
Postbus 22320, 1100 CH Amsterdam.
☎ 20 600 2087

⚥▼ **City Map Produkties**
Postbus 10419, 1001 EK Amsterdam.
☎ 20 626 0702

Publishers: Magazines: Arts
♂▼ *HOMologie*
Postbus 16584, 1001 RB Amsterdam.
☎ 20 618 8045
Published twice a month.

Publishers: Magazines: BDSM
♂▼ *Centurion*
Postbus 93506, 2509 AM Den Haag.

Publishers: Newspapers: Sexuality
♂▼ *De Gay Krant*
Best Publishing Group, Postbus 10, 5680 AA Best.
☎ 49 939 1000 📞 49 937 2638
Covers all of the Benelux. Published every two weeks.

Radio: Sexuality
♂▽ **Stichting Urania**
Postbus 13, 1200 AA Hilversum.

Stores: Books: General
☺□ **De Rooie Rat**
Oude Gracht 65, 3511 AD Utrecht.
☎ 30 231 7189
✉ rooierat@schism.aps.nl
🕐 09:00 - 22:00
Leftist bookshop with gay literature, mainly dutch. International non-fiction: wide variety of social, political & economic issues; coming out signs.

Stores: Clothing: Fetish
☺ **Skin Tight**
Josephstraat 168, 3014 TX Rotterdam.
☎ 10 436 3756 📞 10 436 3756
🕐 Tue - Sat 11:00 - 17:30
Catalogue, FL35, £10. Age statement of 16 is required. English & some French also spoken.

Aalsmeer
Organizations: Sexuality
♂▽ **COC—Meerlanden / Ronde Venen**
Postbus 334, 02977 Aalsmeer.

Akmaar
Organizations: Sexuality
♂▽ **COC—Alkmaar & West Friesland**
Postbus 268, 1800 AG Akmaar.
☎ 72 511 1650

Alkmaar
Stores: Erotica: General
♂▼ **Eros**
Luttik Oudorp 112, Alkmaar.
☎ 72 512 1551
🕐 Mon 13:00 - 18:00, Tue Wed Fri 10:00 - 18:00, Thu 10:00 - 21:00, Sat 10:00 - 17:00

Almelo
Organizations: BDSM
☺□ **Vereniging Studiegroep Sado-Masochisme (VSSM)**
☎ 20 420 2117
✉ vssm@dds.nl
🌐 http://sparkie.riv.net/fetish/vssm
Meets 3rd. Wed of month 20:00
Also uniforms. English & German also spoken.

Amstelveen
Organizations: Sexuality
▽ **Stichting Nederlands Gender Centrum**
Borssenburg 24, 1181 NV Amstelveen.
☎ 20 612 4099
Information & counselling for transsexuals.

Amsterdam
Accommodation: BDSM
♂▼ **Amsterdam House**
Amstel 176a, 1017 AE Amsterdam.
☎ 20 626 2577 📞 20 626 2987
♂▼ **Stablemaster Hotel**

Warmoesstraat 23, 1012 HT Amsterdam.
☎ 20 625 0148
🕐 Bar 17:00 - 24:00

Archives: General
⊕ **IIAV**
Obiplein 4, Amsterdam.
☎ 20 665 0820
🕐 Mon 12:00 - 17:00, Tue 10:00 - 19:00, Wed - Fri 10:00 - 17:00
Extensive women's archives with a large international collection.

☺■ **Museum of Sex**
Damrak 18, 1012 LH Amsterdam.

Archives: Sexuality
♀▽ **Lesbisch Archief**
Eerste Heimstraat 17, Amsterdam.
☎ 20 618 5879
🕐 Mon - Fri 13:00 - 16:30. Telephone Mon - Fri 09:00 - 16:30
Specialises in audio-visual material, with an additional seletion of books, magazines, & photographs.

Bars: BDSM
♂▼ **Anco Bar**
Oudezijds Voorburgwal 55, 1012 EJ Amsterdam.
☎ 20 624 1126 📞 20 620 5275
🕐 10:00 - 22:00

♂▼ **Argos Club**
Warmoesstraat 95, 1012 GZ Amsterdam.
☎ 20 622 6595
🕐 Mon - Thu Sun 21:00 - 03:00, Fri Sat 21:00 - 04:00

♂▼ **The Attic**
Spuistraat 3H, Amsterdam.
☎ 20 638 1695
🕐 12:00 - 02:00

♂▼ **Club Jaecques**
Warmoesstraat 93, 1012 HZ Amsterdam.
☎ 20 622 0323
🕐 20:00 - 02:00

♂▼ **Cockring**
Warmoesstraat 96, 1012 JH Amsterdam.
☎ 20 622 6595
🕐 Mon - Thu Sun 21:00 - 03:00, Fri Sat 21:00 - 04:00

♂▼ **Company**
Amstel 106, Amsterdam.
☎ 20 625 3028
🕐 20:00 - 02:00, Sun 16:00 - 02:00

♂▼ **Cuckoo's Nest**
Nieuwezijds Kolk 6, Amsterdam.
☎ 20 627 1752
🕐 21:00 - 02:00

♂▼ **The Eagle**
Warmoesstraat 86, 1012 HJ Amsterdam.
☎ 20 627 8634
🕐 21:00 - 03:00, Sat 21:00 - 04:00

♂▼ **G-Force**
Oudezijds Armsteeg 7, Amsterdam.
☎ 20 420 1664
🕐 14:00 - 24:00
Friendly café in the red light district for those who are interested in exploring BDSM in a relaxed environment.

♂▼ **De Spijker**
Kerkstraat 4, Amsterdam.
☎ 20 620 5919
🕐 Mon - Thu 13:00 - 01:00, Fri Sat 13:00 - 04:00
Mainly for men, but women are welcome.

♂▼ **Stablemaster Bar**
Warmoesstraat 23, 1012 HT Amsterdam.
☎ 20 625 0148
🕐 Bar 17:00 - 24:00

♂▼ **The Web**
St. Jacobsstraat 6, Amsterdam.
☎ 20 623 6758
🕐 Mon - Thu Sat 14:00 - 01:00, Fri Sat 14:00 - 03:00

Bars: Fetish
☺ **Kinky Club**
Oostelijke Handelskade 21, Amsterdam.
☎ 20 620 5603
Techno-fetishist club.

Counsellors
▽□ **The Free University Hospital**
Department of Endocrinology & Andrology, Postbus 7057, 1007 MB

Amsterdam.
☎ 20 548 9111 Ext.: 199 ✆ 20 548 7502
Professionllly managed full gender dysphoria program.

Distributors: Erotica: General

Scala B. V.
Contactweg 28, 1017 Amsterdam.

Health Services

GG & GD
Venereal Disease Clinic, Groenburgwal 44, Amsterdam.
☎ 20 555 5822
Mon - Fri 08:00 - 10:30
Free testing for EEC citizens. Can arrange anonymous HIV testing for a fee.

Helplines: AIDS

AIDS-Infolijn
☎ 6 022 2220
Mon -Fri 14:00 - 22:00
Free call for information about HIV/AIDS.

Helplines: Sexuality

Gay & Lesbian Switchboard
Postbus 11573, 1001 GN Amsterdam.
☎ 20 623 6565 ✆ 20 638 0407
10:00 - 22:00
Information, counselling, & support about lesbian gay issues.

Manufacturers: Clothing: Fetish

Demask
Regulateurstraat 7, 1033 NB Amsterdam.
☎ 20 620 5603 ✆ 20 492 0393
☎ 20 620 7215 (2nd. facs.)
10:00 - 19:00
Has shops & perhaps the largest manufacturing facility & production of fetish clothing, both rubber & leather in the world. Catalogue, FL30 ($20U.S.). English, German, Italian, Spanish, & Yugoslavian also spoken.

Organizations: Academic: Sexuality

Sociologisch Instituut
Homostudies, Oude Hoogstraat 24, Amsterdam.
☎ 20 525 2226

Organizations: AIDS: Support

HIV-Plusline
☎ 20 685 0055
Mon Wed 13:00 - 16:00, Tue Thu 20:00 - 22:30

Organizations: BDSM

Club LL
Elandsgracht 29-31, 1016 TM Amsterdam.

Stichting SMet…!
Postbus 6, 1000 AA Amsterdam.

Vereniging Studiegroep Sado-Masochisme (VSSM)
Postbus 3570, 1001 AJ Amsterdam.
☎ 20 420 2117
vssm@dds.nl
http://sparkie.riv.net/fetish/vssm
Meets 1st. & 3rd. Sun of month 15:00 for leather & non-leather, 5th. Sat of month (4 times per year) 20:00 for leather only
Contact: Mr. Ed Groenendijk, General Secretary
25-year old BDSM organization with branches throughout the Netherlands. Also uniforms. Publishes *Kerfstok* every two months. English & German also spoken.

Organizations: Bears

Nederbears
Louise Wentstraat 141, 1018 MS Amsterdam.
Contact: Mr. Daniel de Heus

Organizations: Body Size

Girth & Mirth—Amsterdam
Rozenstraat 14, 1016 NX Amsterdam.
☎ 20 625 5128
bigboss@xs4all.nl

Organizations: Motorcycle

MSC Amsterdam
Postbox 3540, 1001 AH Amsterdam.

Organizations: Sexuality

COC—Information Center
Rozenstraat 14, 1016 NX Amsterdam.
☎ 20 623 4079 ✆ 20 626 8300
☎ 20 626 3087 (office)
Every day for different activities. Call for information Mon - Sat 13:00 - 18:00. Office Mon - Fri 09:00 - 17:00

Gay Capital Events
Postbus 17601, 1001 JM Amsterdam.
☎ 20 689 0279 ✆ 20 638 5198
Organises gay events in Amsterdam.

Het Jongensuur
Binnenkadijk 178, 1018 ZH Amsterdam.
☎ 20 622 1710
Female-to-males.

Man-to-Man Gay Information Centre
Spuistraat 21, Amsterdam.
☎ 20 625 8797
12:00 - 24:00
Information about the commercial gay scene in Amsterdam.

Nederlandse Vereniging Humanits
Transsexual Project, Postbus 71, 1000 AB Amsterdam.
☎ 20 626 2445 ✆ 20 622 7367
By appointment only
Contact: Ms. Petra Klene

Nederlandse Vereniging voor Sexuele Hervorming (NVSH)
Blauwburgval 7-9, Amsterdam.
☎ 20 623 9359
Masturbation parties 1st. Thu of month
Society for sexual reform, with groups for tranvestites, transexuals, bisexuals, & pædophiles.

SAD
P. C. Hoofstraat 5, 1071 BL Amsterdam.
☎ 20 662 4206 ✆ 20 664 6069
Information, counselling, & support for lesbians, gays, & bisexuals.

Stichting Bisexualiteit Nederland
Churchill-laan 59d, 1078 DH Amsterdam.
☎ 20 664 2337
stgbined@bi-link.tdcnet.nl

Stichting Gay & Lesbian Association Amsterdam (GALA)
Postbus 15815, 1001 NH Amsterdam.
☎ 20 616 1979 ✆ 20 616 1979
Organises a gay & lesbian festival in Sep.

Stichting Werkgroep Biseksualiteit—Amsterdam
Rozenstraat 14, 1016 NX Amsterdam.
☎ 20 634 0065
☎ 20 684 8250
Meets 2nd. Tue of month 20:00 - 24:00

Organizations: Tattoo

Dutch Tattoo Foundation
Lankgesstraat 3, 10115 AK Amsterdam.

Organizations: Watersports

Rubber Sex Groep
Postbus 12913, 1100 AX Amsterdam.

Photographers: Erotic

Michael Ferron
Weesperzujde 80A, 1091 EJ Amsterdam.

Piercers

Body Manipulations
Stromarkt 11, 1012 SW Amsterdam.
☎ 20 623 3442

Tattooing & Piercing Studio
Kloveniersburgwal 135, 1011 KE Amsterdam.
☎ 20 625 7812

Publishers: Guides: Sexuality

Free Map of Amsterdam
Postbus 43590, 4090 EB Amsterdam.
Published 3 times a year.

Publishers: Information: Sexuality

COC Magazijn
N. V. I. H. COC, Nieuwezidjs Vorburgwal 68 - 70, 1012 SE Amsterdam.
☎ 20 623 4596 ✆ 20 626 7795
nvihcoc@xs4all.nl
http://www.xs4all.nl/~nvihcoc
✓ $
Books & free brochures on coming out & gay, lesbian, & bisexual topics. English also spoken.

Publishers: Magazines: Erotic

☺ **Paragon**
Postbus 23347, 1100 DV Amsterdam.
🏠 $ ⚭ ℓ
Publishes books & magazines. Free catalogue. English & German also spoken.

Publishers: Videos: Erotic

☺ **Paragon**
Postbus 23347, 1100 DV Amsterdam.
🏠 $ ⚭ ℓ
Free catalogue. English & German also spoken.

Radio: General

☺ ■ **Aliens**
Stichting M.V.S. FM 106.8, Cable 103.8, Van Der Hoopstraat, 64HS, 1051 VR Amsterdam.
☎ 20 620 8866 ✆ 20 638 5456
☎ 20 620 0247
🕐 18:00 - 21:00. In English on Sun. See Teletext pp. 601 & 437 on TV Channel 4 for programme details

Stores: Books: General

☺ ■ **The American Book Center**
Kalverstraat 185, 1012 XC Amsterdam.
☎ 20 625 5537 ✆ 20 624 8042
🕐 Mon - Sat 10:00 - 20:00, Thu - 22:00, Sun 11:00 - 18:00
🏠 ▭ ⊙

☺ ■ **Boekhandel Mercurius b.v.**
Hof Van Spaland 31, 3121 CA Shiedam.
☎ 10 471 2313 ✆ 10 471 2313

☺ ■ **Bruna**
Leidsestraat 89, Amsterdam.
☎ 20 622 0578
🕐 09:00 - 22:00
Small gay & lesbian section.

☺▽ **Intermale Gay Bookstore**
Spuistraat 251, 1012 VR Amsterdam.
☎ 20 625 0009 ✆ 20 620 3163
🕐 Mon 12:00 - 18:00, Tue - Sat 10:00 -18:00, Thu - 19:00
🏠 $ ⚭ ▭ ⊙ ⚭ ℓ
The largest bookstore in Amsterdam devoted entirely to books of interest to the gay male. Free catalogue. English & German also spoken.

☺▽ **Vrolijk Boekhandel**
Paleisstraat 135, 1012 ZL Amsterdam.
☎ 20 623 5142 ✆ 20 638 3807
🕐 Mon 11:00 - 18:00, Tue Wed Fri 10:00 - 18:00, Thu 10:00 - 21:00, Sat 10:00 - 17:00

⚇ **Xantippe**
Prinsengracht 290, Amsterdam.
☎ 20 623 5854
🕐 Mon 13:00 - 18:00, Tue - Fri 10:00 - 18:00, Sat 10:00 - 17:00

☺ ■ **Zwart Op Wit**
Utrechtsestraat 149, Amsterdam.
☎ 20 622 8174
🕐 09:30 - 17:00

Stores: Clothing: Fetish

☺ ■ **Ellen Schippers Design**
3rd. Floor, 1E, Jan Steenstraat 112, 1072 NR Amsterdam.
☎ 20 662 3883
Catalogue available.

Stores: Clothing: Leather

☺▽ **Robin & Rik Leathermakers**
Runstraat 30, 1016 GK Amsterdam.
☎ 20 627 8924
🕐 Tue - Sat 11:00 - 18:00
High quality & style leather men's clothes: pants, chaps, jackets, vests, belts, caps, etc.. In stock or made to measure. English, French, & German also spoken.

Stores: Clothing: Rubber

☺ ■ **Stretch**
15 Buiten Oranjestraat, 1013 HX Amsterdam.
☎ 20 627 4305
Custom service also available.

Stores: Erotica: BDSM

☺ **Demask**
Demask Publishing, Zeedijk 64, 1012 BA Amsterdam.
☎ 20 620 5603 ✆ 20 492 0393
☎ 20 620 7215 (2nd. facs.)
🕐 10:00 - 19:00

🏠 ✓ ⚭ ▭ ⊙ ⊙ ▭ ℓ
Has shops & perhaps the largest manufacturing facility & production of fetish clothing, both rubber & leather in the world. Catalogue, FL30 (S20U.S.). English, German, Italian, Spanish, & Yugoslavian also spoken.

☺▽ **Expectations**
Warmoesstraat 32, 1012 JE Amsterdam.
▭ ⊙
Catalogue available.

☺ ■ **G. D. C.**
Nieuwendijk 57-59, Amsterdam.
☎ 20 625 1301
🕐 09:00 - 19:00, Sun 10:00 -18:00

⚇ ■ **Mail & Female**
Amstel 47, 1001 RD Amsterdam.
☎ 20 693 6074 ✆ 20 668 4990
Yearly subscription is Dfl.15.

☺▽ **Master Leathers**
Warmoesstraat 32, 1012 Amsterdam.
☎ 20 624 5573 ✆ 20 624 8747
🕐 12:00 - 18:00, Thu - 20:00, Sat - 17:00

⚇▽ **RoB—Amsterdam**
Weteringschans 253, 1017 XJ Amsterdam.
☎ 20 625 4686 ✆ 20 627 3220
🖳 http://www.euro.net/5thworld/pink/leather.html#rob
🕐 Mon - Fri 11:00 - 18:30, Sat 11:00 - 17:00
Catalogue, Fl25.

☺▽ **Wrapped**
Singel 434, 1017 AV Amsterdam.
☎ 20 420 4022
🕐 Mon 12:00 - 18:00, Tue Wed Fri Sat 10:00 - 18:00, Thu 10:00 - 21:00
🏠 ▭ ⊙
Also tailormade leather & rubber.

Stores: Erotica: General

☺ ■ **Christine Le Duc**
Leidsekruisstraat 33, Amsterdam.
Chain of shops with a lot of fetish & BDSM items. Catalogue available.

☺ ■ **Christine Le Duc**
Spui 6, 1012 WZ Amsterdam.
☎ 20 624 8265
Chain of shops with a lot of fetish & BDSM items. Catalogue available.

☺ ■ **Christine Le Duc**
Oudebrugsteeg 21, 1012 JN Amsterdam.
☎ 20 623 8732
Chain of shops with a lot of fetish & BDSM items. Catalogue available.

☺ ■ **Christine Le Duc**
Reguliersdwarsstraat 107, 1017 BL Amsterdam.
☎ 20 623 1321
Chain of shops with a lot of fetish & BDSM items. Catalogue available.

☺ ■ **Erex**
Nieuwendijk 57-59, Amsterdam.

☺ ■ **Roodhorst**
Ruud, Uitgeverij De Harmonie, Spuistraat 272, 1012 VW Amsterdam.
☎ 20 624 5181 ✆ 20 623 0672

Training: BDSM

⚇▽ **Meester Terry's SM Society & School**
Pienemanstraat 46, 1072 KV Amsterdam.
☎ 20 671 0682
🕐 Meets 4th. Sun of month 15:00
Promotes a wider understanding of BDSM play, explains the intense psychological bond between master & slave, & teaches proper toy usage.

Apeldoorn

Organizations: Fisting

☺▽ **Touch**
193 Kalmoesstraat, 7322 NN Apeldoorn.
🕐 Meets monthly
Contact: Mr. W. W. Salomons
Publishes *Touch* quarterly. Yearly subscription is $10.

Arnhem

Organizations: AIDS: Support

☺ □ **GG & GD**
AIDSverleggroep, Broerenstraat 55, Arnhem.

Organizations: BDSM

☺ □ **Vereniging Studiegroep Sado-Masochisme (VSSM)**
☎ 20 420 2117

Organizations: BDSM

✉ vssm@dds.nl
💻 http://sparkie.riv.net/fetish/vssm
🕐 Meets 1st. Tue of month 20:00
Also uniforms. English & German also spoken.

Organizations: Sexuality

♀♂▽ **COC—Arnhem**
Jacob Cremerstraat 32, Arnhem.
☎ 26 442 3161

Stores: Books: General

☺ ■ **Hijman**
Grote Oord 15, Arnhem.
☎ 26 442 4938
🕐 Mon - Sat 09:00 - 18:00

Stores: Erotica: General

☺ ■ **Christine Le Duc**
Walstraat 55, 6811 BD Arnhem.
Chain of shops with a lot of fetish & BDSM items. Catalogue available.

Baarle Nassau

Stores: Erotica: General

☺ ■ **Fun House**
Nieuwstraat 22, Baarle Nassau.
🕐 10:00 - 22:00

Bergen op Zoom

Organizations: Sexuality

♀♂▽ **COC—Bergen op Zoom**
⬥ Postbus 590, 4000 AN Bergen op Zoom.
☎ 16 425 4235
🕐 Fri 22:00 - 03:00, Sat - 04:00
🚭
English also spoken.

Breda

Organizations: Sexuality

♀♂▽ **COC—Breda**
St. Annastraat 10, Breda.
☎ 76 522 6662

Stores: Erotica: General

☺ ■ **B-1**
Haagdijk 24, Breda.
☎ 76 514 5641
🕐 10:00 - 24:00

☺ ■ **Christine Le Duc**
Haagdijk 14, Breda.
☎ 76 522 5777
🕐 10:00 - 18:00
Chain of shops with a lot of fetish & BDSM items. Catalogue available.

Bussum

Distributors: Erotica: General

☺ **Right Hand Productions**
Postbus 191, 1406 AD Bussum.
☎ 21 591 4288 📞 21 591 4353

Capelle a/d Ijssel

Organizations: Sexuality

⚥▽ **Stichting Reborn**
Maria Daneelserf 10, 2907 BD Capelle a/d Ijssel.
☎ 10 458 3469 📞 10 458 3469
🕐 Mon - Fri 10:00 - 17:00, 2nd. Fri of month 21:00 - 02:00. By appointment only
Contact: Mr. Emmanuel de Vries, Director
Publishes *Syntese*.

Delft

Organizations: Bears

♂▽ **Bears Netherlands**
A. v. d. Leeuwlaan 1062, 2624 MB Delft.
☎ 15 261 4291
Contact: Herr Gerritt Weemekers

Organizations: Sexuality

♀♂▽ **Delftse Werkgroep Homosexualiteit**
Lange Geer, Delft.
☎ 15 214 6893
🕐 Wed Sun 20:00 - 00:30, Fri 21:00 - 02:00

Delfzijl

Organizations: Sexuality

♀♂▽ **Homosum**
☎ 59 661 9823

Den Haag

Organizations: AIDS: Support

☺ □ **The AIDS Speekuur**
Van Beverninkstraat 134, Den Haag.
☎ 70 354 1610
🕐 Tue Thu 19:00 - 21:00

Organizations: Sexuality

♀♂▼ **Stichting Trefcentrum HIG - COC (Basta)**
Scheveningsveer 7, 2514 HB Den Haag.
☎ 70 365 9090
🕐 Closed Mon. Youth group (under 28) 1st. Fri of month 15:00 - 01:30; bisexuals 3rd. Thu of month 20:00 - 00:30; lesbian only Sat 21:00 - 01:30; lesbian, gay, & bisexual (over 40) 1st. Sun of month 15:00 - 19:00; lesbian only (over 35) 2nd Sun of month 15:00 - 19:00

♂ ▽ **Stichting Werkgroep Biseksualiteit—Den Haag**
Scheveningsveer 7, 2514 HB Den Haag.
☎ 70 346 4767
🕐 Meets 3rd. Thu of month 20:00 - 24:00

✉■ **Transformatie**
Postbus 13500, 2501 EM Den Haag.

Stores: Books: General

☺ ■ **The American Book Center**
Lane Poten 23, 2511 CM Den Haag.
☎ 70 364 2742
🕐 Mon - Sat 10:00 - 18:00, Thu - 20:00

☺ ■ **Roode Hand**
Prins Hendrikstraat 138, Den Haag.
☎ 70 364 8861
🕐 Mon - Sat 09:00 - 18:00

☺ ■ **Ruward**
Spui 231, Den Haag.
☎ 70 363 0879

Stores: Erotica: General

☺ ■ **Christine Le Duc**
Piet Heinplein 1, 2518 CA Den Haag.
☎ 20 362 5295
Chain of shops with a lot of fetish & BDSM items. Catalogue available.

Den Helder

Organizations: Sexuality

♀♂▽ **COC—Den Helder**
Postbus 745, Den Helder.
☎ 22 361 6807
☎ 22 363 0732

Doetinchem

Helplines: Sexuality

♀♂▽ **Hulptelefoon**
☎ 31 434 5884

Organizations: Sexuality

♀♂▽ **Werkgroep Homofile Achterhoek**
Postbus 8031, Doetinchem.
☎ 31 436 0811

Dordrecht

Organizations: AIDS: Support

♀♂▼ **AIDS Information**
☎ 78 613 0284
🕐 Mon - Thu 09:00 - 10:00

Organizations: Sexuality

♀♂▽ **COC—Dordrecht**
Postbus 934, 3300 AX Dordrecht.
☎ 78 613 1717
🚭
English also spoken.

Publishers: Books: Fetish

⚤ **De Vaar**
Noordendijk 131, 3311 RN Dordrecht.

Eindhoven

Organizations: BDSM

☺ □ **Vereniging Studiegroep Sado-Masochisme (VSSM)**
 ☎ 20 420 2117
 ✉ vssm@dds.nl
 🌐 http://sparkie.riv.net/fetish/vssm
 🕐 Meets 2nd. Fri of month 20:00
 Also uniforms. English & German also spoken.

Organizations: Sexuality

⚥▽ **COC—Eindhoven**
 Prins Hendrikstraat 54, Eindhoven.
 ☎ 40 245 5700
 🕐 Tue Fri Sat 21:00 - 01:30, Sun 15:00 - 18:00. Lesbian 1st. & 3rd.
 Wed 21:00 - ?

⚥▽ **De Kringen**
 Postbus 6323, 5600 HH Eindhoven.
 🕐 2nd. & 4th.. Sat of month 20:30 - 01:00

▷▽ **Werkgroep Facet**
 Rode Kruislaan 61, 5628 GB Eindhoven.
 ☎ 40 241 5475

Stores: Erotica: BDSM

☺ ■ **Black Box**
 Stratumseind 4, Eindhoven.
 ☎ 40 246 4277

Stores: Erotica: General

☺ ■ **B-1**
 Nieuwestraat 5, Eindhoven.
 ☎ 40 245 1269
 🕐 10:00 - 24:00

☺ ■ **Christine Le Duc**
 Willemstraat 33, Eindhoven.
 ☎ 40 243 9081
 🕐 10:00 - 19:00
 Chain of shops with a lot of fetish & BDSM items. Catalogue available.

☺ ■ **Elise**
 Kleine Berg 40, Eindhoven.
 🕐 Mon - Sat 10:00 -18:00

Emmen

Organizations: Sexuality

⚥▽ **COC—Emmen**
 Postbus 318, Emmen.
 ☎ 59 161 1414
 ☎ 59 162 9144 (infoline)

Enschede

Organizations: Sexuality

⚥▽ **COC—Enschede**
 Walstraat 12-14, Enschede.
 ☎ 53 430 5177

⚥▽ **COC—Twente / Achterhoek**
 Postbus 444, Enschede.

Gemert

Organizations: Sexuality

⚥▽ **Stichting Homo Groep Gemert**
 Postbus 167, 5420 AD Gemert.
 ☎ 49 236 6894
 🕐 Mon 20:00 - 24:00, last Sun of month 15:00 - 18:00

Gorinchem

Organizations: Sexuality

⚥▽ **WIHG**
 Postbus 428, Gorinchem.
 ☎ 18 363 6710

Gouda

Organizations: Sexuality

⚥▽ **COC—Gouda**
 ♿ Postbus 3026, Sperierinastraat 113A, 2800 CC Gouda.
 ☎ 18 252 4634

⚥▽ **Erotheek**
 Waluisstraat 9, Gouda.
 ☎ 18 258 2302
 🕐 10:30 - 22:30, Sat - 21:00

Stores: Erotica: General

☺ ■ **Bureau 700**
 Raam 66, Gouda.
 ☎ 18 251 4381
 🕐 Mon - Sat 13:00 - 18:00

Groningen

Bars: Sexuality

⚣▼ **The Duke**
 Hoogstraat 9, Groningen.
 ☎ 50 313 4609
 🕐 Tue - Sun 21:00 - 01:00

⚣▼ **El Rubio**
 Zwanestraat 26, Groningen.
 ☎ 50 314 0039
 🕐 Sun - Wed 16:00 - ?, Thu Sat 15:00 - ?

Health Services

☺ □ **Academisch Ziekenhuis**
 Oostersingel 59, Groningen.
 ☎ 50 361 2867
 🕐 Mon - Fri 08:30 0 - 12:30

Organizations: BDSM

☺ □ **Vereniging Studiegroep Sado-Masochisme (VSSM)**
 ☎ 20 420 2117
 ✉ vssm@dds.nl
 🌐 http://sparkie.riv.net/fetish/vssm
 🕐 Meets 4th. Sat of month 20:00
 Also uniforms. English & German also spoken.

Organizations: Sexuality

⚥▽ **Abva**
 Postbus 174, Groningen.
 ☎ 50 314 1701

⚥▽ **COC—Groningen**
 Kraneweg 56, Groningen.
 ☎ 50 313 2620
 🕐 Tue Thu Sat 20:00 - 22:00, Fri 16:00 - 01:00, Sun 15:00 - 18:00

Stores: Books: General

☺ ■ **Scholtens**
 Grote Markt 43-44, Groningen.
 ☎ 50 313 9788
 🕐 09:00 - 18:00

Stores: Erotica: General

☺ ■ **Christine Le Duc**
 Zuiderdiep 88, Groningen.
 🕐 Mon - Fri 10:00 - 22:00, Sat 10:00 - 17:00
 Chain of shops with a lot of fetish & BDSM items. Catalogue available.

Haarlem

Health Services

☺ □ **SVGD**
 Zijlweg 2, Haarlem.
 ☎ 23 531 9026
 🕐 Mon - Fri 08:00 -12:00 by appointment only

Organizations: Sexuality

⚥▽ **COC—Kennemerland**
 Postbus 342, 2000 AH Haarlem.
 ☎ 23 532 5453
 ☎ 23 532 7611
 🕐 Mon - Fri 09:00 - 16:30. 24hr. answering machine with
 information

Stores: Books: General

☺ ■ **Agora**
 Zijlstraat 100, Haarlem.
 ☎ 23 531 3182
 🕐 Mon - Sat 09:00 - 18:00

Stores: Clothing: Leather

☺ ■ **Funny Skin**
 Wagenweg 16, 2012 ND Haarlem.
 ☎ 23 542 1870 ✆ 23 421 1538
 🕐 Tue - Sat 10:00 - 17:00
 Catalogue, FL.25, £10, $15U.S..

Stores: Erotica: General

☺ ■ **Christine Le Duc**
 General Cronjistraat 77, 2021 JC Haarlem.
 Chain of shops with a lot of fetish & BDSM items. Catalogue available.

Heereveen

Organizations: Sexuality

⚢▽ **Het Roze Haagie**
Postbus 551, Heereveen.
☎ 51 362 3293
🕘 Meets 2nd. & 4th. Tue

Heerlen

Organizations: Sexuality

⚢▽ **COC—Heerlen**
Honigmanstraat 2, Heerlen.
☎ 45 571 7387
🕘 Tue - Thu 14:00 - 17:00

Stores: Erotica: General

☺ ■ **Christine Le Duc**
Dautzenbergstraat 5, 6411 LA Heerlen.
Chain of shops with a lot of fetish & BDSM items. Catalogue available.

Hendrik Ido Ambacht

Organizations: Sexuality

⚢▽ **ABOP Homogroep**
Tesselschadestraat 214, Hendrik Ido Ambacht.

Hertogenbosch, 's / Den Bosch

Health Services

☺ □ **SVG**
St. Teunislaan 11, 's-Hertogenbosch.
☎ 73 641 4141
🕘 Mon Wed 08:30 - 12:30

Organizations: Body Size

⚢▽ **Girth & Mirth—Big Dutch**
Postbus 1112, 5200 BD 's-Hertogenbosch.
☎ 73 613 5373 — Fax 73 613 5373

Stores: Erotica: BDSM

☺ ■ **Leder Spezial**
Wilgenstraat 18, 5213 SE 's-Hertogenbosch.
☎ 73 612 8849

Stores: Erotica: General

☺ ■ **Christine Le Duc**
Vughterstraat 62-64, 5211 GK s'Hertogenbosch.
Chain of shops with a lot of fetish & BDSM items. Catalogue available.

☺ ■ **Erotic Corner**
Vughterstraat 111, 's-Hertogenbosch.
☎ 73 614 3436
🕘 Mon - Sat 11:00 - 22:00

Hilversum

Health Services

☺ □ **SVG**
☎ 35 629 2475
🕘 Mon 16:00 -17:00 by appointment only

Organizations: Sexuality

⚢▽ **COC—Hilversum**
Postbus 1631, 1200 BP Hilversum.
☎ 35 628 4789

Stores: Erotica: General

☺ ■ **Eros**
Hilvertsweg 43, Hilversum.
☎ 35 623 3588
🕘 13:00 - 20:00

Hoogeveen

Organizations: Sexuality

⚢▽ **COC—Hoogeveen**
Postbus 684, 7900 AR Hoogeveen.
☎ 52 826 7751
☎ 52 826 8385
🕘 Meets 3rd. Thu of month 20:00 - 24:00

Hoogland

Organizations: Sexuality

⚢▽ **Kringen, Regio Amerfoort**
Postbus 28001, 3828 DA Hoogland.
☎ 33 456 1509

Hoorn

Organizations: Sexuality

⚢▽ **Human-Nature & Postorder AEV**
Postbus 453, Hoorn.
☎ 22 923 2994
☎ 22 921 2056

Stores: Books: General

☺ ■ **Bakker**
Nieuwstraat 17-19, Hoorn.
☎ 22 921 4903
🕘 Mon - Sat 09:00 - 18:00

Leeuwarden

Archives: Sexuality

⚢▼ **Anna Blaman Huis**
Postbus 4062, 8901 EB Leeuwarden.
☎ 58 212 1829 — Fax 58 213 9131
🕘 Mon Fri 13:00 - 17:00, Tue Wed 14:00 - 18:00, Thu 14:00 - 21:00
Intercultural information for the gay, lesbian, & women's movement. Located at Zuidvliet 118.

Organizations: Sexuality

⚢▽ **COC—Friesland**
Postbus 708, Leeuwarden.
☎ 58 212 4908
🕘 Thu - Tue 21:00 - 01:00

Leiden

Organizations: Sexuality

⚢▽ **COC—Leiden**
Postbus 11101, Leiden.
☎ 71 522 0640
🕘 Wed Thu 21:00 - 01:00

Radio: Sexuality

⚢▽ ***Freewave Radio***
FM 105.7, Cable 83.1, Oude Rijn 57, 2312 HC Leiden.
☎ 71 512 0110
🕘 Wed 19:00 - 20:00

Stores: Books: General

☺ ■ **Manifest**
Hooglandse Kerkgracht 4, 2312 HT Leiden.
☎ 71 512 5691

Maastricht

Organizations: Sexuality

⚢▽ **COC—Zuid-Limburg**
Bogaardenstraat 43, Maastricht.
☎ 43 321 8337
🕘 Mon Wed Fri 14:00 -17:00

Stores: Books: General

☺ ■ **Tribune**
Kapoenstraat 8, Maastricht.
☎ 43 325 1978
🕘 Tue - Sat 09:00 - 18:00

Middleburg

Organizations: Sexuality

⚢▽ **COC—Middleburg**
Eigenhaardstraat 2, Middleburg.
☎ 11 861 2280
🕘 Wed Fri 21:00 - ?, 2nd. & 4th. Sat of month 21:00 - ?

Nieuw-Vennep

Piercers

☺ ■ **Jan Dehaan**
Postbus 52, 2150 AB Nieuw-Vennep.

Nijmegen

Health Services

☺ □ **SVG**
☎ 80 322 6141
🕘 Mon - Fri

Organizations: Sexuality

⚢▽ **COC—Nijmegen**
Postbus 552, 6500 AN Nijmegen.

☎ 80 323 4237
🕐 Mon 13:30 - 16:00

⚥▽ **Gelders Advies Centrum Homosexualiteit (GACH)**
Postbus 400, Nijmegen.
Counselling, information, & support.

⚥▽ **De Kringen**
Weezenhof 34-37, Nijmegen.
☎ 80 344 0030
Counselling, information, & support.

Organizations: Sexuality: Student

⚥▽ **Homostudies**
Postbus 9108, Nijmegen.
☎ 80 351 2938

Stores: Books: General

☺■ **Dekker / V. d. Vegt**
Plein 1944 #129, Nijmegen.
☎ 80 322 1010
🕐 Mon - Sat 09:00 - 18:00

☺■ **Oude Mol**
Van Broekhuysenstraat 34, Nijmegen.
☎ 80 322 1734
🕐 Mon - Sat 09:00 - 18:00

Stores: Erotica: General

☺■ **B-1**
Bloemenstraat 37, Nijmegen.
☎ 80 323 7453
🕐 09:30 - 23:00, Sun 14:00 - 23:00

☺■ **Christine Le Duc**
Bloemenstraat 78, 6511 EM Nijmegen.
Chain of shops with a lot of fetish & BDSM items. Catalogue available.

Oss

Health Services

☺□ **SVG**
☎ 41 263 4245
🕐 Mon Thu Fri 09:00 - 10:00

Organizations: Sexuality

⚥▽ **COC—Brabant Noordoost**
Postbus 551, Oss.
☎ 41 262 6666
🕐 Mon Wed Fri 14:00 - 17:00

Pijnakker

Organizations: Sexuality

⚥▽ **WHP**
Postbus 66, 2640 AB Pijnakker.
☎ 15 369 7765

Renkum

Organizations: Sexuality

▷▽ **Stichting Ede**
Bennekomseweg 160, 6871 KJ Renkum.
☎ 31 731 8890
Female-to-males. Publishes a newsletter.

Roermund

Bars: BDSM

⚥▼ **Sjinderhannes**
Swalmerstraat 42, Roermund.
☎ 47 533 3119
🕐 Wed Thu Sun 21:00 - 02:00, Fri Sat - 03:00. Leather meeting 2nd. & last Sat of month

Health Services

☺□ **SVG**
☎ 47 532 8112
🕐 Mon - Fri 11:00 - 12:00

Organizations: BDSM

☺■ **The South Goes Mad**
Postbus 435, 6040 AK Roermund.
Organizes periodic BDSM gatherings.

Organizations: Motorcycle

⚥▽ **The Limburg Motorclub**
Postbus 435, 6040 Roermund.
☎ 47 533 3119

⚥▽ **The Rurals MC**

Postbus 561, 6040 AK Roermund.
Publishes *Circuit* every month.

Organizations: Sexuality

⚥▽ **COC—Stadtgroep Roermund**
Postbus 491, Roermund.
☎ 47 532 9257

⚥▽ **Stichting Gay Association**
Swalmerstraat 40-42, Roermund.
☎ 47 533 3119

Roosendaal

Health Services

☺□ **GG & GD**
☎ 16 554 1900
🕐 By appointment only

Organizations: Sexuality

⚥▽ **COC—Roosendaal**
Postbus 1207, 4700 Roosendaal.

Rotterdam

Bars: BDSM

⚥▼ **Shaft**
Schiedamse Singel 137, 3079 DC Rotterdam.
☎ 10 414 1486
🕐 Mon - Thu 20:00 - 02:00, Fri 22:00 - 05:00, Sat 23:00 - 05:00, Sun 17:00 - 02:00

⚥▼ **The Sweet Sixties**
Schiedamsevestl 46, Rotterdam.
☎ 10 213 2032
🕐 Sun - Thu 16:00 - 04:00, Fri Sat 16:00 - 08:00

Health Services

☺□ **Havenzuikhuis**
Haringvliet 2, Rotterdam.
☎ 10 411 2800
🕐 By appointment only

Organizations: BDSM

☺□ **Vereniging Studiegroep Sado-Masochisme (VSSM)**
☎ 20 420 2117
📧 vssm@dds.nl
🌐 http://sparkie.riv.net/fetish/vssm
🕐 Meets 1st. Sun of month 19:30for leather only, 3rd. Tue of month 20:00 for leather & non-leather, & 5th. Fri of month (4 times per year) 20:00
Also uniforms. English & German also spoken.

Organizations: Body Size

⚥▽ **Girth & Mirth—Rotterdam**
Postbus 768, 3000 AT Rotterdam.
☎ 10 414 1555

Organizations: Motorcycle

⚥▽ **MS Rotterdam**
Postbus 22184, 3003 DD Rotterdam.

Organizations: Sexuality

⚥▽ **COC—Rotterdam**
Schiedamse Singel 175, Rotterdam.
☎ 10 414 1555
🕐 Tue Wed 20:00 - 22:00 Thu 22:00 - 01:00, Sat 22:00 - 02:00

⚥▽ **De Kringen**
Platostraat 142, Rotterdam.
☎ 10 419 8310

Publishers: Magazines: BDSM

☺ *Sublime*
M. J. Production, Postbus 61246, 3002 HE Rotterdam.
Small format magazine with information about BDSM clubs & dominants.

Stores: Clothing: Fetish

☺■ **Massad**
⚥ Postbus 3061, Zaagmolendrift 33, 3003 AK Rotterdam. 📞 10 465 9977
☎ 10 466 4368
🕐 Tue - Sat 09:00 - 17:00
Leather manufacturer, bookshop, mail order. Publishes *Massad* every two months. Yearly subscription is $25U.S. incl. s&h.

Stores: Erotica: BDSM

☺■ **My Sin**
Pannekoekstraat 29a, 3011 LC Rotterdam.
☎ 10 404 6568

Stores: Erotica: General

☺ ■ **Christine Le Duc**
Schieweg 108, 3038 BC Rotterdam.
☎ 10 467 9527
Chain of shops with a lot of fetish & BDSM items. Catalogue available.

☺ ■ **Eros**
Zaagmolendrift 10, Rotterdam.
☎ 10 466 8805
⌚ 10:00 - 18:00 Fri - 21:00

☺ ■ **Hans Gay-O-Theek**
Oranjeboomstraat 267, Rotterdam.
☎ 10 485 9079
⌚ 11:00 - 23:00

Terheijden

Organizations: Sexuality

▽ **Stichting Omd**
Postbus 24, 4844 ZG Terheijden.

Terneuzen

Organizations: Sexuality

▽ **COC—Zeeuws Vlaanderen**
Postbus 96, Terneuzen.
☎ 11 563 0654
⌚ Meets Sun 20:00 - 24:00

Tiel

Organizations: Sexuality

▽ **COC—Tiel**
Postbus 223, Tiel.
☎ 34 461 6373

Tilburg

Bars: Sexuality

▼ **The Blue Boy**
Tivolistraat 77, Tilburg.
☎ 13 535 4487
⌚ Wed - Fri 21:00 - ?, Sat 20:00 - ?, Sun 18:00 - ?

Health Services

☺ □ **GG & GD**
☎ 13 463 1515
⌚ Mon - Fri 09:00 - 10:00

Organizations: Sexuality

▽ **COC—Tilburg**
Koestraat 73, Tilburg.
☎ 13 535 9050
⌚ Meets Fri Sat 21:00 - 02:00

Organizations: Sexuality: Student

▽ **Homostudies**
Postbus 90153, Tilburg.
☎ 13 466 9111

Stores: Books: General

☺ ■ **Vrije Boekhandel**
Stadthuisplein 356a, Tilburg.
☎ 13 543 5944
⌚ Mon 13:00 - 18:00, Tue Wed Fri 10:00 - 18:00, Thu - 21:00, Sat - 17:00

Uden

Organizations: Sexuality

▽ **COC—Uden**
Postbus 579, Uden.
☎ 41 326 5821
⌚ Meets 4th. Sun of month

Uithoorn

Organizations: Sexuality

▽ **Homogroep Uithoorn**
Postbus 556, 1422 GB Uithoorn.

Utrecht

Health Services

☺ □ **Academisch Ziekhuis**
Dermatologie, Catharijnensinge 101, Utrecht.
☎ 30 237 2833
⌚ Mon Fri 08:15 - 10:00

Organizations: Academic: AIDS

☺ □ **Bisexuality & AIDS research Group**
Gay & Lesbian Studies Department, The University of Utrecht, Heidelberglaan 1, 3584 CS Utrecht.

Organizations: BDSM

☺ □ **Vereniging Studiegroep Sado-Masochisme (VSSM)**
☎ 20 420 2117
vssm@dds.nl
http://sparkie.riv.net/fetish/vssm
⌚ Meets 2nd. Sun of month 14:30
Also uniforms. English & German also spoken.

Organizations: Fetish: Clothing: Rubber

☺ □ **Club Gum**
c/o NVSH-gebouw, Wittevrouwensingel 100, Utrecht.
☎ 20 420 2117
http://sparkie.riv.nl/fetish/clubgum/party.html
⌚ Meets 4th. Fri of month 20:00 - 01:00. Telephone is VSSM information line

Organizations: Sexuality

▽ **COC—Utrecht**
Postbus 117, Oudegracht 221, 3500 AC Utrecht.
☎ 30 231 8841
⌚ Mon - Fri 13:00 - 17:00
Gives information to homosexual men & lesbian women & gives weekly parties for youth homos & for older gays & lesbians.

▽ **Homostudies Utrecht**
Heidelberglaan 1, Utrecht.
☎ 30 253 4700

▽ **International Lesbian & Gay Association (ILGA)—Utrecht**
Herenweg 93, 3513 CD Utrecht.
☎ 30 234 0912

▽ **Nederlandse Vereniging Humanits**
☎ 54 727 2048
Contact: Mr. & Mrs. Caroline & Aloys Hulshof

Stores: Erotica: General

☺ ■ **Christine Le Duc**
Amsterdamsestraatweg 310, Utrecht.
☎ 30 242 6956
⌚ 10:00 - 23:00
Chain of shops with a lot of fetish & BDSM items. Catalogue available.

■ **Davy's Erotheek**
Amsterdamsestraatweg 197, 3551 CB Utrecht.
☎ 30 243 6815

Valkenswaard

Health Services

☺ □ **SVG**
☎ 40 204 0505
⌚ By appointment only

Veghel

Health Services

☺ □ **SVG**
☎ 41 336 7915
⌚ Mon - Fri 09:00 - 17:00

Venlo

Health Services

☺ □ **GG & GD**
Nijmeegesweg 44, 5900 BD Venlo.
☎ 77 359 8822
☎ 77 354 0408 (24hrs.)
⌚ By appointment only
STD & AIDS information, counselling, testing, & treatment.

☺ □ **SVG**
☎ 77 354 0404
⌚ Mon - Fri 11:00 - 12:00

Venray

Health Services

☺ □ **GG & GD**
Building de Clochert, Venray.
☎ 47 858 5251
⌚ By appointment only

Organizations: Sexuality
♂▽ **COC—Venray**
Postbus 316, Venray.
☎ 47 851 0487
🕐 Wed 20:15 - 00:30

Vlissingen
Organizations: Sexuality
♂▽ **COC—Vlissingen**
Postbus 251, 4380 AG Vlissingen.
☎ 11 841 2248
🕐 21:00 - 24:00, Mon 15:00 - 19:00

Voorburg
Publishers: Videos: BDSM
☺ **West Video**
Postbus 712, 2270 AS Voorburg.
☎ 79 351 3193 ✆ 79 321 0223
One of the biggest BDSM video producers in Holland. Wholesale only,
does not sell to public.

Wageningen
Organizations: Sexuality
♂▽ **Homogroep Wageningen**
Postbus 89, 6700 AB Wageningen.
☎ 31 742 2835
🕐 Meets Fri 21:30 - ?

Weert
Organizations: Sexuality
♂▽ **COC—Weert**
Postbus 194, 6000 AD Weert.
☎ 49 553 3733
🕐 Meets 1st Thu of month

Woerden
Organizations: Sexuality
♂▽ **COC—Woerden**
2nd. Floor, Prins Hendrikkade 114, Woerden.
🕐 Sun 13:00 - 17:00, 4th. Sat of month 20:00 - 01:00

Zoetermeer
Organizations: Sexuality
♂▽ **WHZ**
Postbus 5343, Zoetermeer.
☎ 79 321 0128
☎ 79 331 7111

Zwolle
Health Services
♂▽ **Homogezondheitzentrum**
☎ 38 454 6369
🕐 Tue 19:00 - 21:30

Organizations: Sexuality
♂▽ **COC—Zwolle**
Postbus 1251, Zwolle.
☎ 38 421 0065
🕐 Meets Tue 20:00 - 24:00, Fri 21:00 - 01:00, Sat 22:00 - 03:00

New Zealand

Area: Approximately 271,000 square kilometres
Population: Approximately 3,430,000
Capital City: Wellington
Currency: New Zealand Dollar (NZS)
Official Language: English & Maori
Major Religions: 50% Protestant, 15% Roman Catholic
National Holiday: New Zealand Day, 6th. February
Time zone: GMT plus 12 hours
Country Initials: NZ
Electricity: 230 volts
Country Dialing Code (from elsewhere): 64
Intl. Dialing Prefix (out of the country): 00
Long Distance Dialing Prefix (inside country): 0
Climate: Cool, temperate south, sub-tropical in the north.
Age of consent & homosexuality legislation: Age of consent for
homosexual activity is 16. Homosexual acts were decriminalized in
1986. There still exists discrimination for homosexuals in the military.

NATIONAL RESOURCES
Archives: Sexuality
♂▽ **Lesbian & Gay Archives of New Zealand**
P. O. Box 11695, Wellington.
☎ 4 474 3000 Ext.: 8663
🕐 Appointments preferred
Research library & the national gay & lesbian archive. Housed in the
Alexander Turnbull Library, National Library of NZ, Molesworth Street.
♂▽ **National Gay Rights Coalition (NGRC)**
Gay Tape Library, P. O. Box 68-030, Newton.

Helplines: AIDS
☺☐ **AIDS National Hotline**
☎ 800 802 437
☎ 9 302 2197 (from Auckland)
🕐 24hrs. toll free
Counselling, information, & support for people infected with or affected
by HIV/AIDS.

Helplines: Sexuality
♂▽ **Assault Hotline**
☎ 800 802 437
Last resort phone help in case of assault (through AIDS hotline).

Mailorder: Erotica
♂▼ **Out! Mailorder**
Private Bag 92126, Auckland 1.
☎ 900 51993

Organizations: AIDS: Education
☺☐ **National People Living with AIDS Union**
P. O. Box 2558, Wellington.
☎ 4 382 8791
☎ 4 471 2452 (Collective Thinking)
Publishes *Collective Thinking.*
☺▽ **New Zealand AIDS Foundation—Auckland**
Auckland Community Outreach Centre, 1st. Floor, 44-46 Ponsonby Road,
Ponsonby.
☎ 9 378 9802 ✆ 9 378 9808
☺☐ **New Zealand AIDS Foundation—Head Office**
P. O. Box 6663, Wellesley Street, Auckland.
☎ 4 303 3124 ✆ 4 309 3149
Contact: Mr. Warren Lindburg, Director
☺☐ **Pacific Island AIDS Trust**
P. O. Box 12453, Thordon.
☎ 4 473 4493
HIV/AIDS information & counselling for Pacific islanders.
♂▽ **Te Roopu Tatautoko**
P. O. Box 16050, Wellington.
☎ 4 389 9676
AIDS counselling & information for Maoris.

Organizations: Motorcycle
♂▽ **Mercury Morocycle Club**
P. O. Box 26-335, Epsom.
🕐 Meets 3rd. Fri of month

Organizations: Sexual Politics
♂▽ **Lesbian & Gay Rights Resource Centre**
P. O. Box 11-695, Wellington.

Organizations: Sexuality
♂▽ **Auckland Gay & Lesbian Community Centre**
P. O. Box 5426, Wellesley Street, Auckland.
☎ 9 378 9802 ✆ 9 378 9808
♂▽ **Gay & Lesbian Welfare, Auckland**
⚢ P. O. Box 3132, 45 Anzac Avenue, Auckland.
☎ 9 303 3584 ✆ 9 309 3268
🕐 10:00 - 22:00
Contact: Mr. Neville Creighton, Coordinator / Trainer
Information, support, counselling, referral by 'phone, face-to-face, & in
groups for our queer communities, their families, friends, & hetero
partners. Professionally trained volunteers. French, German, Cantonese,
Mandarin, Japanese, & others also spoken.
♂☐ **Pride & Unity for Male Prostitutes (PUMP)**
P. O. Box 68509, Newton.
Education & promotion of safer sex practices among male sex workers.
♂▽ **Transgender Education, Welfare, & Health
Organization (TEWAHO)**
P. O. Box 6528, Te Aro.
☎ 4 479 2610 ✆ 4 801 5690
Publishes *On TOPs.*

✉▼ **Transvestites Transexuals Group Minorities Trust**
106 Witako Street, Epuni, Lower Hutt.
☎ 4 844 764

Publishers: Magazines: Sexuality

⚥▼ *Express*
 🖎 Cornerstone Publications, P. O. Box 47514, Ponsonby.
 ☎ 9 376 2018 📞 9 376 2019
 🕐 Mon - Fri 09:00 - 17:00
 🚲 ✓ $ 🆅🆂🅰 💳 🖊
 Newspaper to inform & entertain New Zealand's gay, lesbian, bisexual,
 & transsexual community. Express, the national newspaper of gay
 expression. Published every two weeks. Yearly subscription is SNZ35
 local, SNZ100 international.

⚥▼ *Out!*
 Lawrence Publishing Company (NZ) Ltd., Private Bag 92126, Auckland
 1.
 ☎ 9 377 9031 📞 9 377 7767
 Published every two months.

Stores: Books: General

⚥▼ **Out! Bookshop**
 45 Anzac Avenue, Auckland.
 ☎ 9 377 7770 📞 9 377 7767
 🕐 Mon - Wed Sat 11:00 - 18:00, Fri Sat 11:00 - 23:00, Sun 13:00 -
 20:00

Stores: Clothing: Fetish

☺ ■ **L'Amour**
 Saint Kevin's Arcade, Karangahape Road, Auckland 1.
 ☎ 9 379 0497 📞 9 480 1400

Auckland

Health Services

☺ ☐ **Auckland Hospital**
 440 Park Road, Grafton.
 ☎ 9 379 7440

⚥ ▼ **Family Planning Association**
 All Male Clinic, 40 Taharoto Road, Takapuna.
 ☎ 9 486 1014
 🕐 Wed 16:00 - 18:00

Helplines: Sexuality

⚥▽ **Gayline / Lesbianline**
 🖎 P. O. Box 3132, 45 Anzac Avenue, Auckland.
 ☎ 9 303 3584 📞 9 309 3268
 🕐 10:00- 22:00
 Information, support, counselling, referral by 'phone, face-to-face, & in
 groups for our queer communities, their families, friends, & hetero
 partners. Professionally trained volunteers. French, German, Cantonese,
 Mandarin, Japanese, & others also spoken.

♀ ☐ **Womanline**
 ☎ 9 376 5173
 🕐 Mon Fri 11:00 - 20:30

Manufacturers: Clothing: Rubber

☺ ■ **L'Amour—Head Office**
 P. O. Box 5200, Auckland 1.
 ☎ 9 379 0497 📞 9 480 1400
 ☎ 800 508088 (orders)
 Catalogue, AUSS20.

Organizations: AIDS: Education

☺ ▽ **Auckland Community AIDS Services (ACAS)**
 P. O. Box 3702, Auckland 1.
 ☎ 9 309 0156
 Education & community support for the Auckland area.

Organizations: AIDS: Support

☺ ☐ **New Zealand AIDS Foundation—Auckland**
 Burnett Centre & Auckland Support Services, 76 Grafton Road, Auckland.
 ☎ 9 309 5560 📞 9 302 2338
 🕐 Mon Thu 08:00 - 16:30, Wed 08:00 - 17:30, Fri 08:00 - 15:00
 Free information, counselling, & support for people infected with or
 affected by HIV/AIDS.

Organizations: Bears

⚥▽ **Kiwi Bears**
 29 Prospect Terrace, Auckland 3.

⚥▽ **Kubs/Kiwi United Bear Social**
 P. O. Box 5918, Wellesley Street, Auckland.

Organizations: Family

☺ ☐ **Parents of Lesbians & Gays**
 ☎ 9 846 7889

Organizations: Sexuality

♂ ▽ **Auckland Bisexual Group**
 ☎ 9 522 1910
 ☎ 9 631 5236
 🕐 Meets every two weeks

⚥▽ **Auckland Gay & Lesbian Trust**
 P. O. Box 5426, Wellesley Street, Auckland.
 ☎ 9 302 0590
 🕐 Meets 2nd. Wed of month 17:00 - 19:00

⚥▽ **Gays & Lesbians Everywhere in Education (GLEE)**
 ☎ 9 846 1681
 Support for gay & lesbian teachers.

⚥▽ **Hibiscus Coast Men's Support Group**
 ☎ 9 424 8808
 🕐 Regular meetings

♀▽ **Lesbian Coalition**
 P. O. Box 1236, Auckland.

♀▽ **Lesbian Support**
 P. O. Box 3833, Auckland.
 ☎ 8 846 7441
 A safe place for women questioning their sexuality.

⚥▽ **Mutal Gay Mens' Support Group (MGM)**
 P. O. Box 82-144, Highland Park.
 ☎ 9 534 2643

✉▽ **The New Zealand Gender Dysphoria Foundation**
(NZGDF)
 P. O. Box 2827, Auckland.
 Publishes *La Femme* every two months.

☺ ☐ **New Zealand Prostitutes Collective**
 P. O. Box 68-509, Newton 1.
 ☎ 9 366 6106
 Education & promotion of safer sex practices among sex workers.

⚥▽ **Prevention Auckland**
 ☎ 9 357 0415
 Promotes safer sex practices among gay men in Auckland.

✉▽ **Transexual Outreach (TOPPS)**
 P. O. Box 68-501, Auckland.
 ☎ 9 366 6106

⚥▽ **Waiheke Island Gay Support Group**
 ☎ 9 372 7972
 🕐 Meets 2nd. & 4th. Sun of month

Organizations: Sexuality: Student

⚥▽ **Auckland University Gay Students Association**
 c/o Students Union, Auckland University, Auckland.
 🕐 Meets Fri 17:00 - 19:00

⚥▽ **Unitec Gay & Lesbian Support Association**
 ☎ 9 815 0440
 ☎ 9 846 3316

Organizations: Sexuality: Youth

⚥▽ **Howick Gay Youth Group**
 ☎ 9 534 2643

⚥▽ **Icebreakers**
 ☎ 9 376 6633 (Youthline)
 ☎ 9 376 4156 (Rainbow Youth Hotline)
 Free, confidential support for young men & women under 26 who feel
 they may be attracted to members of the same sex.

⚥▽ **Rainbow Youth Trust**
 P. O. Box 5426, Wellesley Street, Auckland.
 ☎ 9 376 4155
 🕐 Mon - Fri 10:00 - 16:00
 Support & informaton for lesbian & gay youth.

Publishers: Documentaries: Sexuality

⚥▼ *Triangle Television, Inc.*
 P. O. Box 78-034, Grey Lynn.
 ☎ 9 376 7385 (Jim Blackman, President)
 ☎ 9 358 0426 (Hans Verluys, Programme Director)
 ✉ hansv@iprolink.co.nz
 Production house making television for the gay, lesbian, & bisexual
 communities.

Publishers: Magazines: Sexuality

♀▼ *Broadsheet Magazine*
 Womanlife, Inc., P. O. Box 56147, Auckland.
 ☎ 9 376 4587
 Published quarterly. Yearly subscription is $27.50NZ.

Publishers: Newspapers: Sexuality

Big Ted & Manu
P. O. Box 5426, Wellesley Street, Auckland.
Newsletter for gay & bisexual youth under 26.

Tamaki Makaurau
P. O. Box 44-056, Herne Bay.
Lesbian newsletter.

Radio: General

Alternative Accent
Sun 13:15
Profiles people who belong to minorities.

SAFE
Every 3rd. Sat
Information & interviews about HIV/AIDS.

Radio: Sexuality

The G & T Breakfast Show
Access Community Radio AM 810, P. O. Box 5609, Auckland.
☎ 9 302 0238 (studio) — Fax 9 302 0237
☎ 9 307 5810 (talkback)
Thu 07:00

In The Pink, The Girls Own Show
95 BFM, c/o AUSA, Private Bag 92019, 34, Princes Street, Auckland.
☎ 9 366 7223 — Fax 9 366 7224
☎ 9 307 3918
Sun 19:00 - 21:00
✓ $
Lesbian & gay program on campus radio station.

This Way Out
Access Community Radio AM 810, P. O. Box 68-030, Newton.
☎ 9 525 8261 — Fax 9 525 8261
☎ 9 302 0238 (studio)
Sat 11:40
International gay & lesbian news magazine.

Stores: Clothing: Fetish

L'Amour
270 Onewa Road, Birkenhead 1.

L'Amour
518 Karangahape Road, Auckland 1.
☎ 9 379 0497 — Fax 9 480 1400

Stores: Erotica: BDSM

Tan Ya Hide Ltd.
413 Mount Eden Road, Auckland.
☎ 9 623 0397 — Fax 9 623 0397

Stores: Military Surplus

Army Surplus Stores
239A Onehunga Mall, Onnga.
☎ 9 634 3792

Television: Sexuality

Triangle Television, Inc.
P. O. Box 78-034, Grey Lynn.
☎ 9 376 7385 (Jim Blackman, President)
☎ 9 358 0426 (Hans Verluys, Programme Director)
hansv@iprolink.co.nz
Production house making television for the gay, lesbian, & bisexual communitites. Currently setting up community access television for Auckland region.

Blenheim

Health Services

Wairau Hospital
Community Health Development Unit, P. O. Box 46, Blenheim.
☎ 3 577 1914
Confidential HIV counselling & testing.

Organizations: Sexuality

Blenheim Gay / Lesbian Contact
P. O. Box 62, Blenheim.
☎ 3 578 2259

Radio: Sexuality

Tea With The Boys
18:00 - 19:00. Lesbian/gay news Thu 09:00 - 10:00

Christchurch

Counsellors

Stuart Currie
☎ 3 3779 4601

Helplines: Sexuality

Gay Information Line
P. O. Box 25-165, Christchurch.
☎ 3 379 3990
24hrs.
Information only.

Gayline
P. O. Box 25-165, Christchurch.
☎ 3 379 4796
Mon 20:00 - 21:00, Sat 19;30 - 22:00
Counselling.

Organizations: AIDS: Education

New Zealand AIDS Foundation—Christchurch
P. O. Box 21-285, Christchurch.
☎ 3 379 3353

Organizations: AIDS: Support

Ettie Rout Centre
P. O. Box 21285, 31 Saint Asaph Street, Christchurch.
☎ 3 379 1953 — Fax 3 365 2477
Mon - Fri 09:00 - 17:00
✓ $
Support, counselling, testing for all people with or affected by HIV. Sexual health counselling for men who have sex with men. Publishes *Ettie Rout Centre News* every month. Yearly subscription is free.

HIV Positive Peer Support Group
☎ 3 379 1953
Meets once a week

Organizations: Sexuality

Lesbian Support Group
P. O. Box 21-069, Christchurch.

Pride & Unity for Male Prostitutes (PUMP)
P. O. Box 13-561, Christchurch.
Education & promotion of safer sex practices among male sex workers.

Organizations: Sexuality: Student

Campus Queers (GUSS)
Canterbury University Students Union Private Bag, Christchurch.

Radio: Sexuality

Lesbian Radio
Mon 21:30
Age statement of 18 is required.

Loud & Queer
Wed 19:00 - 20:00

Stores: Books: General

Out! Bookshop
Colombo Health Club, 661 Colombo Street, Christchurch.
☎ 3 366 7352
Also toys & magazines.

Stores: Erotica: General

Menfriends
P. O. Box 2794, Upstairs, 83 Lichfield Street, Christchurch.
☎ 3 377 1701
7 days per week, from 12:00
Extensive shop for gay & bisexual men. Age statement of 18 is required.

Dunedin

Helplines: Sexuality

Gayline
P. O. Box 1382, Dunedin.
☎ 3 477 2077
Wed 17:30 - 19:30, Fri 19:30: 22:30, answering machine with recording at other times
Information & counselling about gay/lesbian issues.

Organizations: AIDS: Education

New Zealand AIDS Foundation—Dunedin
P. O. Box 1004, Dunedin.
☎ 3 474 7732 — Fax 3 474 7631

Organizations: Sexuality

Gay Boys on Campus
c/o OUSA, P. O. Box 1436, Dunedin.
Meets 2nd. Wed of month 13:00. Call Gayline for details

Pride & Unity for Male Prostitutes (PUMP)
P. O. Box 6407, Dunedin.
Education & promotion of safer sex practices among male sex workers.

Organizations: Sexuality: Youth

⚥▽ **Icebreakers**
 ☎ 3 477 2077
 Confidential group for young men who think they are gay or bisexual.

Publishers: Newspapers: Sexuality

⚥▼ *Pink Express*
 P. O. Box 1382, Dunedin.
 ☎ 3 477 2077
 Gay & lesbian newsletter for Dunedin & area.

Stores: Books: General

☺ ■ **Aberdeen Bookshop**
 185 Hillside, Dunedin.

☺ ■ **Modernway Books**
 331 George Street, Dunedin.
 ☎ 3 477 6636 ✆ 3 488 1139
 ☉ Mon - Thu 09:00 - 17:30, Fri 09:00 - 21:00
 ⚖ ✓ 💳 🆅🅸🆂🅰 🆖 ℓ
 Novelty store selling largest selection of gay magazines, adult gifts, naughty nic-nacs, leather gear, & pipes. Age statement of 18 is required.

☺ ■ **Southern Books**
 225 King Edward Street, Dunedin.

Gisborne

Organizations: Sexuality

⚥▽ **Gisborne Gay Support (GGS)**
 P. O. Box 929, Gisborne.
 ☎ 6 867 9103
 ☉ Wed 19:30 - 21:30
 Please address envelopes to GGS, do NOT address them to Gisborne Gay Support.

Hamilton

Health Services

☺ □ **HIV/STD Clinic**
 ☎ 7 839 9732
 ☉ Wed 15:30 - 18:00

Organizations: AIDS: Education

☺ □ **New Zealand AIDS Foundation—Waikato**
 P. O. Box 41, Hamilton.
 ☎ 7 838 557
 ☎ 7 838 511

Organizations: Sexuality: Student

⚥▽ **Esteem**
 ☎ 7 856 1162
 ☎ 7 856 4085
 Support group for students at university or polytechnical college.

Organizations: Sexuality: Youth

⚥▽ **Icebreakers**
 ☎ 7 856 3161
 Support for young men who are gay/bisexual or think they might be.

⚥▽ **Respect**
 P. O. Box 41, Hamilton.

Radio: Sexuality

⚥▽ *Different Strokes*
 ☎ 7 838 4440
 ☉ Sun 20:00 - 22:00

Stores: Books: General

☺ ■ **Goldmine Bookshop**
 312 Victoria Street, Hamilton.

Hastings

Stores: Books: General

☺ ■ **Stortford Lodge Bookshop**
 1102 Heretaunga Street, Hastings.

Invercargill

Helplines: Sexuality

⚥▽ **Gayline**
 ☎ 3 216 6344
 ☎ 3 477 2077

⚲▽ **Lesbian Line**
 ☎ 3 218 3877

Organizations: Sexuality

⚥▽ **Southland Social Group**

P. O. Box 1567, Invercargill.

Kapiti / Horowhenua

Helplines: Sexuality

⚥▽ **Pride S. I. S.**
 P. O. Box 176, Levin.
 ☎ 6 368 1195
 ☉ Wed - Sun 19:00 - 22:00
 Confidential information & support.

Napier

Helplines: Sexuality

⚥▽ **Gayline**
 ☎ 6 835 7190
 ☉ Wed Fri Sun 19:00 - 22:00

Organizations: AIDS: Education

☺ □ **New Zealand AIDS Foundation—Hawkes Bay**
 P. O. Box 679, Napier.
 ☎ 6 835 5554 ✆ 6 835 5554

Organizations: Sexuality

⚥▽ **Gay Club Hawkes Bay**
 P. O. Box 573, Hastings.

Organizations: Sexuality: Youth

⚥▽ **Icebreakers**
 ☎ 6 835 7190
 ☉ Wed Fri Sun 19:00 - 22:00

Nelson

Health Services

☺ □ **Medical Centre**
 STD Clinic, Rutherford Street, Nelson.
 ☎ 3 546 8881
 HIV testing & counselling.

Organizations: AIDS: Support

☺ □ **Nelson HIV/AIDS Support Network**
 P. O. Box 4022, Nelson South.
 ☎ 3 546 1540 ✆ 3 546 1542
 ☎ 3 547 2827
 ⚖ ✓
 Support, information, education for those concerned about HIV / AIDS, & for those living with HIV / AIDS, their partners, & families.

Organizations: Sexuality

⚥▽ **Spectrum**
 P. O. Box 4022, Nelson South.
 ☎ 3 547 2827
 ☎ 3 548 0814
 ☉ Drop-in centre Thu evening
 ✓
 Support & social group for gay & bisexual men. Publishes *Spectrum Newsletter* every month. Yearly subscription is SNZ20. Age statement of 16 is required.

Radio: Sexuality

⚥▽ *Gaytime FM*
 Spectrum, c/o Spectrum, P. O. Box 4022, Nelson South.
 ☎ 3 525 9781 ✆ 3 525 8779
 ☉ Sun 11:00 - 11:30
 News, views, & interviews of interest to gay & bisexual men. Broadcast on Fresh FM 90.4.

Stores: Erotica: General

☺ ■ **Regal Mag & Toy Shop**
 212 Hardy Street, Nelson.

Palmerston North

Health Services

☺ □ **Public Health STD Centre**
 9 Heretaunga Street, Palmerston North.
 ☎ 6 350 8602 ✆ 6 350 8602
 HIV testing.

Helplines: Sexuality

⚥▽ **Gayline & Lesbianline**
 ☎ 6 358 5378
 Information, counselling, & support.

Organizations: AIDS: Support

☺ □ **AIDS Support Network**
 P. O. Box 1491, Palmerston North.

Organizations: Sexuality

⚥▽ **Manawatu Gay Rights Association Inc.**
P. O. Box 1491, Palmerston North.
🕐 Meets Fri 20:00, Sat 21:30
Call gayline for details.

Rotorua

Helplines: Sexuality

⚥▽ **Gayline**
☎ 87 348 3598
🕐 Tue 19:00 - 21:00

Organizations: AIDS: Support

☺ ☐ **Bay Area AIDS Support Service**
P. O. Box 439, Rotorua.
☎ 7 348 1199 Ext.: 8980

Tauranga

Organizations: Sexuality

⚥▽ **Tauranga Gay Support Group**
P. O. Box 5289, Mount Maunganui.

Stores: Erotica: General

☺ ■ **Nauti Nik Naks**
47B The Strand, Tauranga.

Timaru

Organizations: Sexuality

⚥▽ **Aoraki Lesbian & Gay Group**
P. O. Box 59, Timaru.
☎ 3 615 7668
🕐 Meets 3rd. Sat of month

Wellington

Counsellors

☺ ■ **John Mayesm**
☎ 4 384 5549

Helplines: Sexuality

⚥▽ **Gay Switchboard**
P. O. Box 11-372, Wellington.
☎ 4 385 0674
🕐 19:30 - 22:00
Information & support.

Organizations: AIDS: Education

☺ ☐ **New Zealand AIDS Foundation—Wellington**
P. O. Box 7287, Wellington South.
☎ 4 389 3169 📟 4 389 4207

Organizations: AIDS: Support

☺ ☐ **Awhina AIDS Clinic**
P. O. Box 7287, Wellington South.
☎ 4 389 3169 📟 4 389 4207
Information, counselling, & HIV testing.

☺ ☐ **Body Positive**
P. O. Box 7287, Wellington South.
☎ 4 389 3169 📟 4 389 4207

☺ ☐ **HIV Support Group**
☎ 4 389 3169 📟 4 389 4207
☎ 4 385 9638

Organizations: Motorcycle

⚥▽ **41 South MC**
P. O. Box 27-180, Wellington.

Organizations: Sexuality

⚥▽ **Lesbian Line**
☎ 4 389 8082
🕐 Tue Thu 19:00 - 22:00

☺ ☐ **New Zealand Prostitutes Collective**
P. O. Box 11-412, Wellington.
☎ 4 382 8791 📟 4 801 5690
Education & promotion of safer sex practices among sex workers.

♂ ☐ **Pride & Unity for Male Prostitutes (PUMP)**
☎ 4 382 8791
Education & promotion of safer sex practices among male sex workers.

Organizations: Sexuality: Student

⚥▽ **Lesbian & Gay Student Group**
Private Bag, Victoria University, Wellington.

Organizations: Sexuality: Youth

⚥▽ **Boy Zone**
☎ 4 385 0674
🕐 Meets every two weeks
Call Gay Switchboard for details.

⚥ \ **Icebreakers**
☎ 4 385 0674
Confidential support group for young men who are or think they may be gay/bisexual.

Organizations: Swingers

⚥⚥ ■ **New Zealand Swing Club**
P. O. Box 27-350, Wellington, .
☎ 4 384 8214
Publishes *Linx Adult Shopper.*

Publishers: Directories: Sexuality

⚥▼ **Q Community Events Calendar**
P. O. Box 7287, Wellington South.
☎ 4 389 3169

Publishers: Newspapers: Sexuality

⚥▼ **Awhina**
P. O. Box 7287, Wellington South.
☎ 4 389 3169
Newsletter for the Wellington area.

Radio: Sexuality

⚥▽ **Boy Trouble**
🕐 Wed 19:00 - 20:00

⚥▽ **Gay Broadcasting Collective**
c/o Access AM 873, P. O. Box 12-413, Thorndon.
☎ 4 385 8783
🕐 Sat 11:15 - 12:15

Stores: Books: General

⚥▽ **Out! Bookshop**
1st. Floor, 62 Dixon Street, Wellington.
☎ 4 385 4400
🕐 Mon Tue 10:30 - 18:00, Wed - 19:00, Thu - Sat 10:30 - 20:30
Also toys & magazines.

Whangarei

Health Services

☺ ☐ **Whangarei STD Clinic**
123 Maunu Road, Whangarei.
☎ 9 438 2079

Organizations: AIDS: Support

☺ ☐ **Whangarei Health HIV/AIDS Coördinator**
P. O. Box 742, Whangarei.
☎ 9 438 2070 Ext.: 3543

Northern Ireland

Area: Approximately 244,490 square kilometres for whole of U.K.
Population: Approximately 57,650,000 for whole of U.K.
Capital City: Belfast
Currency: Pound Sterling (£)
Official Language: English & French
Major Religions: 57% Protestant, 13% Roman Catholic
National Holiday: Queen's Birthday, early June
Time zone: GMT
Country Initials: GB
Electricity: 240 volts, 50Hz
Country Dialing Code (from elsewhere): 44
Intl. Dialing Prefix (out of the country): 0101
Long Distance Dialing Prefix (inside country): 0
Climate: Warm, dry summers, cool, wet winters.
Age of consent & homosexuality legislation: Age of consent for sexual activity is 16, but 18 for homosexual activities. Homosexual acts were decriminalized in 1982. In 1992, Homosexual acts are not permitted for the members of the military.
Legal drinking age: 18

NATIONAL RESOURCES

Helplines: AIDS

☺ **AIDS Helpline**
♿ The Centre at The Warehouse, 7 James Street South, Belfast, Antrim BT2 8DN.
☎ 800 137 437 📟 1232 329845
☎ 1232 249268
🕐 Mon - Fri 19:00 - 22:00, Tue Thu 10:00 - 13:00, Sat 14:00 - 17:00

ANTRIM
Belfast
Helplines: Sexuality
♂ **Cara Friend**
P. O. Box 44, Belfast, Antrim BT1 1SH.
☎ 1232 238668

Organizations: AIDS: Support
☺ ☐ **Body Positive—Northern Ireland**
☎ 123 223 5515
🕐 Tue - Fri 14:00 - 16:00
Advice & information about HIV/AIDS & other sexual health issues.

Organizations: Sexuality
♂▽ **Belfast Buttterfly Club**
P. O. Box 210, Belfast, Antrim BT1 1BG.
☎ 158 543 0408
🕐 Call Wed 20:00 - 22:00
Publishes *ITV Magazine*.

Stores: Books: General
☺ **Just Books**
7 Winetavern Street, Belfast, Antrim.
☎ 123 232 5426

LONDONDERRY
Derry
Helplines: Sexuality
♂ **Derry Cara Friend**
c/o 1 Baron's Court, Culmore Road, Derry, Londonderry BT48 7RH.
☎ 150 426 3120

Norway

Area: Approximately 323,880 square kilometres
Population: Approximately 4,300,000
Capital City: Oslo
Currency: kroner (nkr)
Official Language: Norwegian
Major Religions: 88% Lutheran Protestant.
National Holiday: Independence Day, 17th. May
Time zone: GMT plus 1 hour
Country Initials: N
Electricity: 220 volts
Country Dialing Code (from elsewhere): 47
Intl. Dialing Prefix (out of the country): 095
Long Distance Dialing Prefix (inside country): 0
Climate: Climate varies from both north to south and from summer to winter. The northern parts are in the arctic, whereas the southern parts experience a continental climate with warm summers and cold winters.
Age of consent & homosexuality legislation: Age of consent for sexual activity is 16. In 1981, anti-discrimination laws were put in place.

NATIONAL RESOURCES
Helplines: AIDS
☺ ☐ **National Health AIDS-line**
☎ 050 03 4000
Toll-free call.

Organizations: AIDS: Education
☺ ☐ **Landforeningen mot AIDS**
Postboks 9158, 0134 Oslo, Akershus.
☎ 22 17 0700

Organizations: AIDS: Support
♂▽ **Helseutvalget for Homofile**
Rådhusgt. 4, 0151 Oslo, Akershus.
☎ 22 33 7015
🕐 Mon - Fri 09:00 - 15:00
Offices throughout Norway.

☺ ☐ **PLUSS**
Postboks 7879, St. Olavsplass, 0130 Oslo 1, Akershus.
☎ 22 11 4900
A national organization for HIV positive people.

Organizations: BDSM
♂▽ **SMia**
c/o LLH, Postboks 6838, 0130 Oslo, Akershus.
☎ 92 42 0878

☎ 62 42 7466
🕐 Meets monthly on a Fri
☺▽ **SMil Norge**
♿ Postboks 3456, 0406 Bjølsen, Akershus.
☎ 22 17 0501
📧 leifsten@powertech.no
🌐 http://www.powertech.no/SMil/
👍 ✓
Contact: Mr. Leif Stensrud, Editor, Internet home page
Members of other BDSM society visiting Norway are welcome. Home page has telephone number, from which you can get the address. Publishes *SMil Norse bladet* every two months. Age statement of 18 is required.

Organizations: Sexuality
♂ **Landsforeningen for Lesbisk og Homofil Frigjoring (LLH)**
Postboks 6838, St. Olavsplass, 0130 Oslo, Akershus.
☎ 22 36 1948 ✆ 22 11 4745
🕐 Mon - Fri 09:00 - 16:00
Local groups throughout Norway.

Publishers: Magazines: Sexual Politics
♂▼ **Lovetann**
Postboks 752, Sentrum, 0106 Oslo 1, Akershus.
☎ 22 36 0078
Published every two months. Yearly subscription is NK150.

Publishers: Newspapers: Sexuality
♂▼ **Blikk**
Postboks 6838, St. Olavs plass, 0130 Oslo 1, Akershus.
☎ 22 33 4455 ✆ 22 36 2803
🌐 http://www.oslonet.no/home/bjornfk/BLIKK/
Published every month.

AKERSHUS
Hebekk
Organizations: Sexuality
♂▽ **Landsforeningen for Lesbisk og Homofil Frigjoring (LLH)—Akershus**
Postboks 48, 1406 Hebekk, Akershus.

Oslo
Distributors: Books: General
☺ ■ **KAE BokImport**
Schwensensgt 5, 0170 Oslo 6, Akershus.

Helplines: Sexuality
♂▽ **Homofile og Lesbiskes Opplysningstelefon**
Postboks 9054, Grønland, 0190 Oslo, Akershus.
☎ 22 11 3660
☎ 22 11 3360
🕐 Mon - Thu 20:00 - 22:00
Information & support.

Organizations: BDSM
♂▽ **Scandinavian Leather Men (SLM)—Oslo**
Postboks 703, Sentrum, 0106 Oslo, Akershus.
☎ 22 20 2095
🕐 Meets twice a month

Organizations: Sexuality
⚥▽ **Freedom of Personality Expression (FPE)—Northern Europe: Norway**
Postboks 1968, 0125 Vika, Akershus.
📧 jane@oslonett.no
Publishes *Feminform & Intermezzo*.

Piercers
☺ ■ **Oslo Piercing Studio**
Postboks 617, Sentrum, 0106 Oslo, Akershus.
☎ 22 19 9265

Stores: Books: General
☺ ■ **Tronsmo Bokhandel**
Postboks 6754, St. Olavsplass, 0130 Oslo, Akershus.
☎ 22 20 2509 ✆ 20 11 3374
🕐 Mon - Fri 10:00 - 17:00, Thu - 18:00, Sat - 15:00

Stores: Erotica: BDSM
♂▼ **Man Fashion**
Möllergt. 47, 0179 Oslo, Akershus.
☎ 22 36 0603 ✆ 22 35 4586
🕐 Mon - Wed 12:00 - 18:00, Thu Fri 12:00 -19:00, Sat 11:00 -

16:00

☺ ■ **Master Leather**
Storgatan 36, 0184 Oslo, Akershus.
⏲ Mon - Fri 12:00 - 19:00, Sat 12:00 - 15:00

Stores: Erotica: General

⚥▼ **Gay International**
Postboks 9356, Grønland, 0133 Oslo, Akershus.
☎ 22 20 3736 ✆ 22 49 1524
⏲ Mon - Fri 10:00 - 19:00, Sat - 15:00

BUSKERUD

Drammen
Health Services
⚥▽ **Helseavdelingen Helsesjef Th. Hetland**
Strømsøtorg 9, 3002 Drammen, Buskerud.
☎ 32 83 8301
⏲ Mon - Sat 09:00 - 15:00

Hønefoss
Organizations: Fetish: Clothing: Rubber
⚥▽ **Grønn Mann**
Postboks 649, Klekken, Buskerud.
Small rubber club for men.

Kongsberg
Health Services
☺ ☐ **Helseavdelingen Helsesjef Pål Gulbrandsen**
☎ 32 73 1179
Helplines: AIDS
☺ ☐ **Opplysnigstelefon om AIDS**
☎ 32 83 3070

FINNMARK

Kirkenes
Health Services
☺ ☐ **Kirkenes Sykehus Sjefslege Arnt Uchtermann**
☎ 78 99 1701
⏲ Mon - Sat 09:00 - 14:00

HEDMARK

Hamar
Health Services
☺ ☐ **Fylkeslegen i Hamar**
Falsensgate 14, Hamar, Hedmark.
☎ 62 53 0033

HORDALAND

Bergen
Health Services
☺ ☐ **Haukeland Hospital**
☎ 55 20 0944
☎ 55 20 0088
⏲ Wed 15:00 - 18:00
HIV testing.
Organizations: Motorcycle
⚥▽ **Tennklubben**
Postboks 4418, 5028 Bergen, Hordaland.
⏲ Phone HBB for information
Organizations: Sexuality: Student
⚥▽ **Uglesett**
Postboks 1116, 5001 Bergen, Hordaland.
⏲ Call HBB for information

MØRE OG ROMSDAL

Ålesund
Health Services
☺▽ **Helseutvalget**
Postboks 7056, 6022 Åsestranda, Møre og Romsdal.
Organizations: Sexuality
⚥▽ **Homofile Bevegelse—Head Office**

Postboks 665, Centre, 6001 Ålesund, Møre og Romsdal.
☎ 70 12 0915 ✆ 70 12 0915
⏲ Infoline Mon - Thu 18:00 - 22:00, Fri Sat 19:00 - 02:00

Kristiansund
Organizations: Sexuality
⚥▽ **Landsforeningen for Lesbisk og Homofil Frigjøring (LLH)—Kristiansund**
Postboks 775, 6501 Kristiansund, Møre og Romsdal.

Molde
Organizations: Sexuality
⚥▽ **Homofil Bevegelse—Nordmore & Romsdal**
Postboks 71, 6401 Molde, Møre og Romsdal.
☎ 70 12 0915 ✆ 70 12 0915
⏲ Infoline Mon - Thu 18:00 - 22:00, Fri Sat 19:00 - 02:00

NORDLAND

Bodø
Organizations: AIDS: Support
☺ ☐ **Council Physicians AIDS Office**
Verkstedveien, Bodø, Nordland.
☎ 75 52 4210
Organizations: Sexuality
⚥▽ **Landsforeningen for Lesbisk og Homofil Frigjøring (LLH)—Bodø**
Postboks 695, 8001 Bodø, Nordland.
☎ 75 52 2775

Mo
Organizations: Sexuality
⚥▽ **Landsforeningen for Lesbisk og Homofil Frigjøring (LLH)—Mo**
Postboks 109, 8610 Mo, Nordland.

Rana
Health Services
☺ ☐ **Rana Helseråd**
☎ 5 15 2500
Helplines: AIDS
☺ ☐ **Automatisk Telefonsvarer om AIDS**
☎ 75 13 2670
Answering machine with information about AIDS.

OPPLAND

Gjøvik
Health Services
☺ ☐ **Kommuneoverlegen**
Rådhuset, 2800 Gjøvik, Oppland.
☎ 61 17 5600 Ext.: 235

Lillehammer
Health Services
☺ ☐ **Lillehammer Helseråd**
Kirkegate 41, 2600 Lillehammer, Oppland.
☎ 61 25 3540
Organizations: Sexuality
⚥▽ **Landsforeningen for Lesbisk og Homofil Frigjøring (LLH)—Mjøsa**
Postboks 432, 2601 Lillehammer, Oppland.
☎ 61 19 5152 ✆ 62 35 2959
⏲ Regular social meetings
$
One of the local groups of the national organization that fights for lesbian, gay, & bisexual equality in Norway. Publishes a newsletter. English also spoken.

ØSTFOLD

Fredrikstad
Health Services
☺ ☐ **Helsekontor**
☎ 33 31 7010
⏲ 18:00 - 21:00

Moss
Health Services

☺ □ **Fylkeslegen i Ostfold**
☎ 32 25 5589

ROGALAND
Sandnes
Organizations: Sexuality

▽ **Eurofantasia**
Postboks 442, 4301 Sandnes, Rogaland.
☎ 51 662422 — Fax 51 662422
JennyS@transgender.org
http://www.oslonett.no/home/jane/index.html
Week-long event held in May
Contact: Ms. Jenny Sand
All three of the national FPE-NE can be contacted trhough this address.

Sogndal
Organizations: Sexuality

▽ **Homofil Bevegelse—Indre Søre Sogn**
Postboks 58, 5801 Sogndal, Rogaland.
☎ 70 12 0915 — Fax 70 12 0915
Infoline Mon - Thu 18:00 - 22:00, Fri Sat 19:00 - 02:00

Stavanger
Helplines: Sexuality

▽ **Landsforeningen for Lesbisk og Homofil Frigjøring (LLH)—Stavanger**
Postboks 1502, 4004 Kjelvene, Rogaland.
☎ 51 53 1446
Mon 20:00 - 23:00

Organizations: AIDS: Support

☺ □ **AIDS Advisory Office**
☎ 51 56 4977

☺ □ **AIDS-Kontor**
Kongsgate 43, Stavanger, Rogaland.
☎ 51 50 8800
Mon 10:00 - 14:00 15:00 - 19:00, Fri 10:00 - 14:00

Organizations: Sexuality

▽ **Landsforeningen for Lesbisk og Homofil Frigjøring (LLH)—Stavanger**
Postboks 1502, 4004 Kjelvene, Rogaland.
☎ 51 53 1446

SOGN OG FJORDANE
Førde
Organizations: Sexuality

▽ **Homofil Bevegelse—Sogn og Fjordane**
Postboks 367, 6801 Førde, Sogn og Fjordane.
☎ 70 12 0915 — Fax 70 12 0915
Infoline Mon - Thu 18:00 - 22:00, Fri Sat 19:00 - 02:00

SØR TRONDELAG
Trandheim
Organizations: AIDS: Support

☺ □ **Trondheim Helseråd**
St. Elisabeths Hospital, Trandheim, Sør Trondelag.
☎ 73 59 7740
Information & support for people with AIDS.

Tromdheim
Health Services

▽ **Helseutvalget for Homofile**
Postboks 937, 7002 Tromdheim, Sør Trondelag.
☎ 73 52 4557
Mon - Fri 09:00 - 16:00

Trondheim
Helplines: AIDS

☺ □ **Trondeheim Rode Kors**
☎ 73 52 8810
Answering machine with information about HIV/AIDS.

Helplines: Sexuality

▽ **Gay Switchboard**
☎ 73 52 4226
Tue 19:00 - 21:00

Organizations: AIDS: Support

☺ □ **Trondheim AIDS og Infeksjonshelsetjenesten**
☎ 73 99 7990

Organizations: Sexuality

▽ **Landsforeningen for Lesbisk og Homofil Frigjøring (LLH)—Trondheim**
Postboks 937, 7002 Trondheim, Sør Trondelag.
☎ 73 52 4226
10:00 - 14:00

▽ **Rådgivningstjenesten for Homofile**
Møllenberg Lægesenter, Trondheim, Sør Trondelag.
☎ 73 52 3330
Tue 19:00 - 21:00
Information & support for gays & lesbians.

TROMS
Tromsø
Health Services

▽ **Rådgivningstjenesten for Homofile og Lesbiske i Tromsø**
☎ 77 68 5643
Mon 19:00 - 21:00

☺ □ **Sentrum Legekontor**
Storgate 79/83, Tromsø, Troms.
☎ 77 68 2549
Tue 17:00 - 19:00

☺ ▽ **Tromsø Komm. Helsekontor**
☎ 77 62 0485

Organizations: Sexuality

▽ **Landsforeningen for Lesbisk og Homofil Frigjøring (LLH)—Tromsø**
Postboks 500, 9001 Tromsø, Troms.
☎ 77 68 5643
☎ 77 68 2202
Mon - Thu 09:00 - 15:00

VEST-AGDER
Kristiansand
Health Services

☺ □ **Kristiansan Helseråd**
☎ 38 02 9755

☺ □ **Vest-Agder Sentralsykehus**
☎ 38 02 9080

Organizations: Sexuality

▽ **Landsforeningen for Lesbisk og Homofil Frigjøring (LLH)—Kristiansand**
Postboks 4598, Grim, 4602 Kristiansand, Vest-Agder.
☎ 38 02 0048
Mon 18:00 - 21:00

VESTFOLD
Larvik
Health Services

☺ □ **Larvik Helseråd**
Kongegate 15, Larvik, Vestfold.
☎ 33 18 6372
Fri 12:00 - 14:00

Sandefjord
Health Services

☺ □ **Larvik Helseråd**
☎ 33 48 6372
Fri 12:00 - 14:00

Organizations: AIDS: Support

☺ □ **HIV-Kontoret**
☎ 33 46 5390

Tonsberg

Organizations: AIDS: Support

☺ □ **Rådgivningskontoret mot AIDS**
Chr. Frederiksgate 6, Tønsberg, Vestfold.
☎ 33 31 6840
🕘 Thu 18:00 - 21:00

Portugal

Area: Approximately 92,390 square kilometres
Population: Approximately 10,400,000
Capital City: Lisboa (Lisbon)
Currency: Escudo (Esc)
Official Language: Portuguese
Major Religions: 94% Roman Catholic
National Holiday: Independence Day, 1st. December
Time zone: GMT
Country Initials: P
Electricity: 220 volts
Country Dialing Code (from elsewhere): 351
Intl. Dialing Prefix (out of the country): 00
Long Distance Dialing Prefix (inside country): 0
Climate: Wet, mild weather in the north. Less rain in the east & the sub-tropical south.
Age of consent & homosexuality legislation: Age of consent for sexual activity is 14.

NATIONAL RESOURCES

Mailorder: Books: BDSM

☺ **Fernando Cerqueira**
Apartado 223, Oeiras 2780.

Lisboa

Organizations: AIDS: Information

☺ ▽ **Alternativa Positiva**
Apartado 50503, Lisboa 1708.
☎ 795 8296 — Fax 795 8297
Contact: Mr. Júlió Tarragó da Silveira, Presidente da Direcção
National AIDS clearing house.

Organizations: BDSM

⚥ ▽ **GRLP**
Box 52 24, Lisboa 1706.

Publishers: Magazines: Sexuality

⚥ ▼ ***Gaie France en Português***
P. O. Box 22579, Lisboa 1146.
☎ 1 988 9923
Published every month.

⚥ ▼ ***Orbita Gay Macho***
Gay Club I. L. R. E. S., P. O. Box 50224, Lisboa 1706.

Puerto Rico

Area: Approximately 8,900 square kilometres
Population: Approximately 3,600,000
Capital City: San Juan
Currency: U.S. Dollar
Official Language: Spanish & English
Major Religions: 80% Roman Catholic
Time zone: GMT plus 4
Country Initials: PR
Electricity: 120 volts
Country Dialing Code (from elsewhere): 351
Intl. Dialing Prefix (out of the country): 00
Long Distance Dialing Prefix (inside country): 0
Climate: Tropical weather for the whole year.
Age of consent & homosexuality legislation: Officially, homosexuality is illegal, but the authorities are very liberal, particularly in the capital.
Puerto Rico is an autonomous country that recently voted not to become a U.S. state, despite the country's use of the U.S. dollar & legal system.

San Juan

Organizations: AIDS: Education

☺ □ **Instituto de SIDA de San Juan**
1386 Avenida Fernandez Juncos, San Juan 00909.
☎ 809 723 2424

Organizations: Family

☺ □ **Parents & Friends of Lesbians & Gays (PFLAG)—San Juan**
Box 116, 1505 Loiza Street, Santurce 00911.
☎ 809 726 2888

Organizations: Sexuality

⚢ ▽ **Colectivo de Lesbianas Feministas**
Apartado 1003, Estacion Viejo, San Juan 00902.
Publishes *Desde El Ambiente.*

Scotland

Area: Approximately 244,490 square kilometres for whole of U.K.
Population: Approximately 57,650,000 for whole of U.K.
Capital City: Edinburgh
Currency: Pound Sterling (£)
Official Language: English & French
Major Religions: 57% Protestant, 13% Roman Catholic
National Holiday: Queen's Birthday, early June
Time zone: GMT
Country Initials: GB
Electricity: 240 volts, 50Hz
Country Dialing Code (from elsewhere): 44
Intl. Dialing Prefix (out of the country): 0101
Long Distance Dialing Prefix (inside country): 0
Climate: Warm, dry summers, cool, wet winters.
Age of consent & homosexuality legislation: Age of consent for sexual activity is 16, but 18 for homosexual activities. Homosexual acts were decriminalized in 1980. In 1992, Homosexual acts are not permitted for the members of the military.
Legal drinking age: 18

NATIONAL RESOURCES

Helplines: Sexuality

⚥ ▽ **Bisexual Phoneline (Scotland)**
☎ 131 557 3620
🕘 Thu 19:30 - 21:30
Advice & information about HIV/AIDS & other sexual health issues.

BORDERS

County Resources

Helplines: Sexuality

⚥ ▽ **Borders Gay Switchboard**
P. O. Box 3, Hawick, Borders TD9 9RU.
☎ 1450 370 700
🕘 Mon Wed Fri 19:30 - 22:00

CENTRAL

Stirling

Helplines: Sexuality

⚥ ▽ **Dumfries & Galloway L&G Group**
P. O. Box 1299, Dumfries, Dumfries & Galloway DG1 2PD.
☎ 141 221 8372
🕘 19:00 - 22:00
Please address envelopes to DaGLaGG, do NOT address them to Dumfries & Galloway L&G Group.

⚥ ▽ **Forth Friend**
P. O. Box 28, Stirling, Central FK9 5YW.
☎ 1786 471285
🕘 Mon 19:30 - 21:30

Organizations: Sexuality: Student

⚥ **Stirling University LGB Society**
Stirling University, Stirling, Central FK9 4LA.
☎ 178 646 7166
Contact: LGB Officer

Stores: Military Surplus

☺ ■ **Task Force Surplus Supplies**
47 Barton Street, Stirling, Central.
☎ 1786 451136

DUMFRIES & GALLOWAY

County Resources

Helplines: Sexuality

⚥ ▽ **Dumfries & Galloway L&G Group**
P. O. Box 1299, Dumfries, Dumfries & Galloway DG1 2PD.
☎ 141 221 8372
🕘 19:00 - 22:00
Please address envelopes to DaGLaGG, do NOT address them to Dumfries & Galloway L&G Group.

FIFE

Buckhaven

Organizations: AIDS: Support

Fife AIDS Care Through Support (FACTS)
☎ 159 271 5200
Wed 19:30 - 22:00
Advice & information about HIV/AIDS & other sexual health issues.

Kirkcaldy

Helplines: Sexuality

Edinburgh Gay Switchboard
P. O. Box 169, Edinburgh, Lothian EH1 3UU.
☎ 131 556 4049
19:30 - 22:00

Fife Friend
☎ 1592 266688
Fri 19:30 - 22:30
Advice & information about HIV/AIDS & other sexual health issues.

Saint Andew's

Organizations: Sexuality: Student

Saint Andrew's University GaySoc
c/o Chaplaincy Centre, Saint Mary's Place, Saint Andew's, Fife.
Mon 19:30

GRAMPIAN

Aberdeen

Helplines: AIDS

Grampian AIDS Line
☎ 122 457 4000
Advice & information about HIV/AIDS & other sexual health issues.

Helplines: Sexuality

Aberdeen Lesbian, Gay, & Bisexual Switchboard
P. O. Box 174, Aberdeen, Grampian.
☎ 122 458 6869
☎ 122 421 3355 (Minicom)
Wed 19:00-22:00. Minicom Wed Fri 19:00 - 22:00
Advice & information about HIV/AIDS & other sexual health & sexuality issues.

Organizations: AIDS: Support

Aberdeen HIV/AIDS Gay Support Group
P. O. Box 83, Aberdeen, Grampian.

Body Positive—Grampian
☎ 122 440 4408
24hrs.
Advice & information about HIV/AIDS & other sexual health issues.

HIV/AIDS Gay Support Group
P.O. Box 83, Aberdeen, Grampian.

Organizations: Sexuality

Aberdeen LesBiGay Society
Douglas Room, SRC Building, Luthuli House, 50-52 College Bounds, Aberdeen, Grampian.

AGG
P. O. Box 129, Aberdeen, Grampian AB9 6EY.
☎ 122 431 7552
Contact: John
Aberdeen Gay Group meets 3rd. Sunday of the month.

Robert Gordon University LGB Society
RGU Union, Shoe Lane, Aberdeen, Grampian.

Lumphanan

Organizations: Sexuality

Grampian Gender Group (3G)
c/o ADF Editorial Services, Tullochvenus House, Lumphanan, Grampian AB31 4RN.
☎ 133 988 3695
Meets 3rd. Sat of month
Publishes *The Tartan Skirt.*

Publishers: Newspapers: Sexuality

Tartan Skirt
ADF Editorial Services, Tullochvenus House, Lumphanan, Grampian AB31 4RN.

HIGHLAND

Inverness

Helplines: AIDS

Scottish AIDS Monitor (SAM)
28 Huntly Street, Inverness, Highland IV3 5PR.
☎ 146 324 1000
Mon Fri 19:00 - 21:30

Manufacturers: Clothing: General

Kingfisher
Chestnut Cottage, Newton of Petty, Highland IV1 2JQ.
☎ 146 379 1681
Raincoats, jackets, & shirts in latex & rubberized cotton. Catalogue, SAE or IRC.

Organizations: Sexuality

Out & About
P. O. Box 91, Inverness, Highland IV1 2GJ.

Wick

Organizations: Sexuality

Caithness Gay, Bisexual, & Lesbian Connexion
Box 829, Journal Office, 42 Union Street, Wick, Highland KW1 5ED.

LOTHIAN

Edinburgh

Distributors: Books: General

Bookspeed
48 Hamilton Place, Edinburgh, Lothian EH3 5AX.
☎ 131 225 4950 Fax 131 220 6515

Helplines: Sexuality

Edinburgh Gay Switchboard
P. O. Box 169, Edinburgh, Lothian EH1 3UU.
☎ 131 556 4049
19:30 - 22:00

Edinburgh Lesbian Line
P. O. Box 169, Edinburgh, Lothian EH1 3UU.
☎ 131 557 0751
Mon Thu 19:30 - 22:00
Advice & information about HIV/AIDS & other sexual health issues.

Organizations: AIDS: Education

Scottish AIDS Monitor
P.O. Box 248, Edinburgh, Lothian EH6 5NS.
☎ 131 555 4850

Organizations: AIDS: Support

SOLAS
2/4 Abbeymount, Edinburgh, Lothian EH8 8EJ.
☎ 131 659 5116

Organizations: BDSM

Leather Group
Chapps Club Bar, 22 Greenside Place, Edinburgh, Lothian.
☎ 131 558 1270

ORGASM
c/o Gay Scotland, 58 Broughton Street, Edinburgh, Lothian EH1 3SA.

Organizations: Bears

Big Beary Bulky Boys
26b Dublin Street, Edinburgh, Lothian.
☎ 131 538 7775
Meets 4th. Fri of month 20:00 - 22:00

Organizations: Body Size

Four B's Club
c/o D. Caldwell, 7-3 Chessels Court, 240 Canon Gate, Edinburgh, Lothian IH8 8AD.

Organizations: Family

Parent's Enquiry
P. O. Box 169, EH1 5SE, Edinburgh, Lothian EH1 5SE.

Organizations: Motorcycle

MSC Scotland
P. O. Box 28, Head Post Office, Edinburgh, Lothian EH3 5JL.

Organizations: Sexuality

Bisexual Resource Centre

58a Broughton Street, Edinburgh, Lothian EH1 3SA.
☎ 131 557 3620
📧 bifrost@ed.ac.uk
Publishes *Bifrost, The Rainbow Bridge* every month. Yearly subscription is £7.50, £15 outside U.K..

⚥▽ **Dykes Night Out**
P. O. Box 169, Edinburgh, Lothian EH1 3LU.

⚥▽ **Edinburgh College of Art L&G Society**
Edinburgh College of Art SRC, Lauriston Place, Edinburgh, Lothian.
☎ 131 229 1442

⚥▽ **Edinburgh LGB Centre**
58A-60 Broughton Street, Edinburgh, Lothian EH1 3SA.
☎ 131 557 2625

⚥▽ **Lothian LGYM**
P. O. Box 169, Edinburgh, Lothian EH1 3UU.

⚥▽ **Moray House College L&G Society**
c/o SRC, Holyrood Road, Edinburgh, Lothian EH8.
☎ 131 556 5184

⚥▽ **NUS East of Scotland Area LGB Network**
EosANUS, 11 Broughton Market, Edinburgh, Lothian EH3 6NU.
☎ 131 558 1541
Contact: LGB Officer

▷▽ **Trans-Trap**
30/1 Halmyre Street, Edinburgh, Lothian EH6 8QD.
☎ 131 555 6416
Contact: Miss Julie Bradshaw
Please include SAE or IRC for reply. Publishes *Liberty*.

Organizations: Sexuality: Student

⚥ **BLOGS**
c/o Pleasance Bar, Cheviot Room, 60 Pleasance, Edinburgh, Lothian.

⚥ **Queen Margaret College L&G Society**
Students' Association, 36 Clarewood Terrace, Edinburgh, Lothian EH12 8TS.
☎ 131 339 3961
☎ 131 339 1990

⚥ **Heriot Watt University LGB Society**
c/o The Union, Heriot Watt University, Ricarton, Lothian.

Organizations: Sexuality: Youth

⚥▽ **Stonewall Youth Group**
P. O. Box 169, Edinburgh, Lothian EH1 3UU.
☎ 131 556 4040

Piercers

☺▼ **Body Armour Piercing & Tattooing**
Downstairs, 25a Dundas Street, Edinburgh, Lothian EH3 6QQ.
☎ 131 558 3717
① By appoinment only

Publishers: Magazines: Sexuality

⚥▽ *Gay Scotland*
58A Broughton Street, Edinburgh, Lothian EH1 3SA.
☎ 131 557 2625
Published every month.

⚥▼ *Scotsgay*
Pageprint Limited, P. O. Box 666, Edinburgh, Lothian EH7 5YW.
☎ 131 539 0666 📞 131 558 1262
☎ 131 558 1279
📧 scotsgay@drink.demo.co.uk
To subscribe to the Internet version, send e-mail to listserver@drink.demon.co.uk with a body text of: subscribe scotsgay-list.

Publishers: Newspapers: Sexuality

⚥▼ *Scots Scene*
P. O. Box 11, Bathgate, Edinburgh, Lothian EH48 1RX.

Stores: Books: General

☺ **Better Books**
11 Forest Road, Edinburgh, Lothian.
☎ 131 225 1515

☺ **Bobbies Bookshop**
220 Morrison Street, Edinburgh, Lothian.
☎ 131 229 2338

☺ **West & Wilde Bookshop**
25a Dundas Street, Edinburgh, Lothian EH3 6QQ.
☎ 131 556 0079

Stores: Erotica: BDSM

☺ **Drondale Limited**

60 Broughton Street, Edinburgh, Lothian.
☎ 131 556 1471

STRATHCLYDE

County Resources

Helplines: Sexuality

⚥▽ **Ayr Lesbian & Gay Switchboard**
☎ 1292 619000
☎ 141 353 3117 (women)
① 19:00 - 22:00. Women Wed 19:30 - 22:00

⚥▽ **Strathclyde Lesbian & Gay Switchboard**
P. O. Box 38, Glasgow, Strathclyde G2 2QF.
☎ 141 332 8372
① 19:00 - 22:00

Organizations: Sexuality

▷▽ **Crosslynx**
c/o Strathclyde Lesbian & Gay Switchboard, P. O. Box 38, Glasgow, Strathclyde G2 2QF.
☎ 141 332 8372
☎ 141 221 8372
① Meets 2nd. Wed of month

Ayr

Organizations: AIDS: Support

☺ **Ayrshire AIDS Awareness Project Support Group**
P. O. Box 1043, Ayr, Strathclyde KA6 5JQ.

Glasgow

Artists: BDSM

☺ **Anthro**
P. O. Box 186, Glasgow, Strathclyde G3 6DG.

Helplines: AIDS

☺□ **Body Positive—Strathclyde**
☎ 141 332 5010
① Mon - Fri 10:00 - 14:00
Advice & information about HIV/AIDS & other sexual health issues.

Organizations: AIDS: Support

☺ **Scottish AIDS Monitor**
P. O. Box 11, Glasgow, Strathclyde G2 2UT.
☎ 141 353 3133

Organizations: Sexuality: Student

⚥ **Glasgow Caledonian University L&G Society**
Cowcaddens Road, Glasgow, Strathclyde G4 0BA.
☎ 141 332 0681

⚥ **Glasgow University L&G Society**
c/o SRC, John MacIntyre Building, University Avenue, Glasgow, Strathclyde G12 8QQ.
☎ 141 334 9512

⚥ **West of Scotland Area NUS**
Cathcart House, Langside College, 50 Prospecthill Road, Glasgow, Strathclyde G42 9LB.
☎ 141 636 6477
Contact: LGB Officer

Piercers

☺ **Nirvana**
Virginia Galleries, 33 Virginia Street, Glasgow, Strathclyde.
☎ 141 552 5706

Publishers: Magazines: Sexuality

⚥▼ *Harpies & Quines*
P. O. Box 543, Glasgow, Strathclyde G4 9LY.

Stores: Books: General

☺ **Clyde Books**
25 Parnie Street, Glasgow, Strathclyde G1 5RJ.
☎ 141 552 4699

☺ **Glasgow University Shop**
The Hub, Hillhead Street, Glasgow, Strathclyde.

☺ **John Smith**
252 Byres Road, Glasgow, Strathclyde G12.
☎ 141 334 2769

☺ **John Smith**
57 Saint Vincent Street, Glasgow, Strathclyde G2 5TB.
☎ 141 221 7472

☺ **Strathclyde University Union Shop**
90 John Street, Glasgow, Strathclyde.

☺▽ **Trongate Books**
Unit 25, Candleriggs Market, Bell Street, Glasgow, Strathclyde G1 1NU.
☎ 141 552 1545

Stores: Erotica: General
☺ **Third Eye Centre**
350 Sauchihall Street, Glasgow, Strathclyde.

Stores: Military Surplus
☺ ■ **Adventure 1**
38 Dundas Street, Glasgow, Strathclyde G1.
☎ 141 353 3788

☺ ■ **Government Surplus**
26 Green Street, Saltcoats, Strathclyde.
☎ 1294 469343

☺ ■ **Lowson's Army & Navy Store**
385 Paisley Road, Glasgow, Strathclyde G51.
☎ 141 427 0961

☺ ■ **Stewart's Army Surplus**
783 Dumbarton Road, Glasgow, Strathclyde G11.
☎ 141 337 2550

☺ ■ **War & Peace**
60 Bell Street, Glasgow, Strathclyde G1.
☎ 141 552 1101

☺ ■ **War & Peace**
73 Trongate, Glasgow, Strathclyde G1.
☎ 141 552 2240

☺ ■ **War & Peace**
639 Great Western Road, Glasgow, Strathclyde G12.
☎ 141 334 9129

Greenock
Helplines: Sexuality
☺▽ **Dumfries & Galloway L&G Group**
P. O. Box 1299, Dumfries, Dumfries & Galloway DG1 2PD.
☎ 141 221 8372
⏱ 19:00 - 22:00
Please address envelopes to DaGLaGG, do NOT address them to Dumfries & Galloway L&G Group.

Paisley
Publishers: Magazines: Sexuality
☺▼ *Pulse Magazine*
P. O. Box 1248, Paisley, Strathclyde PA3 3YA.
☎ 150 533 5021
✉ pulse@drink.demon.co.uk
Also have an online edition as an Internet mailing list. Send e-mail for details.

TAYSIDE
Dundee
Helplines: Sexuality
☺▽ **Dundee LGB Switchboard Group**
P. O. Box 104, Dundee, Tayside DD1 3YF.
☎ 1382 202620
⏱ Mon 19:00 - 22:00

Organizations: AIDS: Education
☺ **Harm Reduction Centre**
Constitution House, 55 Constitution Road, Dundee, Tayside.
☎ 138 221 0919

☺ **Scottish AIDS Monitor**
c/o SWT Dept., Northern College, Gardyne Road, Broughty Ferry, Tayside.
☎ 138 246 1167

☺ **YMCA**
GALUP, YMCA Drugs & AIDS Project, 76 Bell Street, Dundee, Tayside.
☎ 138 220 0352

Organizations: Sexuality
☺▽ **GLAD**
c/o Students' Association, 158 Marketgait, Dundee, Tayside DD1 1NJ.
☺▽ **Tayfriend**
P. O. Box 182, Dundee, Tayside DD1 9UP.

Organizations: Sexuality: Student
☺ **North of Scotland NUS**
158 Marketgait, Dundee, Tayside DD1 1NJ.
Contact: LGB Officer

Perth
Helplines: Sexuality
☺▽ **Perth Switchboard**
☎ 1738 828840
⏱ Women Mon 19:00 - 22:00

Organizations: Sexuality
☺▽ **Perth Lesbian & Gay Group**
☎ 1738 23917 (men)
☎ 1738 828840 (women)
⏱ Helplines: Men Mon 19:00 - 22:00, women Fri 19:00 - 22:00
Advice & information about HIV/AIDS & other sexual health issues.

South Africa

Area: Approximately 1,221,00 square kilometres
Population: Approximately 35,910,000
Capital City: Pretoria
Currency: Rand (R)
Official Language: Afrikaans, English, & various Bantu languages
Major Religions: Roman Catholic & Protestant
National Holiday: Republic Day, 31st. May
Time zone: GMT plus 2 hours
Country Initials: RSA
Electricity: 250 volts
Country Dialing Code (from elsewhere): 27
Intl. Dialing Prefix (out of the country): 09
Long Distance Dialing Prefix (inside country): 0
Climate: Sunny, temperate climate throughout the country.
Age of consent & homosexuality legislation: President Mandela has stated that discrimination on the basis of sexual orientation is contrary to the spirit freedom in the new South Africa.

NATIONAL RESOURCES
Helplines: Sexuality
☺▽ **Gay & Lesbian Counselling**
P. O. Box 785493, Sandton, Transvaal 2146.
☎ 11 643 2311
⏱ 19:00 - 22:00
Nightly telephone counselling service for all gay issues. Also provides HIV/AIDS information to the community. Runs the gay community house at 38 High street, Berea, Johannesburg. Afrikaans also spoken.

Mailorder: Erotica
☺▽ **Klein Enterprises**
P. O. Box 23225, Joubert Park, Transvaal 2044.
☎ 11 642 8989
Catalogue, R 20.

☺▼ **Nice 'n' Naughty**
P. O. Box 5384, Cape Town, Cape Province 8000.
☎ 21 434 3585 ✆ 21 434 3585

Organizations: Sexuality
✉▽ **The Phœnix Society**
P. O. Box 6433, Parow East, Cape Province 7500.
Publishes *Fanfare*.

Publishers: Magazines: Sexuality
☺▼ *Flash*
c/o Klein Enterprises, P. O. Box 23225, Joubert Park, Transvaal 2044.
☎ 11 642 8989

CAPE PROVINCE
Cape Town
Film Festivals: Sexuality
☺▼ **Out-In-Africa**
P. O. Box 15707, Vlaeberg, Cape Province 8018.
☎ 21 24 1532 ✆ 21 24 1532
✉ jack@aztec.co.za

Health Services
☺ ☐ **City Hospital**
Portswood Road, Green Point, Cape Province.
☎ 21 22 2711

☺ ☐ **Day Hospital**
89 Buitenkant Street, Cape Town, Cape Province.
☎ 21 46 1124

Organizations: Sexuality
☺▽ **Gay Alliance**
P. O. Box 6010, Roggebaai, Cape Province 8012.

☎ 21 21 5420
🕘 24hr. counselling for gay- & lesbian-related issues.
Coördinates resources of the South African gay & lesbian community. HIV/AIDS information & counselling.

Organizations: Sexuality: Student

⚢▽ **Gay & Lesbian Association (GALA)**
c/o SRC, Private Bag, University of Cape Town, Rondebosch, Cape Province 7700.
☎ 21 21 5420

East London

Health Services

☺ □ **Frere Hospital**
☎ 431 27350

Organizations: AIDS: Education

☺ □ **AIDS Action Group**
P. O. Box 1822, East London, Cape Province.
☎ 431 29357
Information & support.

Organizations: Sexuality

⚢▽ **Gay Advice Bureau**
P. O. Box 1822, East London, Cape Province.
☎ 431 26665
☎ 431 29357
Information & counselling for gay & lesbian related issues. Also 431 42 1741.

Johannesburg

Organizations: Sexuality

⚢▽ **Club 30**
P. O. Box 132, Newlands, Cape Province.
☎ 21 23 5794

Kimberly

Organizations: Sexuality

⚢▽ **Gay Association of South Africa (GASA)—Northern Cape**
P. O. Box 705, Kimberly, Cape Province.
☎ 531 31393

NATAL

Durban

Health Services

☺ □ **Addington Hospital**
☎ 31 35 0235

☺ □ **King Edward VIII Hospital**
☎ 31 35 0235

Organizations: AIDS: Support

⚢▽ **AIDS Information & Counselling Service**
P. O. Box 37521, Overport, Natal 4067.
☎ 31 306 0758
🕘 19:00 - 22:00

Organizations: Sexuality

⚢▽ **Natal Gay Community**
P. O. Box 37521, Overport, Natal 4067.
Serves the coastal region of Natal province.

Organizations: Sexuality: Student

⚢▽ **Gay & Lesbian Student Society (GLSS)**
c/o Student Union, Univeristy of Natal, King George V Avenue, Durban, Natal.
☎ 31 22 3800

Stores: Erotica: General

⚢▼ **Fantasies**
1st Floor, Shop 113, 320 West Street, Durban, Natal 4001.
☎ 31 304 1408
Also mail order.

Pietermaritzburg

Organizations: Sexuality

⚢▽ **Gay Association Inland Natal**
P. O. Box 10373, Scotsville, Natal 3209.
☎ 331 47 2109
🕘 10373

ORANGE FREE STATE

Bloemfontein

Health Services

☺ □ **National Hospital**
☎ 51 70411
🕘 24hrs.

Organizations: Sexuality

⚢▽ **Gay Group Bloemfontein**
☎ 51 30 5934
☎ 51 33 2261
Publishes *Liason*.

TRANSVAAL

Johannesburg

Archives: Sexuality

⚢▽ **Gay Library**
38 High Street, Berea, Transvaal 2198.
☎ 11 643 2311
🕘 Tue 19:30 - 21:00, Sat 14:30 - 16:30
Library with over 1,500 gay & lesbian titles.

Bars: BDSM

⚢▼ **Leather Bar**
58 Pretoria Street, Hillbrow, Transvaal.

Health Services

☺ □ **J. G. Strydom Hospital**
☎ 11 726 5128

Helplines: Sexuality

⚢▽ **Gay Switchboard Johannesburg**
10 Hillborough Mansions, Pretoria Street / Klein Street, Hillbrow, Transvaal.
☎ 11 643 2311
Information & counselling by telephone. Also has library.

Organizations: AIDS: Support

☺ □ **AIDS Action Group**
P. O. Box 3330, Johannesburg, Transvaal.
☎ 11 642 5191
🕘 19:00 - 22:00

☺ □ **AIDS Information & Counselling Service**
P. O. Box 503, Parklands, Transvaal 2121.
☎ 11 643 2311
☎ 11 642 5191
🕘 19:00 - 22:00

Organizations: BDSM

⚢▽ **Manpower Network**
P. O. Box 18175, Hillbrow, Transvaal 2038.

Organizations: Bears

⚢▽ **PAWS Social Club**
☎ 11 794 3620
☎ 11 888 1963

Organizations: Motorcycle

⚢□ **Motorcycle Sports Club**
P. O. Box 17029, Hillbrow, Transvaal 2038.
☎ 11 726 1552
☎ 11 640 6354
🕘 Meets 2nd. & 4th. Sun of month
For bike lovers.

Organizations: Sexuality

⚢▽ **Gay Association of South Africa (GASA)—East Rand**
☎ 11 845 2285

⚢▽ **Gay Association of South Africa (GASA)—Johannesburg**
P. O. Box 3330, Johannesburg, Transvaal.
☎ 11 725 4703
🕘 19:00 - 22:00

⚢▽ **Outreach Rand**
☎ 11 643 2311
Support for senior &/or lonely gays & lesbians.

⚢▽ **Rand Gay Organization (RGO)**
P. O. Box 5115, Johannesburg, Transvaal.
☎ 11 932 2713
Information & other services for black gays in Johannesburg & Soweto.

▱▽ **SATRU**
P. O. Box 87283, Houghton, Transvaal 2041.

Publishers: Magazines: Sexuality

☺▼ *Outright*
Liberation Publishers, P. O. Box 2464, Houghton, Transvaal 2041.
☎ 11 648 5032　　　　　📞 11 648 3800
☎ 11 648 9808

Publishers: Newspapers: Sexuality

☺▼ *Exit*
Highland Publications, c. c., P. O. Box 2165, Johannesburg, Transvaal 2000.
☎ 11 614 9866　　　　　📞 11 880 3593
Published every two months. Yearly subscription is R80 in S.A., R100 in Namibia, Zimbabwe, Zambia, Swaziland, Lesotho, Botswana, & Mozambique, S60U.S. elsewhere.

Stores: Books: General

☺ ■ **Phambili Books**
22 Plein Street, Johannesburg, Transvaal 2001.
☎ 11 29 4944

Pretoria
Health Services

☺ ☐ **H. F. Verwoerd Hospital**
☎ 12 42 3211

Organizations: Sexuality

☺▽ **Gay Advice Bureau (GAB)**
P. O. Box 40614, Arcadia, Transvaal 0007.
☎ 11 643 2311
🕐 19:00 - 22:00

☺▽ **Gay Association of South Africa (GASA)— Northern Transvaal**
P. O. Box 40614, Arcadia, Transvaal 0007.
☎ 12 62 1314

Spain

Area: Approximately 504,750 square kilometres
Population: Approximately 39,900,000
Capital City: Madrid
Currency: Peseta (PTS)
Official Language: Spanish
Major Religions: 97% Roman Catholic
National Holiday: National Day, 12th. October
Time zone: GMT plus 1 hour
Country Initials: E
Electricity: 220 volts
Country Dialing Code (from elsewhere): 34
Intl. Dialing Prefix (out of the country): 07
Long Distance Dialing Prefix (inside country): 0
Climate: North west coast is rainiest, but the south east coast is one of the driest areas of Europe. Spain warm, Mediterranean climate everywhere, except the northern mountains, where it is cooler & wetter
Age of consent & homosexuality legislation: Since 1978, the age of consent for sexual activity is 16. The military code still punishes homosexual activity with a prison term of up to six years.

NATIONAL RESOURCES
Mailorder: Clothing: Fetish

☺ ■ **Things**
Apartado 7300, Zaragoza 50080.
☎ 76 44 6362　　　　　📞 76 43 2226

Mailorder: Erotica: BDSM

☺ ■ **S. A. D. E.**
Apartado 12079, Barcelona 08080.
☎ 3 450 4816

Organizations: Sexuality

☺▼ **Instituto Lambda**
2nd. Floor, Passeig Picasso 40, Barcelona 08003.
Publishes *Lambda.*

Publishers: Magazines: Erotic

☺▼ *Chicos*
Studios J. M. R., P. O. Box 23186, Barcelona 08080.
☎ 93 239 6105

Publishers: Newspapers: Sexuality

☺▼ *Infogai*
Publicació Degana del Moviment Gai a Catalunya, c/o Paloma 12 baixos,

Barcelona 08001.
☎ 93 318 1666
🕐 Mon - Sat 19:00 - 21:00

Barcelona
Helplines: Sexuality

☺▽ **Telephono Rosa**
☎ 93 237 7070
🕐 18:00 - 22:00

Organizations: Motorcycle

☺▽ **MSC Barcelona**
P. O. Box 90 63, Barcelona 08080.

☺▽ **MSC Madrid**
P. O. Box 8294, Barcelona 28080.

Publishers: Magazines: BDSM

☺ ■ *S. A. D. E.*
S. A. D. E., Apartado 12079, Barcelona 08080.
☎ 3 450 4816

Stores: Clothing: Footwear

☺ ■ **La Ampurdanesa**
Nou de la Rambla 9, Barcelona 08001.
☎ 3 301 8879
Fetish shoes for men & women.

Stores: Clothing: Sexuality

⚞ **Tina**
Nou de la Rambla 85, Barcelona 08001.

Stores: Erotica: General

☺▼ **Man's BCN**
Tda 1a, C/Valldonzella 49, Barcelona 08030.
☎ 93 301 5419
🕐 Mon - Sat 10:00 - 13:30 17:00 - 20:00

☺ ■ **SBD**
C/Diputacion 155, Entlo F, Barcelona 08011.
☎ 93 451 7564

☺▼ **Sestienda**
C/Rauric 11, Barcelona 08002.
☎ 93 318 8676

Madrid
Bars: BDSM

☺▽ **Leather Bar**
Calle Pelayo 42, Madrid 28000.
☎ 91 308 1462
🕐 Sun - Fri 20:00 - 03:00, Sat - 03:30

Zaragoza
Stores: Clothing: Fetish

☺ ■ **Things**
Predicadores 3, Zaragoza 50003.
☎ 76 44 6362　　　　　📞 76 43 2226

Sweden

Area: Approximately 449,960 square kilometres
Population: Approximately 8,600,000
Capital City: Stockholm
Currency: Swedish Kronen (skr)
Official Language: Swedish
Major Religions: 89% Protestant
National Holiday: Flag Day, 6th. June
Time zone: GMT plus 1 hour
Country Initials: S
Electricity: 220 volts
Country Dialing Code (from elsewhere): 46
Intl. Dialing Prefix (out of the country): 009
Long Distance Dialing Prefix (inside country): 0
Climate: Varied. The temperature is warmer than one might expect for the latitude of the country. 15% of Sweden is within the arctic circle. Midnight sun for two months in the summer, & two months of complete darkness during the winter.
Age of consent & homosexuality legislation: Age of consent for sexual activity is 15. In 1988, a law was passed that made it illegal to discriminate on the basis of sexual orientation.
Legal drinking age: 18

NATIONAL RESOURCES

Mailorder: Books: Erotic

☺ **Black Widow's Web**
Box 11489, 40430 Göteborg, Bohuslän.
31 250839
✓ ₵
Age statement of 18 is required. English also spoken.

Organizations: BDSM

☺ **Black Widow's Web**
Box 11489, 40430 Göteborg, Bohuslän.
31 250839
✓ ₵
Contact: Anders
Age statement of 18 is required. English also spoken.

BOHUSLÄN

Göteborg

Helplines: Sexuality

▽ **Gay Jouren**
☎ 31 11 0104

▽ **Riksförbundet för Sexuellt Likaberättigande (RFSL)—Göteborg**
☎ 31 11 0133

Manufacturers: Piercing Jewelry

☺ ■ **Barbarella**
Postboks 31172, 40032 Göteborg, Bohuslän.
BARBARELLA@algonet.se
http://www.algonet.se/~barbarella/
Tue - Fri 11:00 - 18:00, Sat 11:00 - 14:00
$ ₵
Also piercing studio, shop, & mail order. Free catalogue. English also spoken.

Organizations: AIDS: Support

▽ **Gayhälsen**
☎ 31 60 1874
☎ 31 60 2758

☺ □ **Positivia Gruppen-Väst**
Postboks 11251, 40426 Göteborg, Bohuslän.
☎ 70 760 7092
Tue 10:00 - 12:00

Organizations: BDSM

▽ **Scandinavian Leather Men (SLM)—Göteborg**
c/o Stig Wollbrecht, Postboks 5236, 40224 Göteborg, Bohuslän.
☎ 31 833910
hakan@haxon.se
http://www.skepsis.com/.gblo/bears/CLUBS/scandinavian.html
Contact: Mr. Hakan Hansson

Organizations: Sexuality

▽ **Freedom of Personality Expression (FPE)—Northern Europe: Sweden**
Postboks 49029, 40064 Göteborg, Bohuslän.
Publishes *Feminform & Intermezzo.*

▽ **Friends Club**
Postboks 53025, 40014 Göteborg, Bohuslän.
☎ 31 15 5615

▽ **Riksförbundet för Sexuellt Likaberättigande (RFSL)—Göteborg**
Postboks 2052, 40311 Göteborg, Bohuslän.
☎ 31 11 6151
31 11 3257

Radio: Sexuality

▽ ***Göteborg Gay Radio***
☎ 31 11 1430
Sun Mon 20:00 - 21:00

Stores: Books: General

▼ **Rosa Rummet**
Esperantoplatsen 7-8, 40311 Göteborg, Bohuslän.
☎ 31 11 6151
Thu Sun 19:00 - 22:00

Stores: Erotica: BDSM

☺ ■ **Delta Fashion**
Postboks 47150, 40259 Göteborg, Bohuslän.
31 481026
Also rubber clothing. Catalogue, £6 or ¢12U.S..

☺ ■ **S. Wolbrecht**
Postboks 52536, 40224 Göteborg, Bohuslän.
☎ 31 83 3910
10:00 - 13:00 15:00- 17:00

BORG

Alingsås

Organizations: BDSM

☺ □ **Club Sunrise**
Postboks 314, 44126 Alingsås, Borg.

DALARNA

Falun

Organizations: Sexuality

▽ **Riksförbundet för Sexuellt Likaberättigande (RFSL)—Falun**
Postboks 2021, 79102 Falun, Dalarna.
☎ 23 28485

GÄSTRIKLAND

Gävle

Organizations: Sexuality

▽ **Riksförbundet för Sexuellt Likaberättigande (RFSL)—Gävle**
Fjärde Tvärgatan 55, 80282 Gävle, Gästrikland.
☎ 26 18 0967
26 18 0967
Counselling Sun 19:00- 21:00

GOTLAND

Visby

Organizations: AIDS: Support

☺ □ **Noah's Ark**
☎ 498 21 6850

HALLAND

Halmstad

Helplines: Sexuality

▽ **Gay Jouren**
☎ 35 12 0722
Mon Wed 19:00 - 21:00

Organizations: Sexuality

▽ **Riksförbundet för Sexuellt Likaberättigande (RFSL)—Halland**
Postboks 4092, 30004 Halmstad, Halland.
☎ 35 21 4800
35 12 0722
Mon 14:00 - 21:00
English also spoken.

Stores: Erotica: General

☺ ■ **Erocenter**
Laholmsvägen 25, 30200 Halmstad, Halland.
11:00 - 22:00

JÄMTLAND

Östersund

Organizations: Sexuality

▽ **Riksförbundet för Sexuellt Likaberättigande (RFSL)—Östersund**
Postboks 516, 83126 Östersund, Jämtland.
☎ 63 10 0668

MALMÖHUS IÄN

Malmö

Helplines: Sexuality

▽ **Gay & Lesbian Switchboard**
☎ 40 11 9944
Thu 20:00 - 23:00 for under 23 years, Fri 19:00 - 24:00 for adults over 23

▽ **Riksförbundet för Sexuellt Likaberättigande (RFSL)—Rådgivningen**
Drottninggatan 36, 21141 Malmö, Malmöhus län.

Helplines: Sexuality

☎ 40 611 9950　　　　　　📞 40 971218
☎ 40 611 9951
Organizations: AIDS: Support
☺ ☐ Noahs Ark
Södergatan 13, 21134 Malmö, Malmöhus län.
☎ 40 11 5215
Organizations: Motorcycle
☿▽ Scandinavian Leather Men (SLM)—Malmö
Postboks 2, 20120 Malmö, Malmöhus län.
☎ 40 30 1893　　　　　　📞 40 7 8929
Organizations: Sexuality
☿▽ Riksförbundet för Sexuellt Likaberättigande
(RFSL)—Malmö
Postboks 2, 20120 Malmö, Malmöhus län.
☎ 40 11 9962
Organizations: Sexuality: Youth
☿▽ Qpido
c/o RFSL Malmö, Postboks 2, 20120 Malmö, Malmöhus län.
Radio: Sexuality
☿▽ Gay Radio
⏲ Wed 00:00 - 02:00, Sun 18:00 - 19:30
Stores: Clothing: Lingerie
☺ ■ Foxy Lady
Lundavagen 9, 21218 Malmö, Malmöhus län.
Stores: Erotica: BDSM
☺ ■ Shock
Skomakaregatan 10, Malmö, Malmöhus län.
☎ 40 11 1080
Stores: Erotica: General
☺ ■ Taboo Center
Södra Förstadsgatan 81, 21420 Malmö, Malmöhus län.
☎ 40 97 6410　　　　　　📞 40 97 0181
⏲ Mon - Thu 11.00 - 23:00, Fri - 20:00

MEDELPAD
Sundsvall
Organizations: Sexuality
☿▽ Riksförbundet för Sexuellt Likaberättigande
(RFSL)—Sundsvall
Postboks 3077, 85003 Sundsvall, Medelpad.
☎ 60 17 1330
⏲ 20:00 - 22:00

NARKE
Örebro
Helplines: Sexuality
☿▽ Gay Jouren
☎ 19 12 2550
⏲ Mon 13:00 - 16:00, Wed 20:00 - 23:00
Organizations: Sexuality
☿▽ Riksförbundet för Sexuellt Likaberättigande
(RFSL)—Örebro
Postboks 447, 70148 Örebro, Narke.
☎ 19 14 4232
⏲ Mon - Fri 13:00 - 16:00, Tue 19:00 - 22:00
Radio: Sexuality
☿▽ Kanal Gay
⏲ Wed 21:00 - 22:00, Sat 18:00 - 19:00

NORRBOTTEN
Luleå
Helplines: Sexuality
☿▽ Gay Jouren
☎ 920 17055
⏲ Sun 19:00 - 22:00
Organizations: Sexuality
☿▽ Riksförbundet för Sexuellt Likaberättigande
(RFSL)—Luleå
Postboks 95, 97104 Luleå, Norrbotten.
☎ 920 17055

Piteå
Helplines: Sexuality
☿▽ Riksförbundet för Sexuellt Likaberättigande
ʌ⛓ (RFSL)—Piteå älvdal & norra Västerbotten
Postboks 155, 94124 Piteå, Norrbotten.
☎ 910 22222
🍷 ✓ ✔
Number works from 10 Swedish cities. Age statement of 18 is required.
English also spoken.
Organizations: Sexuality
☿▽ Riksförbundet för Sexuellt Likaberättigande
ʌ⛓ (RFSL)—Piteå älvdal & norra Västerbotten
Postboks 155, 94124 Piteå, Norrbotten.
☎ 911 14440　　　　　　📞 911 92570
☎ 911 22222
🍷 ✓ ✔
Club Polstjärnan open irregularly for beer, wine, & liquor. Contact line
Gayträff Polstjärnan 712 90360. Publishes Paltbladet 8 times a year.
Yearly subscription is 200SEK. Age statement of 18 is required. English
also spoken.

ÖSTERGÖTLAND
Linköping
Helplines: Sexuality
☿▽ Gay Jouren
☎ 13 11 0333
⏲ Tue 19:00 - 22:00
Organizations: AIDS: Support
☺ ☐ Noah's Ark
☎ 13 19 1000
Organizations: Sexuality
☿▽ Riksförbundet för Sexuellt Likaberättigande
(RFSL)—Linköping
Postboks 213, 58102 Linköping, Östergötland.
☎ 13 13 2022
⏲ Meets Fri 20:00 - 24:00 one week, Sat 22:00 - 02:00 the next
Norrköping
Organizations: Sexuality
☿▽ Riksförbundet för Sexuellt Likaberättigande
(RFSL)—Norrköping
Postboks 2042, 60002 Norrköping, Östergötland.
☎ 11 23 8250
☎ 11 23 8250 (counselling)
⏲ Sat 21:00 - ?

SKÅNE
Helsingborg
Organizations: Sexuality
☿▽ Riksförbundet för Sexuellt Likaberättigande
(RFSL)—Helsingborg
Postboks 2118, 25002 Helsingborg, Skåne.
☎ 42 12 3532
Stores: Erotica: General
☺ ■ Erocenter
Järnvägsgatan 27, 25000 Helsingborg, Skåne.
⏲ 11:00 - 22:00
Karlstad
Organizations: Sexuality
☿▽ Riksförbundet för Sexuellt Likaberättigande
(RFSL)—Kristianstad
Postboks 198, 29122 Karlstad, Skåne.
☎ 54 10 6590
⏲ Thu 20:00 - 23:00, Fri 19:00 - 24:00
Lund
Organizations: Sexuality
☿ Gaystudenterna
Postboks 1662, St. Månsgatan 23, 22101 Lund, Skåne.
☎ 46 15 7134
⏲ Wed 20:00 - 24:00
Bar for gay & lesbian students at the university.
☿▽ Riksförbundet för Sexuellt Likaberättigande

(RFSL)—Lund
Postboks1662, 22101 Lund, Skåne.
☎ 46 15 7134
🕐 Sun 19:00 - 22:00
♿

SMÅLAND
Jönköping
Organizations: Sexuality
👁▽ **Riksförbundet för Sexuellt Likaberättigande (RFSL)—Vätterstad**
Postboks 8020, 55008 Jönköping, Småland.
☎ 36 18 8360
👁▽ **SFHR**
Postboks 528, 55117 Jönköping, Småland.
☎ 36 11 4751
Stores: Erotica: General
☺■ **Erocenter**
Vilhem Thams gatan 24, Jönköping, Småland.
Växjö
Health Services
☺☐ **Venhälsan**
☎ 470 88205
Organizations: AIDS: Support
☺☐ **Noah's Ark**
Postboks 98, 35104 Växjö, Småland.
☎ 470 77 0966
🕐 10:00 - 16:00. Telephone answering service Mon Wed Fri 10:00 - 12:00 14:00 - 16:00
Organizations: Sexuality
👁▽ **Riksförbundet för Sexuellt Likaberättigande (RFSL)—Växjö**
Postboks 440, 35106 Växjö, Småland.
☎ 470 20808
🕐 Meets Wed 19:00 - 23:00, last Sat of month 21:00 - 02:00

SÖDERMANLAND
Eskilstuna
Organizations: Sexuality
👁▽ **Riksförbundet för Sexuellt Likaberättigande (RFSL)—Eskilstuna**
Postboks 398, 63106 Eskilstuna, Södermanland.
Nyköping
Organizations: Sexuality
👁▽ **Riksförbundet för Sexuellt Likaberättigande (RFSL)—Nyköping**
Kyrkogatan 15c, 61132 Nyköping, Södermanland.
☎ 155 21 0229

STOCKHOLM
Regional Resources
Stores: Erotica: BDSM
☺ **Läderverkstan**
Box 17098, Rosenlundsgatan 30, 10462 Stockholm.
☎ 8 668 5869 📞 8 658 6953
🕐 Mon - Fri 12:00 - 18:00. Piercing by appointment only
♿
Also piercing & tailormade leathers. Catalogue, 20SEK. English & German also spoken.
Stockholm
Bars: BDSM
☺■ **Hus 1 'Huset**
Sveavägen 57, 11359 Stockholm.
☎ 8 30 8338 📞 8 31 3480
🕐 18:00 - 03:00 daily
☺■ **Kinky Bar**
Polhemsgatan 23, Stockholm.
☎ 8 653 5739
🕐 Fri - Sat - 24:00

BBSs: Sexuality
👁▼ **The Gay Network (TGT)**
📞 8 32 3232. 2400 baud maximum.
Health Services
☺☐ **Venhälsan**
c/o Södersjukhuset Hospital, Ringvägen 52, Stockholm.
☎ 8 616 2500
🕐 Tu Thu 18:00 - 20:00
Free HIV testing & counselling.
Helplines: Sexuality
👁▽ **BHUS-Linjen**
☎ 20 78 3366
🕐 Mon Thu 19:00 - 22:00
Helpline for youth.
👁▽ **Gay Jouren**
☎ 8 24 7465
🕐 20:00 - 23:00
👁▽ **PG-Jouren**
☎ 20 78 4414
👁▽ **Riksförbundet för Sexuellt Likaberättigande (RFSL)—Rådgivningen**
☎ 8 736 0210
🕐 Mon 09:00 - 21:00, Tue - Fri 09:00 - 16:00
Counselling for lesbians, gays, & bisexuals.
Organizations: AIDS: Support
☺☐ **Noah's Ark**
Drottninggatan 61, Stockholm.
☎ 8 23 5060
🕐 Mon - Fri 09:00 - 21:00, Sat 12:00 - 16:00
Part of the Red Cross.
☺☐ **Positiva Gruppen**
Postboks 38055, 10064 Stockholm.
☎ 8 720 1960 📞 8 720 1048
Organizations: BDSM
👁▽ **Scandinavian Leather Men (SLM)—Stockholm**
Box 17241, 10462 Stockholm.
☎ 8 643 3100
🕐 Meets Wed Fri Sat 22:00 - 02:00
Organizations: Bears
👁▽ **Viking Bears**
5 tr, Industrigatan 6, 11246 Stockholm.
✉ twin.bears@tgt.ct.se
🌐 http://www.abc.se/~m8135/viking_b.html
Contact: Mr. Jan Lövbom
Organizations: Fetish: Rubber
👁▽ **Stockholm Rubber Men's Club**
c/o SLM, Box 17241, 10462 Stockholm.
☎ 8 643 3100
🕐 Meets Wed Fri Sat 22:00 - 02:00
Organizations: Piercing
☺■ **IPS**
Postboks 710, 11479 Stockholm.
☎ 8 747 1493 📞 8 747 1493
Organizations: Sexuality
▷▽ **Benjamin**
Postboks 9083, 10271 Stockholm.
☎ 40 611 9923
🕐 Call Tue 19:00 - 21:00
▷▽ **Phi Pi Epsilon—Sverige**
Postboks 529, 10130 Stockholm.
🕐 Meets monthly
👁▼ **Riksförbundet för Sexuellt Likaberättigande (RFSL)**
Postboks 350, 10126 Stockholm.
☎ 8 736 0213 📞 8 30 4730
National gay & lesbian organization with local groups throughout the country.
👁▽ **Stockholm Gay Center**
Postboks 45090, 10430 Stockholm.
☎ 8 736 0212
Organizations: Sexuality: Youth
👁▽ **Föreningen BHUS**
Postboks 19155, 10432 Stockholm.
☎ 8 34 1105
Contact: Mr. Leif Aruhn-Solén

Activities for gay & lesbian youth up to 30 years old.

Publishers: Magazines: Sexuality

⚤▼ ***Reporter***
Postboks 17218, 10462 Stockholm.
☎ 8 669 0012 — Fax 8 669 0424
Published every month.

Radio: Sexuality

⚤▽ ***Stockholm Gay Radio***
☎ 8 736 0216
🕒 Thu Sun 1930

Stores: Books: General

⚤▼ **Agora Bokhandel AB**
Narvavagen 25, 11460 Stockholm.

⚤▽ **Rosa Rummet**
c/o RFSL, Postboks 45090, 10430 Stockholm.
☎ 8 736 0215
🕒 Mon Thu 12:00 - 15:00 18:00 - 21:00 Sat Sun - 15:00

Stores: Clothing: Footwear

☺ ■ **Stiletto Shoes AB**
Postboks 46, 13054 Dalaro, Stockholm.
☎ 750 53237 — Fax 750 53277

Stores: Erotica: BDSM

⚤▼ **Mikes Läder**
Repslagargatan 11, Stockholm.
☎ 8 644 0466
🕒 Tue - Fri 12:00 - 18:00, Sat 12:00 - 16:00

Stores: Erotica: General

⚤▼ **Tass Surtur**
Bergsgatan 47, 12231 Stockholm.

UPPLAND

Uppsala

Helplines: Sexuality

⚤▽ **Gay Jouren**
☎ 18 26 0915
🕒 Mon 19:00 - 21:00

Organizations: Sexuality

⚤▽ **Riksförbundet för Sexuellt Likaberättigande (RFSL)—Uppsala**
Postboks 1147, 75141 Uppsala, Uppland.
☎ 18 23 4750
🕒 Wed 19:00 - 23:00, Fri 20:00 - 02:00, Sun 22:00 - 02:00

Organizations: Sexuality: Student

⚤▽ **Uppsala Gay Studenter (FUGS)**
Postboks 8006, 75237 Uppsala, Uppland.

VÄRMLAND

Karlstad

Organizations: AIDS: Support

☺ □ **Noah's Ark**
☎ 570 11222

Organizations: Sexuality

⚤▽ **Riksförbundet för Sexuellt Likaberättigande (RFSL)—Karlstad**
Postboks 634, 65114 Karlstad, Värmland.
☎ 54 15 2090

VÄSTERBOTTEN

Skellefteå

Helplines: Sexuality

⚤▽ **Switchboard**
☎ 910 22222
🕒 Sun 19:00 - 21:00

Umeå

Organizations: Sexuality

⚤▽ **Riksförbundet för Sexuellt Likaberättigande (RFSL)—Umeå**
Postboks 38, 90102 Umeå, Västerbotten.
☎ 90 11 4710

VÄSTERGÖTLAND

Borås

Organizations: Sexuality

⚤▽ **Riksförbundet för Sexuellt Likaberättigande (RFSL)—Borås**
Postboks 77038, 50007 Borås, Västergötland.
☎ 33 10 6970
🕒 Thu 19:00 - 22:00, Fri 20:00 - 24:00

Stores: Erotica: General

☺ ■ **Erocenter**
Sturegatan 20, Borås, Västergötland.
🕒 11:00 - 22:00

Trollhättan

Organizations: Sexuality

⚤▽ **Riksförbundet för Sexuellt Likaberättigande (RFSL)—Trollhätan**
Postboks 10, 46121 Trollhättan, Västergötland.
☎ 520 11766

VÄSTMANLANDS IÄN

Västerås

Organizations: Sexuality

⚤▽ **Riksförbundet för Sexuellt Likaberättigande (RFSL)—Väterås**
Postboks 12031, 72012 Västerås, Västmanlands län.
☎ 21 11 8041
🕒 Wed 20:00 - 22:00, Sat 21:00 - 02:00

Switzerland

Area: Approximately 41,295 square kilometres
Population: Approximately 6,870,000
Capital City: Bern
Currency: Franc (sfr)
Official Language: German, French, Italian, & Romance
Major Religions: 48% Roman Catholic, 44% Protestant
National Holiday: Confederation Day, 1st. August
Time zone: GMT plus 1 hour
Country Initials: CH
Electricity: 220 volts
Country Dialing Code (from elsewhere): 41
Intl. Dialing Prefix (out of the country): 00
Long Distance Dialing Prefix (inside country): 0
Climate: Continental, but cold winters with plenty of snow for skiing in the mountains. Summer temperatures are approximately 25°C in the summer.
Age of consent & homosexuality legislation: Age of consent for sexual activity is 16, since 1992.
Legal drinking age: 18

NATIONAL RESOURCES

Helplines: Sexuality

⚤▽ **Dialogai**
Boîte Postale 237, 1211 Genève 7.
☎ 22 340 0000 — Fax 22 240 0298
☎ 22 731 8446
🕒 Telephone Wed 19:00 - 22:00, office Wed 20:00 - 22:00
Information, support, & health service. Publishes *Dialogai INFO* every two months.

Mailorder: Clothing: Fetish

☺ ■ **Eccentric Fashion**
Postfach 1, 4857 Riken.
☎ 62 44 2221
Catalogue, £3.

Mailorder: Erotica: BDSM

⚤▼ **Euro-Business Services Inc.**
Schwaendi 63, 6170 Schüpfheim.
☎ 41 485 0081 — Fax 41 485 0090
🕒 Mon - Fri 08:00 - 18:00
Also latex items. Catalogue, free with 2 IRCs.

Mailorder: Erotica

⚤▼ **CEI**
Postfach 3327, 3022 Bern.
☎ 31 42 3666

Catalogue, SFr10.

⌖▼ **David-Versand**
Boîte Postale 308, 9016 Saint-Gallen.

Mailorder: Erotica: Leather

⌖▼ **Macho-Versand**
Engelstraße 62, 8004 Zürich.
☎ 1 241 3215

Mailorder: Erotica

⌖▼ **M-Club**
Postfach 904, 5400 Baden.

⌖▼ **Toy-Versand**
Postfach 555, 8026 Zürich.

Mailorder: Safer Sex Products

☺▼ **The Hot Rubber Company**
Postfach 9869, 8036 Zürich.

Organizations: AIDS: Support

☺☐ **AIDS-Hilfe—Schweiz**
Postfach 141, 8031 Zürich.
☎ 1 273 4242 ✆ 1 273 4263

Organizations: BDSM

⌖▽ **Loge 70 (Schweitz)**
Postfach 725, 8025 Zürich.

Organizations: Bears

⌖ **Bartmänner Schweiz, Barbus de Suisse, Barbuti Svizzeri, Barbus Svissers, Beardmen Switzerland**
Postfach 7560, 8023 Zurich.
Contact: M. Andrea Carlo Polesello, President
More than a club for men & bears: meetings, outings, & brunches monthly. Also contacts with foreign bear clubs. French, Italian, & English also spoken.

Organizations: Fetish: Foot

⌖▽ **Whitesox**
Postfach 235, 5430 Wettingen.
Publishes a newsletter quarterly. Yearly subscription is SFr30. German, French, & English also spoken.

Organizations: Sexuality

⌖▽ **Pink Cross**
Postfach 7512, 3001 Bern.
☎ 31 372 3300 ✆ 31 372 3317

Publishers: Books: Sexuality

⌖▼ **Arcados-Versand**
Rheingasse 69, 4002 Basel.
☎ 61 681 3132 ✆ 61 681 6656
🕐 Tue - Fri 13:00 - 18:30, Sat 12:00 - 17:00
Books about Swiss gay & lesbian history, & other titles.

Publishers: Guides: Sexuality

⌖▼ *Cruiser*
Postfach 109, 8025 Zürich.
☎ 1 261 8200
Free in gay locations.

Publishers: Magazines: Sexuality

⌖▼ *Anderschume / Kontiki*
Postfach 7979, 8023 Zürich.
 ✆ 1 272 8440
German text. Published quarterly.

Stores: Books: General

☺■ **Sec 52 Buchladen & Galerie**
Josefstraße 52, 8005 Zürich.
☎ 1 271 1818 ✆ 1 281 1444
🕐 Mon - Fri 11:00 - 18:30, Sat -16:00
♿
Very large, well chosen assortment of books. The best choice of gay books in Switzerland.

Television: Sexuality

⌖▽ *The Pink Elephant*
Dream Team Productions, Postfach 128, 8957 Spreitenbach.
☎ 77 88 9800 ✆ 56 70 1313
🕐 1st Thu of month
The first regular european GAY-TV programme. Broadcast on a regular public TV station in Switzerland since 1994..

Aarau

Organizations: AIDS: Support

☺☐ **AIDS-Hilfe—Aarau**
Augustin Keller Straße 1, 5000 Aarau.
☎ 64 24 4450
🕐 Mon 08:00 - 12:00, Wed 15:00 - 19:00

Baden

Health Services

☺☐ **Kantonspital**
☎ 56 84 2111
☎ 56 84 2122

Basel / Bâle

Health Services

☺☐ **Kantonsspital Basel**
☎ 61 265 4161
🕐 Mon - Fri 07:30 - 11:30 14:00 - 17:30

Organizations: AIDS: Support

☺☐ **AIDS-Hilfe—Basel**
Claragraben 160, 4057 Basel.
☎ 61 692 2122
🕐 10:00 - 17:00

Organizations: Sexuality

⌖▽ **Homosexuelle Arbeitsgruppen—Basel**
Postfach 1519, 4001 Basel.
☎ 61 692 6655
🕐 Information Wed 20:00, meets 1st. Thu of month 20:00

⌖▽ **Schwule-Lesbische Unigruppe (SLUG)**
Postfach 1519, 4001 Basel.
☎ 61 692 6655
🕐 Wed 20:00

Organizations: Sexuality: Youth

⌖▽ **Jugendgruppe Rose**
Postfach 4520, 4002 Basel.
☎ 61 692 6655
🕐 Meets Mon 19:30. Wed 20:00 telephone only

Publishers: Magazines: Sexuality

⌖▼ *Come Out!*
Gay Media, Postfach 4433, 4002 Basel.
☎ 61 681 3132
Free magazine for the Basel area.

Stores: Clothing: Fetish

☺■ **Crazy Sexy**
Nauenunterfuehrung 10, 4051 Basel.
☎ 61 271 9079

Stores: Erotica: BDSM

☺ **Boutique Fancy**
Postfach 261, 4010 Basel.
☎ 61 271 4656 ✆ 61 271 4720
🕐 Mon - Fri 10:00 - 18:30, Sat 10:00 - 17:00
Leather, latex, PVC, furniture, magazines, books, toys, jewelry, videos, etc.. Location: Elisabethstraße 41 (enter from passageway). Catalogue, SFr40.

Bern

Bars: BDSM

⌖▼ **Ursus Club**
Junkerngasse 1, 3011 Bern.
☎ 31 311 7406
🕐 Fri 21:00 - 03:30 is leather night

Organizations: AIDS: Support

☺☐ **AIDS-Hilfe—Bern**
Wylerstraße 109, 3000 Bern 22.
☎ 31 331 3334 ✆ 31 331 3336
🕐 Mon - Fri 09:00 - 16:00

Organizations: Body Size

⌖▽ **X-Large**
Postfach 407, 3000 Bern 6.
☎ 31 352 7886

Organizations: Sexuality

⌖▽ **Homosexuelle Arbeitsgruppen—Bern**
Postfach 312, 3000 Bern 13.
☎ 31 311 6353

Organizations: Sexuality: Student

⚥▽ **Schwule-Lesbische Unigruppe (SchLUB)—Bern**
c/o SUB, Lerchenweg 32, 3000 Bern.
Gay & lesbian emancipation group at the University of Bern. Organizes dinner, brunches, speeches, etc..

Organizations: Sexuality: Youth

⚥▽ **Jugendgruppe Space**
Postfach 931, 3000 Bern 7.

Stores: Erotica: General

⚥▼ **Loveland**
Postfach 580, 3000 Bern 8.
☎ 31 311 4533 ✆ 31 311 8775
Free catalogue.

Berne

Stores: Clothing: Fetish

☺▼ **Opera**
Zeughausgasse 20, 3011 Berne.
☎ 31 228458

Biel

Organizations: AIDS: Support

☺□ **AIDS-Hilfe—Biel**
Freiestraße 37, 2503 Biel.
☎ 32 42 4342 (Deutsch)
☎ 32 25 0202 (Français)

Chur

Helplines: Sexuality

⚥▽ **Rosa Telefon—Chur**
☎ 81 21 6766
⌚ Tue 19:00 - 21:00

Organizations: AIDS: Support

☺□ **AIDS-Hilfe—Graubünden**
Loestraße 34, 7002 Chur.
☎ 81 22 4900
⌚ Thu 17:00 - 21:00

Frauenfeld

Organizations: Sexuality

⚥▽ **Homosexuelle Organisation Thurgau (HOT)**
Postfach 355, 8501 Frauenfeld.
☎ 54 21 0434

Fribourg / Freiburg

Organizations: AIDS: Support

☺□ **Aide Fribourgeoise Contre le SIDA / AIDS-Hilfe—Fribourg**
Boîte Postale 44, 1705 Fribourg.
☎ 37 21 9678

Genève / Genf

Organizations: AIDS: Support

☺□ **Groupe SIDA Genève**
Boîte Postale 2443, 1211 Genève.
☎ 22 700 1500

Organizations: Sexuality: Student

⚥▽ **Unigaie**
Boîte Postale 311, 1211 Genève 4.
⌚ Meets 15th. of month 20:15 - 19:00

Hinwil

Organizations: Sexuality

⚥▽ **Klick, Schwulengruppe Zürich Oberland**
Postfach 174, 8340 Hinwil.
☎ 55 48 4753

Lausanne

Health Services

☺□ **Hôpital Cantonal**
Service Dermatologie, 17 rue du Bagnon, Lausanne.
☎ 21 314 4141
⌚ 09:00 - 17:00

Organizations: BDSM

⚥▽ **Black Panther's Club**
Case Postale 86, 1010 Lausanne.

Organizations: Motorcycle

⚥▽ **MSC Suisse Romande**
Boîte Postale 3343, 1002 Lausanne.

Stores: Erotica: General

⚥▼ **Pink Shop**
Avenue Tivoli 22, 1007 Lausanne.
☎ 21 311 6969
⌚ 10:00 - 19:00

Liestal

Health Services

☺□ **Kantonspital**
☎ 61 91 9111

Lugano

Organizations: Sexuality

⚥▽ **Associazione Gay Ticino (AGT)**
Casella Postale 5, 6952 Cannobio-Lugano.

Luzern / Lucerne

Helplines: Sexuality

⚥▽ **Sorgentelefon HALU**
☎ 41 51 3532
⌚ Mon 19:00 - 21:00

Organizations: AIDS: Support

☺□ **AIDS-Hilfe—Luzern**
Wesemlinrain 20, 6006 Luzern.
☎ 41 51 6848
☎ 41 51 6960 (counselling)
⌚ Mon 19:00 - 21:00, Wed 09:30 - 11:30, Thu 15:00 - 17:00. Counselling Thu 09:00 - 12:00 14:00 - 17:00

Organizations: Motorcycle

⚥▽ **Zentralschweizer Schwulen-Motorrad-Club (SMC)**
Casella Postale2231, 6002 Luzern.

Organizations: Sexuality

⚥▽ **Homosexuelle Arbeitsgruppe Luzern (HALU)**
Postfach 3112, 6002 Luzern.
☎ 41 51 3532
⌚ Meets Wed

Mammern

Organizations: Sexuality: Youth

⚥▽ **Junge Lesben & Schwule im Thurgau (LuST)**
♿ Postfach 17, 8265 Mammern.
☎ 71 72 3413
⌚ Meets last Tue of month 20:30. Telephone Thu 20:00 - 22:00
Contact: Ms. Toni Cirillo, Secretary
Approximately 30 young (16-35) people in the cantons of Thurgau, Saint Gallen, & Schaffhausen . French, Italian, English (spoken only), & Switzerdeutsch also spoken.

Neuchâtel / Neuenburg

Organizations: AIDS: Support

☺□ **Groupe SIDA Neuchâtel**
6, rue de Verger, 2034 Peseux.
☎ 38 31 4924
⌚ Thu 10:00 - 12:00

Organizations: Sexuality

⚥▽ **Homologay**
Postfach 1719, 2002 Neuchâtel.
☎ 38 31 5726
⌚ Thu 20:00 - ?

Neuenhof

Stores: Clothing: Fetish

☺■ **Arabesque**
Limmerstraße 10, 5432 Neuenhof.
☎ 1 242 9626
Catalogue available.

Rothrist

Stores: Clothing: Fetish

☺■ **Eccentric Fashion**
Bernstraße 215, Rothrist.
Catalogue available.

Saint Gallen

Organizations: AIDS: Support

☺ ☐ **AIDS-Hilfe—Saint Gallen**
Boîte Postale 8, 9001 Saint Gallen.
☎ 71 23 3868
⏰ Tue 09:00 - 12:00 19:00 - 21:00, Thu 19:00 - 21:00, Fri 09:00 - 12:00

Organizations: Sexuality

♂♡▽ **Homosexuelle Arbeitsgruppe Saint Gallen (HASG)**
Postfach 215, 9004 Saint Gallen.

♀▽ **TS-Selbsthilfe Gruppe**
Postfach 92, 9008 Saint Gallen.

Organizations: Sexuality: Youth

♂♡▽ **Jugendgruppe Jackpoint**
Boîte Postale 361, 9004 Saint Gallen.
⏰ Meets Tue 20:00

Stores: Clothing: Fetish

☺ ■ **Dana**
Grossackerstraße 5, 9006 Saint Gallen.
☎ 71 253195
Also body piercing.

Saint Moritz

Organizations: Sexuality: Youth

♂♡▽ **Jugendgruppe WIGWAM**
Casella Postale 3138, 7500 Saint Moritz 3.

Schaffhausen

Organizations: AIDS: Support

☺ ☐ **AIDS-Hilfe—Thurgau / Schaffhausen**
Rathausbogen 15, 8200 Schaffhausen.
☎ 53 25 9338

Sion

Organizations: AIDS: Support

☺ ☐ **Antenne SIDA du Valais Romand**
Boîte Postale 550, 1950 Sion.
☎ 27 22 8757
⏰ Tue 18:00 - 22:00

Solothurn

Organizations: AIDS: Support

☺ ☐ **AIDS-Hilfe—Solothurn**
Postfach 155, 4502 Solothurn.
☎ 65 22 9411

Organizations: Sexuality

♂♡▽ **Homosexuelle Arbeitsgruppe (HASO)**
Postfach 508, 4502 Solothurn.
☎ 65 23 6620
⏰ Meets Mon 20:00

Ticino

Organizations: AIDS: Support

☺ ☐ **Aiuta AIDS Ticino**
Casella Postale 79, 6900 Ticino.
☎ 91 23 1717
⏰ Mon - Thu 10:00 - 17:00

Viganello

Organizations: Sexuality

♂♡▽ **Communita Gay della Svizzera Italiana**
Via Agli Orti 20, Viganello.
Publishes *22%*.

Visp

Organizations: AIDS: Support

☺ ☐ **AIDS-Hilfe—Oberwallis**
St. Martiniplatz 1, 3930 Visp.
☎ 28 46 4668

Winterthur

Helplines: Sexuality

♂♡▽ **Gay Switchboard**
Postfach 281, 8401 Winterthur.

☎ 52 213 8188

Organizations: AIDS: Support

☺ ☐ **AIDS Infostelle Winterthur**
2nd. Floor, Haus zur Eisamkeit, Lagerhuasstraße 5, 8401 Winterthur.
☎ 52 213 8141 ✆ 52 212 8095

Organizations: Sexuality

♂♡▽ **Winterthur Schwule (WISCH)**
Postfach 294, 8401 Winterthur.
☎ 52 213 8188

Stores: Books: General

♂♡▼ **Rainbow Bookshop**
Postfach 281, 8401 Winterthur.
☎ 52 213 8188
⏰ Sat 10:00 - 16:00

Zug

Organizations: AIDS: Support

☺ ☐ **AIDS-Hilfe—Zug**
Zeughausgasse 9, Zug.
☎ 42 22 4865
⏰ Mon 14:00 - 17:00, Tue 09:00 - 13:00, Wed 12:00 - 16:00 17:00 - 21:00, & 1st. Sat of month 09:00 - 15:00

Zürich

Archives: Sexuality

♂♡▼ **Schwule Ausleihbibliothek (HAZ/SOH)**
Postfach 7088, 8023 Zürich.
☎ 1 271 2250
⏰ Tue Wed 19:30 - 21:00

Bars: BDSM

♂♡▼ **Barfüsser**
Spitalgasse 14, 8001 Zürich.
☎ 1 251 4064
⏰ 15:00 - 24:00

♂♡▼ **Phœnix**
Postfach 441, 8026 Zürich.
☎ 1 734 2469

Health Services

☺ ☐ **Städtische Poliklinik für Haut- & Geschlechtskrankheiten**
Hermann Greulich Straße 70, Zürich.
☎ 1241 8900
⏰ Mon - Fri 09:00 - 11:30, Mon - Wed also 15:00 - 17:00, Tue Fri also 15:00 - 19:00

☺ ☐ **University Hospital of Zürich**
Dermatological Clinic, Gloriastraße 31, Zürich.
☎ 1 255 2306
⏰ No appointment needed

Helplines: Sexuality

♂♡▽ **Beratungstelephon für Homosexuelle (HAZZ/SOH)**
Postfach 7088, 8023 Zürich.
☎ 1 271 7011
⏰ Tue 20:00 - 22:00

♂♡▽ **Homosexuelle Arbeitsgruppen Zürich (HAZ)**
Postfach 7088, 8023 Zürich.
☎ 1 271 2250
⏰ Tue - Fri 19:30 - 23:00, Sun 11:00 - 14:00. Tue Women, Wed Youth

Organizations: AIDS: Support

☺ ☐ **AIDS-Hilfe—Zürich**
Birmensdorferstraße 169, 8003 Zürich.
☎ 1 461 1516
⏰ Mon Tue Fri 17:00 - 19:00, Wed 13:00 - 16:00

Organizations: Motorcycle

♂♡▽ **European Confederation of Motorcycle Clubs**
c/o Loge 70 (Schweiz), Postach 725, 8025 Zürich.

♂♡▽ **Leder- & Motorradclub Zürich (LMZ)**
Postfach 3181, 8031 Zürich.
⏰ Meets monthly

Organizations: Sexuality

♂♡☐ **Act-HIV**
Hallwilstraße 78, 8004 Zürich.
☎ 1 291 3720 ✆ 1 241 1562
☎ 1 241 1515 (for PWA)
⏰ Tue Thu 09:00 - 13:00, Wed 19:00 - 22:00

Organizations: Sexuality

⚥▽ **Homosexuelle Arbeitsgruppen Zürich (HAZ)**
Postfach 7088, 8023 Zürich.
☎ 1 271 2250
🕐 Tue - Fri 19:30 - 23:00, Sun 11:00 - 14:00. Office Wed 14:00 - 18:00

⚥▽ **Schweizerische Organisation Homosexuellen (SOH)**
Postfach 4580, 8022 Zürich.
☎ 1 271 7011
🕐 Meets Mon evenings

Organizations: Sexuality: Student

⚥▽ **Zart & Heftig**
Postfach 7218, 8023 Zürich.

Organizations: Sexuality: Youth

⚥▽ **Homosexuelle Arbeitsgruppen Zürich (HAZ)**
Postfach 7088, 8023 Zürich.
☎ 1 273 1177
🕐 Tue - Fri 19:30 - 23:00, Sun 11:00 - 14:00. Tue Women, Wed Youth

Stores: Clothing: Fetish

☺■ **Arabesque**
Brauerstraße 31, 8004 Zürich.
☎ 1 242 9626
Please send letter to the Neuenhoff address. Catalogue available.

Stores: Clothing: Leather

⊕■ **Ale Design**
Segantinistraße 85, 8049 Zürich.

♂ **Erne's Sportlade**
Gasometerstraße 32, 8026 Zürich.
🕐 Tuie Wed Fri 10:00 - 18:00, Thu 10:00 - 21:00 Sat 10:00 - 16:00
Motorbike clothing.

Stores: Erotica: BDSM

⚥▼ **Macho Men's Shop**
Engelstraße 62, 8004 Zürich.
☎ 1 241 3215
🕐 Mon 14:00 - 18:30, Tue Fri 11:00 - 18:30, Sat 10:00 - 16:00

Stores: Erotica: General

⚥▼ **BS-Laden**
Arwandstraße 67, 8004 Zürich.
☎ 1 2241 0441
🕐 16:00 - 18:30, Sat 11:00 - 16:00
Some leather & rubber items.

⚥▼ **Macho City Shop**
Häringstraße 16, 8001 Zürich.
☎ 1 251 1222 ✆ 1 251 1222
🕐 Mon - Fri 11:00 - 18:00, Thu - 21:00, Sat 11:00 - 16:00

☺■ **Sexotica**
Heinrichstraße 122, Zürich.
☎ 1 273 0179
🕐 Mon - Fri 10:00 - 18:30, Sat - 16:00

☺■ **Sexyland**
Brauerstraße 48, Zürich.
☎ 1 242 7989
🕐 Mon - Fri 10:00 - 18:30, Sat - 16:00

Turkey

Area: Approximately 780,000 square kilometres
Population: Approximately 58,400,000
Capital City: Ankora
Currency: Turkish Pound (TL)
Official Language: Turkish
Major Religions: 99% Sunnite Moslem
National Holiday: Republic Day, 29th. October
Time zone: GMT plus 2 hours
Country Initials: TR
Electricity: 220 volts, 50Hz
Country Dialing Code (from elsewhere): 90
Intl. Dialing Prefix (out of the country): 00
Climate: Inland is dry with large temperature variaions, coastal areas are mediterranean.
Age of consent & homosexuality legislation: Age of consent for sexual activity is 15. Sexual activity between men is common, but public showing of a relationship is not common, since men must maintain a masculine façade. Society in general is not tolerant to open displays of homosexuality.

Istanbul

Organizations: Sexuality

⚥▽ **Travesty/Transsexualle**
Lao 176/D.S., Kultur Je Sanat, Siraselviler, Taksim.
☎ 1 578925
German, French & Spanish also spoken. Please address envelopes to Demet Demir, do NOT address them to Travesty/Transsexualle.

U.S.A.

Area: Approximately 9,384,000 square kilometres
Population: Approximately 255,000,000
Capital City: Washington, District of Columbia
Currency: U.S. Dollar (\$U.S.)
Official Language: English
Major Religions: Roman Catholic, Protestant, Jewish
National Holiday: Independence Day, 4th. July
Time zone: GMT minus 5-8 hours. In order from the east, time zones are referred to as Eastern Standard Time (EST), Central Standard Time (CST), Mountain Time, & Pacific Standard Time (PST)
Country Initials: USA
Electricity: 117 volts, 60Hz
Country Dialing Code (from elsewhere): 1
Intl. Dialing Prefix (out of the country): 011
Long Distance Dialing Prefix (inside country): 1
Climate: Most climates are experienced somewhere in this vast country.
Age of consent & homosexuality legislation: Since 1990, homosexuality cannot be used as a reason to bar someone from the United States. Age of consent for sexual activity varies by state. Please see the appropriate state for the information about this subject.
Legal drinking age: 18 in most states, but higher in some.

NATIONAL RESOURCES

Archives: Sexuality

☺▽ **The Happy Foundation**
♿ 411 Bonham, San Antonio, Texas 78205.
☎ 210 227 6451
🕐 By appointment only
Collection of the history of the gay, bisexual, lesbian, & transgender community. Includes art, politics, current concerns, history, sociology, etc..

BBSs: BDSM

☺■ **The Boston Dungeon Society**
✆ 617 397 8844
📟 http://bdsbbs.com or telnet to BDSBBS.COM

♟♟■ **The English Palace**
P. O. Box 213, Hazlet, New Jersey 07730.
☎ 908 739 1354 ✆ 908 739 9402
✆ 908 739 1755
📧 sysop@palace.com
📟 http://palace.com/, & Telnet Palace.com or 199.171.54.2

⚥▼ **Fountains of Pleasure**
P. O. Box 1014, Novi, Michigan 48376-0692.
☎ 810 348 5332
✆ 810 348 7854. 28800 baud maximum.
📧 KVJV70E@Prodigy.com or TheHotLine@aol.com
🕐 24hrs.
♿ ✓ \$ 💳 💳
No charge at the moment, but subject to change. Questions by 'phone invited, but we're in & out, so be persistent. Age statement of 18 is required.

BBSs: Sexuality

⚥▽ **Gay/Lesbian Information Bureau (GLIB)**
c/o Community Educational Services Foundation, P. O. Box 636, Arlington, Virginia 22216.
✆ 703 578 4542

⚥▽ **Gay/Lesbian International News Network (GLINN)**
P. O. Box 93626, Millwaukee, Wisconsin 53203.
☎ 414 289 8780 ✆ 414 289 0789
✆ 414 289 0145

Competitions & Conventions: Sexuality

▽■ **Salishon Society**
P. O. Box 1604, Eugene, Oregon 97440-1604.
☎ 503 688 4282

Counsellors

▽■ **Niela Miller, M.S. Ed., LCSW, LMHC**
People * Systems Potential, 132 Butternut Hollow, Nagog Woods, Massachusetts 01718-1004.
☎ 508 264 4565

✉ niela@world.std.com
⚫ ✓
Counselled crossdressers & transexuals for 13 years. Now training & supervising others working with this population. Book published in 1995.

☞ ■ **National Harry Benjamin Gender Dysphoria Association (HBIGDA)**
P. O. Box 1718, Sonoma, California 95476.
☎ 707 938 2871
Set the standards for treatment of gender dysphoria. Resource for professionals working in this area.

Distributors: Books: Erotic

☺ **Eve Browne Fashions**
17th. Floor, 521 5th. Avenue, New York 10175.
Also does web printing for the adult industry.

Distributors: Magazines: General

☺ **Ubiquity Distributors**
607 Degraw Street, Brooklyn, New York 11217.
☎ 718 875 5491 ✆ 718 875 8047
🕐 Mon - Fri 09:00 - 17:00
✓ $
Wholesaler of specialized alternative periodicals in all subject areas. Sell to retailers only.

Distributors: Videos: Erotic

☞▼ **Sierra Pacific Productions**
P. O. Box 9476, Marina Del Rey, California 90295.
☎ 800 828 4336 ✆ 310 399 4770
☎ 310 399 0557
✓ $ VISA MC
Catalogue published every two months, $10U.S. California residents, $15 elsewhere. Age statement of 21 is required. Spanish also spoken.

Distributors: Videos: Safer Sex

☺ ■ **REW Video**
1404 Arnold Avenue, San José, California 95110-1405.
☎ 800 528 1942 ✆ 800 528 1942
☎ 408 451 9310
✉ rewvideo@aol.com
🕐 Mon -Fri 09:00 - 17:00
⚫ ✓ $ ⚊ VISA MC AMERICAN
Wholesale & retail safer sex, erotic arts, & sexual technique videos. Catalogue, 50¢. Age statement of 18 is required.

Helplines: AIDS

☺ □ **CDC National AIDS Hotline**
c/o The American Social Health Association. P. O. Box 13827, Research Triangle Park, North Carolina 27709-9940.
☎ 800 342 2437 ✆ 919 361 4855
🕐 24hrs. Eastern. 08:00 - 02:00 en español. 10:00 - 22:00 TTY
Up-to-date information about HIV/AIDS. Confidential. 800 243 7889 TTY hotline. Servicio en español 800 344 7432. Spanish also spoken.

Helplines: STDs

☺ □ **CDC National STD Hotline**
c/o The American Social Health Association. P. O. Box 13827, Research Triangle Park, North Carolina 27709-9940.
☎ 800 227 8922
🕐 08:00 - 23:00 Eastern
Up-to-date information, referrals, & educational materials about STDs.

☺ □ **National Herpes Hotline**
c/o The American Social Health Association. P. O. Box 13827, Research Triangle Park, North Carolina 27709-9940.
☎ 800 230 6039
☎ 919 361 8488
🕐 09:00 - 19:00 Eastern
Up-to-date information, referrals to over 90 local support groups in U.S. & Canada, & educational materials about herpes. 800 478 3227 from Canada only. French also spoken.

Helplines: Youth

☺ ■ **National Runaway Switchboard**
☎ 800 621 4000

Mailorder: Adult Toys: Electrical

☺ ■ **P. E. S., Inc.**
1509 West Oakley Boulevard, Las Vegas, Nevada 89102.
☎ 702 474 2991 ✆ 702 474 4088
✉ spidey@accessnv.com
🕸 http://www.webcom.com/~pes
Electrical stimulation toys, bringing human sexuality into the 21st. century.

Mailorder: Books: BDSM

☺ **Blue Moon Books**

P. O. Box 1040, Cooper Station, New York 10276.
☎ 212 505 6880

☞▼ **E-MaleSM**
Liveday Enterprises, P. O. Box 14205, San Francisco, California 94114-0205.
☎ 800 930 9366 ✆ 415 285 2851
☎ 415 285 8520
✉ emalesm@emalesm.com
🕸 http://www.emalesm.com/~emalesm/

♀♀ **Leda**
P. O. Box 35, San Marcos, California 92079.

Mailorder: Books: Erotic

☺ ■ **K. L. Graphics**
Suite 73, 1194 Ala Kapua Street, Kailua-Kona, Hawaii 96740.
☎ 808 325 3157 ✆ 808 325 6326
🕐 Mon - Fri 07:00 - 18:00
⚫ ✓
Lithographs of the BDSM paintings of Sadao Hasegawa. Catalogue, $1. Age statement of 21 is required.

Mailorder: Books: General

⚘ **Berkana Press**
Suite 404, 491 Baltimore Pike, Springfield, Pennsylvania 19064.

☺ ■ **The Eclectic Connection**
Suite 163, 5350 North Broadway, Chicago, Illinois 60640.
International books, magazines, & catalogues.

☺ **The Enclave Book Repository**
P. O. Box 507, Oyster Bay, New York 11771.
☎ 516 922 1169

☺ ■ **Quality Paperback Book Club**
1271 Avenue of the Americas, New York 10020-9991.
☎ 212 522 4200
Sells alternative sexuality publications as well as mainstream ones.

⚘ ▼ **Sisterhood Bookstore**
1351 Westwood Boulevard, Los Angeles, California 90024.
☎ 310 477 7300

☺ ▼ **Womankind Books Inc.**
5 Kivy Street, Huntington Station, Long Island 11746.
☎ 516 427 1289
🕐 09:00 - 20:00
✓ VISA MC
Free catalogue.

⚘ **Women's Word Books**
P. O. Box 387, Springfield, Pennsylvania 19064.

⚘ **Women's Words Books**
902 B Upper Straw Road, Hopkinton, New Hampshire 03229.
☎ 603 228 8000

⚘ **Womontyme Distribution Company**
P. O. Box 50145, Long Beach, California 90815-6145.
☎ 800 247 8903

Mailorder: Books: Sexuality

☞ **Berdache Books**
P. O. Box 9081, Pittsburgh, Pennsylvania 15224.
☎ 412 687 5563

☞ ▼ **A Different Light**
151 West 19th. Street, New York 10011-4116.
☎ 800 343 4002
☎ 212 989 4850
✆ 415 431 6660
✉ adl@atg.org
⚫ ✓ $ VISA MC AMERICAN
Free catalogue published 3 times a year.

☞ **Giovanni's Room**
345 South 12th. Street, Philadelphia, Pennsylvania 19107.
☎ 215 923 2960 ✆ 215 923 0813
🕐 Mon - Sat 10:00 - 19:00
Catalogue available.

☞ **Glad Day Books**
2nd. Floor, 673 Boylston Street, Boston, Massachusetts 02116.
☎ 617 267 3010 ✆ 617 267 5474

⚘ **Heartland Books**
P. O. Box 1105 H, East Corinth, Vermont 05040.
☎ 802 439 5655

☞▼ **Lavendar Jade's**
⚐ P. O. Box 333, Clifton Park, New York 12065-0333.
☎ 518 798 3304

☺ **NSS Seminars, Inc.**
P.O. Box 5001, Ben Lomond, California 95005.
☎ 408 336 9281 ✆ 408 336 9283

✓
Sponsors the National Sexuality Symposium & Exposition in Sep. Publishes a newsletter quarterly.

Oscar Wilde Memorial Bookstore
15 Christopher Street, New York 10014.
☎ 212 255 8097
✓
Free catalogue.

Our World Too
11 South Vandeventer, Saint Louis, Missouri 63108.
☎ 314 533 5322

Paths Untrodden Book Service
P. O. Box 3245, Grand Central Station, New York 10163.
☎ 212 661 5997

People Like Us
1115 West Belmont, Chicago, Illinois 60657.
☎ 312 248 6363 Fax 312 248 1550
plubooks@aol.com
10:00 - 21:00
✓
Free 32-page catalogue published twice a year.

The Real World Emporium
P. O. Box 13125, Lansing, Michigan 48901-3125.
☎ 517 487 6495

Roads Less Travelled
Box 329, 3355 North Five Miles Road, Boise, Idaho 83704.
☎ 208 375 9090

Shaynew Press
P.O. Box 425221, San Francisco, California 94142.
☎ 415 391 9525
shaynew@well.com
http://www.well.com/user/shaynew
09:00 - 21:00
✓
High-quality books of fine art photographs on radical sexuality. Topics include consensual erotic power play, erotic piercings, SM, & non-standard penetration. Catalogue, $1, refundable with purchase. Age statement of 21 is required.

Synergy Book Service
P. O. Box 8, Flemington, New Jersey 08822.
☎ 908 782 101
✓
Publishes *The Whole Sex Catalog.*

Tomes & Treasures
202 South Howard Avenue, Tampa, Florida 33606.
☎ 813 251 9368
Mon - Sat 11:00 - 20:00, Sun 12:00 - 18:00

True Colors
P. O. Box 780969, San Antonio, Texas 78278-0969.
☎ 800 745 0555 Fax 210 408 0707
☎ 210 408 0505

Mailorder: Clothing: Adult Baby

Special Clothes
20 West Masonic View Avenue, Alexandria, Virginia 22301.
☎ 703 683 7343
Manufactures specialty clothing with "easy dressing" features for handicapped adults & children. Much of it looks like toddlers clothing. Not a part of the adult baby scene.

Very Special Clothes
P. O. Box 393, Marathon, Texas 79842.

Mailorder: Clothing: Chainmail

Der Barenhohle
P. O. Box 661521, Sacramento, California 95866.
☎ 916 488 2249
Chainmail hoods, clothings, & accessories. Custom work also available. Catalogue available.

Chain Maille Fashions
1706 Norris Drive, Austin, Texas 78704-2808.
☎ 800 729 4094
☎ 512 447 6040
Mon - Fri 09:00 - 21:00, visits by appointment
✓ $
Primarily medieval styles, but also custom work.

Mailorder: Clothing

Eve Browne Fashions
17th. Floor, 521 5th. Avenue, New York 10175.
Lingerie, TV/TS accessories, magazines, sex education materials, toys, etc..

Mailorder: Clothing: Fetish

ACE Saddle Company
P. O. Box 733, Woodinville, Washington 98702.
Fetish & fantasy leather clothing, whips, etc..

Après Noir
Suite E, 1055 Broadway, Sonoma, California 95476.
☎ 707 935 6595 Fax 707 935 6597
bdyaware@ix.netcom.com
Fetish underwear for men. Catalogue, £2 or $3U.S..

Bootmen Leathers
421 Glovenia Street, Eden, North Carolina 27288.
☎ 800 216 2668 Fax 910 627 7154
☎ 910 627 7154
Mail order also. Catalogue, $5.

Caprice
P. O. Box 27655, Los Angeles, California 90227.

Christopher Briston Enterprises
P. O. Box 332, Elma, New York 14059.
Used firemen's uniforms & other heavy rubber clothing. Catalogue, free with SASE or IRC.

Constance Enterprises
P.O. Box 43079, Upper Montclair, New Jersey 07043.
☎ 201 746 4200 Fax 201 746 4722
☎ 201 746 5466
Tue - Sat 12:00 - 18:00
✓ $

Dream Dresser
P. O. Box 16158, Beverly Hills, California 90209-2158.
☎ 213 848 3480

Fantasies In Lace, Inc.
P. O. Box 100279, Fort Lauderdale, Florida 33310.
☎ 305 581 8412 Fax 305 791 0985
Hosiery & other clothing for crossdressers.

Fantasies Unlimited
P. O. Box 1688, Jupiter, Florida 33468-1688.
☎ 407 743 4244 Fax 407 743 0588
High-heel shoes & stocking, foot fetish supplies, & videos.

Fantasy Fashions
P. O. Box 910, Westmount, Illinois 60559.
Catalogue, $10.

Fashion World International
P.O. Box 277506, Sacramento, California 95827.
☎ 916 631 8777 Fax 916 631 9339
916 985 3307 (free BBS)
bobh@fashion.win.net
http://www.quiknet.com/fashion/fwi.html
24hr. ordering service
✓
64-page catalogue, $20, plus $3 shipping ($8 overseas). Age statement of 21 is required.

Leather & Lust
424 Roselle Street, Linden, New Jersey 07036.
☎ 908 925 7110

Paul C Leather
Suite 959, 2421 West Pratt, Chicago, Illinois 60645.
☎ 312 508 0848 Fax 312 508 0811
☎ 800 338 4740

Raiments
P. O. Box 93095, Pasadena, California 91109.
Historical clothing books, patterns & supplies. NOT in the fetish industry, but they do provide corsetry supplies.

Stanford Hygenic Corp.
P. O. Box 1160, Long Island City, New York 11101.
☎ 718 389 6433 Fax 718 383 0705

Voyages
Dept. AS, P. O. Box 78550, San Francisco, California 94107-8550.
☎ 415 495 4937 (service) Fax 415 896 0933
☎ 415 896 0706 (orders)
Spandex & satin items.

Wardrobes by Carolyn
P. O. Box 183-AS, Melrose, Massachusetts 02176.
☎ 617 662 4432
Also separate adult baby catalogue for $10. Catalogue, $10.

Wicked Ways
P. O. Box 16752, Alexandria, Virginia 22302.
☎ 703 379 4735 Fax 703 379 4735 (call first)
wways@aol.com
Mon - Sat 10:00 - 22:00
✓ $
Catalogue available. Age statement of 18 is required.

Mailorder: Clothing: Footwear

⊕ Aristoc Distributors
P. O Box 9133, Lyndhurst, New Jersey 07071.
Also sells leather, rubber, & PVC clothing. Catalogue, $5.

⊕ Rich Filia
P. O. Box 4188, San Diego, California 92164-4188.
☎ 619 298 1973
Motorcycle, pull-on, lace-up, lineman's, & logger boots.

☺ ■ Sexy Shoes (Leslie Shoe Company)
P. O. Box 48, Rogers City, Michigan 49779-0048.
☎ 517 734 4030
☎ 517 734 3211
⏰ Main number every day 08:00 - 24:00, 2nd. number Mon - Fri 09:00 - 17:00
Catalogue available.

⊕ ■ Shoe Express
P. O. Box 31537, Lafayette, Louisiana 70593-1537.
☎ 800 874 0469 (orders) 📞 318 235 5359
☎ 318 235 5191
⏰ Mon - Fri 09:00 - 18:00, Sat 09:00 - 17:00
✓ $ 💳 💳 💳
20-page catalogue available.

Mailorder: Clothing: General

☺ ■ Amazon Drygoods
2218 East 11th. Street, Davenport, Iowa 52803.
☎ 800 798 7979 📞 319 322 4003
☎ 319 322 6800
⏰ Mon - Fri 09:00 - 17:00, other times by chance
Historical & reproduction clothing & corsets. In addition to main catalogue, have shoe ($5), corset ($17, colour), & sewing pattern ($7) catalogues. Catalogue, $3U.S..

☺ ■ Maitresse
P. O. Box 384, Fairport, New York 14450.
☎ 800 456 8464 📞 716 586 3720
Specialises in gloves, but also carries corsets, girdles, & lingerie.

☺ Noelle Nielson Softwear
P.O. Box 69826, West Hollywood, California 90069.

Mailorder: Clothing: Leather

♂▼ The Bear Man
92 River Drive, Tequesta, Florida 33469.
☎ 407 743 8701
⏰ By appointment only
💳 $ 💳 💳 💳

☺ ■ Black On Black Leathers
P. O. Box 1485, El Cajon, California 92002.
☎ 619 442 6614

☺ ■ World Domination
P. O. Box 1099, New York 10116-1099.
Also custom work by appointment.

Mailorder: Clothing: Lingerie

☺ ■ Frederick's of Hollywood
P. O. Box 229, Hollywood, California 90099-0164.
☎ 818 993 3988

☺ Lady Midnight
#280, 1442-A Walnut Street, Berkeley, California 94709.
☎ 510 845 3823 📞 510 540 1057 Ext. 280

☺ ■ Monique of Hollywood
P. O. Box 85151, Los Angeles, California 90072.
Also sells high-heel boots & shoes, books, magazines, etc..

Mailorder: Clothing: Miscellaneous

☺ ■ Gravity Plus
P. O. Box 2182, La Jolla, California 92038.
☎ 800 383 8056 📞 619 456 8072
☎ 619 454 1626
Gravity boots & other suspension devices.

Mailorder: Clothing: Rubber

☺ ■ Aquala
16 Rubin Road, Rie, New Hampshire 03870.
☎ 603 772 5529
make rubber dry-suits for diving & windsurfing.

☺ ▼ Creative Imageware by J&M
P. O. Box 386, Davison, Michigan 48423.
Catalogue available.

☺ ■ Jerry's Misc. Services
P. O. Box 2064, Fairview Heights, Illinois 62208.
☎ 618 397 2709
Neoprene & leather items. Also rubber fetish videos.

☺ ■ Latex America
14985 South Dixie Highway, Miami, Florida 33176.
Catalogue, $10.

☺ ■ Mariner Wear
6 Hearthwood Drive, Barrington, Rhode Island 02806.
Custom rubber clothing.

☺ ■ Midnight Sun Rainwear
P. O. Box 257, Soldotna, Alaska 99669.
Catalogue, $5.

☺ ▼ Naughty Nancy
P. O. Box 22923, Seattle, Washington 98122-0923.
☎ 206 547 7042
⏰ Mon - Sat 10:00 - 20:00
💳 ✓ $
Custom latex clothing in an amazing array of colours, for those ot you tired of black. French also spoken.

☺ ■ Rainvain
2223 3rd. Avenue South East, Bothell, Washington 98201.
Catalogue, $6.

☺ ■ Wendy's
P. O. Box 85111, Los Angeles, California 90072.
Footwesr & rubber clothing. Catalogue, $6.

Mailorder: Erotica: Adult Baby

♀♂ ■ Annie's Orphans
P.O. Box 1199, Woodstock, New York 12498.
☎ 914 679 4030

☺ ■ Carolyn's Kids
P. O. Box 183-AS, Melrose, Massachusetts 02176.
☎ 617 662 4432
Also $44 video big baby video catalogue; TV catalogue $10. Catalogue, $8.

♀♂ ■ Crissy's Creations
Suite 102-186, 15817 Bernardo Center Drive, San Diego, California 92127.
Catalogue, $5.

♀♂ INCON
P.O. Box 11632, Columbia, South Carolina 29211.
📧 googoob@aol.com
💳 $
Catalogue, free with SASE or IRC. Age statement of 21 is required.

♀♂ ■ JK Perfect Personal Products
P.O. Box 13383, Scottsdale, Arizona 85267-3383.

♀♂ ■ NK Products
P.O. Box 1184, Teaneck, New Jersey 07666-1184.
📧 templer1@ios.com
Publishes *Adult Baby World*.

♀♂ ■ Renas Boutique
76 Bank Street, Seymor, Connecticut 06483.
☎ 203 888 5164

♀♂ ■ Slimwear Of America
P.O. Box 997, Eastsound, Washington 98254.
☎ 360 376 5213 📞 360 376 5231
⏰ Closed Sat - Mon
Hand made full suits, inflatables, TV garments, bloomers, babywear. Catalogue, $17.50U.S. for U.S., $20 elsewhere. Age statement of 21 is required.

♀♂ ■ TAM Design
P.O. Box 1432, Salem, New Hampshire 03079-1432.
☎ 603 898 0316
📧 tamdesign@mv.mv.com
Publishes *Big Baby*.

♀♂ ■ V. I. Products, Inc.
P.O. Box 63, Three Oaks, Michigan 49128.
☎ 616 756 3561 📞 616 756 7382

Mailorder: Erotica

☺ ■ Aladdin Holdings Ltd.
6 Raphune Hill, Saint Thomas, Virgin Islands 00802.
 📞 809 775 7778
⏰ Mon - Sat 09:00 - 19:00 Eastern
💳 ✓
Mail orders honoured only where permitted by island law.

Mailorder: Erotica: BDSM

♂▼ Alternate Marketing
44-489 Town Center Way, Palm Desert, California 92260.
☎ 619 346 7374
Catalogue, $6. Age statement of 21 is required.

♂ Chase Products & FPN6D Services
P.O. Box 1014, Novi, Michigan 48376-0692.

☎ 810 348 8191 — Fax 810 348 8394
KVJV70E@Prodigy.com or TheHotLine@aol.com
✓ $ VISA MC
Erotic bondage supplies, enema equipment, medical instruments & supplies, chain cages, twitches & visible ball crusher, & unusual items. Catalogue, $2; on disk $3. Age statement of 21 is required.

☺ ▼ Chase Products
P. O. Box 1014, Novi, Michigan 48376-1014.
☎ 313 348 8191 — Fax 313 348 5332
🕘 09:00 - 23:00 (however, not always in office)
✓
Catalogue, $2. Age statement of 18 is required.

☺ Decorations by SLAN
Room 139, 825 East Roosevelt Road, Lombard, Illinois 60148-4744.
✓ $
Nipple clamps for well-dressed slaves. Also, some other select erotic toys & tools. Sorry, no telephone orders. Catalogue, $2. Age statement of 21 is required.

☺ ■ Diversified Services
P. O. Box 35737, Brighton, Massachusetts 02135.
☎ 617 787 7426
jwarren@ds.tiac.net
✓ VISA MC
Catalogue, $2. Age statement of 21 is required.

☺ □ Fantasy Island Innovations, Inc.
1304 South West 160th. Avenue, Sunrise, Florida 33326.
☎ 800 785 9955 (orders)
Catalogue, $5.

☺ ■ The Fetish Network
Dept. 600, Suite 4-166, 20533 Biscayne Boulevard, North Miami Beach, Florida 33180.
☎ 800 536 6462
954 370 7007. 28800 baud maximum.
telnet:tfnbbs.com
🕘 Mon - Thu 12:00 - 20:00
✓ $ VISA MC
The largest organization of products & services in the world specializing in BDSM, fantasy, & fetish. A complete catalogue offering fetish & B&D videos, magazines, books, adult leather & toys, novelties, call services, contacts, & on-line BBS services. Quality & discretion with the best products from around the world. $20.00 discounts on orders.. Catalogue published quarterly, $20U.S. (includes free magazine). Age statement of 18 is required. Please see our display advertisement.

☺ ▼ The Finders
50 63rd. Place, Belmont Shore, California 90803.
🕘 07:00 - 17:00
✓
Hard-to-find medical items & other toys. Mail order only.

■ Galleria Diva (DivaNet)
P. O. Box 191576, San Francisco, California 94119-1576.
☎ 415 285 8157 — Fax 415 642 0396
divanet@zoom.com
http://www.zoom.com/divanet/
VISA MC

▼ The Higgins Collection
1950 Abundance Street, New Orleans, Louisiana 70122.
☎ 504 949 0386 — Fax 504 947 7671
AvenueBoys@aol.com
🕘 By appointment only
$ VISA MC
Age statement of 21 is required.

Jaybird's Toybox
P. O. Box 7466, Fort Lauderdale, Florida 33338.

☺ ▼ Laws Leather
3016 Chatham Avenue, Cleveland, Ohio 44113-4029.
☎ 216 961 0939
🕘 By appointment only

☺ The Leather Man, Inc.
111 Christopher Street, New York 10014-4222.
☎ 800 243 5330 — Fax 212 243 5372
☎ 212 243 5339
$ VISA MC
Catalogue available. Age statement of 21 is required. Spanish also spoken.

☺ ■ Leatherhood
4000 Sierra Vista, Sacramento, California 95820.
☎ 916 456 8649 — Fax 916 451 6906
cit&gmt@aol.com
🕘 Evenings
✓ $
Custom work only. Floggers, restraints, paddles, etc.. 8-page catalogue available, published twice a year. Age statement of 18 is required. Spanish also spoken.

☺ ■ Mind Candy Emporium
P. O. Box 931437, Hollywood, California 90093.
☎ 818 907 3199 — Fax 818 886 0017

☺ ■ Morgan's Toybox
P. O. Box 487, Pasadena, Maryland 21122-0104.

▼ Mr. S – Fetters, U.S.A.
310 7th. Street, San Francisco, California 94103.
☎ 800 746 7677 — Fax 415 863 7798
☎ 415 863 7764
🕘 Mon - Sat 11:00 - 19:00
✓ VISA MC
The world's largest leather & latex store & mail order catalogue. Over 2,000 different items in a continually growing inventory. 200-page catalogue, $20U.S. to U.S., $30U.S. foreign. Age statement of 18 is required.

■ San Francisco Dungeon
Suite 263, 110 Pacific Avenue, San Francisco, California 94111-1900.
http://www.sfdungeon.com/

▼ Sandmutopia Supply Company
P. O. Box 410390, San Francisco, California 94141-1314.
☎ 415 252 1195 — Fax 415 252 9574

▼ Scene Gear
512 Observer Highway 1 East/West, Hoboken, New Jersey 07030.
phj@pilot.njin.net
http://www.freedom-subdued.org/forsale/psychie.html
Custom work also available. Please make cheques payable to Patricia Ju.

Larry Townsend
P.O. Box 302, Beverly Hills, California 90213.
☎ 213 463 2333 — Fax 213 655 7314
✓ VISA MC
Catalogue, $2. Age statement of 21 is required. Please see our display advertisement.

☺ ▼ Tuff Stuff
1714 East McDowell Road, Phœnix, Arizona 602 254 9651.
☎ 602 254 9561
🕘 Tue - Fri 09:00 - 18:00, Sat - 15:00

☺ Unique Creations
Suite 13, 3868 Pennwood, Las Vegas, Nevada 98102.
☎ 702 365 1818

The Fetish Network

The largest organization of products and services in the world specializing in SM, Fantasy, Fetish, & Roleplay.

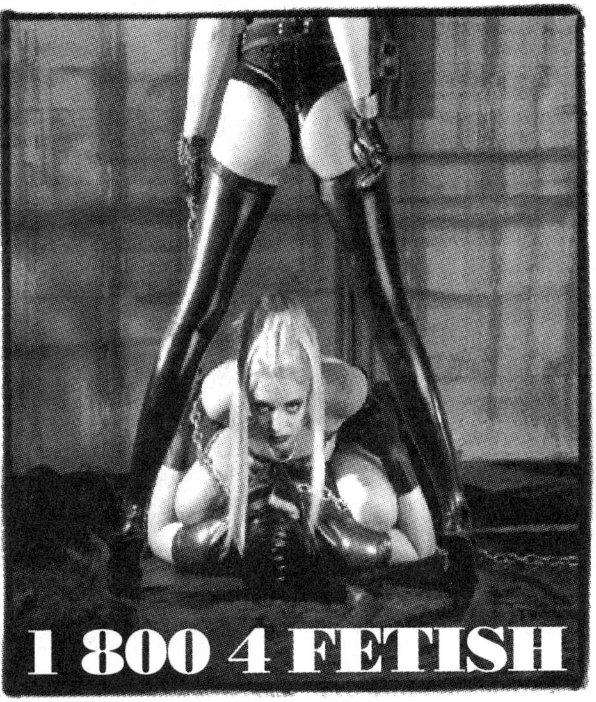

Photo copyright © Todd Friedman

Fetish Videos o Adult Toys o Books
Magazines o Events o BBS
Call Services

Meet others across the nation. The kinkiest connection ever!
Fantasy recordings, classifieds and ONE on ONE!
1 900 745-2953 or 1 800 248-3769 *adults over 18*
Talk to Goddess Dianna Vesta, Lady Beclan, or other well known Domina's for advice, training, consulting or fantasy.
Call **1 800 5 DOMINA**
Major Credit Cards Accepted

Send age statement and SASE for free info:
TFN Research Group, Inc. 20533 Biscayne Blvd. Suite 4-166
Dept.600, North Miami Beach, FL 33180
1 800 4 FETISH, BBS:(954)316-8990, telnet:tfnbbs.com

☺ ■ **Whip Me Raw**
2330 Margo South West, Albuquerque, New Mexico.
☎ 505 873 4981
Custom work also available.

☺ ■ **Zak Designs**
P. O. Box 212, Indiana, Pennsylvania 15701.
☎ 814 445 5319 ✆ 814 446 5755
Catalogue, $5.

Mailorder: Erotica: Bondage

☺ ■ **Lucifer's Armory**
#808, 874 Broadway, New York 10003.

☺ ■ **Male-order Leather**
P. O. Box 787, Danbury, Connecticut 06813.

☺ ■ **Mooring & Mooring**
Suite 116, 7266 Franklin Street, Los Angeles, California 90046.

☺ ■ **Paraphernalia from Beyond Planet X**
P.O. Box 236073, Columbus, Ohio 43223.
☎ 614 272 8984
✓
Mail sales of illustrated bondage-oriented buttons, keychains, "Sold" tags, doorsigns. Primarily female submissive items, expanding to male submissive items. Catalogue free with SAE or IRC. Publishes *Bound To Tease*. Age statement of 18 is required.

☺ ▼ **Spandex from the Imagination of Mark I. Chester**
P. O. Box 422501, San Francisco, California 94142.
☎ 415 621 6294
✉ markic@queernet.org
🕸 http://www.blackiris.com/mchester/michome.html
🕐 Viewing by appointment
🏠 ✓
Unisex spandex bondage gear & fetish clothing: hoods, bodybags, sleepsacks, bondage sacks & catsuits in thick black four-way stretch spandex. Catalogue, $5.

Mailorder: Erotica

☺ **The Christopher Collection**
P. O. Box 5960, Scottsdale, Arizona 85261-5960.
☎ 800 851 0690 ✆ 800 851 0069

☺ **Colt Studios**
P. O. Box 1608, Studio City, California 91614-0608.
☎ 800 445 2758 ✆ 818 985 2145
☎ 818 985 5786

☺ **Condom Wrap**
2038 East 4th. Street, Long Beach, California 90814.
☎ 310 430 3379

☺ ■ **Forbidden Fruit**
♿ 512 Neches, Austin, Texas 78701.
☎ 512 478 8358 ✆ 512 478 8358
🏠 ✓ 💳
Also sells leather items.

Mailorder: Erotica: General

☺▼ **Catalog X**
♿ 850 North East 13th. Street, Fort Lauderdale, Florida 33304.
☎ 954 524 5050 ✆ 954 524 3288
🕐 Mon - Fri 08:00 - 20:00, Sat Sun 12:00 - 17:00
🏠 ✓ 💳
The largest gay & lesbian erotic mail order company in the U.S.. Also the largest retail outlet of its kind in the U.S.. Catalogue, $3. Age statement of 18 is required. Spanish & Portugese also spoken.

☺ ■ **Continental Spectator**
P. O. Box 278, Canal Street Station, New York 10013.
☎ 800 325 4122 ✆ 718 834 8520
🕐 Mon - Fri 09:00 - 17:00
✓ 💳
Catalogue, $3.95.

☺ ▼ **Eve's Garden**
♿ Suite 420, 119 West 57th. Street, New York 10019-2303.
☎ 800 848 3837 ✆ 212 977 4306
☎ 212 757 8651
✉ evesgard@soho.ios.com
🕸 http://www.eve's-garden.com
🕐 Mon - Sat 12:00 -19:00
$ 💳
Women's sexuality mail order company encouraging women to explore & celebrate their sexuality. Catalogue published twice a year, $3, deductible from 1st. purchase. Spanish & French also spoken.

☺ ▼ **Toys in Babeland**
711 East Pike Street, Seattle, Washington 98122.
☎ 800 658 9119 ✆ 206 328 2994
☎ 206 328 2914
✉ babeland@aol.com

🕐 Mon - Fri 10:00 - 18:00, Sat 12:00 - 18:00
✓ $ 💳
Large array of high-quality sex toys, including dildos, vibrators, sensation toys, oils, & other sundries. Also books, videos, & comics. Catalogue, $2U.S..

☺ ■ **Versatile Fashions**
P.O. Box 1051, Tustin, California 92681.
☎ 800 546 2902 ✆ 714 538 7950
☎ 714 538 6498
✉ VFashion@palace.com
🕐 Mon - Sat 11:00 - 19:00
🏠 ✓ 💳
Also corsets for TV & others. Mail order, & shop in Anaheim. Catalogue available. Age statement of 21 is required.

☺ ■ **Windfaire Exxxotic Gifts**
♿ 3885 Buford Highway North East, Atlanta, Georgia 30329.
☎ 404 634 9463
🕐 Mon - Sat 10:00 - 21:00, Sun 13:00 - 18:00

Mailorder: Erotica

⚢ **Heaven Sent Me**
P. O. Box 270, Elbert, Colorado 80106.
☎ 719 495 3000

☺ **Intimate Treasures**
P.O. Box 77902, San Francisco, California 94107-0902.
☎ 415 863 5002 ✆ 415 896 0933
🕐 Mon - Fri 09:00 - 17:00
🏠 ✓ 💳
Erotic products & catalogues. Catalogue, $5. Age statement of 21 is required.

☺ ■ **Klystra**
1194 Ala Kapua Street, Kailua-Kona, Hawaii 96740.
☎ 808 325 3157 ✆ 808 325 6326
🕐 Mon - Fri 07:00 - 18:00
🏠 ✓
Sells enema equipment. Catalogue, $1. Age statement of 21 is required.

Mailorder: Erotica: Leather

☺▼ **Acme Toy Co.**
P. O. Box 1904, Evanston, Illinois 60201-1904.
☎ 312 536 1982 ✆ 708 862 7065
🏠 ✓ $
Catalogue available. Age statement of 26 is required.

☺ **Fantasy Leathers**
P. O. Box, Springfield, Oregon 97477.

☺ ■ **Master Leathers**
P. O. Box 36091, Tucson, Arizona 85740.
✓
Mail order only. Catalogue, $7. Age statement of 21 is required.

☺ ▼ **R. K. Unlimited**
Suite 609, 6606 West Lisbon Avenue, Milwaukee, Wisconsin 53210.
☎ 414 342 1411 ✆ 414 342 4667
Catalogue, $10.

☺ ■ **The Stockroom**
4649-1/2 Russell Avenue, Los Angeles, California 90027.
☎ 800 755 8697 ✆ 213 913 5976
☎ 213 666 2121
✉ jttoys@world.std.com & jttoys@access.digex.net
🕸 http://www.stockroom.com
🕐 Mon - Sat 10:00 - 22:00
🏠 ✓ 💳
32-page catalogue, $15.

☺ **Vyxyn's Leatherworks & Urbane Armory**
P. O. Box 176, Madisonville, Tennessee 37354.
Fantasy armor, belts, boot straps, bracelets, collars, cuffs, & other accessories. Also custom work. Make cheques payable to ISES. Catalogue, $3. Age statement of 21 is required.

🕴 ■ **XTC Leather of New York**
P. O. Box 213, Hazlet, New Jersey 07730.
☎ 908 739 1354 ✆ 908 739 9402
✉ sysop@palace.com
🕸 http://palace.com/xtc/index.htm

Mailorder: Erotica

⚢ **Malibu Sales**
P. O. Box 4371, Los Angeles, California 90078-4371.
☎ 213 871 1225

☺ **Marc Sanders Mail Order**
399 Jayne Avenue, Oakland, California 94610.
☎ 510 444 3204

⚢ **Mercury Mail Order**
Dept. AS, 4084 18th. Street, San Francisco, California 94114-2534.
☎ 415 621 1188

☺ **Montana American West Company**
P. O. Box 6395, Bozeman, Montana 59715.
☎ 800 262 9269

Mailorder: Piercing Jewelry

☺ ■ **Bravo**
P. O. Box 76919, Tampa, Florida 33675-1919.
☎ 813 689 1414 ✆ 813 689 3041
Wholesale enquiries welcome.

☺ ▼ **Gauntlet, Inc. Mail Order & Customer Service**
Box 801, 2215-R Market Street, San Francisco, California 94114.
☎ 800 746 4728 ✆ 415 252 1407
☎ 415 252 1404
✉ kane@gauntlet.com
🌐 http://www.gauntlet.com/
⚫ ✓ $ 💳 💳
Catalogue, $5. Age statement of 21 is required.

☺ ■ **Ringmasters**
P. O. Box 548, Sun Valley, California 91353-0548.

Mailorder: Safer Sex Products

☺ ■ **Adam & Eve**
P. O. Box 900, Carrboro, North Carolina 27510.
☎ 800 274 0333 ✆ 800 794 3318
☎ 919 644 1212
🕐 24hrs.
✓ $ 💳 💳
Free catalogue.

☺ ■ **OPC Supply**
P. O. Box 34463, Omaha, Nebraska 68134-0463.
☎ 402 451 7987 ✆ 402 457 5350
✉ imsl@synergy.net
⚫ ✓ $ 💳 💳
Source of medical supplies for BDSMers. Age statement of 21 is required.

Mailorder: Military Surplus

☺ ■ **Shomer-Tec**
P. O. Box 2039, Bellingham, Washington 98227.
☎ 206 733 6214

Mailorder: Videos: BDSM

♂ ■ **Masta Entertainment**
P. O. Box 411050, San Francisco, California 94141.
☎ 800 996 2782 ✆ 415 695 2936
☎ 415 346 3793
Bringing you the widest selection of BDSM & fetish videos, at the lowest prices you will see anywhere. Catalogue available. Age statement of 21 is required.

♂ ▼ **P. M. Productions**
P. O. Box 4135, West New York, New York 07093.
☎ 800 336 9696

Mailorder: Videos: Body Type

♂ ▼ **Altomar Productions**
#13-114, 1500 West El Camino Boulevard, Sacramento, California 95833.
☎ 916 641 1930
🕐 mon - Fri 09:00 - 18:00 Pacific
✓ 💳 💳 💳
Fantasy sex videos with mostly hairy, uncut, tattooed, mature men (over 40). Free brochure, $5 for full package of information. Mail order only.

Mailorder: Videos: Erotic

♂ ▼ **Atkol Entertainment**
Store 7, 912 South Avenue, Plainfield, New Jersey 07062-1852.
☎ 908 756 2001 ✆ 908 756 0923

☺ **Bijou Video**
1363 North Wells Street, Chicago, Illinois 60610.
☎ 800 932 7111 ✆ 312 337 1270
☎ 312 337 3404
🕐 24hrs., 7 days a week
⚫ ✓ $ ✆ 💳 💳 ⓓ 📧 ℓ
Catalogue published once a year, $32.95U.S.. Age statement of 21 is required.

♂ **Fox Studio**
P. O. Box 641, Venice, California 90294.
☎ 310 399 4770

♂ **Man's Hand Films**
#500, 633 Post Street, San Francisco, California 94109.
☎ 415 771 3918
Catalogue, $3.

♂ **Old Reliable**
Suite 107, 1626 North Wilcox Avenue, Los Angeles, California 90028.

Mailorder: Videos: Fetish

☺ **Concept Imports**
P. O. box 38930, Los Angeles, California 90038.

♂ ■ **Kink Video**
P. O. Box 150790, Brooklyn, New York 11215-0790.
☎ 718 832 3952
✉ nfn@netcom.com

♂♂ **Platinum Video**
4501 Van Nuys Boulevard, Sherman Oaks, California 91403.
☎ 818 503 0280
Videos on foot worship, tickling, enemas, spanking, etc..

Mailorder: Videos: Sexuality

♀ ▼ **Fatale Video**
Box 400, 530 Howard Street, San Francisco, California 94105-3007.
☎ 800 845 4617
☎ 415 861 4723
🕐 Mon - Fri 10:00 - 16:00
⚫ ✓ 💳 💳
Free catalogue. Age statement of 18 is required.

☺ ■ **Lifestyles Organization**
2641 West La Palma Avenue, Anaheim, California 92801-2602.
☎ 714 821 9953 ✆ 714 821 1465
✓ 💳 💳
Publishes *Emerge Playcouple* every two months. Age statement of 18 is required.

Manufacturers: Adult Toys: BDSM

☺ ■ **LifeStyle Leather & Wood**
4378 Whipporwill Road, Gillsville, Georgia 30543.
☎ 706 869 9606
✉ lslw@mindspring.com
🕐 Factory open to visitors. Call for appointment
⚫ ✓ $
Toys of leather, wood, latex, & rubber. Wholesale & retail sales. Special pricing for organizations & clubs. Catalogue, $5. Age statement of 21 is required.

Manufacturers: Clothing: Chainmail

☺ ▼ **Strangeblades & More**
Box 154, 286 Broad Street, Manchester, Connecticut 06040-4034.
☎ 203 645 9394
✉ sblades@aol.com
🕐 11:00 - 23:00
⚫ ✓ $ 💳 💳
We handcraft chain mail fashions & accessories, unique jewelry, custom knives, & some leatherwork. Both a fetish as well as a chain mail & jewelry catalogue will be available in by winter 1995. We also wholesale. Catalogue, $1U.S. Age statement of 18 is required.

Manufacturers: Regalia

☺ ▼ **OLLIE of ORLANDO**
2346 Keystone Drive, Orlando, Florida 32806-4662.
☎ 407 843 5621
🕐 24hrs. answering machine
⚫ $
Wholesale club & run buttons & other item. Mail order only.

Manufacturers: Whips

☺ ■ **Adam's Sensual Whips - Gillian's Toys**
P.O. Box 1146, New York 10156.
☎ 516 842 1711 ✆ 516 842 7518
☎ 212 686 5248
✉ siradam@ix.netcom.com
🌐 http://palace.com/utopian/utopian.htm
✓ 💳 💳
Catalogue, $3.

☺ ▼ **Lashes by Sarah**
Suite 39, 2336 Market Street, San Francisco, California 94114-1521.
☎ 415 621 6048
🕐 11:00 - 21:00
⚫ $ 💳
Cheques payable to S. Jones. Catalogue, $5. Age statement of 21 is required.

☺ **RAWhips**
1980 Lincoln Street, Eugene, Oregon 97405-2602.
✉ RAWhips@aol.com

☺ **San Francisco Whip Company**
P. O. Box 401033, San Francisco, California 94140.
☎ 415 804 7676
Exquisitely handcrafted floggers. Custom made in your choice of leathers. Very reasonable prices. Leather phalluses, harness gags, & other toys.

Organizations: Academic: Psychiatry

☺ □ **The American Association of Sex Educators, Counsellors, & Therapists (AASECT)**
Suite 1717, 435 Michigan Avenue, Chicago, Illinois 60611-4067.
☎ 312 644 0828 ✆ 312 644 8557
⏱ Mon - Fri 08:00 - 17:00 Central
Certifies the professional public as sex educators, therapists, & counsellors. Referral service to the public. Membership $130/year, directory $15, newletter $65/year, journal $30/year.

Organizations: AIDS: Information

☺ **Center for Disease Control**
P. O. Box 830409, Birmingham, Alabama 35283.
☎ 205 991 6920
✉ aidsinfo@cdc-nac.aspensys.com
✉ gopher://cdcnac.aspensys.com:72
Publishes *CDC AIDS Weekly*.

☺ □ **TPA Network**
♿ 1258A West Belmont Avenue, Chicago, Illinois 60657.
☎ 312 404 8726 ✆ 312 472 7505
⏱ Mon - Fri 09:00 - 17:00
✓ VISA MC
HIV/AIDS treatment information & related information & discussion. Publishes *Positively Aware* every two months. Yearly subscription is $15U.S. for U.S., $25 elsewhere.

Organizations: BDSM

♂▽ **BIG**
Box 4, 2336 Market Street, San Francisco, California 94114.
Vaccuum pump club.

♂ **Cosmic Order of KA**
115 East Vine Street, Inverness, Florida 34450-4207.
☎ 904 726 2403
Age statement of 21 is required.

♂▽ **Dads & Sons**
Suite 140, 1278 Glenneyre, Laguna Beach, California 92651.
♨ ✓
Contact: Mr. Kenneth Ulbrich
For daddies & sons who are not related. Age statement of 18 is required.

♂▽ **Mavericks**
P. O. Box 9543, Santa Fe, New Mexico 87504.

Organizations: Bondage

♂▽ **The Foot & Rope Club**
P. O. Box 24173, Speedway, Indiana 46224.

Organizations: Family

☺ □ **Parents & Friends of Lesbians & Gays (PFLAG)— National Office**
P. O. Box 27605, Washington, District of Columbia 20038.
☎ 800 432 6459 ✆ 202 638 0243
☎ 202 638 4200
✉ pflag-talk@vector.casti.com
E-mail address is that of their Internet discussion mailing list. Publishes *PFLAGPole* quarterly.

Organizations: Fetish: Dildo

♂▽ **National Dildo Club**
P. O. Box 29758, Los Angeles, California 90005.

Organizations: Fetish: Foot

♂ ■ **The Foot Fraternity**
P. O. Box 24102, Cleveland, Ohio 44124.
☎ 216 449 4114 ✆ 216 449 0114
⏱ 24hrs.
♨ ✓
Contact: Mr. Doug Gaines
Publishes a newsletter. Yearly subscription is $45. Age statement of 18 is required.

♂▽▼ **The National Foot Network (NFN)**
P. O. Box 150790, Brooklyn, New York 11215-0790.
☎ 718 832 3952
✉ nfn@netcom.com
VISA MC
Publishes *Foot Scene*. Yearly subscription is $30. Age statement of 21 is required.

Organizations: Fetish: Mess

♂ **Club Mud**
P.O. Box 277, Rio Nido, California 95471.
♨ ✓
Contact: Duke
International male membership. Also sells videos, photo sets, etc.. Catalogue, $3. Age statement of 21 is required.

Organizations: Fisting

♂▽ **TRUST (FF National Network)**
c/o ASP, P. O. Box 14543, San Francisco, California 94114.

Organizations: Health

☺ □ **American Social Health Association (ASHA)**
P. O. Box 13827, Research Triangle Park, North Carolina 27709.
☎ 919 361 8400
ASHA is a non-government organization & is the only organization devoted solely to the prevention of STDs.

♂ **National Lesbian & Gay Health Association**
1407 S Street North West, Washington, District of Columbia 20009.
☎ 202 939 7880 ✆ 202 234 1467
Network of lesbian & gay community health centers & health educators, researchers, & service providers.

Organizations: Motorcycle

♂ **Atlantic Motorcycle Coördinating Council**
P. O. Box 6463, JFK Station, Boston, Massachusetts 02114-0017.
☎ 215 634 7156
Contact: Mr. Ed Glaser, President
AMCC is an umbrella organization of 25 clubs from the District of Columbia to Montreal, Québec. Age statement of 21 is required.

Organizations: Scat

♂▽ **Jack's Number Two**
P.O. Box 542253, Houston, Texas 77253.
Publishes a newsletter quarterly.

Organizations: Sexual Politics

☺ □ **The Bar Association for Human Rights**
P. O. Box 1899, Grand Central Station, New York 10163.
☎ 212 431 2156

♀ **National Center for Lesbian Rights**
Suite 570, 870 Market Street, San Francisco, California 94102.
☎ 415 392 6257 ✆ 415 392 8442
Publishes a newsletter quarterly.

♂ **National Center for Lesbian Rights**
Suite 500A, 462 Broadway, New York 10013.
☎ 212 343 9589 ✆ 212 343 9687 (call first)
Publishes a newsletter quarterly.

Organizations: Sexuality

⚲▽ **American Transsexual Education Center (ATEC)**
Suite 584, 1626 North Wilcox Avenue, Los Angeles, California 90028.
☎ 213 389 6938

⚲▽ **Montgomery Medical & Psychological Institute— Georgia**
♿ P. O. Box 33311, Decatur, Georgia 30033.
☎ 404 321 9343
⏱ 12:00 - 18:00
♨ ✓ $ VISA MC
Full service gender programme, including helpline, support, individual & group therapy, professional referrals, seminars, etc. Confidential. Other publications available. Publishes *Insight* quarterly. Yearly subscription is $22. Age statement of 18 is required.

♂ **Partners Task Force for Gay & Lesbian Couples**
P. O. Box 9685, Seattle, Washington 98109-0685.
☎ 206 955 1206
✉ Demian@eskimo.com
✉ http://www.eskimo.com/~demian/partners.html
✓ $ VISA MC
Contact: Mr. Steve Bryant
National resource for same-sex couples. Supporting the diverse community of committed gay & lesbian partners through a variety of media.

Organizations: Shaving

♂ **Clippers**
P.O. Box 5871, Santa Monica, California 90405.

♂▽ **We Enjoy Shaving**
P. O. Box 6316, Reno, Nevada 89513.

Organizations: Tattoo

♂▽ **National Tattoo Association**
P. O. Box 2063, New Hyde Park, New York 11040-0701.

Organizations: Watersports

♂ **Water Boys of San Diego**
#163, 1278 University Avenue, San Diego, California 92103.
☎ 619 525 7755

Piercers

☺ ■ **Body Aware**

Suite E, 1055 Broadway, Sonoma, California 95476.
707 935 6595 — 707 935 6597
bdyaware@ix.netcom.com
Maid's dresses, panties, stockings, camisoles, etc. made to fit men. Catalogue, £1 or $2U.S..

Printers: Adult

Eve Browne Fashions
17th. Floor, 521 5th. Avenue, New York 10175.

Public Speakers: Gender Issues

Niela Miller, M.S. Ed., LCSW, LMHC
132 Butternut Hollow, Nagog Woods, Massachusetts 01718-1004.
508 264 4565
niela@world.std.com
✓
Counselled crossdressers & transexuals for 13 years. Now training & supervising others working with this population. Book published in 1995.

Publishers: Directories: Sexuality

National Shemale Directory
Salishon Society, P. O. Box 1604, Eugene, Oregon 97440-1604.
503 688 4282

Places of Interest
Ferrari Publications, P. O. Box 37887, Phœnix, Arizona 85069.
602 863 2408

Publishers: Guides: Sexuality

Companion Publications
P. O. Box 54, Laguna Hills, California 92653.
714 362 4489
Specializes in lesbian, gay, & bisexual guides to entertainment, legal, medical, & travel topics.

Damron Address Book
Damron Company, P.O. Box 422458, San Francisco, California 94142-2458.
800 462 6654 — 415 703 9049
415 255 0404
Mon - Fri 08:30 - 17:00
✓
Also Woman's Traveller (once a year), a travel guide to North America for lesbians. Published once a year.

Odysseus
Odysseus International Ltd., P. O. Box 1548, Port Washington, New York 11050.
516 944 5330 — 516 944 7540
Mon - Fri 09:00 - 18:00
✓
Published once a year. Yearly subscription is $30.

The Poach Gay Guide
P. O. Box 1014, Novi, Michigan 48376-0692.
810 348 8191 — 810 348 8394
810 348 7854. 28800 baud maximum.
KVJV70E@Prodigy.com or TheHotLine@aol.com
24hrs.
✓ $
Recipients are encouraged to duplicate & distribute copies. Basic listings free. For extended listings, call, write, or e-mail for information. Age statement of 18 is required.

Publishers: Information: Sexuality

QueerAmerica
OutProud!, P. O. Box 24589, San José, California 95154-4589.
info@outproud.org
http://youth.org/outproud/
The national coalition for lesbian & gay youth serves the needs of young men & women by providing advocacy, information, resources, & support.

Publishers: Magazines: Alternative

Electronic Gay Community Magazine
Land of Awes Information Services, P. O. Box 16782, Wichita, Kansas 67216-0782.
316 269 0913 — 316 269 4208
316 269 3172. 19200 baud maximum.
egcm@f9.n291.zl.fidonet.org
http://fn.net/~awes/egcm.htm
18:000 - 22:00
The world's longest running online publication for the gay community, published by gay BBS systems for the Internet. Yearly subscription is free. Age statement of 18 is required.

Publishers: Magazines: BDSM

Dominantly Yours
Continental Spectator, P. O. Box 278, Canal Street Station, New York 10013.
800 325 4122
Mon - Fri 09:00 - 17:00
✓ $
Qaulity magazine with articles, stories, & contact ads. Published twice a year. Age statement of 21 is required.

Publishers: Magazines: Erotic

Black Lace
BLK Publishing Co., P. O. Box 83912, Los Angeles, California 90083-0912.
310 410 0808 — 310 410 9250
newsroom@netcom.com
http://www.blk.com/blk
09:00 - 18:00
✓ $
Published quarterly. Yearly subscription is $20.

BlackFire
BLK Publishing Co., P. O. Box 83912, Los Angeles, California 90083-0912.
310 410 0808 — 310 410 9250
newsroom@netcom.com
http://www.blk.com/blk
09:00 - 18:00
✓ $
Published every two months. Yearly subscription is $30.

Continental Spectator
Continental Spectator, P. O. Box 278, Canal Street Station, New York 10013.
800 325 4122
Mon - Fri 09:00 - 17:00
✓ $
Granddaddy of swingers magazines. Stories, articles, photos, & contact ads. Single copy, latest issue $15U.S. to U.S., $20U.S. elsewhere. Published quarterly. Yearly subscription is $45U.S. to U.S., $60U.S. elsewhere. Age statement of 21 is required.

Publishers: Magazines: Sexuality

BLK
BLK Publishing Co., P. O. Box 83912, Los Angeles, California 90083-0912.
310 410 0808 — 310 410 9250
newsroom@netcom.com
http://www.blk.com/blk
09:00 - 18:00
✓ $
Newsmagazine for the black lesbian & gay community. Published every month. Yearly subscription is $18.

Club TV
Continental Spectator, P. O. Box 278, Canal Street Station, New York 10013.
800 325 4122
Mon - Fri 09:00 - 17:00
✓ $
Stories, articles, photos, & personal ads. Age statement of 21 is required.

He-She Directory
P. O. Box 278, Canal Street Station, New York 10013.
800 325 4122 — 718 834 8520
Mon -Fri 09:00 - 17:00
✓ $
Letters of advice, stories, articles, & contact ads (with photos). Published twice a year. Age statement of 21 is required.

Lavendar Life
Lavendar Enterprises, P. O. Box 898, Binghamton, New York 13902.
607 771 1986 — 607 771 1987
✓ $
Lesbian magazine of fiction, peotry, etc.. Published every month. Yearly subscription is $18.

The Lesbian Calendar
TLC Productions, Box 132, 351 Pleasant Street, Northampton, Massachusetts 01060.
413 586 5514
Monthly listing of events, business & personal ads, & community announcements by, for, & about the lesbian community of Western New England. Northampton's only lesbian publication. Published 11 times a year. Yearly subscription is $25-30U.S. sliding scale.

Publishers: Mailing Lists: Libraries

Willowood Press
P. O. Box 1846, Minot, North Dakota 58702.
701 838 0579 — 701 838 3933
Public, college, high school libraries; college English departments.

Publishers: Newspapers: Sexuality

Kuumba

BLK Publishing Co., P. O. Box 83912, Los Angeles, California 90083-0912.
☎ 310 410 0808 ☏ 310 410 9250
📧 newsroom@netcom.com
🌐 http://www.blk.com/blk
🕐 09:00 - 18:00
🐾 ✓ $ ⚊ VISA 💳 💳 ℓ
Poetry for black lesbians & gay men. Published twice a year. Yearly subscription is $7.50.

♂▼ *Philadelphia Gay News (PGN)*
 ♿ Masco Communication, 505 South 4th. Street, Philadelphia, Pennsylvania 19147.
☎ 215 625 8501 ☏ 215 925 6437
📧 pgn@netaxs.com
🕐 09:00 - 17:00
🐾 ✓ $ ⚊ VISA 💳
Philadelphia's only newspaper of record for the gay, lesbian, & transgendered community. Published every week. Yearly subscription is $110.

Publishers: Videos: Sexuality

♂ Bijou Video
1363 North Wells Street, Chicago, Illinois 60610.
☎ 800 932 7111 ☏ 312 337 1270
☎ 312 337 3404
🕐 24hrs, 7 days a week
🐾 ✓ $ ⚊ VISA 💳 💳 💳 ℓ
Catalogue published once a year, $32.95U.S.. Age statement of 21 is required.

Stores: Books: General

♂▼ Category Six Books
 ⚲ 1029 East 11th. Avenue, Denver, Colorado 80218.
☎ 303 832 6263
🐾 ✓ $ ⚊ VISA 💳 💳

Stores: Clothing: Fetish

☺ SIN
616 East Pine Street, Seattle, Washington 98122.
☎ 800 315 7466 ☏ 206 727 3922
☎ 206 329 0324
📧 sin@aa.net
🌐 http://www.sin-inc.com
🕐 12:00 - 20:00
🐾 ✓ $ ⚊ VISA 💳 💳
Specialties: custom fetish wear & hardware, including shoes, corsets, clothing, literature, body jewelry, piercing, bondage equipment (racks, cages, etc.). We also wholesale & retail our own line of clothing, corsets, & hardware. Catalogue, $5U.S.. Age statement of 18 is required. German also spoken. Please see our display advertisement.

Stores: Erotica: General

☺ Come Again Erotic Emporium
 ♿☺ 353 East 53rd. Street, New York 10022.
☎ 212 308 9394
🕐 Mon - Fri 11:00 - 19:30, Sat 11:00 - 18:00
🐾 $ ⚊ VISA 💳 💳 💳 ℓ
Books & magazines; fetish publications; lingerie up to size 48, including leather & vinyl. Bondage equipment, vibrators, & other novelties. Catalogue, $4.

☺ ▼ Grand Opening!
Suite 32, Arcade Building, 318 Harvard Street, Brookline, Massachusetts 02146.
☎ 617 731 2626 ☏ 617 731 2693
🕐 Mon - Sat 10:00 - 19:00, Sun 12:00 - 17:00
🐾 ✓ $ ⚊ VISA 💳 💳
Boston area's first sexuality boutique especially, but not exclusively for women. BDSM friendly, with toys, books, & videos for everybody. Catalogue available.

Stores: Leatherwork Supplies: General

☺ ■ The Leather Factory
☎ 800 433 3201
☎ 915 858 0477
Over twenty stores throughout the United States.

☺ ■ Tandy Leather Co.
☎ 817 244 6404
Over 300 stores throughout the United States.

Suppliers: Market Research

☺ ▼ Rivendell Marketing Company
P. O. Box 518, Westfield, New Jersey 07091-0518.
☎ 908 232 2021 ☏ 908 232 0521
☎ 212 242 6863
🕐 09:00 - 17:00
🐾 ✓ $
Gay & lesbian marketing specialists since 1979.

Suppliers: Safer Sex Products
☺ ☐ **The Rubber Tree**
 & 4426 Burke Avenue North, Seattle, Washington 98103.
 ☎ 206 633 4750
 ⏲ Mon - Fri 10:00 - 19:00, Sat 10:00 - 18:00
 ⚲ ✓ $ ⚥
 Small non-profit retail store specializing in non-prescription birth control & safer sex supplies, resources, referrals. Education oriented. Catalogue, $1U.S. or 2 IRCs.

ALABAMA
Area: Approximately 131,600 square kilometres
Population: Approximately 4,060,000
Capital City: Montgomery
Time zone: GMT minus 6 hours (CST).

State Resources
Publishers: Newspapers: Sexuality
⚥▽ **The Alabama Forum**
 & Suite 216, 205 32nd. Street South, Birmingham, Alabama 35233-3007.
 ☎ 205 328 9228
 ✉ AlForum@aol.com
 ⚲ ✓ $ ⚥
 Non-profit newspaper, a forum for ideas, concerns, issues of the gay, lesbian, bisexual, transgender community. City, state, national, & international news, features, community events, & directory. Published every month. Yearly subscription is $15U.S..

Anniston
Organizations: AIDS: Support
☺ ☐ **AIDS Services Center, Inc.**
 & P. O. Box 1392, Anniston, Alabama 36202.
 ☎ 205 835 0923

Auburn
Organizations: AIDS: Support
☺ ☐ **Lee County AIDS Outreach**
 P. O. Box 1971, Auburn, Alabama 36831.
 ☎ 205 887 5244
Organizations: Sexuality
⚥▽ **Auburn Gay & Lesbian Association (AGALA)**
 & P. O. Box 821, Auburn, Alabama 36831-0821.
 ⏲ Meets Wed 19:30
Stores: Books: General
☺ ■ **Etc.**
 & 125 North College Street, Auburn, Alabama 36830.
 ✉ 205 821 0080

Birmingham
Archives: Sexuality
⚥▽ **Barnes Memorial Library, Lambda, Inc.**
 P. O. Box 55913, Birmingham, Alabama 35255.
 ☎ 205 326 8600
Counsellors
☺ ■ **Almont Counselling Associates**
 & Suite 112, 956 Montclair Road, Birmingham, Alabama 35213.
 ☎ 205 591 5113
☺ **Jody Gottlieb, Ph.D.**
 2117 16th. Avenue South, Birmingham, Alabama 35205.
 ☎ 205 933 6501
 Individual & couples therapy, including alternative lifestyle issues such as parenting, relationships, homophobia, & supportive clarification of sexual orientation.
☺ **George James, Ph.D.**
 Suite 112, 956 Montclair Road, Birmingham, Alabama 53213.
 Stress, anxiety, depression, gay-related issues, & relationship counselling.
Health Services
☺ ☐ **University of Alabama Hospital**
 619 South 19th. Street, Birmingham, Alabama 35233.
 ☎ 205 975 7545
 HIV & emergency departments.
Helplines: Sexuality
⚥▽ **Gay/Lesbian Information Line**
 & P. O. Box 55913, Birmingham, Alabama 35255.
 ☎ 205 326 8600

⏲ 18:00 - 20:00
TDD available.

Organizations: AIDS: Education
☺ ☐ **Birmingham AIDS Outreach**
 & P. O. Box 55070, Birmingham, Alabama 35255.
 ☎ 205 322 4197
 ⏲ 08:30 - 17:30
 Publishes *Outreach Newsletter.*
Organizations: AIDS: Support
☺ ☐ **AIDS Task Force of Alabama**
 P. O. Box 55703, Birmingham, Alabama 35255.
 ☎ 205 592 2437
 ☎ 205 591 4448 (AIDS/STD hotline)
Organizations: Sexuality
⚥▽ **Lambda Resourcer Center**
 & P. O. Box 55913, Birmingham, Alabama 35255.
 ☎ 205 326 8600
Organizations: Sexuality: Student
⚥▽ **LGB Awareness League**
 P. O. Box A14, Birmingham Southern College, Birmingham, Alabama 35254-0001.
⚥▽ **UAB G/L Student Union**
 P. O. Box 34, Birmingham, Alabama 35294-1150.
Stores: Books: General
☺ ▼ **Lodestar Books**
 & 2020 11th. Avenue South, Birmingham, Alabama 35205.
 ☎ 205 939 3356 ✉ 205 939 3356
Stores: Erotica: General
☺ ■ **Alabama Adult Books**
 & 901 5th. Avenue, Birmingham, Alabama 35203.
 ☎ 205 322 7323
☺ ■ **Birmingham Adult Books**
 7610 1st. Avenue North, Birmingham, Alabama 35206.
 ☎ 205 836 1580

Florence
Publishers: Magazines: BDSM
☺ ■ **The Wild Side**
 TWS Ent., Suite 405, 803 Hermitage Drive, Florence, Alabama 35630.
 Articles & ads for couples, men, & women who enjoy BDSM, bi/gay fantasies, fetishes, TVs/crossdressing, etc.. Yearly subscription is $10U.S. for U.S., $11U.S. elsewhere.

Hoover
Organizations: BDSM
⚥▽ **Pendragons of Birminham**
 Suite 272, 210 Loma Square, Hoover, Alabama 35216.

Huntsville
Health Services
☺ ☐ **Huntsville Hospital**
 101 Sively Road, Huntsville, Alabama 35801.
 ☎ 205 533 8020
Organizations: AIDS: Education
☺ ■ **AIDS Action Coalition**
 & P. O. Box 871, Huntsville, Alabama 35804.
 ☎ 205 533 2437
 Publishes *The Summit.*
Organizations: AIDS: Support
☺ ■ **Davis Clinic**
 & P. O. Box 425, Huntsville, Alabama 35804.
 ☎ 205 533 2437
Organizations: BDSM
☺ ☐ **A.S.B. Munch—Huntsville**
 ✉ wi.159@wizvax.com
 Contact: Dave
Organizations: Sexuality
⚥▽ **The Society for the Second Self (Tri-Ess)—Sigma Rho Gamma**
 P. O. Box 16174, Huntsville, Alabama 35802.
 ⏲ Meets monthly
 Publishes a newsletter every month.

Stores: Books: General

👁️▽ **Opening Books**
ᴷ⅄ 202 Goldsmith Street South East, Huntsville, Alabama 35801-1903.
☎ 205 536 5880

👁️ **Rainbows Ltd.**
Suite 400B, 4321 University Drive, Huntsville, Alabama 35816.
☎ 205 722 9220
🕐 Thu - Sat 10:00 - 22:00, Sun 12:00 - 18:00

Mobile

Health Services

☺ ☐ **Mobile Infirmary Medical Center**
P. O. Box 2144, Mobile, Alabama 36652.
☎ 205 431 2408

☺ ☐ **University of South Alabama Medical Center**
2451 Fillingim Street, Mobile, Alabama 36617.
☎ 205 471 7000

Organizations: AIDS: Support

☺ ☐ **Mobile AIDS Support Services**
⅄ 107 North Ann Street, Mobile, Alabama 36604.
☎ 205 433 6277
☎ 205 432 2437

Organizations: Sexuality

👁️▽ **Mobile Area Lesbian & Gay Assembly (MALAGA)**
⅄ P. O. Box 40326, Mobile, Alabama 36640-0326.
☎ 205 450 0501
Publishes *TQ Guide*.

▷▽ **The Society for the Second Self (Tri-Ess)—Sigma Rho Gamma**
P. O. Box 66286, Mobile, Alabama 36660.
🕐 Meets monthly
Contact: Ms. Lisa Jackson
Publishes *The Continuum* every month.

Organizations: Sexuality: Student

👁️▽ **Gay, Lesbian, & Bisexual Alliance**
University Center Room 280, University of South Alabama, Mobile, Alabama 36688-0002.
☎ 205 666 9824
Send mail to: GLB of USA.

Publishers: Books: Sexuality

👁️ ■ **Factor Press**
P. O. Box 8888, Mobile, Alabama 36689.
☎ 800 304 0077 (24hrs., U.S. orders only)
🕐 24hr. orders only
💳 VISA 💳 MC
Catalogue, $2.

Publishers: Magazines: Sexuality

☺ ■ *Celebrate The Self*
Factor Press, P. O. Box 8888, Mobile, Alabama 36689.
☎ 800 304 0077 (24hrs., orders only)
💳 VISA 💳 MC
Published every two months. Yearly subscription is $12.95.

Montgomery

Health Services

☺ ☐ **Jackson Hospital & Clinic**
1235 Forest Avenue, Montgomery, Alabama 36106.
☎ 205 293 8000

Organizations: AIDS: Education

☺ ☐ **Montgomery AIDS Outreach**
P. O. Box 5213, Montgomery, Alabama 36103.
☎ 205 269 1002

Organizations: Sexuality

▷▽ **Montgomery Medical & Psychological Institute— Alabama**
⅄ P. O. Box 3361, Montgomery, Alabama 36109.
☎ 205 244 9613
Information, support, & referrals.

Pelham

Organizations: BDSM

👁️▽ **Steel City Centurions**
P. O. Box 533, Pelham, Alabama 35124.
☎ 205 664 0609
✉ BhamLeathr@aol.com

Tuscaloosa

Health Services

☺ ☐ **DCH Regional Medical Center**
809 University Boulevard, Tuscaloosa, Alabama 35401.
☎ 205 759 7111

Organizations: AIDS: Education

☺ ☐ **West Alabama AIDS Outreach**
P. O. Box 031947, Tuscaloosa, Alabama 35403.
☎ 205 758 2437

Organizations: Family

☺ ☐ **Parents & Friends of Lesbians & Gays (PFLAG)— Tuscaloosa**
c/o G/LA, P. O. Box 4595, Tuscaloosa, Alabama 35486-4595.
☎ 205 348 7210

Organizations: Sexuality

👁️▽ **Tuscaloosa Lesbian Coalition**
⅄ P. O. Box 6085, Tuscaloosa, Alabama 35486-6085.
☎ 205 333 8227
Publishes *TLC Newsletter*.

Organizations: Sexuality: Student

👁️▽ **University of Alabama Gay & Lesbian Alliance**
⅄ P. O. Box 4595, Tuscaloosa, Alabama 35486-4595.
☎ 205 348 7120
Publishes *Lavendar Tide*.

ALASKA

Area: Approximately 1,480,000 square kilometres
Population: Approximately 570,000
Capital City: Juneau
Time zone: GMT minus 9 hours (PST plus 1 hour). Far islands & Saint Lawrence Island are on Hawaii time of GMT minus 10 hours (PST plus 2 hours).
Climate: Pleasant summers, with an average temperature of approximately 18˚C. Winters are long & cold, with average temperatures of approximately -7˚C.
Age of consent & homosexuality legislation: State has adopted the Model Penal Code or otherwise decriminalized homosexual activities.
Legal drinking age: 21

Anchorage

Health Services

☺ ☐ **Department of Health & Human Services**
⅄ STD Clinic, Room 101, 825 L Street, Anchorage, Alaska 99501.
☎ 905 343 4611

☺ ☐ **Providence Hospital**
3200 Providence Drive, Anchorage, Alaska 99508.
☎ 907 562 2211

Organizations: AIDS: Education

☺ ☐ **Municipality of Anchorage**
⅄ HIV Community Health Educator, P. O. Box 196650, Anchorage, Alaska 99519-66500.
☎ 907 343 4611
☎ 907 343 6872
Free HIV & STD testing & counselling.

Organizations: AIDS: Support

☺ ☐ **Alaskan AIDS Assistance Association (AAAA)**
ᴷ⅄ Suite 100, 730 I Street, Anchorage, Alaska 99501-3423.
☎ 800 478 2437
☎ 907 276 4880

Organizations: Bears

👁️▽ **The Last Frontier**
P. O. Box 202054, Anchorage, Alaska 99520-2054.
✉ tlfmc@micronet.net
🌐 http://www.skepsis.com:80/.gblo/bears/CLUBS/last.frontier.html

Organizations: Sexuality

▷▽ **The Berdache Society**
⅄ P. O. Box 92381, Anchorage, Alaska 99509-2381.
Contact: Ms. Nora Jean York
Publishes *The Berdache Voice*.

Publishers: Newspapers: Sexuality

👁️▼ *Gay Alaska*
P. O. Box 1581, Anchorage, Alaska 99510.

👁️▼ *Identity Newspaper*
Identity, Inc., P. O. Box 200070, Anchorage, Alaska 99520.
☎ 907 258 4777

To improve self & community awareness, understanding, acceptance of individual sexual identities to promote positive attitudes & healthful living for all Alaskans. Also helpline. Published every month. Yearly subscription is a donation.

Klondyke Kontact
#304, 2440 East Tudor Road, Anchorage, Alaska 99507.
907 337 0253
Contributed articles, letters, drawings, poems, cartoon, fiction, & non-fiction, supporting women's culture in many forms. Published every two months. Yearly subscription is a donation.

Stores: Books: General

Alaska Women's Bookstore
Suite 304, 2440 East Tudor Road, Anchorage, Alaska 99507-1129.
907 562 4716 — Fax 907 562 4325
Mon - Thu 11:00 - 19:00, Fri Sat 10:00 - 18:00

Stores: Erotica: General

La Sex Shoppe
305 West Diamond Boulevard, Anchorage, Alaska 99508.
907 522 1987

Swingers Bookstore
710 West Northern Lights, Anchorage, Alaska 99503.
907 561 5039

Chugiak

Organizations: Sexuality

Alaskan Tpeople
P. O. Box 670349, Chugiak, Alaska 99567-0349.
Contact: Ms. Bobbie Wendy Tucey

Juneau

Organizations: Sexuality

South East Alaska Gay & Lesbian Alliance
P. O. Box 211371, Juneau, Alaska 99821-4297.
907 586 4297
Fri 19:00 - 21:00
Publishes *The Perspective*.

ARIZONA

Area: Approximately 295,000 square kilometres
Population: Approximately 3,680,000
Capital City: Phœnix
Time zone: GMT minus 7 hours (Mountain Time)
Climate: Pleasant
Age of consent & homosexuality legislation: All anal & oral sex is illegal in this state.
Legal drinking age: 21

State Resources

Helplines: Sexuality

Lesbian & Gay Community Switchboard
602 234 2762
602 234 0873 (TDD)
10:00 - 22:00

Publishers: Newspapers: Sexuality

Phœnix Resource
Unit 601, 805 North 4th. Avenue, Phœnix, Arizona 85003-1305.
602 256 7476
A rarified look at aspects of queer culture. Published every two weeks. Yearly subscription is $30.

Chloride

Organizations: Polyfidelity

Touchpoint Network for the Non-Monogamous
P. O. Box 408, Chloride, Arizona 86431.

Publishers: Magazines: Polyfidelity

Touchpoint
P. O. Box 408, Chloride, Arizona 86431.

Clarkdale

Manufacturers: Piercing Jewelry

Reactive Metals Studio, Inc.
P. O. Box 890, Clarkdale, Arizona 86324.
602 634 3434
Not piercing oriented, but supplies niobium wire.

Flagstaff

Organizations: Sexuality

Gay & Lesbian Community (GLC)
P. O. Box 183, Flagstaff, Arizona 86002.
602 774 1521

Stores: Books: General

Aradia Books
P. O. Box 266, Flagstaff, Arizona 86002.
602 779 3817

Phœnix

Bars: BDSM

Cattlemen's Exchange Club
138 West Camelback Road, Phœnix, Arizona 85013.
602 266 0875

Counsellors

Conrad Egge, Ph.D.
K Suite 100, 5727 North 7th. Street, Phœnix, Arizona 85014.
602 230 2025
Mon - Fri 08:00 - 18:00
Gay, lesbian, bisexual individuals, couples, families. Gay men's therapy group. HIV/AIDS issues. Instructs Lesbian & Gay Studies at Phœnix College. Age statement of 18 is required.

Sheila Friedeman, Ph.D.
Suite 205, 3930 East Camelback Road, Phœnix, Arizona 85018.
602 956 3006
Clinical psychiatry.

The Lighthouse Center
Suite 290, 9755 North 90th. Street, Scottsdale, Arizona 85258.
602 451 0819

Gary Lovejoy, Ph.D.
Suite 391, 2701 East Camelback Road, Phœnix, Arizona 85016.
602 957 2368 — Fax 602 756 2132
602 756 1669
Mon - Fri 08:00 - 19:00
Also at Suite B 132, 4450 South Rural Road, Tempe Arizona 85282.

Park Central Counselling
Suite 215, 77 East Thomas Road, Phœnix, Arizona 85012-3118.
602 274 0327

Ronald Peterson, Ph.D.
51 East Lexington Avenue, Phœnix, Arizona 85012.
602 234 3500

Health Services

Arizona State Hospital
2500 East Van Buren Street, Phœnix, Arizona 85008.
602 244 1331

Good Samaritan Regional Medical Center
1111 East McDowell Road, Phœnix, Arizona 85006.
602 239 2000

Maricopa Medical Center
2601 East Roosevelt Street, Phœnix, Arizona 85008.
602 267 5011

Scottsdale Memorial Hospital
7400 East Osborn Road, Scottsdale, Arizona 85251.
602 481 4000

Manufacturers: Piercing Jewelry

HTC
Suite 18, 3422 West Wilshire Drive, Phœnix, Arizona 85009.
602 278 1037
Makes surgical steel captive bead rings, & other unusual captive jewelry. Custom work also available.

Mark Jones
602 265 4435
mark545@aol.com
Makes gold & niobium pieces. Catalogue available.

Organizations: Academic: Psychiatry

The American Mental Health Counsellors Association
Gay & Lesbian Task Force, c/o Moon Valley Counselling Associates, 502 East Tam-O-Shanter Drive, Phœnix, Arizona 85022.

Organizations: AIDS: Education

Arizona AIDS Project
4460 North Central Avenue, Phœnix, Arizona 85012.
602 265 3300

Publishes *AAP Happenings*.

Organizations: AIDS: Support

Community AIDS Council
506 East Camelback Road, Phœnix, Arizona 85012-1614.
602 265 2437

Organizations: BDSM

Arizona Power Exchange
P. O. Box 67532, Phœnix, Arizona 85082-7532.
602 415 1123
http://www.xroads.com/apex/
Publishes a newsletter every month.

Copperstate Leathermen Association
P. O. Box 40472, Phœnix, Arizona 85067-0472.
602 274 8194

The National Leather Association (NLA)—Central Arizona
4620 North 7th. Avenue, Phœnix, Arizona 85013.

Universal Brotherhood of Leatherlords
P. O. Box 33844, Phœnix, Arizona 85067-3844.

Organizations: Bears

Desert Bears
Suite 1114, 8787 East Mountain View Road, Scottsdale, Arizona 85258.

Organizations: Motorcycle

Arizona Rangers MC
P. O. Box 13074, Phœnix, Arizona 85002.

Organizations: Sexuality

A Rose
P. O. Box 82813, Phœnix, Arizona 85071-2813.
Publishes *A Rose News*.

V. I. D. A.
P. O. Box 5689, Phœnix, Arizona 85010-5689.
602 938 3932
602 275 3352

Piercers

HTC Body Adornment Studio
Suite 4, 3432 West Wilshire Drive, Phœnix, Arizona 85009.
602 278 1037

Mark Jones
602 265 4435
mark545@aol.com
By appointment only
Catalogue available.

Publishers: Magazines: Fetish

Epidermal Intrusions
#4, 3442 West Wilshire Drive, Phœnix, Arizona 85009.

Publishers: Magazines: Fetish: Raunch

Raunch
Tom's Ranch, P. O. Box 44871, Phœnix, Arizona 85064-4871.
602 241 1604
Published quarterly. Yearly subscription is $12.

Publishers: Newspapers: Sexuality

Echo Magazine
Ace Publishing, Inc., P. O. Box 1808, Phœnix, Arizona 85001.
602 266 0550 602 266 0773
Mon - Fri 10:00 - 17:00
✓
Largest, most-widely distributed news magazine in the south west. Published twice a month. Yearly subscription is $36.

Western Express
P. O. Box 5317, Phœnix, Arizona 85010-5317.
602 254 1324
Since 1981. The oldest, largest gay publication serving the south west. News of local , national interest to the lesbian & gay community, movie reviews, & entertainment.

Stores: Books: General

Changing Hands Bookstore
414 South Mill Avenue, Tempe, Arizona 85281.
602 966 0203

Saint Paul

Publishers: Magazines: Sexuality

At The Crossroads
P. O. Box 112, Saint Paul, Arizona 72760.

Tempe

Counsellors

Counseling Associates
5440 South Clambake, Tempe, Arizona.
85283 602 897 0444

Health Services

Saint Luke's Hospital
1500 South Mill Avenue, Tempe, Arizona 85281.
602 968 9411

Organizations: Bears

Coalition of Ursine Brothers
P. O. Box 25951, Tempe, Arizona 85285-5951.
602 730 8171

Organizations: Body Size

Southwest Men At Large
P. O. Box 25951, Tempe, Arizona 85285-5951.
602 730 8171

Organizations: Sexuality

The Society for the Second Self (Tri-Ess)—Alpha Zeta
P. O. Box 1738, Tempe, Arizona 85280-1738.
Publishes *The Cactus Flower*.

Publishers: Documentaries: Sexuality

Off The Beaten Path
P. O. Box 24435, Tempe, Arizona 85282.
602 839 4771

Texarkana

Organizations: AIDS: Support

Texarkana AIDS Project, Inc.
P. O. Box 3243, Texarkana, Arizona 75504.
501 773 1994
10:00 - 16:00 (emergencies 24hrs.)
Information, support, & counselling about HIV/AIDS.

Tucson

Bars: BDSM

Venture-N
1239 North 6th. Avenue, Tucson, Arizona 85705.
602 882 8224
12:00 - 01:00

Health Services

Tucson Medical Center
5301 East Grant Road, Tucson, Arizona 85712.
602 327 5461

University Medical Center
1501 north Campbell Avenue, Tucson, Arizona 85724.
602 694 0111

Organizations: AIDS: Support

People With AIDS Coalition of Tucson (PACT)
P. O. Box 2488, Tucson, Arizona 85702-2488.
602 770 1710

El Proyecto Arizona-Sonora
801 West Congress Street, Tucson, Arizona 85745.
602 770 1314

Tucson AIDS Project, Inc. (TAP)
Suite 252, 151 South Tucson Boulevard, Tucson, Arizona 85716-5523.
602 326 2437
602 323 9373 (emergencies)
Office number: 602 322 6336.

Organizations: BDSM

Arizona Fellowship Committee
P. O. Box 2542, Tucson, Arizona 85702.

Desert Leathermen
P. O. Box 1586, Tucson, Arizona 85717-1586.

Tucson Arizona Levi/Leathermen
P. O. Box 1774, Tucson, Arizona 85702.

Tucson Knight Owls
P. O. Box 2332, Tucson, Arizona 85702.

Organizations: Bears

Bears of the Old Pueblo
Suite 85, 5052 North Oracle Road, Tucson, Arizona 85704.

520 293 9648
smokey@bearhug.bearclan.com
http://www.csn.net/~jls2/bop/
Meets 2nd. Fri of month

Organizations: Family

Parents & Friends of Lesbians & Gays (PFLAG)—Tucson
5307 East Douglas Street, Tucson, Arizona 85711-5019.

Organizations: Sexuality

The Rainbow People
P. O. Box 36142, Tucson, Arizona 85740-6142.

Wingspan
422 North 4th. Avenue, Tucson, Arizona 85705.
602 624 1779
Tucson's gay, lesbian, & bisexual centre. Publishes *Up Front*.

Organizations: Sexuality: Student

USUA Bisexual, Gay, & Lesbian Association
Room 215, Building 19, University of Arizona, Tucson, Arizona 85721.
602 621 7585 602 621 6147

Publishers: Newspapers: Sexuality

The Observer
P. O. Box 50733, Tucson, Arizona 85703.
602 622 7176
News, views, commentary of, by & for the lesbian & gay comminuty of Arizona. Published every week.

Stores: Books: General

Antigone Books
600 North 4th. Avenue, Tucson, Arizona 85705.
602 792 3715
Mon - Fri 10:00 18:00, Sat 10:00 - 17:00, Sun 12:00 - 17:00 Mountain (Pacific during daylight savings time)
Feminist bookshop with large gay & lesbian section.

ARKANSAS

Area: Approximately 135,000 square kilometres
Population: Approximately 2,360,000
Capital City: Little Rock
Time zone: GMT minus 6 hours (CST))
Climate: Long humid summers with an average temperature of 27°C & cool winters with an average temperature of approximately 4°C.
Age of consent & homosexuality legislation: Anal & oral sex is illegal in this state only between people of the same sex.
Legal drinking age: 21

State Resources

Helplines: Sexuality

Arkansas Gay & Lesbian Task Force Switchboard
P. O. Box 45053, Little Rock, Arkansas 72214.
800 448 8305 (statewide)
501 666 3340 (Little Rock)
18:30 - 22:30

Organizations: AIDS: Support

Arkansas AIDS Foundation
P. O. Box 255007, Little Rock, Arkansas 72205.
501 663 7833
501 666 3340 (AIDS information)
Office: 09:00 - 17:00; information line: 18:30 - 22:30

Helping People With AIDS
P. O. Box 4397, Little Rock, Arkansas 72204.
501 666 6900

Publishers: Magazines: Sexuality

Ozark Feminist Review
P. O. Box 1662, Fayetteville, Arkansas 72701.

Avoca

Organizations: AIDS: Support

Living Pens
P. O. Box 254, Avoca, Arkansas 72711-0254.
Publishes *Living Pens Quarterly Report* quarterly. Yearly subscription is free.

Organizations: Bears

Ozark Mountain Bears
P. O. Box 288, Avoca, Arkansas 72711.

El Dorado

Organizations: AIDS: Education

South Arkansas Fight AIDS
1616 West Block, El Dorado, Arkansas 71730.

Fayetteville

Archives: General

Women's Library
17 North Block Street, Fayetteville, Arkansas 72701-6018.
501 582 4636
Thu 15:30 - 18:30, Sat 12:00 - 02:00

Health Services

Fayetteville Regional Medical Center
1125 North College Avenue, Fayetteville, Arkansas 72703.
501 442 1000

Organizations: AIDS: Support

Washington County AIDS Task Force
P. O. Box 4224, Fayetteville, Arkansas 72702.
501 443 2437
Hotline 07:00 - 19:00

Stores: Books: General

Hays & Sanders Bookstore
25 North Block, Fayetteville, Arkansas 72701.
501 442 0832

Jonesboro

Organizations: Sexuality

The Society for the Second Self (Tri-Ess)—Mu Sigma
P. O. Box 61, Jonesboro, Arkansas 72403-0061.
501 227 8798
501 523 2466
Publishes *Ms. Cotton Belle*.

Publishers: Magazines: Sexuality

Woman To Woman
P. O. Box 137, RR4, Jonesboro, Arkansas 72401-9804.

Little Rock

Counsellors

Psychotherapy Center
Gay Counselling Service, 210 Pulaski, Little Rock, Arkansas 72201.
501 374 3605
Tue 17:00 - 18:30
Free support group.

Health Services

Doctor's Hospital
6101 West Capitol, Little Rock, Arkansas 72205.
501 661 4000

Saint Vincent Infirmary Medical Center
2 Saint Vincent Circle, Little Rock, Arkansas 72205.
501 660 3000

Organizations: AIDS: Support

Psychotherapy Center
AIDS Support Center, 210 Pulaski, Little Rock, Arkansas 72201.
501 374 3605
Contact: Dr. Ralph Hyman

Organizations: Sexuality

Wives'/Partners' Concerns ((SPICE))
P. O. Box 24031, Little Rock, Arkansas 72221.
Contact: Ms. Linda Peacock
Publishes *Sweetheart Connection* quarterly.

Organizations: Sexuality: Youth

People of Alternate Lifestyles (PALS)
210 Pulaski, Little Rock, Arkansas 72201.
501 374 3605
Meets Wed 18:45 - 20:15
Contact: Dr. Ralph Hyman
Youth up to 22 years.

Publishers: Newspapers: Sexuality

Arkansas Advisor
P. O. Box 4397, Little Rock, Arkansas 72214.

Triangle Rising
2311 State Street, Little Rock, Arkansas 72206.

Stores: Books: General

⊕ ■ **Women's Project**
 ⅃ 2224 Main Street, Little Rock, Arkansas 72206.
 ☎ 501 372 5113

North Little Rock

Organizations: BDSM

⚥▽ **The National Leather Association (NLA)—Arkansas**
 P. O. Box 1608, North Little Rock, Arkansas 72115.

⚥▽ **The Officers Club**
 P. O. Box 9343, North Little Rock, Arkansas 72119.

CALIFORNIA

Area: Approximately 404,000 square kilometres
Population: Approximately 29,900,000
Capital City: Sacramento
Time zone: GMT minus 8 hours (PST)
Climate: Pleasant climate in all parts. Cooler in the north. Temperature around 20°-25°C in during summer days, 15°-20° at night. Winter is 5°-10° cooler in most places.
Age of consent & homosexuality legislation: State has adopted the Model Penal Code or otherwise decriminalized homosexual activities. There is legislation in place against discrimination on the basis of sexual orientation.
Legal drinking age: 21

State Resources

Archives: Sexuality

⚥ **Gay & Lesbian Historical Society of Northern California**
 P. O. Box 424280, San Francisco, California 94142.
 ☎ 415 626 0980
 Publishes *Our Stories*.

Manufacturers: Adult Toys: BDSM

☺ ■ **Sportsheets**
 P. O. Box 7800, Huntington Beach, California 92646.
 ☎ 800 484 9954 Ext.: 7962　　　✆ 714 965 7873
 ☎ 714 962 8946
 ✉ sports@deltanet.com
 🌐 http://www.deltanet.com/wlink/sportsheet
 🕑 07:00 - 19:00
 💰 ✓ $ 𝗩𝗜𝗦𝗔 ⬤ ▭
 Soft fantasy restraint that ensures you're only as tied up as you want to be. Free catalogue published twice a year. Age statement of 18 is required. German & Spanish also spoken.

Organizations: Sexuality

⚥▽ **Educational TV Channel (ETVC)**
 ⅃ P. O. Box 426486, San Francisco, California 94142-6486.
 ☎ 510 549 2665
 ☎ 415 334 3439
 ✆ 415 239 8467
 Publishes *The Channel*.

Publishers: Magazines: Sexuality

⚥ *Lesbian News*
 P.O. Box 1430, Twentynine Palms, California 92277.
 ☎ 619 656 0258 Ext.: 113　　　✆ 619 367 3386

⚥▼ *Voice Magazine*
 P. O. Box 632847, San Diego, California 92163-2847.
 ☎ 619 281 8511　　　✆ 619 281 9055

Publishers: Newspapers: Sexuality

⚥ *Gay & Lesbian Times/Uptown*
 P. O. Box 34624, San Diego, California 92163.
 ☎ 619 299 6397　　　✆ 619 299 3430
 Published every week.

⚥▼ *OutNow*
 Suite 124, 45 North 1st. Street, San José, California 95113.
 ☎ 408 991 1873　　　✆ 408 739 3054
 ☎ 415 337 4352
 ✉ news@outnow.com
 🌐 http://www.zoom.com/outnow/
 Published every two weeks. Yearly subscription is $40.

Stores: Erotica: BDSM

☺ **Crypt**
 ⅃ 1515 Washington Street, San Diego, California 92103.
 ☎ 619 692 9499
 🕑 Mon - Thu 11:00 - 23:00, Fri Sat 11:00 - 24:00, Sun 14:00 - 22:00
 💰 ▭ ⬤ ▭

☺ **Crypt On Broadway**
 ⅃ 1712 East Broadway, Long Beach, California 90802.
 ☎ 310 983 6560
 🕑 11:00 - 22:00
 💰 ✓ ▭ 𝗩𝗜𝗦𝗔 ⬤ ▭
 Age statement of 18 is required.

Stores: Erotica: General

☺ **Crypt / North Park Adult Video**
 4094 30th. Street, San Diego, California 92104.
 ☎ 619 284 4724
 🕑 24hrs.
 💰 𝗩𝗜𝗦𝗔 ⬤ ▭ ¢

Agnew

Organizations: Motorcycle

⚥ **Aquila MC**
 P.O. Box 4067, Agnew, California 95054.

Agoura Hills

Publishers: Magazines: Piercing

☺ ■ *Savage*
 Paisano Publications, P. O. Box 1025, Agoura Hills, California 91376-1025.
 ☎ 818 889 8740
 Published quarterly.

Albany

Publishers: Newspapers: Sexuality

⚥ *Aché*
 P. O. Box 6071, Albany, California 94706-0071.
 A journal for black lesbians.

Alpine

Publishers: Magazines: BDSM

⚥⚥ ■ *Behind The Scene*
 P. O. Box 2237, Alpine, California 91903.
 ☎ 619 445 1589
 Also offers spanking & female domination videos. Published 7 times a year. Yearly subscription is $50.

Arcata

Stores: Books: General

☺ ■ **Northtown Books**
 957 H Street, Arcata, California 95521.
 ☎ 707 822 2834

Auburn

Publishers: Magazines: Alternative

☺ ■ **Rip Off Press, Inc.**
 P. O. Box 4686, Auburn, California 95604.
 ☎ 800 468 2669　　　✆ 916 885 8219
 ☎ 916 885 8183
 ✓ 𝗩𝗜𝗦𝗔 ⬤ ▭

Bakersfield

Manufacturers: Whips

☺ ▼ **Draconian Leather**
 #A, 2325 Chester Lane, Bakersfield, California 3304.
 ☎ 805 631 8760
 🕑 Mon - Fri 10:00 - 18:00
 💰 ✓
 Age statement of 21 is required.

Ben Lomand

Organizations: Sexuality

☺ **NSS Seminars, Inc.**
 P.O. Box 5001, Ben Lomand, California 95005.
 ☎ 408 336 9281　　　✆ 408 336 9283
 ✓ 𝗩𝗜𝗦𝗔 ⬤
 Sponsors the National Sexuality Symposium & Exposition in Sep.. Also produces educational sex videos. Free catalogue. Publishes a newsletter quarterly.

Berkeley

Counsellors

⚥▼ **Jim Boland, Ph.D.**
 1466 Hopkins Street, Berkeley, California 94702.
 ☎ 510 524 8540

☺ **Kim Hraca, M.A., MFCC**

Ҟ 2714 Telegraph, Berkeley, California 94705.
☎ 510 601 1859
BDSM-positive therapy.

Health Services

☺ ☐ **Alta Bates Medical Center**
2450 Ashby Avenue, Berkeley, California 94705.
☎ 510 204 1492

☺ ☐ **Berkeley Free Clinic**
⅄ 2339 Durant Avenue, Berkeley, California 94704.
☎ 510 548 2570

Organizations: BDSM

☺ ☐ **Petruchio**
P. O. Box 12182, Berkeley, California 94701.
✉ jaybob@crl.com
⬥
Contact: Mr. Jay Wiseman
Requires SASE or IRC for information or reply. Publishes *The Weather Report.*

Organizations: Sexuality

⚥▽ **Pacific Center—Head Office**
2712 Telegraph Road, Berkeley, California 94705.
☎ 510 841 6224 ✆ 510 548 2983
☎ 510 548 8283
⏱ Mon - Fri 10:00 - 22:00, Sat 12:00 - 16:00 18:00 - 22:00, Sun 18:00 - 21:00
⬥ ✓
Centre for many alternative sexuality groups. Offers HIV/AIDS information & referrals.

☺ ▽ **The Queer Resource Center (QRC)**
⅄ Room 407, 300 Eshleman Hall, University of California - Berkeley, Berkeley, California 94720.
☎ 510 643 8929
⬥ http://www.qrd.org/QRD/www/index.html
Publishes *The Queer Resource Directory.*

Organizations: Sexuality: Student

⚥▽ **Boalt Hall, UC Berkeley School of Law Lesbian, Gay, & Bisexual Caucus**
37 Boalt Hall, University of California - Berkeley, Berkeley, California 94720.

Public Speakers: BDSM

☺ ■ **Jay Wiseman**
P. O. Box 1261, Berkeley, California 94701-1261.
✉ jaybob@crl.com
⬥
Author, speaker, & consultant. Available for interviews, etc.. Mail order for his books.

Publishers: Directories: Naturism

☺ ■ **Bold Type, Inc.**
P. O. Box 1984, Berkeley, California 94701.
☎ 800 624 8433
⏱ Mon - Fri 09:00 - 17:00
✓ 🃏 🃏
Publishes guide to clothing optional locations in California, & some sites in Hawaii, Oregon, & Washington.

Publishers: Magazines: Sexuality

⊚ **Connexions**
P. O. Box 14431, Berkeley, California 94701-5431.
☎ 510 549 3505

⚤▽ **Sinister Wisdom**
Sinister Wisdom, Inc., P. O. Box 3252, Berkeley, California 94703.
⏱ By appointment
✓

☺ ■ **Slippery When Wet**
More! Productions, P. O. Box 3101, Berkeley, California 94703.
☎ 510 845 5457
☎ 510 548 2502
✉ slippery@pobox.com
⬥ http://www2.best.com/~slippery/sww.html
⏱ 24hrs.
⬥ ✓
Electronic magazine. Subscription comes on disk, so specify Mac or IBM PC. Published quarterly. Yearly subscription is $21. Age statement of 21 is required.

Stores: Books: General

⚥▽ **Boadecia's Books**
⅄ 398 Colusa Avenue, Kensington, California 94707.
☎ 510 559 9184
⏱ 11:00 - 21:00, Sun 10:00 - 19:00

☺ ■ **Cody's Books**
⅄ 2454 Telegraph Road, Berkeley, California 94704.
☎ 510 845 7852
⏱ Mon - Thu 10:00 - 21:00, Fri Sat - 22:00

☺ ■ **Gaia Bookstore**
1400 Shattuck, Berkeley, California 94709.
☎ 510 548 4172

Stores: Erotica: General

☺ ■ **F Street—El Cajon**
158 East Main Street, Berkeley, California 92020.
☎ 619 447 0381
⏱ 24hrs.

☺ ▼ **Good Vibrations**
⅄ 2504 San Pablo, Berkeley, California 94702.
☎ 415 974 8980 ✆ 415 974 8989
☎ 510 841 8987
✉ goodvibe@well.sf.ca
⏱ 11:00 - 19:00
⬥ ✓ $ 🃏 🃏 🃏 🃏
Sex toy store with books & videos. Free catalogue. Age statement of 18 is required. Spanish also spoken.

Beverly Hills

Organizations: AIDS: Research

☺ **AIDS & Cancer Research Foundation**
Suite 1800, 8306 Wilshire Boulevard, Beverly Hills, California 90211.
☎ 800 373 4572 ✆ 213 655 1804
HIV/AIDS education. Promotes research for AIDS & cancer.

Photographers: Erotic

☺ ■ **Todd Friedman Photography**
P. O. Box 3737, Beverly Hills, California 90212.
☎ 310 239 4818 ✆ 310 477 5422
Photography of sexuality as an integral part of being, rather than as pornography.

Buena Park

Competitions & Conventions: Sexuality

☺ **Lifestyles**
P. O. Box 7128, Buena Park, California 990622.
☎ 714 821 9953 ✆ 714 821 1465
Annual convention of alternate lifestyles & sexualities.

Publishers: Magazines: Spirituality

☺ ■ **Robert McGinley, Ph.D.**
P. O. Box 5366, Buena Park, California 90622.
☎ 714 821 9939 ✆ 714 821 1465
🃏 🃏 🃏
Yearly subscription is $15. Age statement of 21 is required.

Burbank

Publishers: Directories: Sexuality

⚏ **JMPG**
The Crossdressers International Shopping Guide, P. O. Box 7217, Burbank, California 91510-7217.
Free catalogue.

Camarillo

Counsellors

☺ **Verdantmom**
Ҟ c/o New Beginnings Counselling Center, Suite N, 155 Granada Street, Camarillo, California 93010.
☎ 805 987 3162
✉ Verdantmom@aol.com.
Name is a pseudonym. Adolescents, female & male survivors of incest & molestation, partnerships.

Canoga Park

BBSs: BDSM

☺ ■ **Delos**
☎ 818 348 2365

Organizations: Bears

⚥▽ **Girth & Mirth of LA**
P. O. Box 466, Canoga Park, California 91305.

Organizations: Body Size

⚥▽ **Girth & Mirth—Los Angeles**
P. O. Box 466, Canoga Park, California 91305.
☎ 818 961 7900

Cathedral City
Printers: General
☺▼ **David Printing**
Box 7B, 68-671 Grove Street, Cathedral City, California 92234.
☎ 619 324 4957 ✆ 619 324 2857
🕐 Tue - Fri 08:00 - 17:00, Mon Sat 08:00 - 15:00
⛟ ✓ $ ✉
Full service print headquarters: flyers, brochures, stationary, letterhead, business cards, & all business forms. Will print BDSM-related publications.

Publishers: Newspapers: Sexuality
⚲▼ *David Magazine*
David Enterprises, Box 7B, 68-671 Grove Street, Cathedral City, California 92234.
☎ 619 324 4957 ✆ 619 324 2857
🕐 Tue - Fri 08:00 - 17:00, Mon Sat 08:00 - 15:00
⛟ ✓ $ ✉
Serving the Palm Springs, San Diego, Long Beach, California areas, & Las Vegas, Nevada. Published every two weeks. Yearly subscription is $40U.S..

Stores: Erotica: BDSM
⚲▼ **Black Moon Leather**
#7, 68-449 Perez Road, Cathedral City, California 92234.
☎ 619 770 2925 ✆ 619 328 4440
🕐 Mon - Thu 15:00 - 02:00, Fri - Sun 12:00 - 03:00
⛟ ✓ $ ✉ 💳 💳 💳

Stores: Erotica: General
☺■ **Hidden Joy**
68-424 Commercial Road, Cathedral City, California 92234.
☎ 619 328 1694
🕐 10:00 - 03:00, Fri Sat - 04:00

☺ **Perez Books**
68-366 Perez Road, Cathedral City, California 92234.
☎ 619 321 5597 ✆ 619 321 1597

⚲■ **Worldwide Adult Bookstore**
♿ 68-300 Ramon Road, Cathedral City, California 92234.
☎ 619 321 1313

Chico
Organizations: Family
☺☐ **Parents & Friends of Lesbians & Gays (PFLAG)—Chico**
P. O. Box 1465, Chico, California 95927.
☎ 916 891 5718

Organizations: Sexuality
⚲▽ **Stonewall Alliance of Chico**
♿ P. O. Box 8855, Chico, California 95927.
☎ 916 893 3336
☎ 916 893 3338 (infoline)
Publishes *Centerstone*.

Chula Vista
Stores: Erotica: General
☺■ **F Street—Chula Vista**
1141 Third Avenue, Chula Vista, California 92011.
☎ 619 585 3314

Claremont San Dimas
BBSs: BDSM
☺■ **Throbbs**
✆ 909 626 6831

Compton
BBSs: BDSM
☺■ **Hedonism**
Unit G, 901 West Victoria, Compton, California 90220.
✆ 310 631 7697
🌐 ftp://hedonism.com

Health Services
☺☐ **Mount Diablo Medical Center**
2540 East Street, Compton, California 94520.
☎ 510 682 8200

Publishers: Videos: Bondage
☺■ **Bon Vu Enterprises**
Unit G, 901 West Victoria Street, Compton, California 90220-5801.
☎ 800 827 3787 ✆ 310 631 0415

☎ 310 631 1600
⛟ ✓ $ 💳 💳 💳
Publishes many magazines & videos of sexual fetishes of all sorts. Age statement of 21 is required. Spanish also spoken.

Concord
Organizations: AIDS: Support
☺☐ **Diablo Valley AIDS Center**
2253 Concord Boulevard, Concord, California 94520.
☎ 510 686 3822

Organizations: Fetish: Foreskin
⚲▽ **National Organization of Restoring Men (NORM)**
Suite 209, 3205 Northwood Drive, Concord, California 94520.
☎ 510 827 4077

Organizations: Sexuality
⚲■ **Diablo Valley Girls**
P.O. Box 272885, Concord, California 94527-2885.
☎ 510 937 8432
📧 dvg@rwr13.vip.best.com
🌐 http://www.best.com/~rwr13/.dvg/
🕐 Call Mon - Fri 19:00 - 21:00
Publishes *Devil Woman*.

Stores: Clothing: Sexuality
⚲▼ **Creative Growth Enterprises**
Suite 227, 4480 Treat Boulevard, Concord, California 94521.
☎ 510 798 0922
🕐 Mon - Fri 10:00 - 18:00. Free support Mon - Fri 16:00 - 18:00
$
Complete line of products for female to male transexuals. Also mail order. Free catalogue.

Stores: Erotica: General
☺ **Sarah's Bare Necessities**
1909 Salvio Street, Concord, California 94518.
☎ 510 680 8445
Stripper clothing for men & women. Also erotic leather clothing.

Corona
Artists: BDSM
⚥■ **Brian Viveros**
946 Alta Loma, Corona, California 91720.

Organizations: Sexuality
⚲▽ **Born Free**
P. O. Box 1897, Corona, California 91718.

Corte Madera
Organizations: Sexuality
☺■ **Sunrise Center**
Suite C-200, 45 San Clemente, Corte Madera, California 94925.
☎ 415 924 5483 ✆ 415 924 4214
🕐 Mon Tue Thu Fri 10:00 - 15:00
⛟ ✓ 💳 💳
Contact: Ms. Maggie Kelly
Explorations of Tantra & sexuality.

Culver City
Organizations: Polyfidelity
☺■ **Family Synergy**
P. O. Box 2668, Culver City, California 90231.

Organizations: Sexuality: Youth
⚲ **Lambda Youth Network**
P. O. Box 7911, Culver City, California 90233.

Cypress
Organizations: Sexuality: Student
⚲▽ **Cypress College Lambda Union**
9200 Valley View, Cypress, California 90630.

Daly City
Organizations: Bears
⚲▽ **Golden Gate Connection**
P. O. Box 2328, Daly City, California 94017.
☎ 415 871 7870

Danville
Publishers: Books: Erotic
⚲ **Plastic Cow Productions**

P. O. Box 3081, Danville, California 94526.
☎ 510 736 2153

Publishers: Magazines: Erotic
⊙ *All Your Dreams Fulfilled*
PCP, P. O. Box 3081, Danville, California 94526.

Davis
Organizations: Sexuality: Student
♂♀▽ Bisexual, Gays, & Lesbians at Davis (BGLAD)
& Box 163, UCD Students Activities Office, Davis University, Davis, California 95616.
☎ 916 757 3848
Publishes *The Lavendar Cow*.

Desert Hot Springs
Publishers: Magazines: Erotic
♂▼ *Centaur Magazine*
P. O. Box 621, Desert Hot Springs, California 92240.

El Cajon
BBSs: Adult Baby
☺ ■ The ByteMine Adult Baby BBS
📞 619 443 3915
✉ bill.s@mistress.com
You'll be prompted for a keyword (DIAPER), which allows access to the non-subscriber features. Age statement of 21 is required.

Publishers: Videos: Spanking
♂▼ Studio-7
P. O. Box 1807, El Cajon, California 92022.
☎ 619 440 1020
Age statement of 21 is required.

El Cerrito
Organizations: BDSM
♂♀■ Essemian Press
P.O. Box 1335, El Cerrito, California 94530.
☎ 510 232 1369
🕐 10:00 - 19:00
Contact: Mr. William Westely, Editor
A publication of the Service of Mankind Church exclusively for its contributing members. Publishes *The Essemian Way* quarterly. Age statement of 21 is required.

☺ Service of Mankind Church
P.O. Box 1335, El Cerrito, California 94530.
☎ 510 874 4974 (hotline)
☎ 510 232 1369 (office)
🕐 Office number 10:00 - 19:00
Publishes *Echoes From The Sanctuary* quarterly.

El Toro
Organizations: Family
☺ □ Gay & Lesbian Parents
P. O. Box 1332, El Toro, California 92630.
☎ 714 720 9460

Emeryville
Distributors: Books: General
☺ Publishers Group West
4065 Hollis Street, Emeryville, California 94608.
☎ 510 658 3453

Photographers: Erotic
☺ Craig Morey
Studio 314, 4053 Harlan Street, Emeryville, California 94608.
☎ 510 601 0606 📞 510 601 9326
✉ Morey@Designlink.com
In Japan, contact Mr. Morey's agent: Megapress, Takama Building 2F, 3-24-4 Higashi Shibuya-Ku, Tokyo 150. All others contact Mr. Morey directly.

Publishers: Newspapers: Sexuality
☺ *Spectator Magazine*
Suite 103, 5835 Doyle Street, Emeryville, California 94608.
☎ 800 624 8433 📞 510 658 3326
☎ 510 849 1615
🕐 Mon - Fri 09:00 - 17:00
✓ 💳 💳
Published every week. Yearly subscription is $65. Age statement of 18 is required.

Encino
Counsellors
☺ ■ Michael Perry, Ph.D.
Suite 1120, 16311 Ventura Boulevard, Encino, California 91436.
☎ 818 784 9199 📞 818 784 9212
🕐 Mon - Fri 09:00 - 20:00
♿ ✓

☺ Robin Ribakoff, M.F.C.T.
K Suite 205, 5535 Balboa Boulevard, Encino, California 91316.
☎ 818 957 4065

Escondido
Stores: Erotica: General
☺ ■ F Street—Escondido
237 East Grand Avenue, Escondido, California 92025.
☎ 619 480 6031

Eureka
Stores: Books: General
☺ ■ Booklegger
& 402 2nd Street, Eureka, California 95501.
☎ 707 445 1344

Fairfield
Helplines: Sexuality
♂♀▽ Solano Country Gay & Lesbian Information Line
☎ 7007 448 1010 (recorded message)

Organizations: Sexuality
♂♀▽ Solano Lambda Men's Association (SLMA)
P. O. Box 9, Vacaville, California 95696-0009.
☎ 707 449 1010 (tape recording)

Stores: Books: General
☺ ▼ Vacaville Book Co.
& 315 Main Street, Vacaville, California 95688.
☎ 707 449 0550
🕐 Mon - Sat 10:00 - 20:00

Forestville
Organizations: Spirituality
♂▽ Radical Faerie Circle—Russian River
10656 River Drive, Forestville, California 94436-9752.
☎ 707 887 9851
🕐 Thu 19:00
Contact: Mr. Gordon Redhands

Stores: Books: General
☺ ▼ The Last Word Newsstand
& P. O. Box 1334, Forestville, California 95436-1334.
☎ 707 869 0571

Stores: Clothing: Leather
☺ ■ The Source Leather Shop
P. O. Box 1069, Forestville, California 95436.

Fort Bragg
Stores: Books: General
☺ ■ Windsong Books & Records
& 324 North Main Street, Fort Bragg, California 95437.
☎ 707 964 2050

Fountain Valley
Stores: Erotica: BDSM
☺ ■ Fantasy Lingerie
16112 Harbor Boulevard, Fountain Valley, California 92708.
☎ 714 775 8356

Fresno
Health Services
☺ □ Fresno Community Hospital & Medical Center
P. O. Box 1232, Fresno & R Streets, Fresno, California 93715.
☎ 209 442 6000

☺ □ Valley Medical Center of Fresno
445 South Cedar Avenue, Fresno, California 93702.
☎ 209 453 4000

Organizations: AIDS: Support
☺ □ Central Valley AIDS Team

Organizations: AIDS: Support

 🚻 P. O. Box 4640, Fresno, California 93744.
 ☎ 209 264 2437
 Support, information, & education. Publishes *Team Work*.

Organizations: Bears

☺▽ **Golden State Bears**
 P. O. Box 5561, Fresno, California 97355-5561.
 ☎ 209 496 3875
 ✉ frsnobear@aol.com

Organizations: Sexuality

☺▼ **Valley Woman Books & Gifts**
 🚻 1118 North Fulton, Fresno, California 93728.
 ☎ 209 233 3600
 🕐 10:00 - 21:00, Sat Sun - 18:00
 Publishes *The Inner Word*.

Stores: Books: General

☺■ **Fig Garden Bookstore**
 5148 North Palm Avenue, Fresno, California 93704.
 ☎ 209 226 1845

☺■ **Wildcat Books**
 🚻 1535 Fresno Street, Fresno, California 93706.
 ☎ 209 237 4525

Fullerton
Organizations: Sexuality: Student

☺▽ **Lesbian, Gay, Bisexual Association**
 🚻 UC 243, Box 67, CSU Fullerton, Fullerton, California 92634.
 ☎ 714 773 2067

Stores: Clothing: Rubber

☺■ **Rubber & Rivets**
 2750 Associated Road, Fullerton, California 92635.
 ☎ 714 671 1402
 Also bondage items.

Stores: Erotica: General

☺▼ **Erogenous Zone**
 🚻 343 North State College Boulevard, Fullerton, California 92631-4205.
 ☎ 714 879 3270

Garden Grove
Health Services

☺☐ **Garden Grove Hospital & Medical Center**
 12601 Garden Grove Boulevard, Garden Grove, California 92643.
 ☎ 714 537 5160

Manufacturers: Erotica: Leather

☺■ **Spartacus Centurion**
 13331 Garden Grove Boulevard, Garden Grove, California 92643.
 ☎ 714 971 1113 ☎ 714 971 7406
 ☎ 714 971 0238
 🕐 Office: 09:00 - 17:00, store: mon - Sat 10:00 - 21:00, sun 11:00 - 18:00
 🚻 ✓ 💳 💳
 Store location: Fantasy Lingerie, 16112 Harbor Boulevard, Fountain Valley, California 92708. 714 775 8356, 714 775 0641 facs.. Catalogue published monthly, $3. Age statement of 21 is required.

Organizations: AIDS: Education

☺▽ **AIDS Response Program**
 🚻 12832 Garden Grove Boulevard, Garden Grove, California 92643.
 ☎ 714 534 0961
 🕐 10:00 - 18:00

Organizations: BDSM

☺■ **Orange Coast Leather Assembly (OCLA)**
 c/o The Center OC, Suite A, 12832 Garden Grove Boulevard, Garden Grove, California 92643.
 ☎ 714 534 0862
 🕐 Call 12:00 - 22:00. Meets 3rd. Tue of month 20:00
 Contact: Mr. Brian Dawson

Organizations: Sexuality

☺▽ **Gay & Lesbian Community Services Center of Orange County**
 🚻 #A, 12832 Garden Grove Boulevard, Garden Grove, California 92643.
 ☎ 714 534 0862
 ☎ 714 534 3441 (TDD)
 Publishes *Liason*.

Publishers: Magazines: Fetish

☺▼ *Bizarre*
 Spartacus, 13331 Garden Grove Boulevard, Garden Grove, California

U.S.A.

 92643.
 ☎ 714 971 1113 ☎ 714 971 7406
 $ 💳 💳
 Published quarterly. Yearly subscription is $40. Age statement of 21 is required.

⚥▼ *Transformation*
 Spartacus, 13331 Garden Grove Boulevard, Garden Grove, California 92643.
 ☎ 714 971 1113 ☎ 714 971 7406
 $ 💳 💳
 Published quarterly. Yearly subscription is $40. Age statement of 21 is required.

Sculptor: Fetish

☺■ **Jim Johnson Surplus**
 12932 Ninth Street, Garden Grove, California 92640.
 ☎ 714 534 2973

Stores: Erotica: General

☺■ **East of Eden**
 12065 Garden Grove Boulevard, Garden Grove, California 92643.
 ☎ 714 534 9811

☺■ **Garden of Eden**
 🚻 12061 Garden Grove Boulevard, Garden Grove, California 92643.
 ☎ 714 534 9805

Glendale
BBSs: BDSM

☺■ **Academy**
 📞 818 549 0934

☺■ **Athlete's Bench**
 📞 818 247 2282

Health Services

☺☐ **Glendale Memorial Hospital & Health Center**
 Central & Los Feliz Avenue, Glendale, California 91225.
 ☎ 818 502 2201

Printers: General

☺ **Griffin Printing & Lithograph Co.**
 544 West Colorado Street, Glendale, California 91204-2891.
 ☎ 213 245 3671

Stores: Clothing: Uniforms

☺■ **WearHouse Uniforms**
 3734 San Fernando Road, Glendale, California.
 ☎ 818 243 4440

Gualala
Stores: Books: General

☺■ **Gualala Books**
 🚻 P. O. Box 765, Gualala, California 95445.
 ☎ 707 888 4255
 🕐 Mon - Sat 10:00 - 17:00, Sun 11:00 - 16:00

Guernville
Organizations: BDSM

☺ **The National Leather Association (NLA)—Russian River**
 P. O. Box 548, Guernville, California 93446-0548.

Organizations: Bears

☺▽ **Pacific Bears California LMC—Russian River**
 P. O. Box 1089, Guernville, California 95446.
 ☎ 707 869 3783

Publishers: Directories: Sexuality

☺ *The Directory of Gay & Lesbian Community Publications in the United States & Canada*
 Redwood Empire Agency, P. O. Box 1946, Guernville, California 95466.
 ☎ 707 869 1146

Stores: Books: General

☺■ **By The Books—Russian River**
 16309 Main Street, Guernville, California 95446.
 ☎ 707 869 9031

Hawthorne
Stores: Clothing: Uniforms

☺■ **WearHouse Uniforms**
 13248 Hawthorne Boulevard, Hawthorne, California.
 ☎ 310 676 9180

Hayward

Organizations: BDSM

⚥ ▽ **The Ring**
P. O. Box 192, Hayward, California 94543.
☎ 415 522 9697
📧 The_Ring@ix.netcom.com
Contact: Mr. J. Frazier
Local group for men only.

Healdsburg

Organizations: Family

☺ □ **Parents & Friends of Lesbians & Gays (PFLAG)—**
♿ **Healdsburg**
P. O. Box 1266, Healdsburg, California 95448.
☎ 707 431 8364

Hollywood

Bars: BDSM

⚥▼ **Faultline**
4216 Melrose Avenue, Hollywood, California.
Store is inside the Faultline bar.

☺ **Skin Parlor**
1608 Cosmo Street, Hollywood, California.

Health Services

☺ □ **Hollywood Community Hospital**
6245 De Longpre Avenue, Hollywood, California 90028.
☎ 213 462 2271
HIV & emergency departments.

Organizations: Motorcycle

☺ **Œdipus MC**
P.O. Box 451, Hollywood, California 90028.

Photographers: Erotic

☺ **Ken Marcus Studio**
6916 Melrose Avenue, Hollywood, California 90038.
☎ 213 937 7214 ✆ 213 937 8425

HEARTWOOD
WHIPS OF
Passion

Janette
Heartwood's

Whip Catalog is a must
for anyone who is interested
in whips. - DRUMMER Magazine

Large selection of superbly crafted
FLOGGERS•CATS•FLAT BRAIDS
from stock or custom made
68-page CATALOG w/color photos $6.

412 N. Coast Hwy. #210,
Laguna Beach, CA 92651 (714) 376-9558

Publishers: Magazines: BDSM

♂ ■ *Mistress Jacqueline Magazine*
Pacific Force, Suite 350, 7095 Hollywood Boulevard, Hollywood,
California 90028.

♂ ■ *Power Xchange*
Pacific Force, Suite 350, 7095 Hollywood Boulevard, Hollywood,
California 90028.

Publishers: Newspapers: Sexuality

⚥ *Celebrity Circumcision Survey Master List*
P. O. Box 691024, Hollywood, California 90069.
Newsletter listing the circumcision status of 2,000 celebrities.

⚥ *Update*
P. O. Box 204, Hollywood, California 90028.
Published every week.

Stores: Clothing: Fetish

☺ ■ **Playmates**
6438 Hollywood Boulevard, Hollywood, California 90028.
☎ 213 464 7636
Also sells some BDSM toys.

Huntington Beach

Counsellors

⚥ ▼ **Shiela Benjamin, LCSW**
☎ 714 892 8433

Irvine

Organizations: Sexuality: Student

⚥▽ **UC Irvine GLBSU**
102 University Center, Irvine, California 92717.
☎ 714 856 4260
Publishes *Triangle Times*.

Jenner

Publishers: Mailing Lists: Female

⚲■ **National Women's Mailing List**
P. O. Box 68, Jenner, California 95450.
☎ 707 632 5763

Laguna Beach

Counsellors

⚲▼ **Roxanne Cherry, Ph.D.**
343 3rd. Street, Laguna Beach, California 92651.
☎ 714 497 9925

Manufacturers: Whips

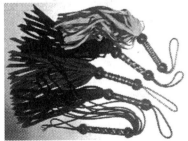

☺ ■ **Heartwood Whips of Passion**
#210, 412 North Coast Highway, Laguna Beach, California 92651.
☎ 714 376 9558
🕐 Mon - Fri during the day, answsing machine at other times
💳 ✓ 💳 💳
Makers of superbly crafted floggers, cats, & flat braids! No store front.
Mail order from stock or custom made. Catalogue, $6, $8 overseas.
Please see our display advertisement.

Organizations: Daddy / Boy

⚥▽ **SCMA**
Suite 140, 1278 Glennerye, Laguna Beach, California 92651.
Contact: Mr. Kenneth Ulbrich
Publishes *Mentor*. Age statement of 21 is required.

Publishers: Magazines: Health

⚥ *Urban Fitness*
Urban Publishing, Inc., Suite 500, 219 Broadway, Laguna Beach,
California 92651.
 ✆ 800 799 8738
☎ 800 797 1998 (subscriptions)
📧 UrbnFitDR@aol.com
A new magazine for a healthy lifestyle. Published every two months.
Yearly subscription is $20.79.

Publishers: Magazines: Sexuality

⚥ *Orange County Blade*
P. O. Box 1538, Laguna Beach, California 92652.
☎ 714 494 4898
Gay, lesbian, & bisexual news magazine. The magazine you pick up if
you are interested in reading. Published every month. Yearly subscription
is $25. Age statement of 18 is required.

Stores: Books: General

☺ ■ **A Different Drummer Bookshop**
♿ #A, 1027 North Coast Highway, Laguna Beach, California 92651.

☎ 714 497 6699
⌚ 10:00 - 19:00, Sat Sun 11:00 - 17:00

Lake Tahoe

Organizations: Sexuality

The Society for the Second Self (Tri-Ess)—Sigma Sigma Beta
P. O. Box 19933, Lake Tahoe, California 96151.

Lakewood

Organizations: Fetish: Smoking

Cigar Studs
P. O. Box 3052, Lakewood, California 90711-3052.

Organizations: Sexuality

Gender Expressions
P. O. Box 816, Lakewood, California 90714-0816.
☎ 310 869 4241 Fax 310 869 5662

Laytonville

Accommodation: BDSM

B&D B&B
P. O. Box 845, Laytonville, California 95454.
☎ 707 984 8343
$
Get away from it all! Beautiful rural setting for a weekend of play. Fully equipped playroom. 4 hours north of SF. Age statement of 21 is required.

Livermore

Artists: BDSM

Jan Moyes
P. O. Box 3217, Livermore, California 94550.
Age statement of 18 is required.

Long Beach

Bars: BDSM

Wolfs
2913 East Anaheim, Long Beach, California.
☎ 310 433 9251

Counsellors

David Mallon, MSW
4116 Sixth Street, Long Beach, California 90814.
☎ 310 434 8236

Barbara Roach, L.C.S.W.
Suite 1, 3490 Linden Avenue, Long Beach, California 90807.
☎ 310 424 1755
Psychological counselling.

Bob Thrasher, M.A.
Suite 920, 249 East Ocean Boulevard, Long Beach, California 90802-4849.
☎ 310 435 1749

Health Services

Long Beach Community Hospital
1720 Termino Avenue, Long Beach, California 90804.
☎ 310 498 1000

Saint Mary Medical Center
1050 Linden Avenue, Long Beach, California 90801.
☎ 310 491 9000

Manufacturers: Furniture: BDSM

Toys For Tops
P. O. Box 15828, Long Beach, California 90815.
☎ 310 425 1070 Fax 310 425 1070
⌚ By appointment only

Organizations: AIDS: Support

Being Alive—Long Beach
1734 East Broadway, Long Beach, California 90802.
☎ 310 495 3422

Organizations: Family

Parents & Friends of Lesbians & Gays (PFLAG)—Long Beach
P. O. Box 8221, Long Beach, California 90808.
☎ 310 984 8335

Organizations: Motorcycle

Council of Southern California Motorcycle Clubs
Suite 201, 2132 Bermuda, Long Beach, California 91804.

LOBOCS MC
P.O. Box 833, Long Beach, California 90801.

Organizations: Sexuality

Bisexual Support Service
The Center, 2017 East 4th. Street, Long Beach, California 908114.
☎ 310 597 2799
⌚ 09:00 - 16:00
✓
Contact: Mr. Gary North

Crossdresser Heterosexual Intersocial Club (CHIC)
P. O. Box 8487, Long Beach, California 90808.
☎ 714 993 7142
CHICSoCal@aol.com
Publishes *CHIC Clippings*.

Organizations: Sexuality: Student

Gay & Lesbian Studies Union
California State University at Long Beach, 1250 Bellflower Boulevard, Long Beach, California 90840.
☎ 310 498 4181

Publishers: Directories: Sexuality

The Long Beach Directory
Turkey Media Services, Suite 621, 4102 7th. Street, Long Beach, California 90804.
☎ 310 434 7129
Published twice a year. Yearly subscription is $4.

The Orange County Directory
Turkey Media Services, Suite 621, 4102 7th. Street, Long Beach, California 90804.
☎ 310 434 7129
Published twice a year. Yearly subscription is $3.

The Palm Springs Directory
Turkey Media Services, Suite 621, 4102 7th. Street, Long Beach, California 90804.
☎ 310 434 7129
Published once a year.

Publishers: Magazines: BDSM

Fundgeon Times
B & D Pleasures, P. O. Box 92889, Long Beach, California 90809-9988.
☎ 800 827 3787 Fax 310 631 0415
☎ 310 631 1600
✓ $ VISA MC AMERICAN EXPRESS
Published every month. Age statement of 21 is required. Spanish also spoken.

Publishers: Magazines: Bondage

Bondage Fantasies
B & D Pleasures, P. O. Box 92889, Long Beach, California 90809-9988.
☎ 800 827 3787 Fax 310 631 0415
☎ 310 631 1600
✓ $ VISA MC AMERICAN EXPRESS
Published every month. Age statement of 21 is required. Spanish also spoken.

Bondage Reader
B & D Pleasures, P. O. Box 92889, Long Beach, California 90809-9988.
☎ 800 827 3787 Fax 310 631 0415
☎ 310 631 1600
✓ $ VISA MC AMERICAN EXPRESS
Published every month. Age statement of 21 is required. Spanish also spoken.

Publishers: Magazines: Fetish

Fetish Bazaar
B & D Pleasures, P. O. Box 92889, Long Beach, California 90809-9988.
☎ 800 827 3787 Fax 310 631 0415
☎ 310 631 1600
✓ $ VISA MC AMERICAN EXPRESS
Published every month. Age statement of 21 is required. Spanish also spoken.

Publishers: Magazines: Sexuality

Bisexuality Newsletter
Gibbin Publications, P. O. Box 20917, Long Beach, California 90801.
☎ 310 597 2799
⌚ 09:00 - 16:00
✓

Cauldron
P. O. Box 14779, Long Beach, California 90803-1345.

Publishers: Newspapers: BDSM

B & D Pleasures

B & D Pleasures, P. O. Box 92889, Long Beach, California 90809-9988.
☎ 800 827 3787 ✆ 310 631 0415
☎ 310 631 1600
🍷 ✓ $ VISA ⬤
Published every month. Age statement of 21 is required. Spanish also spoken.

☺ ■ *Leather Links*
B & D Pleasures, P. O. Box 92889, Long Beach, California 90809-9988.
☎ 800 827 3787 ✆ 310 631 0415
☎ 310 631 1600
🍷 ✓ $ VISA ⬤
Published every month. Age statement of 21 is required. Spanish also spoken.

Publishers: Newspapers: Fetish
☺ ■ *Bizzare Erotic Fantasies*
B & D Pleasures, P. O. Box 92889, Long Beach, California 90809-9988.
☎ 800 827 3787 ✆ 310 631 0415
☎ 310 631 1600
🍷 ✓ $ VISA ⬤
Published every month. Age statement of 21 is required. Spanish also spoken.

Publishers: Newspapers: Sexuality
♂▼ *The Beacon*
Suite 621, 4102 East 17th. Street, Long Beach, California 90804.

Stores: Books: General
☺ ■ **Bluff Park Rare Books**
ᴬᔆ 2535 East Broadway, Long Beach, California 90803.
☎ 310 438 9830 ✆ 310 438 8652

☺ ■ **Chelsea Bookstore**
2501 East Broadway, Long Beach, California 90803.
☎ 310 434 2220

☺▼ **Dodds Bookshop**
⅊ 4818 East 2nd. Street, Long Beach, California 90803.
☎ 310 438 9948

⊕ ▼ **Pearls Booksellers**
⅊ 224 Redondo Avenue, Long Beach, California 90803.
☎ 310 438 8875
⊙ Mon - Fri 11:00 - 19:00, Sat Sun 12:00 - 17:00
Also mail order.

Television: Sexuality
♂▼ **Triangle Express Productions**
P. O. Box 90711, Long Beach, California 90803-0711.
☎ 310 491 1046

Los Angeles
Archives: Sexuality
♂ **Blanche Baker Memorial Library & Archives**
3340 Country Club Road, Los Angeles, California 90019.
☎ 213 735 5252

Bars: BDSM
♂ **Cuffs**
1941 Hyperion Avenue, Silverlake, California 90027.
☎ 213 660 2649

♂▼ **Gauntlet II**
4219 Santa Monica Boulevard, Los Angeles, California 90028.
☎ 213 669 9472
⊙ Daily until 02:00

♂▼ **Griff's**
⅊ 4216 Melrose Avenue, Los Angeles, California 90029.
☎ 213 660 0889
⊙ 18:00 - 02:00, Sun 14:00 - 02:00

♂▼ **Wolfs**
2020 East Artesia Boulevard, Los Angeles, California.

Bars: Fetish
☺ **Vice**
5657 Melrose, Los Angeles, California.
⊙ 21:00 - 02:00
Fetish-friendly dance club operated by the people who bring you the annual Fetish Ball.

Counsellors
☺ **Guy Baldwin, MFCC**
K #6, 2525 Hyperion Avenue, Los Angeles, California 90027.
☎ 213 667 9194
Psychotherapy with an understanding of your lifestyle. Specializes in working with those involved in leather / BDSM / fetish sexuality.

☺ **Susan Manson, MS, MFCC**

K ☎ 213 280 9925
UCLA trained sex therapist. Treatment of sexual problems issues & concerns. Sexual enrichment counselling, education, & consultation.

♂▼ **Jan Reynolds, M.A., MFCC**
⅊ Suite 410, 6310 San Vincente Boulevard, Los Angeles, California 90048.
☎ 213 937 3787

ᐱ▼ **Brad Taylor, M.A.**
Suite 310, 10350 Santa Monica Boulevard, Los Angeles, California 90025.
☎ 310 576 5455

Distributors: Books: General
☺ **Amok Books**
1764 North Vermont Avenue, Los Angeles, California 90027.
☎ 213 665 0956 ✆ 213 666 8105

Health Services
☺ □ **Cedars-Sinai Medical Center**
8700 Beverly Boulevard, Los Angeles, California 90048.
☎ 310 855 5000
HIV & emergency departments.

☺ □ **Century City Hospital**
2070 Century Park East, Los Angeles, California 90067.
☎ 310 553 6211
HIV & emergency departments.

☺ □ **Paul Keith, III, M.D.**
K Suite 1510, 6200 Wilshire Boulevard, Los Angeles, California 90048.
☎ 213 964 1440

☺ □ **Midway Hospital Medical Center**
5925 San Vincente Boulevard, Los Angeles, California 90019.
☎ 213 938 3161
HIV & emergency departments.

☺ **Karen Sandler, D.O.**
K Suite 600, 6464 Sunset Boulevard, Los Angeles, California 90028.
☎ 213 931 1463
Also Suite 420, 5901 West Olympic Boulevard, Los Angeles, California.
213 930 2323.

☺ □ **University of Southern California Medical Center**
1200 North State Street, Los Angeles, California 90033.
☎ 213 226 2622
HIV & emergency departments.

☺ □ **Veterans' Affairs Medical Center**
Wilshire & Sawtelle Boulevards, Los Angeles, California 90073.
☎ 310 478 3711
HIV & emergency departments.

Helplines: Sexuality
♂▽ **Gay & Lesbian Community Services Center**
1213 North Highland Avenue, Los Angeles, California 90038.
☎ 213 464 7400

Manufacturers: Clothing: Chainmail
♂ **Chain Mail Creations**
☎ 213 660 6533
If you can think it, we can link it! Affordable stock & custom designs.

Organizations: AIDS: Education
☺ **People With HIV/AIDS**
3626 West Sunset Boulevard, Los Angeles, California 90026.
☎ 213 667 3262
Publishes *Being Alive*.

Organizations: AIDS: Research
☺ **American Foundation for AIDS Research**
5900 Wilshire Boulevard, Los Angeles, California 90036-5032.
Publishes *AIDS/HIV Clinical Trials Handbook*.

Organizations: AIDS: Support
☺ □ **Aid for AIDS—Los Angeles**
⅊ Suite 200, 8235 Santa Monica Boulevard, Los Angeles, California 90046.
☎ 213 656 1107
Publishes a newsletter.

☺ □ **AIDS Project Los Angeles (APLA)**
⅊ 1313 Vine Street, Los Angeles, California 90028.
☎ 800 922 2437 (hotline)
☎ 213 962 1600
⊙ Mon - Fri 09:00 - 18:00

☺ □ **Being Alive—Los Angeles**
⅊ 3626 West Sunset Boulevard, Los Angeles, California 90026.
☎ 213 667 3262
Publishes *Being Alive*.

☺ **Stop AIDS—Los Angeles**
1213 North Highland Avenue, Los Angeles, California 90038-1254.
☎ 310 659 4778
☎ 310 659 4779 (TDD)

Organizations: BDSM

♂ **Avatar**
#747, 8033 Sunset Boulevard, Los Angeles, California 90046.
☎ 818 563 4626
🕐 Meets 4th. Wed of month

♂ **California B & B Corps**
3455 Garden Avenue, Los Angeles, California 90039.

♂▽ **Leather Corps**
P. O. Box 411332, Los Angeles, California 90041.

♂ **RAP**
#658, 8721 Santa Monica Boulevard, Los Angeles, California 90069.
☎ 213 964 1637
Contact: Mr. Aron Ocho

♂ **Regiment of the Black & Tans**
P.O. Box 291157, Los Angeles, California 90029.
☎ 818 893 1966

♂ **Somandros**
P.O. Box 291338, Los Angeles, California 90029.
☎ 213 465 7589

Organizations: Family

☺☺ **Parents & Friends of Lesbians & Gays (PFLAG)—**
& **Los Angeles**
P. O. Box 24565, Los Angeles, California 90024.
☎ 310 472 8952
🕐 Meets 3rd. Tue of month
Publishes a newsletter.

Organizations: Fetish: Clothing: Rubber

♂▽ **Vulcan America Southern California**
P. O. Box 66306, Los Angeles, California 90066.
✉ VASCInfo@aol.com

Organizations: Fetish: Foreskin

♂▽ **Uncut Club**
P. O. Box 2842, Los Angeles, California 90078.

Organizations: Fetish: Uniforms

♂▽ **Golden State Peace Officers Association**
P. O. Box 46505, Los Angeles, California 90046.

Organizations: Masturbation

♂▽ **Black Jack**
P. O. Box 83515, Los Angeles, California 90083-0515.
☎ 310 338 1516
✓ 💳
Contact: Mr. Jack Black
Safer sex club for black gay men.

Organizations: Motorcycle

♂ **Blue Max MC**
P.O. Box 39522, Los Angeles, California 90039.

♂ **Corps of Rangers**
P.O. Box 1952, Los Angeles, California 90078.
☎ 213 874 0278

♂ **Pacific Coast MC**
P. O. Box 954, Los Angeles, California 90028.

♂ **Satyrs MC**
P.O. Box 1137, Los Angeles, California 90078.
☎ 213 257 0624

♂▼ **Trident—Los Angeles**
#304, 321 South Hobart Boulevard, Los Angeles, California 90020-3613.
☎ 213 383 4866

♂ **Warriors MC**
P.O. Box 2484, Los Angeles, California 90078.

Organizations: Penis Size

⚤ ☐ **The Hung Jury**
P. O. Box 417, Los Angeles, California 90078.
☎ 213 850 3618
Publishes *Measuring Up* quarterly. Yearly subscription is $49.

Organizations: Sexuality

▽ **Androgyny**
P. O. Box 480740, Los Angeles, California 90048.
☎ 213 467 8317

☎ 909 360 5584 (in Riverside)
🕐 Meets Tue 20:00 - 22:00

♂▽ **Gay & Lesbian Community Services Center**
& 1213 Highland Avenue, Los Angeles, California 90038.
☎ 213 464 7400 ✆ 213 463 1702
☎ 213 464 0029 (TDD)
Publishes *Centernews*.

▽ **Gender Awareness League**
P. O. Box 46062, Los Angeles, California 90046.
🕐 Meets Mon 20:00 - 22:00
Contact: Ms. Grace Bredow

▽ **The Society for the Second Self (Tri-Ess)—Alpha**
P. O. Box 36091, Los Angeles, California 90036.
☎ 213 876 6141
🕐 Meets monthly
Publishes *Alpha Bits*.

♂▽ **South Bay Lesbian & Gay Community Center**
& P. O. Box 2777, Redondo Beach, California 90278.
☎ 310 379 2850
Publishes *The Community News*.

Organizations: Sexuality: Student

☺ ▽ **Cal State / Northridge LGBA**
& 18111 Nordhoff Street, Northridge, California 91330.
☎ 818 885 2393

♂▽ **GALA of CSULA**
& Suite 227, 5154 State University Drive, Los Angeles, California 90032.
☎ 213 224 3595

♂▽ **Gay & Lesbian Association UCLA**
500 Kerkhoff Hall, Los Angeles, California 90024.
☎ 213 825 8053
Publishes *Ten Percent*.

♂▽ **Gay & Lesbian Students Union**
Los Angeles Community College, 855 North Vermont Avenue, Los Angeles, California 90028.
☎ 213 669 4306

♂▽ **Lambda Delta Lambda Sorority**
Fraternity & Sorority Relations UCLA, 405 Hilgard Avenue, Los Angeles, California 90024.
☎ 213 825 6322

Organizations: Sexuality: Youth

♂ **Youth Outreach Program**
1213 North Highland Avenue, Los Angeles, California 90038.
☎ 213 464 7400 Ext.: 1702

Piercers

☺ ▼ **Gauntlet, Inc.**
8722 Santa Monica Boulevard, Los Angeles, California 90069.
☎ 310 657 6677 ✆ 310 657 4657
✉ kane@gauntlet.com
🌐 http://www.gauntlet.com/
💰 ✓ $ 💳
Catalogue, $5. Age statement of 21 is required.

☺ ■ **Primeval Body**
4647 Russell Avenue, Los Angeles, California 90027.
☎ 213 666 9601
✉ primeval@pacificnet.net
🌐 http://www.pacificnet.net/~primeval
🕐 12:00 - 19:00 evry day
💰 ✓ 💳

Printers: General

☺ **Merril Company**
1926 East 14th. Street, Los Angeles, California 90021-2891.
☎ 213 231 4133

Publishers: Books: Bondage

♂▼ *The Bondage Book*
1312 North Stanley Avenue, Los Angeles, California 90046.
💰 ✓
Mail order only, no shop front. Published quarterly. Yearly subscription is $32 plus $5 s&h.

Publishers: Directories: Sexuality

♂▼ *Community Yellow Pages*
2305 Canyon Drive, Los Angeles, California 90068.
☎ 800 745 5669
☎ 213 469 4454
A telephone book that serves Southern California from Ventura to San Diego. Published once a year. Yearly subscription is free.

♂▼ **Knight Publishing**

8060 Melrose Avenue, Los Angeles, California 90046-7082.
Publishes directory of gay adult videos, with section on BDSM.

Publishers: Magazines: BDSM

☺ ■ *Wild Times*
S & L Sales Company, Suite 317, 7019 Melrose Avenue, Los Angeles, California 90038.
$ 🏧 ©
Also produces BDSM videos. Mail order only. Published every two months. Yearly subscription is $48. Age statement of 21 is required.

Publishers: Magazines: Erotic

⚢ *Advocate Men*
P. O. Box 4371, Los Angeles, California 90078-4371.
☎ 213 871 1225

Publishers: Magazines: Fetish

☺ ■ *Rubber Rebel*
Gear, Inc., P. O. Box 66306, Los Angeles, California 90066.
☎ 213 683 8313

Publishers: Magazines: Sexuality

⚢ *The Advocate*
Liberation Publications Inc., Tenth Floor, 6922 Hollywood Boulevard, Los Angeles, California 90028.
☎ 213 871 1225 ✆ 213 467 6805
Also owns Alyson Publishing & Publishers Distributing Company.

⚢▼ *Alternatives*
Suite 235, 1283 South La Brea Avenue, Los Angeles, California 90019.
☎ 213 734 2015
For people of colour.

⚤ *The Female FYI*
Suite 2013, 8033 Sunset Boulevard, Los Angeles, California 90046.
☎ 310 859 9488

☺ *Spunk*
Plaza 9, 961 South Irolo Street, Los Angeles, California 90005.
☎ 213 487 9012 ✆ 213 487 3912

Publishers: Newspapers: Literary

☺ *The Los Angeles Times Book Review*
Times Mirror Square, Los Angeles, California 90053.
☎ 213 237 7000
☎ 213 237 7660

Publishers: Newspapers: Sexuality

⚢ *Center News*
c/o Gay & Lesbian Community Center, 1213 North Highland, Los Angeles, California 90038.
☎ 310 464 0029
Published every two months.

⚢▼ *Compass*
Suite 301, 321 South Hobart Boulevard, Los Angeles, California 90020-3613.
☎ 213 739 5891 ✆ 213 739 1786
Free in gay & lesbians locations. Published every two weeks.

⚢ *Edge*
6434 Santa Monica Boulevard, Los Angeles, California 90038.
☎ 213 962 6994 ✆ 213 962 2917
Published every two weeks.

☺ ■ *Faerie Dish Rag (FDR)*
P. O. Box 26807, Los Angeles, California 90026.
Published every month.

⚢ *Ten Percent*
308 Westwood Plaza, Los Angeles, California 900024.

Publishers: Videos: Bondage

⚢▼ *Zeus*
P. O. Box 64250, Los Angeles, California 90064.
✆ 310 474 9645

Publishers: Videos: Sexuality

⚢▼ *Bi Line Productions*
5300 West 104th. Street, Los Angeles, California 90045.
☎ 800 743 8377 ✆ 310 417 5373
☎ 310 412 7084
Also distributes videos.

Radio: Sexuality

⚢▽ *This Way Out*
Overnight Productions, P. O. Box 38327, Los Angeles, California 90038-0327.
☎ 213 874 0874
✉ TWOradio@aol.com
🌐 http://www.qrd.org/qrd/www/media/radio/thiswayout or

ftp://ftp.netcom.com/pub/bn/bnunes.thiswayout
Award-winning internationally distributed weekly gay & lesbian program currently airing on over 85 community stations in eight countries.

Stores: Art Galleries

☺ *Fahey / Klein Art Gallery*
148 North La Brea Avenue, Los Angeles, California 90036.

☺ *La Luz de Jesus*
7400 Melrose Avenue, Los Angeles, California 90046.
☎ 213 651 5875

☺ *Tamara Bane Gallery*
8025 Melrose Avenue, Los Angeles, California 90046.
☎ 213 651 1400 ✆ 310 205 0794

Stores: Books: General

☺ ■ *Author Author*
♿ 1218A Beryl Street, Redondo Beach, California 90277.
☎ 310 798 1230
🕐 Mon - Fri 09:30 - 20:00, Sat - 18:00, Sun - 19:00

☺ ■ *Book Soup*
♿ 8818 Sunset Boulevard, Los Angeles, California 90046.
☎ 310 659 3110 ✆ 310 659 3410
🕐 09:00 - 24:00

☺ ■ *Circus of Books*
4001 Sunset Boulevard, Los Angeles, California 90029.
☎ 213 666 1304

☺ ■ *Either/Or*
♿ 124 Pier Avenue, Hermosa Beach, California 90254.
☎ 310 374 2060

☺ ■ *Globe News*
314 West 6th. Street, Los Angeles, California 90014.
☎ 213 622 4390

⚢▼ *Lavendar Books*
♿ 1213 North Highland Avenue, Los Angeles, California 90038.
☎ 213 464 7400 Ext.: 204
☎ 213 464 0029 (TDD)
🕐 Tue - Sat 10:00 - 17:00

☺ ■ *Universal News Agency*
1655 North Las Palmas Avenue, Los Angeles, California 90028.
☎ 213 467 3850

☺ ■ *World Book & News*
1652 Cahuenga Boulevard, Los Angeles, California 90028.
☎ 213 465 4352 ✆ 213 465 3892

Stores: Clothing: Fetish

☺ ■ *Trashy Lingerie*
402 North La Cienega Boulevard, Los Angeles, California 90048.
☎ 310 652 4543

Stores: Clothing: Rubber

☺ ■ *Syren*
7225 Beverly Boulevard, Los Angeles, California 90036.
☎ 213 936 6693 ✆ 213 936 7586
Catalogue, $5U.S..

Stores: Clothing: Uniforms

☺ ■ *Code-3 Supply Co.*
Suite 5, 965 North Vignes Street, Los Angeles, California 90012.
☎ 213 617 3881
🕐 Mon - Fri 10:00 - 18:00, Sat 10:00 - 16:00
🏧 ©

☺ ■ *Uniforms, Inc.*
2889 West Olympic Boulevard, Los Angeles, California.
☎ 213 383 1395
🏧 ©

Stores: Erotica: BDSM

☺ ■ *Bullock's Leather & Accessories*
#482, 7985 Santa Monica Boulevard, Los Angeles, California 90046-5112.
☎ 213 665 5343
🏧

☺ ■ *Hard Labor Leather*
Suite 47, 3650 Los Feliz Boulevard, Los Angeles, California 90027.

☺ *The Leather Maker*
5720 Melsore Avenue, Los Angeles, California 90038.
☎ 213 461 1095

☺ ▼ *Magick & Fetish Shop*
3934 West Sunset Boulevard, Los Angeles, California.
☎ 213 660 1575 ✆ 213 663 7572
✉ valavic@aol.com
🕐 Tue - Sun 12:00 - 19:00

Fine fetish accessories & occult supplies. Holds monthly BDSM workshops, including instruction, group discussion & participation, & live demos. Age statement of 18 is required.

☺ ▼ **Silverlake Leather**
P. O. Box 27457, Los Angeles, California 90027.
☎ 213 665 5326 ✆ 213 665 1358

☺ ▼ **Spartacus**
7768 3/4 Santa Monica Boulevard, Los Angeles, California 90046.
☎ 213 654 8108
🕐 Tue - Sat 11:00 - 19:00
Catalogue available.

☺ ■ **The Stockroom**
4649-1/2 Russell Avenue, Los Angeles, California 90027.
☎ 800 755 8697 ✆ 213 913 5976
☎ 213 666 2121
✉ jttoys@access.digex.com or jttoys@world.std.com
🖳 http://www.stockroom.com
🕐 Mon - Sat 10:00 - 22:00
♣ ✓ 💳 💳
32-page catalogue, $15.

♂▼ **Tom of Finland Company Inc.**
🅰 1601 Griffith Park Road, Los Angeles, California 90026.
☎ 800 334 6526 ✆ 213 666 2105
☎ 213 666 1052
✉ tomfinland@earthlink.net
🖳 http://www.earthlink.net/~tomfinlandco/
🕐 Mon - Fri 09:00 - 17:00
✓ $ 💳 💳
Sole resource for legendary Tom of Finland works in print, as well as an international source for erotic books, videos, prints, rubberwear, & more. Catalogue, $10. Age statement of 21 is required.

♂▼ **Wayne's LeatheRack**
457 North Fairfax, Los Angeles, California 90036.
☎ 213 655 1016
🕐 Also classes 1st. Thu of month 21:00

Stores: Erotica: General

☺ **Drake's After Midnight Bookstore**
7566 Melrose Avenue, Los Angeles, California 90028.
☎ 213 651 5600 ✆ 213 651 1801

☺ **Highland Books**
6775 Santa Monica Boulevard, Los Angeles, California 90038.
☎ 213 463 0295 ✆ 213 463 3260

☺ ■ **Love Boutique**
2924 Wilshire Boulevard, Santa Monica, California 90403.
☎ 310 453 3459

Stores: Military Surplus

☺ ■ **A. A. Surplus Sales, Inc.**
1700 East Olympic Boulevard, Los Angeles, California 90021.
☎ 213 680 1610

☺ ■ **AA Surplus Sales**
2940 East Olympic Boulevard, Los Angeles, California.
☎ 213 526 3622

Marina Del Rey
Health Services

☺ ☐ **Daniel Freeman Marina Hospital**
4650 Lincoln Boulevard, Marina Del Rey, California 90292.
☎ 310 823 8911
HIV & emergency departments.

Organizations: BDSM

☺ ☐ **Threshold**
Suite 1004, 2554 Lincoln Boulevard, Marina Del Rey, California 90291.
☎ 213 845 0889
🕐 Monthly workshops & discussion groups

Mendocino
Publishers: Magazines: Sexuality

♦ *We Are Visible*
P. O. Box 1494, Mendocino, California 95460.
☎ 707 964 2756

Menlo Park
Piercers

☺ ■ **Fakir Musafar**
P.O. Box 2575, Menlo Park, California 94026-2575.
☎ 415 324 0543
🕐 By appointment only
♣ ✓

Shaman, master piercer & brander. Available for lectures & workshops.

Publishers: Magazines: BDSM

☺ ■ *Body Play & Modern Primitives Quarterly*
Insight Books, P.O. Box 2575, Menlo Park, California 94026-2575.
☎ 415 324 0543
♣ ✓
Also publications on corsetry. Mail order or by appointment. Published quarterly. Yearly subscription is $45U.S. to U.S., $55 elsewhere. Age statement of 21 is required.

Training: BDSM

☺ ■ **Cléo Dubois Academy of SM Arts**
P. O. Box 2345, Menlo Park, California 94026-2345.
☎ 415 322 0124
Weekend courses for dominants & switches. Hands-on experience, philosophy, & techniques. SASE or IRC for reply, please.

Mill Valley
Organizations: Family

☺ ☐ **Parents & Friends of Lesbians & Gays (PFLAG)—Marin County**
P. O. Box 1626, Mill Valley, California 94941.
☎ 415 479 3535

Milpitas
Publishers: Magazines: Fetish

♥♦ ■ *Crib Sheet*
Amber E., P. O. Box 723, Milpitas, California 95035.

Mission Hills
Manufacturers: Clothing: Leather

☺ ▼ **Black Eagle Leather Co.**
♿ P. O. Box 950865, Mission Hills, California 91395-0865.
☎ 818 361 4674 ✆ 213 426 4093
✉ leather@painet.com
🖳 http://www.painet.com/~leather/
🕐 Mon - Fri 10:00 - 19:00
♣ ✓ $ ≻ 💳 💳 🗫 𝄞
On the cutting edge leather chaps, jackets, shorts. Also works in plastic, vinyl thigh-high custom boots. World acclaimed leather masks. Catalogue, $10U.S.. Age statement of 18 is required.

Publishers: Videos: Spanking

♂▼ **Control-T Studios**
P. O. Box 7669, Mission Hills, California 91346-7669.
☎ 818 898 1591 ✆ 818 898 1591
🕐 Mon - Fri 09:00 - 17:00
♣ ✓ 💳 💳

Modesto
Organizations: BDSM

♂▽ **Knights of Malta of California Clubs, Inc.—Motherlode Chapter**
P. O. Box 581133, Modesto, California 95358.

Stores: Books: General

☺ ■ **The Bookstore Ltd.**
♿ 2400 Coffee Road, Modesto, California 95355.
☎ 209 521 0535

☺ ■ **Liberty Books**
♿ 1030 Kansas Avenue, Modesto, California 95354.
☎ 209 524 7603

Monrovia
Sculptor: General

⋈ **Ben Pike**
Suite 107, 401 East Foothill Boulevard, Monrovia, California 91016.
☎ 818 358 9582
Supplies binders for FTMs.

Mountain View
Accommodation: BDSM

☺ **The Backdrop Club**
P.O. Box 390486, Mountain View, California 94039-0486.
☎ 415 965 4499 ✆ 415 964 3879
✆ 415 964 3100. 28800 baud maximum.
✉ info@backdrop.com
🖳 http://www.fantasies.com
♣ ✓ $ 💳 💳 🗫 🗫 𝄞
Playroom rental by the hour or by the night. Age statement of 21 is required. French, Spanish, & Japanese also spoken.

BBSs: Sexuality
☺▼ **The Back Door BBS**
☎ 415 756 2906 (voice, San Francisco)
✆ 415 694 7222. 2400 baud maximum.
🕒 24hr. BBS. Voice 09:00 - 22:00
Hourly rate based on data speed. On-line shopping.

Health Services
☺ ☐ **El Camino Hospital**
2500 Grant Road, Mountain View, California 94040.

Manufacturers: Clothing: Corsets
☺ ■ **B. R. Creations**
P.O. Box 4201, Mountain View, California 94040.
☎ 415 961 5354 ☏ 415 961 5354
🕒 09:00 - 17:00, facs. 24hrs.
🐾 ✓
Publishes *BR Corset Newsletter* every two months. Yearly subscription is $18.

Publishers: Magazines: BDSM
☺ *Common Bonds*
The Backdrop Club, P.O. Box 390486, Mountain View, California 94039-0486.
☎ 415 965 4499 ☏ 415 964 3879
✆ 415 964 3100. 28800 baud maximum.
📧 info@backdrop.com
🌐 http://www.fantasies.com
🐾 ✓ $ ✉ VISA MC ▦ ◨ ℓ
Published twice a year. Yearly subscription is $20. Age statement of 21 is required. French, Spanish, & Japanese also spoken.

Publishers: Magazines: Erotic
✂ *Handjobs*
Avenue Services, P. O. Box 390811, Mountain View, California 94039.
✓
Published every month. Yearly subscription is $45 in U.S., $60 elsewhere.

Napa

Organizations: AIDS: Education
☺ ☐ **Napa Valley AIDS Project**
♿ 601 Cabot Way, Napa, California 94559-4731.
☎ 707 258 2437 ☏ 707 252 1782
🕒 24hr. telephone
Publishes *Gateway.*

Newport Beach

Publishers: Directories: Tattoo
☺ *Tattoo Directory*
P. O. Box 15893, Newport Beach, California 92659.

Publishers: Magazines: BDSM
☺ *The Master's Way*
Church of Epiphany, Suite 339, 4533 MacArthur Boulevard, Newport Beach, California 92660.
Yearly subscription is $20U.S. for U.S., $26U.S. elsewhere.

North Hollywood

BBSs: BDSM
☺ ■ **Oracle**
✆ 818 509 9681
☺▼ **Skinner Jack's Bath House**
✆ 818 760 2147

Health Services
☺ ☐ **Medical Center of North Hollywood**
12629 Riverside Drive, North Hollywood, California 91607.
☎ 818 980 9200
HIV & emergency departments.

Publishers: Magazines: Erotic
✂ *In Touch*
13122 Saticoy Street, North Hollywood, California 91605.
☎ 800 637 0101
☎ 818 764 2288

Publishers: Videos: Erotic
☺ ■ **FM Concepts**
P. O. Box 780, North Hollywood, California 91603.
🐾 ✓ VISA MC
Videos & magazines for foot & stocking fetishists.

Radio: Sexuality
♋▽ *Lesbian Sisters*
🔊 Overnight Productions FM 90.7, c/o KPFK, 3729 Cahuenga Boulevard West, North Hollywood, California 91604.
☎ 818 833 0283

Stores: Books: General
☺ **Exploded Views Books**
5708 Cahuenga Boulevard, North Hollywood, California 91601-2191.
Books of vintage erotic art, photography, etc..

Oakland

BBSs: Sexuality
☺▼ **The Back Door BBS**
☎ 415 756 2906 (voice, San Francisco)
✆ 510 463 2856. 2400 baud maximum.
🕒 24hr. BBS. Voice 09:00 - 22:00
Hourly rate based on data speed. On-line shopping.

Counsellors
✉■ **Rebecca Auge, Ph.D.**
Suite C, 3637 Grand Avenue, Oakland, California 94610.
☎ 415 426 0718
☎ 415 835 9820
Clinical psychologist: gender issues, dysphoria, cross-dressing, etc..

Distributors: Books: General
☺ **Bookpeople**
7900 Edgewater Drive, Oakland, California 94621.
☎ 510 632 4700 ☏ 510 632 1281

Health Services
☺ ☐ **Highland General Hospital**
1411 East 31st. Street, Oakland, California 94602.
☎ 510 437 4397
HIV & emergency departments.
☺ ☐ **Naval Hospital**
HIV & emergency departments.

Manufacturers: Clothing: Corsets
☺ **(sin)ch**
☎ 510 451 7716

Manufacturers: Whips
☺ ■ **Sorodz**
P.O. Box 10692, Oakland, California 94610.
☎ 510 839 2588
🐾 ✓
Catalogue, $3. Age statement of 21 is required.

Organizations: AIDS: Education
☺ **AIDS Project East Bay**
565 16th. Street, Oakland, California 94612.
☎ 510 834 8181
☺ **National Native American AIDS Prevention Center**
Suite A, 2100 Lake Shore Avenue, Oakland, California 94606.
☎ 800 283 2437 (AIDS line) ☏ 510 444 1593
☎ 510 444 2051

Organizations: BDSM
☺▽ **Alameda County Leather Corps**
P. O. Box 11346, Oakland, California 94611-9991.

Organizations: Condoms
☺ **Condom Resource Center**
P.O. Box 30564, Oakland, California 94604.
☎ 510 891 0455
Contact: Mr. Daniel Bao

Organizations: Sexuality
☺ ■ **EroSpirit Research Institute**
P. O. Box 3893, Oakland, California 94609-0893.
☎ 800 432 3767 ☏ 510 652 4354
☎ 510 428 9063
✓ VISA MC
Contact: Mr. Joseph Kramer
✉■ **FTM International**
Suite 142, 5337 College Avenue, Oakland, California 94618.
☎ 510 287 2646 ☏ 510 547 4785
📧 JamisonG@aol.com
🌐 http://www.ftm-intl.org/
✓ $
Contact: Mr. James Green, Director
Publishes *FTM Newsletter* quarterly. Yearly subscription is $15.
✉▽ **The Society for Initiatives & Services in**

Transgender Issues (SISTI)
P. O. Box 30844, Oakland, California 94604-0844.
☎ 510 601 7975

Photographers: Erotic

☺ ■ **Phil Derby**
Suite 191, 6114 LaSalle Avenue, Oakland, California 94611.
☎ 510 486 8960
⚫ ✓
Boudoir & BDSM photography & confidential photodeveloping & photoprinting services.

Piercers

☺ **Raelyn Gallina**
P. O. Box 20034, Oakland, California 94620.
☎ 510 655 2855
Total body jewelry. Exquisite custom jewelry. Catalogue, $2 & large SASE.

☺ ■ **Precision Body Piercing**
4233 Telegraph Avenue, Oakland, California 94609.
☎ 510 547 7751
⬡ http://www.ecsd.com/~casey/
⏱ Tue - Sat 12:00 - 20:00, Sun 12:00 - 17:00
⚫ ✓ 💳 ⬤

Publishers: Newspapers: Sexuality

⚥ *The Family Next Door*
P. O. Box 21580, Oakland, California 94620.
☎ 510 482 5778
Information for lesbian & gay parents about communicating with pediatricians, day care providers, & teachers about gay families & their children's needs, adoption, & other legal matters, family issues, such as grandparents, & other relatives, & starting support groups. Published every two months. Yearly subscription is $50.

⚥ *Gay & Lesbian Quarterly*
459 Boulevard Way, Oakland, California 94610.
☎ 510 869 4544 ✆ 510 893 8378
Quarterly newsletter, summarizing recent psychological & medical research pertiaing to sexual minorities. Free copy upon request. Published quarterly. Yearly subscription is $10.

Stores: Books: General

⊕ ▼ **Mama Bears**
⚫ 6536 Telegraph Road, Oakland, California 94609.
☎ 510 428 9684
Publishes *Mama Bears News & Notes.*

Stores: Erotica: General

☺ **Passion Flower**
4 Yosemite Avenue, Oakland, California 94611.
☎ 510 601 7750 ✆ 510 658 9645

Stores: Military Surplus

☺ ■ **Acme Surplus**
533 8th. Street, Oakland, California 94606.
☎ 415 444 9694

Suppliers: Safer Sex Products

☺ ■ **Mayer Laboratories**
231 Farallon Street, Oakland, California 94607.
☎ 510 452 5555
⏱ Mon - Fri 08:00 - 17:00
✓
Safer sex products to shops, groups, & non-profits organizations.

Training: Spirituality

☺ ■ **Body Electric School**
6527-A Telegraph Road, Oakland, California 94609.
☎ 510 653 1594 ✆ 510 653 4991
⏱ 10:00 - 17:00
⚫ ✓ 💳 ⬤
Workshops in erotic spirituality.

Orange

Health Services

☺ ☐ **University of California Irvine Medical Center**
101 The City Drive, Orange, California 92668.
☎ 714 456 5678

Organizations: Sexuality

⚤ ▼ **BFI Productions**
P. O. Box 3884, Orange, California 92665-0884.
☎ 714 921 1140
⚫ ✓
Publishes *Butt Fun Club* every month. Yearly subscription is $22.50. Age statement of 18 is required.

Stores: Erotica: General

☺ ■ **Versatile Fashions**
Suite C-D, 1010 North Batavia, Orange, California 92667.
☎ 800 546 2902 ✆ 714 538 7950
☎ 714 538 6498
✉ VFashion@palace.com
Also corsets for TV & others.

Pacific Beach

Piercers

☺ ■ **The Cage**
Suite F, 4502 Case Street, Pacific Beach, California.
☎ 619 531 9573

Pacific Grove

Stores: Books: General

⊕ ■ **Raven in the Grove**
Suite 103, 505 Lighthouse Avenue, Pacific Grove, California 93950.
☎ 408 649 6057

Pacifica

Organizations: Sexuality

⚥▽ **The Trangender Forum**
c/o All Together Now Publishing, Box 402, 1277 Linda Mar Center, Pacifica, California 94044.
✉ cindym@zoom.com
⬡ http://www.tgforum.com/
Contact: Ms. Cindy Martin

Palm Springs

Counsellors

⚥▼ **The Prince Institute**
P. O. Box 2916, Palm Springs, California 92263.

Health Services

☺ ☐ **Desert Hospital**
1150 North Indian Canyon Drive, Palm Springs, California 92262.
☎ 619 323 6511
HIV & emergency departments.

Organizations: BDSM

♂▽ **Palm Springs Leather Order of the Desert**
Suite 133, 4741-C East Palm Canyon Drive, Palm Springs, California 92264.
☎ 619 770 3192 ✆ 619 323 9558
Contact: Jay

Publishers: Books: Sexuality

☺ ■ *Penis Power Quarterly*
Added Dimensions Publications, Suite 484, 100 South Sunrise Way, Palm Springs, California 92263.
☎ 619 770 9647 ✆ 619 770 9647
⏱ Mon - Sat 08:00 - 17:00 Pacific
⚫ ✓
Books relating to large endowments, penis enlargement methods, & many other topics related to men's genitals. Published quarterly. Yearly subscription is $19.95. Age statement of 21 is required.

Publishers: Directories: BDSM

☺ ■ *Domination Directory International (DDI)*
Strictly Speaking Publishing Co., P. O. Box 8006, Palm Springs, California 92263.
 ✆ 619 363 6030
Listing of contact ads for dominas world-wide.

Publishers: Magazines: Arts

⚥ *Omega Literary Arts Magazine*
Suite K, 1243 Gene Autrey Trail, Palm Springs, California 92262.
☎ 619 323 0552
Published quarterly.

Publishers: Magazines: Sexuality

⚥▼ *MEGA Scene*
Box 7B, 611 South Palm Canyon Drive, Palm Springs, California 92264.

Publishers: Newspapers: Sexuality

⚥▼ *Bottom Line*
Suite 121-132, 1243 Gene Autrey Trail, Palm Springs, California 92262.
☎ 619 323 0552
Published every two weeks.

⚥▼ *Star Magazine*
Box 7B, 611 South Palm Canyon Drive, Palm Springs, California 92264.
Published every two weeks.

Stores: Books: General

Community Counselling & Consultation, Inc.
750 South Vella Road, Palm Springs, California 92264.
619 323 2118
Mon - Fri 08:30 - 17:30
Publishes *The Forum.*

Palmdale

Stores: Books: General

Sunshine Gifts
38519 Sierra Highway, Palmdale, California 93550.
805 265 0652

Palo Alto

Counsellors

Jeanne West
Suite 50, 450 San Antonio Road, Palo Alto, California 94306.
415 494 2952

Organizations: BDSM

A.S.B. Munch—Palo Alto
wi.199@wizvax.com
Meets Thu 19:30, except Thanksgiving.
Contact: M. Madelaine

Stores: Books: General

Kepler's Books
1007 Elwell Court, Palo Alto, California 94303-4308.
415 324 4321

Stepping Stones
The Artifactory, 226 Hamilton Avenue, Palo Alto, California 94301.
415 583 9685

Pasadena

Counsellors

Aloft
2047 Huntington Drive, South Pasadena, California 91030.
818 441 1789

Health Services

Huntington Memorial Hospital
100 West California Boulevard, Pasadena, California 91105.
818 397 5000
HIV & emergency departments.

Organizations: AIDS: Support

All Saints AIDS Service Center
126 West Del Mar Boulevard, Pasadena, California 91105-2508.
818 796 5633 — 818 796 8198
Mon - Fri 09:00 - 17:00
Publishes *Asklepios.*

Stores: Books: General

Page One
1196 East Walnut Street, Pasadena, California 91106.
818 798 8418
Books by for women.

Petaluma

Distributors: Erotica: General

Kink Distributors
P. O. Box 754, Petaluma, California 94953.
800 805 4657 — 800 805 4657
Humane Restraints & custom bondage items.

Pomona

Organizations: Sexuality

PSGV Transgendered Group
Suite 104, 401 South Main Street, Pomona, California 91765.
909 620 8987
Meets Tue 19:30

Redwood City

BBSs: Sexuality

The Back Door BBS
415 756 2906 (voice, San Francisco)
415 369 1579. 2400 baud maximum.
24hr. BBS. Voice 09:00 - 22:00
Hourly rate based on data speed. On-line shopping.

Health Services

Sequoia Hospital
170 Alameda De Las Pulgas, Redwood City, California 94062.
415 369 5811
HIV & emergency departments.

Organizations: AIDS: Research

AIDS Community Research Consortium
#A, 1048 El Camino Real, Redwood City, California 94063.
415 364 6563

Piercers

Graven Image
846-M Jefferson Avenue, Redwood City, California 94061.
415 369 6365

Stores: Erotica: General

Golden Gate
739 El Camino Real, Redwood City, California 94063.
415 364 6913
24hrs.

Riverside

Organizations: Sexuality: Student

Union of Lesbians, Gays. & Bisexuals
c/o Commons Main Desk, University of California, Riverside, California 92521.
909 787 3337

Stores: Military Surplus

Big John's
5513 Van Buren Boulevard, Riverside, California 92503.
714 939 0723

Sacramento

BBSs: BDSM

Leather First
916 974 1262

Competitions & Conventions: BDSM

Ms. Leather Sacramento
P.O. Box 163044, Sacramento, California 95816.
916 921 1466

Counsellors

Terence O'Brien
2509 Montgomery Way, Sacramento, California 95818.
916 979 3515
Licensed clinical social worker. Sliding scale, general fee $65 / hour, experienced in "perversion," & survivors of abuse. Trained under Guy Baldwin.

Health Services

Sutter General Hospital
2801 L. Street, Sacramento, California 95816.
916 454 2222
HIV & emergency departments.

University of California - Davis Medical Center
2315 Stockton Boulevard, Sacramento, California 95817.
916 734 3096
HIV & emergency departments.

Manufacturers: Piercing Jewelry

Kalake Kaptive Bead
1021 F Street, Sacramento, California 95814.
914 447 9443
Make surgical steel & niobium captive bead rings. Also have large selection of niobium colours & beads. Please specify retail or wholesale. Catalogue, SASE or IRC.

Organizations: AIDS: Education

Sacramento AIDS Foundation
2nd. Floor, 920 20th. Street, Sacramento, California 95814-3133.
916 448 2437

Organizations: BDSM

Living Art Association
P. O. Box 41111, Sacramento, California 95841-0111.
916 339 0331

Sacramento Leather Association
P. O. Box 5789, Sacramento, California 95817.
916 863 3398 (voice mail)
24hr. voice mail
Age statement of 21 is required.

Organizations: Bears

Valley Bears

P. O. Box 189311, Sacramento, California 95820.
☎ 916 484 7840
☎ 916 454 1210
Contact: David

Organizations: Family

☺▽ **Gay Fathers—Sacramento**
P. O. Box 51, Carmichael, California 95609-0051.
☎ 916 924 3237

☺ ☐ **Parents & Friends of Lesbians & Gays (PFLAG)—**
& **Sacramento**
P. O. Box 661855, Sacramento, California 95866.
☎ 916 444 9510

Organizations: Motorcycle

⊕ **Leather & Lace WMC, Inc.**
P.O. Box 163044, Sacramento, California 95816.
☎ 916 452 7469
Contact: Jo

Organizations: Sexuality

☺▽ **Lambda Community Center**
P. O. Box 163654, Sacramento, California 95816.
☎ 916 447 5755
☎ 916 442 0185

▽ **Sacramento Gender Association**
P. O. Box 215456, Sacramento, California 95821-1456.
☎ 916 482 7742
✉ ava4sga@aol.com
Publishes a newsletter.

Organizations: Sexuality: Student

☺▽ **Delta Lambda Phi Fraternity—Sacramento**
& Box 59, 6000 J Street, Sacramento, California 95819.

☺▽ **Gay People's Union**
Sacramento City College, Student Activities, 3835 Freeport Boulevard,
Sacramento, California 95822.
☎ 916 429 7381

Piercers

☺ ■ **The Exotic Body**
1306 1/2 19th. Street, Sacramento, California 95814.
☎ 916 447 6824
Also branding & scarification.

☺ ■ **Don Tullous**
☎ 916 485 5033
⏰ By appointment only

Printers: General

☺ **Griffin Printing/Spilman**
4141 North Freeway Boulevard, Sacramento, California 95839.
☎ 916 649 3511 ✆ 916 649 0238

Publishers: Newspapers: Sexuality

☺ *The Latest Isssue*
P. O. Box 160584, Sacramento, California 95816.
☎ 916 448 8504 ✆ 916 448 8505
Published every month. Yearly subscription is $25.

☺ *Mom Guess What!*
1725 L Street, Sacramento, California 95814.
☎ 916 441 6397
⏰ Mon - Fri 09:00 - 17:00
✓
Serving gays/lesbians in the Sacramento area since 1978 with news,
entertainment, travel, sports, & social events. Published twice a month.
Yearly subscription is $35. Age statement of 18 is required.

Stores: Books: General

☺▼ **Lioness Books**
& 2224 J Street, Sacramento, California 95816.
☎ 916 442 4657
⏰ Mon - Fri 11:00 - 19:00, Sat 12:00 - 18:00, Sun 12:00 - 17:00

☺ ■ **Tower Books**
1600 Broadway, Sacramento, California 95816.
☎ 916 444 6688

Stores: Erotica: General

☺ ■ **Goldies**
201 North 12th. Street, Sacramento, California 95814.
☎ 916 447 5860

☺ ■ **Goldies**
2138 Del Passo Boulevard, Sacramento, California 95815.
☎ 916 922 0103

Suppliers: Travel Arrangements: BDSM

☺▼ **Travel Keys Tours**
P. O. Box 162266, Sacramento, California 95816-2266.
☎ 916 452 5200
⏰ 24hrs.
♠ ✓ $ ⚊ 💳 ● ▬ ▭
Dungeons & Castles of Europe for leathermen in Sept.; antique fairs &
markets for all interested people (not gay-specific). Free catalogue. Age
statement of 21 is required. French, German, & Italian also spoken.

San Anselmo

Counsellors

☺ ■ **Joan Nelson, M.A., Ed.D.**
P. O. Box 2232, San Anselmo, California 94960.
☎ 415 453 6221 ✆ 415 453 4821
♠ ✓
Sex-related counselling.

Organizations: BDSM

℗ **Interchange**
112 San Francisco Boulevard, San Anselmo, California 94960.

℗ **Tannery Row**
112 San Francisco Boulevard, San Anselmo, California 94960.

Organizations: Sexuality

☺ ■ **The National Organization of Circumcision**
Information Resource Centers (NOCIRC)
P. O. Box 2512, San Anselmo, California 94979-2512.
☎ 415 488 9883 ✆ 415 488 9660
Contact: Ms. Marilyn Milos, R.N.
Information on male & female genital modifications of any sort.
Referrals to physicians. Publishes *Nocirc Newsletter* twice a year. Yearly
subscription is $15.

☺▽ **Spectrum**
1000 Sir Francis Drake, San Anselmo, California.
☎ 415 457 1115
Community centre.

San Bernardino

Health Services

☺ ☐ **San Bernardino County Medical Center**
780 East Gilbert Street, San Bernardino, California 92415.
☎ 909 387 8111
HIV & emergency departments.

Helplines: Sexuality

☺▽ **Gay & Lesbian Center, Island Empire**
P. O. Box 6333, San Bernardino, California 92412.
☎ 909 884 5447
⏰ 18:30: 22:00

Organizations: Fetish: Smoking

☺▽ **EBC**
P. O. Box 9927, San Bernardino, California 92427-0927.

Organizations: Sexuality

☺▽ **Gay & Lesbian Center, Island Empire**
& P. O. Box 6333, San Bernardino, California 92412.
☎ 909 884 5447
⏰ 18:30: 22:00

Organizations: Sexuality: Student

☺▽ **Gay & Lesbian Student Union**
& California State University, 5500 University Parkway, San Bernardino,
California 92407.
☎ 090 887 7407

Publishers: Magazines: Body Size

♂ ■ *Squish*
Big Time Publications, Suite 167, 308 East Base Line Street, San
Bernardino, California 92410.
For crush lovers: men being crushed by women.

San Diego

Archives: Sexuality

☺▽ **Lesbian & Gay Historical Society of San Diego**
& P. O. Box 40389, San Diego, California 92164.
☎ 619 260 1522

Bars: BDSM

☺ ■ **Wolfs**
3404 30th. Street, San Diego, California 92104.
☎ 619 291 3730

16:00 - 04:00

BBSs: BDSM

Andros
619 233 6253

Counsellors

Mel Karmen, Ph.D.
4111 Palmetto Way, San Diego, California 92103.
619 296 9442 — 619 295 8668
Mon - Fri 10:00 - 18:00
✓ $
Counselling & psychotherapy to lesbian, gay, bisexual, & transgender community, including people with HIV/AIDS. Also to heterosexual men & women. Age statement of 18 is required.

Al Marks, Ph.D.
3821 Front Street, San Diego, California.
619 296 6134
Psychologist.

John McConnell, Ph.D.
4036 Third Avenue, San Diego, California.
619 296 1216 — 619 296 5027
619 296 8103
✓
Private practice working with individuals & couples. Also works with groups, depending upon demand. Kink-aware & kink-involved.

Health Services

Beach Area Community Health Center
3705 Mission Boulevard, San Diego, California 92109.
619 488 0644

Harbor View Medical Center
120 Elm Street, San Diego, California 92101.
619 235 3102
HIV & emergency departments.

UCSD Medical Center
Owen Clinic, 200 West Arbor Drive, San Diego, California 92103-8681.
619 294 6222

Helplines: Sexuality

Lesbian & Gay Men's Community Center
P. O. Box 3357, San Diego, California 92163.
619 692 4297

Manufacturers: Erotica: BDSM

Crypto Tech Corp.
3132 Jefferson Street, San Diego, California 92110-4421.
800 331 0442
Has 8 of its own stores.

Organizations: AIDS: Education

AIDS Foundation San Diego
4080 Centre Street, San Diego, California 92103.
619 686 5000

Organizations: AIDS: Research

San Diego Community Research Group
3800 Ray Street, San Diego, California 92104.
619 291 2437

Organizations: AIDS: Support

Being Alive—San Diego
720 Robinson Avenue, San Diego, California 92103.
619 281 1400

Organizations: BDSM

Club X
P. O. Box 3092, San Diego, California 92163.
800 598 1859
619 685 5149
Publishes *Chainmail*.

Moonlight Leather Association of the Deaf
P. O. Box 86174, San Diego, California 92138.
Contact: Mr. Jeff Barrett

SandMen
3333 Columbia, San Diego, California 92103.
Contact: Mr. Kelly Thibault

Organizations: Bears

Bears San Diego
P. O. Box 620874, San Diego, California 92162.
619 696 7639
xxltony@crash.cts.com
http://www.skepsis.com/.gblo/bears/CLUBS/Bears_San_Diego/

Organizations: Body Size

Girth & Mirth—San Diego
P. O. Box 86822, San Diego, California 92138-6822.
619 685 8822
GMSD@aol.com
Contact: Mr. Andy Arnoldt, Secretary
Publishes *San Diego at Large*.

Organizations: Family

Parents & Friends of Lesbians & Gays (PFLAG)—San Diego
P. O. Box 82762, San Diego, California 92138.
619 579 7640

Organizations: Fetish: Mess

Mud Buddies
c/o Wolfs, 3404 30th. Street, San Diego, California 92104.

Organizations: Fisting

Red Hankies of San Diego
P. O. Box 3988, San Diego, California 92163.
619 688 8668
619 298 2368
International fisting fisting organization, based in San Diego. For novice to experienced. For contacts of like minds & fetishes. Publishes *RHSD Newsletter* quarterly. Yearly subscription is $20. Age statement of 18 is required.

Organizations: Motorcycle

California Cyclemen MC
P.O. Box 86969, San Diego, California 92138.

Knights on Iron MC
P.O. Box 3992, San Diego, California 92163-1992.

Organizations: Sexuality

Lesbian & Gay Men's Community Center
P. O. Box 3357, San Diego, California 92163.
619 692 4297 (information) — 619 260 3092
619 692 2077 (office)
Publishes *CenterPiece*.

Neutral Corner
P. O. Box 12581, San Diego, California 92112.
619 685 3696
Publishes *Reflections*.

Phœnix Rising
P. O. box 632852, San Diego, California 92163-2852.
Meets weekly
Contact: Ms. Kristen Dixon

San Diego North County Gay & Lesbian Association
P. O. Box 2866, Vista, California 92085-2866.
619 945 2478

Organizations: Sexuality: Student

Lesbian, Gay, & Bisexual Organization
P. O. Box 0077-#18, University of California, San Diego, 9500 Gilman Drive, La Jolla, California 92093-0077.
619 534 4297

Lesbian, Gay, & Bisexual Student Union
P. O. Box 45, Azec Center, San Diego, California 92182.
619 594 2737

Organizations: Sexuality: Youth

Gay Youth Alliance
P. O. Box 83022, San Diego, California 92138.
619 233 9209

Piercers

Claw
709 6th. Avenue, San Diego, California.
619 239 3246

Publishers: Magazines: Erotic

Hotshots
Sunshine Publishing Co., 7060 Convoy Court, San Diego, California 9211.
619 278 9080 — 619 278 9081

Publishers: Magazines: Sexuality

Dream Magazine
Klinger Publications, Klinger Building, 2801 Fouth Avenue, San Diego, California 92103.
Published every month. Yearly subscription is $70.

Publishers: Newspapers: Sexuality

♂▽ *Frontera Gay*
P. O. Box 620 626, San Diego, California 92162.

☺▽ *The North Park Review*
P. O. Box 40174, San Diego, California 92164.
☎ 619 688 0690

♂▽ *Update*
P. O. Box 33148, San Diego, California 92163-3148.
☎ 619 299 0500 ✆ 619 299 6907
Published every week. Yearly subscription is $75.

⊕ ■ *Women's Times*
#1-A-2, 2535 Kettner Boulevard, San Diego, California 92101-1525.
☎ 619 236 9250 ✆ 619 236 8235

Publishers: Videos: Fetish: Uniforms

♂▽ **Bi Coastal Productions (BIC)**
1043 University Avenue, San Diego, California 92103-3392.
☎ 407 655 0558
Publication, wholesale, & mail order of videos.

Stores: Art Galleries

☺ □ **Dove Art**
4060 Morena Boulevard, San Diego, California 92117.
☎ 619 270 7400

☺ ■ **Rita Dean Gallery**
548 5th. Avenue, San Diego, California 92101.
☎ 619 338 8153 ✆ 619 338 0003
Puts on an annual erotic art exhibition.

Stores: Books: General

☺ ■ **Blue Door Bookstore**
3823 5th. Avenue, San Diego, California 92103.
☎ 619 298 8610
🕐 Mon - Sat 09:00 - 21:30, Sun 10:00 - 21:00
🍷 ✓ 💳 ⬭
Shop only, no mail order.

♂▽ **Obelisk The Bookstore**
🚹 1029 University Avenue, San Diego, California 92103.
☎ 619 297 4171
🕐 11:00 - 22:00, Fri Sat - 23:00, Sun 12:00 - 20:00

Stores: Erotica: BDSM

☺ **Crypt**
3404 30th. Street, San Diego, California 92104.
☎ 619 574 1579

☺▽ **Moose Leather**
🚹 2923 Upas Street, San Diego, California 92104.
☎ 619 297 6935
🕐 Tue - Thu 12:00 - 21:00, Fri Sat 12:00 - 22:00
🍷 ✓ $ ⬌ 💳 ⬭
Small leather shop that specializes in custom work, as well as alterations
& repair. All are welcome in our store. Age statement of 18 is required.

Stores: Erotica: General

☺ ■ **Gemini**
5265 University Avenue, San Diego, California 92105.
☎ 619 287 1402

☺ ■ **F Street—Gaslamp**
751 Fourth Avenue, San Diego, California 92101.
☎ 619 236 0841

☺ ■ **F Street—Kearny Mesa**
7865 Balboa Avenue, San Diego, California 92111.
☎ 619 292 8083

☺ ■ **F Street—Mira Mesa**
7998 Miramar Road, San Diego, California 92126.
☎ 619 549 8014

☺ **F Street—North Park**
2004 University, San Diego, California 92104.
☎ 619 298 2644 ✆ 619 298 5807

☺ ■ **F Street—Pacific Beach**
4626 Albuquerque Street, San Diego, California 92109.
☎ 619 581 0400

☺ ■ **F Street—San Ysidro**
4650 Border Villlage Road, San Diego, California 92073.
☎ 619 497 6042
Spanish also spoken.

☺ ■ **F Street—Sports Arena**
3112 Midway Drive, San Diego, California 92110.
☎ 619 221 0075

☺ **Midnight Adult Book & Video**
1407 University Avenue, San Diego, California 92103.

☎ 619 299 7186 ✆ 619 299 3612

☺ **Midnight Adult Book & Video**
3604 Midway Drive, San Diego, California 92110.
☎ 619 222 9973 ✆ 619 222 0866

☺ ■ **Pleasureland**
🚹 836 5th. Avenue, San Diego, California 92101.
☎ 619 237 9056

Stores: Safer Sex Products

☺ **Condoms Plus**
1220 University Avenue, San Diego, California 92103.
☎ 619 291 7406
San Diego county's only condom store. Spanish also spoken.

Television: Sexuality

♂▽ *Our World Television*
3976 Park Boulevard, San Diego, California 92103.
☎ 619 297 4975

San Dimas

Publishers: Magazines: Swingers

☺ ■ *Loving Alternatives*
Omnific Designs West, P. O. Box 459, San Dimas, California 91773.
☎ 909 592 5217 ✆ 818 915 4715
Published every two months. Yearly subscription is $20.

San Francisco

Accommodation: BDSM

☺ **Castlebar**
☎ 415 552 2100
☎ 415 552 6000
🕐 11:00 - 23:00
🍷 ℓ
Two dungeons rented by the hour to couples & small groups. Perfect for
birthdays, anniversaries, & special occasions. Videotaping permitted. Age
statement of 18 is required.

Archives: Sexuality

♂▽ **Harvey Milk Archives**
53-B Manchester Street, San Francisco, California 94110-5214.
☎ 415 824 3449

Bars: BDSM

♂▾■ **Headquarters**
🚹 469 Castro Street, San Francisco, California 94114.
☎ 415 626 5876

♂▾ **Hole In The Wall Saloon**
289 8th. Street, San Francisco, California 94103.
☎ 415 431 4695

♂▾▽ **Jackhammer**
290 Sanchez, San Francisco, California 94114.
☎ 415 252 0290

BBSs: AIDS

☺ ■ **AIDS Info BBS**
P. O. Box 421528, San Francisco, California 94142-1528.
☎ 415 626 124 ✆ 415 626 9415
☎ 415 626 1246
🕐 24 hour service
Computer information system about AIDS. When you use your computer
to log on, you will be asked to register with the BBS. You may use any
name. Free brochure.

BBSs: BDSM

☺ ■ **Backrop**
✆ 415 431 8167

☺ ■ **The Station House**
✆ 415 621 4273

♂▾▽ **Studs**
Box 90, 1800 Market Street, San Francisco, California 94102.
☎ 415 495 1811 ✆ 415 495 0404
✆ 415 495 2929

Competitions & Conventions: BDSM

⊕ **Ms. San Francisco Leather**
Box 490, 2261 Market Street, San Francisco, California 94114.

Counsellors

☺ **Ask Isadora**
K♂✦ #153, 3145 Geary Boulevard, San Francisco, California 94118.
☎ 415 386 5090 ✆ 415 386 5090
🕐 By appointment
🍷 ✓
Syndicated advice columnist on sex & relationships. Private

consultations. Audio tapes on meeting new people, enjoying sex, & improving communication. Age statement of 18 is required.

Michael Bettinger, Ph.D., MFCC
1726 Fillmore Street, San Francisco, California 94115.
415 563 6100 — 415 563 6129
Mon - Fri 12:00 - 21:00
Works with people with any style of life.

Louanne Cole, Ph.D.
#A, 3025 Fillmore Street, San Francisco, California 94123.
415 333 9500
900 773 9463
lcole@netcom.com
24hrs.
900 line has wide selection of information about sexual matters; cost added to your telephone bill.

Dossie Easton, MFCC
406 16th Avenue, San Francisco, California 94118.
415 488 1431
BDSM-aware counsellor experienced with sexual minorities. Individual & couples counselling.

Gender & Self Acceptance Program (GSAP)
P. O. Box 424447, San Francisco, California 94142.
415 558 8058

William Henkin
Suite 111, 1801 Bush Street, San Francisco, California 94109.
415 923 1150 — 415 923 1998
✓ $
Psychotherapy, counselling, & sex education, with special attention to concerns of alternate sex & gender issues. Age statement of 18 is required.

William Horstman, Ph.D.
4328 18th Street, San Francisco, California 94114.
415 431 1790 — 415 863 9031
Psychologist experienced with BDSM / fetish issues, couples counselling, & HIV issues.

Psychology & Counselling Associates
415 863 9559 — 415 863 7447

Margo Rila
415 861 4551

Luanna Rodgers, M.A., MFCC
1609 Church Street, San Francisco, California 94131.
415 641 8890
Mon - Sat by appointment
✓

Maggi Rubenstein, R.N., MFCC, Ph.D.
415 584 0172
12:00 or after 21:00
✓
License MM008794.

Rachel Schochet, Ph.D., MFCC
536 Eureka Street, San Francisco, California 94114.
415 641 1292
Individuals, couples, various issues including HIV, grief & loss, & substance abuse.

David Strout, LSMW
5534 Fulton Street, San Francisco, California 94121-3509.
✓

Distributors: Books: General

Alamo Square Distributors
P.O. Box 14543, San Francisco, California 94114.
415 863 7410 — 415 863 7456

Last Gasp of San Francisco
777 Florida Street, San Francisco, California 94110.
415 824 6636 — 415 824 1836

Distributors Erotica: BDSM

Screaming Leather
Box 810, 2215-R Market Street, San Francisco, California 94114.
Wholesale to retail stores only. Free catalogue.

Health Services

Davies Medical Center
Castro & Duboce Street, San Francisco, California 94114.
HIV & emergency departments.

Kaiser Foundation Hospital
2425 Geary Boulevard, San Francisco, California 94115.
415 202 2000
HIV & emergency departments.

Laguna Honda Hospital
375 Laguna Honda Boulevard, San Francisco, California 94116.
415 664 1580
HIV department.

Lyon-Martin Women's Health Services
#201, 1748 Market Street, San Francisco, California 94102.
415 565 7674 — 415 252 7490
Also has HIV/AIDS information & support.

Charles Moser, Ph.D, M.D.
Suite 125, 45 Castro Street, San Francisco, California 94114.
415 621 4369
Internal & sexual medicine.

Saint Mary's Hospital & Medical Center
450 Stanyan Street, San Francisco, California 94117.
415 668 1000
HIV & emergency departments.

San Francisco General Hospital Medical Center
1001 Potero Avenue, San Francisco, California 94110.
415 206 8000
HIV & emergency departments.

Helplines: AIDS

AIDS/HIV Nightline
415 668 2437

Helplines: Sexual Health

San Francisco Sex Information
P.O. Box 881254, San Francisco, California 94188-1254.
415 989 7374
Mon - Fri 15:00 - 21:00
Free, anonymous, serving all ages & lifestyles.

Helplines: Sexuality

Gay Area Youth Switchboard
P. O. Box 846, San Francisco, California 94101.
415 386 4297

Manufacturers: Clothing: Leather

San Francisco Leather Works
415 566 7376
Wholesale & custom leather.

Manufacturers: Clothing: Footwear

Catherine Coatney
P. O. Box 194492, San Francisco, California 94119-4492.
415 431 7300 — 415 431 7313
Also plastic fetish wear. Catalogue, $4U.S..

Manufacturers: Clothing: Leather

Jacqui
1250 Folsom Street, San Francisco, California 94103.
415 626 6551
Custom leather clothing & costumes.

Manufacturers: Erotica: General

Socket Science Labs
Suite 187, 4104 24th. Street, San Francisco, California 94114.
415 334 1828 — 415 587 7459 (call first)
Mon - Sat 07:00 - 19:00
✓
Wholesale to U.S. & Europe, retail mail order to U.S. & Canada.

Manufacturers: Erotica: Leather

Leather Stitches
P.O. Box 24555, San Francisco, California 94124.
415 546 4075 — 415 822 0500
Mon - Sat 10:00 - 18:00
✓ $
Custom made clothing & accessories in leather. Age statement of 21 is required.

Organizations: AIDS: Education

Bluelights Campaign
Suite 125, 109 Minna Street, San Francisco, California 94105.
415 863 3540

Harvey Milk AIDS Education Project
P. O. Box 14368, San Francisco, California 94114.
415 773 9544
Publishes *Can We Talk?*.

The NAMES Project Foundation
Suite 310, 310 Townsend Street, San Francisco, California 94107-1607.
415 882 5500

National Task Force on AIDS Prevention
631 O'Farrell Street, San Francisco, California 94109.
415 749 6700

Project Inform

Suite 220, 1965 Market Street, San Francisco, California 94103-1012.
800 822 7422 · 415 558 0684
415 558 9051
Mon - Sat 10:00 - 16:00 Pacific
Contact: Mr. Ben Collins

San Francisco AIDS Foundation
P. O. Box 426182, San Francisco, California 94142-6182.
415 864 5855
Also publishes other periodicals. Publishes *Bulletin of Experimental AIDS Treatments (BETA).*

Organizations: BDSM

The 15 Association
P.O. Box 421302, San Francisco, California 94141.
415 673 0452

A.S.B. Munch—San Francisco Bay
bast-request@node.com

Celestial Krewe de Cuir
Suite 201, 155 Haight Street, San Francisco, California 94102-5741.
415 255 4663

Club Domentia
Box 804, 2215-R Market Street, San Francisco, California 94114.

Cogent Warriors
#250, 2261 Merket Street, San Francisco, California 94114.

Organizations: BDSM: Competition

Mr. Drummer
c/o Fantastic Realities Unlimited, Box 490, 2261 Market Street, San Francisco, California 94114.
415 974 1156 · 415 243 8402
✓

Organizations: BDSM

D.L.
P.O. Box 423701, San Francisco, California 94142-3701.

Defenders—San Francisco
c/o Dignity San Francisco, 1329 7th Avenue, San Francisco, California 94117.
415 487 7669
http://www.blackiris.com/SFLeatherMC/SFLclubs/Defenders/Defenders.html

FM
15 Harriett, San Francisco, California 94103.

Golden Gate Guards
P.O. Box 192101, San Francisco, California 94119-2101.
415 431 9475
Contact: Mr. Jack Gooddall

L/SM Round-Up
P. O. Box 425547, San Francisco, California 94142-5547.
415 754 2990
Host the "Bound by Serenity" event in September each year.

LINKS
P.O. Box 420989, San Francisco, California 94142-0989.
415 695 7955
415 255 2157
lthrlinks@aol.com
Contact: Mr. Edward Goehring

Lion's Roar
426 Lux South, San Francisco, California 94080.
415 588 1850

Northern California Leather Association of the Deaf
P. O. Box 641511, San Francisco, California 94164-1511.
Contact: Mr. Patrick Saatzer

Outcasts
P.O. Box 31266, San Francisco, California 94131-0266.
415 668 4622
415 487 5170 (voice mail)
✓ $ ¢
Women to women educational support & social organization for women interested in BDSM between lesbian, bisexual, & transsexual women.

Pervert Scouts
Suite 19, 3288 21st. Street, San Francisco, California 94110.
415 285 7985
PervScouts@aol.com
Meets 2nd. & 4th. Sat of month
Contact: Ms. Beth Carr

S & M Club
583 Grove Street, San Francisco, California 94102.
415 552 7339

San Francisco God-Damned Independents
P.O. Box 192412, San Francisco, California 94119-2412.
415 431 7645
415 91 4256

Sex Magik Faeries Circle
1434 Alemany, San Francisco, California 94112.

Society of Janus
P.O. Box 426794, San Francisco, California 94142-6794.
415 985 7117
415 985 7118 (events line)
janus@blackiris.com
http://www.blackiris.com/SFLeatherMC/janus/Janus.html
Contact: Mr. Jay Wiseman

Sons of Satan
P. O. Box 423701, San Francisco, California 94142-38701.
415 695 2913

Trusted Servants
P.O. Box 14374, San Francisco, California 94114-0374.
415 552 0301
Truserv@blackiris.com
http://www.blackiris.com/SFLeatherMC/SFLclubs/TrustedServants/TShome.html
Contact: Mr. Ken Prag

Organizations: Bears

BearHug Group
Box 160, 2261 Market Street, San Francisco, California 94114-1600.
415 647 9127

Bears of San Francisco
Box 266, 2215-R Market Street, San Francisco, California 94102.
415 541 5000
sfgrizly@quake.net
http://www.q.com/bosf/
Contact: Mr. Richard Polack

Hirsute Fraternity
#3, 26 Church Street, San Francisco, California 94114.

San Francisco Leather Bears
152A Russ, San Francisco, California 94103-4010.

Organizations: Body Size

Affliated Big Men's Clubs
Box 139, 584 Castro Street, San Francisco, California 94114.

Girth & Mirth—San Francisco
176-B Page Street, San Francisco, California 94102.
415 552 1143

Organizations: Bondage

San Francisco Bondage Club
#107, 1800 Market Street, San Francisco, California 94102.

Organizations: Family

Parents & Friends of Lesbians & Gays (PFLAG)—San Francisco
P. O. Box 640223, San Francisco, California 94164-0223.
415 921 8850

Organizations: Fetish: Clothing: Rubber

Rubber Corps
P. O. Box 14407, San Francisco, California 94114.
415 267 7604

Organizations: Fetish: Foreskin

Uncircumcised Society of America (USA)
P. O. Box 26011, San Francisco, California 94126.
Contact: Mr. Bud Berkeley
Dedicated to the appreciation of the foreskin & gneral discussion of the foreskin. SASE or IRC for more information. Publishes *Foreskin Finder List* quarterly.

Uncut
P. O. Box 421263, San Francisco, California 94142-1263.

Organizations: Fetish: Uniforms

Phœnix Uniform Club
P. O. Box 31699, San Francisco, California 94131-0699.
415 863 3127

Organizations: Health

EROS, The Center for Safe Sex
2051 Market Street, San Francisco, California 94114.
415 255 4921
415 864 3767
Call second number for hours
Contact: Mr. Buzz Bense
Age statement of 18 is required.

Organizations: Motorcycle

California Eagles MC
P.O. Box 14665, San Francisco, California 94114-0665.
415 267 0560
CalEagles@aol.com
http://www.blackiris.com/SFLeatherMC/SFLclubs/CalEagles/home.htm
Meets 3rd. Sat of month 15:00

Constantines, Inc., of the Bay Area
P.O. Box 424964, San Francisco, California 94142-4964.
http://www.blackiris.com/SFLeatherMC/SFLclubs/Constantines/Connies.html

Cycle Runners MC
P. O. Box 26737, San Francisco, California 94126-6737.
http://www.blackiris.com/SFLeatherMC/SFLclubs/CRMC/CRMC.html

Knights of Malta of California Clubs, Inc.—Cable Car Chapter
Box 212, 2261 Market Street, San Francisco, California 94114-2588.
komccc@blackiris.com
http://www.blackiris.com/SFLeatherMC/SFLclubs/KofM/KofM.html

La Madrona
P.O. Box 1407, San Francisco, California 94101.

Pacific Bears California LMC—San Francisco
Box 447, 584 Castro Street, San Francisco, California 94114-2500.
415 905 9575

Pegasus Motorcycle Owners Club
242 Diamond Street, San Francisco, California 94114.
415 334 1166
Contact: Chauncy

Rainbow MC
562 Fell Street, San Francisco, California 94102.

Sirens MC San Francisco
P. O. Box 423702, 152A Russ Street, San Francisco, California 94102.
415 530 9328

Warlocks MC
P.O. Box 424365, San Francisco, California 94142-4365.

Women's Motorcycle Contingent
P. O. Box 14781, San Francisco, California 94114-4781.
415 395 8318

Organizations: Piercing

The Association of Professional Piercers
Box 120, 519 Castro Street, San Francisco, California 94114.
app@sfo.com
http://www.sfo.com/~app/index.html

Organizations: Publishing

COSMEP
P. O. Box 703-P, San Francisco, California 94101.
415 922 9490

Organizations: Research: Sexuality

Center for Research & Education in Sexuality
San Francisco State University, San Francisco, California 94132.
415 338 1137
Publishes *The Journal of Homosexuality*.

Organizations: Sexual Politics

The Committee to Preserve Sexual Liberties
P. O. Box 422385, San Francisco, California 94142-2385.
Publishes *The Journal of Sexual Liberty*.

International Gay & Lesbian Human Rights Commission (IGLHRC)
Suite 200, 1360 Mission Street, San Francisco, California 94103.
415 255 8680 Fax: 415 255 8662
iglhrc@igc.apc.org

National Organization to Halt the Abuse & Routine Mutilation of Males (NOHARMM)
P. O. Box 460795, San Francisco, California 94146.
415 826 9351

Organizations: Sexuality

Bay Area Bisexual Network
Suite 24, 2404 California Street, San Francisco, California 94115.
415 703 7977
Contact: Mr. Mark Silver

Digital Queers
Suite 150, 584 Castro Street, San Francisco, California 94114.
415 974 9122 Fax: 415 648 0142
dq@yes.com
24hr. facs. & voicemail
National professional organization serving queers who work in the high technology industry.

EVE Fund
c/o Frameline, 346 9th. Street, San Francisco, California 94103.
415 281 0292
Fund for women who want to produce videos about erotic safe sex.

Film @ Eleven
Box 559, 2215-R Market Street, San Francisco, California 94114.
415 469 2093
Publishes *Hippie Dick!* quarterly. Yearly subscription is $20.

FPSG
P. O. Box 410990, San Francisco, California 94141-0990.
Support group for FTMs of colour only.

International Wavelength, Inc.
Box 829, 2215-R Market Street, San Francisco, California 94114.
415 749 1100 Fax: 415 928 1165
Publishes *Passport*.

Lesbian & Gay Advisory Commission
Suite 800, 25 Van Ness, San Francisco, California 94102-6033.

North American Man Boy Love Association
Suite 8418, 537 Jones Street, San Francisco, California 94102.
415 564 2602
212 631 1194
Publishes *NAMBLA Bulletin*.

San Francisco Gender Information
P.O. Box 423602, San Francisco, California 94142.
Contact: Ms. Christine Beatty
Keeps a database of transgender resources in the San Francisco area.

Organizations: Sexuality: Education

Holiday Associates
P. O. Box 421666, San Francisco, California 94142-1666.
415 863 7326
Mon - Thu 13:00 - 21:00
Contact: Ms. Sybil Holiday
Sex education for safe sex & alternate sexualities.

Organizations: Sexuality: Student

Gay & Lesbian Alliance
c/o Student Activities, San Francisco College, San Francisco, California 94112.
415 239 3212

Gay & Lesbian Alliance San Francisco State University
Room M-100A, 1600 Holloway Avenue, San Francisco, California 94132.

Lesbians In Law (LIL)
c/o Women's Association Law School, Golden Gate College, 536 Mission Street, San Francisco, California 94105.

Gay Law Students at Hastings
Hastings College of the Law, 200 McAllister Street, San Francisco, California 94102.
415 565 4601

Organizations: Sexuality: Youth

Bay Area Sexual Minority Youth Network
P. O. Box 460268, San Francisco, California 94146-0268.
415 487 6870
insideout@igc.apc.org
✓ $
Publishes *InsideOUT*. Yearly subscription is $10 (23 & younger), $20 (24 & older).

Lambda Youth & Family Empowerment
Suite 201, 1748 Market Street, San Francisco, California 94102.
415 565 7681 Fax: 415 252 7490
Support, information, & counselling for youth under 23 & their families.

National Gay Youth Network
P. O. Box 846, San Francisco, California 94101.

Organizations: Watersports

Golden Shower Buddies
Box 395, 584 Castro Street, San Francisco, California 94114.
415 979 0242

Organizations: Wrestling

☺ ■ **Bay Area Boxing Club**
c/o KO, P. O. Box 507, Arlington, Virginia 22314-0507.
☎ 415 585 2365

♂▽ **Northern California Wrestling Club (NCWC)**
Box 504, 584 Castro Street, San Francisco, California 94114.
✉ NCalWrestl@aol.com

♂▽ **Wrasslin' Bears**
Suite 1479, 41 Sutter Street, San Francisco, California 94104-4903.
☎ 415 673 6434
🕐 Meets 3rd. Sun of month. Call in evening
Contact: Mr. Hank Trout

Photographers: Erotic

☺ **Mark Chester**
P.O. Box 422501, San Francisco, California 94114.
☎ 415 621 6294
✉ markic@queernet.org
🌐 http://www.blackiris.com/mchester/michome.html
🕐 Viewing by appointment
🔥 ✓
Sponsors annual erotic art exhibitions: all genders/orientations. Personal work: fine art black & white photographs of gay radical sexuality.

☺ **Charles Gatewood**
P.O. Box 410052, San Francisco, California 94141.
☎ 415 267 7651
✓ VISA MC
Catalogue, $5. Age statement of 21 is required.

Piercers

☺ **Anubis Warpus**
1525 Haight Street, San Francisco, California 94117.
☎ 415 431 2218 ✆ 415 626 1270
🕐 11:00 - 21:00
🔥 ✓ VISA MC ✆
Retail clothing, shoe, magazine & bookshop, with piercing & tattooing. Age statement of 18 is required.

☺ ■ **Body Manipulations**
254 Fillmore Street, San Francisco, California 94117.
☎ 415 621 0408 ✆ 415 621 6926
🕐 Thu - Sat 12:00 - 19:30, Sun - Wed 12:00 - 18:00

☺▼ **Gauntlet, Inc.**
2377 Market Street, San Francisco, California 94114.
☎ 800 746 4728 ✆ 415 431 3170
☎ 415 431 3133
✉ kane@gauntlet.com
🌐 http://www.gauntlet.com/
🔥 ✓ $ VISA MC AMEX
Catalogue, $5. Age statement of 21 is required.

☺ ■ **Nomad**
1881 Hayes Street, San Francisco, California 94117.
☎ 415 563 7771 ✆ 415 563 7771
✉ filagree@sirius.com
🌐 http://www.sirius.com/~stas/NOMAD/nmdhome.html
🕐 11:00 - 19:00 every day
Carries jewelry by Fakir Musafar.

Printers: General

☺ ■ **Norcal Printing**
1595 Farifax Avenue, San Francisco, California 94124.
☎ 415 282 8856 ✆ 415 282 1008
🕐 Mon - Fri 08:00 - 17:00
🔥 ✓
Printers of the Black Book, & other newspapers, magazines, etc..

Public Speakers: Gender Issues

☺ **William Henkin**
K Suite 111, 1801 Bush Street, San Francisco, California 94109.
☎ 415 923 1150 ✆ 415 923 1998
✓ $ ⚥
Sex education, with special attention to concerns of alternate sex & gender issues. Age statement of 18 is required.

Public Speakers: Sexuality

♂▼ **Carol Queen**
P. O. Box 471061, San Francisco, California 94147.
☎ 415 978 0891
Lectures & workshops on all aspects of alternate sexualities.

Publishers: Books: BDSM

♂▼ **Dædalus Publishing Company**
Suite 518, 584 Castro Street, San Francisco, California 94114.
☎ 415 626 1867 ✆ 415 487 1137
✉ 72114.2327@compuserve.com

🌐 http://www.bookfair.com/publishers/daedalus/pbk
✓
Intelligent sexuality publications. Age statement of 21 is required. Please see our display advertisement.

Publishers: Books: Sexuality

☺▼ **Alamo Square Press**
P.O. Box 14543, San Francisco, California 94114.
☎ 415 863 7410 ✆ 415 863 7456

♂▼ **Gay Sunshine Press / Leyland Publications**
P. O. Box 410690, San Francisco, California 94141.
☎ 707 996 6082 ✆ 707 996 8418

♂▼ **Leyland Publications**
P. O. Box 410690, San Francisco, California 94141.
☎ 707 996 6082 ✆ 707 996 8418

Publishers: Directories: Sexuality

♂ **Gaybook**
Box 632, 584 Castro Street, San Francisco, California 94114.
☎ 415 928 1859
A yellow-page type magazine/directory with a comprehensive resource guide, articles of interest, & classified ads for lesbians & gay men in the San Francisco Bay Area. Published twice a year. Yearly subscription is $18.

Publishers: Directories: BDSM

♂▼ **Spunk**
Studio Iguana, #419, 501 1st. Street, San Francisco, California 94107.
 ✆ 415 252 0724
✓
Published every month. Yearly subscription is $5.

Publishers: Films: Sexuality

⊕ ▼ **Feline Films**
P. O. Box 170415, San Francisco, California 94117.
☎ 510 533 6474 ✆ 510 533 6474
🔥 ✓
Erotic films for women. Age statement of 18 is required.

Publishers: Magazines: BDSM

♀▼ **Brat Attack**

P. O. Box 40754, San Francisco, California 94140-0754.
☎ 415 695 0418
🕐 Variable
♿ ✓
Age statement of 18 is required.

🔁▼ **Drummer**
Desmodus, Inc., P. O. Box 410390, San Francisco, California 94141-1314.
☎ 415 252 1195 ✆ 415 252 9574
Published every month. Yearly subscription is $59.

🔁▼ **International Leatherman**
Brush Creek Media, Box 316, 2215-R Market Street, San Francisco, California 94114.
☎ 800 234 3877 ✆ 415 552 3244
☎ 415 552 1506
✉ jwbean@ix.netcom.com
🕐 Mon - Sat 10:30 - 18:00
♿ ✓ $ 💳 💳
Published quarterly. Yearly subscription is $21/year U.S., $29 foreign.
Age statement of 21 is required.

🔁 **Lexicon**
Suite 201, 155 Haight Street, San Francisco, California 94102-5741.
☎ 415 255 4663
Published 17 times a year. Yearly subscription is $20.

🔁▼ **Mach**
Desmodus, Inc., P. O. Box 410390, San Francisco, California 94141-1314.
☎ 415 252 1195 ✆ 415 252 9574

🔁▼ **Venus Infers**
Box 294, 2215-R Market Street, San Francisco, California 94114.
☎ 415 333 1723

Publishers: Magazines: Bears

🔁▼ **Big Ad Productions**
#448, 2966 Diamond Street, San Francisco, California 94131.
☎ 415 695 2327 ✆ 415 695 2327
🕐 Mon - Fri 09:00 - 17:00
♿ ✓

Publishers: Magazines: Erotic

🔁▼ **Girlfriends**
Suite 101, 3415 Cesar Chavez, San Francisco, California 94110-4507.
☎ 415 995 2776 ✆ 415 749 0282
✉ hysteria27@aol.com
🕐 Mon - Fri 08:00 - 17:00, 24hr. voice mail
✓
Published every two months.

🔁▼ **Husky Magazine**
P. O. Box 471030, San Francisco, California 94147.
☎ 415 431 5755

🔁▼ **PowerPlay**
Brush Creek Media, Box 316, 2215-R Market Street, San Francisco, California 94114.
☎ 800 234 3877 ✆ 415 552 3244
☎ 415 552 1506
✉ jwbean@ix.netcom.com
🕐 Mon - Sat 10:30 - 18:00
♿ ✓ 💳 💳
Published quarterly. Yearly subscription is $23. Age statement of 21 is required.

Publishers: Magazines: Fetish

🔁▼ **Foreskin Quarterly**
Brush Creek Media, Box 316, 2215-R Market Street, San Francisco, California 94114.
☎ 800 234 3877 ✆ 415 552 3244
☎ 415 552 1506
✉ jwbean@ix.netcom.com
🕐 Mon - Sat 10:30 - 18:00
♿ ✓ $ 💳 💳
Published quarterly. Yearly subscription is $24/year U.S., $40 foreign.
Age statement of 21 is required.

Publishers: Magazines: Sexuality

🔁▼ **10 Percent**
Browning Grace Communications, Suite 200, 54 Mint Street, San Francisco, California 94103.
☎ 415 905 8590 ✆ 415 227 0463

♀▼ **Anything That Moves**
San Francisco Bay Area Bisexual Network, Suite 24, 2404 California Street, San Francisco, California 94115.
☎ 415 703 7977
Please make cheques payable to BABN. Magazine is sent in discreet packaging. Published quarterly. Yearly subscription is $25.

🔁▼ **Bear Magazine**
Brush Creek Media, Box 316, 2215-R Market Street, San Francisco, California 94114.
☎ 800 234 3877 ✆ 415 552 3244
☎ 415 552 1506
✆ 415 241 9434
✉ jwbean@ix.netcom.com
🕐 Mon - Sat 10:30 - 18:00
♿ $ 💳 💳
Published every two months. Age statement of 21 is required.

🔁▼ **Deneuve**
FRS Enterprises, Suite 15, 2336 Market Street, San Francisco, California 94114.
☎ 415 863 6538 ✆ 415 863 1609
✉ deneuve@cool.com
🕐 Mon - Fri 10:00 - 17:00
♿ ✓ 💳 💳
Published every two months. Yearly subscription is $22.

♀ **Dyke Review**
Box 456, 584 Castro Street, San Francisco, California 94114.
☎ 415 621 3769

⊕ **Feminist Bookstore News**
P. O. Box 882554, San Francisco, California 94188.
☎ 415 626 1556 ✆ 415 626 8970

🔁▼ **Frighten The Horses**
Heat Seeking Publishing, Suite 1108, 41 Sutter Street, San Francisco, California 94104.
☎ 415 824 0282
✉ horses@outright.com
Published quarterly. Age statement of 18 is required.

☺ ■ **Future Sex**
Kundalini Publishing, Inc., Suite 502, 60 Federal Street, San Francisco, California 94107.
☎ 415 541 7725 ✆ 415 541 9860
✉ futursex@well.sf.ca.us
🕐 Mon - Fri 09:00 - 17:00
♿ ✓
Published quarterly. Yearly subscription is $18. Age statement of 18 is required.

⊕ **Girl Jock**
Box 94, 3288 21st Street, San Francisco, California 94110.
☎ 415 206 9230

☺ ■ **Greenery**
Lady Green, #195, 3739 Balboa Avenue, San Francisco, California 94121.
✉ verdant@netcom.com
🕐 Mon - Fri 09:00 - 17:00
♿ ✓
Greenery is only available in the U.S.. Published quarterly. Yearly subscription is $8.

🔁▼ **HOMOture**
P. O. Box 191781, San Francisco, California 94119-1781.
♿ ✓
Irregular publication dates.

⊕ **On Our Backs**
Box 400, 530 Howard Street, San Francisco, California 94105.
☎ 800 845 4617
☎ 415 546 0384
🕐 Mon - Fri 10:00 - 16:00
♿ ✓ 💳 💳
Published every two months. Yearly subscription is $34.95.

Publishers: Magazines: Sexual Politics

☺ ■ **Whorezine**
Suite 19, 2300 Market Street, San Francisco, California 94114.
By & for sex workers & their customers. Published every month. Yearly subscription is $40. Age statement of 21 is required.

Publishers: Magazines: Sexuality

🔁 ■ **CTN Magazine**
P. O. Box 14431, San Francisco, California 94114.
☎ 415 626 9033
✉ CTNMag@aol.com
For the deaf, hard of hearing, & hearing-signing. Published quarterly. Yearly subscription is $30.

🔁▼ **Holy Titclamps**
P. O. box 590488, San Francisco, California 94159-0488.
✉ lroberts@bellas.com
Published quarterly. Yearly subscription is $10.

🔁▼ **Out & About**
Box 290, 2261 Market Street, San Francisco, California 94114.

☎ 415 281 3176

♂▼ *TRUST, The Handballing Newsletter*
Alamo Square Press, P.O. Box 14543, San Francisco, California 94114.
☎ 415 863 7410 📞 415 863 7456
Published quarterly.

♂▼ *wilde*
PDA Press, Inc., Box 400, 530 Howard Street, San Francisco, California 94105.
☎ 800 478 3268
☎ 415 243 3232
Published every two months. Yearly subscription is $31.50.

Publishers: Newspapers: AIDS
☺ *AIDS Treatment News*
P. O. Box 411256, San Francisco, California 94141.
☎ 415 873 2812 📞 415 255 4659
Published quarterly.

Publishers: Newspapers: BDSM
☺▽ *Cuir Underground*
Number 19, 3288 21st. Street, San Francisco, California 94110.
☎ 415 487 7622 (voice mail)
📧 CuirPaper@aol.com or cuiru@black-rose.com
🌐 http://www.black-rose.com/cuiru.html
🕐 24hr. answering machine
🖂 ✓
Newspaper for the San Francisco Bay Area pansexual kink community. Published 10 times a year. Yearly subscription is $20. Age statement of 18 is required. French, Spanish, & Swedish also spoken.

Publishers: Newspapers: Sexuality
♂▼ *Bay Area Reporter*
♿ 395 9th. Street, San Francisco, California 94103.
☎ 415 861 5019
Published every week.

♂ *Dykespeak*
Suite 181, 4104 24th. Street, San Francisco, California 94114.
☎ 415 648 6151
Focused on issues relating to lesbian visibility, interviews with lesbians from all walks of life, entertainment, events, clubs, politics, guest columns, & more. Published every month. Yearly subscription is $20.

♂ *Lavendar Pages*
Box 616, 584 Castro Street, San Francisco, California 94114.
☎ 415 864 4446 📞 415 864 6725
Business directory. Lesbian & gay owned in the heart of S.F.'s Castro. Promotes the patronage of advertisers by rewarding the customer for choosing your business. Published twice a year. Yearly subscription is $11.90.

⊕ *Lesbian Contradiction*
Box 356, 584 Castro Street, San Francisco, California 94114.
Journal of opinion, commentary, humour, & cartoons for women who agree to disagree. Published quarterly. Yearly subscription is $8.

♂ *Odyssey Magazine*
Box 302, 584 Castro Street, San Francisco, California 94114-2500.
☎ 415 621 6514 📞 415 431 7911
Published every two weeks. Yearly subscription is $25.

♂ *Phœnix Rising*
P. O. Box 170596, San Francisco, California 94110.

♂▼ *San Francisco Bay Times*
♿ 288 7th. Street, San Francisco, California 94103.
☎ 415 626 8121
Newspaper & calendar of events for the S.F. Bay Area for the lesbian, gay, & bisexual community. Published every two weeks. Yearly subscription is $54.

♂ *San Francisco Sentinel*
285 Shipley Street, San Francisco, California 94107.
☎ 415 281 3745
California's gay & lesbian newsweekly. Serves the entire San Francisco Bay area & adjoining communities. Published every week. Yearly subscription is $85.

♂▽ *The Slant*
P. O. Box 629, Corte Madera, San Francisco, California 94976.
☎ 415 924 6635 📞 415 927 3670
Published by The Marin Stonewall Alliance to support Marin County's lesbian, gay, & bisexual community. Published every month. Yearly subscription is $18.

♂▼ *White Crane Newsletter*
P. O. Box 170152, San Francisco, California 94117.

Publishers: Videos: BDSM
☺▼ *M & M Productions*
P. O. Box 170415, San Francisco, California 94117.
☎ 510 533 6474 📞 510 533 6474

🖂 ✓
Produce multi-media on topics such as sexual freedom & BDSM. Age statement of 18 is required.

♂▼ Shotgun Video
Box 453, 2215 Market Street, San Francisco, California 94114.
☎ 415 626 5070

Publishers: Videos: Bondage
♂ Grapik Arts Productions
P.O. Box 460142, San Francisco, California 94146-0142.
📞 415 826 2484

Publishers: Videos: Fetish
☺ Starbright Productions
Box 260, 842 Folsom Street, San Francisco, California 94107.
Also mail order.

Publishers: Videos: Piercing & Tattooing
☺ Flash Video
P.O. Box 410052, San Francisco, California 94141.
☎ 415 267 7651
✓ 💳 💳
Catalogue, $5. Age statement of 21 is required.

Publishers: Videos: Sexuality
☺ ■ Erotica S. F.
Suite 307, 499 Alabama Street, San Francisco, California 94110.
☎ 415 861 4101 📞 415 587 0759
🕐 09:00 - 24:00
✓
Catalogue, $3.

Publishers: Videos: Spanking
♠♣ Redboard Video
P. O. Box 2069, San Francisco, California 94126.
☎ 415 296 8712 📞 415 362 1141

Stores: Books: General
☺ ▼ Books & Company
♿ 1323 Polk Street, San Francisco, California 94109-4613.
☎ 415 441 2929

☺ ■ City Lights Bookstore
261 Columbus Avenue, San Francisco, California 94133.
☎ 415 362 8193 📞 415 362 4921

♂▼ A Different Light
♿ 489 Castro Street, San Francisco, California 94114.
☎ 415 431 0891 📞 415 431 0892
📞 415 431 6660
📧 adl@atg.org
🕐 10:00 - 24:00
🖂 ✓ $ 💳 💳 💳 ✐
Free newsletter. Free catalogue published 3 times a year.

☺ ▼ Hog On Ice
♿ 1630 Polk Street, San Francisco, California 94109.
☎ 415 771 7909

☺ ■ The Magazine
♿ 920 Larkin Street, San Francisco, California 94109-7113.
☎ 415 441 7737

☺ Modern Times Bookstore
968 Valencia, San Francisco, California 94110.
☎ 415 282 9246

☺ Old Wives Tales
1009 Valencia Street, San Francisco, California 94110.
☎ 415 821 4675
🕐 11:00 - 19:00, Sun - 18:00
Publishes *Women's Voices Events.*

☺ □ Small Press Traffic
♿ 3599 24th. Street, San Francisco, California 94105.
☎ 415 285 8394

☺ ■ Stacey's Bookshop
♿ 581 Market Street, San Francisco, California 94105.
☎ 415 421 4687 📞 415 777 5017

Stores: Clothing: Fetish
☺ Riga
1391 Haight Street, San Francisco, California 94117.
☎ 415 552 1525 📞 415 552 1665
🕐 11:00 - 19:00 every day
🖂 ✓ 💳 💳 📠 ✐

Stores: Clothing: Leather
♂▼ Image Leather
2199 Market Street, San Francisco, California.

☎ 415 621 7551
☺ ■ **Wendell's Leather Shop**
1623 Polk Street, San Francisco, California 94109.
☎ 415 474 4104
☺ ■ **Worn Out West**
582 Castro Street, San Francisco, California 94114.
☎ 415 431 6020
🕐 Wed - Fri 11:00 - 19:00, Sat Mon Tur 11:00 - 18:00, Sun 12:00 - 17:30
♿ 💳 📷 🚗 ℓ
New & used clothing & leather, rubber, latex, uniforms, boots, fetish toys, cowboy gear, etc.. We also buy, sell, & trade. Spanish also spoken.

Stores: Clothing: Sexuality

⚥■ **Foxy Lady**
2644 Mission Street, San Francisco, California.
☎ 415 285 4980

Stores: Clothing: Uniforms

☺ ■ **Butler's Uniforms**
345 9th. Street, San Francisco, California 94103.
☎ 415 863 8119
Police uniforms & other gear, & Dept. of Corrections uniforms.

Stores: Erotica: BDSM

☺ ▼ **Construction Zone**
2352 Market Street, San Francisco, California 94114.
☎ 415 255 8585
🕐 Mon - Thu 11:00 - 19:00, Fri - Sat 11:00 - 21:00, Sun 12:00 - 18:00
♿ 💳 📷
Also leather repairs & mail order. Age statement of 18 is required.

⚥ **Jaguar**
4057 18th. Street, San Francisco, California 94114.
☎ 415 863 4777
☺ ■ **Leather Etc.**
1201 Folsom Street, San Francisco, California 94103.
☎ 415 864 7558 📞 415 864 7559
🕐 7 days per week
♿ 💳 📷 🚗
Also mail order. Catalogue, $5.

⚥ ▼ **Mr. S – Fetters, U.S.A.**
310 7th. Street, San Francisco, California 94103.
☎ 800 746 7677 📞 415 863 7798
☎ 415 863 7764
🕐 Mon - Sat 11:00 - 19:00
♿ ✓ 💳 📷
The world's largest leather & latex store & mail order catalogue. Over 2,000 different items in a continually growing inventory. 200-page catalogue, $20U.S. to U.S., $30U.S. foreign. Age statement of 18 is required.

☺ ▼ **RoB—San Francisco**
22 Shotwell Street, San Francisco, California.
☎ 415 252 1198 📞 415 252 9574
🕐 Mon 11:00 - 17:00, Tue - Sat 11:00 - 19:00
♿ ✓ 💳 📷 🚗
Age statement of 21 is required.

☺ ▼ **Stormy Leather**
⚥ 1158 Howard Street, San Francisco, California 94103.
☎ 415 626 1672 📞 415 626 4134
🕐 Mon - Thu 12:00 - 18:00, Fri Sat 12:00 - 19:00, Sun 14:00 - 18:00
♿ 💳 📷 🚗
No mail order from store (contact Xandria).

☺ ■ **A Taste of Leather**
317-A 10th. Street, San Francisco, California 94103.
☎ 800 367 0786
☎ 415 252 9166
🕐 12:00 - 20:00
Catalogue, $5. Age statement of 18 is required.

Stores: Erotica: General

⚥ ▼ **The Bear Store**
367 9th. Street, San Francisco, California.
☎ 415 552 1506
🕐 Mon - Sat 11:00 - 18:00
☺ ■ **Books, Etc.**
538 Castro Street, San Francisco, California 94114.
☎ 415 621 8631
🕐 7 days a week
⚥ ■ **Crown Books**
1700 Van Ness, San Francisco, California 94109.
☎ 415 441 7479

☺ ▼ **Good Vibrations**
⚥ Suite 101, 938 Howard Street, San Francisco, California 94103.
☎ 800 289 8423 📞 415 974 8989
☎ 415 974 8990
📧 goodvibe@well.sf.ca
🕐 11:00 - 19:00
♿ ✓ $ ✉ 💳 📷 📧
A clean, well lit store for sex toys & books. Free catalogue. Age statement of 18 is required. Spanish also spoken.

☺ **Open Enterprises, Inc.**
938 Howard Avenue, San Francisco, California 94103.
⚥▼ **Le Salon**
⚥ 4126 18th. Street, San Francisco, California 94124.
☎ 415 552 4213
🕐 08:00 - 02:00
⚥▼ **Le Salon**
⚥ 1118 Polk Street, San Francisco, California.
☎ 415 673 4492
🕐 08:00 - 02:00
☺ **Turk Street News & Video**
66 Turk Street, San Francisco, California 94102.
☎ 415 885 2040

Tattooists

☺ **Everlasting Tattoo**
1939 McAllister, San Francisco, California 94115.
☎ 415 928 6244

Television: Sexuality

⚥▽ **Electric City**
Cable TV, 133 Collingwood, San Francisco, California 94114.
☎ 415 861 7131
☺ ■ **The Erotica Project**
P. O. Box 425481, San Francisco, California 94142-5481.
☎ 415 558 8112 📞 415 863 9771
📧 oddball@SIRIUS.COM
🕐 Mon - Fri 09:00 - 21:00

San José
Health Services

☺ □ **San José Medical Center**
675 East Santa Clara Street, San José, California 95112.
☎ 408 998 3212
☺ □ **Santa Clara Valley Medical Center**
751 South Bascom Avenue, San José, California 95128.
☎ 408 299 5100

Helplines: Sexuality

⚥▽ **Billy De Frank Lesbian & Gay Community Center**
⚥ 175 Stockton Avenue, San José, California 95126-2760.
☎ 408 293 4525
☺ □ **Gay & Lesbian Switchboard**
c/o Billy De Frank Lesbian & Gay Community Center, 175 Stockton Avenue, San José, California 95126-2760.
☎ 408 293 4525

Organizations: AIDS: Education

☺ □ **Aris Project**
⚥ #104, 595 Millich Drive, Campbell, California 95008.
☎ 408 370 3272 📞 408 370 3295
☎ 408 370 3552 (TDD)
Contact: Mr. Tom Myers
Publishes *Pages*.
☺ □ **Santa Clara County Health Department**
⚥ AIDS Program, 976 Lenzen Avenue, San José, California 95126.
☎ 408 299 4151
🕐 Mon - Fri 08:00 - 17:00

Organizations: Fetish: Uniforms

⚥ **South Bay Leather Uniform Group (SLUG)**
175 Stockton, San José, California 95126.
☎ 408 929 7584

Organizations: Sexuality

♂ ▽ **Bisexual Support Group**
c/o Billy De Frank Lesbian & Gay Community Center, 175 Stockton Avenue, San José, California 95126-2760.
☎ 408 293 2429
🕐 Meets 1st. & 3rd. Tue of month 19>00 - 21:00. For information, call weeknights 18:00 - 21:00
✉■ **Rainbow Gender Alliance (RGA)**
P. O. Box 700730, San José, California 95170-0730.
☎ 408 984 4044 (recording)

Organizations: Sexuality

☎ 408 732 1323
✺ http://www.transgender.org/tg/rga/rgapage.html
Publishes *The Rainbow*. Yearly subscription is $10.

✄▼ **Swan's Inner Sorority (SIS)**
P. O. Box 1423, San José, California 95109.
☎ 408 297 1423 ✆ 408 993 8173
🖰 ✓
Contact: Ms. Wendi Seabreeze
Publishes *Swan's Bauble*. Yearly subscription is $25.

Organizations: Sexuality: Student

✎▽ **De Anza Gay & Lesbian Alliance**
21250 Stevens Creek Boulevard, San José, California 95104.
☎ 408 534 4254

✎▽ **West College Gay & Lesbian Student Union**
14000 Fruitvale Avenue, Saratoga, California 95070.
☎ 408 867 2200 Ext.: 358

Organizations: Sexuality: Youth

✎ **National Coalition for Gay, Lesbian, & Bisexual Youth**
P. O. Box 24589, San José, California 95154-4589.
☎ 408 269 6125 ✆ 408 269 5328

Printers: General

☺▼ **Our Print Shop**
P. O. Box 23387, San José, California 95153.
☎ 408 452 0570 ✆ 408 226 0823
🕐 Mon - Fri 11:00 - 18:00 by appointment
🖰 ✓
Print short run books, catalogues, etc. for alternative communities.

Publishers: Newspapers: Sexuality

①▽ **Entre Nous Newsletter**
🖰 P. O. Box 412, Santa Clara, California 95052.
☎ 408 246 1117

✎▼ **Our Paper**
P. O. Box 23387, San José, California 95153.
☎ 408 286 2670
🖰 ✓
Published twice a month.

✎ **Playland Magazine**
Suite 112, 1702 Meridan Avenue, San José, California 95125.
☎ 408 492 9271 ✆ 415 347 6058
Your guide to the Greater Gay & Lesbian Bay Area. Published every month.

✎ **South Bay Times**
Suite 6, 265 Meridan Street, San José, California 95126.

Stores: Art Galleries

☺ **Rycroft Gallery**
168 Serge Avenue, San José, California 95130-1849.

Stores: Books: General

☺ ■ **A Clean Well-Lighted Place for Books**
21269 Stevens Creek Boulevard, Cupertino, California 95014.
☎ 408 255 7600

①▼ **Sisterspirit Bookstore**
🖰 175 Stockton Avenue, San José, California 95126-2760.
☎ 408 293 9372

Stores: Erotica: BDSM

✎■ **Leather Masters**
🖰 969 Park Avenue, San José, California 95126.
☎ 800 417 2636 (outside California) ✆ 408 293 7685
☎ 408 293 7660 (in California)
🕐 Mon - Thu 11:00 - 22:00, Fri 12:00 - 24:00, Sat 12:00 - 18:00
🖰 ✓ 💳 💳
Catalogue, $5. Ago statement of 21 is required.

Suppliers: Diapers

☺■ **Mother's Little Helper Diaper Service**
Suite 153, 5667 Snell Avenue, San José, California 95123.
☎ 800 394 9727
Waterproof diaper cover with pouch.

San Juan Capistrano
Organizations: Sexuality

✄■ **Gender Dysphoria Program of Orange County, Inc.**
Suite 203, 32158 Camino Capistrano, San Juan Capistrano, California 92675.
☎ 714 240 7020
Contact: Mr. William Heard, Ph.D., Director

Evaluation & treatment for gender dysphoric poeple.

San Luis Obispo
Organizations: Sexuality: Student

✎▽ **Gays, Lesbians, & Bisexuals United**
🖰 ASI Box 243, California Polytechnic State University, San Luis Obispo, California 93401.
☎ 805 546 8148
🕐 Recorded message of events

Stores: Books: General

☺ ■ **Coalesce Bookstore**
845 Main Street, Morro Bay, California 93442.
☎ 805 772 2880

☺ ▼ **Volumes of Pleasure**
🖰 1016 Los Osos Valley Road, Los Osos, California 93495.
☎ 805 528 5565

San Marcos
Distributors: Books: General

☺ **Slawson Communications**
15 Vallecitos de Ora, San Marcos, California 92069-1438.
☎ 619 744 2299 ✆ 619 744 0424

Publishers: Videos: Spanking

⚤ **Nu-West Productions**
P. O. Box 1239, San Marcos, California 92079.
☎ 619 630 9979

San Mateo
BBSs: BDSM

☺ ■ **Wally World**
☎ 415 349 6969

BBSs: Bears

✎▼ **PC Bear Lair**
☎ 415 572 9563

BBSs: Sexuality

✎▼ **The Back Door BBS**
☎ 415 756 2906 (voice, San Francisco)
☎ 415 570 7426. 14400 baud maximum.
🕐 24hr. BBS. Voice 09:00 - 22:00
Hourly rate based on data speed. On-line shopping.

Organizations: AIDS: Education

☺ ☐ **San Mateo County AIDS Program**
🖰 3700 Edison Street, San Mateo, California 94403.
☎ 415 573 2588
🕐 Mon - Fri 08:00 - 17:00

Organizations: AIDS: Support

☺ **Eclipse**
173 South Boulevard, San Mateo, California 94402.
☎ 415 572 9702
🕐 Mon - Fri 08:00 - 17:00

Stores: Books: General

⊕ ■ **Two Sisters Bookshop**
🖰 605 Cambridge Avenue, Menlo Park, California 94025.
☎ 415 323 4778

Stores: Erotica: General

☺ ■ **Golden Gate**
🖰 1966 Rumrill Road, San Mateo, California 94806.
☎ 415 620 9639

San Rafael
Counsellors

✄■ **Anne Vitale, Ph.D.**
c/o D Street Counseling Group, 610 D Street, San Rafael, California 94901.
☎ 415 456 4452

Manufacturers: Erotica: Rubber

☺ ■ **Rubberotica**
P. O. Box 10291, San Rafael, California 94912.
Erotic rubber stamps by Michael Manning & Shelley Rae Corner.

Photographers: Erotic

☺ ■ **Boudoir Portraits**
#8, 214 Bayview, San Rafael, California 94901.
☎ 415 721 5480 ✆ 415 545 4031

☺ Mon - Fri 10:00 - 21:00
Publishes a newsletter every two months. Yearly subscription is $30. Age statement of 18 is required.

☺ ■ **Morgan J. Cowin Photography**
5 Windsor Avenue, San Rafael, California 94901.
☎ 415 459 7722
☺ Mon - Sat 09:00 - 18:00
♣ ✓
Teaches erotic photography. Internationally published (e.g. Playboy). Free brochure.

Publishers: Books: Polyfidelity
☺ **Deborah Anapol, IRC**
P. O. Box 150475, San Rafael, California 94915.

Santa Ana
Organizations: Family
☺ □ **Parents & Friends of Lesbians & Gays (PFLAG)—**
♿ **Orange County**
P. O. Box 28662, Santa Ana, California 92799-8662.
☎ 714 997 8047

Stores: Clothing: Uniforms
☺ ■ **Uniforms, Inc.**
8146 Van Nuys Boulevard, Santa Ana, California.
☎ 714 541 3546
🖻 VISA CC

Santa Barbara
Health Services
☺ □ **Santa Barbara Cottage Hospital**
Pueblo Street at Bath Street, Santa Barbara, California 93105.
☎ 805 682 7111

Manufacturers: Adult Toys: Percussion
☺ ■ **Santa Barbara Paddle Company**
P. O. Box 20034, Santa Barbara, California 93120-0034.
☎ 800 569 0971
📧 sbpadl@west.net
🌐 http://www.west.net/~sbpadl/sbpc.htm
VISA CC
The nation's largest mail order supplier of fraternity paddles. Free catalogue.

Organizations: Sexuality
⚥▽ **Gay & Lesbian Resource Center**
♿ #A-17, 126 East Haley, Santa Barbara, California 93101.
☎ 805 963 3636
Publishes *Bulletin*.

Organizations: Sexuality: Student
⚥▽ **Lesbian, Gay, & Bisexual Alliance**
P. O. Box 15048, University of California at Santa Barbara, Santa Barbara, California 93107.
☎ 805 893 4578

Piercers
☺ ■ **Professional Body Piercing by Jack**
☎ 805 962 0296
☺ By appointment
Also sells a wide selection of jewelry.

Printers: General
☺ **Kimberly Press**
5390-P Overpass Road, Santa Barbara, California 93111-2008.
☎ 805 964 6469

Publishers: Books: General
☺ ■ **Para Publishing**
P. O. Box 4232-890, Santa Barbara, California 93140-4232.
☎ 805 968 7277
Publishers of The Self-Publishing Manual.

Publishers: Books: Sexuality
⚥▼ **A. D. Thompson & Co., Publishers**
P. O. Box 20034, Santa Barbara, California 93120.

Stores: Books: General
⚥▽ **Choices Books & Music**
901 De La Vina Street, Santa Barbara, California 93101.
☎ 805 965 5477
♣ ✓ VISA CC
☺ ■ **Earthling Bookstore**
♿ 1137 State Street, Santa Barbara, California 93101-2712.
☎ 805 965 1530

Tattooists
☺ **Ania Metalworks**
P. O. Box 24, Santa Barbara, California 93101.
☺ **Soma Studios**
P. O. Box 24, Santa Barbara, California 93101.
☺ **Tattoo Santa Barbara**
♿ P. O. Box 777, 318 State Street, Santa Barbara, California 93101.
☎ 805 962 7552 ✆ 805 962 1412
📧 stdympna@aol.com
☺ By appointment
♣ $ ⚏ VISA CC 🖃 ℓ
Tattoo artist Pat Fish specializes in celtic knotworks, north west coast american indian images, & birds & fish. Age statement of 18 is required.

Santa Clara
Organizations: BDSM
⚨ **Leather Women Into Sadism Dominance Obedience & Masochism (Leather WISDOM)**
P.O. Box 2519, Santa Clara, California 95055.
Contact: Jill, Founder

Photographers: BDSM
⚥▼ **Ultimate Productions**
P. O. Box 2519, Santa Clara, California 95055.
📧 jillm@netcom.com
Age statement of 18 is required.

Training: BDSM
⚥▼ **J. B. Productions**
P. O. Box 2519, Santa Clara, California 95055.
Education in electric play: TENS units, violet wands with glass probes & electric whips are just a few fun things to explore.

Santa Cruz
Health Services
☺ □ **Dominican Santa Cruz Hospital**
1555 Soquel Drive, Santa Cruz, California 95065.
☎ 408 462 7700

Helplines: AIDS
☺ □ **Santa Cruz AIDS Project**
♿ P. O. Box 557, Santa Cruz, California 95061-0557.
☎ 408 427 4999 (hotline)
☎ 408 427 3900 (office)

Manufacturers: Piercing Jewelry
☺ ■ **Anatometal**
Blanchard Manufacturing, Santa Cruz, California.
☎ 408 462 2366 ✆ 408 464 1254
📧 anatomel@ix.netcom.com
Stainless steel & niobium jewelry. All pieces triple polished.

Organizations: AIDS: Support
⚥▽ **Equinox**
Suite 207-A, 903 Pacific, Santa Cruz, California 95060.
☎ 408 457 1441
☺ Call for hours
Contact: Mr. Josh Wolff

Organizations: BDSM
⚨ ▽ **Power Circle**
P. O. Box 3284, Santa Cruz, California 95063.

Organizations: Sexuality
⚥▽ **Santa Cruz Lesbian, Gay, & Bisexual Community**
♿ **Center**
P. O. Box 8280, Santa Cruz, California 95061-8280.
☎ 408 425 5422

Piercers
☺ ■ **Ken Coyote**
☎ 408 459 8582
☺ By appointment only
Trained by Fakir Musafar.
☺ ■ **Staircase Tattoos**
607 Front Street, Santa Cruz, California.
☎ 408 425 7644
☺ By appointment Wed - Sun 12:00 - late evening

Publishers: Magazines: Sexuality
☺ *Inciting Desire*
343 Soquel Avenue, Santa Cruz, California 95060.

Publishers: Newspapers: Sexuality
☺▽ **Lavendar Reader**
P. O. Box 7293, Santa Cruz, California 95061.

Stores: Books: General
☺ ■ **The Book Loft**
🏠 1207 Soquel Avenue, Santa Cruz, California 95062.
☎ 408 429 1812
☺ ■ **Bookshop Santa Cruz**
♿ 1520 Pacific Avenue, Santa Cruz, California 95060.
☎ 408 423 0900
☺ ■ **Chimney Sweep Books**
419 Cedar Street, Santa Cruz, California 95060.
☎ 408 458 1044
🕐 Mon - Sat 11:00 - 18:00
⊕ ▼ **Herland Book Café**
♿ 902 Center Street, Santa Cruz, California 95060.
☎ 408 429 6636
🕐 10:00 - 18:00
Bookstore with alternative periodicals, books, adult toys, erotic videos, newsletter, monthly events, art gallery, gifts, & music. Age statement of 18 is required.

Suppliers: Needles & Acupuncture Products
☺ ■ **Eastern Currents**
♿ 3040 Childer Lane, Santa Cruz, California 95062.
☎ 800 946 9264
☎ 408 479 8625

Santa Monica
BBSs: BDSM
☺ ■ **X!**
✆ 310 822 9969
Counsellors
▽ **Los Angeles Gender Center (LAGC)**
Suite 100, 3331 Ocean Park Boulevard, Santa Monica, California 90405.
Manufacturers: Piercing Jewelry
☺ ■ **Good Art Company**
218 Pier Avenue, Santa Monica, California 90405.
☎ 800 345 7601
☎ 310 452 7602
Niobium, Titanium, & 316LVM stainless steel captive bead jewelry. Wholesale enquiries welcome. Catalogue, $1.
Organizations: Motorcycle
⊕ □ **Athena Women's MC**
1223 Wilshire Boulevard, Santa Monica, California 90403.
☎ 310 458 3363
Publishers: Newspapers: Sexuality
☺▼ **Lesbian News**
P. O. Box 5128, Santa Monica, California 90405.
☎ 800 458 9888 ✆ 310 452 0562
☎ 310 392 8224
Nations's oldest, largest continuously published lesbian periodical. Features, stories, news, events, & ads.. Published every month. Yearly subscription is $35.
Stores: Art Galleries
☺ **Todd Kaplan Gallery**
220 Pier Avenue, Santa Monica, California 90405.
☎ 310 659 5075 ✆ 310 659 5076
Stores: Erotica: General
☺ ■ **Midnight Special Books**
♿ 1350 Third Street Promenade, Santa Monica, California 90401.
☎ 310 393 2923 ✆ 310 394 6123
🕐 10:30 - 22:00, Fri Sat - 23:00, Sun 11:30 - 22:00

Santa Rosa
BBSs: BDSM
☺ ■ **Rapture**
✆ 707 573 9438/0927
Health Services
☺ □ **Santa Rosa Memorial Hospital**
1165 Montgomery Drive, Santa Rosa, California 95405.
☎ 707 546 3210

Publishers: Newspapers: Sexuality
⊕ **Sonoma County Women's Voices**
P. O. Box 4448, Santa Rosa, California 95402.
☎ 707 575 5654
A community newsjournal by, for, & about women of all sexual orientations, featuring local news, opinions, events, & poetry. Published 10 times a year. Yearly subscription is $10.
☺▽ **We The People**
P. O. Box 8218, Santa Rosa, California 95407.
☎ 707 573 8896
A monthly newsletter distributed throughout the Empire (Sonoma, Napa, & Lake counties). It covers any local news, a local calendar of events, book & theatre reviews, etc.. Published every month. Yearly subscription is $15.
Stores: Books: General
⊕ ▼ **ClaireLight**
♿ Suite 101, 519 Mendocino Avenue, Santa Rosa, California 95401.
☎ 707 575 8879
Publishes a newsletter.
Stores: Erotica: General
☺ ■ **Santa Rosa Adult Books & Video**
3301 Santa Rosa Avenue, Santa Rosa, California 95407.
☎ 707 542 8248

Santee
Organizations: Sexuality
☺▽ **Wishing Well**
P. O. Box 713090, Santee, California 92072.
Publishes *Wishing Well* every two months.

Seal Beach
Stores: Clothing: Rubber
☺ □ **Fit To Be Tied**
Suite D, 222 Main Street, Seal Beach, California 90740.
☎ 310 597 1234 ✆ 310 597 1234
🕐 Sat 11:00 - 16:00 & by appointment
Latex clothing & accessories for men & women. Catalogue, fashions / boots $15; moulded latex $25; video of latex fashions $30.

Sonora
Organizations: AIDS: Education
☺ □ **Sierra AIDS Council**
♿ P. O. Box 1062, Sonora, California 95370.
☎ 209 533 2873
🕐 Mon - Fri 10:00 - 15:00

Soquel
Manufacturers: Piercing Jewelry
☺ ■ **Dakota Steel, Inc.**
Suiite 7, 2827 South Rodeo Gulch Road, Soquel, California 95073.
☎ 800 995 0595 ✆ 408 464 7333
☎ 408 464 7333
Makes "Fakir" jewelry & doubled-bevelled needles. Wholesale enquiries only.
Piercers
☺ ■ **Dakota Steel, Inc.**
Suite 7, 2827 South Rodeo Gulch Road, Soquel, California 95073.
☎ 800 995 0595 ✆ 408 464 7333
☎ 408 464 7333
🕐 By appointment only

Stanford
Organizations: Sexuality
☺ □ **Parents & Friends of Lesbians & Gays (PFLAG)— Mid-Peninsula**
♿ P. O. Box 8265, Stanford, California 94305.
☎ 415 857 1058
☺▽ **Stanford Lesbian, Gay, & Bisexual Community Center**
P. O. Box 8265, Stanford, California 94309.
☎ 415 725 4222 (office)
☎ 415 723 1488 (events)
🕐 Mon - Fri 12:00 - 16:00

Stockton
Organizations: AIDS: Education
☺ □ **San Joaquin AIDS Foundation**
♿ #C-5, 4410 North Pershing, Stockton, California 95207.

☎ 800 367 2437 (hotline)
☎ 209 476 8533
⊕ 24hr. hotline
Publishes *The Voice.*

Organizations: Sexuality
⚥▽ **Gay & Lesbian Association, San Joaquin County**
820 North Madison, Stockton, California 95202.
☎ 209 464 5615 📱 209 464 5615

Studio City
Publishers: Magazines: Sexuality
⚴ **Female Mimics International**
Leoram, Inc., P. O. Box 1622, Studio City, California 91614.
☎ 818 898 1591 📱 818 898 1591
💳 ⬤
Published every two months. Yearly subscription is $52. Age statement of 21 is required.

⚴ **Sissy Exposé**
Leoram, Inc., P. O. Box 1622, Studio City, California 91614.
☎ 818 898 1591 📱 818 898 1591
💳 ⬤
Published every two months. Yearly subscription is $65. Age statement of 21 is required.

Publishers: Magazines: Spanking
☺ **Scene One**
Shadow Lane, Suite 461, 11288 Ventura Boulevard, Studio City, California 91604.
☎ 818 985 9151 📱 818 508 5187
⊕ 24hrs.
✓ 💳 ⬤

Publishers: Videos: Erotic
⚲ **Colt Studios**
P. O. Box 1608, Studio City, California 91614-0608.
☎ 800 445 2758 📱 818 985 2145
☎ 818 985 5786

Stores: Clothing: Sexuality
▷▼ **Jim Bridges' Boutique**
Suite 103, 12457 Ventura Boulevard, Studio City, California 91604.
☎ 818 761 6650
⊕ Wed Thu 14:00 - 20:00, Fri Sat 14:00 - 22:00
⬤ ✓ 💳 ⬤

Sunnyvale
Manufacturers: Piercing Jewelry
☺ ■ **Precision Metal**
Suite 207, 415 South Bernardo Avenue, Sunnyvale, California 94086.
Make steel & niobium captive bead rings.

Organizations: Family
☺ ☐ **Parents & Friends of Lesbians & Gays (PFLAG)—**
& **South Bay**
P. O. Box 2718, Sunnyvale, California 94087.
☎ 408 270 8182

Organizations: Polyfidelity
☺ ■ **South Bay Intinet**
P. O. Box 70203, Sunnyvale, California 94086.
☎ 408 730 9622

Sylmar
Organizations: Tattoo
⚥▽ **Illustrated Men**
P. O. Box 923172, Sylmar, California 91392-3172.
☎ 818 367 3938

Tarzana
Stores: Erotica: General
☺ ■ **Love Boutique**
18637 Ventura Boulevard, Tarzana, California 91356.
☎ 818 342 2400

Topanga
Organizations: Research: Sexuality
☺ **Mariposa Education & Research Foundation**
3123 Schweitzer, Topanga, California 90290.
☎ 818 704 4812
Publishes *Mariposa Newsletter.*

Travis
Stores: Erotica: General
☺ ■ **Parkway Books & Videos**
564 Parker Road, Travis, California 94535.
☎ 707 437 9969

Tucson
Organizations: Sexuality
⚥▽ **Phi, Alpha, Gamma**
Box 347/UCD, Student Activities Office, Davis University, Tucson, California 95616.
☎ 916 753 2090

Tujunga
Manufacturers: Adult Toys: Electrical
☺ **Erotec**
6928 Shadygrove Street, Tujunga, California 91042.
☎ 818 352 4344
Makes electric adult toys, including violet wands.

Tulare
Organizations: Sexuality
▷▽ **The Society for the Second Self (Tri-Ess)**
P. O. Box 194, Tulare, California 93275.
☎ 209 688 9246
Contact: Ms. Carol Beecroft
Publishes *The Femme Mirror* quarterly.

Tustin
Counsellors
⚥▼ **Christopher Street Counseling & Bookstore**
& Suite 102, 14131 Yorba Street, Tustin, California 92680.
☎ 714 731 0224 📱 714 731 2245
☎ 714 731 5445 (hotline)
⊕ Mon - Thu 11:00 - 19:00, Sun 14:00 - 19:00
⬤ ✓ 💳 ⬤
Full continuum of care from a multi-disciplined staff for the concerns of the lesbian, gay, bisexual, & transgendered community. Age statement of 18 is required.

⚥▼ **Gay & Lesbian Counseling Center**
Suite 102, 14101 Yorba Street, Tustin, California 92680.
☎ 714 731 0224 📱 714 731 2245
☎ 714 731 5445 (referral hotline)
⊕ Mon - Thu 11:00 - 13:00 15:00 - 20:30, Fri 11:00 - 15:00
⬤ ✓ 💳 ⬤

Stores: Books: General
⚥▼ **Christopher Street Bookstore**
& Suite 102, 14101 Yorba Street, Tustin, California 92680.
☎ 714 731 0224 📱 714 731 2245
☎ 714 731 5445 (referral hotline)
⊕ Mon - Thu 11:00 - 19:00, Sun 14:00 - 19:00
⬤ ✓ 💳 ⬤
A lavender bookshop, featuring new & used titles, as well as a variety of gift items.

Ukiah
Organizations: Polyfidelity
☺ ■ **Church of All Worlds**
P. O. Box 1542, Ukiah, California 95482.

Stores: Military Surplus
☺ ■ **G. I. Joes**
976 North State Street, Ukiah, California 95482.
☎ 707 468 8834

Universal City
Archives: Sexuality
☺ **Homosexual Information Center**
P. O. Box 8252, Universal City, California 91608-0252.
☎ 318 742 4709

Organizations: Literary
⚲ **Gay & Lesbian Press Association**
P. O. Box 8185, Universal City, California 91608-0185.
☎ 818 902 1476
Publishes *The Media Reporter.*

Upland
Stores: Clothing: Adult Baby
△■ **Especially for Me**
113 North First Avenue, Upland, California 91786.
☎ 909 946 6251 ✆ 909 946 5500
☎ 909 946 6817
🕐 Mon - Sat 09:00 - 21:00, Sun 13:00 - 20:00
🍴 ✓ VISA MC 💳
Sells full line of adult baby clothing for crossdressers. Mail order only.
Publishes *Diapers*. Age statement of 21 is required.

Stores: Erotica: General
☺▼ **Mustang Books & Videos**
⛃ 961 North Central Avenue, Upland, California 91786.
☎ 909 981 0227 ✆ 909 920 3647
🕐 Mon - Thu 08:00 - 01:00, Fri 08:00 - Sun 23:00
🍴 VISA MC
Age statement of 18 is required.

☺■ **Toy Box**
1999 West Arrow Route, Upland, California 91786.
☎ 909 982 9407

Valencia
Printers: General
☺ **Delta Lithograph**
28210-P North Avenue Stanford, Valencia, California 91355-1111.
☎ 805 257 0584 ✆ 805 257 3867

Vallejo
Stores: Books: General
☺■ **Books, Etc.**
⛃ 540 Georgia Street, Vallejo, California 94590.
☎ 707 644 2935

Valley Village
Organizations: Bears
♂▽ **Bears LA**
P. O. Box 4614, Valley Village, California 91617.
☎ 213 850 8958
✉ nerwick@netcom.com
🖧 http://www.skepsis.com/.gblo/bears/CLUBS/Bears_LA/

Van Nuys
Distributors: Videos: BDSM
☺■ **Lyndon Distributors Limited**
15756 Arminta Street, Van Nuys, California 91406.
☎ 818 988 0228

Manufacturers: Prosthetics
☺ **Bodytech**
Suite 145, 13659 Victory Boulevard, Van Nuys, California 91401.
☎ 818 385 0633
Special prosthetics, special effects contact lenses, teeth, etc.. Worked on many blockbuster films. Not scene business, but scene friendly.

Organizations: Polyfidelity
☺■ **Live The Dream**
Suite 150, 6454 Van Nuys Boulevard, Van Nuys, California 91401.
☎ 818 361 6737

Printers: Adult
☺ **Breene Lithograph, Inc.**
5632 Van Nuys Boulevard, Van Nuys, California 91401.
☎ 818 785 8500 ✆ 818 785 0758
Adult printing specialists. Video boxes, catalogues, flyers, etc..

Ventura
Organizations: AIDS: Support
☺☐ **AIDS Care**
P. O. Box 24381, Ventura, California 93002.
☎ 805 683 0446

Organizations: Family
☺☐ **Parents & Friends of Lesbians & Gays (PFLAG)—Ventura County**
P. O. Box 5401, Ventura, California 93005.
☎ 805 644 5863

Organizations: Sexuality
♂▽ **Gay & Lesbian Alliance of Ventura County**
⛃ P. O. Box 3480, Camarillo, California 93011.

☎ 805 963 3636
Publishes *In The Light*.

♂▽ **Gay & Lesbian Resource Center of Ventura County**
⛃ P. O. Box 3480, Camarillo, California 93011.
☎ 805 389 1530

Victorville
Publishers: Magazines: Daddy / Boy
♂ **Chiron Rising**
Chiron Rising Publications, P. O. Box 2589, Victorville, California 92393.
Published every two months. Yearly subscription is $38. Age statement of 18 is required.

Visalia
Printers: General
☺ **Jostens Printing & Publishing**
P.O. Box 991, Visalia, California 93291.
☎ 209 651 3300

Walnut Creek
Organizations: Sexuality
✉▽ **Pacific Center for Human Growth—Walnut Creek**
1250 Pine Street, Walnut Creek, California 94596.
☎ 510 939 7711

Walnut
Publishers: Newspapers: Fetish: Foot
☺■ **In Step**
P. O. Box 386, Walnut, California 91788.
Published every month. Yearly subscription is $32. Age statement of 18 is required.

West Hollywood
Archives: Sexuality
♀▽ **June Mazer Collection & Archive**
626 North Robertson Boulevard, West Hollywood, California 90069.
☎ 310 659 2478

Bars: BDSM
♂▼ **Spike**
7746 Santa Monica Boulevard, West Hollywood, California 90046.
☎ 213 656 9343

Competitions & Conventions: BDSM
☺▼ **Mr. & Ms. Olympus**
Suite 109-368, 7985 Santa Monica Boulevard, West Hollywood, California 90046.
☎ 213 656 5073 ✆ 213 656 3120
✉ tljandcuir@aol.com
🍴 ✓ VISA MC
Age statement of 21 is required.

☺▼ **The Pantheon of Leather**
Suite 109-368, 7985 Santa Monica Boulevard, West Hollywood, California 90046.
☎ 213 656 5073 ✆ 213 656 3120
✉ tljandcuir@aol.com
🍴 VISA MC
Held Spring each year to honour men & women who have made the leather, fetish, & BDSM community what it is today. Age statement of 21 is required.

Counsellors
♂▽ **Gay & Lesbian Adolescent Social Services, Inc.**
⛃ 650 North Robertson Boulevard, West Hollywood, California 90069.
☎ 310 288 1757

Distributors: Videos: BDSM
♂▼ **Close-Up Productions**
P. O. Box 691658, West Hollywood, California 90069.
☎ 800 697 9009 ✆ 213 848 8651
☎ 213 848 2961
🕐 24hr. facs. & 800 line
🍴 ✓ VISA MC
Age statement of 18 is required.

Distributors: Videos: Erotic
♀♂■ **John Floyd Video**
P. O. Box 691658, West Hollywood, California 90069-1658.
☎ 800 697 9009 ✆ 213 848 8651
🕐 24hr. facs. & 800 line
Catalogue, $5. Age statement of 18 is required.

Health Services

⊕ ▼ **The Lesbian Health Project**
Suite 308, 8235 Santa Monica Boulevard, West Hollywood, California 90046.
☎ 213 650 1508

Organizations: Academic: Sexuality

♂♀▽ **The Institute of Gay & Lesbian Education**
626 North Robertson Boulevard, West Hollywood, California 90069.
☎ 310 652 1786
✉ ILGE@aol.com
🌐 http://langevin.usc.edu/~la-motss/ilge.html
✓ VISA MC

Organizations: BDSM

♂♀▽ **Men of All Colors Together (MACT)**
Box 109-136, 7985 Santa Monica Boulevard, West Hollywood, California 90046.

☺ ☐ **The National Leather Association (NLA)—Los Angeles**
Box 109-217, 7985 Santa Monica Boulevard, West Hollywood, California 90046.
☎ 213 856 5643

♀▽ **Women's Leather Network**
P. O. Box 691593, West Hollywood, California 90069.
☎ 213 993 7235

Organizations: Family

♂▽ **Gay Fathers—Los Angeles**
♿ Box 109-346, 7985 Santa Monica Boulvard, West Hollywood, California 90046.
☎ 310 654 0307

Organizations: Sexuality

♀♂▽ **Butch / Femme Network**
P. O. Box 691593, West Hollywood, California 90069.
☎ 213 993 7235

Piercers

☺ ■ **Red Devil Studios**
1149 North La Brea Avenue, West Hollywood, California 90038.
☎ 213 851 0445
🕐 12:00 - 18:00 every day

Publishers: Magazines: BDSM

♂▽ ▼ *Cuir Magazine*
The Leather Journal, Box 109-368, 7985 Santa Monica Boulevard, West Hollywood, California 90046.
☎ 213 656 5073 ✆ 213 656 3120
✉ tjandcuir@aol.com
🕐 Mon - Fri 09:30 - 17:00
♠ ✓ $ 〰 VISA MC
By leather men for leather men. Uninhibited hot fiction, photos, reviews, feature columns, & hot personals. Published every two months. Yearly subscription is $33. Age statement of 21 is required.

Publishers: Magazines: Fetish

☺ ▼ *Fetish*
The Leather Journal, Box 109-368, 7985 Santa Monica Boulevard, West Hollywood, California 90046.
☎ 213 656 5073 ✆ 213 656 3120
✉ tjandcuir@aol.com
🕐 Mon - Fri 09:30 - 17:00
♠ ✓ $ 〰 VISA MC
Southern California's leather/SM/fetish news, features, & ads magazine. Free in Southern California. Published every month. Yearly subscription is $29U.S., $60 overseas. Age statement of 21 is required.

Publishers: Magazines: Sexuality

⚨■ *Dragazine*
P. O. Box 691664, West Hollywood, California 90069-9664.
☎ 310 855 9435
✓
Published twice a year. Yearly subscription is $10.95.

♂▽ ▼ *Military & Police Uniform Association Newsletter*
Military & Police Uniform Association, P. O. Box 69A04, Dept. AS, West Hollywood, California 90069.
☎ 213 650 5112
Men into uniform lifestyle: Military, police, boots, & leather with personal ads, photos, stories, & videos of real marines. SASE or IRC for information. Published quarterly. Yearly subscription is $29.

Publishers: Newspapers: Sexuality

♂▽ ▼ *Frontiers*
Box 109, 7985 Santa Monica Boulevard, West Hollywood, California

90046.
☎ 213 848 2222 ✆ 213 656 8784
🕐 Mon - Fri 09:00 - 18:00
LA's largest, most informative publication. News, commentary, interviews, features, & entertainment. Published twice a month. Yearly subscription is $39.

♂▽ *Planet Homo*
Suite 200, 8380 Santa Monica Boulevard, West Hollywood, California 90069.
☎ 213 848 2220
LA's best & most up-to-date guide to gay happenings in town. Published every two weeks. Yearly subscription is $39.95.

Stores: Books: General

☺ ■ **Circus of Books**
8230 Santa Monica Boulevard, West Hollywood, California 90046.
☎ 213 656 6533 ✆ 213 656 1640

♂▽ ▼ **A Different Light**
8853 Santa Monica Boulevard, West Hollywood, California 90069.
☎ 319 854 6601 ✆ 310 854 6602
♠ ✓ $ 〰 VISA MC AMEX ℓ
Free catalogue published 3 times a year.

♂▽ **Unicorn Bookstore**
8940 Santa Monica Boulevard, West Hollywood, California 90069.
☎ 310 652 6253 ✆ 310 652 6253
🕐 10:30 - 22:30, Fri Sat - 00:30

Stores: Clothing: Fetish

☺ ■ **Dream Dresser**
8444-50 Santa Monica Boulevard, West Hollywood, California 90069.
☎ 213 848 3480
🕐 Mon - Sat 11:00 - 20:00

Stores: Clothing: Leather

☺ **Avalon Leather**
Box 482, 7985 Santa Monica Boulevard, West Hollywood, California 90046.

Stores: Erotica: General

☺ **Drake's After Midnight Bookstore**
9832 Santa Monica Boulevard, West Hollywood, California 90046.
☎ 310 289 8932

☺ **Pleasure Chest**
7733 Santa Monica Boulevard, West Hollywood, California 90046.
☎ 800 753 4536 (orders) ✆ 213 650 1176
☎ 213 650 1022
🕐 10:00 - 01:00
Catalogue, $7.95 + $3 s&h.

Whittier

Suppliers: Diapers

☺ ■ **V. Jensen**
P. O. Box 1201, Whittier, California 90609.
☎ 310 943 8139
Plastic pants in pastel colors & prints. Plain & printed diapers.

Woodland Hills

Organizations: Sexuality

⚨■ **Cross-Talk**
P. O. Box 944, Woodland Hills, California 91365.
 ✆ 818 347 4190
✉ kymmer@xconn.com
🕐 Mon - Fri 09:00 - 17:00
♠ ✓
Contact: Ms. Kymberleigh Richards
Publishes *Cross-Talk* every month.

Publishers: Videos: Erotic

☺ **Rosebud Productions**
22425 Ventura Bouelvard, Woodland Hills, California 91364.
☎ 818 702 8040
Makes videos for those with an anal fetish. Some mail order available.

Publishers: Videos: Sexuality

♂▽ ▼ **Campus Studios**
20929-47 Ventura Boulevard, Woodland Hills, California 91364.
☎ 818 340 7290

Stores: Clothing: Sexuality

⚨■ **Fantasy Fashions**
Suite 196, 22968 Victory Boulevard, Woodland Hills, California 91367.
♠ ✓

Yorba Linda
Organizations: Sexuality
✉▽ **Powder Puffs of California (PPOC)**
P. O. Box 1088, Yorba Linda, California 92686.
☎ 714 779 9013
📧 ppoc@aol.com
🕐 Leave message Mon - Fri 09:00 - 21:00
Publishes *PPOC Girl Talk.*

COLORADO
Area: Approximately 269,000 square kilometres
Population: Approximately 3,310,000
Capital City: Denver
Time zone: GMT minus 7 hours (Mountain Time)
Climate: Mild climate away from the mountains. Great mountains & snow for winter skiing.
Age of consent & homosexuality legislation: State has adopted the Model Penal Code or otherwise decriminalized homosexual activities.
Legal drinking age: 21

State Resources
Organizations: AIDS: Education
☺ ☐ **Colorado AIDS Project**
♿ P. O. Box 18529, Denver, Colorado 80218.
☎ 800 333 2437 (hotline)
☎ 303 837 0166 (office)
🕐 Hotline: Mon - Fri 09:00 - 21:00, Sat - 15:00; Office: Mon - Fri 09:00 - 17:00; TDD: Mon - Fri 09:00 - 21:00, Sat - 15:00
All lines voice & TDD.

Organizations: Sexuality
♂▽ **BiNet—Colorado**
☎ 303 784 5557
📧 cheryl@bbs.tde.com
⚥▽ **The Lesbian Connection**
♿ #E4-233, 2525 Arapahoe Avenue, Boulder, Colorado 80302.
☎ 303 443 1105
Publishes *TLC Newsletter.*

Publishers: Magazines: Sexuality
⚥▼ *Quest Magazine*
Quest Publications, 430 South Broadway, Denver, Colorado 80209.
☎ 303 722 5965 📞 303 698 1183
🍴 ✓ $ 💳 💳 💳
An upscale monthly magazine for the gay & lesbian community of Colorado, featuring news, arts, & entertainment. Published every month. Yearly subscription is $24U.S..

Publishers: Newspapers: Sexuality
⚥▼ *H.*
Quest Publications, 430 South Broadway, Denver, Colorado 80209.
☎ 303 722 5965 📞 303 698 1183
🍴 ✓ 💳 💳 💳
H. is about fun & the joys of being gay in Colorado. Features entertainment, bar shots, & telephone communication. Published twice a month.

Stores: Erotica: BDSM
☺ **The Crypt**
♿ 131 Broadway, Denver, Colorado 80203-3916.
☎ 303 733 3112
🕐 Mon - Sat 10:00 - 22:00, Sun 12:00 - 20:00
♿ 💳 💳 💳
Age statement of 18 is required.

Arvada
Counsellors
✉▼ **The Institute for Gender Study & Treatment**
P. O. Box 126, Arvada, Colorado 80001.
☎ 303 423 9885
Practice is limited to CDs, the gender conflicted, & their partners.

Publishers: Magazines: Sexuality
✉■ *Gender Review*
P. O. Box 126, Arvada, Colorado 80001.
☎ 303 423 9885

Aspen
Organizations: Sexuality
⚥▽ **Aspen Gay & Lesbian Community**
P. O. Box 3143, Aspen, Colorado 81612-3143.
☎ 202 925 9249

Aurora
Organizations: Sexuality
⚥ **National Gay & Lesbian Domestic Violence Victims' Network**
3506 South Ouray Circle, Aurora, Colorado 80013.
☎ 303 266 3477
✉▽ **The Phœnix Project**
Suite 6-178, 1740 South Buckley Road, Aurora, Colorado 80017.
Contact: Ms. Laurie Ciccotello.
☺ ☐ **Teenage Kids of Ts (TAKOTS)**
Suite 6-178, 1740 South Buckley Road, Aurora, Colorado 80017.
Contact: Ms. Laurie Ciccotello
Support for children of transsexual people.

Boulder
Organizations: AIDS: Education
☺ ☐ **AIDS Prevention Program**
♿ 3450 North Broadway, Boulder, Colorado 80304.
☎ 303 441 1160
☺ ☐ **Boulder County AIDS Project**
♿ 2118 14th. Street, Boulder, Colorado 80302-4804.
☎ 303 444 6121

Organizations: BDSM
⚥▼ **Colorado Organization of Dungeon Enthusiasts (CODE)**
P. O. Box 20184, Boulder, Colorado 80308-3184.
☎ 303 499 6757
🕐 Meets once a month
Safe, sane, & consensual environment for education & social contacts. Also has a group in Denver.

Organizations: Sexuality: Student
⚥▽ **Lesbian, Bisexual, & Gay Alliance**
♿ Room 29, UMC at CU, Boulder, Colorado 80309.
☎ 303 492 8567

Publishers: Directories: Sexuality
⚥▼ *Colorado Community Directory*
P. O. Box 2270, Boulder, Colorado 80306.

Publishers: Magazines: AIDS
☺▼ *Positively Friends*
P. O. Box 4262, Boulder, Colorado 80306-4262.
☎ 303 678 5600 📞 303 678 5672
Published quarterly. Yearly subscription is $12. Age statement of 18 is required.

Publishers: Magazines: Sexuality
☺■ *Private Tymes*
Phun Ink Press, P. O. Box 1905, Boulder, Colorado 80306.
☎ 303 575 5652
🕐 24hr. answering machine
For voyeurs & exhibitionists. Also BBS lists & Internet information. Letters & cheques to Stevyn, please. Published quarterly. Yearly subscription is $12. Age statement of 21 is required.

Stores: Erotica: General
☺■ **Newsstand Adult Bookshop**
1720 15th. Street, Boulder, Colorado 80302.
☎ 303 442 9515

Colorado Springs
BBSs: BDSM
⚥▼ **Male Box**
📞 719 471 2244

Counsellors
☺■ **Corky Keeffe, M.A.**
Suite 201, 1425 North Union, Colorado Springs, Colorado 80909.
☎ 719 578 9730
☺▼ **Lifesigns**
♿ Suite 204, 10 Boulder Crescent, Colorado Springs, Colorado 80903.
☎ 719 634 2488 📞 719 633 3513

Health Services
☺ ☐ **Penrose Hospital**
2215 North Cascade Avenue, Colorado Springs, Colorado 80907.
☎ 719 630 5000
HIV & emergency departments.

Helplines: Sexuality

⌖▽ **Pikes Peak Gay & Lesbian Community Center Help Line**
P. O. Box 607, Colorado Springs, Colorado 80901.
☎ 719 471 4429
🕐 Mon - Fri 18:00 - 21:00, Sat 15:00 - 17:00

Organizations: AIDS: Education

☺☐ **Southern Colorado AIDS Poject**
♿ P. O. Box 311, Colorado Springs, Colorado 80901.
☎ 719 578 9092

Organizations: Family

☺☐ **Parents & Friends of Lesbians & Gays (PFLAG)— Colorado Springs**
♿
Suite 204, 10 Boulder Crescent, Colorado Springs, Colorado 80903.
☎ 719 634 2488

Organizations: Sexuality: Student

⌖▽ **Colorado College Gay & Lesbian Alliance**
♿ 902 North Cascade, Colorado Springs, Colorado 80946.
☎ 719 389 6641

Piercers

☺☐ **Pike's Peak Tattoo**
519 South Nevada Avenue, Colorado Springs, Colorado 80903.
☎ 719 632 6141

Publishers: Newspapers: Sexuality

⌖▽ *New Phazes Newsletter*
P. O. Box 6485, Colorado Springs, Colorado 80934-6485.
☎ 719 634 0236
To encourage cohesion in the Pike's Peak region's lesbian community by providing an open forum which stimulates, informs, & entertains. Published 11 times a year. Yearly subscription is $12.

Stores: Books: General

⌖▼ **Abaton Books**
♿ 802 North 25th. Street, Colorado Springs, Colorado 80904-2669.

Stores: Erotica: General

☺▼ **First Amendment**
♿ , 220 East Fillmore Street, Colorado Springs, Colorado 80907.
☎ 719 630 7676
🕐 08:00 - 02:00, Sun - 24:00
💲 ✓ $ 💳 💳

Denver

Archives: Sexuality

⌖▽ **Terry Mangan Library**
P. O. Drawer 18E, Denver, Colorado 80218-0140.
☎ 303 831 6268 📞 303 839 1361

Bars: BDSM

⌖▼ **Buddies**
♿ 2101 Champa Street, Denver, Colorado 80205.
☎ 303 289 9301

⌖▼ **Colorado Triangle**
2036 Broadway, Denver, Colorado 80205.
☎ 303 293 9009

⌖▼ **Compound**
♿ 145 Broadway, Denver, Colorado 80203.
☎ 303 722 7977
🕐 19:00 - 02:00

BBSs: BDSM

☺■ **Denver Exchange**
☎ 303 623 6665
📞 303 458 1227

Counsellors

☺▼ **Gail Bernstein, Ph.D.**
♿ Suite 430, 789 Sherman, Denver, Colorado 80203.
☎ 303 832 5123

⌖▼ **Steven Chain, LCSW**
♿ Suite 300, 360 South Monroe Street, Denver, Colorado 80209.
☎ 303 393 7120

☺■ **Carol Cohen, M.A., LPC**
♿ Suite 634, 2121 South Oneida, Denver, Colorado 80224.
☎ 303 759 5126

☺■ **Daugherty & Associates**
♿ ☎ 303 266 3477

☎ 303 754 7579
Specializes in gender dysphoria.

☺ **Maryann Grundman, Ph.D., LCSW**
♿ New Options Counseling, 682 Grant, Denver, Colorado 80203.
☎ 303 278 4392 📞 303 279 3542
🕐 08:00 - 20:00
💲 ✓ $
Individual, relationship, & group counselling in a safe, supportive environment. Age statement of 18 is required.

☺■ **Judith Rachael Hartman, Ph.D.**
♿ 2160 South Gilpin Street, Denver, Colorado 80210-4615.
☎ 303 722 2212

⌖▼ **Michael Holtby, LSCW**
♿ 309 Cherokee Street, Denver, Colorado 80223.
☎ 303 722 1021
📧 mholtby@aol.com
💲 ✓ 💳 💳

⌖▼ **Betsy Kelso, Psy.D.**
♿ Suite 930, 1873 South Bellair, Denver, Colorado 802222.
☎ 303 757 6969

⌖▼ **John Shell, Ph.D.**
♿ 2250 South Albion Street, Denver, Colorado 80222.
☎ 303 377 6169

▷▽▼ **Deb-Ann Thompson, Ph.D, NCACII, CACIII**
Suite 207, 2755 South Locust Street, Denver, Colorado 80222.
☎ 303 758 6634
Psychotherapy.

⌖▼ **Deb-Ann Thomson**
Suite 290, 2870 North Speer Boulevard, Denver, Colorado 80211.
☎ 303 433 3001 📞 303 433 0111

☺▼ **Robert Vitaletti, Ph.D.**
♿ Suite 567, 1616 17th. Street, Denver, Colorado 880202.
☎ 303 628 5425

Health Services

☺☐ **Colorado Health Action Project**
1615 Ogden, Denver, Colorado 80218.
☎ 303 894 8650

☺☐ **Denver Metro Health Clinic**
605 Bannock Street, Denver, Colorado 80204.
☎ 303 893 7296

☺☐ **Porter Memorial Hospital**
2525 South Downing Street, Denver, Colorado 80210.
☎ 303 778 1955

☺☐ **Provenant Saint Anthony Hospital**
4231 West 16th. Avenue, Denver, Colorado 80204.
☎ 303 629 3511

☺☐ **Saint Joseph Hospital**
1835 Franklin Street, Denver, Colorado 80218.
☎ 202 837 7111

☺☐ **Saint Luke's Medical Center**
1719 East 19th. Avenue, Denver, Colorado 80218.
☎ 303 839 6100

☺☐ **UCHSC**
HIV/STD Testing Clinics, Care Center B, 4200 East 9th. Avenue, Denver, Colorado 80262.
☎ 303 270 8870

Helplines: Sexuality

⌖▽ **Gay & Lesbian Community Center of Colorado, Inc.**
♿ P. O. Drawer 18E, Denver, Colorado 80218-0140.
☎ 303 831 6268 📞 303 839 1361
🕐 Mon - Fri 10:00 - 22:00, Sat - 19:00, Sun 13:00 - 16:00

Manufacturers: Erotica: BDSM

☺ **Zip-Up Leathers**
19 East Bayaud Avenue, Denver, Colorado 80209.
☎ 303 733 7442 📞 303 863 9233
Custom work is available. Catalogue, $3.95.

Manufacturers: Piercing Jewelry

☺■ **Gothic Steel**
P. O. Box 481171, Denver, Colorado 80248.
☎ 303 837 0272
🕐 Piercing by appointment only
Surgical steel, Niobium, & Titanium jewelry with tapered ends. Makes single-use dermal punches. Retail & wholesale mail order.

Organizations: AIDS: Education

☺☐ **Denver AIDS Prevention**
Suite 229, 605 Bannock Street, Denver, Colorado 80204.
☎ 303 893 6300

Organizations: AIDS: Support

☺ □ **PWA Coalition Colorado**
 P. O. Box 300339, Denver, Colorado 80203.
 ☎ 303 837 8214 📞 303 837 9213
 Publishes *Resolute*.

Organizations: BDSM

☺ □ **Colorado Organization of Dungeon Enthusiasts (CODE)**
 Suite 200, 1015 South Gaylord Street, Denver, Colorado 80209.
 Safe, sane, & consensual environment for education & social contacts.

☺ □ **Continental Leather Pride Committee**
 P. O. Box 300747, Denver, Colorado 80203.
 ☎ 303 331 2549
 📧 cdlpride@tde.com
 🌐 http://www.tde.com/~cdlpride

⚥ □ **Defenders—Denver**
 c/o Dignity Denver, P. O. Box 3072, Denver, Colorado 80202.
 ☎ 303 322 8485

☺ □ **Denver Leather Association**
 P. O. Box 300747, Denver, Colorado 80203.
 ☎ 303 331 2549
 📧 cdlpride@tde.com
 🌐 http://www.tde.com/~cdlpride

⚥▽ **Mountain Men of Leather**
 P. O. Box 18876, Denver, Colorado 80218.

⚥▽ **Rocky Mountain Lambda Lions**
 P. O. Box 300416, Denver, Colorado 80203-0416.

Organizations: Bears

⚥▽ **Front Range Bears**
 P. O. Box 101433, Denver, Colorado 80250-1433.
 ☎ 303 331 2705
 📧 jbearj@aol.com
 🌐 http://www.csn.net/~wburdine/frb.htm
 🕐 Meets 2nd. Tue of month

Organizations: Body Size

⚥▽ **Girth & Mirth—Rockies**
 P. O. Box 2315, Denver, Colorado 80201-2315.
 ☎ 303 784 5814

Organizations: Family

☺ □ **Parents & Friends of Lesbians & Gays (PFLAG)—Denver**
 P. O. Box 18901, Denver, Colorado 80218.
 ☎ 303 333 0286

Organizations: Motorcycle

⚥▽ **City Bikers MC**
 P. O. Box 9816, Denver, Colorado 80209-0816.
 ☎ 303 369 0522
 ☎ 303 428 7366

⚥▽ **Rocky Mountaineers MC**
 P. O. Box 2629, Denver, Colorado 80201.
 ☎ 303 733 7047
 🌐 http://www.interealm.com/p/sheyl/rmmc
 Publishes *Dispatch*.

Organizations: Sexuality

⚥▽ **Coming Out / Being Out Group**
 ⚥ 1245 East Colfax Avenue, Denver, Colorado 80218.
 ☎ 303 831 6268

♀♀▽ **Every Woman's Coming Out Group**
 P. O. Drawer 18E, Denver, Colorado 80218-0140.
 ☎ 303 837 1598

⚥♀▽ **Gay & Lesbian Community Center of Colorado, Inc.**
 ⚥ P. O. Drawer 18E, Denver, Colorado 80218-0140.
 ☎ 303 831 6268 📞 303 839 1361
 🕐 Mon - Fri 10:00 - 22:00, Sat - 19:00, Sun 13:00 - 16:00
 Publishes *Centerlines*.

⚥▽ **Men's Coming Out Group**
 1630 East 14th. Avenue, Denver, Colorado 80218.
 ☎ 303 831 6238

⚥▽ **Peer Support Program**
 ⚥ P. O. Drawer 18E, Denver, Colorado 80218-0140.
 ☎ 303 831 6268

☿▽ **The Society for the Second Self (Tri-Ess)—Delta**
 P. O. Box 16208, Denver, Colorado 80216.
 ☎ 303 595 5875
 🕐 Meets monthly
 Publishes *The Femme Mirror*.

Organizations: Sexuality: Student

⚥▽ **Denver University Lesbian, Gay, & Bisexual Alliance (LGBA)**
 8050 East Evans Avenue, Denver, Colorado 80208.
 ☎ 303 871 2321

⚥♀▽ **Lesbian & Gay Resource Center**
 Box 82, Metropolitan State College, Denver, Colorado 80204.
 ☎ 303 629 3317

Organizations: Sexuality: Youth

⚥▽ **Gay & Lesbian Community Center of Colorado, Inc.**
 ⚥ Youth Services, P. O. Drawer 18E, Denver, Colorado 80218-0140.
 ☎ 303 831 6268 📞 303 839 1361
 🕐 Mon - Fri 10:00 - 22:00, Sat - 19:00, Sun 13:00 - 16:00

Piercers

☺ ■ **Bound By Design**
 1326 East Colfax, Denver, Colorado.
 ☎ 303 832 9741
 Also scarification & branding.

Publishers: Magazines: Bears

⚥▼ *American Bear*
 Big Bull, Inc., P. O. Box 300352, Denver, Colorado 80203.
 💰 ✓
 Published every two months.

Publishers: Magazines: Erotic

☺ ■ **Hightail Publishing**
 P. O. Box 11009, Denver, Colorado 80211-0009.
 ☎ 303 458 6653
 🕐 09:00 - 17:00
 Very graphic publications that explore the submissive female. For heterosexual & bisexual men, & all women. Catalogue, $3. Age statement of 21 is required.

Publishers: Magazines: Sexuality

⚥ *Bulk Male*
 Big Bull, Inc., P. O. Box 300352, Denver, Colorado 80203.
 💰 ✓
 Published every two months. Yearly subscription is $32.95.

Publishers: Newspapers: Sexuality

⚢ ▼ *Colorado Woman News*
 P. O. Box 22274, Denver, Colorado 80224.
 ☎ 303 355 9229
 Feminist news magazine. Published every month. Yearly subscription is $25.

♀♀▼ *Lesbians in Colorado*
 P. O. Box 533, 1200 Madison Street, Denver, Colorado 80206-0533.
 ☎ 303 399 3544
 Colorado's only lesbian newspaper. Published 11 times a year. Yearly subscription is $18.

⚥▼ *Out Front*
 244 Washington Street, Denver, Colorado 80203.
 ☎ 303 778 7900
 News & general information for the gay & lesbian communities. Published 25 times a year. Yearly subscription is $60.

⚥▼ *Preferred Stock*
 ⚥ P. O. Box 18515, Denver, Colorado 80218.
 ☎ 303 839 5410 📞 303 727 7751
 News & entertainment - Colorado's best source of gay & lesbian news. Published every two weeks. Yearly subscription is $30.

☺ ■ *The Rocky Mountain Oyster*
 Mountain Top Publishing, P. O. Box 27467, Denver, Colorado 80227.
 ☎ 303 985 3034 📞 303 986 5664
 Published every week. Yearly subscription is $99.

Stores: Books: General

♀♀▼ **Book Garden**
 2625 East 12th. Avenue, Denver, Colorado 80206.
 ☎ 303 399 2004 📞 303 299 6176
 🕐 Mon - Sat 10:00 - 18:00, Sun 12.00 - 17:00
 💰 ✓ 💳 💳 💳

☺ **Tattered Cover Book Store**
 ⚥ 2955 East 1st. Avenue, Denver, Colorado 80206.
 ☎ 800 833 9327 📞 303 399 2279
 ☎ 303 322 7727
 📧 books@tatteredcover.com
 💰 $ ✓ 💳 💳 💳 💳

☺ **Tattered Cover Book Store**
 1628 16th. Street, Denver, Colorado 80202.
 ☎ 800 833 9327 📞 303 399 2279
 ☎ 303 436 1070

✉ books@tatteredcover.com
♣ ✓ $ ⚡ 💳 💲 ⬛

Stores: Clothing: Fetish
☺ ■ **UZI**
508 Colfax, Denver, Colorado 80203.
☎ 303 832 4870
Rubber clothing & bondage gear.

Stores: Erotica: BDSM
☿▽ **Fit 2 A T Leather**
2044 Broadway, Denver, Colorado 80205.
☎ 303 294 9916

Stores: Erotica: General
☺ **Boy Toy**
P. O. Box 13515, Denver, Colorado 80202.
☎ 303 394 4776
☺ ■ **Leather & Lace**
2028 East Colfax Avenue, Denver, Colorado 80206.
☎ 800 441 4695 ✆ 303 333 8141
☎ 303 333 4870
Catalogue, $13 for all four.
☺ ▼ **Pleasures Entertainment Centers, Inc.**
127 South Broadway, Denver, Colorado 80209.
☎ 303 722 5892

Television: Sexuality
☿▽ **The Lambda Report**
KBDI-TV, Channel 12, P. O. Box 9742, Denver, Colorado 80209.
☎ 303 446 2518 ✆ 303 727 7751
🕐 Thu 22:30

Durango
Organizations: Sexuality
☿▽ **Gay & Lesbian Association of Durango**
P. O. Box 1656, Durango, Colorado 81302.
☎ 303 247 7778

Englewood
Counsellors
☺ ■ **Marjorie Bayes, Ph.D.**
♿ Suite B13, 8000 East Prentice, Englewood, Colorado 80111.
☎ 303 377 0246

Fort Collins
Counsellors
☺ ▼ **Ken Hoole, MSW**
101 East Pitkin Street, Fort Collins, Colorado 80524.
☎ 303 221 0272

Organizations: AIDS: Education
☺ ☐ **Northern Colorado AIDS Project**
♿ P. O. Box 182, Fort Collins, Colorado 80522.
☎ 303 223 6227

Organizations: Sexuality
☿▽ **Lambda Community Center**
⬡ 155 North College Avenue, Fort Collins, Colorado 80524.
☎ 303 224 3247

Grand Junction
Organizations: Family
☺ ☐ **Parents & Friends of Lesbians & Gays (PFLAG)—Grand Junction**
P. O. Box 4904, Grand Junction, Colorado 81502.
☎ 303 242 2966

Greeley
Counsellors
☺ ▼ **Marilee Smith, Psy.D.**
♿ Suite 200, 1750 25th. Avenue, Greeley, Colorado 80631.
☎ 303 351 6688

Health Services
☺ ☐ **North Colorado Medical Center**
1801 16th. Street, Greeley, Colorado 80631.
☎ 303 352 4121

Organizations: Bears
☿▽ **Greeley Bears**
P. O. Box 907, Greeley, Colorado 80632.

☎ 970 330 3732 Ext.: 387
Organizations: Sexuality
☿▽ **Greeley Gay, Lesbian, & Bisexual Alliance (GOLBA)**
Student Activities Area, UNC, Greeley, Colorado 80639.
☎ 303 351 1484

Lakewood
Organizations: Sexuality
▽▽ **Gender Identity Center of Colorado, Inc.**
Suite 100, 1455 Ammons Street, Lakewood, Colorado 80215-4993.
☎ 303 202 6466
🌐 http://www.zoom.com/tg/gic/index.html

Printers: Adult
☺ **Mountaintop Design & Typography**
2525 South Wadsworth, Lakewood, Colorado 80232.
☎ 303 985 0202
All forms of design & print services for the adult industry.

Thornton
Tattooists
☺ ■ **Body Graphics Tattoo**
Mission Trace Shipping Center, 3925 B E 120th. Avenue, Thornton, Colorado 80233.
☎ 303 254 4473
🕐 Tue - Thu 11:00 - 19:00, Fri Sat 11:00 - 21:00

CONNECTICUT
Area: Approximately 12,560 square kilometres
Population: Approximately 3,300,000
Capital City: Hartford
Time zone: GMT minus 5 hours (EST)
Climate: Continental climate with temperatures averaging approximately 23°C in the summer, & -2°C in the winter.
Age of consent & homosexuality legislation: State has adopted the Model Penal Code or otherwise decriminalized homosexual activities. There is legislation in place against discrimination on the basis of sexual orientation.
Legal drinking age: 21

State Resources
Manufacturers: Furniture: BDSM
☺ ▼ **Terry Mazurkewicz**
P. O. Box 2476, New Preston, Connecticut 06777.
☎ 203 639 2345
✉ tonkaterry@aol.com
🕐 Evenings, answering machine at other times
♣ ✓
Installs dungeons & makes BDSM equipment.

Organizations: Family
☺ ☐ **Parents & Friends of Lesbians & Gays (PFLAG)—Connecticut**
♿ P. O. Box 16703, Stamford, Connecticut 06905-8703.
☎ 203 544 8724
☎ 203 322 5380

Organizations: Sexuality
▽☐ **Connecticut Outreach Society**
P. O. Box 163, Farmington, Connecticut 06034.
☎ 203 657 4344
Support, education, & outreach. Publishes The Outreach News.

Bridgeport
Organizations: AIDS: Support
☺ ☐ **Family Services Woodfield**
♿ 475 Clinton Avenue, Bridgeport, Connecticut 06605.
☎ 203 368 4291
Information, education, & support for people infected with or affected by HIV/AIDS.

Stores: Books: General
☺ ▼ **Bloodroot**
♿ 85 Ferris Street, Bridgeport, Connecticut 06605.
☎ 203 576 9168

Bristol
Counsellors
☺ ▼ **Wynelle Riley Snow, M.D.**
K♿ Suite 302, 1001 Farmington Avenue, Bristol, Connecticut 06010.
☎ 860 582 1178

Counsellors

🕐 By appointment 08:00 - 18:00
♿ ✓
Board certified psychiatrist, member of the Harry Benjamin International Gender Dysphoria Association. Individual psychotherapy.

Stores: Erotica: General
☺ ▼ **X Factor**
 ♿ 660 Stafford Avenue, Bristol, Connecticut 06010.
 ☎ 203 583 6284
 🕐 Mon - Sat 09:00 - 21:00
X-rated videos for sale & rent, adult magazines, books, newspapers, toys, lotions, bodywear, swinger publications, etc.. Private mailboxes for rent. Catalogue $7.40U.S..

Suppliers: Photoprinting
☺ ▼ **R. L.**
 P. O. Box 2902, Bristol, Connnecticut 06011-2902.
Confidential film processing, & other photographic services where discretion is required.

Colchester
Counsellors
⚥▼ **Janet Peck, M.S.**
 ♿ 244 Main Street, Colchester, Connecticut 06415.
 ☎ 203 537 3977

Danbury
Counsellors
⚥▼ **Suzanne Chapin, M.A.**
 29 Cornell Road, Danbury, Connecticut 06811.
 ☎ 203 792 8423
 🕐 Call in evenings

Health Services
☺ ☐ **Danbury Hospital**
 24 Hospital Avenue, Danbury, Connecticut 06810.
 ☎ 203 797 7000

Organizations: Sexuality
⚥▽ **Gay & Lesbian Alliance of Greater Danbury**
 P. O. Box 2045, Danbury, Connecticut 06810.
 ☎ 203 426 4922
Publishes *GLAD News.*

Organizations: Sexuality: Youth
⚥▽ **Danbury Area Gay, Lesbian, & Bisexual Youth Group**
 P. O. Box 2056, Danbury, Connecticut 06810.
 ☎ 203 798 0863

Stores: Books: General
☺ ■ **Baileywick Books**
 17 Church Street, Milford, Connecticut 06776.
 ☎ 203 354 3865

Stores: Erotica: BDSM
☺ ■ **Fantasy Isle**
 2 Mill Ridge Road, Danbury, Connecticut 06811.
 ☎ 203 743 1792

Darien
Organizations: Sexuality: Youth
⚥▽ **Alternative Youth Club - Tri State Area**
 P. O. Box 2492, Darien, Connecticut 06820.
 ☎ 203 975 9139

Dayville
Counsellors
☺ ☐ **United Services**
 ♿ 1007 North Main Street, Dayville, Connecticut 06241.
 ☎ 203 774 2020

East Hartford
Organizations: BDSM
☺ **Service of Mankind Church—East**
 P.O. Box 28172, East Hartford, Connecticut 06128-1172.
 🕐 Bus. number 10:00 - 19:00
☺ ☐ **United Leatherfolk of Connecticut**
 ♿ P.O. Box 281172, East Hartford, Connecticut 06128-1172.
 ✉ ulofct@aol.com
Contact: Ms. Laura Goodwin
Private, educational BDSM social & support group. Publishes *The Leatherfolk Connection.* Age statement of 18 is required.

Stores: Erotica: BDSM
☺ ▼ **The Leather Harvest**
 ♿ 1165 Main Street, East Hartford, Connecticut 06108.
 ☎ 203 290 8981
 🕐 Mon - Sat 09:00 - 18:00, Thu - 20:00
Catalogue available.
☺ ■ **Water Hole Custom Leather, Inc.**
 982 Main Street, East Hartford, Connecticut 06108-2220.
 ☎ 800 390 6674 📞 860 289 3025
 ☎ 860 528 6195
 ✉ brandrog@netcom.com
 🕐 Mon - Fri 09:00 - 20:00, Sat 09:00 - 18:00, other times by appointment
Leather clothing & toys, & bondage gear. Custom order bondage furniture. Also mail order. Catalogue, $10, refundable on first purchase. Age statement of 18 is required.

Enfield
Stores: Erotica: General
☺ ■ **Bookends**
 ♿ 44 Enfield Street, Enfield, Connecticut 06082.
 ☎ 203 745 3988

Fairfield
Organizations: AIDS: Support
☺ ☐ **Circle of Care**
 ⚥ P. O. Box 338, Fairfield, Connecticut 06430.
 ☎ 203 255 7965

Publishers: Books: BDSM
☺ **Mystic Rose Books**
 P. O. Box 1036, Fairfield, Connecticut 06432.
 ☎ 203 371 6912
 🕸 http://palace.com/rose/mystic2.htm

Greenwich
Organizations: AIDS: Education
☺ ☐ **AIDS Alliance of Greenwich**
 ♿ c/o Department of Health, 101 Field Point Road, Greenwich, Connecticut 06836.
 ☎ 203 622 6460
Publishes *Resource Guide.*

Haddam
Organizations: Sexuality
⚥▽ **P. I. Group**
 P. O. Box 245, Haddam, Connecticut 06438-0245.

Hartford
Counsellors
☺ ■ **Associated Counseling Professionals, Inc.**
 ⚥ P. O. Box 2475, Hartford, Connecticut 06146-2475.
 ☎ 800 654 4320 (in Connecticut)
 ☎ 203 529 2955
☺ ▼ **Creative Counseling Services**
 ⚥ P. O. Box 270408, West Hartford, Connecticut 06127-0408.
 ☎ 203 233 6962
⚥■ **James Koplin, M.Ed., MSW**
 P. O. Box 1465, Hartford, Connecticut 06144.
 ☎ 203 724 4204
☺ ▼ **Timothy Wallace, Ph.D.**
 674 Prospect Avenue, Hartford, Connecticut 06105.
 ☎ 203 233 6229

Health Services
⚥▽ **Gay & Lesbian Health Collective, Inc.**
 ♿ P. O. Box 2094, Hartford, Connecticut 06145-2094.
 ☎ 203 278 4163
Information, counselling, HIV & STD testing, education, & support.
☺ ☐ **Hartford Hospital**
 80 Sseymour Street, Hartford, Connecticut 06102.
 ☎ 203 545 5555
☺ ☐ **Saint Francis Hospital & Medical Center**
 500 Blue Hills Avenue, Hartford, Connecticut 06112.
 ☎ 203 286 6000

Manufacturers: Clothing: Leather
☺ ■ **Leather Creations**

P. O. Box 2212, Hartford, Connecticut 06145.
☎ 203 742 0157
✉ 75730.3031@compuserve.com
Catalogue available.
📠 203 742 0157

Organizations: AIDS: Education

☺ ☐ **AIDS Project Hartford, Inc.**
♿ 30 Arbor Street, Hartford, Connecticut 06106.
☎ 203 247 2437

☺ ☐ **Hartford Health Department**
♿ AIDS Program, 80 Coventry Street, Hartford, Connecticut 06112.
☎ 203 722 6742

Organizations: Family

☺ ☐ **Parents & Friends of Lesbians & Gays (PFLAG)—**
♿ **Hartford**
49 Beechwood Lane, South Glastonbury, Connecticut 06073.
☎ 203 633 7184

Organizations: Motorcycle

⚧ **Hartford Colts, MC**
P. O. Box 4098, Hartford, Connecticut 06147-4098.
☎ 203 278 5616
☎ Phone

Organizations: Sexuality

⚧▽ **Gay, Lesbian, & Bisexual Community Center**
♿ 1841 Broad Street, Hartford, Connecticut 06114-1780.
☎ 203 724 5542
📠 203 724 3443
Publishes *Community Center Update.*

✉☐ **Twenty Club (XX)**
P. O. Box 387, Hartford, Connecticut 06151-0387.
For TS only. Publishes *XX* every month.

Organizations: Sexuality: Student

⚧▽ **Eros**
♿ Box 1385, Trinity College, 300 Summit, Hartford, Connecticut 06106.
☎ 203 297 2408

⚧▽ **Gay & Lesbian Alliance**
♿ c/o Student Association, University of Hartford, West Hartford, Connecticut 06117.

⚧▽ **Lesbian, Gay, & Bisexual Student Alliance**
University of Connecticut School of Social Work, 1800 Asylum Avenue, West Hartford, Connecticut 06117.
☎ 203 523 4841 Ext.: 267

Publishers: Newspapers: Sexuality

⚧ *Metro Line*
1841 Broad Street, Hartford, Connecticut 06114-1780.
☎ 203 236 7813
Award-winning news & features magazine for gay & lesbian community in Connecticut, western Massachusetts, & Rhode Island. News interviews, arts, entertainment calendar, club events, resource guide, health services, & classified. Published every two weeks. Yearly subscription is $35.

Publishers: Videos: BDSM

☺ **Beth Tyler Labs**
P. O. Box 2551, Hartford, Connecticut 06146-2551.
📠 203 871 0293

Stores: Books: General

☺ ■ **Reader's Feast**
529 Farmington Avenue, Hartford, Connecticut 06105.
☎ 203 232 2710

Stores: Erotica: General

☺ ■ **Aircraft News & Books**
349 Main Street, Hartford, Connecticut 06118.
☎ 203 569 2324

☺ ■ **Red Lantern Books**
1247 Main Street, East Hartford, Connecticut 06118.
☎ 203 289 5000

Stores: Military Surplus

☺ ■ **Government Sales, Inc.**
30 Atlantic Street, Hartford, Connecticut 06103.
☎ 203 247 7787

Manchester

Organizations: Sexuality

✉▽ **Gender Identity Clinic of New England**
♿ 68 Adelaide Road, Manchester, Connecticut 06040.
☎ 203 646 8651

Contact: Mr. Clinton Jones, Director
Professional clininc. Scrrening for hormones, etc. Member HBIGDA.

⚧■ **Wesleyan Gay, Lesbian, & Bisexual Alliance (GLBA)**
Box A, 190 High Street, Manchester, Connecticut 06457.
☎ 203 347 9411 Ext.: 2712
🕐 Meets Wed 22:00 during term time

Meriden

Counsellors

☺ **Theresa Porter, Psy.D.**
K #218, 525 Crown Street, Meriden, Connecticut 06450.
☎ 203 237 8978
✉ b2tporter@aol.com

Middletown

Organizations: Sexuality

☺ ☐ **Coalition of Sexuality Organizations**
Wesleyan University, 190 High Street, Middletown, Connecticut 06457.
☎ 203 347 9411 Ext.: 2712

New Britain

Organizations: Sexuality

⚧▽ **Gay & Lesbian Alliance**
Box B-17, CCSU Student Center, Central Connecticut State University, New Britain, Connecticut 06050.

New Haven

Counsellors

☺ **Irwin Krieger, LCSW**
♿ 309 Edwards Street, New Haven, Connecticut 06511.
☎ 203 776 2966

☺▼ **Ellis Perlswig, M.D.**
30 Bryden Terrace, Hamden, Connecticut 06517.
☎ 203 777 1876

Health Services

☺ ☐ **Yale- New Haven Hospital**
20 York Street, New Haven, Connecticut 06519.
☎ 203 785 7200
HIV & emergency departments.

Organizations: AIDS: Education

☺ ☐ **AIDS Project New Haven**
♿ P. O. Box 636, New Haven, Connecticut 06503.
☎ 203 624 2437
☎ 203 624 0947

Organizations: Sexuality: Student

⚧▽ **Lesbian, Gay, & Bisexual Coöperative at Yale**
♿ Box 2031, Yale Station, New Haven, Connecticut 06520.
☎ 203 432 1585

⊙▽ **Yalesbians**
♿ Box 5051, Yale Station, New Haven, Connecticut 06520.
☎ 203 432 0388

Publishers: Magazines: Sexuality

⚧ *Hothead Paisan*
P. O. Box 214, New Haven, Connecticut 06502.

Stores: Books: General

☺ ■ **Bookhaven**
♿ 290 York Street, New Haven, Connecticut 06511.
☎ 203 787 2848

☺ ▼ **Golden Thread Booksellers**
♿ 915 State Street, New Haven, Connecticut 06511.
☎ 203 777 7807
🕐 Mon - Fri 11:00 - 18:00, Thu - 19:00, Sun 13:00 - 17:00

Stores: Erotica: General

☺ ■ **Nu Haven Books & Video**
754 Chapel Street, New Haven, Connecticut 06511.
☎ 203 562 5867

New London

Organizations: AIDS: Education

☺ ☐ **Southeastern Connecticut AIDS Project**
♿ 38 Granite Street, New London, Connecticut 06320-5931.
☎ 203 447 0884

New Preston

Organizations: Bears

⊙⚥▽ **Northeast Ursamen**
P. O. Box 2476, New Preston, Connecticut 06777.
☎ 203 639 2345
✉ skita@bsac.uchc.edu
🌐 http://www.skepsis.com:80/.gblo/bears/CLUBS/Northeast_Ursame
n/

Norwich

Helplines: Sexuality

⊙☐ **Infoline of Eastern Connecticut**
74 Main Street, Norwich, Connecticut 06360.
☎ 203 886 0516
☎ 203 346 9941
🕐 Mon - Fri 08:00 - 21:00

Organizations: Family

⊙☐ **Parents & Friends of Lesbians & Gays (PFLAG)—**
 Norwich
 ♿
☎ 203 822 9216

Rocky Hill

Organizations: Sexuality

⚲▽ **Ye CG Brits**
P. O. Box 106, Rocky Hill, Connecticut 06060-0106.
Open to British-born male-to-females to keep in contact with groups in
Great Britain.

South Windsor

Stores: Clothing: Leather

⊙■ **Good Sports**
1017 Sullivan Avenue, South Windsor, Connecticut 06047.
☎ 800 845 0084
Motorcycle clothing.

Southington

Stores: Books: General

⚥■ **The Source Bookstore**
 ♿ 958 Queen Street, Southington, Connecticut 06489.
☎ 203 621 6255

Stamford

Counsellors

⚥▼ **Diane Hyatt, MSW, CISW**
☎ 203 964 1847

Health Services

⊙☐ **Stamford Hospital**
Shelburne Road & West Broad Street, Stamford, Connecticut 06902.
☎ 203 325 7000

Helplines: Sexuality

⚥▽ **Gay & Lesbian Guideline**
P. O. Box 8185, Stamford, Connecticut 06905.
☎ 203 327 0767

Organizations: AIDS: Education

⊙☐ **Stamford Health Department**
 ♿ AIDS Program, 888 Washington Boulevard, Stamford, Connecticut
06904.
☎ 203 967 2437

Organizations: Sexuality: Student

⚥▽ **Bisexual, Gay, & Lesbian Association**
 ⚥ Box U-8, University of Connecticut, 2110 Hillside Road, Stamford,
Connecticut 06268.
☎ 203 486 3679

Thompson

Organizations: Sexuality

⚲▽ **Images**
P. O. Box 666, Thompson, Connecticut 06241-0666.
☎ 203 779 9708 📞 203 779 9708
Peer support group.

Torrington

Organizations: AIDS: Education

⊙☐ **Northwestern Connecticut AIDS Project**
 ♿ 100 Migeon Avenue, Torrington, Connecticut 06790-4815.

☎ 203 482 1596

Stores: Erotica: General

⊙▼ **Torrington Video Books**
466 Main Street, Torrington, Connecticut 06790.
☎ 860 496 7747
🕐 Mon - Sat 10:00 - 22:00, Sun 12:00 - 20:00
♿ $ 💳 💳
X-rated videos for sale & rent, adult magazines, newspapers, & books,
lotions, etc.. Peep shows 25¢.. Age statement of 18 is required.

Trumbull

Counsellors

⊙▼ **John Emery Istvan, M.S., MSW, LCSW**
K ♿ Suite B-3, Medical Arts Center, 15 Corporate Drive, Trumbull, Connecticut
06611-1378.
☎ 203 268 8858 Ext.: 304 📞 203 268 7399
🕐 By appointment
♿
✓
Psychotherapy for individuals & couples, relationship work, HIV
counselling, recovery work, & consulting. Covered by most insurance. .

Unionville

Organizations: BDSM

⊙☐ **The Society**
P.O. Box 460, Unionville, Connecticut 06085.
☎ 413 592 7239
Publishes a newsletter quarterly.

Waterbury

Stores: Erotica: General

⊙▼ **Video Book & News**
♿ 90 South Main Street, Waterbury, Connecticut 06702.
☎ 203 573 1066
🕐 Mon - Thu 10:00 - 22:00
♿ $ ⚥ 💳 💳
X-rated videos for sale & rent, adult magazines, books, newspapers,
toys, lotions, bodywear, swinger publications, etc.. Private mailboxes for
rent. Catalogue $7.40U.S.. Publishes *Your Meeting Place Magazine*
every month. Yearly subscription is $72U.S.. Age statement of 18 is
required.

Weston

Photographers: Erotic

⊙ **Remy Chevalier**
25 Newton Turnpike, Weston, Connecticut 06883.
☎ 203 227 2065

Willimantic

Stores: Erotica: General

⊙■ **Thread City Book & Novelty**
503 Main Street, Willimantic, Connecticut 06226.
☎ 203 456 8131
🕐 Mon - Sat 11:00 - 21:00, Sun 13:00 - 19:00

Windsor

Publishers: Newspapers: Sexuality

⚥ *WAVES*
P. O. Box 684, Windsor, Connecticut 06095.

DELAWARE

Area: Approximately 5,070 square kilometres
Population: Approximately 670,000
Capital City: Dover
Time zone: GMT minus 5 hours (EST)
Climate: Hot & humid in the summer, with cooler sea breezes. Winters are
 cold with many storms.
Age of consent & homosexuality legislation: All anal & oral sex is
 illegal in this state.
Legal drinking age: 21

Claymont

Organizations: Polyfidelity

⊙■ **Tender Loving Couples**
P. O. Box 322, Claymont, Delaware 19703.

Newark

Organizations: Motorcycle

⚥▽ **Giffins MC**
P. O. Box 7566, Newark, Delaware 19714-7566.

Organizations: Sexuality: Student

☼▽ **Lesbian, Gay, & Bisexual Student Union**
 ♿ Room 201, Student Center, University of Delaware, Newark, Delaware 19716.
 ☎ 302 451 8066

Rehoboth Beach

Organizations: AIDS: Education

☺☐ **Sussex County AIDS Committee**
 c/o D. L. G. H. A., P. O. Box 712, Rehoboth Beach, Delaware 19971.
 ☎ 302 945 3205

Stores: Books: General

☼▼ **Lambda Rising**
 ♿ 39 Baltimore Avenue, Rehoboth Beach, Delaware 19971.
 ☎ 302 227 6969
 ✉ lambdarising@his.com
 🕐 10:00 - 24:00
 Source for every gay, lesbian, bisexual, & transgender book in print (plus thousands out of print) Also videos, music, & gifts.

Willmington

Counsellors

☺▼ **Mary Anne McClemens, M.A., LPCMH**
 ♿ 1804 Millers Road, Arden, Delaware 19810.
 ☎ 302 475 3359

Wilmington

Counsellors

☺■ **David Mozes, Ph.D.**
 Suite 12C, Trolley Square, Wilmington, Delaware 19806.
 ☎ 302 658 3067

☼▼ **Susan Wellington, MC**
 ♿ 908 North Adams Street, Wilmington, Delaware 19801.
 ☎ 302 658 8808

Health Services

☺▽ **Delaware Lesbian & Gay Health Advocates**
 ♿ Suite 5, 601 Delaware Avenue, Wilmington, Delaware 19801-1452.
 ☎ 800 292 0429 (in Delaware only)
 ☎ 302 652 6776
 Free, confidential information, counselling, & HIV/STD testing. Publishes *Working For Health*.

☺☐ **Medical Center of Delaware**
 501 West 14th. street, Wilmington, Delaware 19801.
 ☎ 302 733 1000

Organizations: Sexuality

▽▽ **Renaissance Education Association, Inc.— Delaware**
 P. O. Box 5656, Wilmington, Delaware 19808.
 ☎ 302 995 1396
 ✉ derenais@aol.com
 🕐 Meets 2nd. Sat of month 20:00
 Publishes a newsletter.

Stores: Erotica: General

☺■ **The Smoke Shop**
 ♿ CMS Building, Delaware Avenue, Wilmington, Delaware 19806.
 ☎ 302 655 2861

DISTRICT OF COLUMBIA

Area: Approximately 158 square kilometres
Population: Approximately 610,000
Capital City: Washington
Time zone: GMT minus 5 hours (EST)
Climate: Hot & humid summers. Spring & Autumn have warm days & cool nights. Winters can be cold, with snowstorm activity.
Age of consent & homosexuality legislation: All anal & oral sex is illegal in this state.
Legal drinking age: 21

State Resources

Helplines: Sexuality

☼▽ **Gay & Lesbian Hotline**
 c/o Whitman-Walker Clinic, 1407 S Street North West, Washington, District of Columbia 20009.
 ☎ 202 833 3234
 ☎ 202 332 2192 (Spanish)
 🕐 19:00 - 23:00, Spanish Thu only

Washington

Bars: BDSM

☼▼ **Badlands**
 1415 22nd. Street North West, Washington, District of Columbia 20037.
 ☎ 202 296 0505

☼▼ **Fraternity House**
 2123 Twining Court North West, Washington, District of Columbia 20037.
 ☎ 202 223 4917

Counsellors

☺▼ **Dickinson, Pentz, McCall, Associates**
 Suite 320, 1050 17th. Street North West, Washington, District of Columbia 20036.
 ☎ 202 728 1166

☼▼ **Mindy Jacobs, Ph.D.**
 ♿ Suite C2, 201 Massachusetts Avenue, Washington, District of Columbia 20002.
 ☎ 202 543 0303

☺■ **Joyce Malkin, LCSW-C, LICSW**
 4025 Connecticut Avenue North West, Washington, District of Columbia 20008.
 ☎ 202 363 8119

☼▼ **Philip Silverman, Ph.D.**
 ♿ 3 Washington Circle North West, Washington, District of Columbia 20037.
 ☎ 202 822 0078

☼▽ **Whitman-Walker Clinic**
 ♿ 1407 S Street North West, Washington, District of Columbia 20009.
 ☎ 202 797 3500

Health Services

☺☐ **District of Columbia General Hospital**
 19th. Street & Massachusetts Avenue, Washington, District of Columbia 20003.
 ☎ 202 675 5000
 HIV & emergency departments.

☺☐ **Georgetown University Hospital**
 3800 Reservoir Road North West, Washington, District of Columbia 20007.
 ☎ 202 784 3000
 HIV & emergency departments.

☺☐ **Providence Hospital**
 1150 Varnum Street, Washington, District of Columbia 20017.
 ☎ 202 269 7000
 HIV & emergency departments.

☺☐ **Veterans' Affairs Medical Center**
 50 Irving Street, Washington, District of Columbia 20422.
 ☎ 202 745 8000
 HIV & emergency departments.

Helplines: Sexuality

☼ **Sexual Minority Youth Assistance League**
 Lesbian & Gay Youth Helpline, 3rd. Floor, 333 1/2 Pennsylvania Avenue South East, Washington, District of Columbia 20003-1148.
 ☎ 202 546 5911

Organizations: Academic: Psychiatry

☺ **The American Psychiatric Association**
 1400 K Street, North West, Washington, District of Columbia 20005.

☺☐ **The American Psychological Association**
 Committee on Gay & Lesbian Concerns, 1200 17th. Street North West, Washington, District of Columbia 20036.
 ☎ 202 955 7600

☼ **Society for the Psychological Study of Lesbian & Gay Issues**
 750 1st. Street North East, Washington, District of Columbia 20002-4242.
 ☎ 202 366 6037
 Publishes a newsletter 3 times a year.

Organizations: AIDS: Education

☺ **AIDS Action Council**
 Suite 700, 1875 Connecticut Avenue , Washington, District of Columbia 20009-5728.
 ☎ 202 293 2886
 Publishes *AIDS Action Update*.

☺ **Panos Institute**
 Suite 301, 1717 Massachusetts Avenue North West, Washington, District of Columbia 20036-3001.
 ☎ 202 483 0044 ✆ 202 383 3059

Publishes *WorldAIDS*.

Organizations: AIDS: Information

☺▽ **AIDS Resource Center**
1337 14th. Street, Washington, District of Columbia 20005.
☎ 202 667 0045
Publishes *AIDS Resource Center News*.

Organizations: AIDS: Education

☺ **Carl Vogel Foundation, Inc.**
3rd. Floor, 1413 K Street North West, Washington, District of Columbia
20005.
☎ 202 289 4898 ✆ 202 789 2599

☺ **National Minority AIDS Council**
Suite 400, 300 I Street North East, Washington, District of Columbia
20002-4389.
☎ 202 544 1076 ✆ 202 544 0378

☺ **U.S. Conference of Mayors**
1620 Eye Street North West, Washington, District of Columbia 20006.
☎ 202 293 7330
Publishes *Local AIDS/HIV Services: National Directory*.

Organizations: BDSM

☺☐ **A.S.B. Munch—Washington, D. C.**
✉ ms_mocha@access.digex.net
🕐 Meets 1st. Thu of month 20:00
Contact: Ms. Mocha

♂▽ **Defenders—Washington, D.C.**
P. O. Box 33098, Washington, District of Columbia 22033.
☎ 202 387 4516

♂▽ **GFMC/DC**
c/o DC Eagle, 639 New York North West, Washington, District of
Columbia 20001.

♂ **SigMa**
P.O. Box 11050, Washington, District of Columbia 20008.
☎ 202 728 7589

Organizations: Family

♂▽ **Gay & Lesbian Parents Coalition International
(GLPCI)—Washington, D. C.**
P. O. Box 50360, Washington, District of Columbia 20091.
☎ 202 583 8029 ✆ 201 783 6204
☎ 201 783 6204 (Network)
✉ GLCPINat@ix.netcom.com
Send mail for network to: 538 Park Street, Montclair, New Jersey
07043. Publishes *Network*.

♂▽ **Gay Fathers—Washington, D. C.**
P. O. Box 19891, Washington, District of Columbia 20036-0891.
☎ 301 9900 0638

☺☐ **Parents & Friends of Lesbians & Gays (PFLAG)—
⊕ Washington Metropolitan Area**
Suite 700, 1012 14th. Street North West, Washington, District of
Columbia 20005.
☎ 301 439 3524

Organizations: Fetish: Uniforms

♂▽ **The American Uniform Association (AUA)—Mid-
Atlantic Corps**
P. O. Box 3783, Georgetown Station, Washington, District of Columbia
20007.

Organizations: Fetish: Foreskin

♂▽ **Glans Naked & Unashamed (GNU)**
P. O. Box 6133, Franklin Station, Washington, District of Columbia
20044.

Organizations: Fisting

♂ **FFA/CAC**
P.O. Box 461, Washington, District of Columbia 20044.

Organizations: Library

☺■ **The Library Corporation**
P. O. Box 40035, Washington, District of Columbia 20016.
☎ 800 624 0559 ✆ 202 229 0295
☎ 202 229 0100

☺ **The Library of Congress**
☎ 202 707 6372
☎ 202 707 9790
Contact: Ms. Linda Young

☺ **Registrar of Copyrights**
The Library of Congress, Washington, District of Columbia 20540.

☎ 202 707 6372
☎ 202 707 3000

Organizations: Masturbation

♂▽ **J/O Enthusiasts**
☎ 202 452 5906

Organizations: Motorcycle

♂ **Centaur MC**
P.O. Box 34193, Washington, District of Columbia 20043-4193.
☎ 703 461 0967
☎ 717 236 9271

♂ **Highwaymen TNT**
P. O. Box 545, Washington, District of Columbia 20044.

♂▽ **Potomac MC**
P. O. Box 73266, Washington, District of Columbia 20056.

Organizations: Sexual Politics

♂ **Gay & Lesbian Americans**
P. O. Box 77533, Washington, District of Columbia 20013-7533.
☎ 202 889 5111

♂ **National Gay & Lesbian Task Force**
1734 14th. Street North West, Washington, District of Columbia 20009.
☎ 202 332 6483
Publishes *Task Force Report*.

⊕ **National Organization for Women, Inc.**
Suite 700, 1000 16th. Street North West, Washington, District of
Columbia 20036-5705.
☎ 202 331 0066
Publishes *National NOW Times*.

Organizations: Sexuality

♂▽ **Bi-Ways**
⚥ P. O. Box 959, Washington, District of Columbia 90044.

♂▽ **BiCentrist Alliance**
P. O. Box 2254, Washington, District of Columbia 20013-2254.
Publishes *Bi Centrist*. Yearly subscription is $7.

☺▽ **National Coming Out Day**
P. O. Box 34640, Washington, District of Columbia 20043-4640.
☎ 800 866 6263 ✆ 202 347 5323
☎ 202 628 4160
🕐 Mon -Fri 09:30 - 18:30. 24hr. voice mail
Contact: Ms. Deborah Massa
Coordinates NCOD & is clearing house of coming out information.

♋▽ **Washington - Baltimore Alliance**
P. O. Box 50724, Washington, District of Columbia 20091-0724.
☎ 301 277 5475
🕐 Meets 3rd. Sat of month Sep - Jun, except Dec
Contact: Mr. R. Lewis

Organizations: Sexuality: Student

♂▽ **Duke GALA**
P. O. Box 19375, Washington, District of Columbia 20036-0375.

♂▽ **Georgetown Pride**
⚥ P. O. Box 2239, Hoya Station, Washington, District of Columbia 20057.
☎ 202 687 1592

♂ **National Gay & Lesbian Task Force Campus Project**
1734 14th. Street North West, Washington, District of Columbia 20009.
☎ 202 332 6483

♂▽ **Organization for Lesbian & Gay Student Rights
⚥ (OLGSR)**
UCW 200, The Catholic University of America, Washington, District of
Columbia 20064.
☎ 202 635 5291
☎ 202 332 3142

♂▽ **Yale GALA, DC**
⚥ P. O. Box 15094, Washington, District of Columbia 20003-0094.

Organizations: Sexuality: Youth

♂▽ **Sexual Minority Youth Assistance League**
3rd. Floor, 333 1/2 Pennsylvania Avenue South East, Washington,
District of Columbia 20003-1148.
☎ 202 546 5940
🕐 Mon - Fri 09:00 - 17:00 19:00 - 22:00. Drop-in Mon - Fri 18:00 -
20:00, Sun 15:00 - 18:00
For youth 14 - 21 years old. Publishes *SMYAL News*.

Piercers

☺■ **Perforations Piercing Studio**
900 M Street North West, Washington, District of Columbia.

☎ 202 289 8863
✉ perforat@access.digex.net
🌐 http://www.access.digex.net/~perforat/

Publishers: Guides: Sexuality

♂▽ **Gay & Lesbian Services Guide**
Training By Design, 25 16th. Street South East, Washington, District of Columbia 20003.
☎ 202 546 1549

Publishers: Magazines: Sexuality

♀▼ **Lambda Book Report**
♿ Lambda Rising, Inc., 1625 Connecticut Avenue North West, Washington, District of Columbia 20009-1013.
☎ 202 462 7924 📞 202 462 7257
✉ lambdarising@his.com
🕐 Mon - Thu 10:00 - 18:00
✓ VISA MC AMERICAN
Review of gay & lesbian literature. Reviews virtually every new lesbian & gay book. Also author interviews, & industry news. Published every two months. Yearly subscription is $19.95.

♀♂ **Youth Magazine**
P. O. Box 34215, Washington, District of Columbia 20043.
☎ 202 234 3562

Publishers: Newspapers: Sexuality

⊛ **off our backs**
2423 18th. Street North West, Washington, District of Columbia 20009.
☎ 202 234 8072
The oldest feminist newsjournal still published in the U. S.. 23 years of feminist philosophy & reporting, & still going strong. Published 11 times a year. Yearly subscription is $19.

♀♂ **Open Hands**
P. O. Box 23636, Washington, District of Columbia 20036.

♀♂ **The Washington Blade**
2nd. Floor, 1408 U Street North West, Washington, District of Columbia 20009-3916.
☎ 202 797 7000 📞 202 797 7040
News-oriented - national & Washington area news & features. Published every week. Yearly subscription is $30.

Stores: Books: General

☺▼ **Kramer Books & Afterwords**
♿ 1517 Connecticut Avenue, Washington, District of Columbia 20036.
☎ 202 387 1400

♀■ **Lambda Rising**
♿ 1625 Connecticut Avenue North West, Washington, District of Columbia 20009.
☎ 202 462 6969
☎ 800 621 6969 (for catalogue)
✉ lambdarising@his.com
🕐 10:00 - 24:00
🍷 ✓ VISA MC AMERICAN
Source for every gay, lesbian, bisexual, & transgender book in print (plus thousands out of print) Also videos, music, & gifts. Publishes Lambda Rising News quarterly. Yearly subscription is free.

☺■ **Luna Books**
♿ 2nd. Floor, 1633 P Street North West, Washington, District of Columbia 20036.
☎ 202 332 2543

☺■ **Vertigo Books**
♿ 1337 Connecticut Avenue, Washington, District of Columbia 20036.
☎ 202 429 9272

Stores: Clothing: Leather

☺■ **Felise Leather**
2nd/ Floor, 2613 P Street North West, Washington, District of Columbia.
☎ 202 342 7163
Custom leather clothing.

Stores: Erotica: BDSM

♂▼ **Leather Rack**
1723 Connecticut Avenue, Washington, District of Columbia 20009.
☎ 202 797 7401
🕐 10:00 - 23:00
Also rubber & other BDSM toys.

☺■ **Pleasure Place**
♿ 1710 Connecticut Avenue North West, Washington, District of Columbia 2009.
☎ 202 483 3297 📞 202 483 3297
☎ 800 386 2386 (catalogue & mailorder)
🕐 Mon Tue 10:00 - 22:00, Wed - Sat 10:00 - 24:00, Sun 12:00 - 19:00
🍷 ✓ ✈ VISA MC AMERICAN
Open for 16 years. Leather & latex clothes & toys, lingerie, stockings,

patent thigh-high boots, 6'' heels, engineer boots, etc.. Catalogue, $3. Age statement of 18 is required. Spanish also spoken.

☺ **Pleasure Place**
♿ 1063 Wisconsin Avenue, Washington, District of Columbia 20007.
☎ 202 333 8570 📞 202 333 3997
☎ 800 386 2386 (catalogue & mailorder)
🕐 Mon Tue 10:00 - 22:00, Wed - Sat 10:00 - 24:00, Sun 12:00 - 19:00
🍷 ✓ $ ✈ VISA MC AMERICAN
Open for 16 years. Leather & latex clothes & toys, lingerie, stockings, patent thigh-high boots, 6'' heels, engineer boots, etc.. Catalogue, $3. Age statement of 18 is required. Spanish also spoken.

FLORIDA

Area: Approximately 140,000 square kilometres
Population: Approximately 13,000,000
Capital City: Tallahassee
Time zone: GMT minus 5 hours (EST)
Climate: Florida has a subtropical climate popular with many people from both the U.S. and Canada. Summers are hot & stormy with an average temperature of approximately 27°C. Winters warm by comparison to other states, with an average January temperature of 12°-20°C.
Age of consent & homosexuality legislation: All anal & oral sex is illegal in this state.
Legal drinking age: 21

State Resources

Helplines: AIDS

☺ □ **Florida HIV/AIDS Hotline**
♿ P. O. Box 20169, Tallahassee, Florida 32316.
☎ 800 352 2437
☎ 800 545 7342 (Spanish)
Also 800 243 7101 in Creole.

Organizations: AIDS: Education

☺ □ **Community AIDS Network**
P. O. Box 795, Floral City, Florida 34436-0795.
☎ 904 647 6098

♀♂▽ **Sapphex Learn**
⊛ Suite 206, 14002 Clubhouse Circle, Tampa, Florida 33624.
☎ 813 961 6064 📞 813 961 6064
☎ 813 961 6064 (TDD)
Publishes Sexual Health Enlightenment.

Organizations: Polyfidelity

☺ □ **South Florida Polyamorists**
✉ ceres@gate.net

Organizations: Sexuality

✉□ **Montgomery Medical & Psychological Institute—**
♿ **Florida**
P. O. Box 141133, Gainesville, Florida 32614.
☎ 904 462 4826
🕐 Meets 2nd. & 4th. Fri of month
Publishes Insight quarterly.

Publishers: Newspapers: Sexuality

☺▼ **Community News**
Queer Press, Inc., P. O. Box 14682, Tallahassee, Florida 32317-4682.
☎ 904 671 7982
✉ CommNews@aol.com
🍷 ✓
Florida's largest regional lesbian, gay, bisexual, & trandgendered newspaper. Distributed in 14 cities in Florida, Georgia, & Alabama.

♀♂▽ **Mama Raga**
♿ P. O. Box 1002, Gainesville, Florida 32602.

♀♂▼ **The Weekly News**
901 North East 79th. Street, Miami, Florida 33138.
☎ 305 757 6333 📞 305 756 6488
Gay & lesbian newspaper for south Florida, north Palm Beach, Fort Lauderdale, Miami, & Key West. Published every week. Yearly subscription is $78.

Aventura
Counsellors

✉▼ **Center for Contemporary Counseling**
Suite 607, 299 North East 191 Street, Aventura, Florida 33180.
☎ 305 936 8000

Boca Raton
Organizations: Sexuality

✉■ **Gender Congruity Center**
Suite 404, 9960 Center Park Boulevard South, Boca Raton, Florida 33428.

Organizations: Sexuality

☎ 800 328 2633

Bradenton
Stores: Clothing: Leather
☺ ■ **King's Leathers**
Booths 303 & 304, Red Barn Flea Market, Bradenton, Florida.
☎ 813 751 2167

Brandon
Publishers: Newspapers: Sexuality
♂▼ *Gazette*
P. O. Box 2650, Brandon, Florida 33509-2650.
☎ 813 7566 ✆ 813 654 6995
Florida's gay & lesbian news. No sexually explicit material or adverising. Published every month. Yearly subscription is $21.

Cape Coral
Manufacturers: Piercing Jewelry
☺ ■ **Toucan Productions**
5252 Willow Court, Cape Coral, Florida 33904.
☎ 813 945 3007
Gold body jewelry. Wholesale enquiries welcome.

Clearwater
Publishers: Magazines: BDSM
⚥ *Dominant & Submissive Pleasure*
The Society of O, P. O. Box 4251, Clearwater, Florida 34618.
Published every two months. Yearly subscription is $25. Age statement of 21 is required.
Stores: Erotica: BDSM
♂▽ **Cobra Custom Leather Shop**
Unit 73, 4745 126th. Avenue North, Clearwater, Florida 34622.
☎ 813 553 8884

Coral Springs
Counsellors
▧■ **A Clinical Approach Counseling Center, Inc.**
☎ 305 345 2292
Clinical psychology & counselling.

Crystal Springs
Manufacturers: Piercing Jewelry
☺ ■ **Silver Anchor Enterprises**
P.O. Box 760, Crystal Springs, Florida 33524-0760.
☎ 800 848 7464 (800 Tit Ring) ✆ 813 782 0180
☎ 813 788 0147
⏰ Mon - Fri 09:00 - 17:00
Also mail order. Catalogue, $4. Age statement of 21 is required.

Daytona
Organizations: AIDS: Education
♂▽ **Outreach of Daytona Beach**
1722 North Ridgewood Avenue, Holly Hill, Florida 32117.
☎ 904 672 6069
Publishes *Positive + People*.

Fort Lauderdale
Archives: Sexuality
♂▽ **Stonewall Library & Archives**
330 South West 27th. Street, Fort Lauderdale, Florida 33315.
☎ 954 522 2317
⏰ Sat Sun 10:00 - 12:00
Library & archive of lesbian & gay literature with an emphasis on Florida's gay community. Spanish also spoken.
Bars: BDSM
♂▼ **The Eagle**
1951 Power Line Road, Fort Lauderdale, Florida 33311.
☎ 305 462 6380
♂▼ **The Stud**
1000 West State Road 84, Fort Lauderdale, Florida 33315.
☎ 305 525 7883
⏰ Mon - Fri 16:00 - 02:00, Sat - 03:00, Sun 12:00 - 02:00
BBSs: BDSM
☺ ■ **Underground**
✆ 305 791 3272

U.S.A.

Counsellors
☺▼ **Center For Identity Development South, Ltd.**
4400 West Sample Road, Pompano Beach, Florida 33073.
☎ 305 345 5525
Health Services
☺ □ **Broward General Medical Center**
1600 South Andrews Avenue, Fort Lauderdale, Florida 33316.
☎ 305 355 5610
☺ □ **Florida Medical Center**
5000 West Oakland Park Boulevard, Fort Lauderdale, Florida 33313.
☎ 305 735 6000
HIV & emergency departments.
☺ □ **Imperial Point Medical Center**
6401 North Federal Highway, Fort Lauderdale, Florida 33308.
☎ 305 776 8500
HIV & emergency departments.
☺ □ **STD Clinic**
3698 North West 15th. Street, Fort Lauderdale, Florida 33311.
☎ 305 797 6900
Organizations: AIDS: Education
☺ □ **PWA Coalition—Broward County**
2294 Wilton Drive, Fort Lauderdale, Florida 3305.
☎ 3305 565 9119
Publishes *Coalition Newsline*.
Organizations: AIDS: Support
☺ □ **Center One**
Suite 111, 3015 North Ocean Boulevard, Fort Lauderdale, Florida 33308-7300.
☎ 305 537 4111
Organizations: BDSM
☺ □ **Black Orchid**
P. O. Box 451592, Sunrise, Florida 33345.
✆ 954 437 5176
♂ **FFA - FGC**
P.O. Box 500, Fort Lauderdale, Florida 33302.
☎ 305 761 3961
☎ 305 523 7727
Fisting organization.
☺ □ **The National Leather Association (NLA)—Florida**
P.O. Box 4911, Fort Lauderdale, Florida 33338-1911.
Organizations: Bears
♂▽ **Gold Coast Bears**
c/o W. Willis, 1949 South West Riverside Drive, Fort Lauderdale, Florida 33312.
☎ 305 463 7923
Organizations: Body Size
♂▽ **Girth & Mirth—Florida**
P. O. Box 21022, Fort Lauderdale, Florida 33335.
☎ 305 791 9794
Publishes *Sunshine State Girth & Mirth of Florida*.
Organizations: Motorcycle
♂▽ **Trident—Fort Lauderdale**
Suite 1, 1122 North East 16th. Terrace, Fort Lauderdale, Florida 33304-2321.
Organizations: Sexuality
♂▽ **Gay & Lesbian Community Center**
P. O. Box 4567, Fort Lauderdale, Florida 33338.
☎ 305 763 1530
Publishers: Guides: Sexuality
♂▼ *Hots Spots*
5100 North East 12th. Avenue, Fort Lauderdale, Florida 33334.
☎ 305 928 1862 ✆ 305 772 0142
⏰ Mon - Thu 09:00 - 17:00
Weekly magazine in full colour. We are an entertainment guide to Florida. Published every week. Yearly subscription is $130.
Publishers: Newspapers: Sexuality
🖊 *The Fountain*
Suite 520, 10097 Clearly Boulevard, Plantation, Florida 33324.
♂ *Out Pages*
Suite 528, 1323 South East 17th. Street, Fort Lauderdale, Florida 33316.
☎ 305 524 0547
♂ *Scoop*

Suite 381, 1126 South Federal Highway, Fort Lauderdale, Florida 33326.
☎ 305 764 2323

Radio: Sexuality

☿▽ **Queer Talk**
WFTL Radio, 2100 North West Avenue, Fort Lauderdale, Florida 33311-3426.
☎ 800 874 3454
☎ 305 733 1400

Stores: Books: General

☺ ■ **Broward Adult Books**
⅍ 3419 West Broward Boulevard, Fort Lauderdale, Florida 33312.
☎ 305 792 4991

Stores: Erotica: BDSM

☺ ■ **Fallen Angel**
Store 98 Coral Center, 3045 North Federal Highway, Fort Lauderdale, Florida 33301.
Catalogue, $4.

☺ **Leather Underground, Inc.**
1170 North East 34th. Court, Fort Lauderdale, Florida 33334.
☎ 305 561 3977 ✆ 305 561 4204
⏰ Mon - Sat 09:00 - 18:00
⚙ $ ⚊ 🖅 💳 📠
Also mail order. Catalogue, $20. Age statement of 21 is required.

☺▽ **Trader Tom's Fantasy Depot**
♿ 914 Federal Highway, Fort Lauderdale, Florida 33304.
☎ 305 524 4759

Stores: Erotica: General

☿▼ **Catalog X**
850 North East 13th. Street, Fort Lauderdale, Florida 33304.
☎ 954 524 5050 ✆ 954 524 3288
⏰ Mon - Fri 08:00 - 20:00, Sat Sun 12:00 - 17:00
⚙ ✓ 🖅 💳
Largest gay & lesbian retail outlet of its kind in the U.S.. Also largest gay & lesbian erotic mail order company in the U.S.. Catalogue, $3. Age statement of 18 is required. Spanish & Portugese also spoken.

☺ ■ **Clark's Out of Town News**
♿ 303 South Andrews Avenue, Fort Lauderdale, Florida 33301.
☎ 305 467 1543
⏰ Mon - Fri 08:00 - 20:00, Sat Sun - 19:00

☺ **EJB Enterprises**
Chains, 3370 North East 17th. Avenue, Fort Lauderdale, Florida 33334-5314.
☎ 305 563 9476

☺ ▼ **News - Books - Cards**
⅍ 7126 North University Drive, Tamara, Florida 33321.
☎ 305 726 5544
⏰ Mon - Sat 09:00 - 18:30

☺ ■ **Omni Adult Bookstore**
3224 West Broward Boulevard, Fort Lauderdale, Florida 33312.
☎ 305 584 6825

☺ ■ **Pink Pussycat Boutique**
921 Sunrise Lane, Fort Lauderdale, Florida 33304.
☎ 305 563 4445

Fort Myers

BBSs: General

☺ ■ **The Beach Board**
P. O. Box 181, Fort Myers, Florida 33902.
☎ 813 278 2893 ✆ 813 337 7470
✆ 813 337 4950. 14400 baud maximum.

Health Services

☺ □ **Comprehensive Clinic**
♿ 2231B McGregor Boulevard, Fort Myers, Florida 33901.
☎ 813 334 1448

☺ □ **Lee Memorial Hospital**
2776 Cleveland Avenue, Fort Myers, Florida 33901.
☎ 813 332 1111
HIV & emergency departments.

Piercers

☺ ■ **Leather Tiger**
1412 Bay View Court, Fort Myers, Florida 33901.
☎ 813 334 4084
⏰ Tue - Sun 12:00 - 17:00, 20:00 - 24:00

Publishers: Newspapers: Sexuality

☿ **Support Line**

P. O. Box 546, Fort Myers, Florida 33902.
☎ 813 332 2272
Local newsletter with local information, happenings. Published 10 times a year. Yearly subscription is $10.

Stores: Erotica: General

☺ ■ **Tender Moments / The Other You**
♿ 4635-3 Coronado Parkway, Fort Myers, Florida 33904.
☎ 813 945 1448
⏰ Mon - Fri 10:00 - 18:00, Sat - 16:00

Fort Pierce

Piercers

☺ ■ **Tattoo World**
3550 South Federal Highway, Fort Pierce, Florida 34982.
☎ 407 465 6255

Gainesville

Health Services

☺ □ **Alachua General Hospital**
801 South West Second Avenue, Gainesville, Florida 32601.
☎ 904 372 4321
HIV & emergency departments.

☺ ■ **North Florida Regional Medical Center**
6500 Newberry Road, Gainesville, Florida 32605.
☎ 904 333 4000
HIV & emergency departments.

☺ □ **Shand Hospital at the University of Florida**
1600 South West Archer Road, Gainesville, Florida 32610.
☎ 904 395 0111
HIV & emergency departments.

Helplines: Sexuality

☿▽ **Gay Switchboard**
P. O. Box 12002, Gainesville, Florida 32604-0002.
☎ 904 332 0700
⏰ 18:00 - 23:00, answering system at other times

Organizations: Family

☺ □ **Parents & Friends of Lesbians & Gays (PFLAG)— Gainesville**
P. O. Box 12971, Gainesville, Florida 32604-0971.
☎ 904 377 8131

Organizations: Sexuality: Student

☿▽ **Lesbian, Gay, & Bisexual Student Union of the**
♿ **University of Florida**
P. O. Box 118505, Gainesville, Florida 32611-8505.
☎ 904 332 0700

Organizations: Sexuality: Youth

☿▽ **Gay, Lesbian, & Bisexual Teens**
P. O. Box 12971, Gainesville, Florida 32604-0971.
☎ 904 338 3593

Stores: Books: General

☺ ▼ **Goerings' Book Center**
♿ 1310 West University Avenue, Gainesville, Florida 32603.
☎ 800 726 1487
⏰ Mon - Sat 10:00 - 21:00, Sun - 17:00

♠ ▼ **Iris Books**
♿ 802 West University Avenue, Gainesville, Florida 32601.
☎ 904 375 7477

Stores: Clothing: Lingerie

☺ ■ **French Addiction**
819 West University Avenue, Gainesville, Florida 32601.
☎ 904 373 6628
Catalogue available.

Hernando

Organizations: AIDS: Support

☺ □ **AIDS Network**
P. O. Box 232, Hernando, Florida 34443-0232.

Hollywood

Organizations: Motorcycle

☿▽ **Saber MC**
P.O. Box 14441, Hollywood, Florida 33302.

☿ **Sunrays MC**
2027 Mayo Street, Hollywood, Florida 33020.

Organizations: Sexuality

☆▽ **Serenity**
P. O. Box 307, Hollywood, Florida 33022.
☎ 305 436 9477
🕐 Meets 3rd. Fri of month
Publishes a newsletter.

Publishers: Magazines: BDSM

☺ **Raging Rhino Productions**
P. O. Box 618, Hollywood, Florida 33022.
Publishes BDSM comics.

Jacksonville

Counsellors

☺ ■ **Judith Allison, M.Ed., MSH**
5645 Nettie Road, Jacksonville, Florida 32207.
☎ 904 733 3310

Health Services

☺ ☐ **Duval County Public Health Unit**
STD Clinic, Suite 14, 515 West 6th. Street, Jacksonville, Florida 32206.
☎ 904 633 3620

☺ ☐ **Main Street Clinic**
962 North Main Street, Jacksonville, Florida 32202.
☎ 904 358 3386

☺ ☐ **University Medical Center**
655 West Eighth Street, Jacksonville, Florida 32209.
☎ 904 549 5000
HIV & emergency departments.

Organizations: BDSM

♂▽ **Neue Regel**
6755 Newgate Circle East, Jacksonville, Florida 32244.

Organizations: Motorcycle

♂▽ **Brothers MC, Inc.**
1337 Hubbard Street, Jacksonville, Florida 32206.
☎ 904 353 9973
☎ 904 720 7923 (pager)
⚹ $ ✖ VISA ⦿ ⦿
Contact: Mr. Sherman Hester
Levi/leather club of men who like motorcycles & fun. We party hard, but safely. Hosts out-of-town clubs. Age statement of 21 is required.

Publishers: Books: Sexuality

☺ **Urania Books**
6858 Arthur Court, Jacksonville, Florida 32211.
☎ 904 744 7879

Publishers: Directories: Sexuality

♀▽ *Calendar of Events*
P. O. Box 43335, Jacksonville, Florida 32203.
☎ 904 573 1867
🕐 Irregular hours, answering machine when not in
⚹ ✓ $
Local newsletter informing our lesbian community of social events, politics, films, etc.. Also helps newcomers connect with the local community. Published every month. Yearly subscription is $10.

Key West

Health Services

☺ ☐ **Florida Keys Memorial Hospital**
5900 College Road, Key West, Florida 33040.
☎ 305 294 5531
HIV & emergency departments.

Organizations: BDSM

♂▽ **Key West Wreckers LLC**
P. O. Box 4723, Key West, Florida 33041.
☎ 305 296 3338

Stores: Books: General

☺ ■ **Bargain Books & News Stand**
♿ 1028 Truman Avenue, Key West, Florida 33040.
☎ 305 294 7446
🕐 07:00 - 18:00

☺ ■ **Blue Heron Books**
538 Truman Avenue, Key West, Florida 33040.
☎ 305 296 3508
🕐 Mon - Sat 10:00 - 22:00, Sun - 21:00

♂▼ **A Bookstore Named Desire**
♿ 420 Applerouth Lane, Key West, Florida 33040.
☎ 305 296 1000

☺▼ **Caroline Street Books**
♿ Suite 5, 800 Caroline Street, Key West, Florida 33040.
☎ 305 24 3931

☺ ■ **Key West Island Bookstore**
513 Fleming Street, Key West, Florida 33040.
☎ 305 294 2904

Stores: Erotica: BDSM

☺▼ **Leather Master**
418-A Appelrouth Lane, Key West, Florida 33040.
☎ 305 292 5051
🕐 Mon Tue Thu - Sat 12:00 - 24:00, Wed Sun 12:00 - 18:00
♿ VISA ⦿
Also mail order.

Stores: Erotica: General

☺ ■ **Alligator News & Books**
716 Duval Street, Key West, Florida 33040-7453.
☎ 305 294 4004

Lakeland

Organizations: Fetish: Foot

♂▽ **Foot Guys**
P. O. Box 92931, Lakeland, Florida 33804-2831.

Organizations: Sexuality

♂▽ **Polk Gay & Lesbian Alliance**
♿ P. O. Box 8221, Lakeland, Florida 33802-8221.
☎ 813 644 0085
Publishes *PGLA News*.

Land 'O Lakes

Organizations: BDSM

☺ ☐ **Lifestyle Explorers Club**
P. O. Box 1606, Land 'O Lakes, Florida 34639.

Largo

Organizations: Bondage

♂▽ **Tampa Bay Bondage Club**
P. O. Box 320831, Largo, Florida 33679-2831.
☎ 813 832 2999

Lithis

Organizations: Sexuality

☆▽ **Starburst**
P. O. Box 298, Lithis, Florida 22547-0298.
☎ 813 633 9653
🌐 http://users.aol.com/ashleyar/html/starbrst.html
Publishes *Butterflies*.

Lutz

Organizations: BDSM

♂▽ **Defenders—Tampa Bay**
c/o Dignity, P. O. Box 201, Lutz, Florida 33549.
☎ 813 996 4738

Margate

Publishers: Magazines: BDSM

☺ *Chainmail*
P. O. Box 634945, Margate, Florida 33063.
☎ 305 741 5458

Publishers: Magazines: Sexuality

☺ *The Enamored Writer*
P. O. Box 634945, Margate, Florida 33063.
☎ 305 741 5458

Miami

Artists: Erotic

☺ **Richard Smith**
Suite 692, 6912 North West 72nd. Avenue, Miami, Florida 33166-3036.
☎ 809 541 4500
✉ rsmith@tricom.net
Age statement of 21 is required. Spanish also spoken.

Counsellors

♂▼ **Jorge Arocha, ACSW**
♿ Suite 103, 2000 South Dixie Drive, Miami, Florida 33133.
☎ 305 285 8900

Health Services

☺ □ **Jackson Memorial Hospital**
1611 North West 12th. Avenue, Miami, Florida 33136.
☎ 305 324 8111
HIV & emergency departments.

☺ □ **Mercy Hospital**
3663 South Miami Avenue, Miami, Florida 33133.
☎ 305 854 4400
HIV & emergency departments.

☺ □ **Public Health Clinic**
⅖ 1350 North West 14th. Street, Miami, Florida 33125.
☎ 305 324 2434

☺ □ **South Miami Hospital**
6200 South West 73rd. Street, Miami, Florida 33143.
☎ 305 661 4611
HIV & emergency departments.

☺ □ **Veterans' Affairs Medical Center**
1201 North West 16th. Street, Miami, Florida 33125.
☎ 305 324 4455
HIV & emergency departments.

Helplines: AIDS

☺ □ **Health Crisis Network**
P. O. Box 370098, Miami, Florida 33137-0098.
☎ 800 442 5046 (in Florida)
☎ 305 324 5148 (non-English)
🕐 09:00 - 21:00
Also 305 634 4636 (English).

Helplines: Sexuality

♂♀▽ **Gay, Lesbian, & Bisexual Community Hotline of
Greater Miami**
c/o Lambda Passages, 7545 Biscayne Boulevard, Miami, Florida 33138.
☎ 305 759 3661
🕐 24hr. touch-tone operated answering machine

♂♀▽ **Switchboard of Miami, Inc.**
⅖ 75 South West 8th. Street, Miami, Florida 33130.
☎ 305 358 4357

Organizations: AIDS: Education

☺ □ **Prevention, Education, & Treatment Center (PET)**
⅖ 615 Collins Avenue, Miami Beach, Florida 33139.
☎ 305 538 0525
🕐 Mon - Fri 08:00 - 17:00

Organizations: AIDS: Research

☺ □ **Community Research Initiative of South Florida**
⅗ Suite 200, 1508 San Agnacio Avenue, Miami, Florida 33146-2007.
☎ 305 667 9296 📞 305 667 8686
Publishes *CRI Quarterly* quarterly.

Organizations: AIDS: Support

☺ ▽ **Body Positive Resource Center**
⅖ 187 North East 36th. Street, Miami, Florida 33157.
☎ 305 576 1111
🕐 Mon - Fri 12:00 - 22:00, Sat 13:00 - 16:00
Publishes *Talking Positive.*

☺ □ **PWA Coalition of Dade County**
⅖ 3890 Biscayne Boulevard, Miami, Florida 33137-3731.
☎ 305 576 1111
Publishes *PWAC Monthly Newsletter* every month.

Organizations: BDSM

♂♀▽ **Suncoast Leather Club**
P. O. Box 2772, Coconut Grove, Florida 33731.

Organizations: Body Size

♂♀▽ **XXXLNT**
⅖ P. O. Box 16686, Miami, Florida 33101-6686.
Publishes *XXXLNT.*

Organizations: Sexuality

♀▽ **Animas**
P. O. Box 420309, Miami, Florida 33142.

♂♀▽ **Black & White Men Together (BWMT)—**
⅖ **Tallahassee**
P. O. Box 016686, Miami, Florida 33101-6686.
☎ 800 624 2968 (national line)

♂♀▽ **GLBC, University of Miami**
⅖ c/o Volunteer Services, P. O. Box 249116, Coral Gables, Florida 33124.
☎ 305 284 4483

♂♀▽ **The Lesbian, Gay, & Bisexual Community Center**

⅖ P. O. Box 1717, Miami Beach, Florida 33199-1717.
☎ 305 531 3666

Publishers: Magazines: Sexuality

♀♀ *The Informher*
Friday Night Womyn's Group, P. O. Box 570-132, Miami, Florida 33257.
☎ 305 253 3740
Published every month. Yearly subscription is $12.

Publishers: Newspapers: Sexuality

♂♀ *Planet Homo*
Suite 349, 1521 Alton Road, Miami Beach, Florida 33139.
☎ 305 672 4666

Stores: Books: General

☺ ■ **Book Depot**
1638 Euclid Avenue, Miami, Florida 33139.
☎ 800 438 2750 📞 305 538 7901
☎ 305 538 9666
🕐 11:00 - 19:00

♂♀▽ **GW Miami Beach**
⅖ 718 Lincoln Road Mall, Miami Beach, Florida 33139.
☎ 305 534 4763

♂♀▽ **Lambda Passages**
⅖ 7545 Biscayne Boulevard, Miami, Florida 33138.
☎ 305 754 6900
🕐 Mon - Sat 11:00 - 21:00, Sun 12:00 - 18:00

☺ ■ **Westchester News**
8659 Coral Way, Miami, Florida 33155.
☎ 305 264 6210

Stores: Erotica: General

☺ ■ **Pink Pussycat Boutique**
3419 Main Highway, Coconut Grove, Florida 33133.
☎ 305 448 7656

♂♀■ **Pleasure Chest**
Club Body Center, 2991 Coral Way, Miami, Florida 33133.
☎ 305 448 2214

☺ ■ **Trail Books**
7350 South West 8th. Street, Miami, Florida 33144.
☎ 305 262 4776

Miami Beach

Health Services

☺ □ **Mount Sinai Medical Center**
4300 Alton Road, Miami Beach, Florida 33140.
☎ 305 674 2121
HIV & emergency departments.

☺ □ **South Shore Hospital & Medical Center**
630 Alton Road, Miami Beach, Florida 33139.
☎ 305 672 2100
HIV & emergency departments.

Publishers: Magazines: Sexuality

♀♀▽ *conMOCióN*
Suite 336, 1521 Alton Road, Miami Beach, Florida 33139.
A latina lesbian magazine & information network.

Naples

Organizations: AIDS: Education

☺ □ **Collier AIDS Resource & Education Service, Inc.**
⅖ **(CARES)**
3080 Tamiami Trail North, Naples, Florida 33940-4151.
☎ 813 263 2273 📞 305 263 6751
Publishes a newsletter.

Organizations: Bears

♂♀▽ **Bears of Southwest Florida**
P. O. Box 7992, Naples, Florida 33941-7992.
📧 SWFLBear@aol.com
🌐 http://www.skepsis.com:80/.gblo/bears/CLUBS/sw_fl_bears.html

Printers: General

☺ **Whitehall Company**
4244 Corporate Square, Naples, Florida 33942-4753.
☎ 800 321 9290 📞 941 643 6439
☎ 941 643 6464

Stores: Books: General

☺ ■ **Book Nook**
824 5th. Avenue South, Naples, Florida 33940.
☎ 813 262 4740

⏰ Mon - Sat 08:30 - 18:00, Sun 08:00 - 14:30
⚥▼ **Lavender's**
 Suite 4, 5600 Trail Boulevard, Naples, Florida 33963.
 ☎ 941 594 9499
 ⏰ Tue - Fri 11:00 - 19:00, Sat 11:00 - 16:00
 ♿ ✓
 Also sidelines of pride items.

North Miami Beach
BBSs: BDSM
☺ ■ **The Fetish Network BBS**
 Dept. 600, Suite 4-166, 20533 Biscayne Boulevard, North Miami
 Beach, Florida 33180.
 ☎ 800 536 6462
 📞 954 370 7007. 28800 baud maximum.
 🖥 telnet:tfnbbs.com
 ⏰ Mon - Thu 12:00 - 20:00
 $ 💳 💳
 Owned & operated by lifestyle scene players, including world famous
 Goddess Dianna Vesta. TFN BBS offers full Internet access to on-line
 chat, World Link, newsgroups, & On-line Shopping Mall, which carries all
 their products. Special forums & interest groups that cater to female
 domination, BDSM, fantasy & fetish. Caters to a pan-sexual group
 covering all alternative topics. Yearly subscription is $20. Age statement
 of 18 is required. Please see our display advertisement.

Publishers: Magazines: BDSM
☺ ■ *Attitude*
 The Fetish Network, Dept. 600, Suite 4-166, 20533 Biscayne
 Boulevard, North Miami Beach, Florida 33180.
 ☎ 800 536 6462
 📞 954 370 7007. 28800 baud maximum.
 🖥 telnet:tfnbbs.com
 ⏰ Mon - Thu 12:00 - 20:00
 ✓ $ 💳 💳
 Published by Dianna Vesta, world famous lifestyle Mistress, & The Fetish
 Network. The staff consists of prominent Dominæ from around the
 world, offering special tribute to the dominant woman & those who
 adore Her. Contains lesbian themes, as well as DS couples who want to
 incorporate loving rôle-play into their relationship. Intelligent,
 informative, & REAL! Single issues are $14.50. Published every two
 months. Yearly subscription is $75U.S. (add 20% for overseas postage).
 Age statement of 18 is required. Please see our display advertisement.

Publishers: Magazines: Sexuality
☺ ■ *Eclectic Attitudes*
 The Fetish Network, Dept. 600, Suite 4-166, 20533 Biscayne
 Boulevard, North Miami Beach, Florida 33180.
 ☎ 800 536 6462
 📞 954 370 7007. 28800 baud maximum.
 🖥 telnet:tfnbbs.com
 ⏰ Mon - Thu 12:00 - 20:00
 ✓ $ 💳 💳
 Publisher of Attitude magazine & owners of The Fetish Network, Eclectic
 Attitudes is a perfect bound journal. "EA" provides an intelligent,
 realistic, & loving look into the world of sexual alternatives, BDSM,
 fantasy, fetish, rôleplay, & many other topics. $20.00 per issue (allow
 2 to 3 weeks). Published quarterly. Yearly subscription is $80U.S. (add
 20% for overseas postage). Age statement of 18 is required. Please see
 our display advertisement.

Training: BDSM
☺ ■ **Dianna Vesta**
 ☎ 800 433 8474
 Owner of The Fetish Network & world famous lifestyle mistress offers
 training, teaching, & consulting for couples wanting to explore BDSM,
 fantasy, & fetish. Located in south Florida, Goddess Vesta offers
 telephone consultations, live sessions, & workshops. Age statement of
 18 is required.

Ocala
Organizations: BDSM
☺ □ **A.S.B. Munch—Florida**
 📧 tymedwn1st@aol.com

Olaca
Organizations: Sexuality
⚥▽ **Alternate Lifestyle Alliance of Olaca**
 P. O. Box 71291, Olaca, Florida 32671.
 ☎ 904 624 3779

Orlando
Bars: BDSM
♂▼ **Full Moon Saloon**
 ♿ 500 North Orange Blossom Trail, Orlando, Florida 32805.

☎ 407 648 8725
⚥ **Orlando Eagle**
 3400 South Orange Blossom Trail, Orlando, Florida 32805.
 ☎ 407 843 6334

Competitions & Conventions: BDSM
⚥♀ ■ **Domination**
 P. O. Box 574977, Orlando, Florida 32857.
 ☎ 407 678 3388 ✆ 407 678 9553
 ♿ ✓ $
 Yearly event held in February. Age statement of 21 is required.

Health Services
☺ □ **Lucerne Medical Center**
 818 South Main Lane, Orlando, Florida 32801.
 ☎ 407 649 6111
☺ □ **Orlando Regional Medical Center**
 1414 Kuhl Avenue, Orlando, Florida 32806.
 ☎ 407 841 5111
☺ □ **Princeton Hospital**
 1800 Mercy Drive, Orlando, Florida 32808.
 ☎ 407 295 5151

Organizations: AIDS: Support
☺ □ **Fight For Life**
 1875 Boggy Creek Road, Kissimmee, Florida 33744.
 ☎ 407 932 4482

Organizations: BDSM
☺ □ **Domination**
 P. O. Box 574977, Orlando, Florida 32857.
 ☎ 407 678 3388 ✆ 407 678 9553
 ♿ ✓ $
 Yearly event held in February. Age statement of 21 is required.
☺ □ **People Exchanging Power—Central Florida**
 ☎ 407 678 3388 ✆ 407 678 9553
⚥▽ **Saint Crispin L/L Fraternity**
 ♿ 2346 Keystone Drive, Orlando, Florida 32806-4662.
 ☎ 407 843 5621
 Contact: Ollie

Organizations: Bears
⚥▽ **Bears of Central Florida**
 P. O. Box 647, Orlando, Florida 32802.
 ☎ 407 240 0814
⚥▽ **Florida Bear Hunters**
 5270 Lawndale Frive, West Orlando, Florida 32808-6129.

Organizations: Family
⚥▽ **Gay & Lesbian Parents Coalition International**
 ♿ **(GLPCI)—Florida**
 P. O. Box 561504, Orlando, Florida 32856-1504.
 ☎ 407 420 2191
☺ □ **Parents & Friends of Lesbians & Gays (PFLAG)—**
 ♿ **Orlando**
 P. O. Box 141321, Orlando, Florida 32814-1312.
 ☎ 407 896 0689
 ☎ 407 236 9177 (voice mail)

Organizations: Motorcycle
⚥▽ **Challengers International MC**
 ♿ P.O. Box 883, Orlando, Florida 32802-0883.
 ☎ 407 425 9836
⚥▼ **Conquistadors MC**
 P.O. Box 555591, Orlando, Florida 32855-5591.
 ☎ 407 423 1546
 ✓

Organizations: Sexuality
⚥▽ **Fantasia**
 c/o GLCS, P. O. Box 533446, Orlando, Florida 32853-3446.
 ☎ 407 425 4527
 ⏰ Meets twice a month

Piercers
☺ ■ **Leather Tiger**
 122 North Orange Avenue, Orlando, Florida 32801.
 ☎ 407 839 0710
 ⏰ Tue - Sun 12:00 - 17:00

Publishers: Newspapers: Sexuality
⚥ *The Triangle*
 P. O. Box 533446, Orlando, Florida 32853-3446.
 ☎ 407 425 4527

The main source of news & information for central Florida's lesbigay community. Published every month. Yearly subscription is $10.

☞ *A Friendly Voice*
Suite 21, 410 North Orange Blossom Trail, Orlando, Florida 32805.
☎ 407 872 2213
☎ 813 855 5108 (in Tampa)

Stores: Books: General

☺■ **Out & About Books**
⚢ 930 North Mills Avenue, Orlando, Florida 32803.
☎ 407 896 0204
⏰ Mon - Sat 11:00 - 20:00, Sun 13:00 - 18:00

Stores: Erotica: BDSM

☺▼ **Absolute Leather**
3400 South Orange Blossom Trail, Orlando, Florida 32809.
☎ 800 447 4820
☎ 407 843 8168

☞ **The Leather Closet**
498 Orange North Blossom Trail, Orlando, Florida 32805. ✆ 407 649 4116
☎ 407 649 2011
⏰ 12:00 - 03:00 everyday
🔥 ✓ $ ✈ VISA 💳 📷 🅳 💳 ℓ
Custom leatherwork, pride items, swimwear. Seamstresses on staff. Also mail order. Age statement of 21 is required.

Stores: Erotica: General

☺■ **The Original Bookstore**
Ꮶ 2203 South Orange Blossom Trail, Orlando, Florida 32805.
☎ 407 648 4546
⏰ Sun - Wed 08:00 - 02:30, Thu - Sat 24hrs

Tattooists

☺■ **Deana's Skin Art Studio**
Suite B, 14180 East Colonial Drive, Orlando, Florida 32826.
☎ 407 281 1228
⏰ 12:00 - 20:00
🔥 VISA 💳

Panama City

Organizations: AIDS: Education

☺□ **Bay Area Services & Information Coalition (BASIC)**
P. O. Box 805, Panama City, Florida 32402.
☎ 904 785 1088

Pensacola

Bars: BDSM

☞■ **Numbers Pub**
Ꮶ 200 South Alcaniz, Pensacola, Florida 32501.
☎ 904 438 9004
Some leather.

BBSs: BDSM

☺■ **Titan**
✆ 904 476 1270

Health Services

☺■ **West Florida Regional Medical Center**
8383 North Davis Highway, Pensacola, Florida 32523.
☎ 904 494 5000

Organizations: AIDS: Education

☺□ **AIDS/DTD Program**
⚢ P. O. Box 12604, Pensacola, Florida 32574-2604.
☎ 904 444 8654
⏰ Mon - Fri 08:00 - 17:00

Organizations: Family

☺□ **Parents & Friends of Lesbians & Gays (PFLAG)—Pensacola**
⚢
P. O. Box 34479, Pensacola, Florida 32507-4479.
Phone contacts & information send upon request.

Pompano Beach

Organizations: Sexuality

☜▽ **The Eden Society**
P. O. Box 1692, Pompano Beach, Florida 33061-1692.
☎ 305 784 9316
⏰ Meets 2nd. Sat of month
Publishes a newsletter.

Saint Petersburg

Counsellors

⊕■ **Sue Brewer, MSW, LCSW**
Ꮶ Suite 109, 1700 Park Street North, Saint Petersburg, Florida 33170.
☎ 813 347 3680

☜▼ **Judith Meisner, Ph.D., LCSW, LMFT**
Suite 209, 3530 First Avenue North, Saint Petersburg, Florida 33713.
☎ 813 327 1672
⏰ By appointment only

Health Services

☺□ **Bayfront Medical Center**
701 Sixth Street South, Saint Petersburg, Florida 33701.
☎ 813 823 1234

☺□ **Saint Anthony's Hospital**
1200 Seventh Avenue, Saint Petersburg, Florida 33705.
☎ 813 825 1100

Helplines: Sexuality

☞▽ **The Line**
P. O. Box 14323, Saint Petersburg, Florida 33733.
☎ 813 586 4297
⏰ 19:00 - 23:00, computer information system at other times

Organizations: BDSM

☞ **Adventurers - Sun Coast**
P.O. Box 8043, Saint Petersburg, Florida 33738.

Organizations: Sexuality

☜▽ **Enchanté**
1801 69th. Avenue South, Saint Petersburg, Florida 33712.
☎ 813 972 2617
☎ 813 866 0438
Contact: Mr. J. Hores
Publishes a newsletter.

Organizations: Wrestling

☞▽ **Tampa Bay Wrestling Club**
P. O. Box 21552, Saint Petersburg, Florida 33742-1552.

Publishers: Newspapers: Sexuality

☞ **Womyn's Words**
P. O. Box 15524, Saint Petersburg, Florida 33733.

Stores: Erotica: General

☺■ **Fourth Street Bookmart**
⚢ 1427 4th. Street South, Saint Petersburg, Florida 33704.
☎ 813 821 8824

Stores: Military Surplus

☺■ **The Army Navy Store**
6000 66th. Street, Saint Petersburg, Florida.
☎ 813 544 8004

☺■ **Hap's Militaria & Collectibles**
6620 4th. Street North, Saint Petersburg, Florida.
☎ 813 527 9532
⏰ Tue - Fri 10:00 - 17:00, Sat 12:00 - 17:00
Daggers, swords, helmets, medals, uniforms, patches, etc..

☺■ **Lormer Military Shop**
6643 49th. Street North, Saint Petersburg, Florida.
☎ 813 527 2721
Daggers, swords, helmets, medals, patches, etc..

Sarasota

Counsellors

☺■ **Carol Twitchell, Psy.D.**
⚢ Suite 222, 73 South Palm Avenue, Sarasota, Florida 34236.
☎ 941 365 9424
🔥
Second office at Suite 103, 401 Johnson Lane, Venice, Florida 34292.

Distributors: Books: General

☺ **Bookworld Services**
1933 Whitfield Loop, Sarasota, Florida 34243. ✆ 813 753 9396
☎ 813 758 8094

Health Services

☺□ **Sarasota Memorial Hospital**
1700 South Tamiami Trail, Sarasota, Florida 34239.
☎ 813 955 1111

Manufacturers: Erotica: Leather

☺■ **Shadowfax Leathercraft**

P. O. Box 10451, Sarasota, Florida 34278-0451.
☎ 941 371 5242
✉ MShadowfax@aol.com
🕐 Call eves.. By appointment only
🐾 ✓ $
Custom leatherwork: restraints, whips, specialty apparel, dungeon furnishings, theatrical props, & costuming. Creative design & conceptualization services. Original artwork by Charon. Catalogue, $10U.S.. Age statement of 18 is required.

Organizations: Sexuality
⚥▽ **Gay & Lesbian Alliance**
P. O. Box 15851, Sarasota, Florida 34277.

Stores: Books: General
☺ ■ **Read All Over**
2245 Bee Ridge Road, Sarasota, Florida 34239.
☎ 813 923 1340

Stores: Erotica: General
☺ ■ **Adult Pursuits**
5759 Beneva Road, Sarasota, Florida 34233.
☎ 813 923 2815
🕐 Mon - Sat 09:00 - 21:00
Also stocks leather & BDSM items.

☺ ■ **Adult Pursuits**
3480 17th. Street, Sarasota, Florida 34235.
☎ 813 366 3501
🕐 Mon - Sat 09:00 - 21:00
Also stocks leather & BDSM items.

South Beach
Publishers: Newspapers: Sexuality
☺ ■ *Wire*
1638 Euclid Avenue, South Beach, Florida 33139.

Sunrise
Artists: BDSM
☺ **Preston Graphics**
P. O. Box 451592, Sunrise, Florida 33345.

Tallahassee
Health Services
☺ □ **Leon County Health Department**
♿ VD Clinic, P. O. Box 2745, Tallahassee, Florida 32316.
☎ 904 487 3155

☺ □ **Tallahassee Memorial Regional Medical Center**
Miccosukee Road & Magnolia Drive, Tallahassee, Florida 32308.
☎ 904 681 1155

Organizations: Sexuality
⚥▽ **The Society for the Second Self (Tri-Ess)—Tau Lambda**
P. O. Box 3426, Tallahassee, Florida 32315-3426.

Organizations: Sexuality: Student
⚥▽ **Lesbian, Gay, & Bisexual Student Union**
♿ FSU Box 65914, Florida State University, Tallahassee, Florida 32313-5914.
☎ 904 644 8804

Printers: General
☺ **Rose Printing**
P.O. Box 5078, Tallahassee, Florida 32314-5078.
☎ 904 576 4151 ✆ 904 576 4153

Publishers: Miscellaneous
⚥ **Naiad Press, Inc.**
P. O. Box 10543, Tallahassee, Florida 32302.
☎ 904 539 5965

Stores: Books: General
☺▼ **Rubyfruit Books**
♿ 666-4 West Tennessee Street, Tallahassee, Florida 32304.
☎ 904 222 2627 ✆ 904 222 0411
🕐 Mon - Sat 10:30 - 18:30, Thu - 20:00, Sun 12:00 - 17:00
🐾 ✓ $ 💳 MC
Also carries music & pride items, & rent videos. Get community resource information here! Also mail order.

Tampa
Counsellors
☺▼ **Busch Counseling Center, Inc.**

AS 1404 West Busch Boulevard, Tampa, Florida 33612.
☎ 813 933 6904

☺ ■ **Counseling Services of Brandon**
uite G, 107 East Robertson, Brandon, Florida 33511.
☎ 813 654 0166

☺▼ **Chase McEwen, ACSW, LCSW**
♿ Suite A, 104 East Fowler Avenue, Tampa, Florida 33612.
☎ 813 932 9300

Health Services
☺ □ **Memorial Hospital of Tampa**
2901 Swann Avenue, Tampa, Florida 33609.
☎ 813 873 6400
HIV & emergency departments.

☺ □ **Saint Joseph's Hospital**
3001 Martin Luther King Boulevard, Tampa, Florida 33607.
☎ 813 870 4000
HIV & emergency departments.

☺ □ **Tampa General Healthcare**
Davis Islands, Tampa, Florida 33606.
☎ 813 251 7000
HIV & emergency departments.

Helplines: Sexuality
⚥▽ **Gay Hotline, Inc.**
♿ Suite 608, 1222 South Dale Mabry Highway, Tampa, Florida 33629.
☎ 813 229 8839

Manufacturers: Erotica: BDSM
☺ ■ **James Bondage**
7926 Woodvale Circle, Tampa, Florida 33616.

Organizations: AIDS: Support
☺ □ **PWA Coalition of Tampa Bay**
♿ P. O. Box 9731, Tampa, Florida 33674-9731.
☎ 813 238 2887

☺ □ **Tampa AIDS Network**
♿ 11215 North Nebraska Avenue, Tampa, Florida 33612.
☎ 813 978 8683

Organizations: BDSM
☺ □ **D. S. S. G.**
P. O. Box 30, Valrico, Florida 33594-0030.
☎ 813 689 7999

⚥▽ **Tampa Bay Trailblazers**
Suite 370, 8206 West Waters, Tampa, Florida 33615.
✉ Oberontpa@aol.com

Organizations: Bears
⚥▽ **West Florida Growlers**
P. O. Box 22801, Tampa, Florida 33622-2801.
☎ 813 821 1075
✉ growlers@aol.com
🌐 http://www.skepsis.com:80/.gblo/bears/CLUBS/west.florida.growl ers.html

Organizations: Sexuality: Student
⚥▽ **University of South Florida Gay, Lesbian, & Bisexual Coalition**
♿ CTR 2466, 4202 East Fowler Avenue, Tampa, Florida 33620.
☎ 813 974 4297

Organizations: Spanking
☺ **P. M. Club**
P. O. Box 1251604, Tampa, Florida 33614.

Piercers
☺ ■ **Bravo**
Suite C-307, 333 Fulkenburg RoadNorth, Tampa, Florida 33619.
☎ 813 689 1414 ✆ 813 689 3041
Large selection of jewelry, & will do custom work.

☺ ■ **Leather Tiger**
1411 7th. Avnue, Tampa, Florida 33602.
☎ 813 248 8814
☎ 813 831 6482
Also make jewelry in Niobium, stainless steel, & other precious metals. Catalogue, $3.

Publishers: Newspapers: Sexuality
⚥ *Encounter*
Suite 913, 1222 South Dale Mabry Highway, Tampa, Florida 33629.
☎ 8113 877 7913

Stores: Books: General

Three Birds Bookstore
1518 7th. Avenue, Tampa, Florida 33605.
813 247 7041

Tomes & Treasures
202 South Howard Avenue, Tampa, Florida 33606.
813 251 9368
Mon - Sat 11:00 - 20:00, Sun 12:00 - 18:00

Stores: Erotica: BDSM

Christine's Lingerie Inc.
11124B North 30th. Street, Tampa, Florida 33512.
813 979 0154
64-page catalogue, $3.

Exotique
Northwest Plaza, 4023 West Waters Avenue, Tampa, Florida 33614.
813 889 9477
Catalogue, $10U.S. for U.S., $10U.S. elsewhere.

Stores: Military Surplus

Army-Navy Store of Tampa, Inc.
1312 North Tampa Street, Tampa, Florida.
813 229 2172

Command Post, Inc.
3402 Dale Mabry Highway South, Tampa, Florida.
813 831 9245

Headquarters Military Surplus, Inc.
1450 Bears Avenue East, Tampa, Florida.
813 759 0459

West Palm Beach

Counsellors

Keith Allen Platt, LCSW
Suite 212, 2601 North Flagler Drive, West Palm Beach, Florida.
407 835 3934

Health Services

Good Samaritan Medical Center
Flagler Drive at Palm Beach Lakes Boulevard, West Palm Beach, Florida 33401.
407 655 5511

Palm Beach County AIDS Clinic
3518 Broadway, West Palm Beach, Florida 33407.
407 845 4444

Palm Beach County Health Department
P. O. Box 29, West Palm Beach, Florida 33402-0029.
407 837 3090

Palm Beaches Medical Center
2201 45th. Street, West Palm Beach, Florida 33407.
407 842 6141

Saint Mary's Hospital
901 45th. Street, West Palm Beach, Florida 33407.
407 844 6300

Organizations: AIDS: Education

Comprehensive AIDS Program
P. O. Box 18887, West Palm Beach, Florida 33416-8887.
407 881 9040

Organizations: AIDS: Support

PWA Coalition of Palm Beach
P. O. Box 19855, West Palm Beach, Florida 33416-4855.
407 697 8033

Organizations: Motorcycle

Eagle MC
3311 Liddy Avenue West, West Palm Beach, Florida 33316.

Publishers: Newspapers: Sexuality

Community Voice
P. O. Box 17975, West Palm Beach, Florida 33416.
407 471 1528
News & views magazine for gays, lesbians, & bisexuals. Published every month. Yearly subscription is $18.

Stores: Books: General

Changing Times Bookstore
Suite 806, 911 Village Boulevard, West Palm Beach, Florida 33409.
407 640 0496

Stores: Erotica: BDSM

Eurotique, Inc.
Suite 341, 4521 P. G. A. Boulevard, Palm Beach Gardens, Florida 33410.
407 624 5609 — 407 624 5609

Winter Park

Organizations: Sexuality

The Society for the Second Self (Tri-Ess)—Phi Epsilon Mu
P. O. Box 3261, Winter Park, Florida 32790-3261.
ggsandra@aol.com
Meets 1st. Sat of month
Publishes a newsletter every month.

Zephyrs Hills

Piercers

Jack Yount
813 783 7377

GEORGIA

Area: Approximately 150,000 square kilometres
Population: Approximately 6,500,000
Capital City: Atlanta
Time zone: GMT minus 5 hours (EST)
Climate: Hot summers of approximately 29°C & very high humidity. Winters are cool at approximately -4°C.
Age of consent & homosexuality legislation: All anal & oral sex is illegal in this state.
Legal drinking age: 21

State Resources

Organizations: Bears

Dixie Bears
dobywood@ix.netcom.com or hosstnr@aol.com
http://www.skepsis.com:80/.gblo/bears/CLUBS/Dixie_Bears/
Meets 3rd. Sat of month

Athens

Stores: Books: General

Barnett's Bookstore
147 College Avenue, Athens, Georgia 30601.
706 353 0530

Tattooists

Midnight Iguana Tattoing, Inc.
283 West Broad Street, Athens, Georgia 30601.
706 549 0190
midiguana@aol.com
Mon - Sat 11:00 - 23:00
Ultra-modern, hospital-sterile, professional, experienced, nationally published tatto studio. All styles of tattoo art, including custom & portrait. Also body piercing. Age statement of 18 is required. German also spoken.

Atlanta

Bars: BDSM

Atlanta Eagle
306 Ponce de Leon Avenue North East, Atlanta, Georgia 30308-2013.
404 873 2453
Wed - Sun 18:00 - 03:00

Bars: General

Mon Cherie's The Chamber
2115 Faulkner Road, Atlanta, Georgia 30324.
404 248 1612 — 404 577 7460
Thu Fri 22:00 - 04:00, Sat 10:00 - 03:00
VISA
Also put on BDSM & fetish shows. Age statement of 21 is required.

BBSs: BDSM

Annette's Castle
404 843 9751

Health Services

Crawford Long Hospital of Emory University
550 Peachtree Street North East, Atlanta, Georgia 30365.
404 686 4411

Grady Memorial Hospital
80 Butler Street, Atlanta, Georgia 30335.
404 616 4307
HIV & emergency departments.

Piedmont Hospital
1968 Peachtree Road, Atlanta, Georgia 30309.
404 605 5000

☺ □ **Saint Joseph's Hospital of Atlanta**
5665 Peachtree Dunwoody Road North East, Atlanta, Georgia 30342.
☎ 404 851 7001

☺ **Mark Tanner, M.D.**
K 1935 Howell Mill Road, Atlanta, Georgia 30318.
☎ 404 355 2000
Internal medicine.

☺ □ **West Paces Medical Center**
3200 Howell Road North West, Atlanta, Georgia 30327.
☎ 404 351 0351

Helplines: Sexuality

⚥▽ **Atlanta Gay Center Helpline**
♿ 63 12th. Street, Atlanta, Georgia 30309.
☎ 404 892 0661 (TDD capable)

Organizations: AIDS: Education

☺ □ **AID Atlanta**
AS 1438 West Peachtree Street North West, Atlanta, Georgia 30309.
☎ 404 000 0600 ✆ 404 875 6799
Publishes *Infolines*.

Organizations: BDSM

☺ □ **A.S.B. Munch—Atlanta**
✉ dna@law.emory.edu or an169847@anon.penet.fi

⚥▽ **Atlanta S&M Solidarity (ASS)**
P. O. Box 8361, Atlanta, Georgia 30306-0361.
☎ 404 521 3829 (voice mail)
🕐 Meets monthly, plus educational presentations

☺ □ **Headspace**
✉ headspce@law.emory.edu
Mailing list for BDSMers in Atlanta.To subscribe, send e-mail with Subscribe in the subject line. Regular updates of Atlantamunch times & locations.

⚥▽ **The Leathermen**
P. O. Box 8595, Atlanta, Georgia 30306.

☺ □ **The National Leather Association (NLA)—Atlanta**
P. O. Box 7941, Atlanta, Georgia 30357-0941.
☎ 404 624 1676 (24hr. recording)
✉ kyle@crl.com
🕐 Meets Sat 20:00

⚥▽ **Panther LL, Inc.**
P. O. Box 191286, Atlanta, Georgia 31119-1286.
✉ 73671.2350@CompuServe.com

☺ □ **People Exchanging Power (PEP)—Atlanta**
P. O. Box 921291, Norcross, Georgia 30092.
☎ 404 621 7961 (voice mail)
🕐 Meets Sat 20:00
Contact: Lady D
Friendly, informative organization. Usually has one or more local toy stores or vendors represented at its meetings. Publishes *Tops & Bottoms*.

⚥▽ **TDA - Atlanta**
P. O. Box 8051, Atlanta, Georgia 30306.

Organizations: Bears

⚥▽ **Southern Bears**
P. O. Box 13964, Atlanta, Georgia 30324.
☎ 404 908 3381
✉ mhr@ursa-major.spdcc.com
🌐 http://www.skepsis.com/.gblo/bears/CLUBS/Southern_Bears/
🕐 Meets 2nd. Sat of month 20:00

Organizations: Family

☺ □ **Parents & Friends of Lesbians & Gays (PFLAG)—Atlanta**
♿
P. O. Box 8482, Atlanta, Georgia 30306.
☎ 404 691 4729

Organizations: Fetish: Uniforms

⚥▽ **The American Uniform Association (AUA)—Atlanta Brigade**
1553 Johnson Road, Atlanta, Georgia 30306.
Contact: Mr. Frank Puckett

Organizations: Motorcycle

⚥▽ **Atlantis MC**
P. O. Box 54642, Atlanta, Georgia 30308.

Organizations: Sexuality

⚥▽ **Atlanta Gay Center**
♿ 63 12th. Street, Atlanta, Georgia 30316.
☎ 404 876 5372 (office)
☎ 404 892 0661 (helpline, TDD capable)

🕐 18:00 - 23:00
Publishes *The News*.

⚥▽ **Atlanta Gender Exploration (AGE)**
P. O. Box 77562, Atlanta, Georgia 30357.
☎ 404 875 9846
🕐 Meets twice a month
Publishes *Atlanta Gender Chronicle*.

♀▽ **BiAtlanta**
P. O. Box 5240, Atlanta, Georgia 30307.
☎ 404 256 8992

♀▽ **Bisexual Atlanta Resource Center (BARN)**
☎ 404 908 3413

☺ **The National Organization of Sexual Enthusiasts (NOSE)**
P. O. Box 8733, Atlanta, Georgia 30306.
☎ 404 377 5760 ✆ 404 377 6962
Publishes *The Sexual Enthusiast* quarterly. Yearly subscription is $20.

Organizations: Sexuality: Student

⚥▽ **Agnes Scott Lesbian & Bisexual Alliance**
P. O. Box 501, Decatur, Georgia 30030.
☎ 404 373 1632

⚥▽ **Alliance of Lesbian, Gay, & Bisexual Students**
♿ Box 1817, University Center, Georgia State University, Atlanta, Georgia 30303.
☎ 404 605 7681

⚥▽ **Emory Lesbian & Gay Organization (ELGO)**
♿ P. O. Box 23515, Atlanta, Georgia 30322.
☎ 404 727 6692

⚥▽ **Georgia Tech's Gay & Lesbian Alliance**
♿ P. O. Box 50291, Georgia Tech Station, Atlanta, Georgia 30332-0548.
☎ 404 497 0684

Organizations: Shaving

⚥ **Philly Hair Razors**
P. O. Box 725044, Atlanta, Georgia 31139-9044.
☎ 215 784 7140
Contact: Mr. Ed Johnson

Piercers

☺ ■ **The Piercing Experience**
1654 McLendon Avenue, Atlanta, Georgia 30307.
☎ 800 646 0393 ✆ 404 378 0027
☎ 404 378 9100
🕐 12:00 - 22:00
💳 VISA CC 💲
The only full-service body piercing studio in the state. Age statement of 18 is required.

☺ ■ **Urban Tribe**
1131 Euclid Avnue, Little Five Points, Georgia 30307.
☎ 404 365 2407

Publishers: Guides: Sexuality

⚐ *Crossdressers InfoGuide*
P. O. Box 566065, Atlanta, Georgia 30356.
☎ 404 333 6455

Publishers: Magazines: Corsets

⚐■ *Corset Digest*
4514 Chamblee-Dunwoody Road, Atlanta, Georgia 30338.

Publishers: Magazines: Sexuality

⚥ *Sage*
P. O. Box 42741, Atlanta, Georgia 30311-0741.
☎ 404 223 7528

⚥■ *The Transsexual Voice*
P. O. Box 16314, Atlanta, Georgia 30321.

Publishers: Newspapers: Sexuality

⚥▽ *Etcetera Magazine*
♿ P. O. Box 8916, Atlanta, Georgia 30306.
☎ 404 525 3821 ✆ 404 525 1908
The Southeast's leading lesbian & gay weekly, since 1985. Provides news & entertainment for Georgia, Florida, North Carolina, South Carolina, Alabama, & Tennessee. Published every week. Yearly subscription is $52.

⚥▼ *Southern Voice*
P. O. Box 18215, Atlanta, Georgia 30316.
☎ 404 876 1819
A full service gay & lesbian newspaper, serving the southeast. Published every week. Yearly subscription is $58.

Radio: Sexuality

👁▽ **Southern Gay Dreams**
WRFG, P. O. Box 5332, Atlanta, Georgia 30307.
☎ 404 523 3471

Stores: Books: General

☺ ■ **Borders Book Shop**
⅋ 3655 Roswell Road, Atlanta, Georgia 30342.
☎ 404 237 0707

☺ ▼ **Brushstrokes**
1510 Piedmont Avenue North East, Atlanta, Georgia.
☎ 404 876 6567 ✆ 404 233 9557
🕐 Mon - Thu 10:00 - 22:00, Fri - Sat 10:00 - 23:00, Sun 12:00 -
22:00
▣ ✓ 𝗩𝗜𝗦𝗔 𝗠𝗖
Many BDSM & fetish publications. No mail order.

⊕ ▼ **Charis Books & More**
⅋ 1189 Euclid Avenue North East, Atlanta, Georgia 30307.
☎ 404 524 0304

👁▼ **Outwrite Bookstore & Coffeehouse**
⅋ Suite A-108, 931 Monroe Drive, Atlanta, Georgia 30308-1778.
☎ 404 607 0082 ✆ 404 607 0092
✉ outwritekd@aol.com
🕐 Mon - Thu 10:00 - 22:00, Fri Sat - 23:00, Sun 12:00 - 22:00
▣ ✓ $ 𝗩𝗜𝗦𝗔 𝗠𝗖 𝗔𝗠𝗘𝗫 ▤
Gay & lesbian selections. Also most BDSM texts currently available. Also
mail order.

☺ ■ **Oxford Books**
2345 Peachtree Road North East, Atlanta, Georgia 30305.
☎ 404 262 3332

Stores: Clothing: Fetish

☺ ■ **Throb**
1140 Euclid Avenue North East, Atlanta, Georgia.
☎ 404 522 0355 ✆ 404 577 7254
▣ 𝗩𝗜𝗦𝗔 𝗠𝗖
Latex, leather, adult novelties, corsets, wigs, & much more. Catalogue
available.

Stores: Clothing: Leather

☺ ■ **Midnight Blue**
394-D Cleveland Avenue, Atlanta, Georgia.
☎ 404 766 6288

☺ **Warlords, Inc.**
⅋ 2111 Faulkner Road, Atlanta, Georgia 30324.
☎ 404 315 9000 ✆ 404 315 9000 (call first)
🕐 Tue - Fri 11:00 - 19:00, Sat - 21:00
▣ $ 𝗩𝗜𝗦𝗔 𝗠𝗖

Stores: Erotica: BDSM

☺ ▼ **593 Group**
593 Westminster Drive, Atlanta, Georgia 30324.
☎ 404 853 5109
🕐 Mon - Thu 11:00 - 18:00, Fri Sat 19:00, Sun 13: -17:00
▣ ✓ $ ⅋ 𝗩𝗜𝗦𝗔 𝗠𝗖 ▤ Ⅾ
Free catalogue.

👁▼ **The Leather Post / Taz Men**
842 Highland Avenue North East, Atlanta, Georgia 30306.
☎ 404 873 5080

👁▼ **Mohawk Leather**
c/o The Eagle, 306Ponce De Leon Avenue North East, Atlanta, Georgia.
☎ 404 874 4732
🕐 Wed - Sun 18:00 - 03:00
Inside The Eagle bar.

☺ ■ **The Pleasure Zone**
1329 Brocket Road, Clarkston, Georgia.
☎ 404 414 1137

☺ ■ **The Poster Hut**
2175 Cheshire Bridge Road, Atlanta, Georgia.
☎ 404 633 7491
Also piercing jewelry.

Stores: Erotica: General

☺ ■ **Nine & A Half Weeks**
1023 West Peachtree Street North East, Atlanta, Georgia.
☎ 404 815 9622
🕐 Daily - 02:00
Carries BDSM books, magazines, videos, & toys.

☺ ■ **Uptown Novelties**
1893 Cheshire Bridge Road, Atlanta, Georgia.
☎ 404 875 9210
Some BDSM literature & toys.

Stores: Military Surplus

☺ ■ **Army Surplus Sales Inc.**
342 Peachtree Street North East, Atlanta, Georgia.
☎ 404 521 2227
Catalogue available.

Suppliers: Travel Arrangements: BDSM

☺ ■ **Ambassador World Travel**
✉ inanna@netcom.com
Leigh Ann specializes in discreet travel arrangements for alternate
sexuality communities.

Tattooists

☺ ■ **Sacred Heart Tattoos**
Suite 5, 483 Moreland Avenue, Atlanta, Georgia 30307.
☎ 404 222 0393

Buford

Organizations: BDSM

☺ □ **Atlanta Power Exchange**
P. O. Box 183, Buford, Georgia 30518.
☎ 404 945 0154

Decatur

Helplines: Sexuality

✉■ **American Educational Gender Information Services,
Inc. (AEGIS)**
P. O. Box 33724, Decatur, Georgia 30033.
☎ 404 939 2128 ✆ 404 939 1770
✉ aegis@mindspring.com
🌐 http://www.cdspub.com/AEGIS.html
Publishes *Chrysalis Magazine* quarterly.

Doraville

Counsellors

☺ **Brenda Hawkins, Ed.D.**
K Suite A-2, 3684 Stewart Road, Doraville, Georgia 30340.
☎ 404 986 4247
🕐 By appointment

Lithonia

BBSs: Sexuality

☺ ▼ **Graffiti**
P. O. Box 3176, Lithonia, Georgia 30058.
☎ 404 972 9709
✆ 404 972 4999

Macon

Organizations: AIDS: Education

☺ ▽ **Central City AIDS Network**
⅋ 530 First Street, Macon, Georgia 31201.
☎ 912 750 8080

Organizations: AIDS: Information

☺ ▽ **The Rainbow Center**
⅋ 530 First Street, Macon, Georgia 31201.
☎ 912 750 8080

Marietta

Health Services

☺ □ **Kennestone Hospital**
677 Church Street, Marietta, Georgia 30060.
☎ 404 793 5000

Manufacturers: Furniture: BDSM

☺ ■ **Pegasus Leatherworks**
P. O. Box 670191, Marietta, Georgia 30066.
Whips & BDSM furniture.

Suppliers: Diapers

☺ ■ **Medical Disposables Company**
1165 Hayes Industries Drive, Marietta, Georgia 30062-2428.
☎ 404 422 3036
☎ 800 241 8205
Disposable diapers, diaper liners, & waterproof pants.

Norcross

Suppliers: Diapers

☺ ■ **Contenta, Inc.**
Suite C, 3343 Peachtree Corners Circle, Norcross, Georgia 30092.
☎ 404 446 2235

Liners & cloth diapers.

Rosewell

Organizations: Sexuality

☿▽ **The Society for the Second Self (Tri-Ess)—Sigma Epsilon**
P. O. Box 272, Rosewell, Georgia 30077-0272.
☎ 404 552 4415 (helpline)
⊕ Meets monthly
Publishes *The Southern Belle*.

Savannah

Organizations: Sexuality

☿▽ **First City Network, Inc.**
P. O. Box 2442, Savannah, Georgia 31401.
☎ 912 236 2489
Publishes *Network News*.

Valdosta

Organizations: Sexuality

♂▽ **Valdosta State College Gay & Lesbian Association**
VSC Box 7097, Valdosta, Georgia 31698.
☎ 912 247 0181
✉ dcarver@grits.valdosta.peachnet.edu
Contact: Mr. Doug Carver

HAWAII

Area: Approximately 16,650 square kilometres
Population: Approximately 1,100,000
Capital City: Honolulu
Time zone: GMT minus 10 hours (PST minus 2 hours)
Climate: Sub-tropical climate keeps summer day temperatures at approximately 28°C & winter temperatures at 20°C. Night time temperature are low, due to the trade winds that blow most of the time.
Age of consent & homosexuality legislation: State has adopted the Model Penal Code or otherwise decriminalized homosexual activities.
Legal drinking age: 21

State Resources

Helplines: Sexuality

☿▽ **Gay Community Directory**
& P. O. Box 37083, Honolulu, Hawaii 96837-0083.
☎ 808 521 6000 (24hr. tape listing)

Organizations: AIDS: Education

☺ ☐ **AIDS Project Hawaii**
P. O. Box 8425, Honolulu, Hawaii 96815.
☎ 808 926 2122

Organizations: AIDS: Support

☺ ☐ **PWA Coalition—Hawaii**
P. O. Box 11752, Honolulu, Hawaii 96828.
☎ 808 948 4792
Publishes *Living Now News*.

Publishers: Guides: Sexuality

☿ **The Pages**
Lifestyle Publishing Inc., Suite A, 2851 Kihei Place, Honolulu, Hawaii 96816-1355.
☎ 808 737 6400 ☏ 808 735 8825
The most comprehensive gay & lesbian guide to Hawaii. Published once a year. Yearly subscription is $4.

Publishers: Magazines: Sexuality

☿▼ **Island Lifestyle Magazine**
Lifestyle Publishing Inc., Suite A, 2851 Kihei Place, Honolulu, Hawaii 96816-1355.
☎ 808 737 6400 ☏ 808 735 8825
✓ VISA MC
The magazine serving the gay & lesbian community of Hawaii. Published every month. Yearly subscription is $16.50.

Publishers: Newspapers: Sexuality

☿▽ **Gay Community News**
& P. O. Box 37083, Honolulu, Hawaii 96837-0083.
☎ 808 521 6000
Hard news, complete Hawaii (all island) territory, books, entertainment, reviews, & editorial. Published every month. Yearly subscription is $25.

☿▼ **Island Lesbian Connection**
P. O. Box 356, Suite 171, Paia, Hawaii 96779.
☎ 808 575 2681 ☏ 808 579 8556
⊕ 09:00 - 21:00 every day
🍺 ✓ $ ⚊

All-island newsletter with information by & for lesbians in Hawaii. Published every month. Yearly subscription is $16.50.

☿▽ **The Jungle Vine**
P. O. Box 4056, Hilo, Hawaii 96720.

Tattooists

☺ **Skin Deep Tattoo**
626 Front Street, Lahaina, Hawaii 96761.
☎ 808 661 8531 ☏ 808 661 8288
✉ skindp@aol.com
⊕ 10:00 - 22:00
🍺 ✓ $ VISA MC

Hawaii (Big Island)

Organizations: AIDS: Education

☺ ☐ **AIDS Project**
P. O. Box AO, Kailua Kona, Hawaii 96745.
☎ 808 969 6626 (hotline)
☎ 808 326 2391 (office)
⊕ Hotline 24hrs.

Organizations: Polyfidelity

☺ ☐ **Abundant Love Institute**
P. O. Box 6306, Oceanview, Hawaii 96737.
☎ 808 929 9691 ☏ 809 929 9831
✉ RyamPEP@aol.com
🕸 http://www.wp.com/Lovemore
⊕ Mon - Fri 09:00 - 17:00
🍺 ✓ $ ⚊ VISA MC
Contact: Ms. Ryam Nearing
National organization & resource for people who believe in loving more than one person at a time responsibly, intimately, & in integrity. Publishes *Loving More Magazine* quarterly. Yearly subscription is $30.

Organizations: Sexuality

☿▽ **Gay & Lesbians of Hawaii Island (GALOHI)**
P. O. Box 639, Kailua Kona, Hawaii 96745.
☎ 808 329 0049
Publishes a newsletter.

Publishers: Magazines: Sexuality

☿▽ **Outspoken**
& Kalani Honua, Inc., P. O. Box 4500, R. R. 2, Kehena Beach, Hawaii 96778.
☎ 808 965 7828 ☏ Call first
✉ kh@ILHawaii.net
🕸 http://www.maui.net/~randm/kh2.html or http://www.virtualcities.com/~virtual
🍺 ✓ $ ⚊ VISA MC ⚊ ℯ
Educational news service for the Hawaiian gay. lesbian, bi community. Arranges monthly meetings & annual gatherings, welcoming vistors to the islands. Published every two months. Yearly subscription is $12.

Maui

Organizations: Sexuality

☿▽ **Both Sides Now**
P. O. Box 5042, Kahului, Hawaii 96732.
☎ 808 572 1884
Publishes *Both Sides Now*.

Organizations: Sexuality: Youth

☿▼ **Maui Lesbian/Gay Youth Project**
& P. O. Box 356, Suite 171, Paia, Hawaii 96779.
☎ 808 575 2681 (Karen) ☏ 808 579 8556
☎ 808 573 1093 (Joe)
⊕ Meets weekly
🍺 ✓ $ ⚊
Contact: Ms. Karen Anna
Support group for youth to 21 years. Presentations for teachers & youth workers.

Oahu

Competitions & Conventions: Sexuality

▨■ **Sexual Identity Center (SIC)**
P. O. Box 3224, Honolulu, Hawaii 96801-3244.
☎ 808 926 1000

Counsellors

☿▼ **Michael Bridge, Ph.D.**
Suite 2605, 1188 Bishop Street, Honolulu, Hawaii 96813.
☎ 808 526 2605

Health Services

☺ ☐ **Kaiser Foundation Hospital**
3288 Moanalua Road, Honolulu, Hawaii 96819.

☎ 808 834 5333
☺ ☐ **Queen's Medical Center**
1301 Punchbowl Street, Honolulu, Hawaii 96813.
☎ 808 538 9011
HIV & emergency departments.
☺ ☐ **Saint Francis Medical Center**
2230 Liliha Street, Honolulu, Hawaii 96817.
☎ 808 547 6011

Organizations: BDSM
☺ ☐ **People Exchanging Power (PEP)—Paradise**
c/o Mistress Athena, P. O. Box 22959, Honolulu, Hawaii 96826.

Organizations: Body Size
⚤▽ **Big Men of Hawaii**
c/o GLCC Room 8, 1820 University Avenue, Honolulu, Hawaii 96826.

Organizations: Sexuality
⚤▽ **Gay & Lesbian Community Center**
& 2nd. Floor, 1820 University Avenue, Honolulu, Hawaii 96801.
☎ 808 951 7000 ✆ 808 926 1000
Publishes *Honolulu Outlook.*
⚲▽ **Hawaii Transgender Outreach**
P. O. Box 4530, Honolulu, Hawaii 96812.
☎ 808 923 4270
🕐 Meets bi-weekly
Publishes a newsletter.
⚲▽ **Lesbian Support Group**
c/o GLCC, 2nd. Floor, 1820 University Avenue, Honolulu, Hawaii 96826.
☎ 808 951 7000

Organizations: Sexuality: Youth
⚤▽ **Gay & Lesbian Teen Task Force**
c/o GLCC, 1820 University Avenue, Honolulu, Hawaii 96826.
☎ 808 951 7000

Publishers: Guides: Sexuality
⚥ *Pocket Guide to Hawaii*
c/o Pacific Ocean Holidays, P. O. Box 88245, Honolulu, Hawaii 96830.
☎ 808 923 2400
Designed especially for gay visitors to Hawaii. Descriptive listings of gay & gay-friendly businesses. Detailed maps of Waikiki & the gay district. Published 3 times a year. Yearly subscription is $15U.S..

Stores: Books: General
☺ ■ **Pacific Book House**
435 Atkinson Drive, Honolulu, Hawaii 96814-4729.
✆ 808 942 2242
☺ ■ **Walden Books**
212 Waikiki Shopping Plaza, 2250 Kalakaua Avenue, Honolulu, Hawaii 96815.
☎ 808 922 4154

Stores: Erotica: BDSM
☺ ■ **Submission**
Suite 110, 1831 Ala Moana Boulevard, Honolulu, Hawaii 96815.
☎ 808 942 0670
🕐 Mon - Sat 14:00 - 22:00

IDAHO
Area: Approximately 215,000 square kilometres
Population: Approximately 1,010,000
Capital City: Boise
Time zone: GMT minus 7 hours (Mountain Time)
Age of consent & homosexuality legislation: All anal & oral sex is illegal in this state.

State Resources
Helplines: AIDS
☺ ☐ **Idaho AIDS Foundation**
P. O. Box 421, Boise, Idaho 83701.
☎ 800 677 2437 ✆ 208 345 4579
☎ 208 345 2277
🕐 Helpline Mon - Fri 18:00 - 21:00. Office Mon - Fri 08:00 - 12:00

Organizations: AIDS: Education
☺ ☐ **Idaho AIDS Foundation**
P. O. Box 421, Boise, Idaho 83701.
☎ 800 677 2437 ✆ 208 345 4579
☎ 208 345 2277
🕐 Helpline Mon - Fri 18:00 - 21:00. Office Mon - Fri 08:00 - 12:00
☺ ☐ **North Idaho AIDS Coalition**
Panhandle Health District, 2195 Ironwood Court, Coeur D'Alene, Idaho 83814.

☎ 800 677 2437
☎ 208 769 3533

Organizations: Sexuality
⊕ **Idaho Women's Network**
P. O. Box 1385, Boise, Idaho 83701.
☎ 208 344 5738

Publishers: Newspapers: Sexuality
⚥▽ *Diversity*
P. O. Box 323, Boise, Idaho 83701.
☎ 208 336 3870
Diversity is the only gay & lesbian newspaper in Idaho. We include news, opinion, & features. 20% subscription, 75% distribution. Published 11 times a year. Yearly subscription is $10.

Boise
Health Services
☺ ☐ **Saint Alphonsus Regional Medical Center**
1055 North Curtis Road, Boise, Idaho 83706.
☎ 208 378 2121

Organizations: BDSM
⚥▽ **The Lion Regiment**
P. O. Box 1721, Boise, Idaho 83706.
☎ 208 322 8174

Organizations: Sexuality
⚥▽ **The Community Center (TCC)**
P. O. Box 323, Boise, Idaho 83701.
☎ 208 336 3870

Publishers: Books: Spanking
☺ ▼ **BoisLine**
P. O. Box 8182, Boise, Idaho 83707.
🔥 ✓
Age statement of 18 is required.

Caldwell
Stores: Erotica: General
☺ ■ **Adult Shop**
716 Arthur Avenue, Caldwell, Idaho 83605.
☎ 208 454 2422

Moscow
Organizations: Sexuality
⚥▽ **Inland Northwest Gay People's Alliance**
P. O. Box 8135, Moscow, Idaho 83843.
☎ 208 882 8034
Publishes a newsletter.

Pocatello
Stores: Erotica: General
☺ ■ **Pegasus Unusual Books**
246 West Center Street, Pocatello, Idaho 83204.
☎ 208 232 6493
☺ ■ **Silver Fox**
143 South 2nd. Avenue, Pocatello, Idaho 83201-6446.
☎ 208 234 2477

ILLINOIS
Area: Approximately 144,000 square kilometres
Population: Approximately 11,500,000
Capital City: Springfield
Time zone: GMT minus 6 hours (CST)
Climate: Hot & humid summers, but cold winters with a lot of snow. Temperatures can reach 32°C in the summer & -18°C in the winter.
Age of consent & homosexuality legislation: State has adopted the Model Penal Code or otherwise decriminalized homosexual activities.
Legal drinking age: 21

Alton
Publishers: Newspapers: Sexuality
⚥ *This Week in Saint Louis (TWISL)*
Kacmer Publishing Co., P. O. Box 8068, Alton, Illinois 62002-8068.
☎ 618 465 9370

Arlington Heights
Stores: Books: General
⊕ ■ **Prairie Moon**
8 North Dunton, Arlington Heights, Illinois 60005.
☎ 708 342 9608

Aurora
Stores: Erotica: General
☺ **Denmark Books**
 1300 US Rt 30, Aurora, Illinois 60504.
 ☎ 708 898 9838 📠 708 898 1087

Belleville
Organizations: AIDS: Education
☺ ☐ **Bethany Place**
 ♿ 224 West Washington Street, Belleville, Illinois 62222.
 ☎ 618 234 0291

Bloomington
Health Services
☺ ☐ **Saint Joseph's Medical Center**
 2200 East Washington Street, Bloomington, Illinois 61701.
 ☎ 309 622 3311

Manufacturers: Adult Toys: BDSM
☺ ▼ **Silver Smoke**
 Box 101, 156A East Lake Street, Bloomington, Illinois 60108.
 ☎ 708 653 1287
 ⊕ ✓ $ ✈ VISA MC AMERICAN 💳
 Free catalogue.

Organizations: Sexuality: Student
⚥♂▽ **Gay & Lesbian Alliance**
 ♿ Illinois State University, Normal, Illinois 61761-6901.
 ☎ 309 438 2429
 ⏱ Mon - Fri 11:00 - 17:00

Publishers: Magazines: Body Size
⚹ ■ **Wilson Barber's Quarterly**
 Oakhaus, 910 West Division, Normal, Illinois 61761.
 ☎ 309 454 2128
 About admiration of fat women. Published quarterly. Yearly subscription is $20.

Publishers: Magazines: Bondage
♂ ▼ **Bi Monthly Bondage**
 Subnormal, P. O. Box 602, Normal, Illinois 61761.
 Published every two months. Yearly subscription is $15.

Stores: Books: General
☺ ▼ **Once Upon a Time (OUT)**
 311 North Main Street, Bloomington, Illinois 61701.
 ☎ 309 828 3998 📠 309 828 8879
 ⏱ Mon Wed Fri 16:00 - 20:00, Sat 10:00 - 20:00, Sun 12:00 -
 17:00
 ⊕ ✓ $ ✈ VISA MC

Carbondale
Organizations: Sexuality: Student
⚥♂▽ **Gays, Lesbians, Bisexuals, & Friends**
 ♿ OSD, 3rd. Floor, Student Center, Southern Illinois University, Carbondale,
 Illinois 62901.
 ☎ 618 453 5151
 ⏱ Mon - Fri 17:00 - 21:00

Champaign / Urbana
Helplines: Sexuality
⚥♂▽ **Lesbian, Gay, & Bisexual Switchboard**
 ♿ 284 Illini Union, 1401 West Green Street, Urbana, Illinois 61801.
 ☎ 217 384 8040
 ⏱ Mon - Fri 20:00 - 22:00

Organizations: AIDS: Education
☺ ☐ **Gay Community AIDS Project**
 P. O. Box 713, Champaign, Illinois 61824-0713.
 ☎ 217 351 2437

Organizations: BDSM
☺ **The Group with No Name**
 805 East Green Street, Urbana, Illinois 61801.
 ☎ 217 384 7333
 ✉ folo@firefly.prairienet.org
 🌐 http://uiulsi.uiuc.edu/~steele/gnn.html
 Contact: Mr. Folo Watkins
 Association of people in central Illinois who are interested in the DBSM /
 leather sexuality. Monthly meetings & play parties. Publishes The Crop
 Report every month. Yearly subscription is free. Age statement of 18 is
 required.

Organizations: Sexuality
♂ ▽ **Champaign-Urbana Bisexual Network**
 c/o The McKinley Foundation, 809 South Fifth Street, Champaign, Illinois
 61820.
 Publishes The Bi Monthly 10 times a year. Yearly subscription is $10.

Organizations: Sexuality: Student
⚥♂▽ **People for Lesbian, Gay, & Bisexual Concerns**
 ♿ 264 Illini Union, 1401 West Green Street, Urbana, Illinois 61801.
 ☎ 217 333 1187
 ⏱ Mon - Fri 20:00 - 22:00

Publishers: Newspapers: Sexuality
⚥♂ **Lavendar Prairie News**
 P. O. Box 2096, Champaign, Illinois 61825-2096.
 ☎ 312 769 9009

Stores: Books: General
☺ ■ **Horizon Bookstore**
 1115 1/2 West Oregon Street, Urbana, Illinois 61801-3715.
 ☎ 217 328 2988
⚧ ■ **June Addams Book Shop**
 ♿ 208 North Neil Street, Champaign, Illinois 61820.
 ☎ 217 356 2555
 ⏱ Mon - Fri 10:00 - 17:00, Sun 13:00 - 17:00
 Publishes Women's Newsletter.

Chicago
Archives: Sexuality
⚥♂▽ **Gerber/Hart Library & Archives**
 ♿ 3352 North Paulina Street, Chicago, Illinois 60657.
 ☎ 312 883 3003

Bars: BDSM
♂▽▼ **Cell Block**
 ♿ 3702 North Halsted Street, Chicago, Illinois.
 ☎ 312 665 8064
♂▽▼ **Chicago Eagle**
 ♿ 5015 North Clark Street, Chicago, Illinois 60640.
 ☎ 312 728 0050
 ⏱ 20:00 - 04:00, Sat - 05:00, Sun 17:00 - 04:00
♂▽▼ **Dëeks**
 ♿ 3401 North Sheffield, Chicago, Illinois 60657.
 ☎ 312 549 3335
 ⏱ Wed - Fri 21:00 - 02:00, Sat 21:00 - 03:00, Sun 19:00 - 02:00
 ⊕ VISA MC
♂▽▼ **Manhandler Saloon**
 1948 North Halsted Street, Chicago, Illinois.
 ☎ 312 871 3339
 ⏱ Sun - Fri - 04:00, Say - 05:00
♂▽■ **Manhole**
 3458 North Halsted Street, Chicago, Illinois 60657.
 ☎ 312 975 9244
♂▽▼ **Touché**
 6412 North Clark Street, Chicago, Illinois.
 ☎ 312 465 7400 📠 312 465 8856
 ⏱ Mon - Fri 17:00 - 02:00, Sat 12:00 - 03:00, Sun - 02:00

BBSs: BDSM
♂▽▼ **Cockpit**
 ☎ 312 337 2410
☺ ■ **Common Bonds**
 ☎ 312 227 3910
☺ ■ **Final Frontier**
 ☎ 312 334 8638
☺ ■ **Outer Limits**
 ☎ 708 259 0410
 ☎ 708 289 7958. 14400 baud maximum.
☺ ■ **The Zoo**
 ☎ 312 743 9791

Counsellors
☺ **Thom Baxley**
 K #1, 1949 West Winona, Chicago, Illinois 60640-2675.
 ☎ 312 275 0130 📠 312 883 3904
 Therapist.
☺ ☐ **Community Counseling Centers of Chicago**
 ♿ 4740 North Clark, Chicago, Illinois 60640.
 ☎ 312 769 0205
⚥▽ **Randi Ettner, Ph.D.**

1214 Lake Street, Evanston, Illinois 60201.
☎ 708 328 3433
Clinical Psychologist.

⚥▼ **Hannah Frisch, Ph.D.**
⚲ 4933 South Dorchester, Chicago, Illinois 60615.
☎ 312 924 5057

☺ **Norton Knopf, Ph.D.**
K Suite 807, 151 North Michigan Avenue, Chicago, Illinois 60601-7543.
☎ 312 363 5011

☺▼ **John Power, MSW**
K 718 West Melrose, Chicago, Illinois 60657-3418.
☎ 312 327 9886
🕐 By appointment
⚲ ✓ $ ⚞
Individual hypnotherapy for stress management, problem resolution, & health maintenance. Self-hypnosis taught for pain & habit control. Age statement of 18 is required.

Distributors: Books: General

☺ **Independent Publishers Group (IPG)**
814 North Franklin Avenue, Chicago, Illinois 60610.
☎ 312 337 0747 ✆ 312 337 5985

☺ **Login Publishers Consortium**
1426 West Randolf Street, Chicago, Illinois 60607.
☎ 312 733 8228 ✆ 312 666 2680

Health Services

☺☐ **Cook County Hospital**
1835 West Harrison Street, Chicago, Illinois 60612.
☎ 312 633 6000
HIV & emergency departments.

⚥▽ **Howard Brown Health Center**
⚲ 945 West George Street, Chicago, Illinois 60657.
☎ 312 871 5777
STD & HIV testing counselling.

☺☐ **Illinois Masonic Medical Center**
836 West Wellington Avenue, Chicago, Illinois 60657.
☎ 312 975 1600
HIV & emergency departments.

☺☐ **Northwestern Memorial Hospital**
Superior Street & Fairbanks Court, Chicago, Illinois 60611.
☎ 312 908 2000
HIV & emergency departments.

☺☐ **Rush-Presbyterian-Saint Luke's Medical Center**
1653 West Congress Parkway, Chicago, Illinois 60612.
☎ 312 942 5000
HIV & emergency departments.

☺☐ **Saint Joseph Hospital & Medical Center**
2900 North Lake Shore Drive, Chicago, Illinois 60657.
☎ 312 665 3000
HIV & emergency departments.

Helplines: Miscellaneous

☺☐ **In Touch Hotline**
c/o Counseling Center (MLC 333), University of Illinois at Chicago, 601 South Morgan, Chicago, Illinois 60657.
☎ 312 996 5535
🕐 18:00 - 03:00

Helplines: Sexuality

⚥▽ **Lesbian & Gay Helpline**
⚲ c/o Horizons Community Services, 961 West Montana, Chicago, Illinois 60614.
☎ 312 929 4357
☎ 312 327 4357 (TDD)
🕐 18:00 - 22:00

Helplines: Youth

☺☐ **Chicago Runaway Switchboard**
3080 North Lincoln, Chicago, Illinois 60657.
☎ 800 621 3230

Manufacturers: Clothing: Corsets

☺■ **Paul C Leather**
Suite 959, 2421 West Pratt, Chicago, Illinois 60645.
☎ 312 508 0848 ✆ 312 508 0811
☎ 800 338 4740

Manufacturers: Erotica: Leather

☺■ **Paul C Leather**
Suite 959, 2421 West Pratt, Chicago, Illinois 60645.
☎ 312 508 0848 ✆ 312 508 0811
☎ 800 338 4740
Also makes corsets to order.

Manufacturers: Whips

☺ **Stella McKayne**
☎ 312 905 1941
Makes horsehair whips.

☺■ **Joe Wheeler**
Suite 101, 1559 North La Salle, Chicago, Illinois 60610.
☎ 312 835 3468 ✆ 312 477 6044
🕐 08:00 -17:00 every day
⚲ ✓ $ ⚞
Custom made, individually balanced whips & floggers meticulously crafted in a wide variety of textures & exotic leathers. Age statement of 21 is required.

Organizations: Academic: Sexuality

♁▽ **The Institute of Lesbian Studies**
P. O. Box 25568, Chicago, Illinois 60625.

Organizations: AIDS: Education

☺☐ **AIDS Education Project**
2045 West Washington Street, Chicago, Illinois 60614.
☎ 312 477 4709

☺☐ **AIDS Foundation of Chicago**
⚲ Suite 303, 1332 North Halsted Street, Chicago, Illinois 60622-2632.
☎ 312 642 5454

☺ **Dental Alliance for AIDS/HIV**
Suite 200, 101 West Grand Avenue, Chicago, Illinois 60610.
☎ 312 645 4891 ✆ 312 222 0329

☺ **Physicians Association for AIDS Care**
Suite 200, 101 West Grand Avenue, Chicago, Illinois 60610.
☎ 312 222 1326 ✆ 312 222 0329
Publishes *PAACNotes*.

☺ **Plusvoice**
Suite 1150, 29 South Lasalle Street, Chicago, Illinois 60603.
☎ 312 929 9761

☺ **The Riemer Foundation**
Suite 1000, 3023 North Clark Street, Chicago, Illinois 60657.
☎ 312 935 7233 ✆ 312 288 4844

☺☐ **Stop AIDS Chicago**
909 North Belmont Avenue, Chicago, Illinois 60657.
☎ 312 871 3300
🕐 Mon - Thu 10:00 - 22:00, Fri 10:00 - 18:00
Publishes *Stop AIDS in Action*.

Organizations: AIDS: Support

☺▽ **Family & Friends of PWA's Support Network**
⚲ Holy Covenant MCC, 17 West Maple, Hinsdale, Illinois 60521-3495.
☎ 708 325 8488

☺☐ **National Association of People With AIDS— Chicago**
⚲ Suite 303, 1332 North Halsted Street, Chicago, Illinois 60622-2632.

Organizations: BDSM

☺☐ **A.S.B. Munch—Chicago**
✉ kchap@ripco.com
Contact: Dryada

⚥ **Chest Men of America**
P. O. Box 138551, Chicago, Illinois 60613.
☎ 312 975 9593

⚥ **Chicago Hellfire Club**
P.O. Box 5426, Chicago, Illinois 60680.
☎ 312 486 2436
Contact: Mr. David Igasaki, Secretary

☺ **Chicagoland Discussion Group**
Suite 806, 3023 North Clark Street, Chicago, Illinois 60657-5205.
☎ 312 281 1097 (24hr. infoline)
🕐 Meets monthly. 24hr. information line
⚲ ✓
Contact: Ms. Diane Barker
Publishes *CDG Dungeoneer* quarterly.

⚥▽ **Enigma**
2329 North Leavitt Street, Chicago, Illinois 60647.

☺☐ **Leather United - Chicago**
P.O. Box 7635, Round Lake Beach, Illinois 60073.

⚥▼ **Mid-America Fists In Action (MAFIA)**
P.O. Box 2230, Chicago, Illinois 60610-2230.
☎ 312 539 1669
Contact: Mr. Paul Laws
Fisting organization.

☺☐ **Sober, Safe, Sane, Consensual Club - Chicago (S3C3)**

#3A, 4558 North Dover, Chicago, Illinois 60604.
✉ S3C3@aol.com
Contact: Mr. David Katzenberg, Club Administrator
Educational & social outlet for people involved in or supportive of a 12-step recovery program. Send SASE or IRC for reply.

Organizations: Bears

☞♡ **Chi Town Society**
P. O. Box 416825, Chicago, Illinois 60641.

☞♡ **Great Lakes Bears—Chicago**
♿ P. O. Box 578840, Chicago, Illinois 60647.
☎ 312 509 5135

Organizations: Body Size

☞♡ **Girth & Mirth—Chicago**
♿ P. O. Box 14384, Chicago, Illinois 60614.
☎ 312 776 9223

Organizations: Family

☺ ☐ **Children of Lesbians & Gays Everywhere (COLAGE)**
P. O. Box 121, 3023 North Clark Street, Chicago, Illinois 60657.
☎ 312 583 8029 ✆ 312 783 6204
✉ KidsOfGays@aol.com
Publishes *Just For Us.*

☺ ☐ **Parents & Friends of Lesbians & Gays (PFLAG)—Chicago**
♿ P. O. Box 11023, Chicago, Illinois 60611.
☎ 312 472 3079

☺ ☐ **Parents & Friends of Lesbians & Gays (PFLAG)—Hinsdale**
♿ c/o Holy Covenant MCC, 17 West Maple, Hinsdale, Illinois 60521-3495.
☎ 708 325 8488

Organizations: Fetish: Uniforms

☞♡ **The American Uniform Association (AUA)—Chicago Brigade**
P. O. Box 804675, Chicago, Illinois 60680.

Organizations: Literary

☞♡ **The American Library Association**
Gay & Lesbian Task Force, c/o O. L. D. S., 50 East Huron Street, Chicago, Illinois 60611-2795.

Organizations: Masturbation

☞ **Chicago Jacks**
P.O. Box 408084, Chicago, Illinois 60640.

Organizations: Motorcycle

☞♡ **Open Road Riders of Chicagoland**
P.O. Box 14033, Chicago, Illinois 60614.
☎ 708 795 1803

☞ **Rodeo Riders**
3516 North Bosworth, Chicago, Illinois 60657.

Organizations: Sexuality

☞ **American College Personnel Association**
Standing Committee for Lesbian, Gay, & Bisexual Awareness, Campus Housing M/C579, Room 317 SRH, 818 South Wolcott Street, Chicago, Illinois 60612-3727.
Contact: Ms. Jo Campbell

♂ ♡ **Bi Chicago**
P. O. Box 408808, Chicago, Illinois 60640.
☎ 312 275 0186
Publishes a newsletter every month.

☞♡ **Black & White Men Together (BWMT)—Chicago**
♿ 2863 North Clark Street, Chicago, Illinois 60657.
☎ 312 334 2012 ✆ 312 907 0083
☎ 800 624 2968 (national line)
Publishes a newsletter.

↘♡ **Chicago Gender Society**
♿ P. O. Box 578005, Chicago, Illinois 60657.
☎ 312 863 7714
⏰ Meets 2nd. Tue, 4th. Tue, & 4th. Sat of month
Publishes *The Primrose.*

☞♡ **Fox Valley Gay Association**
♿ P. O. Box 393, Elgin, Illinois 60120.
☎ 708 931 1110
⏰ Mon - Fri 19:00 - 22:00
Publishes *Fox Tales.*

☞♡ **Gay & Lesbian Community Center of Chicago**
♿ 2863 North Clark Street, Chicago, Illinois 60657.
☎ 312 665 5300 ✆ 312 665 5329

☞♡ **Horizons Community Services, Inc.**
♿ 961 West Montana, Chicago, Illinois 60614.
☎ 312 472 6469
☎ 312 929 4357 (helpline)
⏰ Mon - Thu 09:00 - 22:00; helpline 18:00 - 22:00. TDD 312 327 4357

☞♡ **Midwest Men's Center, Chicago**
P. O. Box 2547, Chicago, Illinois 60690.
☎ 312 348 3254
Publishes *Men Nurturing News.*

☞♡ **North Suburban Gay Association**
♿ P. O. Box 465, Wilmette, Illinois 60091.
☎ 708 251 8853

↘♡ **The Sunday Society**
P. O. Box 478850, Chicago, Illinois 60647.
☎ 312 486 3126
☎ 312 252 7024
⏰ Meets 3rd. Sun of month
Contact: Ms. Sheila L.
Support group.

Organizations: Sexuality: Student

☞♡ **Northwestern University Bisexual, Gay, & Lesbian Alliance**
♿ 1999 Sheridan Road, Evanston, Illinois 60201.
☎ 708 491 2375

☞♡ **Pride at UIC**
♿ P. O. Box 4348 M/C 118, Chicago, Illinois 60680.
☎ 312 996 4424
⏰ Mon - Fri 09:00 - 17:00

☞♡ **University of Chicago Gay & Lesbian Alliance**
♿ Room 207, 1212 East 59th. Street, Chicago, Illinois 60637.
☎ 312 702 9734

Organizations: Spirituality

☺ ☐ **Radical Faerie Circle—Chicago**
Coach House, 812 North Noble, Chicago, Illinois 60622-5352.
☎ 312 235 8315
Publishes a newsletter every two months. Yearly subscription is $5.

Photographers: Erotic

☺ **Steinmeier Photography**
Suite 712 S, 680 North Lake Shore Drive, Chicago, Illinois 60611.
☎ 312 642 4707 ✆ 312 951 0920
Catalogue, $5.

Photographers: Fetish

☺ **Steve Abrams**
P. O. Box 14239, Chicago, Illinois 60614.
☎ 312 868 1542

Piercers

☺ **Hank Bangćok**
613 West Briar, Chicago, Illinois 60657.
☎ 312 404 5838

☺ ■ **Body Basics**
613 West Briar, Chicago, Illinois 60657.
☎ 312 404 5838 ✆ 312 404 5898
✉ bbasics@interserv.com
🌐 http://www.io.org/~bbasics/
⏰ Tue - Sat 14:00 - 22:00
💳 💲 ▨▨ MC

☺ ■ **Chris**
☎ 312 404 6107
⏰ By appointment only

☺ ■ **House of Whacks**
1800 West Cornelia, Chicago, Illinois.
☎ 312 761 6969 ✆ 312 761 4375
✉ Whacks1@interaccess.com
🌐 http://www.interaccess.com/Secrets/Whacks.html
⏰ Fri 16:00 - 20:00, Sat 14:00 - 20:00
💳 💲 ▨▨ MC
Catalogue, $12U.S., $15U.S. foreign. Age statement of 18 is required.

Printers: General

☺ **Adams Press**
Suite 1920, 500 North Michigan Avenue, Chicago, Illinois 60611.
☎ 708 676 3426 ✆ 312 326 3838

☺ **R. R. Donnelly & Sons**
2223 Martin Luther King Drive, Chicago, Illinois 60616.
☎ 312 326 8000 ✆ 312 326 8543

Publishers: Directories: Sexuality

✪ **Alternative Phone Book**
Suite 114, 425 West Surf Street, Chicago, Illinois 60657.

✪▽ **The Directory of Bookstores Specializing in Gay, Lesbian, & Feminist Books**
American Library Association, Gay & Lesbian Task Force, c/o O. L. D. S., 50 East Huron Street, Chicago, Illinois 60611.

☺ ▽ **The Directory of Professional Groups of Gays & Lesbians**
American Library Association, Gay & Lesbian Task Force, c/o O. L. D. S., 50 East Huron Street, Chicago, Illinois 60611.

✪▼ **The Lesbian & Gay Pink Pages, Chicago**
DAC Marketing, Inc., Suite 779, 3023 North Clark Street, Chicago, Illinois 60657.
☎ 800 982 4717
☎ 312 549 3709

✪▼ **OUT! Resource Guide**
Lambda Publications, Suite 2-D, 1115 West Belmont Avenue, Chicago, Illinois 60657.
☎ 312 871 7610 ✆ 312 871 7609
✉ outlines@interaccess.com
✓
Lesbian, gay, & bisexual resources in the Chicago area. Published twice a year.

Publishers: Magazines: BDSM

✪▼ **Red Plaid**
The James Publishing Group, Inc., P. O. Box 148005, Chicago, Illinois 60614-8005.
Extreme BDSM art, stories, & photos. Published quarterly. Yearly subscription is $28. Age statement of 21 is required.

Publishers: Magazines: Sexuality

✪ **Open Hands**
3801 North Keeler Avenue, Chicago, Illinois 60641.
☎ 312 736 5526 ✆ 312 736 5475

♂ **Playboy**
680 North Lake Shore Drive, Chicago, Illinois 60611.
☎ 312 751 8000
🌐 http://www.playboy.com/

Publishers: Newspapers: General

☺ ■ **Chicago Tribune**
435 North Michigan Avenue, Chicago, Illinois 60611-4041.
☎ 312 222 5991 ✆ 312 222 3650

Publishers: Newspapers: Sexuality

✪ **Concord**
P. O. Box 10461, Chicago, Illinois 60610.

✪▽ **Gay Chicago Magazine**
🖘 Ultra Ink, Inc., 3121 North Broadway, Chicago, Illinois 60657-4522.
☎ 312 327 7271 ✆ 312 327 0112
An arts & entertainment guide to Chiago's gay & lesbian community. Published every week. Yearly subscription is $96.

✪ **Nightlines**
Lambda Publications, Suite 2-D, 1115 West Belmont Avenue, Chicago, Illinois 60657.
☎ 312 871 7610 ✆ 312 871 7609
✉ outlines@interaccess.com
✓
Weekly entertainment, calendar, sports, & humour guide for Chicago gays & lesbians. Published every week. Yearly subscription is $48.

✪▼ **Outlines**
Lambda Publications, Suite 2-D, 1115 West Belmont Avenue, Chicago, Illinois 60657.
☎ 312 871 7610 ✆ 312 871 7609
✉ outlines@interaccess.com
✓
Monthly news, entertainment, & features. Chicago, national, & international information for gays & lesbians. Published every month. Yearly subscription is $32.

✪ **Plus Voice**
1258 West Belmont Avenue, Chicago, Illinois 60657-3207.

✪▼ **Windy City Times**
Sentury Publications, 2nd. Floor, 970 West Montana Street, Chicago, Illinois 60614.
☎ 312 935 1790 ✆ 312 935 1853

Stores: Barber Supplies

☺ **Valentine & Son, Inc.**
34 West Van Buren Street, Chicago, Illinois 60604.
☎ 312 939 3221

☎ 312 922 6881
Barber shop that usually has violet wands in stock.

Stores: Books: General

☺ **Barbara's Bookstore**
3130 North Broadway, Chicago, Illinois 60657.
☎ 312 477 0411
☎ 312 281 2333

☺ ▼ **Left Bank Bookstall**
♿ 104 South Oak Park Avenue, Oak Park, Illinois 60302.
☎ 708 383 4700

✪▼ **People Like Us**
1115 West Belmont, Chicago, Illinois 60657.
☎ 312 248 6363 ✆ 312 248 1550
✉ plubooks@aol.com
🕙 10:00 - 21:00
💳 ✓ 💳 💳 💳
Free 32-page catalogue published twice a year.

✪▼ **The Pride Agenda Bookshop**
♿ 1109 Westgate, Oak Park, Illinois 60301.
☎ 708 524 8429

☺ ■ **Unabridged Books**
3251 North Broadway, Chicago, Illinois 60657.
☎ 312 883 9119
🕙 Mon - Fri 10:00 - 22:00, Sat Sun 10:00 - 20:00
💳 ✓ 💳 💳 💳

Stores: Clothing: Fetish

☺ ■ **Dressed To Kill**
3635 North Broadway, Chicago, Illinois 60613.
☎ 312 248 1860

Stores: Clothing: Leather

☺ ▼ **The Alley**
858 West Belmont Avenue, Chicago, Illinois 60657.
☎ 312 883 1800
🕙 Mon - Fri 10:00 - 22:00, Sat 10:00 - 01:00, Sun 12:00 - 21:00
💳 ✓ 💳 💳 💳

☺ ■ **Carline Leathers**
5328 North Wayne Avenue, Chicago, Illinois 60640.
☎ 312 334 1444 ✆ 312 334 1470

Stores: Clothing: Rubber

☺ **House of Whacks**
♿ 4017 North Damen Avenue, Chicago, Illinois 60618.
☎ 312 761 6969 ✆ 312 761 4375
✉ Whacks1@interaccess.com
🌐 http://ww.interaccess.com/Secrets/Whacks.html
🕙 Fri 16:00 - 20:00, Sat 14:00 - 20:00
💳 $ ✓ 💳 💳 💳
Catalogue, $12U.S., $15U.S. foreign. Age statement of 18 is required.

Stores: Clothing: Sexuality

⚤ **Translucere**
♿ 2652 North Lincoln Street, Chicago, Illinois 60614.
☎ 312 477 6006 ✆ 312 477 6044
🕙 Tue - Sat 12:00 - 19:00
💳 $ ✓ 💳 💳
Clothing, makeovers, breastforms, 5''-7'' high-heels, books, wigs, corsets, etc. for cross-dressers. Catalogue available, published once a year. Spanish also spoken.

Stores: Clothing: Uniforms

☺ ■ **Advance Uniform Co.**
1132 South Wabash, Chicago, Illinois.
☎ 312 922 1797
🕙 Mon - Fri 08:00 17:30, Sat 08:00 - 15:00
Manufactures uniforms of all sorts.

☺ ■ **VGC Uniforms**
5050 West Irving Park Road, Chicago, Illinois.
☎ 312 545 3676

☺ ■ **VGC Uniforms**
10626 South Western Avenue, Chicago, Illinois.
☎ 312 779 6121

Stores: Erotica: BDSM

☺ **The Black Market**
116 North Milwaukee Avenue, Chicago, Illinois 60612.
☎ 312 278 6780
✉ bmc@texcat.com
🕙 Tue - Fri 12:00 - 20:00, Sat Sun 11:00 - 17:00

☺ ▼ **Caliber**
♿ 5015 North Clark Street, Chicago, Illinois 60640.
☎ 312 728 7228 (retail)

☎ 312 878 3038 (studio)
Inside the Eagle bar.

☺ ▼ **Male Hide Leathers**
⚥ 2816 North Lincoln Avenue, Chicago, Illinois 60657.
☎ 312 929 0069 ✆ 312 348 5493
🕐 Tue - Sat 12:00 - 20:00, Sun 13:00 - 17:00
✓ 🚗 💳 🖃

☺ **Px3**
P. O. Box 388361, Chicago, Illinois 60638.
☎ 312 854 6172
Catalogue, $2, applied to first order.

Stores: Erotica: General

☺ ■ **99th. Floor**
33406 North Halsted Street, Chicago, Illinois 60657.
☎ 312 348 7781 ✆ 312 348 1405
🕐 Mon - Fri 12:00- 20:00, Fri Sat 12:00 - 22:00, Sun 12:00 - 18:00
⚙ 💳 💳
General clothing store with extensive fetsih collection.

☺ ■ **Cupid's Treasures**
⚥ 3519 North Halsted, Chicago, Illinois 60657.
☎ 800 287 4370 ✆ 312 348 0976
☎ 312 348 3884
🕐 Sun - Thu 11:00 - 24:00, Fri Sat 11:00 -01:00
⚙ ✓ ✔ 💳 💳 🖃 🖃
An erotic love boutique. Catalogue, $7U.S.. Age statement of 18 is required.

☺ ▼ **Pleasure Chest**
⚥ 3143 North Broadway, Chicago, Illinois 60657.
☎ 312 525 7151

⚥ ■ **Quimby's Queer Store**
⚥ 1328 North Damen Avenue, Chicago, Illinois 60622.
☎ 312 342 0910
🕐 Mon - Sat 11:00 - 22:00, Sun 12:00 - 20:00
⚙ ✓ 💳 💳
Catalogue, $2. Age statement of 18 is required.

☺ ■ **Ram Bookstore**
3511 1/2 North Halsted, Chicago, Illinois 60657.
☎ 312 525 9528

☺ **Taboo Tabou**
⚥ 852 West Belmont Avenue, Chicago, Illinois 60657.
☎ 312 548 2266
☎ 312 723 3739
🕐 11:00 - 21:30
⚙ ✓ 💳 💳 🖃
Full fetish store, carrying latex, leather, PVC, & corsets.

Stores: Military Surplus

☺ ■ **Army Navy Surplus U.S.A.**
3100 North Lincoln, Chicago, Illinois.
☎ 312 348 8930

☺ ■ **Belmont Army Surplus**
945 West Belmont, Chicago, Illinois.
☎ 312 975 0626

☺ ■ **Dugout Ltd.**
5214 West Irving Park Road, Chicago, Illinois.
☎ 312 777 1496
Uniforms & other military supplies.

☺ ■ **United Army Surplus**
1544 West Howard, Chicago, Illinois.
☎ 312 671 8610

Suppliers: Market Research

⚥ **Overlooked Opinions, Inc.**
Suite 277, 3712 North Broadway, Chicago, Illinois 60613.
Publishes *In Full View*.

Tattooists

☺ ■ **No Hope * No Fear**
#306, 1579 North Milwaukee Avenue, Chicago, Illinois 60622.
☎ 312 772 1960
🕐 Tue - Sat 12:00 - 20:00
⚙
Piercing also available. Age statement of 18 is required.

Television: AIDS

☺ **HIV Update**
c/o PAAC, Suite 200, 101 West Grand Avenue, Chicago, Illinois 60610.
☎ 312 222 1326

De Kalb

Organizations: Motorcycle

⚥▽ **Trident—Windy City**

P. O. Box 180, De Kalb, Illinois 60115.
Contact: Mr. Robert Ridinger.

Organizations: Sexuality: Student

⚥▽ **Lesbian, Gay, & Bisexual Coalition**
⚥ Room 256A, Holmes Student Center, Northern Illinois University, De Kalb, Illinois 60115.
☎ 815 753 0584
Publishes *Prideletter*.

Des Plaines

Publishers: Newspapers: Sexuality

⚥ **Suburban Network**
P. O. Box 1770, Des Plaines, Illinois 60017-1770.

Edwardsville

Organizations: Sexuality: Student

⚥▽ **Gay & Lesbian Association of Students at SIU-E**
⚥ P. O. Box 1168, Edwardsville, Illinois 62026.
☎ 618 692 2686

Galesburg

Organizations: Sexuality: Student

⚥▽ **Gay & Lesbian Community Alliance**
Box K1648, Knox College, Galesburg, Illinois 61401.

Stores: Erotica: General

☺ ■ **Galesburg Adult Book & Video**
595 North Henderson Street, Galesburg, Illinois 61401.
☎ 309 342 7019

Glen Ellyn

Organizations: Sexuality

⚥▽ **West Suburban Gay Association**
P. O. Box 161, Glen Ellyn, Illinois 60138.
☎ 708 790 9742 (info hotline)
🕐 Mon - Thu 19:00 - 22:30
⚙ ✓
Publishes *WSGA News*. Age statement of 21 is required.

Highland Park

Counsellors

⚥▽ **Ronald Baron, M.D.**
2120 Sheridan Road, Highland Park, Illinois 60035.
☎ 708 432 7007
Psychiatrist.

Lake Bluff

Distributors: Books: General

☺ **Quality Books**
918 Sherwood Drive, Lake Bluff, Illinois 60044-2204.
☎ 708 295 2010 ✆ 708 295 1556

Lake Villa

Manufacturers: Chastity Belts

☺ **Chastete**
25302 Columbia Bay Drive, Lake Villa, Illinois 60046.
☎ 708 356 8300
Catalogue, $5U.S..

Monticello

Manufacturers: Adult Toys: Masturbation

☺ ■ **Abco Research Associates**
P. O. Box 354, Monticello, Illinois 61856.
☎ 217 762 2141 ✆ 217 762 7500
🕐 Mon - Fri 09:00 - 22:00 Central
Produces high tech masturbation devices for men & women. Catalogue, $3. Age statement of 21 is required.

Peoria

Health Services

☺ ☐ **Peoria City County Health Department**
⚥ 2116 North Sheridan Road, Peoria, Illinois 61604.
☎ 309 679 6028
Anonymous STD & HIV testing.

Riverside

Photographers: Fetish

⚥ **Ron Volanti**

P. O. Box 236, Riverside, Illinois 60546.
☎ 708 484 8412

Rock Island
Organizations: Motorcycle
☼ **Blackhawk MC**
313 20th. Street, Rock Island, Illinois 61201.
☎ 309 788 7389

Rockford
Organizations: AIDS: Education
☺ ☐ **AIDS Care Network**
♿ Suite 165, 221 North Longwood Street, Rockford, Illinois 61107-4171.
☎ 815 968 2437
Publishes *Bridges*.

Organizations: Bears
☼▽ **Rock Valley Bears**
P. O. Box 4341, Rockford, Illinois 61110.
☎ 815 963 7962
✉ ilbear@aol.com
🕸 http://www.geopages.com/WestHollywood/1065/

South Bend
Distributors: Books: General
☺ **the distributors**
702 South Michigan, South Bend, Illinois 46618-1622.
☎ 219 232 8500 📞 219 233 3607
☎ 219 232 8500 Ext. 27

Springfield
Organizations: Sexuality
♋▽ **Springfield Area Lesbian Outreach (SALO)**
☊ P. O. Box 5487, Springfield, Illinois 62705.
☎ 217 525 4297

Stores: Books: General
☺▼ **Sundance**
1428 East Sangamon Avenue, Springfield, Illinois 62702.
☎ 217 788 5243 📞 217 788 5243

Villa Park
Organizations: Sexuality
☺▼ **Review**
P. O. Box 7406, Villa Park, Illinois 60131.
☎ 708 620 6946
🕐 21:00 - 23:00. Meets 2nd. Tue of month 19:30
Contact: Mr. Jerry Walters
Support & information for gay & bisexual married men.

Washington
Organizations: Sexuality
♋☐ **Central Illinois Gender Association (CIGA)**
P. O. Box 182, Washington, Illinois 61571.
☎ 309 444 9918
🕐 Best to call between 19:00 - 21:30
Contact: Ms. Joann Fraser, Secretary
Support group for transgendered & gender-conflicted people. Publishes
Finesse every month. Yearly subscription is $20.

Wheaton
Organizations: Polyfidelity
☺■ **Alternatives to Monogamy**
P. O. Box 4172, Wheaton, Illinois 60189-4172.
☎ 708 510 7027
✉ nudist@rci.ripco.com

Winfield
Organizations: BDSM
☼ **D. A. D. S.**
P.O. Box 573, Winfield, Illinois 60190.

Winnetka
Stores: Erotica: General
☺■ **Glove Me Tender**
1007 Green Bay Road, Winnetka, Illinois 60093.
☎ 708 501 2880
Every imaginable kind of glove.

Wood Dale
Organizations: Sexuality
♋▽ **The Society for the Second Self (Tri-Ess)—Chi**
P. O. Box 40, Wood Dale, Illinois 60191-0040.
☎ 708 364 9514
Publishes a newsletter.

Woodridge
Publishers: Magazines: BDSM
⚧■ *Passion, Our Leather Soul*
Diamond, Suite 54A, 8280 James Avenue, Woodridge, Illinois 60517.
For femdoms.

INDIANA
Area: Approximately 93,000 square kilometres
Population: Approximately 5,560,000
Capital City: Indianapolis
Time zone: GMT minus 5/6 hours (both EST & CST)
Climate: Warm & humid summers with temperatures averaging approximately 24°C. Winters are cold & potentially snowy, with temperatures averaging -2°C in mid-winter.
Age of consent & homosexuality legislation: State has adopted the Model Penal Code or otherwise decriminalized homosexual activities.
Legal drinking age: 21

State Resources
Organizations: AIDS: Education
☺☐ **Indiana CARES, Inc.**
Suite 101, 3951 North Meridian Street, Indianapolis, Indiana 46208.
☎ 317 630 9075

Organizations: Bears
☼▽ **Hoosier Bears of Indiana**
P. O. Box 531311, Indianapolis, Indiana 46254-1311.
☎ 317 293 4394
✉ dallas@indy.win.net
🕸 http://www.skepsis.com:80/_gblo/bears/CLUBS/Hoosier_Bears/
🕐 Meets 2nd. Sun of month 14:00
Publishes *Bear-Trax*. Age statement of 21 is required.

Organizations: Sexuality
♋☐ **Indiana Crossdressers Society (IXE)**
♿ P. O. Box 20710, Indianapolis, Indiana 46220.
☎ 317 781 0834
☎ 812 876 5635
Mainly heterosexual members, but some gays. Publishes a newsletter every month.
♋▽ **Out & About Indiana**
☊ Suite 105, 133 West Market Street, Indianapolis, Indiana 46204-2801.
☎ 317 925 9126 📞 317 925 2401
Out & About Indiana is the state's largest, most active social & recreational organization for gay men, lesbian women, & their friends. Publishes *OUTlines* every month. Yearly subscription is $12.
♋▽ **Tri-State Alliance**
☊ P. O. Box 2901, Evansville, Indiana 47728-0901.
☎ 812 484 4853

Publishers: Newspapers: Sexuality
☼▼ *Indiana Word*
Word Publications, Suite 2800, Tower 1, 225 East North Street, Indianapolis, Indiana 46204-1349.
☎ 317 579 3075 📞 317 687 8840
🕐 24hr. answering machine
✍
Men-oriented, three state editions (Kentucky, Ohio, & Indiana). No 900 ads or nudity. Published every month.

Bloomington
Health Services
☺☐ **Bloomington Hospital**
601 West Second Street, Bloomington, Indiana 47403.
☎ 812 336 6821

Organizations: Research: Sexuality
☺ **The Kinsey Institute**
Morrison Hall 313, Bloomington, Indiana 47405-2501.
☎ 812 855 7686 📞 812 855 8277
✉ libknsy@indiana.edu
🕸 gopher://lib-gopher.lib.indiana.edu:7040/1/1/kinsey

Organizations: Sexuality: Student
♋▽ **OUT**

Room 48-G, Indiana Memorial Union, Indiana University, Bloomington,
Indiana 47405.
☎ 812 855 5688

Radio: General

☻ □ **WFHB**
P. O. Box 1973, Bloomington, Indiana 47402.
☎ 812 323 1200

Stores: Books: General

☻ ▼ **Aquarius Books**
306 South Washington Street, Bloomington, Indiana 47401-3529.
☎ 812 336 0988
⏱ 11:00 - 18:00, Sat 10:00 - 17:00, Sun 13:00 - 16:00

Eldridge

Printers: General

☺ **Bawden Printing, Inc.**
400 South 14th. Avenue, Eldridge, Indiana 52748.
☎ 319 285 4800 📞 319 285 8240

Evansville

Health Services

☺ ☐ **Saint Mary's Medical Center of Evansville**
3700 Washington Avenue, Evansville, Indiana 47714.
☎ 812 479 4000

Organizations: AIDS: Education

☺ □ **AIDS Resource Group of Evansville, Inc.**
⑃ Suite 301, Old Courthouse, 201 North West 4th. Street, Evansville,
Indiana 47708-1357.
☎ 812 421 0059

Organizations: Family

⚥▽ **Evansville Gay & Lesbian Parents Coalition**
P. O. Box 2794, Evansville, Indiana 47728.
☎ 812 422 4075

Stores: Books: General

☺ ▼ **A. A. Michael Books**
⑃ 1541 South Green River Road, Evansville, Indiana 47700.
☎ 812 479 8979

Fishers

Piercers

☺ ■ **Body Accents**
☎ 317 842 0569
⏱ By appointment
Above the belt piercing only.

Fort Wayne

Counsellors

☺ ▼ **Family Study Institute of Fort Wayne**
⑃ Suite 220, 909 North Coliseum Boulevard, Fort Wayne, Indiana 46805.
☎ 219 424 2455

Health Services

☺ □ **Parkview Memorial Hospital**
2200 Randallia Drive, Fort Wayne, Indiana 46805.
☎ 219 484 6636

☺ □ **Saint Joseph Medical Center**
700 Broadway, Fort Wayne, Indiana 46802.
☎ 219 425 3000

☺ □ **STD Clinic**
⑃ Room 505, City Council Building, 1 East Main Street, Fort Wayne,
Indiana 46802.
☎ 219 428 7504
STD & HIV testing by appointment.

☺ □ **Veterans' Affairs Medical Center**
2121 Lake Avenue, Fort Wayne, Indiana 46805.
☎ 219 426 5431

Helplines: Sexuality

⚥▽ **Gay & Lesbian Helpline**
☎ 219 744 1199
⏱ Mon - Thu 19:00 - 22:00, Fri Sat - 24:00, Sun - 21:00

Organizations: AIDS: Education

☺ □ **AIDS Task Force, Inc.**
⑃ P. O. Box 13527, Fort Wayne, Indiana 46869.
☎ 219 744 1144

Organizations: Bears

⚥▽ **Old Fort Bears**
P. O. Box 6535, Fort Wayne, Indiana 46896.

Organizations: Sexuality

⚲▽ **Ladies After Dark**
P. O. Box 4389, Fort Wayne, Indiana 46895.

⚥▽ **Up The Stairs Community Center**
3426 Broadway, Fort Wayne, Indiana 46807.
☎ 219 744 1144
⏱ Mon - Thu 19:00 - 22:00, Fri Sat - 24:00, Sun 19:00 - 21:00

Goshen

Organizations: AIDS: Education

☺ □ **Oaklawn**
⑃ P. O. Box 46526, Goshen, Indiana 46527.
☎ 219 533 1234

Greenwood

Organizations: Polyfidelity

☺ ■ **Loving Alternatives**
P. O. Box 1322, Greenwood, Indiana 46162.
✉ poli@holli.com

Indianapolis

Archives: Sexuality

⚥▽ **Fort Wayne Gay & Lesbian Resource Center &
Archives**
c/o Up The Stairs Community Center, 3426 Broadway, Indianapolis,
Indiana 46807.
☎ 219 744 1144

BBSs: BDSM

☺ □ **B&D Comm**
📞 317 784 6975

Counsellors

☺ ■ **Eric Applegate, PC, MS, NACA II, AAMFT, CST**
⑃ Suite 18, 2625 North Meridian, Indianapolis, Indiana 46208.
☎ 317 925 1881

Health Services

☺ □ **Indiana University Medical Center**
550 North University Boulevard, Indianapolis, Indiana 46202.
☎ 317 274 5000
HIV & emergency departments.

☺ □ **Infectious Diseases Clinic**
⑃ Free Anonymous Test Site, 1101 West 10th. Street, Indianapolis,
Indiana 46202.
☎ 317 635 8378

☺ □ **Methodist Hospital of Indiana**
I-65 at 21st. Street, Indianapolis, Indiana 46202.
☎ 317 929 2000

☺ □ **Richard Roudebush Veterans' Affairs Medical
Center**
1481 West Tenth Street, Indianapolis, Indiana 46202.
☎ 317 635 7401

☺ □ **Saint Vincent Hospital & Health Care Center**
2001 West 86th. Street, Indianapolis, Indiana 46202.
☎ 317 338 2345

☺ □ **William Wishard Memorial Hospital**
1001 West Tenth Street, Indianapolis, Indiana 46202.
☎ 317 639 6671
HIV & emergency departments.

Helplines: AIDS

☺ □ **Indiana AIDS Hotline**
P. O. Box 2152, Indianapolis, Indiana 46206.
☎ 317 257 4673
⏱ 19:00 - 23:00

Helplines: Sexuality

⚥▽ **Gay & Lesbian Switchboard**
P. O. Box 2152, Indianapolis, Indiana 46206.
☎ 317 639 5937
⏱ 19:00 - 23:00

Organizations: AIDS: Education

☺ □ **Damien Center**
⑃ 1350 North Pennsylvania, Indianapolis, Indiana 46202.
☎ 317 632 0123

Organizations: BDSM

☺ □ **A.S.B. Munch—Indianapolis**
📧 kalee@indy.net
Contact: Monika

⚥▽ **The National Leather Association (NLA)—
Indianapolis**
1310 North Oakland Avenue, Indianapolis, Indiana 46201.
☎ 317 634 4272

Organizations: Bears

⚥ **Omikron**
P.O. Box 44234, Indianapolis, Indiana 46244-0234.

Organizations: Sexuality

⚥▽ **Black & White Men Together (BWMT)—
Indianapolis**
P.O. Box 88784, Indianapolis, Indiana 46208.
☎ 317 253 4297

Organizations: Sexuality: Student

⚥▽ **The IUPUI Advocate**
♿ Box 37m University Library O06A, 815 West Michigan Street,
Indianapolis, Indiana 46202.
☎ 317 274 0079

Organizations: Sexuality: Youth

⚥▽ **Indianapolis Youth Group**
P.O. Box 20716, Indianapolis, Indiana 46220-0716.
☎ 317 541 8726
☎ 800 347 8336 (teen hotline)
Publishes *IYG Reachout*.

Piercers

☺ ■ **Future Shock**
6323 Ferguson, Indianapolis, Indiana 46220.
☎ 317 251 6957

Stores: Books: General

☺ ▼ **Bookland**
♿ 137 West Market Street, Indianapolis, Indiana 46204.
☎ 317 639 9864

☺ ■ **Borders Book Shop**
♿ 5612 Castleton Corner Lane, Indianapolis, Indiana 46250.
☎ 317 849 8660
🕐 09:00 - 21:00, SUN 11:00 - 17:00

♿ ▼ **Dreams & Swords**
6503 Ferguson Street, Indianapolis, Indiana 46220-1148.
☎ 800 937 2706
☎ 317 253 9966
Free catalogue.

Stores: Erotica: General

⚥▼ **Body Works Shop**
4120 North Keystone Avenue, Indianapolis, Indiana 46205.
☎ 317 547 9210

Lafayette

Organizations: AIDS: Education

☺ ▽ **Project AIDS Lafayette (PAL)**
♿ P.O. Box 5375, Lafayette, Indiana 47903.
☎ 800 524 3229 (in state)
☎ 317 742 2305

Organizations: Sexuality: Student

⚥▽ **The Network**
Box 512, Purdue Memorial Union, West Lafayette, Indiana 47906.

⚥▽ **Purdue Gay Alliance**
Box 687, Stewart Center, Purdue University, Lafayette, Indiana 47907.
☎ 812 497 2712

Michigan City

Stores: Clothing: Fetish

☺ ■ **Naughty But Nice**
104 West US Highway 30, Michigan City, Indiana 46360.
☎ 219 879 6363

Mishawaka

Organizations: BDSM

⚥ **Firekeepers of Indiana**
P.O. Box 1043, Mishawaka, Indiana 46546.

Muncie

Organizations: Sexuality: Student

⚥▽ **Gays & Lesbians at Notre Dame / Saint Mary's
♿ College**
P.O. Box 194, Muncie, Indiana 46556.

⚥▽ **Lesbian & Gay Student Association**
Box 400, Student Center, Muncie, Indiana 47306.

Richmond

Organizations: Sexuality: Student

⚥▽ **Earlham Lesbian, Bisexual, & Gay People's Union**
P.O. Drawer 279, Earlham College, Richmond, Indiana 47374.
☎ 317 983 1436

Piercers

☺ ■ **Red Ring Studios**
139 1/2 South 5th. Street, Richmond, Indiana 47374.
☎ 317 966 4667
🕐 By appointment only

South Bend

Health Services

☺ □ **Memorial Hospital of South Bend**
615 North Michigan Street, South Bend, Indiana 46601.
☎ 219 234 9041

☺ □ **Saint Joseph County Health Department**
♿ 9th. Floor, County-City Building, 227 West Jefferson Boulevard, South
Bend, Indiana 46601.
☎ 219 284 9725

☺ □ **Saint Joseph's Medical Center**
801 East LaSalle, South Bend, Indiana 46617.
☎ 219 237 7111

Organizations: AIDS: Education

☺ ▽ **Michiana AIDS Support Group**
♿ P.O. Box 1521, South Bend, Indiana 46634.
☎ 219 232 6930

Organizations: Sexuality

⚥▽ **Open Arms**
P.O. Box 845, Mishawaka, Indiana 46544.
🕐 Meets monthly

Organizations: Sexuality: Student

⚥▽ **OUT**
♿ Room U100F, IUSB Student Association, 1700 Mishawaka Avenue,
South Bend, Indiana 46615.
☎ 219 237 4125

Stores: Erotica: General

☺ ▼ **Little Denmarks Books**
3002 Western Avenue, South Bend, Indiana 46619.
☎ 219 233 9538

Terre Haute

Organizations: Sexuality: Student

⚥▽ **Lambda Group**
c/o Box 18, Hulman Memorial Student Union, Indiana State University,
Terre Haute, Indiana 47809.

IOWA

Area: Approximately 145,000 square kilometres
Population: Approximately 2,900,000
Capital City: Des Moines
Time zone: GMT minus 6 hours (CST)
Climate: Hot, humid summers, with average highs of approxiamtely 24°C.
Cold winters with average lows of approximately -7°C.
Age of consent & homosexuality legislation: State has adopted the
Model Penal Code or otherwise decriminalized homosexual activities.
Legal drinking age: 21

State Resources

Publishers: Magazines: Sexuality

♀ □ ***Iowa Woman Magazine***
Iowa Woman Endeavors, Inc., P.O. Box 680, Iowa City, Iowa 52244-
0680.
📧 rbailey@blue.weeg.uiowa.edu
Grassroots organization with educational mission to provide a public
forum for communication among women. Literature & visual art by
women. Published quarterly. Yearly subscription is $20U.S..

Ames

Helplines: Sexuality

☿▽ **Lesbian, Gay, & Bisexual Alliance**
 ᕫ 39 Memorial Union, Ames, Iowa 50011.
 ☎ 515 294 2104

Organizations: Sexuality

☿▽ **Gays, Lesbians, & Bisexuals of Ames (GLBA)**
 ᕫ P. O. Box 1761, Ames, Iowa 50010-1761.
 ☎ 515 233 5000
 Publishes *GLB Ames Newsletter*.

Organizations: Sexuality: Student

☿▽ **Lesbian, Gay, & Bisexual Alliance**
 ᕫ 39 Memorial Union, Ames, Iowa 50011.
 ☎ 515 294 2104
 Publishes *The Rainbow Connection*.

Piercers

☺ ■ **Lasting Impressions**
 111 Main Street, Ames, Iowa.
 ☎ 515 233 2819

Stores: Erotica: General

☺ ■ **Pleasure Palace II**
 117 Kellogg Street, Ames, Iowa 50010.
 ☎ 515 232 7717

Cedar Rapids

Organizations: AIDS: Education

☺ ☐ **Rapids AIDS Project**
 ᕫ American Red Cross, 3601 42nd. Street North East, Cedar Rapids, Iowa 52402-7111.
 ☎ 319 393 9579

Organizations: Sexuality

☿▽ **Gay & Lesbian Resource Center**
 ᕫ P. O. Box 1643, Cedar Rapids, Iowa 52406.
 ☎ 319 366 2055

☿▽ **Iowa Artistry**
 P. O. Box 75, Cedar Rapids, Iowa 52406.
 ✉ scottm@ins.infonet.net
 Support group. Publishes a newsletter every two months.

Piercers

☺ ■ **Arbuckle's Tattoo & piercing Emporium**
 97 1/2 16th. Avnue South West, Cedar Rapids, Iowa 52404.
 ☎ 319 363 1242

Council Bluffs

Organizations: BDSM

☿ **Midlands Communication Network**
 Box 103B, RR3, Council Bluffs, Iowa 51503-9427.
 Contact: Mr. Tom Winfield

Organizations: Sexuality

☿▽ **River City Gender Alliance (RCGA)**
 P. O. Box 680, Council Bluffs, Iowa 51502-0680.
 Meets monthly. Publishes *The Transformer* every two months.

Stores: Erotica: General

☺ ■ **Off Broadway Emporium**
 3216 1st. Avenue, Council Bluffs, Iowa 51501.
 ☎ 712 328 2673

Davenport

Organizations: AIDS: Education

☺ ☐ **Quad Cities AIDS Coalition**
 Suite 6A, 605 North Main Street, Davenport, Iowa 52803-5245.
 ☎ 319 324 8638

Organizations: Sexuality

☿▽ **Quad-City Society for Sexuality Education**
 1236 West 8th. Street, Davenport, Iowa 52802.
 ☎ 319 324 6941
 🕐 Call 18:00 - 21:00. Meets 1st. Sun of month 18:00

Publishers: Newspapers: Sexuality

☺ ■ *River Bend Vision*
 P. O. Box 408, Davenport, Iowa 52808-4078.

Des Moines

Counsellors

☿▼ **Central Iowa Gender Institute**
 P. O. Box 12164, Des Moines, Iowa 50312-9403.
 ☎ 515 277 7754

Health Services

☺ ☐ **Broadlands Medical Center**
 1801 Hickman Road, Des Moines, Iowa 50314.
 ☎ 515 282 2200

Organizations: BDSM

☿▽ **Cornhaulers L & L Club**
 P.O. Box 632, Des Moines, Iowa 50303-0632.

Organizations: Sexuality

☿▽ **Gay & Lesbian Resource Center**
 ᕫ 4211 Grand Avenue, Des Moines, Iowa 50312.
 ☎ 515 279 2110
 🕐 Mon - Fri 16:00 - 22:00
 Publishes *GLRC Report*.

☺ ☐ **Parents & Friends of Lesbians & Gays (PFLAG)—**
 ᕫ **Des Moines**
 c/o GLRC, 4211 Grand Avenue, Des Moines, Iowa 50312.
 ☎ 515 274 4851
 🕐 Mon - Fri 09:30 - 16:00

Organizations: Sexuality: Student

☿▽ **Drake University Alternative Lifestyles**
 ᕫ c/o GLRC, 4211 Grand Avenue, Des Moines, Iowa 50312.
 ☎ 515 274 4851
 🕐 Mon - Fri 09:30 - 16:00

Publishers: Newspapers: Sexuality

☿▼ *For You*
 P. O. Box 35092, Des Moines, Iowa 50315-0301.

Stores: Books: General

☺ ■ **Borders Book Shop**
 1821 22nd Street, West Des Moines, Iowa 50265.
 ☎ 515 223 1620

Stores: Erotica: General

☺ ■ **Batchelor's Library**
 2020 East Euclid, Des Moines, Iowa 50317.
 ☎ 515 266 7992

☺ ■ **Gallery Bookstore**
 1114 Walnut Street, Des Moines, Iowa 50309-3426.
 ☎ 515 245 9164

Suppliers: Diapers

☺ ■ **Briggs Corporation**
 P. O. Box 1698, 7887 University Blvd., Des Moines, Iowa 50303-1698.
 ☎ 800 247 2343
 ☎ 800 222 1996
 Health care goods for hospitals, but will sell to the public. Catheters, underpads, rubber sheeting, & cloth & disposable diapers. 712-page catalogue available.

Dubuque

Organizations: AIDS: Education

☺ ☐ **Dubuque Regional AIDS Coalition**
 1016 Rhomberg Avenue, Dubuque, Iowa 52001-3461.
 ☎ 319 589 4181

Evansdale

Organizations: Sexuality

☿▽ **Evansdale Men's Support Group**
 P. O. Box 3133, Evansdale, Iowa 50707-0133.
 ☎ 319 233 4766

Grinnell

Organizations: Sexuality: Student

☺ ▽ **Queer Community**
 ᕫ Office of Student Affairs, P. O. Box 805, Grinnell, Iowa 50112-0810.

Iowa City

Health Services

☺ ☐ **Mercy Hospital**
 500 East Market Street, Iowa City, Iowa 52245.
 ☎ 319 339 0300

Helplines: Sexuality
⚥▽ **LesBiGayline**
⅄ University of Iowa Memorial Union, Iowa City, Iowa 52242.
☎ 319 335 3215

Organizations: Academic: AIDS
⚥▽ **Iowa Center AIDS Resources & Education (ICARE)**
⅄ P. O. Box 2989, Iowa City, Iowa 52244-2989.
☎ 319 338 2135

Organizations: AIDS: Education
☺☐ **AIDS Project**
⅄ 1105 Gilbert Court, Iowa City, Iowa 52240.
☎ 319 356 6040

Organizations: BDSM
⚥▽ **The Ursine Group**
P. O. Box 1143, Iowa City, Iowa 52240.
📟 319 338 5810
✉ IowaBears@avalon.net or cmdltm@mhvax.weeg.uiowa.edu
🌐 http://www.avalon.net/~iowabears/tug/TheUrsineGroup.html

Organizations: Bears
⚥▽ **Bear Paws of Iowa**
P.O. Box 2774, Iowa City, Iowa 52244-2774.
✉ bearjeff@aol.com
🌐 http://www.skepsis.com:80/.gblo/bears/CLUBS/bear_paws.html
Contact: Jeff

Organizations: Sexuality: Student
☺▽ **Spectrum**
⅄ University of Iowa Memorial Union, SAC, Iowa City, Iowa 52242.
☎ 319 354 1703

Piercers
☺■ **Moon Mystique**
Suite 16, 114 1/2 East College, Iowa City, Iowa 52240.
☎ 319 338 5752

Publishers: Newspapers: Sexuality
♋ *Common Lives, Lesbian Lives*
P. O. Box 1553, Iowa City, Iowa 52244.
Seeks to document the experience & thoughts of lesbians as we claim our past, name out present, & envision our evolving futures. Published quarterly. Yearly subscription is $15.

Stores: Books: General
☺▼ **Grassroots Books**
P. O. Box 984, Iowa City, Iowa 52244-0984.
☎ 319 339 4678
🕐 Tue - Sun afternoons & evenings
☺■ **Prairie Lights Bookstore**
⅄ 15 South Dubuque Street, Iowa City, Iowa 52240.
☎ 319 337 2681
🕐 Mon - Fri 09:00 - 21:00, Sat Sun - 17:00
☺■ **University Bookstore**
⅄ University of Iowa, Iowa City, Iowa 52242.
☎ 319 335 3179

Stores: Erotica: General
☺■ **Pleasure Palace I**
315 Kirkwood, Iowa City, Iowa 52244.
☎ 319 351 9444

Iowa Falls
Organizations: Sexuality
⚥▽ **GLNCI / North Central Iowa**
RR3 Box 249, Iowa Falls, Iowa 50126-9421.
Publishes a newsletter.

Mason City
Organizations: AIDS: Education
☺☐ **North Iowa AIDS Project**
⅄ 232 2nd. Street South East, Mason City, Iowa 50401-3906.
☎ 515 423 0025

Mount Vernon
Organizations: Academic: Sexuality
☺ **Society for Scientific Study of Sex**
P.O. Box 208, Mount Vernon, Iowa 52314.
☎ 319 895 8407
📟 319 895 6203
🌐 gopher://lib-gopher.lib.indiana.edu
Contact: Mr. Howard Ruppel

Organizations: Sexuality: Student
⚥▽ **Cornell Gay & Lesbian Alliance**
Old Sem Cornell College, Mount Vernon, Iowa 52314-1098.
☎ 319 895 4224

Waterloo
Organizations: AIDS: Education
☺☐ **AIDS Coalition of North East Iowa**
P. O. Box 1680, Waterloo, Iowa 50704-1680.
☎ 319 234 6831

Organizations: Family
☺☐ **Parents & Friends of Lesbians & Gays (PFLAG)— Waterloo**
317 Hartman Avenue, Waterloo, Iowa 50701-2332.
☎ 319 234 6531

Organizations: Sexuality: Student
⚥▽ **University of Northern Iowa Gay & Lesbian**
⅄ **Outreach (UNIGLOW)**
c/o Counseling Center, SSC 213, Cedar Falls, Iowa 50613.
☎ 319 273 2676

Stores: Erotica: General
☺■ **Danish Book World II**
⅄ 1507 Laporte Road, Waterloo, Iowa 50702.
☎ 319 234 9340
🕐 24hrs.

KANSAS
Area: Approximately 212,000 square kilometres
Population: Approximately 2,490,000
Capital City: Topeka
Time zone: GMT minus 6 hours (CST)
Age of consent & homosexuality legislation: Anal & oral sex is illegal in this state only between people of the same sex.
Legal drinking age: 21

State Resources
Organizations: AIDS: Education
☺▽ **Positive Action Coalition of Kansas, Inc. (PACK)**
P. O. Box 2144, Topeka, Kansas 66601.

Publishers: Newspapers: Sexuality
⚥▼ *Parachute*
P. O. Box 11347, Wichita, Kansas 67202.
☎ 800 536 6519
☎ 316 651 0500

Kansas City
Health Services
☺☐ **University of Kansas Hospital**
3901 Rainbow Boulevard, Kansas City, Kansas 66160.
☎ 913 588 1270

Publishers: Magazines: Sexuality
♂ *Changing Men*
P. O. Box 3121, Kansas City, Kansas 66103-0121.

Stores: Erotica: BDSM
☺■ **Lazy J Leather**
P. O. Box 2702, Kansas City, Kansas 66110.
☎ 913 287 7432
📟 913 287 7432
✓
Publishes *AHS B/D Newsletter* every month.

Kechi
Organizations: Sexuality
☿▽ **Wichita Transgender Alliance**
P. O. Box 315, Kechi, Kansas 67067.
Publishes a newsletter.

Lawrence
Organizations: Sexuality: Student
⚥▽ **LesBiGay Services of Kansas**
⅄ Box 13, University of Kansas, 410 Kansas Union, Lawrence, Kansas 66045.
☎ 913 864 3091
Publishes *The Vanguard*.

Leavenworth
Organizations: Sexuality
▷▽ **CD Research Center**
418 Lyn Street, Leavenworth, Kansas 66048-3437.
Contact: Ms. Rebecca Gail Croslove

Lindsborg
Publishers: Books: Sexuality
☺ **Barbo Carlson Enterprises**
P. O. Box 364, Lindsborg, Kansas 67456.
☎ 913 227 3276

Manhattan
Helplines: Sexuality
⌔▽ **Flint Hills Alliance**
P. O. Box 2018, Manhattan, Kansas 66502-0023.
☎ 913 587 0016

Overland Park
Organizations: Sexuality
▷▽ **Crossdressers & Friends**
P. O. Box 4092, Overland Park, Kansas 66204.
☎ 913 791 3847
🕐 Meets 1st. Thu & 3rd. Sat of month
Male-to-female support. Publishes a newsletter.

Shawnee Mission
Stores: Erotica: BDSM
⌔▼ **The Leather Shop**
Suite 101, 7602 Goddard, Shawnee Mission, Kansas 66214.
☎ 913 268 3652

Topeka
Helplines: Sexuality
⌔▽ **Gay Rap Telephone Line of Topeka**
P. O. Box 223, Topeka, Kansas 66601.
☎ 913 233 6558
🕐 21:00 - 24:00, recorded message at other times

Organizations: AIDS: Education
☺▽ **Topeka AIDS Project**
&. 1915 South West 6th. Street, Topeka, Kansas 66606.
☎ 913 232 3100

Wichita
Health Services
☺▢ **Saint Francis Regional Medical Center**
929 North Saint Francis Street, Wichita, Kansas 67214.
☎ 316 268 5000
HIV & emergency departments.
☺▢ **Wesley Medical Center**
550 North Hillside Avenue, Wichita, Kansas 67214.
☎ 316 688 2468

Helplines: Sexuality
⌔▽ **Wichita Gay Info Line**
P. O. Box 16782, Wichita, Kansas 67216-0782.
☎ 316 269 0913 ✆ 316 269 4208
🕐 12:00 - 22:00

Organizations: AIDS: Education
☺▢ **AIDS Referral Services (ARS)**
Suite E, 1809 North Broadway Street, Wichita, Kansas 67214-1146.
☎ 316 264 2437

Organizations: Bears
⌔▽ **Hirsute Pursuit**
P. O. Box 16782, Wichita, Kansas 67216-0782.
☎ 316 269 0913 ✆ 316 269 4208
☎ 316 269 3172
✉ awes@fn.net
🖥 http://www.fn.net/~awes/hp

Organizations: Sexuality
⌔▽ **Wichita Gay & Lesbian Alliance**
P. O. Box 2845, Wichita, Kansas 67201.
☎ 316 267 1852

Publishers: Newspapers: Sexuality
⌔ *Emerald City News*

P. O. Box 16782, Wichita, Kansas 67216.
☎ 316 269 0913 ✆ 316 269 4208
Published every month.
⌔ *Personally Speaking*
P. O. Box 16782, Wichita, Kansas 67216-0782.

Stores: Books: General
⌔▼ **Visions & Dreams**
&. 3143 West Maple, Wichita, Kansas 67213.
☎ 316 942 6333
🕐 10:00 - 20:00, Sun 12:00 - 18:00

Stores: Erotica: General
☺■ **Adult Entrée**
220 East 21st. Street, Wichita, Kansas 67213.
☎ 316 832 1816
☺■ **Christie's Toy Box**
1445 North Rock Road, Wichita, Kansas 67206.
☎ 913 226 3004
☺■ **Plato's Bookstore**
1306 East Harry Street, Wichita, Kansas 67211.
☎ 316 269 9036
☺■ **T. B.'s Camelot**
1515 South Oliver, Wichita, Kansas 67218.
☎ 316 688 5343

KENTUCKY
Area: Approximately 103,000 square kilometres
Population: Approximately 3,700,000
Capital City: Frankfort
Time zone: GMT minus 5/6 hours (both EST & CST)
Age of consent & homosexuality legislation: All anal & oral sex is illegal in this state.
Legal drinking age: 21

State Resources
Organizations: AIDS: Education
☺▢ **Northern Kentucky AIDS Consortium**
610 Covington Drive, Covington, Kentucky 41017.
☎ 606 291 0770

Organizations: AIDS: Support
☺▽ **Kentuckiana People With AIDS Coalition (KIPWAC)**
&. 810 Barret Avenue, Louisville, Kentucky 40204.
☎ 502 574 5493
Publishes *KIPWAC Update*.

Organizations: Sexuality
⌔▽ **Kentucky Gay & Lesbian Educational Center**
P. O. Box 4264, Louisville, Kentucky 40204.
☎ 502 636 0935

Publishers: Newspapers: Sexuality
⌔▼ *Kentucky Word*
Word Publications, Suite 2800, Tower 1, 225 East North Street, Indianapolis, Indiana 46204-1349.
☎ 317 579 3075 ✆ 317 687 8840
🕐 24hr. answering machine
&. ✓
Three state editions (Indiana, Kentucky, & Ohio). No 900 ads, no nudity. Published every month.
⌔▼ *The Letter*
The Letterhead, P. O. Box 3882, Louisville, Kentucky 40201.
☎ 502 772 7570 ✆ 502 635 6469
☎ 502 636 0935
✉ WillNich@aol.com
🕐 10:00 - 17:00
&. ✓ $ ➥
To inform the gay & lesbian communities of political, AIDS, & entertainment that concerns them locally, statewide, & internationally. Published every month. Yearly subscription is $25. Age statement of 18 is required.

Bowling Green
Organizations: Sexuality: Student
⌔▽ **Western Kentucky University Lambda**
P. O. Box 8335, Bowling Green, Kentucky 41101.

Suppliers: Diapers
☺■ **Dripride / Weyerhaeuser**
P. O. Box 1198, Bowling Green, Kentucky 42104.
☎ 502 843 1070
☎ 800-253-3078
Disposable diapers.

Lexington

Bars: BDSM

♂▼ **Crossings**
117 North Limestone Street, Lexington, Kentucky 40507.
☎ 606 233 7266
🕐 Mon - Sat 16:00 -01:30
Also has leather / latex shop.

Health Services

☺ ☐ **Saint Joseph's Hospital**
One Saint Joseph Street, Lexington, Kentucky 40504.
☎ 606 278 3436

☺ ☐ **Veterans' Affairs Medical Center**
2250 Leestown Pike, Lexington, Kentucky 40511.
☎ 606 233 4511

☺ ☐ **Veterans' Affairs Medical Center**
800 Zorn Avenue, Lexington, Kentucky 40206.
☎ 502 895 3401

Organizations: BDSM

♂▽ **Bluegrass C. O. L. T.s**
P. O. Box 12403, Lexington, Kentucky 40583-2403.
C. O. L. T.s: Circle Of Leathermen Together.

♂▽ **Knight Cruisers**
P. O. Box 11002, Lexington, Kentucky 40512-1002.
☎ 606 225 4315
☎ 606 255 9966
✉ KnightCru@aol.com

Organizations: Sexuality

♂▽ **Lexington Gay & Lesbian Services Organization**
♿ P. O. Box 11471, Lexington, Kentucky 40575.
☎ 606 231 0335
🕐 Wed - Fri Sun 20:00 - 23:00
Publishes *GLSO News.*

Organizations: Sexuality: Student

♂▽ **UK Lambda**
♿ P. O. Box 647, University of Kansas Main Station, Lexington, Kentucky 40506.

Publishers: Newspapers: Sexuality

♂ **GLSO News**
P. O. Box 11471, Lexington, Kentucky 40575.
☎ 606 266 8887
GLSO News serves the needs of the central Kentucky, bluegrass lesbigay community. Published every month. Yearly subscription is $10.

Stores: Books: General

☺ ■ **Joseph-Beth Booksellers**
♿ 3199 Nicholasville Road, Lexington, Kentucky 40503.
☎ 606 273 2911 📱 6060 272 6948
🕐 Mon - Thu 09:00 - 21:00, Fri Sat - 22:00, Sun 12:00 - 18:00

Stores: Clothing: Uniforms

☺ ■ **Gall's, Inc.**
2680 Palumbo Drive, Lexington, Kentucky 40555-4658.
☎ 800 477 7766
☎ 606 266 7227
Police equipment & clothing store. Not BDSM friendly. Catalogue available.

Stores: Erotica: BDSM

♂▼ **The Rack**
Lower Level, c/o Crossings, 117 North Limestone Street, Lexington, Kentucky 40507.
☎ 606 233 7266
🕐 Mon - Sat 16:30 - 01:00

Stores: Erotica: General

☺ ▼ **The Phœnix Bookstore**
♿ 933 Winchester Road, Lexington, Kentucky 40505.
☎ 606 255 9881

Louisville

Organizations: AIDS: Education

☺ ▽ **Community Health Trust, Inc.**
♿ P. O. Box 4277, Louisville, Kentucky 40204.
☎ 502 625 5496
Publishes *Heart Beat.*

Organizations: BDSM

☺ ☐ **A.S.B. Munch—Louisville**

P. O. Box 17054, Louisville, Kentucky 40217-0054.
✉ craftman@iglou.com
🕐 Usually meets 2nd. Sat of month 19:00

♂▽ **Louisville Nightwings**
P. O. Box 32051, Louisville, Kentucky 40232-2051.

Organizations: Bears

♂▽ **Bluegrass Bears**
P. O. Box 37001, Louisville, Kentucky 40233-7001.
☎ 502 569 1889
✉ luckyrj@iglou.com
🌐 http://www.skepsis.com:80/.gblo/bears/CLUBS/bluegrass.bears.ht
ml

Organizations: Family

☺ ☐ **Parents & Friends of Lesbians & Gays (PFLAG)—Louisville**
P. O. Box 5002, Louisville, Kentucky 40255-0002.
☎ 502 589 3316

Organizations: Sexuality

♂ **Black & White Men Together (BWMT)**
Suite 1, 222 East Ormsby Avenue, Louisville, Kentucky 40203.
☎ 502 637 3781
☎ 800 624 2968 (national line)
Publishes *NABWMT Journal.*

♂▽ **Black & White Men Together (BWMT)—Louisville**
P. O. Box 1838, Louisville, Kentucky 40201.
☎ 502 772 3025

⚥▽ **Louisville Gender Society**
P. O. Box 5458, Louisville, Kentucky 40255-0458.
☎ 812 944 5570
☎ 502 458 8028
✉ dawnw@transgender.org
Contact: Ms. Dawn Wilson

Organizations: Sexuality: Student

♂▽ **Gay, Lesbian, Or Bisexual Alliance (GLOBAL)**
♿ SAC W301, University of Louisville, Louisville, Kentucky 40292.
☎ 502 852 4556
☎ 502 852 3918

Publishers: Magazines: Sexuality

☺ *Disability Rag*
P. O. Box 145, Louisville, Kentucky 40201.

Stores: Books: General

☺ ■ **Carmichael's Bookstore**
♿ 1295 Bardstown Road, Louisville, Kentucky 40204.
☎ 502 456 6950

☺ ■ **Hawley-Cooke**
♿ Gardiner Lane Center, Louisville, Kentucky 40205.
☎ 502 546 6660

☺ ■ **Hawley-Cooke**
♿ 27 Shelbyville Road Plaza, Louisville, Kentucky 40207.
☎ 502 893 0133

Stores: Clothing: Cowboy

☺ ■ **The Leatherhead Shop**
1601 Bardstown Road, Louisville, Kentucky.
Not scene people, so be discreet when visiting the shop.

Stores: Clothing: Fetish

☺ ■ **Worn To Be Wild**
7511 Appletree Way, Louisville, Kentucky 40228-2236.

Stores: Clothing: Leather

☺ **Sun Leather & Lace**
1501 1/2 South 7th. Street, Louisville, Kentucky 40208.
☎ 502 634 4705
🕐 12:00 - 20:00 💳 VISA MC

Stores: Erotica: BDSM

☺ ■ **D. A. B.**
1501 South 7th. Street, Louisville, Kentucky.

Newport

Organizations: AIDS: Education

☺ ☐ **Northern Kentucky AIDS Task Force**
Northern Kentucky District Health Department, 401 Park Avenue, Newport, Kentucky 41071.
☎ 606 491 6611

Owensboro

Organizations: AIDS: Support

☺ □ **Kentuckiana People With AIDS Coalition (KIPWAC)**
P. O. Box 109, Owensboro, Kentucky 42302.
☎ 502 683 2438
☎ 502 443 3225 (in Paducah)

LOUISIANA

Area: Approximately 113,000 square kilometres
Population: Approximately 4,240,000
Capital City: Baton Rouge
Time zone: GMT minus 6 hours (CST)

State Resources

Archives: Sexuality

☺ □ **Homosexual Information Center**
115 Monroe Street, Bossier City, Louisiana 71111-4539.
Publishes a newsletter.

Publishers: Newspapers: Sexuality

⚢▼ ***Ambush***
P. O. Box 71291, New Orleans, Louisiana 70172-1291.
☎ 504 522 8049 Fax 504 522 0907
Gulf South entertainment & news guide since 1982. Published 27 times a year. Yearly subscription is $45.

⚢▼ ***Impact***
P. O. Box 52079, New Orleans, Louisiana 70152.
☎ 504 944 6722
🕒 Mon - Fri 10:00 - 17:00
News (local & national), entertainment, plus reviews of books, films, & theatres for New Orleans & the Gulf Coast for seven years. Published every two weeks. Yearly subscription is $50.

Alexandria

Organizations: AIDS: Education

☺ □ **Central Louisana AIDS Support Services (CLASS)**
♿ 824 16th. Street, Alexandria, Louisiana 71301.
☎ 800 444 7993
☎ 318 442 1010
🕒 Mon - Fri 08:30 - 15:00
Free, anonymous HIV testing.

Baton Rouge

Organizations: AIDS: Education

☺ □ **Friends For Life—Capital Area AIDS Services, Inc.**
♿ Suite 13, 4521 Jamestown Avenue, Baton Rouge, Louisiana 70808-3234.
☎ 504 923 2277

Publishers: Newspapers: Sexuality

⚢ ***Voices Magazine***
P. O. Box 66703, Baton Rouge, Louisiana 70896.
☎ 504 665 7815

Stores: Books: General

☺ ■ **Hibiscus Books**
635 Main Street, Baton Rouge, Louisiana 70802.
☎ 504 387 4264
🕒 Call for opening hours

Gretna

Publishers: Newspapers: Sexuality

⚢ ***Tattler***
P. O. Box 211, Gretna, Louisiana 70045-0211.

Lafayette

Organizations: AIDS: Education

☺ □ **Lafayette CARES**
♿ P. O. Box 91446, Lafayette, Louisiana 70509.
☎ 318 233 2437
🕒 Hotline 24hrs.. Office Mon - Fri 08:00 - 15:00
Publishes *CARES News*.

Organizations: Family

☺ □ **Parents & Friends of Lesbians & Gays (PFLAG)—Lafayette**
P. O. Box 31078, Lafayette, Louisiana 70503.
☎ 318 984 2216

Organizations: Sexuality

⚣▽ **Krewe of Apollo de Lafayette**
♿ P. O. Box 53251, Lafayette, Louisiana 70505-3251.

Stores: Erotica: General

☺▼ **Loveworks**
♿ 3607C Ambassador Caffery Parkway, Lafayette, Louisiana 70503.
☎ 318 988 5000

Lake Charles

Organizations: AIDS: Education

☺ □ **Southwest Louisiana AIDS Council**
435 10th. Street, Lake Charles, Louisiana 70601-6092.
☎ 318 439 5145
☎ 800 256 5145 (outside Lake Charles)

Stores: Books: General

☺ ■ **Pappy's**
2627 Ryan Street, Lake Charles, Louisiana 70601.
☎ 318 436 2819

Monroe

Organizations: AIDS: Education

☺ □ **GO CARE**
2121 Justice Street, Monroe, Louisiana 71201.
☎ 318 325 1092

Organizations: Sexuality

⚢▽ **Lambda of Northeast Louisiana**
P. O. Box 4407, Monroe, Louisiana 71211.
☎ 318 387 0442

New Orleans

Artists: BDSM

☺ ■ **Matt**
903 Spain Street, New Orleans, Louisiana 70117.

Bars: BDSM

⚢▼ **The Country Club**
♿ 634 Louisa Street, New Orleans, Louisiana 70117.
☎ 504 945 0742
Some leather.

⚣▼ **The Phœnix Men's Room**
941 Elysian Fields, New Orleans, Louisiana 70117.
☎ 504 945 9264
🕒 24hrs.

⚣▼ **Rawhide**
740 Burgundy Street, New Orleans, Louisiana 70116.
☎ 504 525 8106

Counsellors

⚢▼ **Terry Mayers, M.Ed., BCSW, ACSW**
♿ 1412 Thalia, New Orleans, Louisiana 70130.
☎ 504 524 5973

☺ ■ **Liz Simon, BCSW**
♿ Suite 209, 3500 Saint Charles Avenue, New Orleans, Louisiana 70115.
☎ 504 899 6024

Health Services

☺ □ **Children's Hospital**
200 Henry Clay Avenue, New Orleans, Louisiana 70118.
☎ 504 8999 9511
Emergency & HIV outpatient departments.

☺ □ **Medical Center of Louisiana at New Orleans**
1532 Tulane Avenue, New Orleans, Louisiana 70140.
☎ 504 568 3201
HIV & emergency departments.

☺ □ **Tulane University Hospital & Clinincs**
1415 Tulane Avenue, New Orleans, Louisiana 70112.
☎ 504 588 5263
Emergency & HIV outpatient departments.

☺ □ **Veterans' Affairs Medical Center**
1601 Perdido Street, New Orleans, Louisiana 70146.
☎ 504 568 0811
HIV & emergency departments.

Organizations: AIDS: Education

☺ □ **NO/AIDS Task Force**
♿ 1407 Decatur Street, New Orleans, Louisiana 70116.
☎ 800 992 4379 (hotline)
☎ 504 944 2437 (hotline)
🕒 Mon - Fri 14:00 - 24:00, Sat Sun - 22:00
Office number: 504 945 4000. Publishes *Newsline*.

☺ □ **Northwest Louisiana AIDS Task Force**

P. O. Box 832, New Orleans, Louisiana 71162-0832.
☎ 318 221 8219

Organizations: AIDS: Support

☺ ☐ **New Orleans PWA Coalition**
P. O. Box 2616, New Orleans, Louisiana 70176-2616.
☎ 504 944 3663

☺ ▽ **Project Lazarus**
& P. O. Box 3606, New Orleans, Louisiana 70177-3606.
☎ 504 949 3609

Organizations: BDSM

⚢▽ **Knights d'Orleans**
P. O. Box 50812, New Orleans, Louisiana 70150.

⚢▽ **Lords of Leather**
P. O. Box 712105, New Orleans, Louisiana 70172.
☎ 602 233 9042 Ext.: 270 📱 602 233 9042

⚢▽ **The National Leather Association (NLA)—New Orleans**
P. O. Box 50133, New Orleans, Louisiana 70150-0133.

Organizations: Bondage

⚢▽ **New Orleans Bondage Club**
P. O. Box 57901, New Orleans, Louisiana 70157-7901.

Organizations: Family

☺ ☐ **Parents & Friends of Lesbians & Gays (PFLAG)— New Orleans**
& P. O. Box 15515, New Orleans, Louisiana 70175.
☎ 504 895 3936
Publishes *The Banner.*

Organizations: Sexuality

⚲▽ **Gulf Area Gender Alliance**
P. O. Box 870213, New Orleans, Louisiana 70187-1300.
🕐 Meets 2nd. Sat of month
Publishes *The Flip Side.*

⚢▽ **Lesbian & Gay Community Center of New Orleans**
816 North Rampart Street, New Orleans, Louisiana 70172.
☎ 504 522 1103

Piercers

☺ ■ **Art Accent Tattooing**
1014 North Rampart, New Orleans, Louisiana 70116.
☎ 514 581 9812
☎ 514 949 5377

☺ ■ **Rings of Desire**
1128 Decatur Street, New Orleans, Louisiana 70116.
☎ 504 524 6147
🕐 Wed - Sun 12:00 - 20:00

Publishers: Guides: Sexuality

⚢ *This Week Guide*
704 Touro Street, New Orleans, Louisiana 70116.
☎ 504 948 7814

Stores: Books: General

⚢▼ **Faubourg-Marigny Bookstore**
600 Frenchmen Street, New Orleans, Louisiana 70116.
☎ 504 943 9875

☺ ■ **Sidney's Newstand**
917 Decatur Street, New Orleans, Louisiana 70116.
☎ 504 524 6872

Stores: Erotica: BDSM

⚢▼ **Second Skin**
& 521 Philip Street, New Orleans, Louisiana 70116.
☎ 504 561 8167
🕐 12:00 - 22:00, Sun - 18:00

Stores: Erotica: General

☺ ■ **Airline Books**
1404 26th. Street, Kenner, Louisiana 70062.
☎ 504 468 2931

☺ ■ **Lenny's News**
& 5420 Magazine Street, New Orleans, Louisiana 70115.
☎ 504 897 0005
🕐 07:00 - 22:00

☺ ▽ **Lenny's News**
& 622 South Carrollton Avenue, New Orleans, Louisiana 70118.
☎ 504 866 5127
🕐 08:00 - 23:00

☺ ▽ **Panda Bear**

& 415 Bourbon Street, New Orleans, Louisiana 70130.
☎ 504 529 3593

☺ ■ **Tom's Toybox**
907 Bourbon Street, New Orleans, Louisiana 70116.
☎ 504 523 7827

Television: Sexuality

⚢▽ *Just For The Record*
Public Access Television, P. O. Box 35373, Dallas, Texas 75235-0373.
☎ 214 351 1901 📱 214 351 6099

Shreveport

Organizations: AIDS: Education

☺ ☐ **Philadelphia Center**
& P. O. Box 44454, Shreveport, Louisiana 71134-4454.
☎ 318 222 6633

⚥ ☐ **YWCA AIDS Minority Outreach**
& 700 Pierre Avenue, Shreveport, Louisiana 71103.
☎ 504 226 8717

Thibodaux

Publishers: Magazines: Sexuality

⚲ *Alternate Woman*
Lonnie Marshall Publications, P. O. Box 6002, Thibodaux, Louisiana 70302-6002.
☎ 504 369 6976

MAINE

Area: Approximately 80,000 square kilometres
Population: Approximately 1,230,000
Capital City: Augusta
Time zone: GMT minus 5 hours (EST)
Climate: Continental climate moderated by the Atlantic ocean. summers reach a high temperature of approximately 24°C, winters a low of -1°C. There is plenty of rain here.
Age of consent & homosexuality legislation: State has adopted the Model Penal Code or otherwise decriminalized homosexual activities.
Legal drinking age: 20

State Resources

Film Festivals: Sexuality

⚢■ **Maine Gay & Lesbian Film Festival**
c/o Out & Out Productions, P. O. Box 7982, Portland, Maine 04112.

Helplines: Sexuality

⚢▽ **Gay & Lesbian Phoneline**
c/o P. O. Box 990, Caribou, Maine 04736.
☎ 207 498 2088
🕐 19:00 - 21:00

Organizations: AIDS: Education

☺ ☐ **The AIDS Project (TAP)**
& 5th. Floor, 22 Monument Square, Portland, Maine 04101.
☎ 800 851 2437
☎ 207 774 6877

☺ ☐ **Waldo-Knox AIDS Coalition**
& P. O. Box 956, Belfast, Maine 04915.
☎ 207 338 1427

Organizations: AIDS: Support

☺ ☐ **PWA Coalition of Maine**
& 377 Cumberland Avenue, Portland, Maine 04101.
☎ 207 773 8500

Organizations: Sexuality

⚢▽ **Fruits of Our Labors**
P. O. Box 125, Belfast, Maine 04915.
☎ 207 338 2913

Publishers: Newspapers: Sexuality

⚢▽ *Apex*
Phœnix Press, P. O. Box 4743, Portland, Maine 04112.
☎ 207 282 8091
We are a radical queer news journal, loving to publish controversy & creativity. Published 11 times a year. Yearly subscription is $20.

⚢▼ *Community Pride Reporter*
& Suite 623, 142 High Street, Portland, Maine 04101.
☎ 207 879 1342 📱 207 879 1342
✉ CPRPride@aol.com
🕐 Mon - Fri 09:00 - 17:00
💲 $
Serving the lesbian, gay, bisexual, & transgendered communities of Maine & New Hampshire. A&E, resources, news, information, op-ed,

features, etc.. Published every month. Yearly subscription is $25.

Auburn
Counsellors
☺▼ **Norma Kraus Eule, LCSW**
 ♿ 10 Minot Avenue, Auburn, Maine 04210.
 ☎ 207 784 8747

Augusta
Counsellors
▷▽ **Theseus Counseling Services**
 K Suite 222, 126 Western Avenue, Augusta, Maine 04330.
 ☎ 207 621 0858 📞 207 621 0858
 🕐 Mon - Fri afternoons & evenings
 💷 ✓ VISA MC
 Therapist & public speaker. French, German, Spanish, Italian, & Greek
 also spoken.

Bangor
Health Services
☺☐ **Eastern Maine Medical Center**
 489 State Street, Bangor, Maine 04401.
 ☎ 207 945 7000

Organizations: AIDS: Education
☺☐ **Eastern Maine AIDS Network (EMAN)**
 ♿ P. O. Box 2038, Bangor, Maine 04402-2038.
 ☎ 207 990 3626
 🕐 Mon - Fri 08:30 - 16:30
 Publishes *Network News*.

Organizations: Sexuality
☿▽ **Downeast Lesbian & Gay Organization (DELGO)**
 Unitarian Church, 126 Union Street, Bangor, Maine 04401.
 ☎ 207 942 6503
☿▽ **Gay & Lesbian Network**
 P. O. Box 212, Bangor, Maine 04401.
 ☎ 207 862 5907
 ☎ 207 941 2189
▷▽ **Maine Gender Resource & Support Service**
 P. O. Box 1894, Bangor, Maine 04402-1894.
 Contact: Ms. Jean Churchill
 Information, referrals, support. NOT a support group.

Biddeford
Organizations: Sexuality
♀▽ **Out Among Friends**
 P. O. Box 727, Biddeford, Maine 04055.
 ☎ 207 799 0297

Brunswick
Organizations: AIDS: Education
☺☐ **Merrymeeting AIDS Support Services**
 ♿ P. O. Box 57, Brunswick, Maine 04011-0057.
 ☎ 207 725 4955

Damariscotta
Publishers: Magazines: Sexual Politics
♂ *Maine Progressive*
 P. O. Box 1048, Damariscotta, Maine 04543.
 ☎ 207 563 1668
 An alternative voice for people committed to achieving a democratic
 society in which everyone can live in dignity & peace. Published 11
 times a year. Yearly subscription is $12.

Stores: Books: General
☺▼ **Laughing Moon Bookstore**
 P. O. Box 1084, Damariscotta, Maine 04543.
 ☎ 207 563 5537
 🕐 Tue - Sat 10:00 - 17:00

East Waterboro
Organizations: Sexuality
♀▽ **Out For Good**
 P. O. Box 153, East Waterboro, Maine 04031.
 ☎ 207 247 3461

Ellsworth
Organizations: AIDS: Education
☺☐ **Down East AIDS Network (DEAN)**

♿ 114 State Street, Ellsworth, Maine 04605.
 ☎ 207 667 3506

Gardiner
Counsellors
☺■ **Karen Molvig, Psy.D.**
 103 Brunswick Avenue, Gardiner, Maine 04345.
 ☎ 207 582 1559

Hallowell
Organizations: Family
☺☐ **Parents & Friends of Lesbians & Gays (PFLAG)—
Hallowell**
 23 Winthrop Street, Hallowell, Maine 04347.
 ☎ 207 623 2349

Lewiston
Organizations: AIDS: Education
☺☐ **Androscoggin Valley AIDS Coalition (AVAC)**
 ♿ P. O. Box 7977, Lewiston, Maine 04243-7977.
 ☎ 207 786 4697

Stores: Erotica: General
☺■ **Adult Bookstore**
 314 Lisbon Street, Lewiston, Maine 04240.
 ☎ 207 784 5961
☺▼ **Paris Adult Bookstore**
 297 Lisbon Street, Lewiston, Maine 04240.
 ☎ 207 784 6551
 ☎ 207 783 6677

Portland
Bars: BDSM
♂▼ **The Chart Room Saloon**
 ♿ P. O. Box 7435, Portland, Maine 04101.
 ☎ 207 774 9262

Counsellors
♂▼ **Bellville Counseling Associates**
 ♿ P. O. Box 186, Portland, Maine.
 ☎ 207 729 8727
☺ **Cheryl Fuller, M.A., LCPC**
 K 813 Brighton Avenue, Portland, Maine 04102.
 ☎ 207 774 4436
 Licensed psychotherapist.
☺■ **Jacob Watson, M.A., L.C.P.C.**
 ♿ Watson Counselling, 491 Stevens Avenue, Portland, Maine 04103.
 ☎ 207 870 8656
 ☎ 207 761 2522
 🕐 08:00 - 18:00
 💷 ✓
 Specializing in terminal illness, death & dying, loss & transition, grief &
 bereavement. International workshops: "Grief, Loss, & Transition". Age
 statement of 18 is required.

Health Services
☺☐ **Maine Medical Center**
 22 Bramhall Street, Portland, Maine 04102.
 ☎ 207 871 0111

Organizations: BDSM
♂▽ **HarborMasters**
 P. O. Box 4044, Station A, Portland, Maine 04101.

Organizations: Family
☺☐ **Parents & Friends of Lesbians & Gays (PFLAG)—
Portland**
 P. O. Box 8742, Portland, Maine 04104.
 ☎ 207 766 5158

Organizations: Sexuality
♂▽ **Gay & Lesbian Alliance**
 University of Southern Maine, 88 Winslow Street, Portland, Maine
 04103.
 ☎ 207 874 6956
♂▽ **Matlovich Society**
 P. O. Box 942, Portland, Maine 04104.
 ☎ 203 773 1209
♂▽ **Time Out**
 P. O. Box 11502, Portland, Maine.

☎ 207 871 9940
✉□ **Transupport**
🏳 P. O. Box 17622, Portland, Maine 04112.
Publishes *Trans-Talk*.

Organizations: Sexuality: Student
⚥▽ **Alliance for Sexual Diversity**
University of Southern Maine, Portland, Maine.
☎ 207 774 4919

Organizations: Sexuality: Youth
⚥▽ **Outright**
P. O. Box 5370, Portland, Maine 04101-1070.
☎ 207 774 4357

Publishers: Miscellaneous
⚤ **Astarte Shell Press**
P. O. Box 3648, Portland, Maine 04101-3648.
☎ 207 828 1992

Stores: Books: General
☺■ **Bookland Of Mill Creek**
♿ Mill Creek Shopping Center, South Portland, Maine 04106.
☎ 207 799 2659
☺■ **Books, Etc.**
38 Exchange Street, Portland, Maine 04101.
☎ 207 774 0626
🕐 09:30 - 18:00, Dec & Summer - 21:00, Sun 12:00 - 17:00

Stores: Erotica: General
☺■ **Congress Book Shop**
♿ 668 Congress Street, Portland, Maine 04101.
☎ 207 774 1377
☺■ **Treasure Chest**
♿ 2A Pine Street, Portland, Maine 04101.
☎ 207 772 2225

Waterville
Organizations: Sexuality: Student
⚥▽ **The Bridge**
♿ c/o Stu-A, Colby College, Waterville, Maine 04901.
☎ 207 872 3000
🕐 Wed 19:00 - 22:00

Stores: Erotica: General
☺■ **Priscilla's**
18 Water Street, Waterville, Maine 04901.
☎ 207 873 2774
☺■ **Treaure Chest II**
5 Sanger Avenue, Waterville, Maine 04901-4851.
☎ 207 873 7411

MARYLAND
Area: Approximately 25,350 square kilometres
Population: Approximately 4,800,000
Capital City: Annapolis
Time zone: GMT minus 5 hours (EST)
Climate: Warm summers with an average temperature of approximately 25°C. Winters average 1°C. All the weather here is influenced by the nearby oceans. In the late summer & early Autumn, severe storms & hurricanes usually pass through the area.
Age of consent & homosexuality legislation: All anal & oral sex is illegal in this state.
Legal drinking age: 21

State Resources
Organizations: Motorcycle
⚥▽ **Spartan MC**
P. O. Box 23623, Alexandria, Virginia 22304-9362.

Annapolis
Organizations: Family
☺□ **Parents & Friends of Lesbians & Gays (PFLAG)—Annapolis**
P. O. Box 722, Crownsville, Maryland 21432.
☎ 410 849 3524

Stores: Erotica: General
☺■ **20-20 News**
2020 West Street, Annapolis, Maryland 21401.
☎ 410 266 0514

Stores: Erotica: Spanking
☺■ **Naughty Victorian**
2315-B Forest Drive, Annapolis, Maryland 21401.
☎ 410 626 1879
🕐 09:00 - 21:00
✓ 💳 💳 💳
Catalogue, $5.

Baltimore
Bars: BDSM
⚥▼ **The Baltimore Eagle**
2022 North Charles Street, Baltimore, Maryland 21218.
☎ 410 823 2453
♿ 💳 💳
Leather store inside.
⚥▼ **P. T. Max**
1735 Maryland Avenue, Baltimore, Maryland 21201.
☎ 410 539 6965
Some leather.

BBSs: BDSM
☺■ **Harbor Bytes**
📞 410 235 6753

Counsellors
⚥▼ **Chesapeake Psychological Services**
♿ Suite 1304, 28 West Allegheny Avenue, Towson, Maryland 21204-3919.
☎ 410 321 1091
☺▼ **Gregory Lehne, Ph.D.**
♿ 4419 Falls Road, Baltimore, Maryland 21211.
☎ 410 366 0642
✉▼ **Martin Malin, Ph.D.**
Suite 3, 2114 North Charles Street, Baltimore, Maryland 21218.
☎ 410 528 1638

Health Services
⚥▽ **The Chase Brexton Clinic**
♿ Suite 211, 101 West Read Street, Baltimore, Maryland 21201.
☎ 410 837 2050
🕐 Mon - Thu 09:00 - 21:00, Fri - 16:00
HIV counselling & testing, & other support services.
☺□ **Johns Hopkins Hospital**
600 North Wolfe Street, Baltimore, Maryland 21287.
☎ 410 955 5000
HIV & emergency departments.
☺□ **Sinai Hospital of Baltimore**
2401 West Belvedere Avenue, Baltimore, Maryland 21215.
☎ 410 578 5678
☺□ **University of Maryland Medical System**
22 South Greene Street, Baltimore, Maryland 21201.
☎ 410 328 8667
☺□ **Veterans' Affairs Medical Center**
10 North Greene Street, Baltimore, Maryland 21201.
☎ 410 605 7001

Helplines: Sexuality
⚥▽ **Gay & Lesbian Switchboard**
241 West Chase Street, Baltimore, Maryland 21201. 📞 410 837 8512
☎ 410 837 8888
☎ 410 837 8529 (TDD)
🕐 19:00 - 22:00

Manufacturers: Furniture: BDSM
☺■ **Stocks & Bonds**
P. O. Box 3592, Baltimore, Maryland 21214.
☎ 410 426 8158
Custom made BDSM furniture. Also items from stock.

Organizations: AIDS: Education
⚥▽ **AIDS Action Baltimore, Inc.**
2105 North Charles Street, Baltimore, Maryland 21218.
☎ 410 837 2437

Organizations: AIDS: Information
⚥□ **Health Education Resource Organization, Inc.**
Suite 825, 101 West Read Street, Baltimore, Maryland 21201.
☎ 410 685 1180 📞 410 752 3353

Organizations: AIDS: Support
☺□ **People With AIDS Coalition**
♿ Suite 808, 101 Read Street, Baltimore, Maryland 21201.

Organizations: AIDS: Support

☎ 410 625 1677
Publishes *News & Views*.

Organizations: BDSM

♂ **COMMAND**
P.O. Box 23764, Baltimore, Maryland 21203-5164.

☺ **The D&S Society of Baltimore**
P.O. Box 20248, Baltimore, Maryland 21204.
☎ 410 385 3331
☎ 410 377 0123

♀ ☐ **Females Investigating Sexual Terrain (FIST)**
P. O. Box 41032, Baltimore, Maryland 21203-6032.
☎ 410 675 0856

♂▼ **Shipmates of Baltimore, Inc.**
P.O. Box 13434, Baltimore, Maryland 21203.
✉ stine@ibm.net

Organizations: Family

☺ ☐ **Parents & Friends of Lesbians & Gays (PFLAG)—**
♿ **Baltimore**
P. O. Box 5637, Baltimore, Maryland 21210.
☎ 410 433 3524

Organizations: Motorcycle

♂▽ **Trident—Baltimore**
P. O. Box 211, Clinton, Maryland 20735.

Organizations: Polyfidelity

☺ ■ **Potomac Area Lifestyles**
509 East 42nd. Street, Baltimore, Maryland 21218-1202.

Organizations: Sexuality

♂▽ **Baltimore Lambda Alliance of the Deaf**
P. O. Box 22444, Baltimore, Maryland 21203-4444.
☎ 410 523 8396 (TTY/TDD)

♂▽ **Black & White Men Together (BWMT)—Baltimore**
♿ P. O. Box 33186, Baltimore, Maryland 21218.
☎ 410 542 6218
☎ 410 336 3767

▷▽ **The Bridge Club**
P. O. Box 11737, Baltimore, Maryland 21206-0337.
🕐 Meets monthly
Contact: Ms. Michelle Gerald
Publishes a newsletter.

♂▽ **Gay & Lesbian Community Center**
♿ 241 West Chase Street, Baltimore, Maryland 21201.
☎ 410 837 5445 ✆ 410 837 8512
☎ 410 837 8529 (TDD)

♂▽ **J/OE**
♿ P. O. Box 22181, Baltimore, Maryland 21203.

▷▽ **Renaissance Education Association, Inc.—**
Baltimore
P. O. Box 39189, Baltimore, Maryland 21212.

♂▽ **Takoma Park Lesbians & Gays (TPLAG)**
♿ P. O. Box 5243, Baltimore, Maryland 20913.
☎ 301 891 3953

▷▽ **Transgender Support Group of Baltimore**
c/o Gay & Lesbian Community Center, 241 West Chase Street,
Baltimore, Maryland 21201.
☎ 410 837 5445 ✆ 410 837 8512
☎ 410 837 8529 (TDD)
🕐 Meets monthly

Organizations: Sexuality: Student

♂ **American College Personnel Association**
UMBC, Baltimore, Maryland 21228.
Contact: Ms. Liz Prince, Director of Susquehanna Hall
Publishes *Out On Campus*.

♂▽ **Bisexual, Gay, & Lesbian Alliance at JHU**
♿ SAC, Johns Hopkins, 3400 North Charles Street, Baltimore, Maryland
21218.
☎ 410 516 4088

♂▽ **Lesbian, Gay, & Bisexual Alliance of UMBC**
♿ University Center Box 26, 5401 Wilkens Avenue, Baltimore, Maryland
21228-5394.
☎ 410 788 8765
Publishes *Closet Space*.

♂▽ **Towson State University Gay & Lesbian Outreach**
Suite 404, 7800 York Road, Towson, Maryland 21204.
☎ 410 830 4007

U.S.A.

Organizations: Sexuality: Youth

♂▽ **Sufficient As I Am (SAIM)**
♿ 241 West Chase Street, Baltimore, Maryland 21201.
☎ 410 837 5445
For youth 14 - 24 years.

Publishers: Magazines: Daddy / Boy

♂ *Daddy Magazine*
Ganymede Press, Inc., 1735 Maryland Avenue, Baltimore, Maryland
21201.
☎ 410 727 5241
Age statement of 18 is required.

Publishers: Magazines: Sexuality

♂ *Tribe*
Columbia Publishing Company, 234 East 25th. Street, Baltimore,
Maryland 21218.
☎ 410 366 7070

Publishers: Newspapers: Sexuality

♂▼ *Baltimore Alternative*
P. O. Box 2351, Baltimore, Maryland 21203.
☎ 410 235 3401
Serving the Baltimore & Washington communities since 1986. Published
every month. Yearly subscription is $24.

♂▽ *Baltimore Gay Paper*
241 West Chase Street, Baltimore, Maryland 21203.
☎ 410 837 7748 ✆ 410 837 8512
Published every two weeks.

◯▽ *Amazon Times*
P. O. Box 135, Owing Mills, Maryland 21170-0135.
Published quarterly.

Stores: Books: General

☺ ■ **Atomic Books**
229 West Read Street, Baltimore, Maryland 21201.
☎ 410 728 5490 ✆ 410 669 4179
✆ 410 889 3543
✉ atomicbk@clark.net
🌐 http://www.atomicbooks.com/atomicbk/
🕐 Mon - Thu 12:00 - 18:00, Fri Sat 12:00 - 19:00, Sun 12:00 -
17:00
Literary finds for mutated minds.

♂▼ **Lambda Rising**
♿ 241 West Chase Street, Baltimore, Maryland 21201.
☎ 410 234 0069
✉ lambdarising@his.com
🕐 10:00 - 22:00
♿ ✓ $ 🔲 VISA ⬤ AMEX
Source for every gay, lesbian, bisexual, & transgender book in print
(plus thousands out of print) Also videos, music, & gifts.

♀ ▼ **Lammas Women's Books & More**
♿ 1001 Cathedral Street, Baltimore, Maryland 12101.
☎ 410 752 1001
🕐 Sun - Wed 11:00 - 18:00, thu - Sat 11:00 - 22:00
♿ ✓ 🔲 VISA ⬤ 🔲
Book & gift store. Also mail order, special orders. Wide selection: books,
gifts, toys for & about women. Video club.

☺ ■ **Mystery Loves Company**
♿ 1730 Fleet Street, Baltimore, Maryland 21231.
☎ 410 276 6708
🕐 Tue - Sat 11:00 - 18:00, Sun 12:00 - 17:00

Stores: Clothing: Leather

☺ ■ **Firefly**
3714 Eastern Avenue, Baltimore, Maryland 21224.
☎ 410 732 1232
🕐 Mon - Fri 11:00 - 21:00, Sat 11:00 - 20:00

Stores: Erotica: BDSM

♂▼ **Leather Underground**
136 West Read Street, Baltimore, Maryland 21201.
☎ 410 528 0991
🕐 Mon - Sat 10:00 - 18:00

Stores: Erotica: General

☺ ■ **Book Nook, Inc.**
1825 North Charles Street, Baltimore, Maryland 21201.
☎ 410 752 5778

☺ ■ **Broadway News Center**
301 South Broadway, Baltimore, Maryland 21231.
☎ 410 342 9590

Bethesda

Counsellors
▷▼ **Rusty Lynn, BD, MSW, LCSW**
4835 Del Ray Avenue, Bethesda, Maryland 20814.
☎ 301 652 6448

Health Services
☺ ☐ **National Institutes of Health**
Clinical Center, 9000 Rockville Pike, Bethesda, Maryland 20892.
☎ 301 496 3227
HIV department. No emergency department.

Publishers: Newspapers: Sexuality
Coming Out Pagan
P. O. Box 30811, Bethesda, Maryland 20824-0811.
A celebration of LesbiGay spirituality with a focus on nature religions, the joy of being alive, & deep conection with the Divine. Published quarterly. Yearly subscription is $11.

Stores: Books: General
☺ ■ **Borders Book Shop**
11301 Rockville Pike, North Bethesda, Maryland 20895-1021.
☎ 301 816 1067
⏰ 09:00 - 23:00, Sun 11:00 - 20:00

Charlestown

Stores: Erotica: BDSM
♂▼ **Mike's Custom Leathers**
P. O. Box 287, Charlestown, Maryland 02129.
☎ 617 241 8968
☎ 617 742 4084
⏰ Main number: 12:00 onwards, second number: Wed - Sun 22:00 onwards
⚙ ✓ VISA ⊙
Two locations: one in The Sling, Boston, one in The Brig, North Dartmouth. Age statement of 21 is required.

Chicopee

Organizations: BDSM
☺ ☐ **The Society**
P.O. Box 844, Chicopee, Maryland 01021.
☎ 413 592 7239
Publishes a newsletter quarterly.

College Park

Organizations: Sexuality: Student
♂▽ **Lesbian, Gay, & Bisexual Aliance**
♿ 3107 Adele Stamp Union, University of Maryland, College Park, Maryland 20742.
☎ 301 314 8467
Publishes *LGBA Newsletter*.

Publishers: Magazines: Sexuality
Feminist Studies
University of Maryland, College Park, Maryland 20742.
☎ 301 405 7415

Tattooists
☺ ■ **Great Southern Tattoo Company**
9403 Baltimore Boulevard, College Park, Maryland 20740.
☎ 301 474 8820
⏰ Mon - Fri 15:00 - 21:00, Sat Sun 12:00 - 20:00
VISA ⊙ AMEX

Columbia

Organizations: AIDS: Education
☺ ☐ **AIDS Alliance of Howard County**
c/o Hospice Services, Suite 433, 5537 Twin Knolls Road, Columbia, Maryland 21045.
☎ 410 313 2333

Organizations: Sexuality
♂▽ **Gay & Lesbian Community of Howard County**
P. O. Box 2115, Columbia, Maryland 21045.

Deer Park

Organizations: Sexuality
▷▽ **Tri-State Transgendered Club**
P. O. Box 3102, Deer Park, Maryland 21550-1002.
☎ 301 453 3538
⏰ Meets monthly
Contact: Ms. Diane Terrant

Fort Meade

Stores: Erotica: General
☺ ■ **Annapolis Road Books**
1656 Old Annapolis Road, Fort Meade, Maryland 21113.
☎ 301 674 9414

Frederick

Stores: Books: General
☺ ■ **Bradley Books**
318 North Market Street, Frederick, Maryland 21701.
☎ 301 662 9886

Gaithersburg

Organizations: Family
☺▽ **Gay & Lesbian Parents Coalition (GLPC—MW)**
♿ 14908 Piney Grove Court, Gaithersburg, Maryland 20878.
☎ 301 762 4828

Publishers: Magazines: Fetish
☺ ■ *Black Leather Times*
CBLT, 3 Calabar Court, Gaithersburg, Maryland 20877-1036.
☎ 301 975 7092
Yearly subscription is $8. Age statement of 18 is required.

☺ ■ *Blue Blood*
CBLT, 3 Calabar Court, Gaithersburg, Maryland 20877-1036.
☎ 301 975 7092
Yearly subscription is $20 U.S., $33 elsewhere.

Glen Burnie

Organizations: Tattoo
☺ ☐ **The Alliance of Professional Tattooists, Inc.**
Suite 205, 7477 Baltimore-Annapolis Boulevard, Glen Burnie, Maryland 21061.
☎ 410 768 1963 ☏ 410 760 1880

Greenbelt

Organizations: Motorcycle
♂▽ **Trident—Washington, D.C.**
P. O. Box 1255, Greenbelt, Maryland 20768-1255.
☎ 301 297 7539

Hyattsville

Stores: Erotica: General
☺ ■ **Silver News**
2488 Cillum Road, Hyattsville, Maryland 20782.
☎ 301 779 1024

Langley Park

Organizations: Sexuality
♂▽ **BiNet—USA**
P. O. Box 7327, Langley Park, Maryland 20787.
☎ 202 986 7186
✉ rain@glib.org
⚙ ✓
Publishes *BiNet USA News* quarterly. Yearly subscription is $10 U.S..

Lanham

Distributors: Books: General
☺ **National Book Network**
Suite A, 4720 Boston Way, Lanham, Maryland 20706-4310.
☎ 301 459 8696 ☏ 301 459 2118

Laurel

Organizations: Sexuality
♂▽ **Gay People of Laurel**
♿ P. O. Box 25, Laurel, Maryland 20725.
☎ 301 776 6891

Stores: Books: General
☺ ■ **Indecent Exposure**
14631 Baltimore AVenue, Laurel, Maryland 20707.
☎ 301 725 5683

☺ ■ **Laurel News Agency**
106 Washington Boulevard, Laurel, Maryland 20707.
☎ 301 725 9671

Rockville

Manufacturers: Erotica: Leather

☺ **Robert Grimes**
1923 Rockland Avenue, Rockville, Maryland 20851.
☎ 301 816 3251
✉ grimes@unix.tpe.com
🕐 13:00 - 24:00
♿ ✓ $
Custom leather BDSM designs. No clothing. Also mail order.

Publishers: Magazines: Daddy / Boy

✑ *Daddybear*
P. O. Box 2483, Rockville, Maryland 20847.
☎ 800 344 1175
☎ 301 681 3938
Age statement of 18 is required.

Suppliers: Travel Arrangements: BDSM

☺▼ **Atlas Travel East**
12100 Nebel Street, Rockville, Maryland 20852.
☎ 800 357 4190
☎ 301 984 9060

Salisbury

Stores: Erotica: General

☺■ **Salisbury News Agency**
616 South Salisbury Road, Salisbury, Maryland 21801.
☎ 410 543 4469

Silver Spring

Counsellors

⚥▼ **Robyn Zeiger, Ph.D., CPC**
9920 Cottrell Terrace, Silver Spring, Maryland 20903.
☎ 301 445 7333

Organizations: Polyfidelity

☺■ **Potomac Area Polyamory Network**
P. O. Box 8162, Silver Spring, Maryland 20907.
☎ 301 587 1193
✉ videonut@ix.netcom.com

Stores: Erotica: General

☺■ **Max Wonder**
♿ 9421 Georgia Avenue, Silver Spring, Maryland 20910-1435.
☎ 301 585 3333
🕐 08:00 - 23:00
♿ ✓ $ ⚥ 💳 💳 💳 💳

Tattooists

☺■ **Capitol Tattoo**
7920 Georgia Avenue, Silver Spring, Maryland.
☎ 301 585 3483
Also do some piercing.

Temple Hills

Stores: Books: General

☺■ **Marlow Heights Periodicals**
4518 Saint Barnabas Road, Temple Hills, Maryland 20748.
☎ 301 899 6458

Walkersville

BBSs: BDSM

☺■ **The Power Exchange**
P. O. Box 714, Walkersville, Maryland 21793.
☎ 703 749 9150
🖥 ftp://tpe.ncm.com or ftp://tpe.ds.ncm.com
💳 💳
Contains the resource directory of the SM/Leather/Fetish Community
Outreach Project. Age statement of 21 is required.

Wheaton

Counsellors

☺▼ **Richard Ruth, Ph.D.**
K ♿ Suite 1, 11303 Amherst Avenue, Wheaton, Maryland 20902.
☎ 301 933 3072 📞 301 933 0118
🕐 By appointment
♿ ✓
Spanish also spoken.

MASSACHUSETTS
Area: Approximately 20,000 square kilometres

Population: Approximately 6,025,000
Capital City: Boston
Time zone: GMT minus 5 hours (EST)
Climate: Warm summers with an average temperature of approximately 24°C.
Winters are cold with a lot of snow, & temperatures averaging
approximately -2°C. Provincetown has a milder temperature than that of
Boston.
Age of consent & homosexuality legislation: All anal & oral sex is
illegal in this state (no prosecutions if the activity is in private.) There is
legislation in place against discrimination on the basis of sexual
orientation.
Legal drinking age: 21

State Resources

Internet Mailing Lists: Sexuality

♂▽ **BIVERSITY**
☎ 617 338 9595
✉ biversity-request@gnu.ai.mit.edu
Announcements (not discussion) of events of interest to the bisexual
community in New England.

Manufacturers: Erotica: BDSM

☺ **Leather by Danny (& Cohorts)**
☎ 617 288 2203
✉ dantan@ace.com
Custom leather restraints. Specialises in cuffs & collars accented with
colour.

Manufacturers: Furniture: BDSM

☺ **Dragon's Design**
☎ 508 465 5185
Also rubber clothing, toys, & restraints.

Organizations: AIDS: Education

☺☐ **AIDS Action Committee**
♿ 131 Clarendon Street, Boston, Massachusetts 02116.
☎ 800 235 2331 (in Massachusetts only)
☎ 800 788 1234 (youth only)
Hotline also: 617 437 6200.

☺☐ **AIDS Allies**
♿ 93 Mill Park, Springfield, Massachusetts 01108.
☎ 413 747 5144

☺☐ **AIDS Information Collective**
Hampshire College, Amherst, Massachusetts 01002.
☎ 413 539 4600
Publishes *AIDSnews*.

☺☐ **American Red Cross**
♿ Berkshire AIDS Coalition, 480 West Street, Pittsfield, Massachusetts
01201.
☎ 800 332 2030
☎ 413 442 1506

Organizations: AIDS: Support

☺▽ **Affected by AIDS Support Group**
⚥ 175 Wendell Avenue, Pittsfield, Massachusetts 01201.
☎ 413 443 7905
☎ 413 442 1838

Organizations: Sexuality

⚥▽ **Gender Identity Support Services for Transexuals
(GISST)**
☎ 617 720 3413
Support & referral.

Allston

Piercers

☺■ **Rites of Passage**
107 Brighton Avenue, Allston, Massachusetts.
☎ 617 783 1918
🕐 Mon - Wed Fri 14:30 - 19:00, Sat 12:30 - 19:00

Amherst

Counsellors

⚥▽ **Lesbian, Bisexual, & Gay Men's Counseling
Collective**
Student Union Box 41, University of Massachusetts, Amherst,
Massachusetts 01003.
☎ 413 545 2645

Organizations: Family

☺☐ **Parents & Friends of Lesbians & Gays (PFLAG)—
Pioneer Valley**
P. O. Box 55, South Hadley, Massachusetts 01075-0055.
☎ 413 532 4883

Organizations: Sexuality: Student

♂▽ **Hampshire College Gay & Bisexual Men's Alliance**
Hampshire College, Amherst, Massachusetts 01002.
☎ 413 549 4600
⏲ Meets weekly

♂▽ **Lesbian, Bisexual, Gay Alliance (LBGA)**
♿ Student Union Box 66, University of Massachusetts, Amherst, Massachusetts 01003.
☎ 413 545 0154

♂▽ **Program for Gay, Lesbian, & Bisexual Concerns**
Crampton House/SW, University of Massachusetts, Amherst, Massachusetts 01003.
☎ 413 545 4824
☎ 413 545 2632
⏲ 24hr. telephones

Publishers: Magazines: Sexuality

⊕ *Trivia*
P. O. Box 9606, Amherst, Massachusetts 01059-9606.

Publishers: Newspapers: Sexuality

⊕ ▽ *Valley Women's Voice*
♿ 321 Student Building, University of Massachusetts, Amherst, Massachusetts 01003.
☎ 413 545 2436

Radio: Sexuality

☺☐ *Women's Media Project*
♿ WMUA, 102 Campus Center, University of Massachusetts, Amherst, Massachusetts 01003.
☎ 413 545 2876

Stores: Books: General

☺▽ **Food For Thought Books**
♿ 106 North Pleasant Street, Amherst, Massachusetts 01002-1703.
☎ 413 253 5432

Andover

Counsellors

☺ **Raymond Arsenault, Ph.D.**
Κ #201, 138 Haverhill Street, Andover, Massachusetts 01810.
☎ 508 475 7171
Psychologist.

Attleboro Falls

Organizations: Sexuality

♂▽ **Triborough Triangles**
♿ P. O. Box 2751, Attleboro Falls, Massachusetts 02763.
☎ 508 223 4636

Avon

Distributors: Books: General

☺ **Golden Lee Distributors**
75 Stockton Drive, Avon, Massachusetts 02322.
☎ 508 586 3900 📞 508 588 5352

Belmont Center

Counsellors

▽ **Dennis Pearne, Ed.D.**
9 Alexander Avenue, Belmont Center, Massachusetts 02178.
☎ 617 484 0013
Clinical psychologist.

Boston

Artists: Erotic

☺■ **Q. W. Hq. P.**
P. O. Box 281, Astor Station, Boston, Massachusetts 02123.
👝 ✓
Creates b&w art of any fantasy. Also publishes small magazine. Make cheques payable to cash. Publishes *D. B. VelVeeda Presents*. Age statement of 18 is required.

Bars: BDSM

♂▼ **The Boston Eagle**
520 Tremont Street, Boston, Massachusetts.
☎ 617 542 4494

♂▼ **Club 119**
119 Merrimac Street, Boston, Massachusetts.
☎ 617 367 0713

♂▼ **Ramrod**
1254 Boylston Street, Boston, Massachusetts 02215.

☎ 617 266 2986
Women welcome.

☺▼ **The Sling**
228 Cambridge Street, Boston, Massachusetts.
☎ 617 742 4084

BBSs: BDSM

☺■ **Bound for Pleasure**
☎ 617 374 9255

Counsellors

☺☐ **Focus, Inc.**
186 1/2 Hampshire Street, Cambridge, Massachusetts 02139.
☎ 617 876 4488

♂▽ **Joel Hencken, Ph.D.**
45 Lincoln Street, Watertown, Massachusetts 02127-1950.
☎ 617 864 7711

♂▼ **Mass Bay Counseling Associates**
5th. Floor, 321 Columbus Avenue, Boston, Massachusetts 02116.
☎ 617 739 7832

▽ **Elke O'Donnell, Ph.D.**
43 Roberts Road, Cambridge, Massachusetts 02138.

♂▼ **Miriam Rosenberg, M.D., Ph.D.**
♿ ☎ 508 358 7512

☺▼ **Madeline Spadola, Ms.Ed, CADAC**
♿ 108 Summer Street, Somerville, Massachusetts 02143.
☎ 617 625 0761

▽ **Theseus Counseling Services**
Κ P. O. Box 390861, Cambridge, Massachusetts 02139-0861.
☎ 617 868 3157
⏲ Mon - Fri afternoons & evenings
👝 ✓ 💳 💳
Therapist & public speaker. French, German, Spanish, Italian, & Greek also spoken.

Health Services

☺☐ **Boston City Hospital**
818 Harrison, Boston, Massachusetts 02118.
☎ 617 534 5000

⊕ ☐ **Brigham Women's Hospital**
75 Saint Francis Street, Boston, Massachusetts 02115.
☎ 617 732 5500

☺☐ **Cambridge Hospital**
1493 Cambridge Street, Cambridge, Massachusetts 02139.
☎ 617 498 1000

♂▽ **Fenway Community Health Center**
7 Haviland Street, Boston, Massachusetts 02115.
☎ 617 267 0900
Services include HIV education & testing.

☺☐ **Massachusetts General Hospital**
32 Fruit Street, Boston, Massachusetts 02114.
☎ 617 726 2000
HIV & emergency departments.

☺☐ **New England Deaconess Hospital**
185 Pilgrim Road, Boston, Massachusetts 02215.
☎ 6177 632 2000

☺☐ **New England Medical Center**
750 Washington Street, Boston, Massachusetts 02111.
☎ 617 956 5000

☺☐ **Saint Elizabeth's Medical Center of Boston**
☎ 617 789 3000

☺☐ **Veterans' Affairs Medical Center**
150 South Huntington Avenue, Jamaica Plain, Massachusetts 02130.
☎ 617 232 9500

Helplines: Sexuality

♂▽ **Boston Gay & Lesbian Helpline**
☎ 617 267 9001 (voice or TTY)
⏲ Mon - Fri 16:00 - 23:00, Sun 18:00 - 23:00

Internet Mailing Lists: Sexuality

♦♦☐ **POLY-BOSTON**
✉ Majordomo@world.std.com
Non-Monogamous Relationships Discussion List. Discussion of non-monogamy, polyfidelity, & group marriage in the Boston area. To subscribe, send e-mail to: Majordomo@world.std.com with body text of: subscribe poly-boston.

Manufacturers: Clothing: Rubber

♂▼ **Rubberworks**
♿ 1254 Boylston Street, Boston, Massachusetts 02215.
☎ 617 734 9582 📞 617 734 2212

☎ 617 266 0151
🕐 12:00 - 20:00
🏠 ✓ $ ⚡ ₵
Custom rubber clothing & repairs.

Manufacturers: Erotica: BDSM

☺ **Brigid's Trove**
Suite 2, 72 Church Street, Somerville, Massachusetts 02143.
☎ 617 666 9390
Custom clothing, toys, whips, floggers, etc..

Organizations: Academic: Psychiatry

⚥▼ **The American Group Psychotherapy Association**
Gay, Lesbian, & Bisexual Interest Group, c/o Joel Frost, Suite 214, 520 Commonwealth Avenue, Boston, Massachusetts 02215.
☎ 617 266 1616

Organizations: BDSM

☺ ☐ **A.S.B. Munch—Boston**
✉ davo@max.tiac.net

⚥▽ **Ambassadors**
Suite 2, 262 Shawmut, Boston, Massachusetts 02118.

⚥ ▼ **Common Bond**
P. O. Box 390313, Boston, Massachusetts 02139.

⚥▽ **Defenders—Boston**
55 East Springfield Street, Boston, Massachusetts 02118.
☎ 617 437 0998

⚥ **dreizehn**
P. O. Box 1486, Boston, Massachusetts 02117.

⚥▽ **Leather Knights**
P. O. Box 1969, Boston, Massachusetts 02105-1969.

Organizations: Bears

⚥▽ **New England Bears**
P. O. Box 873, Cambridge, Massachusetts 02140-0008.
☎ 617 762 7821 Ext.: 4
✉ nebnews@aol.com or dhorton@spdcc.com
🌐 http://ptown.com/neb/

Organizations: Body Size

⚥▽ **Girth & Mirth—New England**
P. O. Box 6041, Boston, Massachusetts 02209.
☎ 617 387 0762
Publishes a newsletter.

Organizations: Family

☺ ☐ **Parents & Friends of Lesbians & Gays (PFLAG)—Boston**
P. O. Box 44-4, Boston, Massachusetts 02144.
☎ 617 547 2440

Organizations: Fetish: Clothing: Rubber

☺▽ **The Boston Rubber Club**
1254 Boylston Street, Boston, Massachusetts 02215.
☎ 617 734 9582 ✆ 617 734 2212
☎ 617 266 0151
🕐 Meets 4th. Fri. of month 20:30
Contact: Mr. Wayne Goguen, President
Social fetish club. Publishes a newsletter every two months.

Organizations: Fetish: Foreskin

☺ ▽ **The Circumcision Resource Center**
P. O. Box 232, Boston, Massachusetts 02133.
☎ 617 523 0088
Catalogue, free with SASE or IRC.

Organizations: Motorcycle

⚥ **Entre Nous MC**
P.O. Box 984, Boston, Massachusetts 02103.

⚥ ☐ **Moving Violations**
P. O. Box 2356, Cambridge, Massachusetts 02238-2356.
☎ 617 695 8093

⚥▽ **Riders MC**
P.O. Box 519, Boston, Massachusetts 02258.

⚥▽ **Vikings MC**
P. O. Box 6464, JFK Station, Boston, Massachusetts 02114-6464.
☎ 617 451 5377
Contact: Mr. Joe Laing

Organizations: Polyfidelity

☺ ■ **Family Tree**
P. O. Box 441275, Somerville, Massachusetts 02144.
✉ ftree@contra.org
🌐 http://www.contra.org/ftree/

Publishes a newsletter every month.

Organizations: Sexuality

⚥▽ **AXA**
P. O. Box 380547, Cambridge, Massachusetts 02238.
🕐 Wed 18:30

♂ ▽ **Bisexual Community Resource Center**
♿ P. O. Box 639, Cambridge, Massachusetts 02139.
☎ 617 338 9595
✉ brc@panix.com
🌐 http://www.qrd.org/QRD/www/BRC/brc-toc.html

♂ ▽ **Biversity Boston**
♿ P. O. Box 639, Boston, Massachusetts 02139.
☎ 617 338 9595
Publishes *Biversity Calendar*.

⚥▽ **Black & White Men Together (BWMT)—Boston**
GCN Box 1, 25 West Street, Boston, Massachusetts 02111-1213.

⚥ ▽ **Boston Bisexual Women's Network**
♿ c/o The Center, P. O. Box 639, Cambridge, Massachusetts 02140.
☎ 617 3389595
Publishes *Bi-Women* every two months.

⚥▽ **Boston Lesbian & Gay Community Center**
♿ P. O. Box 69, West Medford, Massachusetts 02156-0069.
☎ 617 247 2927
🕐 10:00 - 22:00
Publishes *The Center Times*.

⚥▽ **Chiltern Mountain Club**
P. O. Box 407, Boston, Massachusetts 02117-0407.
☎ 617 859 2843

⚥▽ **Dorchester Gay & Lesbian Alliance (GALA)**
♿ P. O. Box 329, Dorchester, Massachusetts 02122.
☎ 617 825 3737

♂ ▽ **East Coast Bisexual Network**
P. O. Box 639, Cambridge, Massachusetts 02140.

⚥▽ **Enterprise**
P. O. Box 629, Jamaica Plain, Massachusetts 02130.
☎ 617 983 3264
Group for female-to-males & intersexes.

⚥▽ **Gays & Lesbians of Watertown (GLOW)**
⚥ P. O. Box 384, Watertown, Massachusetts 02272-0384.

⚥▽ **International Foundation for Gender Education (IFGE)**
P. O. Box 229, Waltham, Massachusetts 02154-0229.
☎ 617 899 2212 ✆ 617 899 5703
☎ 617 893 8340
🌐 http://www.transgender.org/tg/ifge/index.html
🕐 14:00 - 18:00
✓ 💳 💳
Contact: Ms. Merrissa Sherril Lynn, Founding Director
Also has library open to public. Free catalogue of publications. Publishes *TV-TS Tapestry Journal* quarterly. Yearly subscription is $40.

⚥▽ **The Society of Cross-Dressing Hardware Engineers (SCHE)**
Suite L, 276 Pearl Street, Cambridge, Massachusetts 02139.
Publishes *SCHE Mail*.

⚥▽ **Transgendered Alliance**
P. O. Box 38-1005, Cambridge, Massachusetts 02238.

Organizations: Sexuality: Student

⚥▽ **Babson Gay & Lesbian Alliance**
P. O. Box 631, Babson Park, Wellesley, Massachusetts 02157.

⚥▽ **Boston University Gay, Lesbian, & Bisexual Caucus**
♿ Boston University School of Law, 765 Commonwealth Avenue, Boston, Massachusetts 02115.
☎ 617 353 8974

⚥▽ **Brandeis Triskelion**
♿ Box 32-L, Brandeis University, Waltham, Massachusetts 02254-9110.
☎ 617 736 4761

⚥▽ **Gay Men & Lesbian Alliance**
♿ c/o Dr. P. Korn, Suffolk University, Beacon Hill, Massachusetts 02114.
☎ 617 573 8226

⚥▽ **Gays & Lesbians at Andover Newton Theological School (GLANTS)**
210 Herrick Road, Boston, Massachusetts 02159.

⚥▽ **Gays, Lesbians, Bisexuals, & Friends at MIT (GAMIT)**
MIT 50-306, 142 Memorial Drive, Cambridge, Massachusetts 02139.
☎ 617 253 5440

☟▽ **Harvard Gay & Lesbian Caucus**
P. O. Box 1809, Cambridge, Massachusetts 02238.
Publishes *The Harvard Gay & Lesbian Review* quarterly. Yearly subscription is $16.

☟▽ **Lesbian, Gay, & Bisexual Caucus**
& Northeastern School of Law, 400 Huntington Avenue, Boston, Massachusetts 02115.

☟▽ **Lesbian, Gay, & Bisexual Center**
& University of Massachusetts, 100 Morrissey Boulevard, Dorchester, Massachusetts 02125-3393.
☎ 617 287 7983
Publishes a newsletter.

☟▽ **Lesbian, Gay, & Bisexual Community at Boston College**
Box L-112, Boston College, Chestnut Hill, Massachusetts 02167.
☎ 617 552 2979

Photographers: Erotic

☺ **Laura Graff**
P. O. Box 2353, Jamaica Plain, Massachusetts 02130-0020.

Publishers: Books: Erotic

☺▼ **Circlet Press**
Suite 278, 1770 Massachusetts Avenue, Cambridge, Massachusetts 02140.
☎ 617 864 0492 ✆ 617 864 0492
✉ circlet-info@circlet.com
⊕ http://www.circlet.com/circlet/home.html
♠ ✓ $ ▭ ▭
Erotic science fiction & fantasy with alternate sexuality themes. Age statement of 18 is required.

Publishers: Books: Sexuality

☟▼ **Alyson Publications, Inc.**
40 Plympton Street, Boston, Massachusetts 02118.
☎ 617 542 5679 ✆ 617 542 9189
✓ ▭ ▭
Publishers since 1980, now owned by Liberation Publications, Inc..

Publishers: Directories: Sexuality

♂▼ **International Directory of Bisexual Groups**
Bisexual Community Resource Center, P. O. Box 639, Cambridge, Massachusetts 02139.
☎ 617 338 9595
✉ brc@panix.com
⊕ http://www.qrd.org/QRD/www/BRC/brc-toc.html
Published every two months.

Publishers: Guides: Sexuality

☟▼ **The Guide**
P. O. Box 593, Boston, Massachusetts 02199.
☎ 617 266 8557 ✆ 617 266 1125
⏰ 09:00 - 17:00
✓
Published every month. Yearly subscription is $25.

Publishers: Magazines: BDSM

⚲▼ **Bad Attitude**
Phantasia Productions, P. O. Box 390110, Cambridge, Massachusetts 02139-0110.
Published quarterly. Yearly subscription is $30.

⚲ **Mastery Magazine**
Alternate Woods Publishing, Suite 355-028, 89 Massachusetts Avenue, Boston, Massachusetts 02115.
✉ aidan@blp.com

Publishers: Magazines: Erotic

☺ **Paramour Magazine**
P. O. Box 949, Cambridge, Massachusetts 02140-0008.
☎ 617 499 0069
Published quarterly. Yearly subscription is $18. Age statement of 21 is required.

Publishers: Magazines: Literary

☺■ **The Boston Book Review**
4th. Floor, 30 Brattle Street, Cambridge, Massachusetts 02138.
☎ 617 497 0344 ✆ 617 497 0394
✉ BBReview@shore.net
Yearly subscription is $20, outside U.S. $38.

Publishers: Magazines: Sexuality

☺■ **EIDOS Magazine**
Brush Hill Press, P.O. Box 96, Boston, Massachusetts 02137-0096.
☎ 800 403 4367 ✆ 617 364 0096
☎ 617 262 0096

⏰ 24hr. voice mail
♠ ✓ ▭ ▭
Published quarterly. Yearly subscription is $55. Age statement of 21 is required.

☟▼ **Gayme Magazine**
Zymurgy, P. O. Box 15645, Boston, Massachusetts 02215.
☎ 617 695 8015
♠ ✓
Published twice a year. Yearly subscription is $10U.S. for U.S., $14U.S. for Cdn..

☟ **Polished Knob**
Planet 23 Productions, P. O. Box 487, Boston, Massachusetts 02134-0004.
✉ pk@planet23.com
Published quarterly. Yearly subscription is $12. Age statement of 21 is required.

Publishers: Mailing Lists: General

☺■ **Resources Mailing Lists**
P. O. Box 1067, Harvard Square Station, Cambridge, Massachusetts 02138-1067.
☎ 617 825 8895

Publishers: Newspapers: General

⊕ **Sojourner - The Women's Forum**
42 Seaverns Avenue, Boston, Massachusetts 02130.
☎ 617 524 0415
A feminist news journal that includes features, opinion pieces, reviews, & original fiction & poetry. Published every month. Yearly subscription is $19.

Publishers: Newspapers: Sexuality

☟ **Alliance of Massachusetts Asian Lesbians and Gay Men**
P. O. Box 543, Boston, Massachusetts 02199.

☟▼ **Bay Windows**
& 1523 Washington Street, Boston, Massachusetts 02111.
☎ 617 266 6670
Published every week.

☟ **Fag Rag**
P. O. Box 331, Kenmore Station, Boston, Massachusetts 01060.

☟ **Gay Community News**
Bromfield Street Educational Foundation, 29 Stanhope Street, Boston, Massachusetts 02118.
☎ 617 262 6969
Published every week.

☟ **Gay Review**
39 East Concord Street, Boston, Massachusetts 02118.
☎ 617 262 2101

☟ **IN Newsweekly**
IN Publications, 258 Shawmut Drive, Boston, Massachusetts 02118-8246.
☎ 617 292 0212 ✆ 617 426 8264
New England's largest gay & lesbian newspaper. Covers news, politics, health, arts, & entertainment, & the club scene for our eclectic readers. Published every week. Yearly subscription is $125.

Stores: Books: General

☺■ **Brookline Booksmith**
& 279 Harvard Street, Brookline, Massachusetts 02146.
☎ 617 566 6660

☺■ **Buddenbrooks**
2nd. Floor, 755 Boylston Street, Boston, Massachusetts 02116.
☎ 617 536 4433

☺▼ **Crone's Harvest**
& 761 Jamaica Street, Jamaica Plain, Massachusetts 02130.
☎ 617 983 9530
⏰ 10:00 - 19:00, Sun 12:00 - 18:00

☟▼ **Glad Day Bookshop**
673 Boylston Street, Boston, Massachusetts 02116.
☎ 617 267 3010

☺■ **Harvard Book Store**
& 1256 Massachusetts Avenue, Cambridge, Massachusetts 02138.
☎ 617 661 1515
⏰ 09:30 - 23:00, Sun 12:00 - 18:00

⊕■ **New Words**
& 186 Hampshire Street, Cambridge, Massachusetts 02139.
☎ 617 876 5310
☎ 617 876 3340 (TDD)
⏰ Mon - Fri 10:00 - 20:00, Sat - 18:00, Sun 12:00 - 18:00

☺■ **Redbook**

Stores: Books: General

📖 3 Central Square, Cambridge, Massachusetts 02139-3310.
　☎ 617 522 1464
　🕐 Tue - Fri 12:00 - 19:00, Sat Sun 12:00 - 17:00
☺ ▼ **Unicorn Books**
　🖇 1210 Massachusetts Avenue, Arlington, Massachusetts 02174.
　☎ 617 646 3680
☺ ■ **Wordsworth**
　30 Brattle Street, Cambridge, Massachusetts 02138.
　☎ 617 354 5201

Stores: Clothing: Uniforms

☺ ■ **AAA Police Supply**
　900 Providence Highway, Dedham, Massachusetts.
　☎ 617 326 8845

Stores: Erotica: BDSM

☺ ■ **Hubba Hubba**
　932 Massachusetts Avenue, Cambridge, Massachusetts 02139.
　☎ 617 492 9082
　Also has high-heeled shoes in all sizes.
⚥▼ **Innovations**
　c/o The Boston Ramrod, 1245 Boylston Street, Boston, Massachusetts
　02215.
☺ ■ **Marquis de Sade**
　73 Berkeley Street, Boston, Massachusetts.
　☎ 617 426 2120

Stores: Erotica: General

☺ ■ **Lifestyles for the 90's**
　269 Moody Street, Waltham, Massachusetts 02154.
　☎ 617 891 6060
☺ ■ **Love Toy Books**
　646 Washington Street, Boston, Massachusetts 02111.
　☎ 617 451 2168

Stores: Leatherwork Supplies: General

☺ ■ **Berman Leathercraft**
　25 Melcher Street, Boston, Massachusetts 02210-1599.
　☎ 617 426 0870

Stores: Military Surplus

☺ ■ **Massachusetts Army Navy Store**
　895 Boylston, Boston, Massachusetts.
　☎ 617 267 1559
☺ ■ **Melrose Army Navy Store**
　488 Main Street, Melrose, Massachusetts.
　☎ 617 665 9729
☺ ■ **Stoughton Army Navy Center**
　763 Washington, Stoughton, Massachusetts.
　☎ 617 341 0769
☺ ■ **Winthrop Army Navy Store**
　462 Shirley, Winthrop, Massachusetts.
　☎ 617 539 0617

Boylston

Organizations: BDSM

⚥ **Boston Ducks**
　P.O. Box 81, Boylston, Massachusetts 01505-0081.
　☎ 617 783 5298
　Contact: Mr. Gene Lawrence

Bridgewater

Organizations: Sexuality

⚥▽ **South Shore Gay & Lesbian Alliance**
　P. O. Box 712, Bridgewater, Massachusetts 02324.
　☎ 508 293 5183

Burlington

Organizations: Sexuality

▽ **Nightlife**
　P. O. Box 1132, Burlington, Massachusetts 02803.
　☎ 508 658 4421

Charlestown

Organizations: BDSM

⚥▽ **Boston Unified Leather Legion (BULL)**
　P. O. Box 287, Charlestown, Massachusetts 02129-0002.
　☎ 617 241 8968
　🕐 Call in afternoon
⚥ **Mike's Men**

　P.O. Box 287, Charlestown, Massachusetts 02129.
　☎ 617 241 8968
　Contact: Mr. Mike Miller
⊕ **Wanda's Wenches**
　P. O. Box 287, Charlestown, Massachusetts 02129.

Dennisport

Printers: General

☺ **Crane Duplicating**
　P.O. Box 99, Dennisport, Massachusetts 02639.
　☎ 508 760 1601　　　　　📠 508 760 1544

Dorchester

Organizations: Motorcycle

⚥ **Iron Eagles MC**
　#3, 381 Adams Street, Dorchester, Massachusetts 02122-1240.

East Dedham

Organizations: Sexuality

▽ **Reflections**
　P. O. Box 4002, East Dedham, Massachusetts 02026.
　🕐 Meets 4th. Sat of month 15:00 - 17:00
　Publishes a newsletter.

Framingham

Health Services

☺ □ **Metrowest Medical Center**
　115 Lincoln Street, Framingham, Massachusetts 01701.
　☎ 508 383 1020

Organizations: Sexuality: Student

⚥▽ **Framingham State College Gays, Lesbians, &**
　Friends (GLAF)
　College Center 508, 100 State Street, Framingham, Massachusetts
　01701.

Organizations: Sexuality: Youth

⚥▽ **Framingham Regional Alliance of Gay & Lesbian**
　🖇 **Youth (FRAGLY)**
　P. O. Box 426, Framingham, Massachusetts 01701.
　☎ 508 655 7183

Stores: Books: General

☺ ■ **Borders Book Shop**
　🚹 85 Worcester Road, Framingham, Massachusetts 01701.
　☎ 508 875 2321

Gloucester

Stores: Books: General

☺ ■ **The Bookstore**
　61 Main Street, Gloucester, Massachusetts 01930.
　☎ 508 281 1548

Great Barrington

Publishers: Magazines: Sexuality

⊕ *Hikané*
　P. O. Box 841, Great Barrington, Massachusetts 01230.

Greenfield

Organizations: Sexuality

▽ **After Surgery Support Exchange for Transexuals**
　(ASSET)
　P. O. Box 3121, Greenfield, Massachusetts 01302.
　📧 asset@crocker.com

Stores: Books: General

☺ ■ **World Eye Bookshop**
　🚹 60 Federal Street, Greenfield, Massachusetts 01301.
　☎ 413 772 2186
　🕐 09:00 - 19:00, Fri - 21:00, Sun 12:00 - 17:00

Hadley

Organizations: Sexuality

▽ **Sunshine Club**
　P. O. Box 149, Hadley, Massachusetts 01035-0149.
　Contact: Ms. Roberta Steel
　Publishes a newsletter every month.

Haverhill

Organizations: BDSM

☺ **The Femina Society International**
P.O. Box 1873, Haverhill, Massachusetts 01831-1873.
☎ 718 648 8215
✉ infinity@palace.com
🕐 Mon - Fri 11:00 - 20:00
👗 ✓ $
Contact: Ms. Charlene Deering, F. S.
Networking & education in matriarchal female domination, goddess spirituality. The Panty Institute e-mail broadcast forum on Delphi. Telephone consultation . Publishes *Femina*. Yearly subscription is $10. Age statement of 21 is required.

Lowell

Counsellors

☺ ■ **Merrimack Valley Counseling**
♿ 184 Pleasant Valley Street, Methuen, Massachusetts 01844-5855.
☎ 508 687 4383

Organizations: Sexuality

♁▽ **Shared Times**
P. O. Box 8822, Lowell, Massachusetts 01853.
☎ 508 441 9081

Organizations: Sexuality: Student

♂▽ **Gay Outreach Association for Lowell Students (GOALS)**
South Box 59, 1 University Avenue, Lowell, Massachusetts 01854.
☎ 508 452 3679

Printers: General

☺ **Courier Corporation**
165 Jackson Street, Lowell, Massachusetts 01852-2195.
☎ 508 458 6351

Stores: Erotica: General

☺ ■ **Tower Newsstand**
101 Gorham Street, Lowell, Massachusetts 01852.
☎ 508 452 8693
🕐 06:00 - 01:00, Fri Sat - 03:00

Malden

Publishers: Books: Sexuality

♂▽ **Purple Stone Press & Productions**
P. O. Box 249, Malden, Massachusetts 02148.
☎ 617 321 3569 ✆ 617 321 9901
🕐 Mon - Fri 09:00 - 17:00 Eastern

Books & educational videos about gay, lesbian, bisexual, & transgender youth & adults in schools. Mail order only.

Stores: Military Surplus

☺ ■ **GI Joe's Genuine Surplus**
196-198 Ferry Road, Malden, Massachusetts.
☎ 617 322 8600
👗 💳

☺ ■ **Jerry's Army & Navy Store**
415 Main Road, Malden, Massachusetts.
☎ 617 324 6990

Marblehead

Organizations: Sexuality

♂▽ **North Shore Gay & Lesbian Alliance**
P. O. Box 806, Marblehead, Massachusetts 02945.
☎ 617 745 3848

Marlborough

Organizations: Sexuality

♁▽ **West of Boston Lesbians (Wobbles)**
♿ P. O. Box 292, Marlborough, Massachusetts 01752.
☎ 508 386 7737
Publishes a newsletter.

Medfield

Suppliers: Diapers

☺ ■ **Support Plus**
P. O. Box 500, 99 West Street, Medfield, Massachusetts 02052.
☎ 800 229 2910
☎ 508 359 8372
Carry Depends, Dignity, & Curity adult disposable diapers.

Middleboro

Organizations: BDSM

♂▽ **Black Eagle MC**
285 West Grove Street, Middleboro, Massachusetts 02346.
Contact: Mr. Dennis Samson

Millis

Organizations: Bears

♁ **T-Bears of Boston**
72 Van Kleek Road, Millis, Massachusetts 02054.
☎ 508 376 5892
Contact: Ms. Catherine Kuhlman

Natick

Publishers: Magazines: Sexuality

✉▼ **Transgendered Magazine**
P. O. Box 2085, Natick, Massachusetts 01760.
Magazine on DOS diskette. Published quarterly. Yearly subscription is $45.

Needham Heights

Organizations: Swingers

☺ ☐ **Sterling**
P. O. Box 542, Needham Heights, Massachusetts 02194.
☎ 508 586 4442
SASE or IRC required. When calling, a female must be present. Dances & parties for couples & single women only. Publishes a newsletter.

Newburyport

Organizations: Sexuality

♁▽ **Merrimack Valley Lesbians**
☎ 508 521 2239

Newton Centre

Organizations: BDSM

☺ ☐ **The National Leather Association (NLA)—New England**
9100-164, 831 Beacon Street, Newton Centre, Massachusetts 02159.
✉ nla-ne@id.wing.net
Contact: Mr. John Klein
Publishes *Scarlet Leather* every two months. Yearly subscription is $6.

Nonantum

Stores: Clothing: Sexuality

✉ **Vernon's Specialties, Inc.**
♿ P. O. Box 95189, Nonantum, Massachusetts 02195-5189.
☎ 617 894 1744 ✆ 617 647 4082
🕐 Mon Tue 10:00 - 17:00, Wed Thu Sat 10:00 - 18:00, Fri 10:00 - 20:00
👗 ✓ 💳 💳 💳 💳
Also mail order. Catalogue, $10.

Stores: Erotica: BDSM

✉ **Inclinations**
P. O. Box 95189, Nonantum, Massachusetts 02195-5189.
☎ 617 893 4597 ✆ 617 647 4082
🕐 Mon Tue 10:00 - 17:00, Wed Thu Sat 10:00 - 18:00, Fri 10:00 - 20:00
👗 ✓ 💳 💳 💳 💳
Also mail order. Catalogue, $10.

Northampton

Health Services

☺ ☐ **Veterans' Affairs Medical Center**
Route 9, Northampton, Massachusetts 01060.
☎ 413 584 4040
HIV department. No emergency department.

Organizations: BDSM

♁ ▽ **Shelix**
♿ P.O. Box 416, Northampton, Massachusetts 01060-1416.
Publishes a newsletter.

Organizations: Sexuality

✉☐ **East Coast FTM Group**
P. O. Box 60585, Florence Station, Northampton, Massachusetts 01060.

Organizations: Sexuality: Student

☻▽ **Smith College Lesbian, Gay, & Bisexual Alliance**
Stoddard Annex, Smith College, Northampton, Massachusetts 01063.
☏ 413 585 4907

Piercers

☺ ■ **Adam Meyerson**
3 Horn Face, 45 Olive Street, Northampton, Massachusetts 01060.
☏ 413 582 0424
◷ By appointment only

Stores: Books: General

☺ ■ **Beyond Words Bookshop**
189 Main Street, Northampton, Massachusetts 01060.
☏ 413 586 6304
◷ 09:30 - 21:00, Fri Sat - 22:30, Sun 12:00 - 17:00

☼ ▼ **Lunaria Feminist Bookstore**
90 King Street, Northampton, Massachusetts 01060.
☏ 413 586 7851 (voice & TDD)
◷ Tue Wed Fri 10:00 - 18:00, Thu - 20:00, Sat - 17:00, Sun 12:00 - 17:00

Stores: Erotica: BDSM

☺ ■ **Primitive Leather**
267 Pleasant Street, Northampton, Massachusetts 01060.
Also do piercings.

Orleans

Organizations: Sexuality

✉▽ **Innvestments**
P. O. Box 2194, Orleans, Massachusetts 02653.
◷ Meets 1st. Tue of month, except in the summer
Support group. Publishes a newsletter.

Publishers: Magazines: Sexual Politics

☼ *Women of Power Magazine*
P. O. Box 2785, Orleans, Massachusetts 02653.
☏ 508 240 7877

Palmer

Suppliers: Diapers

☺ ■ **Health Tec, Inc.**
First Street, Palmer, Massachusetts 01069-0720.
☏ 413 289 1221
☏ 800 343 1205
Liners & disposable diapers.

Pittsfield

Counsellors

✉▽ **Josefina Speckert, M.Ed.**
Suite 3, 30 East Housatonic Street, Pittsfield, Massachusetts 01201.
Psychotherapist.

Organizations: Family

☺ □ **Parents & Friends of Lesbians & Gays (PFLAG)—Berkshire**
Box 241, RR2, Lee, Massachusetts 01238.
☏ 413 243 2382
☏ 413 458 5171
Publishes a newsletter.

Provincetown

Organizations: AIDS: Support

☺ □ **Provincetown Positive PWA Coalition**
P. O. Box 1465, Provincetown, Massachusetts 02657.
☏ 508 487 3998

Organizations: BDSM

☻▽ **Mates**
P. O. Box 883, Provincetown, Massachusetts 02657-0883.
☏ 508 487 3732

Organizations: Motorcycle

☻▽ **Mooncussers MC**
P. O. Box 4404, Provincetown, Massachusetts 02657.

Publishers: Magazines: Sexuality

☻■ *Provincetown Advocate*
P. O. Box 93, Provincetown, Massachusetts 02657.
☏ 508 487 1170

Publishers: Mailing Lists: Sexuality

☻▼ **Provincetown Purchase Company**
104 Bradford Street, Provincetown, Massachusetts 02657.
☏ 508 487 3232 ✆ 508 487 1605

Publishers: Newspapers: Sexuality

☺ *Provincetown Magazine*
14 Center Street, Provincetown, Massachusetts 02657.
☏ 508 487 3384
Provincetown's town paper (gay & straight) for 13 years. Popular with both tourists & locals. Published every week. Yearly subscription is $64.

Stores: Books: General

☺ ■ **The Little Store**
205 Commercial Street, Provincetown, Massachusetts 02657.
☏ 508 487 0208

☻▼ **Now Voyager**
P. O. Box 751, Provincetown, Massachusetts 02657.
☏ 508 487 0848
◷ 11:00 - 23:00 during season

☺ ■ **Provincetown Bookshop**
246 Commercial Street, Provincetown, Massachusetts 02657.
☏ 508 487 0964

Stores: Erotica: General

☺ ▼ **1st. Old Store**
227 Commercial Street, Provincetown, Massachusetts 2657.
☏ 508 487 1010

Randolph

Organizations: BDSM

☻▽ **The Esoterica Society**
P. O. Box 37, Randolph, Massachusetts 02368.

Shawseen

Organizations: Sexuality

✉▽ **Tayland House**
P. O. Box 3128, Shawseen, Massachusetts 01810-0804.
◷ Weekly meetings

Springfield

Helplines: Sexuality

☻▽ **Gay & Lesbian Info Services**
P. O. Box 891, Springfield, Massachusetts 01138-0891.
☏ 413 731 5403

Organizations: Sexuality

☻▽ **Lesbian, Gay, & Bisexual Support Group**
P. O. Box 891, Springfield, Massachusetts 01138-0891.
☏ 413 458 4273

☻▽ **Valley Gay Alliance**
P. O. Box 80051, Springfield, Massachusetts 01138-0051.
☏ 413 736 2324
◷ Meets 1st. Tue of month 19:30
Publishes *VGA Gayzette*.

Stores: Erotica: General

☺ ■ **Springfield Books & Video**
292 Worthington Street, Springfield, Massachusetts 01103.
☏ 413 781 6833

Swansea

Stores: Books: General

☺ ■ **Newsbreak**
Stuarts Plaza, Route 6, Swansea, Massachusetts 02777.
☏ 508 675 9380

Thorndike

Printers: General

☺ ■ **Van Volumes Limited**
400 High Street, Thorndike, Massachusetts 01079.
☏ 413 283 8556 ✆ 413 283 7884

Vineyard Haven

Organizations: Sexuality

☻□ **Island Lesbian & Gay Association**
P. O. Box 1809, Vineyard Haven, Massachusetts 02568.
☏ 508 693 3563
Publishes *Stone Walls*.

Waltham
Health Services
☺ ☐ **Walthamweston Hospital & Medical Center**
Hope Avenue, Waltham, Massachusetts 02254.
☎ 617 647 6000
Organizations: Spanking
⚢☐ **Northeast Erotic Spanking Society (NESS)**
14 Russell Street, Waltham, Massachusetts 02154.
Contact: Mr. Tom Elliott
Exclusively for couples who love to spank. Primarily erotic spanking, not BDSM. Send SSAE (4 IRCs outside U.S.) for information. Publishes *N. E. S. S. News* quarterly. Yearly subscription is $20. Please address envelopes to Tom Elliot, do NOT address them to Northeast Erotic Spanking Society or N. E. S. S. News.

Watertown
Manufacturers: Erotica: BDSM
☺ **Eclectic Engineering / Consensual Leather**
P. O. Box 745, Watertown, Massachusetts 02172.
Custom leathers, from floggers to slings.

Wayland
Counsellors
▽ **Diane Ellaborn, LICSW, NASW**
Suite 205, 16 Boston Post Road, Wayland, Massachusetts 01778.
☎ 508 877 9671
Psychotherapist.
Organizations: Sexuality
▽ **The Adam Society**
P. O. Box 367, Wayland, Massachusetts 01778-0367.
Contact: Mr. Dan Riley
Support for female-to-males & Sos. Publishes *Adam's Word*.

West Medford
Counsellors
▽ **Services for Men (& Their Families)**
66 Wyman Street, West Medford, Massachusetts 02155.
☎ 617 395 2450
Professional clinic.

West Newton
Organizations: Sexuality
▽ **Getting Real**
P. O. Box 194, West Newton, Massachusetts 02165.
Support for hermaphrodites, intersexes, & primary transexuals.

Westford
Printers: General
☺ **Courier Westford Inc.**
1 Pleasant Street, Westford, Massachusetts 01886.
☎ 508 692 6321

Weymouth
Stores: Military Surplus
☺ ■ **Army Navy Store**
532 Pond Way, Weymouth, Massachusetts.
☎ 617 331 4249

Williamstown
Organizations: Sexuality
▽ **The Myriad Network**
P. O. Box 288, Williamstown, Massachusetts 01267.
Publishes *The Myriad Network* quarterly.
Organizations: Sexuality: Student
▽ **Bi-The-Way**
SU Box 322, Williams College, Williamstown, Massachusetts 01267.
▽ **Gay, Lesbian, & Allied Student Society**
North Adams State College, North Adams, Massachusetts 01247.
☎ 413 664 4511
▽ **Williams Bisexual, Gay, & Lesbian Union**
Student Union Box 3209, Williams College, Williamstown, Massachusetts 01267.
☎ 413 597 2413
Publishers: Newspapers: Sexuality
▽ *Berkshire Alternatives*

P. O. Box 508, North Adams, Massachusetts 01247-0508.

Woburn
Organizations: Sexuality
▽ **Tiffany Club of New England, Inc. (TCNE)**
P. O. Box 2283, Woburn, Massachusetts 01888-0483.
☎ 617 891 8325
🕐 Answered Tue 19:00 - 22:00, voice mail at other times
Publishes *Rosebuds*.
▽ **Tiffany Club Wives' Support Group**
P. O. Box 2283, Woburn, Massachusetts 01888-0483.
☎ 617 891 9325
🕐 Meets monthly
Publishes *Rosebuds*.

Worcester
Health Services
☺ ☐ **Health Awareness Services**
71 Elm Street, Worcester, Massachusetts 01609.
☎ 508 756 7123
Education & outreach related to HIV/AIDS.
☺ ☐ **University of Massachusetts Medical Center**
55 Lake Avenue, Worcester, Massachusetts 01655.
☎ 508 856 0011
HIV & emergency departments.
Organizations: Sexuality
▽ **Worcester County Lesbian & Gay Alliance**
P. O. Box 427, Worcester, Massachusetts 01614-0427.
☎ 508 829 9898
Organizations: Sexuality: Student
▽ **Clark University Bisexual, Lesbian, & Gay Alliane (BLAGA)**
Box 5-B, 950 Main Street, Worcester, Massachusetts 01610-1477.
☎ 508 793 7287
Organizations: Sexuality: Youth
▽ **Supporters of Worcester Area Gay & Lesbian Youth**
P. O. Box 592, West Side Station, Worcester, Massachusetts 01602.
☎ 508 755 0005
Stores: Books: General
☺ ■ **Myrtle Bookstore**
42 Myrtle Street, Worcester, Massachusetts 01608.
☎ 508 755 7541
Stores: Erotica: General
☺ ■ **United Book**
290 Main Street, Worcester, Massachusetts 01608.
☎ 508 752 9293

MICHIGAN
Area: Approximately 147,000 square kilometres
Population: Approximately 9,300,000
Capital City: Lansing
Time zone: GMT minus 5 hours (EST)
Climate: Summers are warm with an average temperature of approximately 21°C. Winters are cold and very snowy, with an average temperature of approximately -1°C.
Age of consent & homosexuality legislation: All anal & oral sex is illegal in this state.
Legal drinking age: 21

State Resources
Organizations: AIDS: Education
☺ ☐ **HIV/AIDS Advocacy Project**
Suite 210, 106 West Allegan, Lansing, Michigan 48933-1706.
☎ 800 288 5923
Organizations: BDSM
☺ **Michigan Society for Domination & Submission (MSDS)**
LdyVette@aol.com
Organizations: Motorcycle
▽ **Trident—Michigan**
P. O. Box 5614, Dearborn, Michigan 48128-4901.
☎ 313 271 4901
Publishers: Newspapers: Sexuality
▽ *Between The Lines*

Diva & Empress Publications, Inc., 1632 Church Street, Detroit, Michigan 48216.
☎ 313 961 4862
✉ Between.The.Lines@um.cc.umich.edu
Michigan's lesbigay newspaper. News, interviews, entertainment, events, columns, & a calendar featuring local personalities & points of view. Published every month. Yearly subscription is $20.

Allendale

Organizations: Sexuality: Student
⚥▽ **Ten Percent of U**
Grand Valley State University, 1 Campus Drive, Allendale, Michigan 49401.
☎ 616 895 6611

Ann Arbor

Counsellors
⚥▽ **Lesbian & Gay Male Advocates**
& 3116-18 Michigan Union, University of Michigan, 530 State Street, Ann Arbor, Michigan 48109.
☎ 313 763 4186
☎ 313 662 1977

▽▽ **Sandra Samons, ACSW**
c/o Homestead Counseling Center, 1480 Shevchenko, Ann Arbor, Michigan 48103.
☎ 313 663 7871

☺ ■ **Lynne Tenbusch, Ph.D.**
Suite C-1, 2301 South Horon Avenue, Ann Arbor, Michigan 48104-5133.
☎ 313 973 3232

☺ ▼ **Jim Wilton, MSW, CSW**
♨ 513 Oswago, Ann Arbor, Michigan 48104-2624.
☎ 313 663 5021

Health Services
☺ □ **University of Michigan Hospitals**
1500 East Medical Center Drive, Ann Arbor, Michigan 48109.
☎ 313 936 4000

☺ □ **Veterans' Affairs Medical Center**
2215 Fuller Road, Ann Arbor, Michigan 48105.
☎ 313 761 5458

Organizations: BDSM
⚤ ▽ **Ultra-Sex Alliance**
P. O. Box 7621, Ann Arbor, Michigan 48107.

Organizations: Family
☺ □ **Parents & Friends of Lesbians & Gays (PFLAG)—**
& **Ann Arbor**
P. O. Box 7471, Ann Arbor, Michigan 48107-7471.
☎ 313 769 1684

Organizations: Sexuality: Student
⚥▽ **University of Michigan**
Lesbian, Gay, & Bisexual Programs Office, 3116 Michigan Union, Ann Arbor, Michigan 48109.
☎ 313 763 4186
🌐 http://www.umich.edu/~inqueery/

Printers: General
☺ ■ **Braun-Brumfield**
P.O. Box 1203, Ann Arbor, Michigan 40106-1203.
☎ 313 662 3291 ✆ 313 662 1667

☺ ■ **Cushing-Malloy**
P.O. Box 8632, Ann Arbor, Michigan 48107-8632.
☎ 313 663 8554 ✆ 313 663 5731

☺ **Edwards Brothers**
2500 South State Street, Ann Arbor, Michigan 48106-1007.
☎ 313 769 1000 ✆ 313 769 1756

☺ **Malloy Lithographing**
P.O. Box 1124, Ann Arbor, Michigan 49106-1124.
☎ 313 665 6113 ✆ 313 665 2326

☺ **Shear-Davis**
715 West Ellsworth Road, Ann Arbor, Michigan 48108-3320.
☎ 313 741 0123

Stores: Books: General
☺ ■ **Borders Book Shop**
303 South State Street, Ann Arbor, Michigan 38104.
☎ 313 668 7652

⚥▼ **Common Language**
& 215 South Fouth Street, Ann Arbor, Michigan 48104.
☎ 313 663 0036

🕐 12:00 - 20:00, Sun - 16:00

☺ ■ **Community Newscenter #4**
& 330 East Liberty, Ann Arbor, Michigan 48104.
☎ 313 663 6168

☺ ■ **Crazy Wisdom Bookstore**
& 206 North 4th. Avenue, Ann Arbor, Michigan 48104.
☎ 313 665 2757

Tattooists
☺ ■ **Creative Tattoo**
307 East Liberty, Ann Arbor, Michigan.
☎ 313 662 2520
🕐 Piercing by appointment only

Bay City

Organizations: BDSM
⚥▽ **L & L Society—Bay City**
P. O. Box 2145, Bay City, Michigan 48707.
☎ 517 982 8054

Organizations: Sexuality
⚥▽ **Tri-Cities Gay & Lesbian Alliance**
P. O. Box 303, Bay City, Michigan 48707.
☎ 517 799 2583

Benton Harbor

Printers: General
☺ ■ **Patterson Printing**
1550 Territorial Road, Benton Harbor, Michigan 49022-1937.
☎ 616 925 2177 ✆ 616 925 6057

Berkeley

Counsellors
☺ **Dale Ross**
2366 Earlmont, Berkeley, Michigan 48072.
☎ 313 544 7041

Organizations: BDSM
⚥▽ **Icon Detroit**
P. O. Box 725421, Berkeley, Michigan 48072-5421.
☎ 313 831 1852

Chelsea

Printers: General
☺ **Bookcrafters**
P.O. Box 370, 613 East Industrial Drive, Chelsea, Michigan 48118-0370.
☎ 313 475 9145 ✆ 313 475 7337
☎ 313 475 9145 Ext. 371

Publishers: Magazines: Sexual Politics
⚥ *Libertarians for Gay & Lesbian Concerns*
Newsletter
P. O. Box 447, Chelsea, Michigan 48118.
☎ 313 475 9792
The goal is to promote the libertarian political philosophy to the gay community. Published quarterly. Yearly subscription is $15.

Dearborn

Organizations: BDSM
⚥▽ **Wolf Pack S&M**
P. O. Box 5066, Dearborn, Michigan 48128.

Detroit

Bars: BDSM
⚥▼ **Chains**
& 6228 Michigan, Detroit, Michigan.
☎ 313 897 3650

⚥▼ **Detroit Eagle**
& 1501 Holden, Detroit, Michigan 48208.
☎ 810 873 6969

⚥▼ **Sam's Tiffany's on the Park**
17436 Woodward Avenue, Detroit, Michigan.

Counsellors
⚥▽ **East Side Ministry of Social Services**
♨ 9162 Crane, Detroit, Michigan 48213.
☎ 313 331 0033

☺ ▼ **Kevin Kinsel, MSW, CSW, PC**
108 East 5th. Street, Royal Oak, Michigan 48067.

☎ 810 541 6830

Health Services

☺ ☐ **Harper Hospital**
3990 John R, Detroit, Michigan 48201.
☎ 313 745 8303
HIV & emergency departments.

☺ ☐ **Henry Ford Hospital**
2799 West Grand Boulevard, Detroit, Michigan 48202.
☎ 313 876 2600
HIV & emergency departments.

Helplines: Sexuality

⚥▽ **Affirmations**
☎ 313 398 4297
☎ 313 398 7105 (office)
🕐 Mon - Fri 18:00 - 23:00

Organizations: AIDS: Education

☺ ☐ **Midwest AIDS Prevention Project (MAPP)**
P. O. Box 20031, Ferndale, Michigan 48220.
☎ 313 545 1435

Organizations: BDSM

☺ ☐ **A.S.B. Munch—Detroit**
📧 Illowen@netcom.com
🕐 Meets 3rd. Sat of month 18:00
Contact: Lon

⚥ **Baccus - Detroit**
P.O. Box 04552, Detroit, Michigan 48204.
☎ 313 933 9344

⚥▽ **Countrymen**
16801 Plymouth Road, Detroit, Michigan 48227.
☎ 313 836 2324

Organizations: Family

⚥▽ **Our Kids**
c/o Pandora Books for Open Minds, 226 West Lovell, Detroit, Michigan 49007.
☎ 616 388 5656
For gay & lesbian parents.

☺ ☐ **Parents & Friends of Lesbians & Gays (PFLAG)—**
♿ **Detroit**
P. O. Box 145, Farmington Hills, Michigan 48332.
☎ 810 478 8408

Organizations: Motorcycle

⚥ **Trident—Detroit**
P.O. Box 19436, Old Redford Station, Detroit, Michigan 48219.

Organizations: Sexuality

⚥▽ **Affirmations Lesbian & Gay Community Center**
Suite 110, 195 West Nine Mile Road, Ferndale, Michigan 48220.
☎ 313 398 4297

⚥▽ **Black & White Men Together (BWMT)—Detroit**
♿ P. O. Box 24831, Detroit, Michigan 48224-8831.
☎ 313 569 8595

⚥☐ **Detroit Area Gay / Lesbian Council (DAG/LC)**
♿ P.O. Box 4425, Troy, Michigan 48099-4425.
☎ 810 853 2488

⚲▽ **National Gender Dysphoria Organization &
Support Group (NGDO)**
P.O. Box 02732, Detroit, Michigan 48202.
☎ 313 842 5228
Contact: Ms. Justina Williams
Suppport & education. Publishes *NGDO Key To Freedom.*

⚥▽ **The Triangle Foundation**
♿ 19641 West Seven Mile Road, Detroit, Michigan 48219-2721.
☎ 313 537 3323

Printers: General

☺ **Harlo Press**
50-P Victor Avenue, Detroit, Michigan 48203-3193.
☎ 313 883 3600

Publishers: Magazines: Sexuality

⚥ *Kick! Magazine*
Kick Publishing Company, P. O. Box 2225, Detroit, Michigan 48231.
☎ 313 438 0704 📞 313 963 4627
Magazine for black gay & lesbian culture. Published every month. Yearly subscription is $15U.S. for U.S., $38U.S. for Cdn..

Stores: Erotica: General

⚥■ **Escape Bookstore**
18728 West Warren, Detroit, Michigan 48228.
☎ 313 336 6558

☺ ■ **Worldwide Magazines**
16140 Woodward Avenue, Highland Park, Michigan 48203.
☎ 313 866 6020

Dexter

Printers: General

☺ **Thomson-Shore, Inc.**
7300 West Joy Road, Dexter, Michigan 48130-0305.
☎ 313 426 3939 📞 313 426 6216
🌐 http://www.tshore.com

Douglas

Organizations: AIDS: Education

☺ ☐ **Holland AIDS Resource Center**
56 Wall Stree, Douglas, Michigan.
☎ 616 396 3538
☎ 616 227 3421
🕐 Meets 1st. & 3rd. Thu of month 19:00

Dowagiac

Counsellors

☺ **Brian Rendel, M.A, NCC**
🄺 c/o The Family Center, Inc, 216 Pennsylvania Avenue, Dowagiac, Michigan 49047.
☎ 616 782 9811
📧 76327.3035@compuserve.com
Ask to be seen by Brian Rendel only. No need to mention to secretary reason for counselling.

East Landing

Stores: Books: General

☺ ■ **Grand River Books**
515 East Grand River, East Landing, Michigan.
☎ 517 333 3666

Ferndale

Manufacturers: Furniture: BDSM

☺ ■ **Nocturne Productions**
640 Wordsworth, Ferndale, Michigan 48067.
☎ 810 542 7980
💳 ✓ $ VISA 💳 💳
Catalogue, $5.

Organizations: Motorcycle

⚥ **International Roadmasters**
3146 Grayson, Ferndale, Michigan 48220.

Stores: Books: General

⚲ **A Woman's Prerogative**
175 West Nine Mile Road, Ferndale, Michigan.
☎ 810 545 5702
🕐 Tue Wed Fri Sat 12:00 - 19:00, Thu 12:00 - 21:00, Sun 12:00 - 17:00

Flint

Counsellors

☺ ■ **Kenneth Kreger, MA, CSW, LPC**
Northbank Center, 400 North Saginaw Street, Flint, Michigan 48502.
☎ 810 234 3658

☺ ■ **Susan Wedda, MSW, ACSW, BCD**
Northbank Center, 400 North Saginaw Street, Flint, Michigan 48502.
☎ 810 234 3658

Health Services

☺ ☐ **Hurley Medical Center**
One Hurley Plaza, Flint, Michigan 48503.
☎ 810 257 9000

☺ ☐ **McLaren Regional Medical Center**
401 South Ballenger Highway, Flint, Michigan 48532.
☎ 810 762 2000

Organizations: Family

☺ ☐ **Parents & Friends of Lesbians & Gays (PFLAG)—**
Flint
P. O. Box 90722, Burton, Michigan 48509-0722.
☎ 313 631 4910

Stores: Books: General

☺ ■ **Young & Welshans Books**
G-4270 Miller Road, Flint, Michigan 48507.
☎ 800 366 8290
☎ 810 732 0620
⊕ Mon - Thu Sat 09:30 - 21:00, Fri - 22:00, Sun 11:00 - 17:00

Grand Rapids

Health Services

☺ □ **Metropolitan Hospital**
P. O. Box 1352, 1919 Boston Street, Grand Rapids, Michigan 49506.
☎ 616 247 7200
HIV & emergency departments.

☺ □ **Saint Mary's Health Services**
P. O. Box 1352, 200 Jefferson Avenue South East, Grand Rapids, Michigan 49503.
☎ 616 774 6399

Manufacturers: Erotica: Leather

☺ ▼ **Wolfmark Woodworks**
The Cell, 76 South Division, Grand Rapids, Michigan 49503.
☎ 616 774 9518 ✆ 616 459 1786
⊕ Mon - Sat 09:00 - 18:00
▦ ✓ $ ⚞
Age statement of 18 is required.

Organizations: AIDS: Education

☺ □ **Grand Rapids AIDS Resource Center**
⅃ P. O. Box 6603, Grand Rapids, Michigan 49516.
☎ 616 459 9177 ✆ 616 459 4031
Information, referral, & other services. Publishes *Communiqué*.

Organizations: BDSM

⚥ **Grand Rapids Rivermen**
P.O. Box 3497, Grand Rapids, Michigan 49501-3497.

⚥ **Nimbus**
P.O. Box 68123, Grand Rapids, Michigan 49516-8123.

Organizations: Family

☺ □ **Parents & Friends of Lesbians & Gays (PFLAG)— Grand Rapids**
Grace Episcopal Church, Grand Rapids, Michigan.
☎ 616 285 9133
Meets 2nd. Sun of month 14:00.

Organizations: Sexuality

⚥▽ **IME of Western Michigan**
P. O. Box 1153, Grand Rapids, Michigan 49501.
⊕ Meets monthly

⚥▽ **The Lesbian & Gay Community Network of Western Michigan**
909 Cherry Street, Grand Rapids, Michigan 49506-1403.
☎ 616 458 3511
Publishes *Network News*.

Organizations: Sexuality: Student

⚥▽ **State University Association of Lesbians & Gays**
P. O. Box 84, Rankin Center, Grand Rapids, Michigan 49307.

Organizations: Sexuality: Youth

⚥▽ **Windfire**
P. O. Box 1352, Grand Rapids, Michigan 49501.
☎ 616 459 5900
⊕ Meets Thu 19:00

Printers: General

☺ **Eerdmans Printing Company**
231 Jefferson Avenue South East, Grand Rapids, Michigan 49503-4569.
☎ 616 451 0763

Stores: Books: General

☺ ■ **Community Newscenter / Webster's**
⅃ 3848 28th. Street South East, Grand Rapids, Michigan 49512-1804.
☎ 616 285 7055

⚥▼ **Sons & Daughters**
⅃ 962 Cherry Street South East, Grand Rapids, Michigan 49506.
☎ 616 459 8877
⊕ Mon - Fri 12:00 - 24:00, Sat Sun 10:00 - 24:00

Holland

Organizations: AIDS: Education

☺ □ **Holland AIDS Resource Center**
c/o American Red Cross, 270 James Street, Holland, Michigan 49424.

☎ 616 396 6545

Jackson

Suppliers: Diapers

☺ ■ **Camp International, Inc.**
P. O. Box 89, Jackson, Michigan 49204.
☎ 517 787 1600
☎ 800 492 1088
Waterproof pants.

Kalamazoo

Health Services

☺ □ **Borgess Medical Center**
1521 Gull Road, Kalamazoo, Michigan 49001.
☎ 616 383 7000

☺ □ **Bronson Methodist Hospital**
252 East Lovell Street, Kalamazoo, Michigan 49007.
☎ 616 341 6000

Helplines: Sexuality

⚥▽ **Lesbian / Gay Resource Line**
c/o Kalamazoo Gay / Lesbian Center, P. O. Box 1532, Kalamazoo, Michigan 49005.
☎ 616 345 7878
Publishes a newsletter.

Organizations: AIDS: Education

☺ □ **Community AIDS Resource & Education Service (CARES)**
⅃ 628 South Park Street, Kalamazoo, Michigan 49007.
☎ 616 381 2437

Organizations: BDSM

⚥ **Mall City Cruisers**
1718 Alamo, Kalamazoo, Michigan 49006.

Organizations: Sexuality

⚥▽ **Kalamazoo Gay / Lesbian Center**
P. O. Box 1532, Kalamazoo, Michigan 49005.
☎ 616 345 7878
Publishes a newsletter.

Organizations: Sexuality: Student

⚥▽ **Alliance for Bisexual, Lesbian, & Gay Support**
⅃ P. O. Box 226, Faunce Student Services, Western Michigan University, Kalamazoo, Michigan 49008.
☎ 616 387 2134

⚥▽ **Gay & Lesbian Support Group**
Kalamazoo College, 1200 Academy Street, Kalamazoo, Michigan 49006-3291.

Organizations: Sexuality: Youth

⚥▽ **Lesbian, Gay, & Bisexual Teen Support Group**
First Presbyterian Church, 321 West South Street, Kalamazoo, Michigan.
☎ 616 327 8107
⊕ Meets Thu 19:00

⚥▽ **Windfire**
c/o WMU ALGS, Kalamazoo, Michigan.

Publishers: Newspapers: Sexuality

⚥▽ *Lavendar Morning*
P. O. Box 729, Kalamazoo, Michigan 49005.
☎ 616 685 5377
Published every month.

Stores: Books: General

⚥▼ **Pandora Books for Open Minds**
⅃ 226 West Lovell, Kalamazoo, Michigan 49007.
☎ 616 388 5656

Stores: Erotica: General

⚥▼ **Triangle World & Leather Palace**
⅃ 551 Portage Road, Kalamazoo, Michigan 49007.
☎ 616 373 4005
⊕ Tue - Sun 12:00 - 22:00
▦ ⚞ ▦ 𝗩𝗜𝗦𝗔 ●● ⚞
Gift store with leather, magazines, videos, books, novelties, cards, & jewelry. Age statement of 18 is required.

Keego Harbor

Publishers: Books: Bondage

☺ **Shunga Comix**
P. O. Box 281, Keego Harbor, Michigan 48320.

Bondage comics & art.

Lansing

Counsellors

☺ ■ **Julie Railey, ACSW**
1218 Red Oak Lane, East Lansing, Michigan 48823.
☎ 517 332 1449

Health Services

☺ □ **Lansing General Hospital**
2727 South Pennsylvania Avenue, Lansing, Michigan 48910.
☎ 517 372 8220

☺ □ **Sparrow Hospital**
1215 East Michigan Avenue, Lansing, Michigan 48912.
☎ 517 482 2700

Organizations: Family

☺ □ **Parents & Friends of Lesbians & Gays (PFLAG)—**
⅋ **Lansing**
P. O. Box 35, Okemis, Michigan 48805.
☎ 517 349 3612

Organizations: Sexuality

♁▽ **Ambitious Amazons / Lesbian Center**
P. O. Box 811, East Lansing, Michigan 48826.
☎ 517 371 5257

♂▽ **Capitol Men's Club**
P. O. Box 4361, East Lansing, Michigan 48826-4361.
☎ 517 484 6342
Publishes a newsletter.

♁▽ **Lesbian Alliance (GLWA)**
⅋ P. O. Box 6423, East Lansing, Michigan 48826.
☎ 517 394 1454 (TDD available)
Publishes a newsletter.

Organizations: Sexuality: Student

♂▽ **Alliance of Lesbian-Bi-Gay Students (ALBGS)**
⅋ 442 Student Union Building, Michigan State University, East Lansing, Michigan 48824.
☎ 517 353 9795
☎ 517 353 5225

Publishers: Magazines: Sexuality

♁▽ *Lesbian Connection*
P. O. Box 811, East Lansing, Michigan 48826.
☎ 517 371 5257

Stores: Books: General

☺ ■ **Community Newscenter #1**
Frandor Shopping Center, Lansing, Michigan 48912.
☎ 517 351 7562

Livonia

Counsellors

▽ **Lee Padula, Ph.D.**
Suite 110, 37677 Professional Center Drive, Livonia, Michigan 48145.
☎ 313 953 3333

Madison Heights

Printers: General

☺ **National Reproductions Corporation**
29400 Stephenson Highway, Madison Heights, Michigan 48071.
☎ 313 298 7900

Publishers: Newspapers: Sexuality

♂▼ *Metra*
P. O. Box 71844, Madison Heights, Michigan 48071-0844.
☎ 313 543 3500
Entertainment for gays & lesbians on the midwest. Published twice a month. Yearly subscription is $34.

Marquette

Health Services

☺ □ **Marquette County Health Department**
⅋ Continuum of Care Program, AIDS Service, 184 US Highway 41, Negaunee, Michigan 49866.
☎ 906 475 7651

Organizations: Sexuality: Student

♂▽ **10% Society at NMU**
Box 95, University Center, Marquette, Michigan 49855.

Mount Morris

Organizations: Bears

♂♁▽ **Mid-Michigan Bears**
P. O. Box 483, Mount Morris, Michigan 48458.
☎ 810 687 5927

Mount Pleasant

Organizations: Sexuality: Student

♂▽ **Central Michigan University Lesbian & Gay Alliance**
P. O. Box 34, Warriner Hall, Central Michigan University, Mount Pleasant, Michigan 48859.
☎ 517 774 3822

Muskegon

Organizations: AIDS: Education

☺ □ **Muskegon Area AIDS Resource Services**
Suite 211, 1095 3rd. Street, Muskegon, Michigan 49441.
☎ 616 722 2437

New Baltimore

Publishers: Audio Tapes: BDSM

♂ ■ **Skye**
P. O. Box 365, New Baltimore, Michigan 48047.
Audio tapes for submissive men. Age statement of 21 is required.

Novi

Organizations: BDSM

♂♁▽ **Order of the Marquis & Chevalier**
P.O. Box 1014, Novi, Michigan 48376-1014.
☎ 810 348 5332 　 ✆ 810 348 8394
✉ KVJV70E@Prodigy.com
⏰ SM workshops last Wed of month. Algolagnic Atelier (weekend SM workshops) last weekend Jan
Contact: Mr. Mark Ensinger, Grand Marquis
Age statement of 18 is required.

♂♁▽ **STUDS-30, Inc.**
P.O. Box 692, Novi, Michigan 48376-0692.
☎ 810 348 5332 　 ✆ 810 348 8394
✉ KVJV70E@Prodigy.com
⏰ Meets 3rd. Sat of month
Contact: Mr. Mark Ensinger, Treasurer
Supports local gay charities, bar nights, social events, out of town trips. Famous for Jailhouse Rocks & Leather Ice Cream socials. Age statement of 18 is required.

Publishers: Books: BDSM

☺ **SAK Publishing**
Suite 131, 434322 West Oaks Drive, Novi, Michigan 48377.
Fiction & true stories of BDSM & cross dressing.

Petosky

Organizations: Sexuality

▽ **Northwest Michigan Gender Society**
P. O. Box 271, Petosky, Michigan 49770.
⏰ Monthly meetings
Contact: Ms. Tricia Marie Benton
Publishes a newsletter every month.

Pontiac

Organizations: Bears

♂ **Great Lakes Bears—Pontiac**
P.O. Box 431666, Pontiac, Michigan 48343.
☎ 313 338 1991
🌐 http://www.geopages.com/colosseum/1496/

Organizations: Motorcycle

♂ **Motorcity Men of Leather**
P.O. Box 431843, Pontiac, Michigan 48343-1843.
☎ 313 352 0182

Portage

Organizations: Family

☺ □ **Parents & Friends of Lesbians & Gays (PFLAG)—Kalamazoo**
P. O. Box 1201, Portage, Michigan 49801-1201.
☎ 616 327 8107
⏰ Meets 4th. Sun of month 14:00

☺ □ **Parents & Friends of Lesbians & Gays (PFLAG)—**

ᕃ **Portage**
P. O. Box 1201, Portage, Michigan 49081-1201.

Redford

Organizations: Body Size

♂▽ **Girth & Mirth—Detroit**
P. O. Box 39523, Redford, Michigan 48239.
☎ 313 531 3907

Royal Oak

Health Services

☺◯ ■ **William Beaumont Hospital**
3601 West Thirteen Mile Road, Royal Oak, Michigan 48073.
☎ 810 551 5000

Organizations: BDSM

☺▽ **Metro Leather Society**
1101 South Woodward, Royal Oak, Michigan 48067.
☎ 313 547 8919

Organizations: Bears

♂▽ **Motor City Bears**
P. O. Box 1894, Royal Oak, Michigan 48068.
☎ 810 988 0227
✉ mcbinfo@aol.com
🕸 http://webspace.com/~krussweb/mcbears/index.htm

Organizations: Sexuality

⚥▽ **Crossroads**
P. O. Box 1245, Royal Oak, Michigan 48068-1245.
☎ 313 537 3267
Publishes *Crossroads Chatter.*

Publishers: Documentaries: Sexuality

♂▽ **Voice & Vision Productions**
P. O. Box 1242, Royal Oak, Michigan 48068.

Publishers: Magazines: Sexuality

♂▼ *Cruise Magazine*
Rome Enterprises, Inc., P. O. Box 398, Royal Oak, Michigan 48068.
☎ 810 545 9040 ✆ 810 545 1073
🕐 Tue - Fri 11:00 - 17:00
🍽 ✓
Weekly news & entertainment magazine serving Michigan, Ohio, &
Windsor, Ontario, Canada. Published 50 times a year. Yearly subscription
is $35.

Stores: Books: General

♂▽ **Chosen Books**
120 West 4th. Street, Royal Oak, Michigan 48067.
☎ 800 453 5758 ✆ 810 543 6159
☎ 810 543 5758
🕐 12:00 - 22:00

Stores: Erotica: BDSM

☺ ■ **Noir Leather**
ᕃ 415 South Main Street, Royal Oak, Michigan 48067.
☎ 810 541 3979 ✆ 810 541 4147
🕐 Mon - Sat 11:00 - 20:00, Sun 13:00 - 17:00 (closes one hour later
in summer)
🍽 ✓ $ ⚐ VISA MC ▭
Also wholesale. Catalogue, $2.

Saginaw

Organizations: Sexuality: Student

♂▽ **Saginaw Valley State College Gay & Lesbian
Alliance**
Student Government, University Center, Saginaw, Michigan 48710.

Saline

Printers: General

☺ **McNaughton & Gunn**
960 Woodland Drive, Saline, Michigan 48176.
☎ 313 429 5411 Ext.: 265 ✆ 313 429 4033

Southfield

Organizations: BDSM

☺◯ **The National Leather Association (NLA)—Detroit**
P.O. Box 2844, Southfield, Michigan 48037-2844.
☎ 810 354 5841
🍽 ✓ $
Age statement of 18 is required.

Publishers: Books: BDSM

⚐ **On Your Knees**
Suite 423, 19785 West 12 Mile, Southfield, Michigan 48076.

Southgate

Publishers: Books: Spanking

☺ ■ **Diamond Distribution**
P. O. Box 1813, Southgate, Michigan 48195.
Spanking artwork books.

Publishers: Magazines: Spanking

☺ *Awakenings*
BB Publications, P. O. Box 1813, Southgate, Michigan 48195.

Traverse City

Distributors: Books: General

☺ **Publishers Distribution Service (PDS)**
Suite 203, 121 East Front Street, Traverse City, Michigan 49684.
☎ 616 929 0733 ✆ 9293808

Organizations: Sexuality

♂▽ **Friends North**
ᕃ P. O. Box 562, Traverse City, Michigan 49685-0562.
☎ 616 946 1804
Publishes *Networking 45 North.*

Organizations: Sexuality: Youth

♂▽ **Windfire**
902 West Front Street, Traverse City, Michigan 49685.
☎ 616 922 4800

Stores: Books: General

☺▼ **Bookie Joint**
ᕃ 120 South Union Street, Traverse City, Michigan 49684.
☎ 616 946 8862
🕐 10:00 - 20:00, Fri Sat - 22:00

Warren

Stores: Erotica: BDSM

☺ ■ **J & S Sports Products**
ᕃ 23146 Van Dyke Avenue, Warren, Michigan 48089.
☎ 810 754 6971 ✆ 810 754 6971
🕐 Mon - Fri 12:00 - 20:00, Sat Sun 12:00 - 18:00
🍽 ✂ VISA MC ▭
Age statement of 18 is required.

Ypsilanti

Organizations: Sexuality: Student

♂▽ **Lesbian, Gay, & Bisexual Student Association
(LGBSA)**
c/o Office of Campus Life, 221 Goodison Hall, Ypsilanti, Michigan
48197.

Stores: Erotica: General

♂▼ **Magazine Rack**
ᕃ 515 West Cross, Ypsilanti, Michigan 48197.
☎ 313 482 6944

MINNESOTA

Area: Approximately 207,000 square kilometres
Population: Approximately 4,380,000
Capital City: Saint Paul
Time zone: GMT minus 6 hours (CST)
Climate: Continental weather with a temperature difference between summer
& winter. Plenty of rain in the summer, & plenty of snow in the winter.
Tornadoes are occur here fairly often.
Age of consent & homosexuality legislation: All anal & oral sex is
illegal in this state.
Legal drinking age: 21

State Resources

Organizations: AIDS: Education

☺◯ **Minnesota AIDS Project**
ᕃ⚐ 1400 Park Avenue South, Minneapolis, Minnesota 55404.
☎ 612 341 2060 ✆ 612 341 4057
☎ 800 248 2437 (hotline)
Publishes a newsletter.

Organizations: Family

☺◯ **Parents & Friends of Lesbians & Gays (PFLAG)—
Minnesota**
P. O. Box 8588, Minneapolis, Minnesota 5408-0588.

☎ 612 458 3240
Publishes a newsletter.

☺ ☐ **Parents & Friends of Lesbians & Gays (PFLAG)—**
♿ **Southern Minnesota**
2205 Elton Hills Drive North West, Rochester, Minnesota 55901-1564.
☎ 507 282 0484

Organizations: Fetish: Clothing: Leather
♂▽ **Minnesota Leather Den**
Women's Group, P. O. Box 29348, Brooklyn Center, Minnesota 55430.
☎ 612 292 0542
Not BDSM oriented.

Publishers: Magazines: Sexuality
⚥▼ **Outlooks Magazine**
P. O. Box 80637, Minneapolis, Minnesota 55408.
☎ 612 377 8141 ✆ 612 374 2170

Publishers: Newspapers: Sexuality
⚥▽ **Equal Time**
♿ Suite 1600, 121 South 8th. Street, Minneapolis, Minnesota 55402-
2833.
☎ 612 823 3836
A respected source of information for the lesbigay communities
throughout the 5-state region. One of the top news papers in the
burgeoning gay press nationwide. Published every week. Yearly
subscription is $34.

⚥▽ **Gaze Magazine**
♿ Suite 130, 2344 Nicollet Avenue, Minneapolis, Minnesota 55404.
☎ 612 871 7472 ✆ 612 871 0525

⚥▽ **WomenWorks**
⚥ P. O. Box 300106, Minneapolis, Minnesota 55403.
☎ 612 377 9114

Albert Lea
Organizations: Sexuality
⚥▽ **Albert Lea Lesbian & Gay Outreach**
⚥ P. O. Box 341, Albert Lea, Minnesota 56007.

Brooklyn Center
Organizations: Fetish: Clothing: Leather
⊕▽ **Minnesota Leather Den**
P. O. Box 29348, Brooklyn Center, Minnesota 55430.
☎ 612 561 6526
Not oriented to BDSM.

Concord
Publishers: Newspapers: Sexuality
⊕▽ **WomenWise**
⚥ c/o Concord Feminist Health Center, 38 South Main Street, Concord,
Minnesota 03301.
☎ 603 225 2739
Women's health journal with a feminist philosophy. International
distribution. Published quarterly. Yearly subscription is $10.

Duluth
Health Services
☺ ☐ **Duluth Community Health Center**
♿ 2 East 5th. Street, Duluth, Minnesota 55805.
☎ 218 722 1479

☺ ☐ **Miller-Dawn Medical Center**
502 East Second Street, Duluth, Minnesota 55805.
☎ 218 727 8762

☺ ☐ **Saint Mary's Medical Center**
407 East Third Street, Duluth, Minnesota 55805.
☎ 218 726 4000
HIV & emergency departments.

Organizations: AIDS: Education
☺ ▽ **Minnesota AIDS Project**
⚥ Suite 300, 8 North 2nd. Avenue, Duluth, Minnesota 55802.
☎ 218 727 2437

Organizations: Sexuality
⚥▽ **Aurora, A Northland Lesbian Center**
Suite 210, 8 North 2nd. Avenue, Duluth, Minnesota 55802.
☎ 218 722 4903
⏰ Mon Wed Thu 11:00 - 17:30, Fri - 19:00
Publishes a newsletter.

Organizations: Sexuality: Student
⚥▽ **University Lesbian, Gay, & Bisexual Alliance**

Kirby Student Center, University of Minnesota at Duluth, 10 University
Drive, Duluth, Minnesota 55812.

Eagan
Stores: Clothing: Footwear
☺▼ **Wholesale Boot Supply**
3711 South Hills Lane, Eagan, Minnesota 55123.
☎ 612 452 4695
⏰ 08:00 - 20:00
⚥ ✓ $ ⚏
Specializes in motorcycle & heavy work boots.

Eden Prairie
Printers: General
☺ ■ **Viking Press/Banta**
7000 Washington Avenue South, Eden Prairie, Minnesota 55344.
☎ 612 941 8780 ✆ 612 941 2154

Mankato
Counsellors
⚥▽ **Alternative Lifestyles Office**
♿ MSU Box 4, Mankato, Minnesota 56002-8400.
☎ 507 389 1455

Organizations: Sexuality
⚥▽ **Gay, Lesbian, & Bisexual Activities**
P. O. Box 3511, Mankato, Minnesota 56002.
☎ 507 345 7799

Marsall
Organizations: AIDS: Education
☺ ☐ **Minnesota AIDS Project**
109 South 5th. Street, Marsall, Minnesota 56258.
☎ 507 532 3825

Minneapolis / Saint Paul
Counsellors
☺ ▼ **Mindy Benowitz, Ph.D.**
⚥ Suite 205, 1730 Clifton Place, Minneapolis, Minnesota 55403.
☎ 612 870 0398

⚥▽ **Family & Children's Services**
♿ Gay & Lesbian Counselling Program, 414 South 8th. Street, Minneapolis,
Minnesota 55404.
☎ 612 339 9101 ✆ 612 339 9150
⏰ By appointment only

☺ ■ **Frederickson & Associates**
⚥ 821 Raymond Avenue, Saint Paul, Minnesota 55114.
☎ 612 646 8373

⚥☐ **Midway Family Services**
♿ Gay, Lesbian, Bisexual, Transgender Counseling Program, Suite 200,
166 4th. Street, Saint Paul, Minnesota 55101-1400.
☎ 612 222 0311

Health Services
☺ ☐ **Abbott Northwestern Hospital**
800 East 28th. Street, Minneapolis, Minnesota 55407.
☎ 612 863 4000
HIV & emergency departments.

☺ ☐ **Hennepin County Medical Center**
701 Park Avenue South, Minneapolis, Minnesota 55415.
☎ 612 347 2121

☺ ☐ **Red Door Clinic**
♿ 525 Portland Avenue, Minneapolis, Minnesota 55415.
☎ 612 348 6363

☺ ☐ **University of Minnesota Hospital**
Harvard Street & East River Street, Minneapolis, Minnesota 55455.
☎ 612 626 3000

☺ ☐ **Veterans' Affairs Medical Center**
One Veterans Drive, Minneapolis, Minnesota 55417.
☎ 612 725 2000
HIV & emergency departments.

Helplines: Sexuality
⚥▽ **Gay & Lesbian Hotline**
☎ 612 822 8661
⏰ Mon - Sat 16:00 - 24:00

Organizations: Bears
⚥▽ **North Country Bears**
P. O. Box 580473, Minneapolis, Minnesota 55458-0473.

Organizations: Bears

☎ 612 588 2506
✉ ncbears@rplace.mn.org
🌐 http://www.primenet.com:80/~rstbear/ncb/ncbears.htm

Organizations: Body Size

⚥▽ **Girth & Mirth—Twin Cities**
♠ P. O. Box 4288, Hopkins, Minnesota 58343.
☎ 612 938 8551

Organizations: BDSM

☺□ **A.S.B. Munch—Minnesota**
✉ Dan.Brady@tcl.mmbbs.mn.org
⏱ Meets 3rd. Thu of month 19:30
Also known as Minnesota Links.

⚥▽ **Atons of Minneapolis**
P. O. Box 2311, Loop Station, Minneapolis, Minnesota 55402-0311.
☎ 612 333 4458
✉ AtonsMpls@aol.com

⚥▽ **Black Guard**
P. O. Box 8989, Minneapolis, Minnesota 55408-8989.

⊕ ▽ **Knights of Leather**
♿ P. O. Box 582601, Minneapolis, Minnesota 55458-2601.
☎ 612 870 7473 (answering machine)

⚥▽ **Minnesota Leather Encounter, Inc.**
P. O. Box 8784, Minneapolis, Minnesota 55458-0784.

Organizations: Bondage

⚥▽ **Twin Cities Bondage Association (TCBA)**
P. O. Box 141151, Minneapolis, Minnesota 55414.

Organizations: Bears

⚥▽ **MnBears**
Box 107, 54 South Ninth Street, Minneapolis, Minnesota 55402.
☎ 612 220 1382
✉ MnBear@onldiver.com

Organizations: Family

☺□ **Parents & Friends of Lesbians & Gays (PFLAG)—Saint Cloud**
P. O. Box 7641, Saint Cloud, Minnesota 56302.
☎ 612 259 4238

Organizations: Sexuality

♂ ▽ **Bisexual Connection**
♠ P. O. Box 13158, Minneapolis, Minnesota 55414.

☺ **Brian Coyle Community Center**
♿ 420 15th. Avenue South, Minneapolis, Minnesota 55454.
☎ 612 338 5283 ✆ 612 338 8421
⏱ Mon - Fri 09:00 - 20:00, Sat 10:00 - 17:00

▷▽ **City Lakes Crossgender Community (CLCC)**
P. O. Box 16265, Minneapolis, Minnesota 55416.
☎ 612 229 3613
🌐 gopher://rodent.cis.umn.edu.:11132/00/all-files/M-City%20of%20Lakes%20Crossgender%20Community
⏱ Monthly meetings

⚥▽ **Gays South of Lake Street**
P. O. Box 8663, Minneapolis, Minnesota 55408.

▷▽ **Gender Education Center (GEC)**
P. O. Box 186, Minneapolis, Minnesota 55311.
☎ 612 425 5445 ✆ 612 425 8595
Contact: Ms. Debbie Davis, Director
Educational outreach, support, resource, workshops, & education.

⚥' ▽ **The Men's Center**
♿ Suite 55, 3255 Hennepin Avenue, Minneapolis, Minnesota 55408.
☎ 612 822 5892
Publishes *Men Talk*.

▷▽ **Minnesota Freedom of Gender Expression (MFGE)**
P. O. Box 17945, Saint Paul, Minnesota 55117.
☎ 612 220 9027 (voice mail)
Publishes a newsletter every two months.

▷▽ **New Men & Women of Minnesota**
P. O. Box 6432, Minneapolis, Minnesota 55406-0432.
☎ 612 220 1920
Publishes a newsletter.

⚥▽ **North Woods Radical Faerie Circle**
Suite 3, 1807 Elliot Avenue, Minneapolis, Minnesota 55404.
☎ 612 334 1948

⚥▽ **Northland Gay Men's Center**
Suite 309, 8 North 2nd. Avenue, Minneapolis, Minnesota 55802.
☎ 218 722 8585
⏱ Mon Wed Thu 11:00 - 17:30, Fri - 19:00
Publishes a newsletter.

▷▽ **The Society for the Second Self (Tri-Ess)—Beta Gamma**
P. O. Box 8591, Minneapolis, Minnesota 55408.

▷▽ **TSSG**
P. O. Box 13659, Saint Paul, Minnesota 55113.
☎ 612 653 7936

▷▽ **University of Minnesota**
Gender Dysphoria Program, c/o Program in Human Sexuality, Suite 180, 1300 South 2nd. Street, Minneapolis, Minnesota 55454.
☎ 612 625 1500 ✆ 612 626 8311
Professionally managed gender program. Member of HBIGSA.

⊕ **Women's Studies**
Ford 492, University of Minnesota, Minneapolis, Minnesota 55455.
☎ 612 624 9326
Publishes *Matrices*.

Organizations: Sexuality: Student

⚥▽ **The 10% Group**
P. O. Box 5855, Saint John's University, Collegeville, Minnesota 56321.
☎ 612 363 2734

⚥▽ **Delta Lambda Phi Fraternity—Minnesota**
♿ P. O. Box 13122, Minneapolis, Minnesota 55414-5122.
☎ 612 336 4196

⚥▽ **Lesbian, Gay, & Bisexual Resource Center (LGBRC)**
♿ Women's Center, Saint Cloud University, 720 South 4th. Avenue, Saint Cloud, Minnesota 56301-4498.
☎ 612 654 5166

⚥▽ **Macalester Gays, Lesbians, & Bisexuals United**
♿ Macalester College Union 205, 1600 Grand Avenue, Saint Paul, Minnesota 55105.
☎ 612 696 6248

⚥▽ **Normandale Community College Lesbian & Gay Network**
♿ 9700 France Avenue South, Bloomington, Minnesota 55431.
☎ 612 832 6544

⚥▽ **United Theological Seminary Lesbian & Gay Caucus**
♿ 3000 5th. Street North West, New Brighton, Minnesota 55112.
☎ 612 633 8703

⚥▽ **University Bi Community**
♿ 235 Coffman Union, 300 Washington Avenue South East, Minneapolis, Minnesota 55455.
☎ 612 626 2344

⊕▽ **University Lesbians**
♿ c/o U-YW, 244 Coffman Union, 300 Washington Street South East, Minneapolis, Minnesota 55455.
☎ 612 625 1611

⚥▽ **University of Minnesota**
♿ Gay, Lesbian, Bisexual, & Transgender Programs Office, 429 Walter Library, 117 Pleasant Street South East, Minneapolis, Minnesota 55455.
☎ 612 626 9765

⚥▽ **University of Minnesota Lesbian & Gay Law Students Association**
University of Minnesota Law Center, 229 19th. Avenue South, Minneapolis, Minnesota 55454.
☎ 612 625 1000

⚥▽ **William Mitchell College of Law Gay & Lesbian Association**
875 Summit Avenue, Saint Paul, Minnesota 55454.
☎ 612 646 3966

Organizations: Sexuality: Youth

⚥▽ **District 202**
2524 Nicollet Avenue, South Minneapolis, Minnesota 55408.
☎ 612 871 5559
Aslo for transgender youth.

Printers: Adult

☺ **Mindanao Printing Company**
1222 Hazel Street North, Saint Paul, Minnesota 55119-4500.
☎ 612 774 3768 ✆ 612 771 9772
Small printer that specialises in 4-colour inserts for cassettes & brochures.

Printers: General

☺ **Academic Bookbinding**
153 26th. Avenue South East, Minneapolis, Minnesota 55414.
☎ 612 331 6381 ✆ 612 331 2409
Custom book binding (no printing). Will bind fetish & BDSM titles.

Publishers: Magazines: Arts

♂♀▽ *The Evergreen Chronicles*
The Evergreen Chronicles, P. O. Box 8939, Minneapolis, Minnesota 55408-0939.
☎ 612 649 4982
✉ bergx021@maroon.tc.umn.edu
🕐 Mon - Fri 09:00 - 17:00
Published 3 times a year. Yearly subscription is $20.

Publishers: Magazines: Sexuality

♀ *Hurricane Alice*
207 Church Street South East, Minneapolis, Minnesota 55455.
☎ 612 625 1834

⚥ *Sing Heavenly Muse!*
P. O. Box 13320, Minneapolis, Minnesota 55414.

Publishers: Magazines: AIDS

☺▽ **PWAlive Publications, Inc.**
♿ P. O. Box 80216, Minneapolis, Minnesota 55408-8216.
☎ 612 640 7927

Publishers: Magazines: Sexuality

☺ *Man Bag*
The ARTpolice Agency, P. O. Box 6313, Minneapolis, Minnesota 55406.
☎ 612 291 0718
Art magazine with emphasis on drawing our deepest, sickest sex dreams. Published twice a year. Yearly subscription is $6. Age statement of 18 is required.

Publishers: Magazines: Fetish: Raunch

♂▼ *Your Ass & My Face*
P. O. Box 80089, Minneapolis, Minnesota 55408.

Publishers: Miscellaneous

⚥ **Spinsters Ink**
P. O. Box 300170, Minneapolis, Minnesota 55403.
☎ 612 558 9655

♂ **Womyn's Braille Press, Inc.**
P. O. Box 8475, Minneapolis, Minnesota 55408.
☎ 612 872 4352
☎ 612 822 0549 eves. & weekends

Publishers: Newspapers: Literary

♂▼ *The James White Review*
P. O. Box 3356, Traffic Station, Minneapolis, Minnesota 55403.
☎ 612 339 8317
The James White Review is a gay literary quarterly which has published the work of established & well-known authors, as well as emerging writers. Published quarterly. Yearly subscription is $12 in U.S., $14 in Cdn., $17 elsewhere.

Publishers: Newspapers: Sexuality

♂▼ *Bifocal*
P. O. Box 13158, Minneapolis, Minnesota 55414.

♂ *Maize*
P. O. Box 8742, Minneapolis, Minnesota 55408-0742.

⚥ *Minnesota Womens' Press*
771 Raymond Avenue, Saint Paul, Minnesota 55114.
☎ 612 646 3968

Radio: Sexuality

♂□ *Fresh Fruit*
♿ KFAI FM 90.3, 1808 Riverside Avenue, Minneapolis, Minnesota 55454-1035.
☎ 612 341 3144
🕐 Thu 19:00 - 20:00

Stores: Books: General

♂▼ **A Brother's Touch**
2327 Hennepin Avenue, Minneapolis, Minnesota 55405.
☎ 612 377 6279
🕐 Mon Tue 11:00 - 19:00, Wed - Fri - 21:00, Sat - 18:00, Sun 12:00 - 17:00

☺■ **Dream Haven Books Uptown**
♿ 1403 West Lake Street, Minneapolis, Minnesota 55408.
☎ 612 825 4720
🕐 Mon Thu Dri 11:00 - 21:00, Tue Wed Sat 11:00 - 19:00, Sun 12:00 - 17:00
⚥ ✓ $ 💳 🆔 💳 💳
Specialties: fringe & alternative culture; fiction, non-fiction, comics, & some audio-visual. Mail order fetish magazines, BDSM literature, & independent comics. Catalogue, 2 IRCs or 1st. class stamps. Age statement of 21 is required.

Stores: Erotica: General

⚥▼ **Amazon Bookstore, Inc.**
♿ 1612 Harmon Place, Minneapolis, Minnesota 55403.
☎ 612 338 6560

☺■ **Broadway Book & Video**
♿ 901 Hennepin Avenue, Minneapolis, Minnesota 55403.
☎ 612 338 7303

☺ **Fantasy House**
81 South 10th. Street, Minneapolis, Minnesota 55403.
☎ 612 333 6313

☺■ **Sex World**
♿ 241 2nd. Avenue North, Minneapolis, Minnesota 55401.
☎ 612 672 0556

Suppliers: Photoprinting

☺■ **Venus Photography**
Suite 348, 54 South 9th. Street, Minneapolis, Minnesota 55402.
☎ 612 338 1302 ✆ 612 339 1159
🕐 08:00 - 21:00
⚥ ✓
Confidential, discreet developing & printing. Mail order only.

Television: Sexuality

♂♀▽ *Green & Yellow TV*
P. O. Box 40, Eagle Lake, Minnesota 56024.
☎ 800 821 5456
🕐 Weekly one hour cable TV program

Moorhead

Organizations: Academic: Sexuality

♂♀ **Society for Lesbian & Gay Philosophy**
Moorhead State University, Moorhead, Minnesota 56563.
☎ 218 236 4087
Contact: Professor Chekola

Organizations: AIDS: Education

☺□ **Clay County Health Department**
♿ West Central AIDS Project, 914 8th. Avenue North, Moorhead, Minnesota 56560.
☎ 218 299 5220

Organizations: Sexuality

♂♀▽ **Priarie Lesbian & Gay Community**
P. O. Box 83, Moorhead, Minnesota 56560.
☎ 701 237 0556
Publishes *Communiqué*.

Organizations: Sexuality: Student

♂♀▽ **10% Society**
♿ MSU Box 266, Moorhead, Minnesota 56563.
☎ 218 236 2227

Northfield

Organizations: Sexuality: Student

♂♀▽ **Lesbian, Gay, & Bisexual Community, Carleton**
♿ **College**
Carleton College, Northfield, Minnesota 55057.
☎ 507 663 4154

☺□ **Olaf Lesbian & Gay Alliance (OLAGA)**
Student Counseling Center, Saint Olaf College, Northfield, Minnesota 55057.
☎ 507 663 2305

Reno

Publishers: Newspapers: Sexuality

♂ *Sierra Voice*
P. O. Box 1191, Reno, Minnesota 89504.
☎ 702 355 1628
Newspaper serving the estimated 60-90,000 members of the gay & lesbian community in Northern Nevada & Eastern Sierra. Features, news, etc.. Published every month. Yearly subscription is $20.

Rochester

Organizations: AIDS: Education

☺□ **Minnesota AIDS Project**
♿ Suite 200-B, 1500 North East 1st. Avenue, Rochester, Minnesota 55906.
☎ 507 282 8771

Organizations: Sexuality

♂♀▽ **Gay & Lesbian Community Services**

Organizations: Sexuality

 ⅏ P. O. Box 454, Rochester, Minnesota 55903.
 ☎ 507 281 3265

Saint Cloud
Organizations: Sexuality: Student
⚥▽ **Lambda**
 ⅏ Colbert Hall North, Saint Cloud State University, Saint Cloud, Minnesota
 56301.
 ☎ 612 654 5166
 🕐 Thu 19:00 - 21:00

Waseca
BBSs: BDSM
☺■ **Minnesota Underground**
 ✆ 507 835 8001

Winona
Publishers: Newspapers: Sexuality
⚥ *In Step Magazine*
 Winona Daily News, Winona, Minnesota 55987.

MISSISSIPI
Area: Approximately 122,000 square kilometres
Population: Approximately 2,600,000
Capital City: Jackson
Time zone: GMT minus 6 hours (CST)
Age of consent & homosexuality legislation: All anal & oral sex is
 illegal in this state.

State Resources
Counsellors
⚥▽ **Gay & Lesbian Counseling Services of the United**
 ⅏ **Community Church**
 P. O. Box 7654, Jackson, Mississipi 39284-7654.
 ☎ 601 373 8610
 🕐 Mon - Sat 18:00 - 23:00

Helplines: AIDS
☺ **AIDS Hotline**
 ⅏ P. O. Box 8342, Jackson, Mississipi 39284-8342.
 ☎ 601 371 1318

Helplines: Sexuality
⚥▽ **Community Services Network, Inc.**
 P. O. Box 7737, Jackson, Mississipi 39284-7737.
 ☎ 601 373 8610
 🕐 24hrs.

Organizations: Sexuality
⚥▽ **Mississippi Gay & Lesbian Task Force (MGLTF)**
 308 Caillavet Street, Biloxi, Mississipi 39530.
 ☎ 601 435 2398
⚥▽ **Mississippi Phoenix Coalition, Inc.**
 P. O. Box 7737, Jackson, Mississipi 39284-7737.
 ☎ 601 373 8610
 🕐 08:30 - 22:00

Publishers: Newspapers: Sexuality
✉□ *Grace & Lace Letter*
 P. O. Box 31253, Jackson, Mississipi 39286-1253.
 ☎ 601 982 7678

Biloxi
Health Services
☺□ **Veterans' Affairs Medical Center**
 400 Veterans Avenue, Biloxi, Mississipi 39531.
 ☎ 601 388 5541

Organizations: AIDS: Education
☺□ **South Mississipi AIDS Task Force**
 466 Caillavet Street, Biloxi, Mississipi 39530.
 ☎ 601 435 1234

Organizations: Sexuality
⚥▽ **GL Friendly**
 308 Caillavet Street, Biloxi, Mississipi 39530.
 ☎ 601 435 2398

Greenville
Stores: Books: General
☺■ **The Bookstore**
 ⅏ 323 Washington Avenue, Greenville, Mississipi 38701.

 ☎ 601 332 2665

Hattiesburg
Organizations: Sexuality: Student
⚥▽ **Gay, Lesbian, & Bi Student Organization (GLBSO)**
 USM P. O. Box 8471, Hattiesburg, Mississipi 39406.
 ☎ 601 583 7997

Jackson
Health Services
☺□ **University Hospitals & Clinics**
 University of Mississippi Medical Center, 2500 North State Street,
 Jackson, Mississipi 39216.
 ☎ 610 984 1000
☺□ **Veterans' Affairs Medical Center**
 1500 East Woodrow Wilson Drive, Jackson, Mississipi 39216.
 ☎ 610 362 4471

Organizations: Sexuality
⚨▽ **The Society for the Second Self (Tri-Ess)—Beta**
 Chi
 P. O. Box 31253, Jackson, Mississipi 39286-1253.
 ☎ 601 982 7678
 Contact: Ms. Lee Frances, Secretary
 Publishes *Premiere*.

Publishers: Newspapers: Sexuality
⚥▽ *The Mississippi Voice*
 P. O. Box 7737, Jackson, Mississipi 39284-7737.
 ☎ 601 373 8610
⚥ *This Month in Mississipi*
 P. O. Box 8342, Jackson, Mississipi 39204.
 ☎ 601 353 7611
 Published every month.

MISSOURI
Area: Approximately 179,000 square kilometres
Population: Approximately 5,150,000
Capital City: Jefferson City
Time zone: GMT minus 6 hours (CST)
Age of consent & homosexuality legislation: All anal & oral sex is
 illegal in this state.

State Resources
Counsellors
☺ **Pat Murrell, MSW, LCSW**
 K P. O. Box 23305, Saint Louis, Missouri 63156.
 ☎ 314 569 5795
 ☎ 618 462 4051
 💰 $ —
 Counselling for sexuality, gender identity, crisis, AIDS, sexual abuse, &
 trauma issues. Age statement of 18 is required.

Organizations: AIDS: Education
☺□ **AIDS Project of the Ozarks**
 ⅏ 1722 South Glenstone Avenue, Springfield, Missouri 65804-1508.
 ☎ 417 881 1900
 🕐 Mon - Fri 09:00 - 17:00, helpline - 21:00
☺□ **Mid-Missouri AIDS Project**
 ⅏ Suite 305, 811 Cherry Street, Columbia, Missouri 65201-4892.
 ☎ 413 875 2437 ✆ 314 442 0058

Publishers: Newspapers: Sexuality
⚥▽ *News-Telegraph*
 Piasa Publishing Company, P. O. Box 14229-A, Saint Louis, Missouri
 63178.
 ☎ 800 301 5468 ✆ 314 664 6303
 ☎ 314 664 6411
 📧 Newstele@aol.com
 💰 ✓ $
 News, entertainment, advertising, etc., for the lesbian & gay community
 in Missouri, Kansas, Southern Illinois, Arkansas, & Western Tennessee.
 Published twice a month. Yearly subscription is $48.

Ava
BBSs: BDSM
☺■ **Laura's Lair**
 ✆ 417 683 5534

Cape Giradeau
Organizations: Sexuality: Student
⚥▽ **Gay & Lesbian Student Association**

& SG Office, 2nd. Floor UC, South Missouri State University, Cape Girardeau, Missouri 63701.
☎ 314 651 2996
⏱ 24hr. recorded message

Stores: Books: General
☺ ■ **Metro News**
415 Broadway, Cape Girardeau, Missouri 63701.
☎ 314 335 8633

Columbia
Health Services
☺ ☐ **Harry S. Truman Memorial Veterans' Hospital**
800 Hospital Drive, Columbia, Missouri 65201.
☎ 314 443 2511
☺ ☐ **University & Childrens' Hospital**
One Hospital Drive, Columbia, Missouri 65212.
☎ 314 882 8000

Helplines: Sexuality
⚲▽ **Lesbian & Gay Helpline**
☎ 314 449 4477

Organizations: Sexuality
⚲▽ **Coming Out Collective**
⚲ P. O. Box 48, Columbia, Missouri 65205-0048.
☎ 314 442 4174
Publishes *Coming Out Newsletter*.

Organizations: Sexuality: Student
⚲▽ **Triangle Coalition**
& A022 Brady Commons, University of Missouri, Columbia, Missouri 65211.
☎ 314 882 4427

Radio: Sexuality
⚲■ *The Gaydar Show*
&& KOPN FM 89.5, 915 East Broadway, Columbia, Missouri 65201.
☎ 314 874 5676
⏱ Wed 22:00 24:00

Stores: Erotica: General
☺ ■ **Eclectics**
& 1122-A Wilkes Boulevard, Columbia, Missouri 65201.
☎ 314 443 0873
⏱ 11:00 - 24:00
☺ ■ **Midwest Adult Bookstore**
101 East Walnut, Columbia, Missouri 65201-4164.
☎ 314 442 6622

Ferguson
Suppliers: Diapers
☺ ■ **Home Delivery Incontinent Supplies Co., Inc.**
325 Paul Ave., Ferguson, Missouri.
☎ 800 538 1036
☎ 314 997 8771
[VISA] ⊙⊙
Disposable diapers available discreetly by UPS. Sample packs available.

Independence
Organizations: Polyfidelity
☺ ■ **Glendower**
P. O. Box 520291, Independence, Missouri 64052.

Kansas City
Counsellors
⚲▼ **Lambda Counseling Services**
& 5128 Brookside Boulevard, Kansas City, Missouri 64112-2736.
☎ 816 531 7133
☺ **Mark McCarthy, M.S., LPC**
Suite 200, 4520 Madison, Kansas City, Missouri 64111.
☎ 816 931 0011

Health Services
☺ ☐ **Kansas City Free Health Clinic**
& Second Floor, 2 East 39th. Street, Kansas City, Missouri 64111.
☎ 816 753 5144
Publishes *Free Health Clinic Newsletter*.
☺ ☐ **Research Medical Center**
2316 East Meyer Boulevard, Kansas City, Missouri 64132.
☎ 816 276 4000
☺ ☐ **Truman Medical Center**

2301 Holmes Street, Kansas City, Missouri 64108.
☎ 816 556 3000
☺ ☐ **Veterans' Affairs Medical Center**
4801 Linwood Boulevard, Kansas City, Missouri 64128.
☎ 816 861 4700

Organizations: AIDS: Education
☺ ☐ **Heartland AIDS Resource Council**
& 600 East 31st. Street, Kansas City, Missouri 64109-1436.

Organizations: BDSM
⚲▽ **Kansas City Pioneers**
P. O. Box 413025, Kansas City, Missouri 64141.
☺ ☐ **The National Leather Association (NLA)—Kansas City**
P.O. Box 414545, Kansas City, Missouri 64141.
✉ dsplnaryn@aol.com

Organizations: Bears
⚲▽ **Kansas City Cave Bears**
P. O. Box 45161, Kansas City, Missouri 64171.
☎ 816 986 9696

Organizations: Family
⚲▽ **Gay & Lesbian Parents Coalition (GALA)**
&& 6241 Blue Ridge Boulevard, Kansas City, Missouri 64133-4107.
☎ 816 356 9589

Organizations: Sexuality
♂▽ **Black & White Men Together (BWMT)—Kansas City**
P. O. Box 412432, Kansas City, Missouri 64141.
☎ 816 931 4470
Publishes *MACT/KC*.
⚲▽ **Gay & Lesbian Services Network**
P. O. Box 32592, Kansas City, Missouri 64111.
☎ 816 374 5910
⏱ Telephone is Gay Talk 17:00 - 01:00
⚲▽ **Gender Dysphoria Support**
P. O. Box 45124, Kansas City, Missouri 63111.
☎ 816 241 1411
⏱ Meets every other Fri
Contact: Ms. Joan Cunningham

Photographers: BDSM
☺ ■ **Janet Ryan**
P. O. Box 32732, Kansas City, Missouri 64171.
B&W photos of the leather, fetish, BDSM community.

Piercers
☺ ■ **Extremus Body Arts**
& 4037 Broadway, Kansas City, Missouri 64111.
☎ 816 756 1142
✉ EXTREMUS@aol.com
⏱ Mon - Sat 12:00 - 20:00
⚲
Full service body piercing studio. Midwest's largest selection of fine body jewelry. Walk-ins welcome. Branding & scarification by appointment. Age statement of 18 is required.

Publishers: Newspapers: Sexuality
⚲▽ *News-Telegraph*
Piasa Publishing Company, P. O. Box 10085, Kansas City, Missouri 64171.
☎ 800 303 5468 ✆ 816 561 2623
☎ 816 561 6266
✉ NewsTele@aol.com
⚲ ✓ $
Kansas city office. See state resources for main office. Published twice a month. Yearly subscription is $48.

Stores: Books: General
☺ ■ **Borders Book Shop**
& 9108 Metcalf, Overland Park, Missouri 66212.
☎ 913 642 3642
⏱ 08:00 - 22:00, Fri Sat - 23:00, Sun 11:00 - 19:00
☺ ▼ **Phœnix Books**
5710 North East 50th. Street, Kansas City, Missouri 64119-3812.
☎ 816 931 5794
⏱ 10:00 - 18:00, Sun 10:00 - 17:00
☺ ■ **Ray's Playpen**
&& 3235 Main Street, Kansas City, Missouri 64111.
☎ 816 753 7692

Printers: General

U.S.A.

Marceline
Printers: General
☺ **Walsworth Publishing Company**
306 North Kansas Avenue, Marceline, Missouri 64658.
☎ 816 376 3543
☎ 816 376 3543 Ext. 3342 ✆ 816 258 7798

Saint Charles
Stores: Erotica: General
☺ ■ **Bargain Books**
3010 North Highway 94, Saint Charles, Missouri 63301.
☎ 800 834 4127
☎ 314 723 9598

Saint Louis
Bars: BDSM
♂▼ **Clementine's**
♠ 2001 Menard Street, Saint Louis, Missouri 63104.
☎ 314 664 7869

BBSs: BDSM
☺ ■ **Hotflash**
✆ 314 771 6060

Counsellors
☺▼ **Linda Rogers, Ph.D.**
♠ Suite 925, 231 South Berniston Avenue, Clayton, Missouri 63105.
☎ 314 727 1907
☺ **Robert Snyder, Ph.D.**
K ♿ Suite 321T, 225 South Merramac, Saint Louis, Missouri 63105.
☎ 314 727 9088
☼ By appointment
♠ ✓ $ ⚥
Counselling & psychotherapy for individuals & couples (child, adolescent, & adult).
☺▼ **Dick Wagner, MSW, ACSW**
♿ 10349 Watson Road, Saint Louis, Missouri 63127.
☎ 314 965 1942

Health Services
☺ ☐ **Barnes Hospital**
One Barnes Plaza, Saint Louis, Missouri 63110.
☎ 314 362 5000
☺ ☐ **Christian Hospital Northeast**
11133 Dunn Road, Saint Louis, Missouri 63136.
☎ 314 355 2300
☺ ☐ **Christian Hospital Northwest**
1225 Graham Road, Saint Louis, Missouri 63031.
☎ 314 839 3800
☺ ☐ **Veterans' Affairs Medical Center**
☎ 314 984 6661

Helplines: Sexuality
♂▽ **Gay & Lesbian Hotline**
Challenge Metro, P. O. Box 23227, Saint Louis, Missouri 63156.
☎ 314 367 0084
☼ 18:00 - 22:00

Organizations: AIDS: Education
☺ ☐ **Doorways**
♿ P. O. Box 4652, Saint Louis, Missouri 63108.
☎ 314 454 9599
☺ ▽ **Saint Louis Effort for AIDS (EFA)**
♿ Suite 104E, 5622 Delmar, Saint Louis, Missouri 63112-2646.
☎ 314 367 2382
Publishes *Frontline*.

Organizations: BDSM
♂♀ ☐ **Gyncrocrat Alliance**
P. O. Box 13034, Saint Louis, Missouri 63144.
♂▽ **Tartarus**
P. O. Box 24243, Saint Louis, Missouri 63130.

Organizations: Bears
♂▽ **Show Me Bears**
P. O. Box 8192, Saint Louis, Missouri 63156-8192.
☎ 314 995 2690
✉ showmebear@aol.com

Organizations: Body Size
♂▽ **Girth & Mirth—Saint Louis**

P. O. Box 63163, Saint Louis, Missouri 63163.

Organizations: Family
☺ ☐ **Parents & Friends of Lesbians & Gays (PFLAG)—**
♿ **Saint Louis**
7443 Cromwell Drive, Saint Louis, Missouri 63105.
☎ 314 821 3524

Organizations: Motorcycle
♂ **Blue Max Cycle Club**
P.O. Box 233, Main Station, Saint Louis, Missouri 63166.
♂ **Gateway MC**
P.O. Box 14055, Saint Louis, Missouri 63178.

Organizations: Polyfidelity
☺ ■ **Saint Louis Lifestyles**
P. O. Box 411010, Saint Louis, Missouri 63141.
✉ lvl@inlink.com

Organizations: Sexuality
♂▽ **Men's Support Group**
c/o Metropolitan Community Church, 1120 Dolman Avenue, Saint Louis, Missouri 63104.
☎ 314 231 9100
☼ Tue 19:30
♂▽ **Mid-America Gender Group Information Exchange (MAGGIE)**
c/o Saint Louis Gender Foundation, P. O. Box 9433, Saint Louis, Missouri 63117.
☎ 314 997 9897
Contact: Ms. Jennifer Richards
♂▽ **Saint Louis Gender Foundation (LGS)**
P. O. Box 9433, Saint Louis, Missouri 63117.
☎ 314 997 9897 (voice mail)
☎ 314 367 4128
Publishes *Gateway Femmes Gazette*.

Organizations: Sexuality: Student
♂▽ **Gay & Lesbian Olin Business School Alliance**
♿ **(GLOBAL)**
Campus Box 1133, Washington University, 1 Brookings Drive, Saint Louis, Missouri 63130.
☎ 314 935 6315
♂▽ **Gay, Lesbian, & Bisexual Community Alliance**
♠ Campus Box 1128, Washington University, 1 Brookings Drive, Saint Louis, Missouri 63130.
☎ 314 935 5349
♂▽ **Lesbian & Gay Campus Organization**
267 University Center, 8001 Natural Bridge Road, Saint Louis, Missouri 63121-4499.
☎ 314 553 5380

Publishers: Newspapers: Sexuality
♀▼ **Lestalk**
Rose Publications, 3314 Magnolia Avenue, Saint Louis, Missouri 63118-1233.
☎ 314 773 3220

Stores: Books: General
☺ ■ **Books-N-Things**
♿ 1 South Old Orchard, Saint Louis, Missouri 63119.
☎ 314 961 3755
☺ ■ **Daily Planet News**
♠ 243 North Euclid, Saint Louis, Missouri 63108.
☎ 314 367 1333
☺▼ **Left Bank Books**
♠ 399 North Euclid, Saint Louis, Missouri 63108.
☎ 314 367 6731
♂■ **Pages Video & More**
♠ 10 North Euclid, Saint Louis, Missouri 63108.
☎ 314 361 3420

Springfield
Stores: Books: General
☺ ■ **Renaissance Books**
1337 East Montclair, Springfield, Missouri 65804.
☎ 417 883 5161
☺ ■ **Sunshine News**
3537 West Sunshine, Springfield, Missouri 65807.
☎ 417 831 2298

284

Wentzville

BBSs: BDSM

☺ ■ **Throbnet**
 ✆ 314 327 LUST

MONTANA

Area: Approximately 377,000 square kilometres
Population: Approximately 804,000
Capital City: Helena
Time zone: GMT minus 7 hours (Mountain Time)
Age of consent & homosexuality legislation: Anal & oral sex is illegal in this state only between people of the same sex.

State Resources

Organizations: AIDS: Education

♂♀▽ **Criticare**
 P. O. Box 1253, Billings, Montana 59103.
 ☎ 406 255 7467

Organizations: Sexuality

♀▽ **Montana Lesbian Coalition (MLC)**
 P. O. Box 131, Helena, Montana 59624.
 Please address envelopes to MLC, do NOT address them to Montana Lesbian Coalition.

♂♀▽ **Pride, Inc.**
 P. O. Box 775, Helena, Montana 59624-0775.
 ☎ 406 549 4466

Billings

Health Services

☺ □ **Deaconess Medical Center**
 2800 Tenth Avenue North, Billings, Montana 59101.
 ☎ 406 657 4141

Organizations: AIDS: Education

☺ □ **Yellowstone AIDS Project**
 P. O. Box 1748, Billings, Montana 59103.
 ☎ 406 252 1212

Stores: Erotica: General

☺ ■ **Adult Bookstore**
 2702 Minnesota Avenue, Billings, Montana 59101.
 ☎ 406 245 4293

Bozeman

Organizations: Sexuality: Student

♂♀▽ **Lambda Alliance of Gay Men & Lesbians**
 ♿ c/o Women's Center, Hamilton Hall 15, Bozeman, Montana 59717.
 ☎ 406 994 3836
 ◷ Mon - Fri 09:00 - 16:00, recording at other times

Stores: Erotica: General

☺ ▼ **Ms. Kitty's Adult Shop**
 12 North Willson Street, Bozeman, Montana 59715.
 ☎ 406 586 6989

Butte

Organizations: AIDS: Education

☺ □ **Butte AIDS Support Services**
 ♿ P. O. Box 382, Butte, Montana 59703.
 ☎ 406 494 6125
 ◷ 24hrs.

Missoula

Stores: Books: General

☺ □ **University Center Bookstore**
 ♿ University of Montana, Campus Drive, Missoula, Montana 59806.
 ☎ 406 4921

Stores: Erotica: General

☺ ■ **Fantasy for Adults Only**
 ♿ 210 East Main Street, Missoula, Montana 59801.
 ☎ 406 543 7760
 ◷ 08:00 - 01:30, Fri Sat - 03:00, Sun 10:00 - 24:00

☺ ■ **Fantasy for Adults Only**
 2611 Brooks Street, Missoula, Montana 59801.
 ☎ 406 543 7510
 ◷ 08:00 - 01:30, Fri Sat 24hrs.

NEBRASKA

Area: Approximately 199,000 square kilometres
Population: Approximately 1,600,000
Capital City: Lincoln
Time zone: GMT minus 6/7 hours (both CST & Mountain Time)
Age of consent & homosexuality legislation: State has adopted the Model Penal Code or otherwise decriminalized homosexual activities.

State Resources

Organizations: AIDS: Education

☺ □ **Nebraska AIDS Project**
 ♿ 3624 Leavenworth Street, Omaha, Nebraska 68105.
 ☎ 800 782 2437
 ☎ 402 342 4233
 ◷ Mon - Fri 09:00 - 17:00, daily 18:00 - 23:00

Organizations: BDSM

☺ □ **Omaha Players Club**
 P. O. Box 34463, Omaha, Nebraska 68134-0463.
 ☎ 402 451 7987 ✆ 402 457 5350
 ✉ imsl@synergy.net
 Contact: Ms. Amy Marie Meek
 Pansexual educational & social club. Publishes *Chain Mail*. Age statement of 21 is required.

Publishers: Newspapers: Sexuality

♂♀▼ **The New Voice**
 P. O. Box 3512, Omaha, Nebraska 68103.
 ☎ 402 451 4737
 Comunicating to lesbigay & transgender readers with local, regional, & national news. Published every month. Yearly subscription is $19.

♂♀▼ **Times of the Heartland**
 P. O. Box 3586, Omaha, Nebraska 68103-0586.
 ☎ 402 341 6900

Lincoln

Organizations: Family

☺ □ **Parents & Friends of Lesbians & Gays (PFLAG)—**
 ♿ **Lincoln**
 P. O. Box 4374, Lincoln, Nebraska 68504.
 ☎ 402 467 4599
 ◷ 24hrs. telephone

Organizations: Sexuality: Student

♂♀▽ **Gay & Lesbian Resource Center (GLSA)**
 ♿ Room 234, Nebraska Union, Lincoln, Nebraska 68588-5644.
 ☎ 402 472 5644

♂♀▽ **Gay Men's Support Group**
 ♿ Room 213, University Health Center, Lincoln, Nebraska 68588-0618.
 ☎ 402 472 7450
 Confidential counselling & support from trained counsellors.

Stores: Books: General

♂♀▼ **Arbor Moon Alternative Bookstore**
 ♿ 440 South 44th. Street, Lincoln, Nebraska 68510-1861.
 ☎ 402 477 5666
 ◷ Mon - Fri 12:00 - 20:00, Sat - 18:00

Omaha

BBSs: BDSM

☺ ■ **Mirrored Dragon's Dream**
 ✆ 402 734 2073

Health Services

☺ □ **University of Nebraska Medical Center**
 600 South 42nd. Street, Omaha, Nebraska 68198.
 ☎ 402 559 7400

Organizations: BDSM: Competition

♂♀▽ **International Mr. Fantasy**
 Fantasy Productions, P. O. Box 8203, Omaha, Nebraska 68108-8203.
 Age statement of 21 is required.

Organizations: BDSM

♂♀▽ **OMEN**
 4515 South 16th. Street, Omaha, Nebraska 68107-2128.

Organizations: Family

☺ □ **Parents & Friends of Lesbians & Gays (PFLAG)—**
 ♿ **Omaha**
 2912 Lynnwood Drive, Omaha, Nebraska 68123.
 ☎ 402 291 6781

Organizations: Motorcycle

🛇 ☐ **Two Wheelers Auxiliary Troop**
P. O. Box 3216, Omaha, Nebraska 69103.

Organizations: Sexuality: Youth

♂☐ **Parents & Friends of Lesbians & Gays (PFLAG)—**
♿ **Omaha**
Youth Support Group, 2912 Lynnwood Drive, Omaha, Nebraska 68123.
☎ 402 291 6781

Publishers: Newspapers: Sexuality

♀▼ *Womenspace*
P. O. Box 24712, Omaha, Nebraska 68124-0721.

NEVADA

Area: Approximately 285,000 square kilometres
Population: Approximately 1,206,000
Capital City: Carson City
Time zone: GMT minus 8 hours (PST)
Climate: Hot, dry desert weather. Average summer temperature is approximately 32˚C. Average winter temperature is approximately 10˚C. Temperatures are approximately 10˚C cooler in the north of the state.
Age of consent & homosexuality legislation: Anal & oral sex is illegal in this state only between people of the same sex.
Legal drinking age: 21

State Resources

Organizations: AIDS: Education

☺ ☐ **Aid for AIDS (AFAN)—Nevada**
♿ 1111 Desert Lane, Las Vegas, Nevada 89102-2305.
☎ 702 474 2437 (hotline)
☎ 702 382 2326
Publishes *AFANews.*

Organizations: Sexuality

♂▽ **Southern Nevada Association of Pride (SNAP)**
⚥ P. O. Box 70807, Las Vegas, Nevada 89170-0807.
☎ 702 798 9455

♀▽ **Women United of Nevada**
P. O. Box 12956, Las Vegas, Nevada 89112-0956.
☎ 702 366 8421

Publishers: Newspapers: Sexuality

♂▼ *Las Vegas Bugle*
P. O. Box 14580, Las Vegas, Nevada 89114-4580.
☎ 702 369 6260 ✆ 702 369 9325
✓
The Bugle is news, events, entertainment, & advertising for Las Vegas & Nevada. Bugle Night Beat is classified, 900-numbers, & entertainment advertising. Published every month. Yearly subscription is $35.

Henderson

Organizations: Sexuality

⚧▽ **The Society for the Second Self (Tri-Ess)—Theta Upsilon Gamma**
P. O. Box 91871, Henderson, Nevada 89009-1871.

Las Vegas

Artists: BDSM

☺ **T. Roman Panasewicz**
P. O. Box 29083, Las Vegas, Nevada 89126-3083.

Bars: BDSM

♂▼ **The Buffalo**
4640 Paradise, Las Vegas, Nevada 89109.
☎ 702 733 8355

Health Services

☺ ☐ **University Medical Center**
1800 West Charleston Boulevard, Las Vegas, Nevada 89102.
☎ 702 383 2000

☺ ■ **Valley Hospital Medical Center**
620 Shadow Lane, Las Vegas, Nevada 89106.
☎ 702 388 4000
HIV & emergency departments.

Manufacturers: Whips

☺ ■ **Mark Allen Productions**
#14, 3750 S. Valley View, Las Vegas, Nevada 89103.
☎ 800 858 5568 ✆ 702 873 1100
☎ 702 873 0216
🕐 08:30 - 17:00

Western arts equipment: bullwhips, knives & tomahawks, & videos & books. Not scene friendly, be discreet.

Organizations: BDSM

♂▽ **CB&V**
P. O. Box 97694, Las Vegas, Nevada 89193.

☺ ☐ **Eroticism through Sensual Conduct, Attitude, & Power Exchange (Escape)—West**
Suite 106, 330 South Decatur, Las Vegas, Nevada 89107.
☎ 702 226 5441 (voicemail)

♂♀☐ **The Orb & Scepter**
c/o New Visionary Press, Suite 483, 252 Convention Center Drive, Las Vegas, Nevada 89109.
☎ 702 251 7201

Organizations: Bears

♂▽ **Blackjack Bears of Las Vegas**
P. O. Box 29307, Las Vegas, Nevada 89126-3307.
☎ 702 225 4513
📧 bearcublv@aol.com or bearinlv@aol.com

♂▽ **Las Vegas Bears**
P. O. Box 34263, Las Vegas, Nevada 89133.
☎ 702 658 7548

Organizations: Family

☺ ☐ **Parents & Friends of Lesbians & Gays (PFLAG)—Las Vegas**
P. O. Box 20145, Las Vegas, Nevada 89112.
☎ 702 369 8700

Organizations: Motorcycle

♂▽ **Desert Brotherhood MC**
P. O. Box 71145, Las Vegas, Nevada 89170.

♂▽ **Satyricons MC**
P. O. Box 19357-0357, Las Vegas, Nevada 89132.
☎ 702 733 8355

Organizations: Sexuality

♂▽ **The Center**
P. O. Box 60301, Las Vegas, Nevada 89160.
☎ 702 733 9800

Organizations: Sexuality: Student

♂ ▽ **Delta Lambda Phi Fraternity—Las Vegas**
♿ Box 60301, University of Nevada at Las Vegas, 912 East Sahara, Las Vegas, Nevada 89160.
☎ 702 733 9800
Send IRC or stamps to ensure reply.

Photographers: Erotic

☺ **Richard Mueller**
P. O. Box 19425, Las Vegas, Nevada 89132.
☎ 702 796 9592

Piercers

☺ ■ **Alter Ego**
☎ 702 796 8054 ✆ 702 389 2967

Stores: Books: General

♂▼ **Get Booked**
♿ 4643 Paradise Road, Las Vegas, Nevada 89109.
☎ 702 737 7780 ✆ 702 792 2712
🕐 Mon 10:00 - 24:00, Tue - Sun 10:00 - 02:00
⚥ ✓ VISA MC

Stores: Erotica: BDSM

☺ ▼ **Lock, Stock, & Leather**
♿ Number 10, 4640 Paradise Road, Las Vegas, Nevada.
☎ 702 796 9801 ✆ 702 248 1954
🕐 Tue - Sun 16:00 - 23:00, Fri Sat - 02.00
$ $ — VISA MC
Alternative family store. Leather & rubber in the back. Custom work available.

Stores: Erotica: General

☺ ■ **Desert Adult Books**
♿ 4350 Las Vegas Boulevard North, Las Vegas, Nevada 89115.
☎ 702 643 7982

☺ ■ **Erotica Plus**
4029 West Sahara, Las Vegas, Nevada 98102.
☎ 702 362 0079
Some leather & BDSM items.

Reno

Counsellors

🔗▼ **Caring Counseling**
2061 Market Street, Reno, Nevada 89502.
☎ 702 322 7771

Health Services

☺ ☐ **Saint Mary's Regional Medical Center**
235 West Sixth Street, Reno, Nevada 89520.
☎ 702 323 2041

☺ ☐ **Washoe Medical Center**
77 Pringle Way, Reno, Nevada 89520.
☎ 702 328 4100

Organizations: BDSM

♂▽ **Knights of Malta MC—Western**
P. O. Box 7726, Reno, Nevada 89510.

Publishers: Newspapers: Sexuality

♀▼ **Lesbian Voices**
P. O. Box 33004, Reno, Nevada 89533-3004.

♂ **Reno Informer**
Suite 213-185, 5150 Mae Anne Avenue, Reno, Nevada 89523.
☎ 702 826 2257 📞 702 826 2257
Local news, national news via Gaynet News Service, AIDS information, classifieds, political information, local writers. Also distributed in Carson City, Lake Tahoe, & Sacramento. Yearly subscription is $25.

Stores: Books: General

☺ ■ **Bold Print**
♿ 3432 Lakeside Drive, Reno, Nevada 89509.
☎ 702 829 2653
🕐 10:00 - 20:00, Sat Sun - 18:00

♂▼ **Grapevine Books**
♿ 1450 South Wells Avenue, Reno, Nevada 89502-2971.
☎ 702 786 4869

Stores: Erotica: BDSM

☺ **Fantasy Faire**
1298 South Virginia Street, Reno, Nevada 98502.
☎ 702 323 6969

Sparks

Organizations: BDSM

⚥ ▽ **Reno's Leather Underground**
P. O. Box 6093, Sparks, Nevada 89432.

♂▽ **Silver State Leather Association**
P. O. Box 50762, Sparks, Nevada 89435.
☎ 702 331 7059

Organizations: Sexuality

🔗▽ **Jennifer & Friends**
P. O. box 1284, Sparks, Nevada 89432.
🕐 Meets monthly

NEW HAMPSHIRE

Area: Approximately 23,250 square kilometres
Population: Approximately 1,115,000
Capital City: Concord
Time zone: GMT minus 5 hours (EST)
Climate: Pleasant summer with temperatures averaging approximately 21°C. Winters can be long & harsh, with plenty of snow.
Age of consent & homosexuality legislation: State has adopted the Model Penal Code or otherwise decriminalized homosexual activities.
Legal drinking age: 20

State Resources

Helplines: Sexuality

♂▽ **Gay Info Line of New Hampshire**
♿ Box 181, 26 South Main Street, Concord, New Hampshire 03301.
☎ 603 224 1686
Information about local organizations & professionals who want to be of service to the lesbian & gay community. Publishes a calendar of events.

Organizations: AIDS: Education

☺ ☐ **AIDS Community Resource Network (ACORN)**
♿ P. O. Box 2057, Lebanon, New Hampshire 03766.
☎ 603 448 2220

Organizations: BDSM

♂▽ **The Norsemen**
P.O. Box 556, Manchester, New Hampshire 03105-0556.

☎ 603 641 3450

Organizations: Family

♂▽ **New Hampshire Gay Parents**
P. O. Box 5981, Manchester, New Hampshire 03108-5981.
☎ 603 527 1082

☺ ☺ **Parents & Friends of Lesbians & Gays (PFLAG)—**
🐘 **New Hampshire**
18 Hobbs Road, Kensington, New Hampshire 03833.
☎ 603 623 6023
Publishes *PFLAG NH Newsletter.*

Amherst

Organizations: Sexuality: Youth

♂▽ **Tir-State Gay / Lesbian Awareness Dialogue Group**
☎ 603 673 5391

Bartlet

Organizations: Sexuality

♀▽ **Northern Voice**
P. O. Box 26, Bartlet, New Hampshire 03812.
☎ 603 374 1833

Campton

Organizations: Sexuality

♀▽ **The Lakes - Mountains Coinnection**
P. O. Box 164, Campton, New Hampshire 03223.
☎ 603 726 3667

Concord

Counsellors

☺▼ **Lyn Foley, ACSW**
30 South Main Street, Concord, New Hampshire 03301.
☎ 603 224 5600

Health Services

☺ ☐ **New Hampshire Hospital**
105 Pleasant Street, Concord, New Hampshire 03301.
☎ 603 271 5200

Organizations: Sexuality

♀▽ **NH Lambda**
P. O. Box 1043, Concord, New Hampshire 03302.
☎ 603 627 8675

Publishers: Newspapers: Sexuality

♂ **Breathing Space**
P. O. Box 730, Concord, New Hampshire 03302-0730.

Conway

Organizations: Sexuality

♂▽ **Mountain Valley Men**
P. O. Box 36, Conway, New Hampshire 03813-0036.
☎ 207 925 1034

Durham

Organizations: Sexuality: Student

♂▽ **The Alliance**
♿ Room 7, Memorial Union Building, University of New Hampshire, Durham, New Hampshire 03802.
☎ 603 862 4522

Francestown

Organizations: Sexuality: Youth

♂▽ **Monadnock Outright**
731 Bennington Road, Francestown, New Hampshire 04043.
☎ 603 547 2545

Hanover

Organizations: Sexuality: Student

♂▽ **Dartmouth Gay & Lesbian Organization (DAGLO)**
Hinman Box 5057, Collis Center, Hanover, New Hampshire 03755.
☎ 603 646 3636

Keene

Counsellors

🔗☐ **Cheshire Counseling Associates**
P. O. Box 1124, Keene, New Hampshire 03431.

Counsellors

☎ 603 357 5544

Organizations: Family

⚥▽ **Monadnock Area Lesbian / Gay Parents**
47 Adams Street, Keene, New Hampshire 03431.
☎ 603 352 6741

Organizations: Sexuality

▽ **Gender Talk North**
P. O. Box 211, Keene, New Hampshire.
☎ 603 924 8828
Support group.

⚥▽ **Monadnock Area Womyn (MAW)**
P. O. Box 6345, Keene, New Hampshire 03431.
☎ 603 352 6741

⚥▽ **Monadnock Gay Men (MGM)**
⚴ P. O. Box 1124, Keene, New Hampshire 03431.
☎ 603 357 5544
Publishes *MGM Newsletter*.

Organizations: Sexuality: Student

⚥▽ **Lesbian Bisexual Gay Alliance**
Keene State College, Keene, New Hampshire 03431.
☎ 603 352 1909

Manchester

Counsellors

⚥▼ **Patricia Barr, Ph.D.**
⚴ 61 North Street, Manchester, New Hampshire 03104.
☎ 603 647 2366

⚥▼ **Denise Lamothe, Psy.D.**
♿ 311 Highlander Way, Manchester, New Hampshire 03103.
☎ 603 627 3739

⚥▼ **Joyce Whiting, ACSW**
♿ Suite 518, 795 Elm Street, Manchester, New Hampshire 03101.
☎ 603 666 4299

Health Services

☺□ **Veterans' Affairs Medical Center**
718 Smyth Road, Manchester, New Hampshire 03104.
☎ 603 624 4366

Organizations: BDSM

⚥ **Bottoms-Up**
P.O. Box 556, Manchester, New Hampshire 03105-0556.
☎ 603 367 8304

Organizations: Sexuality: Youth

⚥▽ **Teen Options Clinic**
976 Elm Street, Manchester, New Hampshire.
☎ 603 429 1616

Merrimack

Organizations: Sexuality: Youth

⚥ ▽ **Merrimack Valley Youth Group**
☎ 603 424 7759

Nashua

Organizations: Sexuality

⚥▽ **Alternative Lifestyles Fellowship**
Suite 332, 131 DW Highway, Nashua, New Hampshire 03060-5245.

Organizations: Sexuality: Youth

⚥▽ **Southern New Hampshire Gay & Lesbian Youth (SNHAGLY)**
P. O. Box 294, Nashua, New Hampshire 03060.
☎ 603 672 0792

Plymouth

Counsellors

▽ **Nasncy Strapko, Ph.D.**
P. O. Box 157, Plymouth, New Hampshire 03264.
☎ 603 536 1306
Psychotherapist.

Organizations: Sexuality: Student

⚥▽ **Alternative Lifestyles Support Organization (ALSO)**
♿
Plymouth State College, P. O. Box 492, Plymouth, New Hampshire 03264-0492.
☎ 603 535 2796

Portsmouth

Organizations: AIDS: Education

⚥▽ **AIDS Response of the Seacoast**
Suite 3, 10 Vaughn Hall, Portsmouth, New Hampshire 03801.
☎ 603 433 5377

Organizations: Sexuality

⚥▽ **Out & About**
P. O. Box 332, Portsmouth, New Hampshire 03802-0332.
☎ 603 659 2139

⚥▽ **Seacoast Gay Men (SAG)**
P. O. Box 1394, Portsmouth, New Hampshire 03802-1394.
☎ 603 898 1115
⊕ Mon 19:00 (except holidays)

Organizations: Sexuality: Youth

⚥▽ **Seacost Outright**
P. O. Box 842, Portsmouth, New Hampshire 03802.
☎ 800 639 6095 (teenline)
☎ 603 431 1013

Stores: Books: General

⚥ ■ **Lady Iris**
Suite 1, 25 Melbourne Street, Portsmouth, New Hampshire 03801-4817.
☎ 603 436 3634

Stores: Erotica: General

☺ ■ **The Fifth Wheel**
Route 1 Bypass North, Portsmouth, New Hampshire 03801.
☎ 603 436 1504

☺ ■ **Peter's Palace**
♿ Route 1 Bypass North, Portsmouth, New Hampshire 03801.
☎ 603 436 9622
⊕ 09:00 - 23:00

Salem

Counsellors

☺ **Raymond Arsenault, Ph.D.**
K 19 Main Street, Salem, New Hampshire 03079.
☎ 603 898 5105
Psychologist.

Sanbornville

Suppliers: Diapers

☺ ■ **Edley Enterprises, Inc.**
P. O. Box 429, Sanbornville, New Hampshire 03872.
☎ 603 473 2539
Cloth diapers & waterproof pants. Discreet shipping.

Weirs Beach

Tattooists

☺ ■ **Sign Of The Wolf Tattoo**
☎ 603 366 2557
Piercing also available.

West Franklin

Publishers: Magazines: Sexuality

▽■ *TV-TS Confidential*
Writer's Etc., P. O. Box 6211, West Franklin, New Hampshire 03235.
☎ 603 934 3379
⊕ 11:00 - 21:00
✓
Non-sexual publication for transgender & transvestite. Published every month. Yearly subscription is S36. Age statement of 21 is required.

NEW JERSEY

Area: Approximately 19,250 square kilometres
Population: Approximately 7,750,000
Capital City: Trenton
Time zone: GMT minus 5 hours (EST)
Climate: Summer temperatures can reach 28°C, winter lows can reach -2°C. The Atlantic ocean has a moderating influence on the coastal areas.
Age of consent & homosexuality legislation: State has adopted the Model Penal Code or otherwise decriminalized homosexual activities. There is legislation in place against discrimination on the basis of sexual orientation.
Legal drinking age: 21

State Resources

Film Festivals: Sexuality

⚥▽ **New Jersey Lesbian & Gay Film Festival**

c/o Gay & Lesbian Arts Society (GALAS), P. O. Box 1291, Montclair, New Jersey 07042.

Health Services
☺ □ **HIV Confidential Testing Service**
 ⚹ Annex, Community Service Building, Route 31, Flemington, New Jersey 08822.
 ☎ 908 806 4893

Helplines: AIDS
⚥▽ **Gay Helpline of New Jersey**
 ☎ 201 285 1595
 ⏱ 19:30 - 22:30
 For Morris County.

Helplines: Sexuality
⚥▽ **Gay Helpline of New Jersey**
 P. O. Box 1734, South Hackensack, New Jersey 07606.
 ☎ 201 692 1794
 ⏱ 19:30 - 22:30

Organizations: AIDS: Education
☺ □ **AIDS Coalition of Southern New Jersey**
 Suite 210, 900 Hadden Avenue, Collingswood, New Jersey 08108.
 ☎ 800 229 2437
 ☎ 609 854 7578
☺ □ **Hyacinth AIDS Foundation**
 ⚹ 3rd. Floor, 103 Bayard Street, New Brunswick, New Jersey 08901.
 ☎ 800 433 0254 (in New Jersey)
 ⏱ Office: Mon - Fri 09:00 - 17:00; hotline: Mon Fri 10:00 - 22:00, Sat 11:00 - 17:00

Organizations: AIDS: Support
☺ □ **AIDS Benefit Committee of New Jersey**
 P. O. Box 1443, Plainfield, New Jersey 07061.
 ☎ 908 561 4359

Organizations: Family
☺ □ **Parents & Friends of Lesbians & Gays (PFLAG)— North Jersey**
 P. O. Box 244, Belleville, New Jersey 07109.
 ☎ 201 267 8414

Organizations: Sexuality
⚥▽ **Delaware Valley Gay Neighbors**
 P. O. Box 11161, Yardville, New Jersey 08620.
 Publishes *DVGN Quarterly Newsletter*. Please address envelopes to DVGN, do NOT address them to Delaware Valley Gay Neighbors or DVGN Quarterly Newsletter.
⚥▽ **New Jersey Lesbian & Gay Coalition**
 ⚹ P. O. Box 1431, New Brunswick, New Jersey 08903.
 ☎ 201 763 0668
⚥▽ **Ocean (County) Lesbian-Gay Alliance, Inc.**
 ⚹ P. O. Box 421, Seaside Park, New Jersey 08752-0421.
 ☎ 908 793 3603
⚥▽ **Organization for Gay Awareness**
 P. O. Box 1291, Montclair, New Jersey 07042.
 ☎ 201 746 6196

Organizations: Sexuality: Youth
⚥▽ **Gay & Lesbian Youth in New Jersey (GALY-NY)**
 ⚹ P. O. Box 127, Convent Station, New Jersey 07961-0137.
 ☎ 201 285 1595
 ⏱ Helpline 19:30 - 22:30. Meets Sat 13:30 - 16:30
 For youth 16 - 21 years.

Publishers: Newspapers: Sexuality
⚥▼ *Lavendar Express*
 P. O. Box 514, Harrison, New Jersey 07029.
 ☎ 201 439 1593 ✆ 201 385 1916
 ✉ HCKK46A@Prodigy.com
 ⚹ ✓ $ 💳 ⚹ ⚹
 New Jersey's lesbian journal. Published since 1978. The best way to find out what's happening in new Jersey & the surrounding areas. Published every month.
⚥▼ *Network for the 10% Plus*
 P. O. Box 10372, New Brunswick, New Jersey 08906.
 ☎ 908 873 0266
 Our motto is: Every day issues for every day gays. Published every month. Yearly subscription is $29.95.

Asbury Park
BBSs: BDSM
⚥▼ **Backroom II**
 ☏ 908 774 6069

Organizations: Family
☺ □ **Parents & Friends of Lesbians & Gays (PFLAG)— Monmouth / Ocean Counties**
 P. O. Box 1542, Asbury Park, New Jersey 07712.
 ☎ 908 905 6823
 ⏱ Meets 2nd. Wed of month 20:00

Organizations: Sexuality
⚥▽ **Jersey Shore Gay & Lesbian Community Center**
 ⚹ Suite 7, 529 Bangs Avenue, Asbury Park, New Jersey 07712.
 ☎ 908 493 0730
 Please address envelopes to JSGL Community Center, do NOT address them to Jersey Shore Gay & Lesbian Community Center.

Atlantic City
Bars: BDSM
⚥▼ **Rendezvous Lounge**
 137 South New York Avenue, Atlantic City, New Jersey 08401.
 ☎ 609 347 8539
 ⏱ 15:00 - 03:00

Health Services
☺ □ **Atlantic City Medical Center**
 1925 Pacific Avenue, Atlantic City, New Jersey 08401.
 ☎ 609 344 4081

Organizations: AIDS: Education
☺ ▽ **South Jersey AIDS Alliance**
 ⚹ 1301 Atlantic Avenue, Atlantic City, New Jersey 08401-7247.
 ☎ 800 281 2437 (in New Jersey)
 ☎ 609 347 8799
 ⏱ 800 number is 24hrs.

Stores: Erotica: General
☺ ■ **Atlantic News Agency**
 101 South Illinois Avenue, Atlantic City, New Jersey 08401.
 ☎ 609 344 9444

Suppliers: Miscellaneous
✉▽ ■ **Genie Trimmers**
 326 Spencer Building, Atlantic City, New Jersey 08411-0009.
 Supplies waist trimmers & rib belts for FTMs.
✉▽ ■ **Spencer Gifts**
 326 Spencer Building, Atlantic City, New Jersey 08411-0009.
 Supplies waist trimmers & rib belts for FTMs.

Berlin
Stores: Erotica: General
☺ ■ **Red Barn Adult Bookstore**
 Route 73, Berlin, New Jersey 08009.
 ☎ 609 767 1525

Blackwood
Counsellors
☺ ▼ **Focused Counseling Services, Inc.**
 ⚹ 8 North Black Horse Pike, Blackwood, New Jersey 08102.
 ☎ 609 228 8910

Blairstown
Stores: Clothing: Fetish
☺ **Dark Alley**
 3 Route 94, Blairstown, New Jersey 07825.
 ☎ 908 362 8728

Brick
Counsellors
☺ ▼ **Dianne Garcia, MSW, Ph.D.**
 478 Manchester Avenue, Brick, New Jersey 08723-5225.
 ☎ 908 920 8110 ✆ 908 920 4432
 ⏱ Mon - Thu 12:00 - 20:00
 ⚹ ✓ $
 Stress management, psychotherapy, & hypnosis by holistic practitioner in comfortable provacy of her home office.

Brick Town
Stores: Erotica: General
☺ ■ **Unisex Adult Bookstore**
 2148 Route 88E, Brick Town, New Jersey 08723.
 ☎ 908 295 0166

Bridgewater

Distributors: Books: General

☺ ■ **Baker & Taylor Books**
652 East Main Street, Bridgewater, New Jersey 08807.
☎ 908 218 0400

Butler

Tattooists

☺ ■ **Tattoo Factory**
94 Main Street, Butler, New Jersey 07405.
☎ 201 838 7828
⏱ Mon - Sat 15:00 - 21:00
🔗 VISA MC
Also makes custom DBSM equipment in wood or iron.

Chatham

Printers: General

☺ **Multiprint, Inc.**
80 Longhill Lane, Chatham, New Jersey 07928.
☎ 201 635 6400 📠 201 635 6402

Cherry Hill

Counsellors

☺ ■ **Joellyn Ross, Ph.D.**
♿ J-49 Executive Mews, 1930 East Marlton Pike, Cherry Hill, New Jersey 08003.
☎ 609 424 1065

Stores: Clothing: Wigs

▽ **Wig Service Shop**
Barclay Towers, 1200 East Mrlton Pike, Cherry Hill, New Jersey 08034.
☎ 609 428 8448
⏱ Mon - Sat 11:00 - 16:00

Denville

Counsellors

☺▽ **Norma Lafferty, MSW**
♿ ☎ 201 586 3694

Stores: Books: General

☺▽ **Perrin & Treggett Booksellers**
♿ 3130 Route 10 West, Denville, New Jersey 07834.
☎ 800 770 8811 📠 201 328 0999
☎ 201 328 8811

Dover

Accommodation: BDSM

☺ ■ **Fantasy Inn**
P. O. Box 321, Dover, New Jersey 07801.

Organizations: AIDS: Education

☺ □ **AIDS Center at Hope House**
♿ 19-21 Belmont Avenue, Dover, New Jersey 07801.
☎ 201 361 7443 (AIDS Hopeline)
☎ 201 361 7555
Publishes *The Olive Branch*.

Dunellen

BBSs: BDSM

☺ ■ **gLiTcH**
📞 908 968 4349
✉ jod@glitch.com

East Rutherford

Publishers: Magazines: Sexuality

☺ *TRASH*
c/o D&W Enterprises, P.O. Box 292, East Rutherford, New Jersey 07073.

Edison

Stores: Erotica: General

☺ ■ **Adult Bookstore**
1851 State Highway, Edison, New Jersey 08817.
☎ 908 985 9619

Egg Harbor City

Stores: Erotica: General

☺ ■ **Adult World**
25 White Horse Pike, Egg Harbor City, New Jersey 08215.
☎ 609 965 1110

Fort Lee

Television: General

☺ **CNBC Real Personal**
2200 Fletcher Avenue, Fort Lee, New Jersey 07024.
☎ 201 585 2622 📠 201 585 6276

Hackensack

Suppliers: Diapers

☺ ■ **Duro-Med Industries, Inc.**
301 Lodi Street, Hackensack, New Jersey 07602.
☎ 201 488 5055
Disposable diapers, liners, & waterproof pants.

Hawthorne

Piercers

☺ ■ **Pleasurable Piercings, Inc.**
417 Lafayette Avenue, Hawthorne, New Jersey 07506.
☎ 201 238 0305 📠 201 238 9564
☎ 800 774 6086 (in New Jersey)
✉ needleboy@aol.com
⏱ Tue - Sat 12:00 - 20:00, Sun Mon 12:00 - 17:00
🔗 ✓ VISA MC
Catalogue, $5. Age statement of 18 is required. Spanish also spoken.

Stores: Erotica: BDSM

☺ ■ **Pleasurable Alternatives**
7 Garfield Avenue, Hawthorne, New Jersey 07506.
☎ 201 238 0305 📠 201 238 9564
☎ 800 774 6086 (in New Jersey)
✉ needleboy@aol.com
🔗 ✓ VISA MC
Catalogue, $5. Age statement of 18 is required. Spanish also spoken.

Highland

Performers: Music: BDSM

☺ **Genitorturers**
68 Highland Avenue, Highland, New Jersey 07732.
Group that includes SM as part of its stage persona.

Hoboken

Counsellors

☺▽ **Tod Bergman, MSW**
♿ 324 Garden Street, Hoboken, New Jersey 07030.
☎ 201 795 4050

Howell

Stores: Erotica: General

☺ ■ **Howell Adult Book Store**
6825 Highway 9 North, Howell, New Jersey 07731-3327.
☎ 908 363 9680

Tattooists

☺ ■ **Images in Ink**
Howell Mall, Route 9 South, Howell, New Jersey.
☎ 908 901 6205
Piercing also available.

Huntington

Publishers: Videos: Sexuality

☺ ■ **Focus International**
1160 East Jericho Turnpike, Huntington, New Jersey 11743.
☎ 516 549 5320 📠 516 549 2066
⏱ 09:00 - 17:00
✓ VISA MC
Self-help & sex education videos.

Irvington

Stores: Erotica: General

☺ ■ **Best Adult Bookstore**
166 Prospect Avenue, Irvington, New Jersey 07111.
☎ 201 372 0130

Jersey City

Counsellors

☺▽ **Margaret Nichols, Ph.D.**
♿ 281 Pavonia Avenue, Jersey City, New Jersey 07302.
☎ 201 798 5926

Publishers: Magazines: BDSM

Bandanna
P. O. Box 13090, Jersey City, New Jersey 07303-4090.
☎ 201 216 0552 Fax 201 963 2409
Published every two months. Yearly subscription is $24 (incl s&h).

Linden

Stores: Clothing: Fetish

A Woman's Touch
124 Wood Avenue, Linden, New Jersey 07036.
☎ 908 486 8022

Lyndhurst

Publishers: Magazines: Sexuality

The Unforgettable Fire
P. O. Box 388, Lyndhurst, New Jersey 07071.

Mays Landing

Organizations: Sexuality

Rennaissance—South Jersey
P. O. Box 189, Mays Landing, New Jersey 08330.
☎ 609 435 5401
☎ 609 641 3782
Meetings & support.

Metuchen

Printers: General

Scarecrow Press
52 Liberty Street, Metuchen, New Jersey 08840.
☎ 201 548 8600

Middlesex

Suppliers: Diapers

Geri-Care Products
252 Wagner Street, Middlesex, New Jersey 08846.
☎ 908 469 7722
Cloth diapers, cloth contoured diapers, & waterproof pants.

Millburn

Counsellors

Betty Levin, MA
117 Sagamore Avenue, Millburn, New Jersey 07041.
☎ 201 763 1035

Montclair

Competitions & Conventions: Fetish: Clothing

Dressing For Pleasure Gala
P. O. Box 43079, Upper Montclair, New Jersey 07043.
☎ 201 746 4200 Fax 201 746 4722
☎ 201 746 5466
Held in mid-October. Call Tue - Sat 12:00 - 18:00
✓ $ VISA MC AMERICAN EXPRESS

Counsellors

Alternative Approach Counseling & Psychotherapy Center
☎ 201 736 8785

Center For Identity Development
31 Trinity Place, Montclair, New Jersey 07042.
☎ 201 744 6386

Diane Giachetti, CSW, ACSW
☎ 201 998 7705

Rosemarie Kopacsi, Ph.D., ACSW
Suite 209, 460 Bloomfield Avenue, Montclair, New Jersey.
☎ 201 338 4834

Beth Lewinter, MSW, CSW
Suite 303, 37 North Fullerton Avenue, Montclair, New Jersey 07042.
☎ 201 783 6351

Montclair State College
☎ 201 893 5271
24hrs.
Walk-in & telephone counselling & referrals.

Gwen Wolverton, Psy.D.
1 Upper Mountain Avenue, Montclair, New Jersey 07042.
☎ 201 746 1414

Manufacturers: Piercing Jewelry

Rings & Things
7 Midland Avnue, Montclair, New Jersey 07042.
☎ 201 783 9633
Steel, Niobium, gold jewelry in geometric designs with bi-coloured Niobium. Free catalogue.

Organizations: AIDS: Education

New Jersey AIDS Connection
P. O. Box 162, Montclair, New Jersey 07042.
☎ 201 481 1412

Organizations: Sexuality

Always On Sunday
P. O. Box 1708, Montclair, New Jersey 07042.
☎ 201 783 1419

Stores: Clothing: Fetish

Dressing For Pleasure
590 Valley Road, Upper Montclair, New Jersey 07043.
☎ 201 746 4200 Fax 201 746 4722
☎ 201 746 5466
Tue - Sat 12:00 - 18:00
✓ VISA MC
The elite boutique strictly for the exotic shopper. Also mail order books, magazine, videos, & more. Catalogue, $3U.S..

Moorestown

Distributors: Books: General

Koen Book Distributors
P. O. Box 600, Moorestown, New Jersey 080547.
☎ 609 235 4444 Fax 609 727 6914
Mon - Fri 09:00 - 17:00

Morristown

Counsellors

Allen Wells Center for Psychotherapy & Healing
102 Ogden Place, Morristown, New Jersey 07960.
☎ 201 539 0301

Organizations: Sexuality

Renaissance Education Association, Inc.—Northern New Jersey
P. O. Box 9192, Morristown, New Jersey 07960.
☎ 201 663 0772
Contact: Ms. Lynda Frank

Neptune

Organizations: AIDS: Education

AIDS Support Team
71 Davis Avenue, Neptune, New Jersey 07753.
☎ 908 776 4700
Mon - Fri 09:00 - 17:00

New Brunswick

Counsellors

Insitute for Personal Growth
8 South 3rd. Avenue, Highland, New Jersey 08904-2510.
☎ 908 246 8439

Organizations: Sexuality

Lesbians & Gay MEn of New Brunswick
P. O. Box 1949, New Brunswick, New Jersey 08903-1949.
☎ 908 247 0515
Meets 2nd. & 4th. Tue of month 20:00

More Than You Can Count
P. O. Box 4178, Highland Park, New Jersey 08904.
☎ 908 819 0601

Publishers: Books: General

Rutgers University Press
109 Church Street, New Brunswick, New Jersey 08901.
Have published books about BDSM-related topics, such as gay police.

Publishers: Newspapers: Sexuality

Gay GAIA
267 Sanford Street, New Brunswick, New Jersey 08901.

Radio: Sexuality

Gay Spirit
WRSU FM 88.7, 126 College Avenue, New Brunswick, New Jersey 08903.
☎ 908 932 8800
Tue 21:00 - 23:00

Stores: Books: General

Chapter One Books

128 Raritan Avenue, Highland Park, New Jersey 08904.
908 828 7648
10:30 - 23:00

New Providence

Organizations: Polyfidelity

Tri-State Polyamory
P. O. Box 625, New Providence, New Jersey 07974-0625.

Publishers: Directories: Books

R. R. Bowker
ABI Department, 121 Chanlon Road, New Providence, New Jersey 07974.
908 665 2883

Newark

Health Services

Newark Beth Israel Medical Center
201 Lyons Avenue, Newark, New Jersey 07112.
201 926 7000

United Hospitals Medical Center
15 South Ninth Street, Newark, New Jersey 07107.
201 268 8000
HIV & emergency departments.

University Hospital
University of Medicine & Dentistry of New Jersey, 150 Bergen Street, Newark, New Jersey 07103.
201 982 4300
HIV & emergency departments.

Helplines: AIDS

AIDS Helpline
Saint Michael's Medical Center, 268 M. L. King Boulevard, Newark, New Jersey 07102.
201 877 5525
Mon - Fri 08:30 - 16:30

Organizations: AIDS: Education

Newark Community Health Centers, Inc.
P. O. Box 1960, Newark, New Jersey 07101.
201 565 0355

Organizations: Motorcycle

Cycles MC
P.O. Box 25191, Newark, New Jersey 07102.
Contact: Mr. Gustave Trenker

Photographers: Erotic

John Santerineross
247 New Jersey Railroad Avenue, Newark, New Jersey 07105.
201 743 6290

North Bergen

Printers: General

Book Mart Press
2001 Forty Second Street, North Bergen, New Jersey 07047.
201 864 1887 212 594 3344

North Brunswick

Suppliers: Diapers

Humanicare International, Inc.
1200 Airport Road, North Brunswick, New Jersey 08902.
201 214 0660
800 631 5270
Dignity pants & pads.

North Haledon

Stores: Books: General

Pandora Book Peddlars
885 Belmont Avenue, North Haledon, New Jersey 07508.
201 427 5733

Oakland

Organizations: Sexuality

Feminine Connection
201 337 7506

Piscataway

Organizations: BDSM

Locker Jocks
P. O. Box 8221, Piscataway, New Jersey 08855.

Plainfield

Counsellors

Beryl Cohn, RNC, MSW
908 757 8981

Sylvia Walker, MSW, ACSW
908 561 6073

Organizations: Sexuality

Central Jersey Alliance of Gay, Lesbian, & Bisexual People
P. O. Box 909, Plainfield, New Jersey 07061.
908 756 4955

Stores: Books: General

Cutting Edge
695 West 7th. Street, Plainfield, New Jersey 07060.
908 769 3250

Princeton

Counsellors

Bunker Hill Consultation Center
Box 570, Road 1, Princeton, New Jersey 08540.
609 497 0899

Judith Dean, Ed.D., M.Div., M.S.
Creative Psychotherapy Associates, Suite 110, 55 Princeton-Hightsown Road, Princeton Junction, New Jersey 08550.
609 275 6556

Organizations: Sexuality

Gay People Princeton
P. O. Box 2303, Princeton, New Jersey 08543.

Organizations: Sexuality: Student

Lesbian, Gay, & Bisexual Alliance
Princeton University, 306 Aaron Burr Hall, Princeton, New Jersey 08544.
609 258 4522

Red Bank

Counsellors

Daphnee Banks, MSW, CSW, ACSW
248 Broad Street, Red Bank, New Jersey 07701.
908 530 8483

Organizations: Sexuality

East Coast Couples Network (ECCN)
c/o Monmouth Ocean Group, P. O. Box 8243, Red Bank, New Jersey 07701.
Publishes *Monmouth-Ocean News*.

Monmouth Ocean Transgender Group (MOTG)
P. O. Box 8243, Red Bank, New Jersey 07701.
Meetings & support. Publishes *Monmouth-Ocean News*.

Publishers: Miscellaneous

Lavendar Circle Press
P. O. Box 8932, Red Bank, New Jersey 07701.

Stores: Books: General

Earth Spirit
16 West Front Street, Red Bank, New Jersey 07701.
908 842 3855

River Edge

Organizations: Sexuality

The Society for the Second Self (Tri-Ess)—Chi Delta Mu
P. O. Box 1, River Edge, New Jersey 07661-0001.
201 663 0772

Roselle

Publishers: Magazines: Erotic

Pump It Up!
Mirza, Inc., 139 West 4th. Avenue, Roselle, New Jersey 07203.
908 245 5323 908 241 6152
09:00 - 21:00
Published quarterly. Yearly subscription is $16. Age statement of 21 is required.

Stores: Erotica: BDSM

Master's Toychest
139 West 4th. Avenue, Roselle, New Jersey 07203.

908 245 5223 908 241 6153
Age statement of 21 is required.

Sewell

Organizations: Sexuality: Student

IMRU of Gloucester County College
P. O. Box 227, Sewell, New Jersey 08080.
609 468 5000 Ext.: 750

Somerville

Counsellors

Virginia Stein, MA
357 William Street, Somerville, New Jersey 08876.
908 722 6343

Stone Harbor

Distributors: Erotica: Chastity Belts

Tim Swig Associates Group
P. O. Box 234, Stone Harbor, New Jersey 08247.
609 368 2482
Distributes both Posey & Humane Restraints products.

Sussex

Organizations: Sexuality

The Loving Brotherhood
P. O. Box 556, Sussex, New Jersey 07461.
201 875 4710
Publishes *Loving Brotherhood Newsletter*. Yearly subscription is $12.

Teaneck

Counsellors

Roz Yager Kupferman, BS, MA, Psy.A.
304 Winthrop Road, Teaneck, New Jersey 07666.
201 837 6381

Publishers: Magazines: Erotic

First Hand
P. O. Box 1314, Teaneck, New Jersey 07666.
201 836 9177

Guys Magazine
P. O Box 1314, Teaneck, New Jersey 07666.
201 836 9177 201 836 5055

Titusville

Suppliers: Diapers

Nikky / Natural Baby Co., Inc.
Box 160, RD 1, Titusville, New Jersey 08560.
609 737 2895
Flannel diapers, waterproof pants, diaper covers, & bed-wetter pants. Up to 110lb sizes.

Toms River

Counsellors

Fran Hepburn, MSW, CADC
Suite 5, 1518 Highway 37E, Toms River, New Jersey 08753.
908 270 2952

Organizations: Sexuality

Transexual Organization Self Help
6 Firehorn Way, Toms River, New Jersey 08755.
Contact: Mr. A. J. Gilberti
Support for male-to-females.

Trenton

Organizations: Sexuality

The Society for the Second Self (Tri-Ess)—Sigma Nu Rho
P. O. Box 9255, Trenton, New Jersey 08650.
609 586 1351

Union City

Publishers: Documentaries: BDSM

Since May Productions
P. O. Box 351, Union City, New Jersey 07087.
201 864 7837 201 864 7837

Washington Township

Counsellors

Donna Gordon, MA, NCPsyA
63 Horizon Court, Washington Township, New Jersey 07675.
201 652 2957

Wayne

Counsellors

H.E.L.P, Inc.
1065 Alps Road, Wayne, New Jersey 07470-37007.
201 666 7246
201 305 6738

Organizations: Sexuality: Student

Coalition of Lesbians, Gay, & Friends
Student Center, William Patterson College, Wayne, New Jersey 07440.
201 595 3427

Westmount

Counsellors

Walter Dean Hicks, Ph.D., CAS
Suite 608, 216 Haddon Avenue, Westmount, New Jersey 08108-2814.
609 854 3155

Wildwood

BBSs: BDSM

Inferno
609 886 6818

Woodbridge

Organizations: BDSM

Pocono Warriors
P. O. Box 1483, Woodbridge, New Jersey 07095-0970.

Woodcliff Lake

Counsellors

David Panozzo, CSW

NEW MEXICO

Area: Approximately 315,000 square kilometres
Population: Approximately 1,520,000
Capital City: Santa Fe
Time zone: GMT minus 7 hours (Mountain Time)
Climate: Dry, continental weather. Average summer highs are approximately 35°C, winter lows are approximately 2°C.
Age of consent & homosexuality legislation: State has adopted the Model Penal Code or otherwise decriminalized homosexual activities.
Legal drinking age: 21

State Resources

Organizations: AIDS: Education

New Mexico AIDS Services
Suite D, 4200 Silver Avenue South East, Albuquerque, New Mexico 87108.
505 266 0911
Publishes *Volunteer*.

Organizations: AIDS: Support

New Mexico Association of People Living With AIDS (NMPLA)
111 Montclaire South East, Albuquerque, New Mexico 87108.
505 266 0342
10:00 - 17:00
Publishes *HIV in New Mexico*.

New Mexico Association of People Living With AIDS (NMPLA)
1915A Rosina, Santa Fe, New Mexico 87108.
505 982 5995
10:00 - 17:00

Publishers: Newspapers: Sexuality

Mavericks
P. O. Box 9543, Santa Fe, New Mexico 87504.
Newsletter for gay cowboys & their admirers. Published quarterly. Yearly subscription is $25.

Signals
P. O. Box 1713, Santa Fe, New Mexico 87504.

Albuquerque

Accommodation: BDSM

⌖▼ **Dave's B&B on the Rio Grande**
 ⚹ P. O. Box 27214, Albuquerque, New Mexico 87125-7214.
 ☎ 505 247 8312 ✆ 505 842 0733
 ✉ davesbb@Rt66.com
 🌐 http://www.Rt66.com/~DAVESBB
 🕐 07:00 - 23:00
 ⚹ ✓ $ ✈ 🚃 💳 💷
 Casual & private for gays & leatherfolk.. Age statement of 18 is required.

Bars: BDSM

⌖▼ **The Ranch & Cuffs**
 8900 Central Avenue South East, Albuquerque, New Mexico 87123.
 ☎ 505 275 1616
 🕐 Mon - Sat 11:00 - 02:00, Sun 12:00 - 24:00
 ♿

Health Services

☺ ☐ **Saint Joseph Medical Center**
 601 Grand Avenue North East, Albuquerque, New Mexico 87102.
 ☎ 505 848 8000

☺ ☐ **University Hospital**
 2211 Lomas Boulevard North East, Albuquerque, New Mexico 87106.
 ☎ 505 843 2121

☺ ☐ **Veterans' Affairs Medical Center**
 2100 Ridgecrest Drive South East, Albuquerque, New Mexico 87108.
 ☎ 505 265 1711

Helplines: Sexuality

⌖▽ **Common Bond Gay & Lesbian Information Line**
 P. O. Box 26836, Albuquerque, New Mexico 87125.
 ☎ 505 266 8041
 🕐 19:00 - 22:00

Organizations: BDSM

☺ ☐ **A. E. L.**
 P. O. Box 80676, Albuquerque, New Mexico 87198.
 ☎ 505 345 6484

⌖▽ **Hijos del Sol**
 1529 Parsifal North East, Albuquerque, New Mexico 87112.

⌖▽ **Sandia Leathermen**
 8900 Central South East, Albuquerque, New Mexico 87123.

Organizations: Bears

⌖▽ **Bears of Mañana**
 6804 4th. North West, Albuquerque, New Mexico 87107.
 ☎ 505 343 0430

Organizations: Motorcycle

⌖▽ **Motorcyclemen of New Mexico**
 P. O. Box 35844, Albuquerque, New Mexico 87176-5844.
 ☎ 505 247 8312
 Contact: Mr. Dave Bedford, President

Organizations: Sexuality

⌖▽ **Lesbian Support Rap Group**
 ⚹ c/o Full Circle Books, 2205 Silver Avenue South East, Albuquerque, New Mexico 87106.
 ☎ 505 266 0022

⌖▽ **Men's Rap Group**
 ⚹ c/o Common Bond, 4013 Silver Avenue South East, Albuquerque, New Mexico 87106.
 ☎ 505 266 8041
 🕐 Wed 19:00 - 21:00

⌖▽ **The Society for the Second Self (Tri-Ess)—Phi**
 Suite 241, 8200 Montgomery North East, Albuquerque, New Mexico 87109.
 🕐 Meets monthly
 Publishes *Fiesta!*

Organizations: Sexuality: Student

⌖▽ **Gay & Lesbian Student Union**
 ⚹ P. O. Box 100, Room 215, Student Union Building, University of New Mexico, Albuquerque, New Mexico 87131.
 ☎ 505 277 6739

Organizations: Sexuality: Youth

⌖▽ **Out Reach**
 P. O. Box 682, Albuquerque, New Mexico 87103-0682.

 ☎ 505 255 3552

Piercers

☺ ■ **Hardware, Inc.**
 2622 Central South East, Albuquerque, New Mexico 87106.

☺ ■ **Ritual**
 ☎ 505 255 1549

☺ ■ **Rob Scoville**
 ☎ 505 843 7435

☺ ■ **Sachs**
 3112 Central South East, Albuquerque, New Mexico 87106.
 ☎ 505 266 1661

☺ ■ **Sine Qua Non**
 147 Harvard Drive South East, Albuquerque, New Mexico 87106.

Publishers: Magazines: Sexuality

⌕ *Lesbian Ethics*
 P. O. Box 4723, Albuquerque, New Mexico 87196.

☺ ■ *Tantra Magazine*
 P. O. Box 10268, Albuquerque, New Mexico 87184.
 ☎ 505 384 2292
 ✓
 Published quarterly. Yearly subscription is $18. Age statement of 21 is required.

Publishers: Newspapers: Sexuality

⌕ *Common Bond*
 P. O. Box 26836, Albuquerque, New Mexico 87215.

⌕ *Out! Magazine*
 P. O. Box 27237, Albuquerque, New Mexico 87125. ✆ 505 842 5114
 ☎ 505 243 2540
 Published every month. Yearly subscription is $15.

⌕ *Proud Out Loud*
 P. O. Box 25191, Albuquerque, New Mexico 87125.
 ☎ 505 275 9721
 Published quarterly.

Publishers: Newswire Services: Sexuality

⌖▽ **GayNet**
 P. O. Box 25524, Albuquerque, New Mexico 87125-0524.
 ☎ 505 842 5112 ✆ 505 842 5114

Stores: Books: General

⌖▼ **Full Circle Books**
 ⚹ 2205 Silver Avenue South East, Albuquerque, New Mexico 87106.
 ☎ 800 951 0053
 ☎ 505 266 0022
 🕐 Mon - Fri 10:00 - 18:00, Sat Sun - 17:00

☺ ■ **Living Batch Bookstore**
 ⚹ 106 Cornell Drive South East, Albuquerque, New Mexico 87106.
 ☎ 505 262 1619

☺ ■ **Newsland Bookstore**
 ⚹ 2112 Central Avenue South East, Albuquerque, New Mexico 87106.
 ☎ 505 242 0694

⌖▼ **Sisters' & Brothers' Bookstore**
 ⚹ 4011 Silver Avenue South East, Albuquerque, New Mexico 87108-2643.
 ☎ 505 266 7317

Stores: Erotica: BDSM

☺ **The Leather Shoppe**
 4217 Central North East, Albuquerque, New Mexico 87108.
 ☎ 505 266 6690

Stores: Erotica: General

☺ ■ **Harris Newsstand**
 ⚹ 5319 Menaul North East, Albuquerque, New Mexico 87110.
 ☎ 505 880 8696

Clovis

Organizations: Sexuality

⌖▽ **Clovis/Portales Common Bond**
 ⚹ P. O. Box 663, Clovis, New Mexico 88101.
 ☎ 505 356 2656
 🕐 Mon Wed 20:00 - 21:00, answering machine at other times

Las Cruces

Organizations: Sexuality

⌕▽ **Sabra Lesbian Coalition**
 ⚹ c/o P. O. Box 992, Mesilla, New Mexico 88046.
 🕐 Meets twice a month in Las Cruces

Organizations: Sexuality: Student
☿▽ **Gay & Lesbian Student Association**
P. O. Box 4639, New Mexico State University, Las Cruces, New Mexico 88003.

Publishers: Newspapers: Sexuality
♐▽ *Matrix*
P. O. Box 992, Mesilla, New Mexico 88046.
Published every month.

Santa Fe
Health Services
☺☐ **Saint Vincent Hospital**
455 Saint Michael's Drive, Santa Fe, New Mexico 87501.
☎ 505 983 3361

Organizations: AIDS: Education
☺☐ **AIDS Wellness Program & Clinic**
✦ VNS, 811 Saint Michael's Drive, Santa Fe, New Mexico 87501.
☎ 505 983 1822

☿▽ **Gay Men's Health Project**
✦ Suite C, 1223 South Saint Francis Drive, Santa Fe, New Mexico 87501-4033.
☎ 505 984 0911

Organizations: BDSM
☿▽ **Hearts of the West**
P. O. Box 674, Santa Fe, New Mexico 87504-0674.

Stores: Books: General
☺■ **Galisteo News**
✦ 201 Galisteo Street, Santa Fe, New Mexico 87501.
☎ 505 984 1216

Serafina
Publishers: Magazines: Sexuality
♐ *Maize*
P. O. Box 130, Serafina, New Mexico 87569.

Taos
Stores: Erotica: General
☺▼ **Taos Book Shop**
✦ 122D Kit Carson Road, Taos, New Mexico 87571.
☎ 505 758 3733
⏰ 09:00 - 18:00

Tesuque
Counsellors
☺ **Raymond Hillis, Ph.D.**
K P.O. Box 818, Tesuque, New Mexico 87574.
☎ 505 983 3549
✉ ray@nets.com.
Also maintains practices in Santa Fe, New Mexico & Los Angeles, California.

University Park
Organizations: Sexuality
☿▽ **Gay Men's Support Group**
P. O. Box 4639, University Park, New Mexico 88003.

NEW YORK
Area: Approximately 125,000 square kilometres
Population: Approximately 18,.000 ,000
Capital City: Albany
Time zone: GMT minus 5 hours (EST)
Climate: Hot, very humid summers with highs averaging 32°C. Winters are cold with average lows of -3°C. Snow storms can close a city down for a day or two. Coastal areas have weather moderated by the Atlantic ocean.
Age of consent & homosexuality legislation: State has adopted the Model Penal Code or otherwise decriminalized homosexual activities. There is legislation in place against discrimination on the basis of sexual orientation.
Legal drinking age: 21

State Resources
Counsellors
☿▼ **Eileen Walsh, M.S.**
K ✦ 34 Old Route 22, Pawling, New York 12564.
☎ 914 855 5306
♠ ✓ $ ⚊

Organizations: AIDS: Education
☺☐ **AIDS Community Services of Western New York**
✦ 121 West Tupper Street, Buffalo, New York 14201-2142.
☎ 716 847 2441
⏰ 09:00 - 21:00
Publishes *The AIDS Newsletter*.

☺☐ **AIDS Task Force of Central New York**
✦ 627 West Genessee Street, Syracuse, New York 13204.
☎ 315 475 2430

☺▽ **AIDS Treatment Data Network**
✦ 9th. Floor, 259 West 30th. Street, New York 10001-2809.
☎ 212 268 4196 ✆ 212 268 4199
☎ 212 643 0870 (español)
Publishes *Treatment Directory*.

☺☐ **New York State Division of Human Rights**
✦ Office of Discrimination Issues, 12th. Floor, 55 West 125th. Street, New York 10027.
☎ 800 532 2437
☎ 212 870 8624

☺☐ **Southern Tier AIDS Program, Inc.**
✦ 122 Baldwin Street, Johnson City, New York 13790-2148.
☎ 800 333 0892
☎ 607 798 1706
⏰ 09:00 - 17:00

Organizations: BDSM
☺■ **Marci & Friends**
✉ MarciCram@aol.com
Pansexual BDSM group in central New YOrk state.

Organizations: Sexuality
☿▽ **Governor's Office of Lesbian & Gay Concerns**
✦ Executive Chamber, State Capitol, Albany, New York 12224.
☎ 518 486 3168

☿▽ **New York State Division of Human Rights**
✦ Office of Gay & Lesbian Concerns, 55 West 125th. Street, New York 10027.
☎ 212 870 8604

Publishers: Newspapers: Sexuality
♁☐ *Common Ground*
1155 Orchard Park Road, West Seneca, New York 14224.
☎ 716 675 1433

☿▼ *In The Life*
✦ P. O. Box 921, Wappingers Falls, New York 12590.
☎ 914 227 7456 ✆ 914 226 5313
✉ ITLifenews@aol.com
⏰ 09:00 - 17:00
♠ ✓ $ ⚊ ▭ ⬡ ⬛
Newspaper covering news, national, regional, local - columnists, review of music, books, videos, & much more. Published every month. Yearly subscription is \$22U.S.. Age statement of 18 is required.

☿▽ *Sappho's Isle*
960 Willis Avenue, Albertson, New York 11507.
☎ 516 747 5417
Published every month. Yearly subscription is \$20.

Albany
Counsellors
♁■ **Captial District Center for Dissociative Disorders**
P. O. Box 9136, Albany, New York 12209.
☎ 518 462 0213
✉ 71231,3713@compuserve.com

☺▼ **Katherine Eustis Crouch, CSW**
127 North Allen Street, Albany, New York 12203.
☎ 518 456 5845

☺■ **John Crowe, CRC, CAC**
305 Hamilton Street, Albany, New York 12210.
☎ 518 436 1578

☺▼ **Arlene Istar, CSW, CAC**
K ✦ Choices Counselling Associates, 266 Delaware Avenue, Delmar, New York 12054.
☎ 518 439 9270
Transgender welcome.

♁■ **Maureen O'Brien, CSW, ACSW**
P. O. Box 9136, Albany, New York 12209.
☎ 518 462 0213
☎ 518 447 5715

Health Services
☺☐ **Albany Medical Center**
43 New Scotland Avenue, Albany, New York 12208.

518 262 3125
HIV & emergency departments.

Veterans' Affairs Medical Center
113 Holland Avenue, Albany, New York 12208.
518 462 3311

Organizations: AIDS: Education

AIDS Council of Northeastern New York
88 4th. Avenue, Albany, New York 12202-1422.
518 434 4686

Organizations: Motorcycle

STARS MC
P.O. Box 2484, Albany, New York 12220-0484.

Organizations: Sexuality

Capital District Lesbian & Gay Community Center
P. O. Box 131, Albany, New York 12201-0131.
518 462 6138
Mon - Thu 19:00 - 22:00, Fri Sat - 23:00, Sun 14:00 - 22:00
Publishes *Community News.*

Transgenderists' Independence Club (TGIC)
P. O. Box 13604, Albany, New York 12212-3604.
518 436 4513
Call Thu 19:00 - 21:00, voice mail at other times
Publishes a newsletter every two months.

Organizations: Sexuality: Student

Lesbian, Gay, & Bisexual Alliance SUNY Albany (LGBA)
CC116 1400 SUNY, Albany, New York 12222.
518 442 5672
Meets Tue 20:30

Lesbian, Gay, & Bisexual Caucus
SASU, 300 Lark Street, Albany, New York 12210.
518 465 2406

Rensselaer Gay, Lesbian, & Bisexual Alliance
P. O. Box 146, Troy, New York 12181-0146.
518 271 2655 518 276 6920
Publishes *People First.*

Organizations: Sexuality: Youth

Lesbian & Gay Youth Group
P. O. Box 131, Albany, New York 12201.
518 462 6138

Publishers: Magazines: AIDS

Art & Understanding
Suite 205, 25 Monroe Street, Albany, New York 12210-2743.
518 426 9010 518 436 5354

Publishers: Newspapers: Sexuality

Community
P. O. Box 131, Albany, New York 12201.
The Capital District's only lesbian & gay news journal, publised by the Capital District Gay & Lesbian Community. Published every month. Yearly subscription is free.

Women Centered News
P. O. Box 3057, Albany, New York 12203.

Stores: Books: General

Lifestyle Books
37 Central Avenue, Albany, New York 12210.
518 433 1290
10:00 - 22:00

Stores: Erotica: General

Adult Education Books
1115 State Street, Schenactady, New York 12308.

Another World
145 Erie Boulevard, Schenactady, New York 12308.

Continental Books
1455 State Street, Schenactady, New York 12308.

Savage Gifts & Leather
88 Central Avenue, Albany, New York 12208.
518 434 2324

Amityville

Publishers: Magazines: BDSM

Capitulation
Fantastic Books Publications, P. O. Box 34, Amityville, New York 11701-0034.
516 753 2677 516 753 2423
Also publish other titles in the femdom area.

Publishers: Magazines: Fetish

Leg Tease
Rem-mer Ltd., P. O. Box 34, Amityville, New York 11701-0034.
516 753 2677 516 753 2423
Published every month. Yearly subscription is $75.

Annandale on Hudson

Organizations: Sexuality

Sexual Minorities Alligned for Community, Education, & Support (SM Aces)
Bard College, Annandale on Hudson, New York 12504.
LiamTu@aol.com
Contact: Mr. Liam Tumulty
University group focussed on maintaining a community of people interested in deviant sexuality, & educating the wider community about these practices.

Organizations: Sexuality: Student

Bard Bisexual, Lesbian, & Gay Alliance
Bard College, Annandale on Hudson, New York 12504.
914 758 6822

Babylon

Publishers: Newspapers: Sexuality

Parlee Plus/ Equal Time the News
P. O. Box 430, Babylon, New York 11702.
516 587 8669
Published every month.

Bay Shore

Bars: BDSM

Long Island Eagle
94 North Clinton, Bay Shore, New York 11706.
516 968 2750

Health Services

Southside Hospital
301 East Main Street, Bay Shore, New York 11706.
516 968 3000

Manufacturers: Piercing Jewelry

Body Designs
Suite 1014, 1319 Elayne Avenue, Bay Shore, New York 11706.
516 968 0141
516 968 8847 (catalogue & mail order)
Makes surgical steel, Niobium, & gold Jewelry. Retail & wholesale available. Catalogue available.

Organizations: BDSM

Long Island Ravens
c/o Long Island Eagle, 94 North Clinton, Bay Shore, New York 11706.
516 666 6091

Piercers

Body Designs
1746 Sunrise Highway, Bay Shore, New York 11706.
516 968 0141
Catalogue available.

School of Professional Body Piercing
1746 Sunrise Highway, Bay Shore, New York 11706.
516 968 0141
Catalogue available.

Bayside

Publishers: Magazines: Penis Size

Small Gazette
Small Etc., P. O. Box 610294, Bayside, New York 11361-0294.
Published quarterly. Yearly subscription is $30.

Binghamton

Archives: Sexuality

Latina Lesbian History Project
P. O. Box 678, Binghamton, New York 13905-0678.

Health Services

Binghamton General Hospital
20-42 Mitchell Avenue, Binghamton, New York 13903.

☎ 607 762 2200

Organizations: Sexuality: Student

♂▽ **Lesbian, Gay, & Bisexual Union SUNY (LGBU)—**
& **Binghamton**
c/o Box 2000, Binghamton, New York 13901.
☎ 607 777 2202
Publishes a newsletter.

Publishers: Newspapers: Sexuality

♂▽ *Amethyst*
SYOL Ltd., P. O. Box 728, Binghamton, New York 13905.
☎ 607 723 5790
To inform & educate about gay activities & issues - try to be a lesbian,
gay & bi-inclusive. Published every two months. Yearly subscription is
$10 donation.

⚥ *Hera*
The Women's Community Center, P. O. Box 354, Binghamton, New
York 13902.
☎ 607 724 3462
News, reviews, & analysis for feminists & lesbians in Binghampton &
ventral New york. Carries lesbian & gay news. Published 10 times a
year. Yearly subscription is $10.

Stores: Erotica: General

☺■ **Allies Boulevard Bookstore Downtown**
P. O. Box 452, Binghamton, New York 13902.
☎ 607 724 8659

☺■ **Allies Boulevard Bookstore East**
& 483 Court Street, Binghamton, New York 13904.
☎ 607 724 9749

☺■ **North Street Bookshop**
17 Washington Avenue, Endicott, New York 13760.
☎ 607 785 9606

Brentwood

Stores: Erotica: General

♂▼ **Heaven Sent Me**
& 108 Cain Drive, Brentwood, New York 11717.
☎ 516 434 4777 ✆ 516 435 0808
⏰ 24hrs.

Bronx

Bars: BDSM

♂▼ **Cellblock 28**
⚷ #ST1, 3021 Briggs Avenue, Bronx, New York 10458.
☎ 718 733 3144 ✆ 718 733 3115 (call first)
☎ 718 367 7484
⏰ Mon - Wed 20:00 - 02:30, Sun 16:00 - 24:00
A leathermen's BDSM & JO safe sex club. Monthly parties put on by
local BDSM clubs & others. Age statement of 21 is required.

Health Services

☺□ **Bronx Lebanon Hospital Center**
1276 Fulton Avenue, Bronx, New York 10456.
☎ 718 590 1800
HIV & emergency departments.

☺□ **Bronx Municipal Hospital Center**
Pelham Parkway & Eastchester, Bronx, New York 10461.
☎ 718 918 8141
HIV & emergency departments.

☺□ **Lincoln Medical & Mental Health Center**
234 East 149th. Street, Bronx, New York 10451.
☎ 718 579 5700

☺□ **Montefiore Medical Center**
111 East 210th. Street, Bronx, New York 10467.
☎ 718 920 4321
HIV & emergency departments.

☺□ **North Central Bronx Hospital**
3424 Kossuth Avenue, Bronx, New York 10467.
☎ 718 519 3500

☺□ **Veterans' Affairs Medical Center**
130 West Kingsbridge Road, Bronx, New York 10468.
☎ 718 584 9000

Organizations: Sexuality

♀▽ **The Society for the Second Self (Tri-Ess)—Chi**
Delta Mu
P. O. Box 477, Co-op Station, Bronx, New York 10475.
☎ 201 663 0772
⏰ Meets 2nd. Sat of month

Publishers: Directories: Books

☺ *The Cumulative Book Index*
H. W. Wilson Company, 950 University Avenue, Bronx, New York
10452.
☎ 212 588 8400

Publishers: Newspapers: BDSM

⚥■ *Whips*
Thor Publications, P. O. Box 950, Parkchester Station, Bronx, New York
10462.
Age statement of 21 is required.

Stores: Clothing: Uniforms

☺■ **F & J Police Equipment, Inc.**
378 East 161st. Street, Bronx, New York.
☎ 718 665 4535

Brooklyn

BBSs: Sexuality

♂▼ **Backroom**
TOSS, Inc., Suite 2517, 1412 Avenue M, Brooklyn, New York 11230.
☎ 718 951 8998
✆ 718 951 8256
Gay & lesbian community BBS with leather areas.

Counsellors

☺ **Michael Bernet**
Κ ☎ 718 284 4162
Manhattan & Brooklyn, New York locations.

☺■ **Shelley Juran, Ph.D.**
☎ 718 625 6526

Distributors: Erotica: General

☺ **Xclusiv Distributors, Inc.**
451 50th. Street, Brooklyn, New York 11220.
☎ 718 439 1271 ✆ 718 439 1272

Health Services

☺□ **Brookdale Hospital Medical Center**
Linden Boulevard at Brookdale Plaza, Brooklyn, New York 10456.
☎ 718 240 5000
HIV & emergency departments.

☺□ **Brooklyn Hospital Center**
121 De Kalb Avenue, Brooklyn, New York 11201.
☎ 718 250 8005
HIV & emergency departments.

☺□ **Kings County Hospital Center**
451 Clarkson Avenue, Brooklyn, New York 11203.
☎ 718 245 3131

☺□ **Veterans' Affairs Medical Center**
800 Poly Place, Brooklyn, New York 11209.
☎ 718 630 3500

Organizations: AIDS: Education

☺□ **Brooklyn AIDS Task Force**
CSP, 465 Dean Street, Brooklyn, New York 11217.
☎ 718 783 0883

⚥ **Women & AIDS Resource Network**
Suite 212, 30 3rd. Avenue, Brooklyn, New York 11217.
☎ 718 596 6007 ✆ 718 596 6041

Organizations: BDSM

☺■ **New York Metro D&S Singles**
#2J, 3395 Nostrand Avenue, Brooklyn, New York 11229.
☎ 718 648 8215
⏰ Meets 3rd. Fri of month. 24hr. answering machine
Contact: Ms. G. Artemis
Send SASE or IRC for reply. Publishes a newsletter quarterly. Age
statement of 21 is required.

Organizations: Sexuality

♂▽ **Gay & Lesbian Alliance at Brooklyn College**
& Brooklyn College Student Activities, James Hall, Brooklyn, New York
11210-2889.
☎ 718 951 4234

▷□ **Girls Night Out**
P. O. Box 350369, Brooklyn, New York 112350007.
☎ 201 794 1665 Ext.: 2021
Contact: Ms. Barbara Fortune
Publishes *Lipstick & Lace*.

♀▽ **Shades of Lavendar**
295 9th. Street, Brooklyn, New York 11215.
☎ 718 499 0352

Publishes *Lavendar Notes.*

Organizations: Sexuality: Student

⚥▽ **Gay, Lesbian, & Bisexual Alliance**
OSA, Pratt Hall, Pratt Institute, Brooklyn, New York 11205.
☎ 718 636 3790

⚥▽ **Gay, Lesbian, & Bisexual Alliance of Kingsborough**
2001 Oriental Boulevard, Brooklyn, New York 11235.
☎ 718 368 5400

Organizations: Sexuality: Youth

♀♀▽ **Brooklyn Lesbian Youth Sisters**
c/o Shades of Lavendar, 295 9th. Street, Brooklyn, New York 11215.
☎ 718 499 0352

Photographers: Erotic

☺ **Efrain Gonzales**
392 First Street, Brooklyn, New York 11215.

Stores: Books: General

☺■ **Community Bookshop**
143 7th. Avenue, Brooklyn, New York 11215.
☎ 718 783 3075

Stores: Erotica: BDSM

☺■ **S. A. M. Co.**
Box 514, 9728 3rd. Avenue, Brooklyn, New York 11029.
☎ 718 748 7593
🕐 By appointment only
Custom work & dungeon also available. Catalogue available.

Stores: Leatherwork Supplies: General

☺■ **Veterans Leather**
204 25th. Street, Brooklyn, New York 11232-9970.
☎ 718 768 0300

Buffalo

BBSs: BDSM

☺■ **Multicom4**
☎ 716 442 1669
✆ 716 733 1111. 14400 baud maximum.
Age statement of 21 is required.

Counsellors

⚥▼ **Greg Bodekor, MS, CAC**
☎ 716 884 8670

Health Services

☺☐ **Buffalo General Hospital**
100 High Street, Buffalo, New York 14203.
☎ 716 845 5600

☺☐ **Erie County Medical Center**
463 Grider Street, Buffalo, New York 14215.
☎ 716 898 3000

☺☐ **Sheenan Memorial Hospital**
425 Michigan Avenue, Buffalo, New York 14203.
☎ 716 848 2000

Organizations: AIDS: Education

☺☐ **AIDS Alliance of Western New York**
367 Delaware Avenue, Buffalo, New York 14202.
☎ 716 852 6778

Organizations: BDSM

⚥▽ **Buffalo Fetish & Leather Organization (BFLO)**
P. O. Box 3, Niagara Station, Buffalo, New York 14201-0003.

Organizations: Family

☺☐ **Parents & Friends of Lesbians & Gays (PFLAG)—Western New York**
P. O. Box 861, Buffalo, New York 14225.
☎ 716 883 0384

Organizations: Sexuality

▽ **Buffalo Transition Support**
P. O. Box 320, Buffalo, New York 14220.
☎ 716 629 5421
🕐 Meets 4th. Sat of month 16:00 -18:00
Contact: Vicki

▽ **Crossroads of Buffalo**
Suite 102, 2316 Delaware Avenue, Buffalo, New York 14216.

⚥▽ **Gay Positive Buffalo**
P. O. Box 287, Station C, Buffalo, New York 14209.
☎ 716 884 8670

Organizations: Sexuality: Student

⚥▽ **Graduate Gay & Lesbian Alliance**
♿ 362 Student Union, SUNY-Buffalo, Amherst, New York 14260.
☎ 716 645 3063

⚥▽ **Lesbian, Gay, & Bisexual Alliance**
Buffalo State College, 130 Elmwood Avenue, Cassety, New York 14222-1095.
☎ 716 645 3063 ✆ 716 645 2112

Organizations: Sexuality: Youth

⚥▽ **Gay & Lesbian Youth Services**
♿ 190 Franklin Street, Buffalo, New York 14202.
☎ 716 855 0221
🕐 24hr. hotline Mon Wed, Fri 18:00 - 21:00, Sat 13:00 - 17:00

Publishers: Guides: Sexuality

⚥▼ *Western New York Sentinel*
P. O. Box 2136, Buffalo, New York 14240-2136.
☎ 716 894 6657
Premiere bar guide for the gay & lesbian community of western New York. Published every month. Yearly subscription is $14.

Publishers: Magazines: Sexuality

⚥▼ *Pride Path Magazine*
Suite 117, 266 Elmwood Avenue, Buffalo, New York 14222.
☎ 716 876 3881

Publishers: Newspapers: Sexuality

⚥ *Alternate Expressions*
P. O. Box 446, Buffalo, New York 14205-0446.

⚥ *Volumé*
P. O. Box 106, Buffalo, New York 14213.

⚥▼ *Outwords*
P. O. Box 443, Buffalo, New York 14209.
☎ 716 883 4814

Stores: Books: General

☺▼ **Four Corner News**
1079 Hertel Avenue, Buffalo, New York 14216.
☎ 716 877 4344

☺■ **Talking Leaves... Books**
♿ 3158 Main Street, Buffalo, New York 14214.
☎ 716 837 8554 ✆ 716 837 3861
🕐 Mon - Sat 10:00 - 18:00, Wed Thu - 20:00
💰 ✓ 💳 💳 💳

☺■ **Village Green Bookstore**
3670 McKinley Parkway, Blasdell, New York 14219-2658.
☎ 716 827 5895

☺■ **Village Green Bookstore**
♿ 765A Elmwood Avenue, Buffalo, New York 14222-1600.
☎ 716 884 1200 ✆ 716 884 3007

Stores: Erotica: General

☺■ **Book-And**
83 West Chippewa, Buffalo, New York 14202.
☎ 716 856 8936

☺■ **Village Book & News**
♿ 3102 Delaware Avenue, Kenmore, New York 14217.
☎ 716 887 5027

Centereach

Organizations: Sexuality

▽ **New York Girl & Partner**
P. O. Box 456, Centereach, New York 11720.

Chatham

Accommodation: BDSM

☺ **The Country House**
P. O. Box 200, Chatham, New York 12037-0200.
☎ 518 392 6209

Coram

Organizations: Fetish: Foot

☺☐ **Lotus Foot Love Club**
Drawer G, Coram, New York 11727.

Cortland

Stores: Books: General

☺■ **Basil's Bookstore**
12 1/2 Main Street, Cortland, New York 13045.

☎ 607 756 9409

Deer Park
Stores: Erotica: General
☺ ■ **Cupid's Video Boutique**
786 Grand Boulevard, Deer Park, New York 11729.
☎ 516 586 0066　　　　　　　　✆ 516 586 0092

East Hampton
Public Speakers: Sexuality
☺ ■ **Annie Sprinkle**
P. O. Box 2650, East Hampton, New York 11937.
☎ 516 329 9020　　　　　　　　✆ 516 329 3720
☎ 212 265 3796
⏱ Mon - Fri 10:00 - 18:00

East Meadow
Piercers
☺ ■ **Long Island Connection**
2087 Hempstead Turnpike, East Meadow, New York 11554.

East Setauket
Publishers: Magazines: Spanking
⚥ ■ *Men Under Control*
CF Publications, Box 706, East Setauket, New York 11733.
☎ 516 689 6743　　　　　　　　✆ 516 689 6755
For dominant women & the men they spank. Published every two months. Yearly subscription is $60.

Elmhurst
Health Services
☺ □ **Elmhurst Hospital Center**
☎ 718 334 4000

Elmira
Stores: Erotica: General
☺ ■ **Deluxe Book Bargains**
123 Lake Street, Elmira, New York 14901.
☎ 607 734 9656

Fairport
Stores: Books: General
☺ ■ **Village Green Bookstore**
587 Moseley Road, Fairport, New York 14450-3347.
☎ 716 425 7950　　　　　　　　✆ 716 425 4968

Far Rockaway
Health Services
☺ □ **Saint John's Episcopal Hospital - South Shore**
327 Beach 19th. Street, Far Rockaway, New York 11691.
☎ 718 868 7000

Fayetteville
Counsellors
☺ ■ **Alison Deming**
♿ 208 Redfield Avenue, Fayetteville, New York 13066.
☎ 315 637 8990

Forest Hills
Publishers: Magazines: Sexuality
⚤ *On The Issues*
Choices Women's Medical Center, Inc., 97-99 Queens Boulevard, Forest Hills, New York 11374.
☎ 718 275 6020　　　　　　　　✆ 718 997 1206
🖂 onissues@echonyc.com
🖧 http://www.echonyc.com/~onissues

Fredonia
Organizations: Sexuality: Student
⚢▽ **Gay, Lesbian, & Bisexual Union (GLBSU)**
SUC Fredonia, Campus Center, Fredonia, New York 14063.

Great Neck
Suppliers: Diapers
☺ ■ **First Quality Products, Inc.**
Suite 302, 40 Cotter Mill Road, Great Neck, New York 11021.
☎ 516 829 3030
Disposable diapers & waterproof pants.

Hampstead
Stores: Medical Equipment
☺ ■ **Alfa Medical**
59 Madison Avenue, Hampstead, New York 11550.
☎ 800 762 1586　　　　　　　　✆ 516 773 4339
Used autoclaves & sterilizers bought, repaired, sold. Also new equipment. Not part of the scene, so be discreet.

Huntington Station
Publishers: Miscellaneous
⚥▼ **Rising Tide Press**
5 Kivy Street, Huntington Station, New York 11746.
☎ 516 427 1289
⏱ 09:00 - 20:00

Island Park
Suppliers: Diapers
☺ ■ **Woodbury Products, Inc.**
4410 Austin Boulevard, Island Park, New York 11558.
☎ 516 431 4242
☎ 800 879-3427
Various types of disposables diapers. Free samples available.

Ithaca
Organizations: Sexuality
⚢▽ **Ithaca Gay & Lesbian Activities Board (IGLAB)**
P. O. Box 6634, Ithaca, New York 14851.
⚢▽ **Ithaca Lesbian, Gay, & Bisexual Task Force**
♿ P. O. Box 3951, Ithaca, New York 14852-3951.
☎ 607 347 4605
🖂 jsp1@cornell.edu
Contact: Mr. Jeff Popow
News, features, opinion pieces, regular columns, & more. Emphasizes local, regional, & state stories. Publishes *Outlines* quarterly.

Organizations: Sexuality: Student
⚢▽ **Cornell Lesbian, Gay, & Bisexual Alliance**
P. O. Box 45, 207 Willard Stright Hall, Ithaca, New York 14852.
☎ 607 255 6482

Stores: Books: General
☺ ■ **Book Sale Gallery**
103 West State Street, Ithaca, New York 14850.
☎ 607 272 9882
☺ ▼ **Borealis Bookstore**
♿ 113 North Aurora Street, Ithaca, New York 14850-4301.
☎ 607 272 7752
⚤ ■ **Smedley's Bookshop**
307 West State Street, Ithaca, New York 14850.
☎ 607 273 2325
⏱ Tue - Fri 10:00 - 18:00, Sat 10:00 - 17:00

Kingston
Stores: Books: General
☺ ■ **Author Author**
89 Broadway Roundout, Kingston, New York 12401.
☎ 914 339 1883
☎ 914 339 1889

Mattydale
Stores: Erotica: General
☺ **Salt City Book & Video**
♿ 2807 Brewerton Road, Mattydale, New York 13211.
☎ 315 454 0629
⏱ 24hrs.
💰 ✂ 💳 💳
Age statement of 18 is required.

Nassau
BBSs: BDSM
☺ ■ **Long Island Connection**
✆ 516 794 5959

New Paltz
Organizations: Sexuality: Student
⚢▽ **Bisexual, Gay, & Lesbian Alliance at New Paltz (BiGAYLA)**
♿ Room 332, Student Union Building, New Paltz, New York 12561.
☎ 914 257 3097

☎ 914 257 5081

New York
Archives: Sexuality
ⓒ▽ **The Lesbian Herstory Webweaving Collective**
P. O. Box 1258, New York 10116.
☎ 718 768 3953
✉ kgs@intac.com
🌐 http://www.intac.com/~kgs/lha/index.html
Publishes *Lesbian Herstory Archives News*.

Artists: BDSM
☺ **Mercy**
P. O. Box 1028, New York 10028.
Private commissions. Send SASE with enquiry.
☺ **Ira Smith**
P. O. Box 1085, New York 10276.
☎ 212 260 6396 ✆ 917 969 7340
🕐 By appointment only
♣ ✓ $ ✈
Catalogue available. Age statement of 21 is required.

Bars: BDSM
♂▼ **Boots & Saddle**
♿ 76 Christopher Street, New York 10014.
☎ 212 929 9684
🕐 08:00 - 04:00, Sun 12:00 - 04:00
♂▼ **Candle Bar**
309 Amsterdam Avenue, New York 10023.
☎ 212 874 9155
🕐 14:00 - 04:00
♂▼ **Eagle's Nest**
♿ 142 11th. Avenue, New York 10011.
☎ 212 691 8451
🕐 22:00 - 04:00
♂▼ **The L. U. R. E.**
409 West 13th. Street, New York.
☎ 212 741 3919
🕐 Mon - Fri 20:00 - 04:00, Sat Sun 17:00 - 04:00. Some women Wed & Sat. Leather, Uniform, Rubber, Etc. dress code on weekends. The Noose leather store open Wed eve & WE eve
☺■ **Maze**
Upstairs, 28 10th. Avenue, New York.
🕐 Thu - Sat
☺■ **Paddles**
540 West 21st. Street, New York.
☎ 212 463 8599
♂▼ **Rawhide**
212 8th. Avenue, New York 10011.
☎ 212 242 9332
♂▼ **The Spike**
120 11th. Avenue, New York 10011.
☎ 212 243 9688
🕐 15:00 - 04:00, Sun brunch 13:00 - 17:00
♂♀■ **The Vault**
28 10th. Avenue, New York.
☎ 212 255 6758
🕐 Thu - Sat
Sex club equipped with BDSM equipment.

Bars: Sexuality
♀▼ **Club Edelweiss**
580 11th. Avenue, New York 10036.
☎ 212 629 1021
♀▼ **Sally's II**
The Carter Hotel, 252 West 43rd. Street, New York 10036.
☎ 212 944 6000 Ext.: 212

BBSs: BDSM
☺■ **Cyberoticomm**
✆ 212 233 4328
☺■ **Moon Dog**
✆ 718 692 2498
♂▼ **The Nightstick**
✆ 718 898 9195
System password: S&M.
☺■ **The Wall**
✆ 718 278 2120

BBSs: General
☺■ **Erotic Visions**
P. O. Box 203, New York 11013.

✆ 212 296 8151

BBSs: Sexuality
♂▼ **The Malestop**
✆ 212 721 4180
Mainly chat. Has leather area.

Counsellors
♂▽ **Robert Allmen, MS, M.Div.**
P. O. Box 436, Central Islip, New York 11722.
☎ 516 723 0348
☺■ **Carolyn Asnien, MA**
☎ 212 749 4171
☺▼ **John Aspinall, CSW**
♿ 18 Karen Court, Oyster Bay, New York 11771.
☎ 516 922 6155
♂▼ **Hedda Begelman, MSW, RCSW**
☎ 516 795 1320
☺▽ **Bisexual Information & Counseling Service**
♿ Suite 1-A, 599 West End Avenue, New York 10024.
☎ 212 874 7937
☺▼ **Ralph Blair**
Suite 1G, 311 East 72nd. Street, New York 10021.
☎ 212 517 3171
☺▼ **Daniel Bloom, JD, CSW**
35 West 9th. Street, New York 11011.
☎ 212 674 0404
☺▼ **Sue Blume, CSW**
☎ 516 379 4731
♂▼ **Mildred Borras, Ph.D.**
♿ 18 East 93rd. Street, New York 10128.
☎ 212 505 8371
☺■ **Mildred Byrum, Ph.D.**
26 West 9th. Street, New York 10011.
☎ 212 674 1091
☺▼ **Joseph Canarelli, CSW**
Suite 313, 222 East 5th. Street, New York 10003.
☎ 212 529 8940
☺■ **Julie Capone, CSW**
6 Meadow Ridge, Woodbury, New York 11797.
☎ 516 367 1016
☺■ **Thomas Capone, Ph.D.**
6 Meadow Ridge, Woodbury, New York 11797.
☎ 516 367 1016
♂▼ **Stephen Capson, Psy.D.**
412 6th. Avenue, New York 10011.
☎ 212 769 8299
☺▽ **Center for Non-Traditional Families**
♿ 111 West 90th. Street, New York 10024.
☎ 212 721 1012
♂▼ **Chelsea Psychotherapy Associates**
♿ Suite 1305, 80 8th. Avenue, New York 10011.
☎ 212 206 0045
♂▼ **Judith Clarke, MSW, ACSW, BCD**
☎ 212 254 7256
☺▼ **Clare Cross, CSW**
♿ ☎ 212 662 4609
♂▼ **Jane D'Amico, MSW, CSW, CAC**
Suite C, 333 Main Street, Roslyn, New York 11576.
☎ 516 621 3033
♂▼ **Robert Driscoll, CSW**
8 Stuyvesant Oval, New York 10009.
☎ 212 228 2745
☺▼ **Carl Eden, CSW**
Suite 5W, 80 Charles Street, New York 10014.
☎ 212 929 7178
☺■ **Edith Eisenberg, ACSW**
Suite 110, 21 73rd. Road, Forest Hills, New York 11375.
☎ 718 263 0779
♂■ **Elaine Felshin, Ph.D.**
☎ 212 533 4092
☺■ **Robert Fontanella, CSW**
Room 807, 80 5th. Avenue, New York 10011-8002.
☎ 212 741 2739
♂▼ **Susan Frankel, CSW, BCD**
♿ Suite PHA, 710 West End Avenue, New York 10025-6808.
☎ 212 877 5114
☺■ **Susan Gair, MSW, CSW**

315 Central Park West, New York 10024.
☎ 212 799 5436

⚥ ▼ **Gay Counseling Center of Long Island**
P. O. Box 1133, Massapequa, New York 11758.
☎ 516 795 0151

⚥ ▼ **Gay Men's Psychotherapy Referral Service**
☎ 212 388 2738

⚥ ▼ **Gay Psychological Services**
♿ 412 Avenue of the Americas, New York 10011.
☎ 212 265 1974

⚥ ▼ **Paul Giogianni, CSW**
♿ 165 East 32nd. street, New York 10016.
☎ 212 532 2599

☺ ■ **Jonathan Goldberg, Ph.D.**
♿ Suite 1A, 342 West 85th. Street, New York 10024.
☎ 212 496 0535

⚥ ▼ **Gotham Psychotherapy Associates**
♿ ☎ 212 903 4033

☺ ▼ **Robert Grabowski, CSW, ACSW**
Suite 109, 23 71st Road, Queens, New York.
☎ 718 261 1346

☺ ■ **Sally Graham, Ph.D.**
Suite 601, 24 East 12th. Street, New York 10003.
☎ 212 807 0543
☎ 212 803 5412

⚥ ▼ **David Lindsey Griffin, CSW, CAC**
935 8th. Avenue, New York 10019.
☎ 212 582 1881

☺ ▼ **Scott Hatley, MS, CSW**
♿ Suite 916, 200 Park Avenue South, New York 10003.
☎ 212 674 4706

⚥ ▼ **Richard Horwitz, CSW, CAC**
♿ Suite 15N, 175 West 12th. Street, New York 10011.
☎ 212 780 9400

⚥ ▽ **Institute for Human Identity**
First Floor, 118 West 72nd. Street, New York 10023.
☎ 212 799 9432

☺ ▼ **Robert Isaacs, CSW**
♿ Suite 4, 115 Washington Place, New York 10014.
☎ 212 229 0090

☺ ▼ **Kent Jarratt, ACSW**
Suite 1D, 26 West 9th. Street, New York 10011.
☎ 212 674 7370

⚥ ▼ **Linda Jones, CSW, ACSW**
♿ Suite 1003, 80 East 11th. Street, New York 10003.
☎ 212 982 9232
☎ 201 858 4743

☺ ■ **Lee Kassan, MA**
♿ Suite 12H, 56 7th. Avenue, New York 10011.
☎ 212 989 3613

⚥ ▼ **Bruce Kerner, Psy.D.**
Suite 315, 230 Park Avenue, New York 10169.
☎ 212 682 1288

☺ ▼ **Mark Koppel, Ph.D.**
172 West 79th. Street, New York 10024.
☎ 212 362 7027
☎ 914 277 7809

☺ ▼ **Patricia Landry, CSW, BCD**
271 Merrick Avenue, East Meadow, New York 11554-1549.
☎ 516 794 2626

☺ ■ **Brian Lathrop, NCPsy.A.**
♿ Suite 4A, 63 Downing Street, New York 10014.
☎ 212 727 9797
🕐 By appointment

⚥ ▼ **Kathryn Lesko, Ph.D.**
Suite 6B, 60 West 10th. Street, New York 10011.
☎ 212 598 4090

⚥ ▼ **Joyce Liechenstein, Ph.D.**
♿ Suite 7H, 444 East 20th. Street, New York 10009.
☎ 212 673 4427

☺ ■ **Susan Lippman, CSW**
☎ 718 639 5969

☺ ▼ **Manhattan Psychotherapy**
Suite 1103, 20 West 72nd. Street, New York 10023.
☎ 212 724 8767

☺ ■ **Rick Marschall, CSW, CAC**
161 West 16th. Street, New York 10011.
☎ 212 620 7155

☺ ▼ **Maureen McGovern, MSW**
247 West 15th. Street, New York 10011.
☎ 212 929 1498

■ **Metamorphosis**
♿ P. O. Box 6260, Broadway Station, Long Island City, New York 11106-0260.
☎ 718 728 4615
🕐 By appointment. Call Mon - Fri 11:00 - 17:00
Professional psychotherapy & evaluation.

☺ **Wynn Miller, MSW, CSW**
K ☎ 212 989 4641
Serving the leather / BDSM community, short term counselling, & crisis intervention.

☺ ▼ **Kenneth Noone, CSW, CAC**
☎ 718 820 39700

⚥ ▼ **Gerrie Nussdorf, Ph.D.**
☎ 212 691 1818

⚥ ▼ **Ken Page, CSW**
♿ Suite 1717, 853 Broadway, New York 10003.
☎ 212 420 0394

⚥ ▼ **Michael Pantaleo, CSW, CAC**
Suite 3C, 222 West 14th. Street, New York 10011.
☎ 212 691 2312

⚥ ▼ **Passages Counseling Center**
♿ 3680 Route 112, Coram, New York 11727-4133.
☎ 516 698 9222

⚥ ▼ **Vincent-John Patti, ACSW**
K ♿ Suite 3, 226 East 13th. Street, New York 10003-5623.
☎ 212 473 3623
🕐 Mon Wed Thu10:00 - 23:00
Private practice specializing in sexual & gender identity issues, non-traditional families, AIDS, & the BDSM community. Age statement of 18 is required.

☺ ■ **Michael Quadland, Ph.D.**
Suite 1P, 10 Downing Street, New York 10014-4737.
☎ 212 691 1617

⚥ ▼ **Jerry Raphael, Ph.D.**
☎ 212 982 6135

⚥ ▼ **Lynne Roberts, CSW, ACSW**
♿ ☎ 212 749 1596

☺ ▼ **Nino Romano, CSW, MSW**
♿ Suite 503, 24 East 12th. Street, New York 10003.
☎ 212 242 2896

⚢ ▼ **Lydia Rosa, ACSW**
922 Harmon Drive, Larchmont, New York 10538-1800.
☎ 914 834 2128

☺ ▼ **Jerome Ruderman, JD, MS**
♿ Suite 25A, 140 West End Avenue, New York 10023.
☎ 212 877 7344

☺ ▼ **Linda Saegert**
☎ 516 825 2289

⚥ ▼ **Robert Scherma, Psy.D.**
Suite 500, 412 Avenue of the Americas, New York 10011.
☎ 212 969 0988

⚥ ▼ **Michael Schernoff, CSW, ACSW**
♿ Suite 1305, 80 8th. Avenue, New York 10011.
☎ 212 675 9563

☺ ▼ **Jay Schlesinger, Ph.D.**
13 North Dorado Circle, Haupauge, New York 11788.
☎ 516 582 2188

☺ ■ **Beverly Schmidt, RCSW**
♿ Suite 3M, 145 4th. Avenue, New York 10003.
☎ 516 329 0474

▼ **C. Schooler**
425 West 23rd. Street, New York 10011.
☎ 212 243 1224
Services include pre-operative treatment for transgender clients.

☺ ▼ **Conrad Sernier, ACSW, CSW**
♿ 301 East 22nd. Street, New York 10010.
☎ 212 260 2590

⚥ ▼ **Nanette Shaw, Ph.D.**
♿ ☎ 212 505 7869
☎ 516 725 5945

⚥ ▼ **Charles Silverstein, Ph.D.**
233 West 83rd. Street, New York 10024.
☎ 212 799 8574

⚥ ▼ **Gregory Verhey, MSW, CSW**

1346 Victory Boulevard, Staten Island, New York 10301.
☎ 212 447 3473

☺ ■ **Kenneth Weene, Ph.D.**
114 Kathleen Drive, Syosset, New York 11791-5816.
☎ 516 496 8023
⚲ ✓ $ ⚭
Individual, group, family, & relationship therapy.

♂⚥▼ **Mark Williams, Ph.D.**
♿ Suite 916, 200 Park Avenue South, New York 10003.
☎ 212 254 0529

♂⚥▼ **Mark Wind, MA, CAC, NCAC II**
Suite 609, 10 West 15th. Street, New York 10011-6821.
☎ 212 929 4390

☺▼ **Joy Witchel, CSW, CAC**
☎ 212 477 8258

⚲■ **Miriam Yelsky, Ph.D.**
♿ 350 West 24th. Street, New York 10011.
☎ 212 243 0261

☺ ■ **Irene Zelterman, CSW**
☎ 718 832 3739
⏱ Eve, some WE

Distributors: Erotica: General

♂⚥▼ **Executive Imports International**
Suite 1102, 210 Fifth Avenue, New York 10010.
Distributor of femdom glossies, paperbacks, & videos. Also some maledom, TV, & fetish-fashion.

Distributors: Videos: Erotic

☺ **First Run Features**
153 Waberly Place, New York 10014.
☎ 212 243 0600

☺ **Noble Distributors**
Suite 180, 245 8th. Avenue, New York 10011.
☎ 800 662 5372
Also does 4-colour printing.

Film Festivals: Sexuality

♂⚥ **Lesbian/Gay Film Festival**
Suite 510, 462 Broadway, New York 10013-2618.
☎ 212 966 5656
Publishes *Positive Projections*.

Health Services

☺ ☐ **Bayley Seton Hospital**
75 Vanderbilt Avenue, Staten Island, New York 10304.
☎ 718 390 6000

☺ ☐ **Bellevue Hospital Center**
First Avenue & 27th. Street, New York 10016.
☎ 212 561 4141
HIV & emergency departments.

☺ ☐ **Beth Israel Medical Center**
First Avenue & 16th. Street, New York 10128.
☎ 212 420 2000
HIV & emergency departments.

☺ ☐ **Coler Memorial Hospital**
Franklin D. Roosevelt Island, New York 10044.
☎ 212 848 6000
HIV & emergency departments.

♁ ▽ **Guttman Breast Diagnostic Institute**
55 5th. Avenue, New York 10003.
☎ 212 463 8733

☺ ☐ **Harlem Hospital Center**
506 Lenox Avenue, New York 10037.
☎ 212 939 1340
HIV & emergency departments.

☺ ☐ **Lenox Hill Hospital**
100 East 77th. Street, New York 10021.
☎ 212 434 2000
HIV & emergency departments.

☺ ☐ **Metropolitan Hospital Center**
1901 First Avenue, New York 10029.
☎ 212 230 6262

☺ ☐ **Mount Sinai Medical Center**
One Gustave L. Levy Place, New York 10029.
☎ 212 241 6500
HIV & emergency departments.

♀♂ ☐ **New York City Department of Health**
♿ Lesbian Health Project, Office of Gay & Lesbian Health Concerns, Box 67, 125 Worth Street, New York 10013.
☎ 212 788 4315 ☎ 212 788 5243

♀♂▽ **New York City Department of Health**
♿ Office of Gay & Lesbian Health Concerns, Box 67, 125 Worth Street, New York 10013.
☎ 212 788 4315 ☎ 212 788 5243

♀♂ ▽ **New York City Department of Health**
♿ Provider Education Project, Office of Gay & Lesbian Health Concerns, Box 67, 125 Worth Street, New York 10013.
☎ 212 788 4399 ☎ 212 788 5243
Training & consultation for health care providers on lesbian, gay, & bisexual issues.

☺ ☐ **New York Downtown Hospital**
170 William Street, New York 10038.
☎ 212 312 5000
HIV & emergency departments.

☺ ☐ **The New York Hospital**
525 East 68th. Street, New York 10021.
☎ 212 746 5454
HIV & emergency departments.

☺ ☐ **North General Hospital**
1879 Madison Avenue, New York 10035.
☎ 212 424 4000

☺ ☐ **Presbyterian Hospital in the City of New York**
Columbia-Presbyterian Medical Center, New York 10032.
☎ 212 305 2500
HIV & emergency departments.

☺ ☐ **Queens Hospital Center**
82-68 164th. Street, Jamaica, New York 11432.
☎ 718 883 3000

☺ ☐ **Roosevelt Hospital**
1000 Tenth Avenue, New York 10019.
☎ 212 523 4000
HIV & emergency departments.

☺ ☐ **Saint Clare's Hospital & Health Center**
415 West 51st. Street, New York 10019.
☎ 212 586 1500
HIV & emergency departments.

☺ ☐ **Saint Luke's Hospital Center**
1111 Amsterdam Avenue, New York 10025.
☎ 212 523 4000
HIV & emergency departments.

♁ ▽ **Saint Marks Women's Health Collective**
♿ P. O. Box A711, New York 10163-0711.
☎ 212 228 7482
⏱ Clinic 09:00

☺ ☐ **Saint Vincents' Medical Center of Richmond**
355 Bard Avenue, Staten Island, New York 10310.
☎ 718 876 1234

☺ ☐ **Veterans' Affairs Medical Center**
423 East 23rd. Street, New York 10010.
☎ 212 686 7500
HIV & emergency departments.

☺ ☐ **Youth Health Services**
14th. Floor, Draper Hall, 1918 1st. Avenue, New York 10029.
☎ 212 230 7408

Helplines: Miscellaneous

☺ ☐ **Response of Suffolk County**
P. O. Box 300, Stony Brook, New York 11790.
☎ 516 751 7500
⏱ 24hrs.

Helplines: Sexuality

♀♂▽ **Gay & Lesbian Hotline**
♿ P. O. Box 1905, White Plains, New York 10602.
☎ 914 948 4922
⏱ 19:00 - 22:00

♀♂▽ **Gay & Lesbian Switchboard**
☎ 212 777 1800

♀♂▽ **Gay & Lesbian Switchboard of Long Island (GLSB of LI)**
P. O. Box 1312, Ronkonkoma, New York 11779.
☎ 516 737 1615
⏱ 19:00 - 23:00

♀♀▽ **Lesbian Switchboard**
☎ 212 741 2610
⏱ Mon - Fri 18:00 - 22:00

♀♂☐ **Long Island Crisis Center**
Pride For Youth, 2740 Martin Avenue, Bellmore, New York 11710.
☎ 516 679 1111 (hotline) ☎ 516 781 8306
☎ 516 826 0244 (office)

🕐 24hrs. hotline
Formerly Middle Earth Crisis Center. Also weekly coffee house, free short-term counselling, support, & community education to those under 24.

Manufacturers: Erotica: Leather

☞▼ **David Menkes**
Suite 3, 144 Fifth Avenue, New York 10011.
☎ 212 989 3706 ✆ 212 229 0184
🕐 By appointment only
🛍 ✓
Catalogue, $5.

Manufacturers: Piercing Jewelry

☺■ **Dan Natkiel**
Room 306, 7th. Street Residence, 40 East 7th. Street, New York 10003.
Niobium, surgical steel, & Titanium jewelry.

☺■ **Venus Modern Body Arts, Inc.**
199 East 4th. Street, New York 10009.
☎ 212 473 1954
🕐 12:00 - 21:00
Make large selection of Niobium, Titanium, surgical steel, & gold jewelry.

Organizations: Academic: Sexology

☺ **The Sex Institute**
513 Broadway, New York 10012.
☎ 212 674 7111
📧 rjnoonan@bway.net or rjn@is.nyu.edu
🌐 http://www.bway.net/~rjnoonan/
Contact: Mr. Raymond Noonan, Director

Organizations: Academic: Sexuality

☞▽ **Center for Lesbian & Gay Studies**
c/o Duberman, Graduate Center, CUNY, 33 West 42nd. Street, New York 10036-8099.
☎ 212 642 2924
Publishes *The Directory of Lesbian & Gay Scholarship.*

☞▽ **Gay Academic Union**
P. O. Box 480, Lenox Hill Station, New York 10021-0033.
☎ 212 864 0361
Publishes *Gai Saber Monographs.*

Organizations: AIDS: Education

☺□ **AIDS Resource Center (ARC)**
♿ 12th. Floor, 275 7th. Avenue, New York 10001.
☎ 212 633 2500
🕐 09:30 - 17:30

☺□ **AIDS Center of Queens County (ACQC)**
♿ Suite 1220, 97-45 Queens Boulevard, Rego Park, New York 11374.
☎ 718 896 2500 ✆ 718 275 2094
☎ 718 896 2985
🕐 Mon - Fri 09:00 - 21:00, Sat 10:00 - 16:00
Publishes *ACQC Journal.*

☺□ **AIDS Services of Lower Manhattan**
Suite405, 80 5th. Avenue, New York 10011.
☎ 212 645 0875

☺□ **Bronx AIDS Services**
Suite 903, 1 Fordham Plaza, Bronx, New York 10458.
☎ 718 295 5605

☺□ **Bronx Lesbian AIDS Task Force**
♿ P. O. Box 1738, Bronx, New York 10451.

☺□ **Columbia University**
Gay Health Advocacy Project, 400 John Jay Hall, Columbia University, New York 10027.
☎ 212 854 2878

☞▽ **Community Health Project**
208 West 13th. Street, New York 10011.
☎ 212 675 3559

☞▽ **Hetrick-Martin Institute**
♿ 2 Astor Place, New York 10003.
☎ 212 674 2400 ✆ 212 674 8650
☎ 212 674 8695
🕐 Mon - Fri 09:00 - 19:00
Training & education about HIV/AIDS & sexual orientation.

☺□ **Long Island Association for AIDS Care, Inc. (LIAAC)**
♿ P. O. Box 2859, Huntington Station, Long Island, New York 11746.
☎ 516 385 2437
☎ 516 385 2451 (office)

☺□ **Stamp Out AIDS**
240 West 44th. Street, New York 10036.
☎ 212 354 8899

☺□ **Staten Island AIDS Task Force**

♿ 29 Hyatt Street, Staten Island, New York 10301.
☎ 718 981 3366

☺□ **Upper Manhattan Task Force on AIDS**
♿ Suite 1940, 475 Riverside Drive, New York 10115.
☎ 212 870 3352

Organizations: AIDS: Research

☺ **American Foundation for AIDS Research**
Suite 123, 733 3rd Avenue, New York 10017-3204.
Publishes *AIDS/HIV Treatment Directory.*

Organizations: AIDS: Support

☺□ **AIDS Center of Queens County (ACQC)**
♿ 175-61 Hillside Avenue, Jamaica, New York 11432.
☎ 718 739 2525 ✆ 718 275 2094
☎ 718 896 2985
🕐 Mon Thu Fri 09:00 - 18:00, Tue Wed 09:00 - 20:00

☺ **Gay Men's Health Crisis**
129 West 20th. Street, New York 10011.
☎ 212 807 6665 (hotline)
☎ 212 807 6664 (Office)
Contact: Mr. David Klotz, Coördinator, AIDS Prevention Programs
Publishes *The Volunteer; Treatment Issues; & AIDS Clinical Update.*

☺□ **People With AIDS Coalition of Long Island, Inc.**
1170 Route 109, Lindenhurst, New York 11757-1002.
☎ 516 225 5797 ✆ 516 225 5796
☎ 516 225 5700 (life line)
🕐 Mon - Fri 10:00 - 18:00, Sat 11:00 - 15:00

☺□ **PWA Coalition of New York, Inc.**
♿ 8th. Floor, 50 West 17th. Street, New York 10011.
☎ 800 828 3280 (hotline) ✆ 212 647 1419
☎ 212 647 1415
Publishes *Coalition Newsline.*

Organizations: BDSM

☺□ **A.S.B. Munch—Applemunch**
📧 vixen@panix.com
🕐 Meets 2nd. Thu of month 19:00

☞▽ **Amalgamated American Male**
P. O. Box 2096RM, New York 10013.

☞▽ **Brothers In Leather**
GPO Box 1035, New York 10116.
Contact: Mr. D. Perry
Leather men of colour.

⚲ **Clit Club**
432 West 14th. Street, New York.
🕐 Meets Fri Sat 22:00

☞ **Defenders—New York**
P.O. Box 1146, Old Chelsea Station, New York 10011.
☎ 908 324 6475

☺□ **The Eulenspiegel Society (TES)**
P.O. Box 2783, Grand Central Station, New York 10163-2783.
☎ 212 388 7022 (recorded message)
📧 tes@dorsai.org or LolitaTES@aol.com
🕐 Meets Tue 20:00
Publishes *Prometheus* quarterly. Yearly subscription is $20. Age statement of 21 is required.

☞▽ **Gay Male SM Activists**
Box D23, 332 Bleeker Street, New York 10014-2818.
☎ 212 727 9878
🕐 Usually meets 2nd. & 4th. Wed of month
✓
Publishes *Newslink.*

☞▽ **GOAL**
Suite 11, 510 East 20th. Street, New York 10009.

👫□ **Hellfire Club**
28 9th. Avenue, New York.
☎ 212 647 0063
🕐 Thu - Sun 20:00 - 03:00

⚲▽ **Lesbian Sex Mafia**
♿ P.O. Box 993, Murray Hill Station, New York 10156.
☎ 212 222 9329
📧 LCub@aol.com
🕐 Meets monthly
Publishes a newsletter.

☞▽ **Men of Discipline**
Suite 177, 18 Greenwich Avenue, New York 10011.
☎ 212 366 0861

☺□ **The National Leather Association (NLA)—Metro New York**
P.O. Box 488, Triborough Station, New York 10035-0488.

☎ 212 802 9295
⏱ Call for information
Publishes a newsletter.

⚥▽ **New York Strap & Paddle Association**
Box F4, 496A Hudson Street, New York 10014.
☎ 718 367 7484
⏱ Meets 2nd. & 4th. Mon of month
Age statement of 21 is required.

⚥▽ **The Renegades**
P. O. Box 1457, Canal Street Station, New York 10013.
☎ 201 217 1646 (recorded message)
⏱ Meets twice a month
Also Slave Trainers of New York (STONY).

Organizations: BDSM: Student

☺■ **Conversio Virium**
Columbia University, Ferris Booth Hall, New York 10027.
☎ 212 316 6479
📧 conversio@columbia.edu
🌐 http://www.columbia.edu/cu/cv/
BDSM organization on campus.

Organizations: Bears

⚥▽ **Bergenfield Bears**
P. O. Box 980, New York 10113.
📧 colt@panix.com
🌐 http://www.panix.com/~colt/bbl.html

⚥▽ **New York Bears**
Box F4, 332 Bleeker Street, New York 10014-2818.
☎ 212 367 7484
Age statement of 21 is required.

Organizations: Bondage

⚥▽ **New York Bondage Club**
P. O. Box 7280, JAF Station, New York 10118.
☎ 212 315 0040
⏱ Meets 1st. & 3rd. Fri of month. Doors open 20:00 - 21:00.
Newsletter not regular
🏳 ✓
Publishes a newsletter. Age statement of 18 is required.

Organizations: Daddy / Boy

⚥▽ **New York Boys & Dads**
Box F4, 332 Bleeker Street, New York 10014-2818.
Age statement of 21 is required.

Organizations: Family

⚥▽ **Gay Fathers I**
194 Riverside Drive, New York 10025.
☎ 212 874 7727
Contact: Mr. R. Boxer

⚥▽ **Gay Fathers of Greater New York**
& P. O. Box 1321, Midtown Station, New York 10018-0725.
☎ 212 721 4216
Publishes a newsletter.

⚥▽ **Gay Fathers of Long Island**
P. O. Box 2483, Patchogue, New York 11772-2483.
☎ 516 282 9478

⚥▽ **Gay Fathers of Westchester (GFW)**
P. O. Box 686, Croton Falls, New York 10519.
☎ 914 948 4922

☺☐ **Parents & Friends of Lesbians & Gays (PFLAG)—**
& **Long Island**
109 Browns Road, Huntington, New York 11743.
☎ 516 938 8913

☺☐ **Parents & Friends of Lesbians & Gays (PFLAG)—**
New York City
P. O. Box 553, Lenox Hill Station, New York 10021.
☎ 212 463 0629
Publishes a newsletter.

☺☐ **Parents & Friends of Lesbians & Gays (PFLAG)—**
& **Queens**
Suite 4E, 167-10 Crocheron Avenue, Flushing, New York 11358.
☎ 718 460 4064
⏱ Meets 3rd. Sun of month 13:00

☺☐ **Parents & Friends of Lesbians & Gays (PFLAG)—**
Westchester
3 Leatherstocking Lane, Mamaroneck, New York 10543.
☎ 914 698 3619
Contact: Ms. Rose Dinolfo

Organizations: Fetish: Foot

⚥▽ **Foot Friends**

P. O. Box 304, Village Station, New York 10014.
☎ 212 675 7352
⏱ Meets quarterly in New York City

Organizations: Health

☺ **Sex Information & Education Council (SIECUS)**
#25FL, 130 West 42nd. Street, New York 10036-7901.
☎ 212 819 9770
Publishes *SIECUS Reports.*

Organizations: Literary

☺ **The Book Industry Study Group**
Suite 604, 160 Fifth Avenue, New York 10011.
☎ 212 929 1393

☺ **ISBN Agency**
245 West 17th. Street, New York 10011.
☎ 212 337 6975

Organizations: Masturbation

⚥▽ **J's Hangout**
Ground Floor, 675 Hudson Street, New York.
☎ 212 242 9292
Enter at east side of building at junction of 14th. & 9th..

Organizations: Motorcycle

⚥▽ **Cycle/Wheels MC**
P. O. Box 615, New York 10116.

⚥▽ **Empire City MC**
P.O. Box 7951, New York 10116-4634.
Founded in 1964.

⚥▽ **Excelsior MC**
P.O. Box 1386, Bowling Green Station, New York 10274-1130.

⚔ **Iron Guard BC NYC**
P.O. Box 1475, Old Chelsea Station, New York 10013.
☎ 908 245 5323 ☏ 908 241 6152

⚧▽ **Sirens MC**
c/o Gay & Lesbian Community Center, 208 West 13th. Street, New York 10011.
☎ 212 807 8211
☎ 212 696 2872
⏱ Meets 3rd. Tue of month

⚔ **Trident—New York, #2**
400 Parker Street, Newark, New Jersey 07104.

⚔ **Wheels MC**
P.O. Box 615, GPO, New York 10001.

Organizations: Penis Size

⚔ **Nine Plus Club, Inc.**
P.O. Box 1267, Ansonia Station, New York 10023.

Organizations: Research: Sexuality

⚥ **National Council for Research on Women**
10th. Floor, 530 Broadway, New York 10012.
☎ 212 274 0730 ☏ 212 274 0831

Organizations: Sexual Politics

☺☐ **American Civil Liberties Union**
132 West 43rd. Street, New York 10036.
☎ 212 944 9800

⚲▽ **Transgender Rights**
☎ 212 979 8547
Publishes *Rights News.*

Organizations: Sexuality

♀▽ **Bisexual Women of Color Group**
P. O. Box 497, New York 10108.
☎ 212 459 4784

⚥▽ **Black & White Men Together (BWMT)—New York**
♿ P. O. Box 1518, Ansonia Station, New York 10023.
☎ 212 330 7678
Publishes *MACT/NY Information Bulletin.*

⚥▽ **Bridges**
P. O. Box 1084, Shoreham, New York 11786.
☎ 516 744 2512

⚲▽ **The F2M Fraternity**
P. O. Box 509, Lenox Station, New York 10021.
☎ 908 298 8797
☎ 212 570 1260

⚥▽ **Gay & Lesbian Community Center**
208 West 13th. Street, New York 10011-7702.
☎ 212 620 7310
🌐 http://www.panix.com/~dhuppert/gay/center/

⊙ 09:00 - 23:00
Publishes *Center Voice*.

⚥▽ **Gay & Lesbian Alliance in Orange County**
⅃ P. O. Box 1557, Greenwood Lake, New York 10925.
☎ 914 782 1525
⊙ Meets Tue 20:00

⚥▽ **Gay Men of the Bronx**
⅃ P. O. Box 511, Bronx, New York 10451.
☎ 718 792 8078
☎ 718 378 3497 (Spanish)
Publishes *GMOB Update*.

⚥▽ **Gay Men's Alliance of Hudson Valley**
P. O. Box 1513, White Plains, New York 10602.
☎ 914 948 4922

⚥▽ **Gaymen & Lesbians in Brookhaven (GLIB)**
⅃ P. O. Box 203, Brookhaven, New York 11719-0203.
☎ 516 286 6867
⊙ Men meet 1st. & 3rd. Sun of month 16:00, women meet 1st. &
3rd. Thu of month 20:00
Publishes *GLIB News*.

✉☐ **Gender Identity Project for Transsexuals**
The Lesbian & Gay Community Services Center, 208 West 13th. Street,
New York 10014.
☎ 212 620 7310
⊙ By appointment
Support, counselling, advocacy, & referral service.

✉☐ **Greater New York Gender Alliance**
Suite 3H, 330 West 45th. Street, New York 10036.
☎ 212 765 3561
⊙ 18:00 - 22:00
Contact: Ms. Lynda Frank

⚲▽ **Imperial Queens of New York & Long Island**
⅃ Suite 120, 80-A Greenwich Avenue, New York 10011.
☎ 212 580 9862 (New York City)
☎ 516 889 1980 (Long Island)
⊙ Meets 1st. Fri of month 20:15
Publishes *Imperially Yours*.

⚥▽ **Lambda Association of Staten Island**
P. O. Box 665, Staten Island, New York 10314.
☎ 718 979 8890

☺▽ **Lavendar & Lace**
Box F4, 332 Bleeker Street, New York 10014-2818.
☎ 212 255 6758

⚥▽ **Lavendar Heights**
⅃ Cornerstone Center, 178 Bennett Avenue, New York.
☎ 212 569 2023
Publishes *Lavendar Heights News*.

☺☐ **The Loft Lesbian & Gay Community Services
Center, Inc.**
P. O. Box 1513, White Plains, New York 10602.
☎ 914 948 4922
Publishes *The Loft Community News*.

⚥▽ **Long Island Gay Men's Group**
P. O. Box 433, Levittown, New York 11756.
☎ 516 694 2407
Publishes *L. I. Male*.

⚥▽ **Long Island Gay Men's Social Group**
☎ 516 334 2773
☎ 516 364 6894
⊙ Call 19:00 - 23:00

⚥▽ **Mayor's Office for the Lesbian & Gay Community**
⅃ Room 311, 52 Chambers Street, New York 10007.
☎ 212 788 2706

✉▽ **Metropolitan Gender Network**
P. O. Box 45, 561 Hudson Street, New York 10014.
☎ 201 794 1665 Ext.: 332
☎ 718 461 9050
⊙ Meets 2nd. Sun of month
Publishes *City Lights*.

♂▽ **New York Bisexual Network**
P. O. Box 497, Times Square Station, New York 10108.
☎ 212 459 4784

✉☐ **New York City Gender Alliance (NYCGA)**
⅃ c/o Fem Fashions, Suite 7R, 9 West 31st. Street, New York 10001.
☎ 212 570 7389
⊙ By appointment
Contact: Ms. Kristine James, Director

⚥▽ **New York Femmes**
P. O. Box 580281, Station A, Flushing, New York 11358.
☎ 212 388 2736

⚥▽ **North American Man Boy Love Association
(NAMBLA)**
P. O. Box 174, Midtown Station, New York 10018.
☎ 212 807 8578

⚥▽ **Queens Gay & Lesbians United (Q-GLU)**
⅃ P. O. Box 4669, Sunnyside, New York 11104.
☎ 718 639 4951

⚥▽ **Rockland Lesbian Gay Alliance (RLGA)**
P. O. Box 549, Nyack, New York 10960.
☎ 914 353 6925

✉▽ **Survivors of Transexuality Anonymous**
☎ 212 969 0888 (voice mail)
⊙ Meets Tue 18:30 - 20:00, Sun 18:30 - 22:00

Organizations: Sexuality: Student

⚥▽ **Bisexual, Lesbian, & Gay Alliance at City College
⅃ New York**
Finley Student Center, Convent Avenue, New York 10031.
☎ 212 650 8234

⚥▽ **Cardozo Gay & Lesbian Law Student Alliance**
55 5th. Avenue, New York 10003.

⚥▽ **College of Staten Island Lesbian, Gay, & Bisexual
Alliance**
Room 217, Campus Center, 2800 Victory Boulevard, Staten Island, New
York 10314.

⚥▽ **Columbia Lesbian, Bisexual, & Gay Coalition**
303 Earl Hall, Columbia University, New York 10027.
☎ 212 854 1488
Publishes a newsletter.

⚥▽ **Einstein Association of Gays & Lesbians (EAGL)**
Department of Molecular Genetics, Albert Einstein College of Medicine,
Bronx, New York 10461.
Contact: Dr. Frank Lilli

⚥▽ **Gay & Lesbian Union at NYU**
⅃ Loeb Student Center, Suite 810, 566 La Guardia, New York 10012.
☎ 212 998 4938

⚥▽ **Gay & Lesbian Union at Queens College**
⅃ Student Union Building Room 210, 65-30 Kissena Boulevard, Flushing,
New York 11367-0904.
☎ 718 520 1866

⚥▽ **Gay Students Alliance at Baruch College**
Box 321, 137 East 22nd. Street, New York 10010.

⚥▽ **Gay, Lesbian, & Bisexual Union**
⅃ c/o Campus Life, SUNY Purchase, 735 Anderson Road, Purchase, New
York 10577-1400.
☎ 914 251 6976

⚥▽ **Hofstra Gay & Lesbian Student Association**
c/o SGA Office, Hofstra University, Hempstead, New York 11550.
☎ 516 560 6960

⚥▽ **Lambda Lesbian & Gay Student Association**
⅃ John Jay College, 445 West 59th. Street, New York 10019.
☎ 212 237 8738
☎ 212 237 8732

⚥▽ **Lesbian & Gay Law Student at NYU**
240 Mercer Street, New York 10012.

⚥▽ **Lesbian & Gay Students Association**
⅃ New York Law School, 57 Worth Street, New York 10013.
☎ 212 431 2100

⚥▽ **Lesbian & Gay Support Group, Fordham University**
Box 480, Station 37, Bronx, New York 10458.

⚥▽ **Lesbian, Gay, & Bisexual Alliance**
⅃ Student Union 045A, SUNY at Stony Brook, Stony Brook, New York
11794.
☎ 516 632 6469

⚥▽ **Lesbians at Queens College**
⅃ Student Union Building, 65-30 Kissena Boulevard, Flushing, New York
11367.
☎ 718 263 5668

⚥▽ **The New School Gay, Lesbian, Bisexual Collective**
66 West 12th. Street, New York 10011.

⚥▽ **Queensboro Community College Lesbian & Gay
Male Alliance**
Queensboro Community College of CUNY, Bayside, New York 11364.
☎ 718 631 6212

⚥▽ **Saint John's University Lesbian, Gay, & Bisexual
Alliance**
P. O. Box 55, Carlstadt, New Jersey 07072.
☎ 718 390 8829

Organizations: Sexuality: Youth

Bisexual, Gay, & Lesbian Youth of New York
The Center, 208 West 13th. Street, New York 10011.
212 620 7310
Meets Sat 13:00 - 18:00
Publishes *OutYouth.*

Community Health Project Outreach to Teens
The Center, 208 West 13th. Street, New York 10011.
212 255 1673
Mon - Fri 10:00 - 19:00

Gay & Lesbian Youth of Hudson Valley
P. O. Box 216, Congers, New York 10920.
914 948 4922

Hetrick-Martin Institute
2 Astor Place, New York 10003.
212 674 2400 — Fax 212 674 8650
212 674 8695
Mon - Fri 09:00 - 19:00
Publishes *HMI Report Card.*

Long Island Gay & Lesbian Youth, Inc.
P. O. Box 977, Levittown, New York 11756.
516 627 3340
516 579 6382

Mayor's Office for the Lesbian & Gay Community
Educational Coalition on Lesbian & Gay Youth, Room 311, 52 Chambers Street, New York 10007.
212 788 2706

Twentysomething
P. O. Box 396, Old Chelsea Station, New York 10011.
212 967 7711 Ext.: 3163

Organizations: Watersports

Golden Shower Association
Box K-95, 332 Bleeker Street, New York 10014-2818.

Rainmakers Club
c/o AAM, P. O. Box 2096RM, New York 10013.

Organizations: Wrestling

Knights Wrestling Club
P. O. Box 161, Jackson Heights, New York 11372.
718 639 5141

Metro Gay Wrestling Alliance, Inc. (MGWA)
Suite 14F, 500 West 43rd. Street, New York 10036.
212 563 7066
Publishes *Wrestlespeak.*

Photographers: Erotic

Barbara Alper
c/o Secret, Boîte Postale 1400, 1000 Bruxelles 1.
212 316 6518 — Fax 212 316 1259

Vince Gabrielly
Number 1, 785 Eighth Avenue, New York 10036.
212 977 5433 (studio) — Fax 212 977 9400
212 974 1996

Thomas Glover
c/o J. Schall, Suite 4B, 20 East 9th. Street, New York 10003.

Doris Kloster
Suite 8B, 144 East 24th. Street, New York 10010.
212 614 6621 — Fax 212 982 2009

David Morrow
212 645 6797

Photographers: Fetish

Eric Kroll
P. O. Box 464, Grand Central Station, New York 10017.
212 684 2465

Piercers

Gauntlet, Inc.
2nd Floor, 144 Fifth Avenue, New York 10011.
212 229 0180 — Fax 212 229 0184
kane@gauntlet.com
http://www.gauntlet.com/
✓ $ VISA MC AMERICAN EXPRESS
Catalogue, $5. Age statement of 21 is required.

Shaman Body Piercing
212 505 8488
http://128.122.132.159:9999/~thebin/shaman.html
By appointment only

Venus Modern Body Arts, Inc.
199 East 4th. Street, New York 10009.
212 473 1954
12:00 - 21:00
Catalogue available.

Printers: General

Port City Press, Inc.
500 Fifth Avenue, New York 10110.
212 921 9166 — Fax 212 921 9173

Quebecor America Book Group
1185 Sixth Avenue, New York 10036.
212 827 2700 — Fax 212 302 5869

Publishers: Books: Erotic

Badboy Books
801 Second Avenue, New York 10017.
800 458 9640 (credit card orders) — Fax 212 687 2993
212 661 7878 (editorial)
VISA MC

Hard Candy Books
801 Second Avenue, New York 10017.
800 458 9640 (credit card orders) — Fax 212 687 2993
212 661 7878 (editorial)
VISA MC

NBM Publishing
Suite 1504, 185 Madison Avenue, New York 10016.
800 886 1223 — Fax 212 545 1227
212 545 1223
Mon - Fri 09:00 - 18:00
✓ VISA MC
Mail order only. Catalogue, free with stamp or IRC. Age statement of 21 is required.

Richard Kasak Books
801 Second Avenue, New York 10017.
800 458 9640 (credit card orders) — Fax 212 687 2993
212 661 7878 (editorial)
VISA MC

Publishers: Books: Sexuality

JH Press
P. O. Box 1243, New York 10023-1243.

Masquerade Books
801 Second Avenue, New York 10017.
800 458 9640 (credit card orders) — Fax 212 687 2993
212 661 7878 (editorial)
VISA MC

Rhinocerous Books
801 Second Avenue, New York 10017.
800 458 9640 (credit card orders) — Fax 212 687 2993
212 661 7878 (editorial)
VISA MC

Routledge Press
29 West 35th. avenue, New York 10001.

St. Martin's Press
175 Fifth Avenue, New York 10010.

Publishers: Directories: Books

K. G. Saur Publishing Company
c/o Gale Research, 150 East 50th. Street, New York 10022.
212 751 3033

Literary Market Place
245 West 17th. Street, New York 10011.
212 645 9700

Publishers: Directories: Booksellers

American Booksellers Association
137 West 25th. Street, New York 10001
212 463 8450

Publishers: Directories: Sexuality

Gayellow Pages
Renaissance House, P. O. Box 533, Village Station, New York 10014-0533.
212 674 0120 — Fax 212 420 1126
Directory of resources for lesbians & gay men. Published once a year.

Publishers: Guides: Sexuality

Columbia Fun Maps
118 East 28th. Street, New York 10016.
212 447 7877 — Fax 212 447 7876
09:00 - 17:00
Free guides to 63 North American locations.

HX (Homo Xtra)
Suite 703, 19 West 21st. Street, New York 10010.
☎ 212 627 0747
The largest & most popular gay publication in New York. Focuses on nightlife & entertainment listing. Published 51 times a year. Yearly subscription is $99.

Publishers: Magazines: AIDS
POZ
P. O. Box 1279, New York 10113-1279.
☎ 212 242 2163 ✆ 212 675 8505

Publishers: Magazines: BDSM
☺ ■ Black Leather In Color (BLIC)
BLIC Collective, #808, 874 Broadway, New York 10003.
☎ 212 229 2502 ✆ 212 777 5349
🖂 ✓
For people of color in the leather, BDSM, & fetish community. Published quarterly. Yearly subscription is $10.

☺ ■ De Sade's World
Executive Imports International, P. O. Box 1839, New York 10116.
Published quarterly.

☺ ■ Domina
Suite 1166, 305 Madison Avenue, New York 10165.
Fetish magazine with two sections in colour. Stories, articles, photos, listings, & mail order. U.S. office of U.K. magazine. Published quarterly. Yearly subscription is $100.

☺ Sandmutopia Guardian
The Utopian Network, P.O. Box 1146, New York 10156.
☎ 516 842 1711 ✆ 516 842 7518
🖥 http://palace.com/utopian/utopian.htm
🕐 Mon - Fri 11:00 - 21:00
Yearly subscription is $24.

Publishers: Magazines: Erotic
Blueboy Magazine
28 West 25th. Street, New York 10010.
☎ 212 647 0222 ✆ 212 647 0236

Honcho
MMG Services Inc., Suite 4100, 462 Broadway, New York 10013.
☎ 212 966 8400 ✆ 212 966 9366

Jock
28 West 25th. Street, New York 10010.
☎ 212 647 0222 ✆ 212 647 0236

Machismo
28 West 25th. Street, New York 10010.
☎ 212 647 0222 ✆ 212 647 0236

Mandate
MMG Services Inc., Suite 4000, 462 Broadway, New York 10013.
☎ 212 966 8400 ✆ 212 966 9366

Numbers
28 West 25th. Street, New York 10010.
☎ 212 647 0222 ✆ 212 647 0236

Obsession
28 West 25th. Street, New York 10010.
☎ 212 647 0222 ✆ 212 647 0236

♣ Penthouse
Penthouse International, Ltd., 1965 Broadway, New York 10023-5965.
☎ 212 496 6100
🖥 http://www.penthousemag.com/

♣ Playgirl
801 Second Avenue, New York 10017.
☎ 212 986 5100

Playguy
MMG Services Inc., Suite 4000, 462 Broadway, New York 10013.
☎ 212 966 8400 ✆ 212 966 9366

Stars
28 West 25th. Street, New York 10010.
☎ 212 647 0222 ✆ 212 647 0236

▼ Straight to Hell (The Manhattan Review of Unnatural Acts)
P. O. Box 20424, New York 10023.
Published 3 times a year. Yearly subscription is $9.

Torso
MMG Services Inc., Suite 4000, 462 Broadway, New York 10013.
☎ 212 966 8400 ✆ 212 966 9366

Publishers: Magazines: General
Details
632 Broadway, New York 10012.
☎ 212 420 0689

Publishers: Magazines: Literary
☺ The Library Journal
249 West 17th. Street, New York 10011.
☎ 212 645 0067

☺ The New York Review of Books
250 West 57th. Street, New York 10107.
☎ 212 757 8070

☺ Publishers Weekly
249 West 17th. Street, New York 10011.
☎ 212 645 9700 ✆ 212 645 0067

Publishers: Magazines: Piercing
☺ ■ In The Flesh
OB Enterprises, Suite 2305, 450 Seventh Avenue, New York 10123-0101.
Published twice a year.

Publishers: Magazines: Sexual Politics
⊕ Heresies
P. O. Box 1306, Canal Street Station, New York 10013.
☎ 212 227 2108

Publishers: Magazines: Sexuality
Colorlife!
210 Riverside, New York 10025.

▼ Dirty
P. O. Box 1697, New York 10009.
☎ 212 780 2151 ✆ 212 979 8637
🖂 Riotboyyy@aol.com
🖂 ✓
Sample copies are $3.75.

Iniquity
28 West 25th. Street, New York 10010.
☎ 212 647 0222 ✆ 212 647 0236

▼ Masquerade Erotic Newsletter
Masquerade Books, 801 Second Avenue, New York 10017.
☎ 800 458 9640 (credit card orders) ✆ 212 687 2993
☎ 212 661 7878 (editorial)
[VISA] [MC]
Published every two months. Yearly subscription is $15. Age statement of 21 is required.

▼ Metrosource
Suite 5F, 622 Greenwich Street, New York 10014.
☎ 212 691 5127

▼ Michael's Thing Magazine
& Suite 4D, 240 West End Avenue, New York 10023.
☎ 212 724 3691

▼ My Comrade
Suite 15, 326 East 13th. Street, New York 10003.

Out
Out Publishing, Inc., Suite 800, 110 Greene Street, New York 10012.
☎ 212 334 9119 ✆ 212 334 9227
🕐 Mon - Fri 09:00 - 17:00
🖂 [VISA] [MC]
Published every month. Yearly subscription is $24.95.

▼ Out & About
Out & About, Inc., Suite 401, 8 West 19th. Street, New York 10011.
☎ 800 929 2268 ✆ 212 645 6785
☎ 212 645 6922
🖂 outandabout@aol.com
[VISA] [MC]
Published 10 times a year. Yearly subscription is $49.

☺ Paradise
P. O. Box 2116, New York 10116.
☎ 212 630 0242

▼ Paws Magazine
2nd. Floor, 349 West 12th. Street, New York 10014.

Penthouse Forum
& General Media Inc., 277 Park Avenue, New York 10172.
☎ 212 702 6000
🕐 09:00 - 17:00
Articles, reviews, & erotic fiction, plus explicit reader letters. Also publishes special issues. Published 13 times a year. Yearly subscription is $29.97.

Screw Magazine
Goldstein Publications, 4th Floor, 116 West 14th., New York 10011.
☎ 212 989 8001
Published every week. Yearly subscription is $26.

Publishers: Magazines: Youth
☺ Project X

Suite 1007, 27 West 20th. Street, New York 10011.
☎ 212 266 6603 📠 212 645 5489

Publishers: Mailing Lists: Sexuality

Renaissance House
P. O. Box 533, Village Station, New York 10014-0533.
☎ 212 674 0120 📠 212 420 1126

Strubco, Inc.
P. O. Box 1274, Old Chelsea Station, New York 10113-0920.
☎ 212 242 1900 📠 212 242 1963

Publishers: Miscellaneous

Gay Presses of New York
P. O. Box 294, Village Station, New York 10014.

Pagan Press
26 Saint Marks Place, New York 10003.
☎ 212 674 3321

Publishers: Newsletters: Sexual Politics

In Your Face
c/o Riki Anee Wilchins, 274 West 11th. Street, New York 10014.
Riki@PipeLine.Com or nrn@world.std.com
Published twice a year.

Publishers: Newspapers: BDSM

Dominant Domain
New Esoteric Press, P. O. Box 300684, JFK Station, Jamaica, New York 11430.
☎ 718 846 1140 📠 718 849 9311
VISA MC
Coverage also includes cross dressing, infantilism, & foot worship. Published 13 times a year. Yearly subscription is $47U.S. for U.S., $57U.S. elsewhere. Age statement of 21 is required.

Dominant Mystique
New Esoteric Press, P. O. Box 300689, JFK Station, Jamaica, New York 11430.
☎ 718 846 1140 📠 718 849 9311
VISA MC
Coverage also includes cross dressing, infantilism, & foot worship. Published 13 times a year. Yearly subscription is $47U.S. for U.S., $57U.S. elsewhere. Age statement of 21 is required.

Feminine Illusion
New Esoteric Press, P. O. Box 300684, JFK Station, Jamaica, New York 11430.
☎ 718 846 1140 📠 718 849 9311
VISA MC
Coverage also includes cross dressing, infantilism, & foot worship. Published 13 times a year. Yearly subscription is $47U.S. for U.S., $57U.S. elsewhere. Age statement of 21 is required.

Publishers: Newspapers: Fetish

Fetish World
New Esoteric Press, P. O. Box 300689, JFK Station, Jamaica, New York 11430.
☎ 718 846 1140 📠 718 849 9311
VISA MC
Coverage also includes cross dressing, infantilism, & foot worship. Published 13 times a year. Yearly subscription is $47U.S. for U.S., $57U.S. elsewhere. Age statement of 21 is required.

Publishers: Newspapers: General

Women's Studies Quarterly
Feminist Press at The City University of New York, 311 East 94th. Street, New York 10128.
☎ 212 360 5790
Published quarterly.

Publishers: Newspapers: Literary

Voice Literary Supplement
The Village Voice, 36 Cooper Square, New York 10003.
☎ 212 475 3300

Publishers: Newspapers: Sexuality

Christopher Street
P. O. Box 1475, New York 10008-1475.

Gay Scene
P. O. Box 247, Grand Central Station, New York 10163.

The New York Native
That New Magazine, P. O. Box 1475, Church Street Station, New York 10008.
☎ 212 627 2120
Published every week.

On The Wilde Side
106 Cain Drive, Brentwood, New York 11717.
☎ 516 435 0005 📠 516 435 0005

A valuable resource guide distributed throughout the tri-state area. If it's important news regarding the gay & lesbian community, it's in here. Published every month. Yearly subscription is $35.

Out Magazine
Suite 800, 110 Greene Street, New York 10012.
☎ 212 334 9119

Radical Chick
The Center, 208 West 13th. Street, New York 10011.
Lesbian chic analysed; humour, reviews, video, art, political news, poetry, & fiction. Published quarterly. Yearly subscription is $20.

The Record
311 East 72nd. Street, New York 10021.

Senior Action in a Gay Environment (S. A. G. E.)
16th. Floor, 305 Fashion Avenue, New York 10001-6008.
☎ 212 741 2247

Stonewall News
That New Magazine, P. O. Box 1475, Church Street Station, New York 10008.
☎ 212 627 2120

Publishers: Videos: BDSM

O Productions
P. O. Box 866, Peter Stuyvesant Station, New York 10009.
☎ 212 243 3700 Ext.: 412 📠 212 614 9059
🕘 10:00 - 22:00
✓
Age statement of 21 is required.

Publishers: Videos: Bondage

Star Maker Video
P. O. Box 289, Canal Street Station, New York 10013.
☎ 212 541 6877 📠 212 541 4397
Catalogue, $5. Age statement of 21 is required.

Radio: Sexuality

Gay & Lesbian Independent Broadcasters (GLIB)
c/o WBAI, Box 18, 505 8th. Avenue, New York 10018.
☎ 212 473 1689

Lavendar Wimmin
WUSB FM 90.1, SUNY at Stony Brook, Stony Brook, New York 11794.
☎ 516 632 6901
🕘 Thu 18:00 - 19:00

Stores: Art Galleries

Ditury & David
149 Mercer Street, New York 10021.

Erotics Gallery
Suite 1011, 41 Union SquareWest, New York 10003.
☎ 212 633 2241

Neikrug Photographica, Ltd.
224 East 68th. Street, New York 10021.
☎ 212 288 7741

Stores: Books: General

Book Gallery
P. O. Box 2070, Saint James, New York 11780-0603.
☎ 516 862 7982

Book Hampton
14 Main Street, East Hampton, New York 11937.
☎ 516 324 4939

Book Hampton
93 Main Street, Southampton, New York 11968.
☎ 516 283 0270

A Different Light
151 West 19th. Street, New York 10011-4116.
☎ 212 989 4850 📠 212 989 2158
🕘 10:00 - 24:00
VISA MC
Free catalogue published 3 times a year.

Les Hommes Bookshop
2nd. Floor, 217 West 80th. Street, New York 10024.

Judith's Room
681 Washington Street, New York 10014.
☎ 212 727 7330

Lee's Mardi Gras Boutique
565 10th. Avenue, New York 10036.
☎ 212 947 7773
Also stocks wigs, corsets, lingerie, make-up, etc.. Catalogue available.

Mags 'R' Us
116 Christopher Street, New York 11014.
☎ 212 627 2245

12:30 - 24:00

Mosaic Books
167 Avenue B, New York 10009.
212 475 8623
Tue - Sun 12;00 - 20:00

Oscar Wilde Memorial Bookstore
15 Christopher Street, New York 10014.
212 255 8097
11:30 - 20:00
Free catalogue.

Saint Marks Bookshop
12 Saint Marks Place, New York 10003.
212 260 7853 — Fax 212 598 4950

Shakespeare & Co.
716 Broadway, New York 10003.
212 529 1330 — Fax 212 979 5711

Three Lives & Co., Ltd.
154 West 10th. Street, New York 10014.
212 741 2069

Wendell's Magazines
22 8th. Avenue, New York 10014.
212 645 1197

Stores: Clothing: Fetish

Ian's
5 Saint Marks Place, New York 10003.
212 420 1857
Mon - Sat 11:00 - 19:00
$
Subversive evening wear.

Ian's
1151 2nd. Avenue, New York 10021.
212 838 3969
Mon - Sat 11:30 - 20:00
$
Subversive evening wear.

Mud Honey
124 East 4th. Street, New York 10002.
212 995 5593

Purple Passion
P. O. Box 1139, New York 110113.
212 807 0486
hiltontes@aol.com
Thu - Sun 11:00 - 19:00, Mon - Wed by appointment
Fetish clothing, toys, magazines, & books. Store at 242 West 16th. Street. Free catalogue.

Stores: Clothing: Sexuality

Fem Fashions, Inc.
Suite 7R, 9 West 31st. Street, New York 10001.
212 629 5750
By appointment only
Catalogue, $10.

Lee's Mardi Gras Boutique
P. O. Box 843, New York 10108.
212 645 1888

Unique Quality Products, Inc.
Suite 3307, 2170 Broadway, New York 10024.
212 580 4335
Clothing & hoods. Catalogue, $5.

Stores: Clothing: Uniforms

Dornan Uniforms
653 11th. Avenue, New York.
212 247 0937
Catalogue available.

Stores: Erotica: BDSM

Body Worship
102 East 7th. Street, New York.
212 614 0124

The Leather Man, Inc.
111 Christopher Street, New York 10014.
800 243 5330 — Fax 212 243 5372
212 243 5339
12:00 - 24:00
$
Catalogue available. Age statement of 21 is required. Spanish also spoken.

The Noose
261 West 19th. Street, New York 10011.
212 807 1789
Tue - Sat 11:00 - 20:00, Sun 13:00 - 20:00. In Dec, also Mon 11:00 - 20:00

The Noose II
c/o the Lure, 409 West 13th. Street, New York.
212 807 1789
Wed eve & Sat Sun eve

Tino Trevino's Leather Den
Studio 1F, 25 West 16th. Street, New York 10011.
212 620 0828 — Fax 212 620 0828 (call first)
By appointment only 10:00 - 18:00

Stores: Erotica: General

Adult Entertainment Center
488 8th. Avenue, New York 10001.
212 947 1590

Adult Shop
6083 Sunrise Highway, Holbrook, New York 11741.
516 472 9519 — Fax 516 472 4063

Ann Street Adult Entertainment Center
21 Ann Street, New York 10038.
212 267 9760

Courageous Books
250 West 42nd. Street, New York 10036.
212 944 1050

Etcetera News
337 Bleeker Street, New York 10014.
212 675 7952

Eve's Garden
Suite 420, 119 West 57th. Street, New York 10019-2303.
800 848 3837 — Fax 212 977 4306
212 757 8651
evesgard@soho.ios.com
http;//www.eve's-garden.com
Mon - Sat 12:00 -19:00
$
Women's sexuality boutique encouraging women to explore & celebrate their sexuality. 36-page catalogue published twice a year, free to store customers. Spanish & French also spoken.

G & D Merchandise
113 West 42nd. Street, New York 10036.
212 221 8947

Gaiety Burlesk
201 West 46th. Street, New York 10036.
212 221 8868

Gay Pleasures / Gay Treasures
546 Hudson Street, New York 10014.
212 255 5756
212 944 7561
11:00 - 24:00

Pink Pussycat Boutique
167 West 4th. Street, New York 10014.
212 243 0077 — Fax 212 627 7193
Sun - Thu 10:00 - 02:00, Fri Sat 10:00 - 03:00

Pleasure Chest
156 7th. Avenue South, New York 10014.
212 242 2158
212 242 4185
13:00 - 01:00

Pleasure Palace
733A 8th. Avenue, New York 10036.
212 265 5213
24hrs.

Stilletto
59 West 8th. Street, New York.

Xtasy Down Under Male Emporium
691 8th. Avenue, New York 10036.
212 262 0178
24hrs.

Stores: Military Surplus

Federal Bargain Stores
580 Broadway, New York 10012.

Trader
364 Canal Street, New York 10013.

Television: Sexuality

The Closet Case Show
P. O. Box 790, New York 10108.

♋ *Dyke TV*
Sang Froid, P. O. Box 88, New York 10002-9998.
☎ 212 343 9335 ✆ 212 343 9337

♂♋ **Gay Cable Network**
Suite 703, 150 West 26th. Street, New York 10001.
☎ 212 727 8850 ✆ 212 229 2347

♂▽ *Out In The Nineties*
♂⚲ Gay Broadcasting System, Suite A3, 178 7th. Avenue, New York 10011.
☎ 212 243 1570
Manhattan cable channel 16.

Niagara Falls
Organizations: Sexuality

♂▽ **Gay & Lesbian Support (GALS)**
♂⚲ P. O. Box 1464, Niagara Falls, New York 14302.

Stores: Erotica: General

☺ ■ **Unique News**
1907 Main Street, Niagara Falls, New York 14305.
☎ 716 282 9282

Oneonta
Organizations: Sexuality

☺▽ **Lesbian & Gay Concerns Network (LGCN)**
c/o Unitarian Universalist Church, Oneonta, New York 13820.
☎ 607 432 1289

♋▽ **The Society for the Second Self (Tri-Ess)—Lambda Chi Lambda**
P. O. Box 870, Oneonta, New York 13820.
☎ 607 547 4118
🕐 Meets monthly
Contact: Ms. Sharon Ann Stuart
Publishes *Cornbury's Closet.*

Organizations: Sexuality: Student

♂▽ **Gay Organization for Alternative Lifestyles (GOAL)**
c/o Student Association, Hunt Union Building, SUNY, Oneonta, New York 13820.

Oswego
Organizations: Sexuality: Student

♂▽ **Gay & Lesbian Alliance SUC-Oswego**
♂ c/o Student Association, Room 225, Hewitt Union, Oswego, New York 13126.
☎ 315 341 2955

Pelham
Organizations: Body Size

♂▽ **Girth & Mirth—New York**
P. O. Box 10, Pelham, New York 10803.
☎ 914 699 7735
Publishes *Fat Apple Review.*

Plattsburgh
Organizations: Sexuality: Student

♂▽ **Lesbian, Gay, & Bisexual Alliance at Plattsburgh**
♂ Angell College Center, SUNY Plattsburgh, Plattsburgh, New York 12901.
☎ 518 564 3200

Port Chester
Publishers: Magazines: Sexuality

♂ ■ *Options Magazine*
AJA Publishing Corp., P. O. Box 470, Port Chester, New York 10573.
Published 10 times a year. Yearly subscription is $21.

Potsdam
Helplines: Miscellaneous

☺ □ **Reachout of Saint Lawrence County, Inc.**
P. O. Box 5051, Potsdam, New York 13676.
☎ 315 265 2422

Organizations: Sexuality: Student

♂▽ **Lesbian, Gay, & Bisexual Association at SUNY Postdam**
♂ Barrington Student Union, Potsdam, New York 13676.
☎ 315 267 2184

Poughkeepsie
Counsellors

☺ ▼ **Audrey Steinhorn**
♂ 24 Davis Avenue, Poughkeepsie, New York 12603.
☎ 914 452 0374

Health Services

☺ □ **Vassar Brothers Hospital**
Reade Place, Poughkeepsie, New York 12601.
☎ 914 454 8500

Organizations: Family

☺ □ **Parents & Friends of Lesbians & Gays (PFLAG)—Mid-Hudson**
P. O. Box 880, Pleasant Valley, New York 12569.
☎ 914 221 9559

Organizations: Sexuality

♋▽ **Transgender Network**
P. O. Box 1611, Southg Road Annex, Poughkeepsie, New York 12601-0611.
🕐 Meets 1st. & 3rd. Fri of month

Organizations: Sexuality: Student

♂▽ **Poughkeepsie Gay & Lesbian Alliance (GALA)**
♂ P. O. Box 289, Hughsonville, New York 12537.
☎ 914 473 1500
☎ 914 431 6756

♂▽ **Vassar Gay People's Alliance**
♂ Box 271, Vassar College, Poughkeepsie, New York 12601.
☎ 914 437 7203

Stores: Erotica: General

☺ ■ **Hamilton Book**
216 North Hamilton Street, Poughkeepsie, New York 12601.
☎ 914 473 1776

Rego Park
Publishers: Newspapers: BDSM

⚥ ■ *Whipping Post*
La Carnivale, P. O. Box 8027, Rego Park, New York 11374.
☎ 212 689 6397
Published every month. Yearly subscription is $30.

Rochester
Bars: BDSM

♂▼ **Batchelor Forum**
670 University Avenue, Rochester, New York 14607-1232.
☎ 716 271 6930

BBSs: BDSM

☺ ■ **Multicom4**
☎ 716 442 1669
✆ 716 473 4070. 14400 baud maximum.
Age statement of 21 is required.

Health Services

☺ □ **Genessee Hospital**
224 Alexander Street, Rochester, New York 14607.
☎ 716 263 6000

☺ □ **Rochester General Hospital**
1425 Portland Avenue, Rochester, New York 14621.
☎ 716 338 4000

☺ □ **Strong Memorial Hospital of the University of Rochester**
601 Elmwood Avenue, Rochester, New York 14642.
☎ 716 275 2100
HIV & emergency departments.

Organizations: AIDS: Education

☺ □ **AIDS Rochester, Inc.**
♂ Suite C, 1350 University Avenue, Rochester, New York 14607-1622.
☎ 716 442 2220
☎ 716 442 2200 (hotline)
🕐 Hotline 24hrs. Both lines voice & TDD

Organizations: AIDS: Support

☺ □ **Helping People With AIDS (HPA)**
P. O. Box 1543, Rochester, New York 14603-1543.
☎ 716 987 1853

Organizations: Family

☿▽ **Gay Fathers Group**
AS P. O. Box 25525, Rochester, New York 14625.
☎ 716 924 4397

☿▽ **Gay Married Men's Support Group**
P. O. Box 10041, Rochester, New York 14610.

☺ ☐ **Parents & Friends of Lesbians & Gays (PFLAG)—Rochester**
c/o Gay Alliance, Genesee Valley, 179 Atlantic Avenue, Rochester, New York 14607-1255.
☎ 716 436 7051
Publishes a newsletter.

Organizations: Masturbation

☿▽ **T.O.M.**
P.O. Box 10514, Rochester, New York 14610.
🕐 Meets about every three weeks
🔥 ✓

Organizations: Motorcycle

☿▽ **Rochester Rams MC**
P.O. Box 1727, Rochester, New York 14603.
☎ 716 244 9812

☿ **Trident—Rochester**
P.O. Box 40655, Midtown Station, Rochester, New York 14604.

Organizations: Sexuality

⚥☐ **CD Network**
AS P. O. Box 92055, Rochester, New York 14692.
☎ 716 251 2132
🕐 24hr. answering machine. Meets monthly
Publishes CD News every two months. Yearly subscription is $25.

☿▽ **Gay Alliance, Genesee Valley**
♿ 179 Atlantic Avenue, Rochester, New York 14607-1255.
☎ 716 244 9030
The oldest gay & lesbian newspaper in New York state, published by the non-profit Gay Alliance, Genesee Valley. Publishes The Empty Closet 11 times a year. Yearly subscription is $10.

Organizations: Sexuality: Student

☿▽ **Bisexual, Gay, & Lebian Association of RIT**
♿ c/o Student Directorate / Ritreat, 1 Lombard Memorial Drive, Rochester, New York 15623.
☎ 716 475 3296

☿▽ **Gay, Lesbian, Bisexual, & Friends Association (GLBFA)**
#101J, Wilson Commons, University of Rochester, New York 14627.
☎ 716 275 9379

Organizations: Sexuality: Youth

☿▽ **Lesbian & Gay Youth of Rochester**
c/o Gay Alliance, Genesee Valley, 179 Atlantic Avenue, Rochester, New York 14607-1255.
☎ 716 251 9604

Stores: Books: General

☺▼ **Silkwood Books, Inc.**
♿ 633 Monroe Avenue, Rochester, New York 14607.
☎ 716 473 8110
🕐 Tue Wed 11:00 - 18:00, Thu - Sat - 21:00, Sun 12:00 - 17:00

☺■ **Village Green Bookstore**
AS 766 Monroe Avenue, Rochester, New York 14607-3296.
☎ 716 442 1151

☺■ **Village Green Bookstore**
AS 1954 West Ridge Road, Rochester, New York 14626.
☎ 716 723 1600 📞 716 723 1669

☺■ **Worldwide News**
100 Saint Paul Street, Rochester, New York 14604.
☎ 716 546 7140

Stores: Clothing: Leather

☺ **Pride Leathers**
728 South Avenue, Rochester, New York 14620.
☎ 716 242 7840
Distinctive tailored leather made to your specifications.

Stores: Erotica: BDSM

☿▼ **Rochester Custom Leathers**
Village Gate Square Mall, 274 North Goodman Street, Rochester, New York 14607-1154.
☎ 800 836 9047 📞 716 242 7978
☎ 716 442 2323

🕐 11:00 - 21:00
🔥 ✓ VISA MC AMERICAN
Catalogue, $2. Age statement of 21 is required.

Stores: Erotica: General

☺■ **Dundalk News**
561 State Street, Rochester, New York 14608.
☎ 716 325 2248
🕐 24hrs.
Alternative lifestyle resource center.

☺■ **Hudson Video & News**
♿ 1462 Hudson Avenue, Rochester, New York 14621.
☎ 716 342 8310
🕐 24hrs.

☺■ **New Clinton Book Mart**
115 Clinton Avenue North, Rochester, New York 14604-1411.
☎ 716 325 9322

☺■ **North End News**
♿ 490 Monroe Avenue, Rochester, New York 14607.
☎ 716 271 1426

☺■ **State Street Bookstore**
AS 109 State Street, Rochester, New York 14614.
☎ 716 263 9919

☺■ **Times Square Books**
57 Mortimer Street, Rochester, New York 14604-1317.
☎ 716 325 9570

Ronkonkoma

Organizations: Sexuality

⚥▽ **Long Island Femme Expression (LIFE)**
P. O. Box 3015, Ronkonkoma, New York 11779-0417.
☎ 516 283 1333
Support for heterosexual cross dressers. Publishes Lifelines.

Publishers: Newspapers: BDSM

👥■ **Female Supremacy**
Tiffany Enterprises, Suite 541, 3333 Veterans Highway, Ronkonkoma, New York 11779.
☎ 516 467 0480
Published 8 times a year. Yearly subscription is $20. Age statement of 18 is required.

Publishers: Newspapers: Bondage

👥■ **Bondage Times**
Tiffany Enterprises, Suite 541, 3333 Veterans Highway, Ronkonkoma, New York 11779.
☎ 516 467 0480
Published 8 times a year. Yearly subscription is $20. Age statement of 18 is required.

Publishers: Newspapers: Spanking

👥■ **Spanking Times**
Tiffany Enterprises, Suite 541, 3333 Veterans Highway, Ronkonkoma, New York 11779.
☎ 516 467 0480
Published every two months. Yearly subscription is $20. Age statement of 18 is required.

Saranac Lake

Organizations: Sexuality

☿▽ **Adirondack GALA**
P. O. Box 990, Saranac Lake, New York 12983-0990.

Saratoga Springs

Stores: Books: General

☺■ **Nahani**
♿ 482 Broadway, Saratoga Springs, New York 12866.
☎ 518 587 4322

Schenectady

Stores: Clothing: Fetish

☺■ **Regalia**
1521 State Street, Schenectady, New York 12304.
☎ 518 374 1900
Catalogue available.

Stony Brook

Radio: Sexuality

☿▽ **The Word is OUT!**
WUSB FM, Student Union Building, University at Stony Brook, Stony Brook, New York 11794.

☎ 516 632 6500

Syracuse
Health Services
☺ ☐ **Community-General Hospital of Greater Syracuse**
Broad Road, Syracuse, New York 13215.
☎ 315 492 5011

☺ ☐ **University Hospital**
SUNY Health Science Center, 750 East Adams Road, Syracuse, New York 13210.
☎ 315 464 5540
HIV & emergency departments.

☺ ☺ ☐ **Veterans' Affairs Medical Center**
Irving Avenue & University Place, Syracuse, New York 13210.
☎ 315 476 7461
No emergency department.

Helplines: Sexuality
⚢▽ **Gayline**
P. O. Box 738, Syracuse, New York 13201-0738.
☎ 315 422 5732
⏲ Mon - Fri 19:30 - 21:30

⚢▽ **Gayphone**
c/o Syracuse University Gay, Lesbian, Bisexual Student Association, 750 Ostrom Avenue, Syracuse, New York 13244-4350.
☎ 315 443 3599
⏲ 19:00 - 23:00

Organizations: AIDS: Education
☺ ☐ **The Boys From Syracuse**
P. O. Box 6728, Syracuse, New York 13217-6728.
☎ 315 474 3616

Organizations: BDSM
⚥ **Black Fire Association**
P.O. Box 354, University Station, Syracuse, New York 13210.
☎ 315 471 4563
Contact: Mr. Ted H.

Organizations: Sexuality
⚢☐ **Expressing Our Nature (EON)**
523 West Onondaga Street, Syracuse, New York 13204-3226.
☎ 315 475 7013 (office)
☎ 315 475 5611 (voice mail)

⚢▽ **Gay & Lesbian Alliance**
826 Euclid Avenue, Syracuse, New York 13210.
☎ 315 422 5732

⚢▽ **Gay & Lesbian Alliance of Syracuse (GLAS)**
P. O. Box 1675, Syracuse, New York 13201.
☎ 315 422 5732

Organizations: Sexuality: Student
⚢▽ **Gay & Lesbian & All Student Association**
& Onondaga Community College, Route 173, Syracuse, New York 13215.

⚢▽ **Syracuse University Gay, Lesbian, Bisexual Student Association**
750 Ostrom Avenue, Syracuse, New York 13244-4350.
☎ 315 443 3599
⏲ Gayphone operates 19:00 - 23:00

Organizations: Sexuality: Youth
⚢▽ **Lambda Youth Services**
& P. O. Box 6103, Syracuse, New York 13217.
☎ 315 422 9741

Publishers: Newspapers: Sexuality
⚢▼ *The Pink Paper*
P. O. Box 6462, Syracuse, New York 13217-6462.

Stores: Books: General
⚲ ■ **My Sisters' Words**
304 McBride Street, Syracuse, New York 13203.
☎ 315 428 0227

Stores: Erotica: General
☺ ■ **Burnet Bookstore**
303 Burnet Avenue, Syracuse, New York 13203.
☎ 315 471 9230

Teaneck
Publishers: Magazines: Erotic
⚥ *Manscape*
P. O. Box 1314, Teaneck, New York 07666.

☎ 201 836 9177

⚥ *Manshots*
P. O. Box 1314, Teaneck, New York 07666.
☎ 201 836 9177

Troy
Radio: Sexuality
⚢▽ *Homo Radio*
WRPI FM 91.5, c/o WRPI FM 91.5, 1 WRPI Plaza, Troy, New York 12180.
☎ 518 276 6248 ✆ 516 276 6920
☎ 518 276 2655 (machine)

Utica
Organizations: AIDS: Education
☺ ☐ **Mid-New York AIDS Coalition**
1644 Genessee Street, Utica, New York 13502-5428.
⏲ Mon Wed Fri 11:00 - 02:00

Organizations: Motorcycle
⚢▽ **Utica Tri's, MC**
& P.O. Box 425, Utica, New York 13503.
✉ mastersvox@aol.com

Organizations: Sexuality
⚥ **Greater Utica Lambda Fellowship**
P. O. Box 122, Utica, New York 13503-0122.
Newsletter serving members of Greater Utica Lambda Fellowship & the lesbigay community of Utica, New York. Publishes *Gulf Gayzette* every month. Yearly subscription is $7.50.

Publishers: Magazines: Sexuality
⚢▽ *Lesbian Interest Press (LIP)*
⚥ P. O. Box 761, Utica, New York 13503.
☎ 315 942 4035
☎ 315 336 3197 (warmline)

Stores: Erotica: General
☺▼ **Adult World**
& 319 Oriskany Boulevard, Yorkville, New York 13495.

Vestal
Organizations: Sexuality
⚥▽ **Cross Expressions**
P. O. Box 931, Vestal, New York 13851.
☎ 607 862 3203
✉ lyssa@unix.tpe.com
Contact: Mr. Daniel Stephens
Peer support for heterosexual cross dressers.

Webster
Manufacturers: Restraints: BDSM
☺ ■ **Fantasy World Products**
P.O. Box 609, Webster, New York 14580-0609.
⏲ Mon - Fri 09:00 - 17::00
⚥ ✓ $ ⚲
We manufacture Cathy's Cuffs, soft restraints, whips, blindfolds, spankers, collars, & leashes. High quality adult products since 1981. Catalogue, free with SASE or IRC. Age statement of 21 is required.

Williamsville
Organizations: Sexuality
⚢☐▽ **The Society for the Second Self (Tri-Ess)—Nu Phi Chi**
Box 197, 7954 Transit Road, Williamsville, New York 14221-4100.
Also known as the Buffalo Belles.

Woodside
Organizations: Sexuality
☺ ☐ **The Skinnydippers**
51-04 39th. Avenue, Woodside, New York 11377-3145.
☎ 718 651 4689 ✆ 718 424 1883
Publishes *Skinnydipping*.

Woodstock
Piercers
☺ ■ **Pat's Tats**
102 Mill Hill Road, Woodstock, New York 12498.
☎ 914 679 4429
⏲ By appointment Mon - Thu, walk-in on Sun

Stores: Books: General

☺ ■ **Golden Notebook**
 & 29 Tinker Street, Woodstock, New York 12498.
 ☎ 914 679 8000
 🕑 11:00 - 19:00, Summer - 21:00

NORTH CAROLINA

Area: Approximately 126,000 square kilometres
Population: Approximately 6,600,000
Capital City: Raleigh
Time zone: GMT minus 5 hours (EST)
Age of consent & homosexuality legislation: All anal & oral sex is
illegal in this state.

State Resources

Organizations: Bears

♂♥▽ **Carolina Bear Lodge**
 P. O. Box 37103, Charlotte, North Carolina 28237.
 ☎ 704 529 2891

 Statewide social group for bears & bear lovers that provides a wide
 variety of activities for members. Publishes a newsletter every month.
 Age statement of 21 is required.

Publishers: Magazines: Erotic

♂♥▼ **Blue Nights**
 & Pride Publishing & Typesetting, Inc., P. O. Box 221841, Charlotte, North
 Carolina 28222.
 ☎ 704 531 9988 ✆ 704 531 1361
 ✉ prdtype@cybernetics.net
 🌐 $ VISA ● 💳
 Guide to adult entertainment, with erotic fiction, reviews of latest videos,
 witty advice column, & over 5 pages of personals. Published every two
 weeks. Yearly subscription is $30U.S.. Age statement of 18 is required.

Asheville

Counsellors

♂♥▼ **James Harrison, Ph.D.**
K & 172 Asheland Avenue, Asheville, North Carolina 28801.
 ☎ 704 253 3055
 🕑 09:00 - 19:00 & by appointment
 ✆ $ ✉ VISA ●
 Gay affirmative psychological services.

Helplines: Sexuality

♂♥▽ **Asheville Gay & Lesbian Information Line**
 c/o SALGA, P. O. Box 197, Asheville, North Carolina 28802.
 ☎ 704 253 2971

Organizations: AIDS: Education

☺ □ **Mountain AIDS Coalition**
 & P. O. Box 1862, Asheville, North Carolina 28802.
 ☎ 704 253 4647

☺ □ **Western North Carolina AIDS Project**
 & P. O. Box 2411, Asheville, North Carolina 28802.
 ☎ 704 252 7489

Organizations: AIDS: Support

☺ ▽ **PWA Support Groups**
 & c/o All Souls Episcopal Church, P. O. Box 5978, Asheville, North Carolina
 28813.
 ☎ 704 277 7815
 ☎ 704 669 2635

Organizations: Family

☺ ▽ **Parents & Friends of Lesbians & Gays (PFLAG)—**
 & **Western North Carolina**
 P. O. Box 5978, Asheville, North Carolina 28813.
 ☎ 704 277 7815
 ☎ 704 669 2635

Organizations: Sexuality

♂♥▽ **Southern Appalachian Lesbian & Gay Alliance**
 & **(SALGA)**
 P. O. Box 197, Asheville, North Carolina 28802.
 ☎ 704 645 5908

▽□ **Phœnix Transgender Support**
 P. O. Box 18332, Asheville, North Carolina 28814.
 ☎ 704 259 9428
 Publishes *Gender Quest*.

Organizations: Sexuality: Youth

♂♥▽ **OutFit**
 & c/o All Souls Episcopal Church, P. O. Box 5978, Asheville, North Carolina

28813.
 ☎ 704 277 7815
 ☎ 704 669 2635

Publishers: Newspapers: Sexuality

♂♥▽ **Community Connections**
 P. O. Box 18088, Asheville, North Carolina 28814.
 ☎ 704 252 4037

Stores: Books: General

☺ ▼ **Downtown Books & News**
 & 67 North Lexington Street, Asheville, North Carolina 28801.
 ☎ 704 253 8654
 🕑 08:00 - 18:00, Sun - 16:00

☺ ▼ **Malaprop's Bookstore**
 & 61 Haywood, Asheville, North Carolina 28801.
 ☎ 704 254 6734
 🕑 09:00 - 20:00, Fri Sat - 22:00, Sun 12:00 - 17:00

Boone

Organizations: AIDS: Support

♂♥▽ **Hope HIV Support Group**
 Box 549A, Boone, North Carolina 28607.
 ☎ 704 264 4109

Organizations: Family

☺ □ **Parents & Friends of Lesbians & Gays (PFLAG)—**
 Boone
 Box 549A, Boone, North Carolina 28607.
 ☎ 704 264 4109

Organizations: Sexuality: Student

♂♥▽ **SAGA**
 ASU Box 8979, Boone, North Carolina 28608.
 ✆ 704 265 2636

Chapel Hill

Organizations: AIDS: Education

☺ ▽ **AIDS Service Agency**
 P. O. Box 16572, Chapel Hill, North Carolina 27516.
 ☎ 919 990 1101

Organizations: Sexuality: Student

♂♥▽ **Bisexuals, Gay Men, Lesbians, & Allies for**
 & **Diversity (B-GLAD)**
 Box 39, Carolina Union CB5210, Chapel Hill, North Carolina 27599.
 ☎ 919 962 4401

Printers: General

☺ ■ **Professional Press**
 P.O. Box 4371, Chapel Hill, North Carolina 27515-4371.
 ☎ 919 942 8020 ✆ 919 942 3094

Stores: Books: General

☺ ■ **Internationalist Books**
 & P. O. Box 951, Chapel Hill, North Carolina 27514.
 ☎ 919 942 1740
 🕑 Mon Wed Fri 12:00 - 18:00, Tue Thu 12:00 - 20:00, Sat 10:00 -
 18:00

⊕ ■ **Southern Sisters**
 102 Groomsbridge Court, Chapel Hill, North Carolina 27516-1103.
 ☎ 919 682 0739

Charlotte

Bars: BDSM

♂ **Brass Rail**
 3707 Wilkinson Boulevard, Charlotte, North Carolina.
 ☎ 704 399 8413
 🕑 Mon - Sat 17:00 - 02:30, Sun 15:00 - 02:30

BBSs: BDSM

☺ ■ **The Exchange**
 ✆ 704 342 2333

Health Services

☺ ☺ **Carolinas Medical Center**
 100 Blythe Avenue, Charlotte, North Carolina 28203.
 ☎ 704 355 2000

☺ ☺ **Presbyterian Hospital**
 200 Hawthorne Lane, Charlotte, North Carolina 28204.
 ☎ 704 384 4942

Helplines: Sexuality

Gay & Lesbian Switchboard of Charlotte
P. O. Box 11144, Charlotte, North Carolina 28220.
☎ 704 535 6277 (also TDD)
TDD also available on this number.

Organizations: AIDS: Education

Metrolina AIDS Project
P. O. Box 32662, Charlotte, North Carolina 28232.
☎ 800 289 2437
☎ 704 333 2437
Mon - Fri 09:30 - 18:30. Office: 704 333 1435 Mon - Fri 09:00 - 17:00

Outreach UFS
United Way Building, 301 South Brevard Street, Charlotte, North Carolina 28202.
☎ 704 332 9034

Organizations: AIDS: Support

The Refuge
P. O. Box 31564, Charlotte, North Carolina 28231.
☎ 704 372 5499

Organizations: BDSM

Tradesmen, Inc.
P. O. Box 36712, Charlotte, North Carolina 28204.

Organizations: Bears

Confederate Bears
Suite 304D, 300 Sharon Amity, Charlotte, North Carolina 28211.

Organizations: Family

Parents & Friends of Lesbians & Gays (PFLAG)—Charlotte
5815 Charing Place, Charlotte, North Carolina 28211.
☎ 704 364 1474

Organizations: Sexuality

Alternative Gender-Oriented (AGO)
1235-E East Boulevard, Charlotte, North Carolina 28203.

Black & White Men Together (BWMT)—Charlotte
P. O. Box 411734, Charlotte, North Carolina 28241.
☎ 704 563 0067

Carolina Trans-Sensual Alliance
P. O. Box 25347, Charlotte, North Carolina 28229-5347.
☎ 704 531 8838
Publishes *All The Beautiful People*.

Married Men's Group
P. O. Box 19524, Charlotte, North Carolina 28219.

Metrolina Community Service Project
P. O. Box 11144, Charlotte, North Carolina 28220.
☎ 704 535 6277 (also TDD)

The Society for the Second Self (Tri-Ess)—Kappa Beta
P. O. Box 12101, Charlotte, North Carolina 28220.
Meets every 3rd. WE
Publishes *The Pink Slip*.

WOW!
P. O. Box 12072, Charlotte, North Carolina 28220.
☎ 704 364 5435

Organizations: Sexuality: Youth

Time Out Youth
P. O. Box 11122, Charlotte, North Carolina 28220.
☎ 704 377 3399

Printers: General

Delmar Printing & Publishing
P.O. Box 1013, Charlotte, North Carolina 28201-1013.
☎ 704 847 9801 Fax 704 845 1218

Publishers: Miscellaneous

Integrity Indexing
Suite 1, 2012 Queens Road West, Charlotte, North Carolina 28207.
☎ 704 335 9936

Publishers: Newspapers: Sexuality

Q Notes
Pride Publishing & Typsetting, Inc., P. O. Box 221841, Charlotte, North Carolina 28222.
☎ 704 531 9988 Fax 704 531 1361
pridtype@cybernetics.net
Mon - Fri 13:00 - 17:00
✓
The Carolinas' most comprehensive gay & lesbian newspaper. No 900 phone sex ads. Distributed all over North & South Carolina. Published every month. Yearly subscription is $15.

Stores: Books: General

Independence News
3205 The Plaza, Charlotte, North Carolina 28205.
☎ 704 332 8430

Paper Skyscraper
300 East Boulevard, Charlotte, North Carolina 28203.
☎ 704 333 7130

Rising Moon Books & Beyond
316 East Boulevard, Charlotte, North Carolina 28203.
☎ 704 332 7473
Mon - Thu 10:00 - 19:00, Fri Sat - 18:00, Sun 13:00 - 18:00
✓ $ VISA MC
Multicultural focus, including gay, lesbian, bisexual, transexual, African - Native - Asian, American. Jewelry, music, cards, T-shirts, buttons, etc.. some French also spoken.

White Rabbit Books
314 Rensselaer Avenue, Charlotte, North Carolina 28203.
☎ 704 377 4067

Dallas

Organizations: Family

Parents & Friends of Lesbians & Gays (PFLAG)—Southeast Region
P. O. Box 722, Dallas, North Carolina 28034.
☎ 704 922 9273

Durham

Counsellors

Androgyny Center
Suite 186, 3325 Chapel Hill Road, Durham, North Carolina 27707.
☎ 919 489 8753

Health Services

Lesbian & Gay Health Project
P. O. Box 3203, Durham, North Carolina 27715-3203.
☎ 919 286 4107
Publishes a newsletter.

Helplines: Sexuality

Lesbian & Gay Health Project
☎ 919 286 4107

Organizations: AIDS: Education

The AIDS Services Project
P. O. Box 3203, Durham, North Carolina 27715-3203.
☎ 919 268 7475

Organizations: AIDS: Research

Duke AIDS Research & Treatment Center
P. O. Box 3284, Duke University Medical Center, Durham, North Carolina 27710.
☎ 919 684 5260

Organizations: AIDS: Support

People With HIV/AIDS Support Group
c/o Lesbian & Gay Health Project, P. O. Box 3203, Durham, North Carolina 27715-3203.
☎ 919 286 4107
☎ 919 286 7475

Organizations: Sexuality

Black & White Men Together (BWMT)—Durham
P. O. Box 3411, Durham, North Carolina 27702-3411.
Publishes a newsletter.

Triangle Lesbian & Gay Alliance
P. O. Box 3295, Durham, North Carolina 27705-1295.
☎ 919 929 4053

Organizations: Sexuality: Youth

Outright
P. O. Box 3203, Durham, North Carolina 2715-3203.
☎ 800 879 2300 (within NC)
☎ 919 286 2396
Triangle area gay, lesbian, & bisexual youth (13 - 22).

Stores: Books: General

Bull Durham's News

North Gate Mall, Durham, North Carolina 27705.
☎ 919 286 4054

Regulator Bookshop
720 9th. Street, Durham, North Carolina 27705.
☎ 919 286 2700

Fayetteville

Bars: BDSM

Oz
2540 Gillespie Street, Fayetteville, North Carolina 28306.
☎ 910 485 2037
Some leather.

Health Services

Cape Fear Valley Medical Center
1638 Owen Drive, Fayetteville, North Carolina 28304.
☎ 910 609 4000

Organizations: Sexuality

Lambda Association of Fayetteville
P. O. Box 53281, Fayetteville, North Carolina 28305.
☎ 910 484 7337

Stores: Erotica: General

Fort Video & News
4431 Bragg Boulevard, Fayetteville, North Carolina 28303.
☎ 910 868 9905
24hrs.

President News
3712 Bragg Boulevard, Fayetteville, North Carolina 28303.

Flat Rock

Organizations: Family

Parents & Friends of Lesbians & Gays (PFLAG)—Flat Rock
Box 105L, Route 2, Flat Rock, North Carolina 28731.
☎ 704 696 8250

Gastonia

Stores: Erotica: General

321 News & Video
1410 North Chester Street, Gastonia, North Carolina 28052.
☎ 704 866 0075

Greensboro

Health Services

Moses H. Cone Memorial Hospital
1200 North Elm Street, Greensboro, North Carolina 27401.
☎ 910 574 7000

Helplines: Sexuality

Alternative Resources of the Triad
P. O. Box 4442, Greensboro, North Carolina 27404.
☎ 910 274 2100
☎ 910 748 0031

Organizations: AIDS: Education

Triad Health Project
P. O. Box 5716, Greensboro, North Carolina 27435.
☎ 910 275 1654

Organizations: BDSM

Tarheel Leather Club
P. O. Box 16457, Greensboro, North Carolina 27416-0457.
☎ 910 288 4709
masterwolf@aol.com
Weekday evenings until 24:00. Organizes a run 4th. Jul
✓
Contact: Mr. Frank Sabino
Publishes *Tar & Feathers* every month. Age statement of 21 is required.

Organizations: Body Size

Girth & Mirth—North Carolina
P. O. Box 38032, Greensboro, North Carolina 27438.
☎ 704 274 2100
Publishes *Carolina Chubby Review*.

Great Triad Men
P. O. Box 38032, Greensboro, North Carolina 27438.

Organizations: Family

Parents & Friends of Lesbians & Gays (PFLAG)—Greensboro
P. O. Box 4442, Greensboro, North Carolina 27404.
☎ 910 274 2100

Organizations: Sexuality

Black & White Men Together (BWMT)—Greensboro
P. O. Box 14327, Greensboro, North Carolina 27415.

Triad Gender Association
P. O. Box 78082, Greensboro, North Carolina 27427-8082.
Meets monthly
Contact: Ms. Louise Hahn, MA, NCC

Organizations: Sexuality: Student

Gay & Lesbian Student Association
Box 27, Elliott University Center, University of North Carolina at Greensboro, Greensboro, North Carolina 27412.
☎ 910 334 5110

Organizations: Sexuality: Youth

GLASS
P. O. Box 4442, Greensboro, North Carolina 27404.
☎ 910 274 2100

Stores: Books: General

White Rabbit Books & Things
1833 Spring Garden Street, Greensboro, North Carolina 27403-2286.
☎ 910 272 7604 Fax 910 272 9015
Mon - Sat 10:00 - 19:00, Sun 13:00 - 18:00
✓ VISA MC

Stores: Erotica: General

Gents
3722 High Point Road, Greensboro, North Carolina 27407.
☎ 910 855 9855

Treasure Box Video & News
1203 East Bessemer Avenue, Greensboro, North Carolina 27405.
☎ 910 373 9849
24hrs.

Hickory

Organizations: AIDS: Education

AIDS Leadership Foothills Area (ALFA)
P. O. Box 2987, Hickory, North Carolina 28603.
☎ 704 322 1447

Raleigh

Counsellors

Androgyny Center
P. O. Box 31165, Raleigh, North Carolina 27622.
☎ 919 848 0500

Health Services

Dorothea Dix Hospital
820 South Boylan Avenue, Raleigh, North Carolina 27603.
☎ 919 733 5324

Rex Hospital
4420 Lake Boone Trail, Raleigh, North Carolina 27607.
☎ 919 783 3100

Helplines: Sexuality

Gay & Lesbian Helpline of Wake County
P. O. Box 36207, Raleigh, North Carolina 27606-6207.
☎ 919 821 0055
1900 - 22:00

Organizations: AIDS: Education

AIDS Service Agency of Wake County
P. O. Box 12583, Raleigh, North Carolina 27605.
☎ 919 834 2437
Mon - Fri 09:00 - 17:00

Wake County Department of Health
10 Sunnybrook Road, Raleigh, North Carolina 27620-4049.
☎ 919 250 3950 (counselling & testing) Fax 919 250 0443
☎ 919 250 3999 (HIV early intervention)
Also: AIDS Case Management 919 250 4510.

Organizations: BDSM

Triangle Area Power Exchange (TAPE)
P. O. Box 89708, Raleigh, North Carolina 27624.

Organizations: Family

Parents & Friends of Lesbians & Gays (PFLAG)—Raleigh

P. O. Box 10844, Raleigh, North Carolina 27605-0844.
☎ 919 380 9325

Organizations: Sexuality: Student

North Carolina State Lesbian / Gay Student Union
P. O. Box 7314, North Carolina State University, Raleigh, North Carolina 27695.
☎ 929 829 9553

Organizations: Sexuality: Youth

A Safer Place Youth Network (ASPYN)
P. O. Box 12831, Raleigh, North Carolina 27605-2831.
☎ 929 851 9544

Piercers

Fleshworks
☎ 919 782 5548

Publishers: Newspapers: Sexuality

Front Page
P. O. Box 27928, Raleigh, North Carolina 27611.
☎ 919 829 0181 Fax 919 829 0830
Mon - Fri 13:00 - 21:00
✓
Gay men & lesbians in North & South Carolina. Published twice a month. Yearly subscription is $35. Age statement of 18 is required.

Stores: Erotica: BDSM

Innovations
517 Hillsborough Street, Raleigh, North Carolina 27603.
☎ 919 833 4833
Wed - Sat 11:00 - 19:00, Sun 13:00 - 19:00
✓ $ VISA MC

Stores: Erotica: General

Our Place
327 West Hargett Street, Raleigh, North Carolina 27601.
☎ 919 833 8968

Pegasus
6804 Davis Circle, Raleigh, North Carolina 27612.
☎ 919 782 2481

Ramseur

Stores: Leatherwork Supplies: General

Zack White Leather
1515 Main Street, Ramseur, North Carolina 27316.
☎ 800 633 0396

Salisbury

Organizations: Sexuality

GDANC Support Group
P. O. Box 305, Salisbury, North Carolina 28145.
☎ 704 642 1914
Meets 3rd. Sat of month

Sanford

Organizations: AIDS: Education

Lee County AIDS Task Force (LCATF)
P. O. Box 4262, Sanford, North Carolina 27331-4262.

Stores: Erotica: General

Sanford Video & News
667 Homer Boulevard, Sanford, North Carolina 27330.
☎ 919 774 9124

Wilmington

Health Services

New Hanover Regional Medical Center
2131 South 17th. Street, Wilmington, North Carolina 28401.
☎ 910 343 7000

Helplines: Sexuality

Gay & Lesbian Switchboard
c/o GROW, Suite 182, 341-11 South College Road, Wilmington, North Carolina 28403.
☎ 910 675 9222

Organizations: AIDS: Education

GROW
Suite 182, 341-11 South College Road, Wilmington, North Carolina 28403.
☎ 910 675 9222

University of North Carolina - Wilmington
Committee on AIDS, 601 South College Road, Wilmington, North Carolina 28403.
☎ 910 395 3119

Organizations: BDSM

Menamore Levi / Leather Club
P. O. Box 7364, Wilmington, North Carolina 28406.
☎ 910 675 9222 Ext.: 534
Menamore@aol.com
Contact: Mr. Chris Zimmerman
Age statement of 21 is required.

Organizations: Family

Parents & Friends of Lesbians & Gays (PFLAG)—Wilmington
☎ 910 392 6475
Contact: Mr. Alvin Landy

Organizations: Sexuality

Between Ourselves
2148 Harrison Street, Wilmington, North Carolina 28401-6922.

Publishers: Newspapers: Sexuality

Between Ourselves
2148 Harrison, Wilmington, North Carolina 28401.

Winston-Salem

Counsellors

Louise Hahn, MA, NCC
940 Hutton Street, Winston-Salem, North Carolina 27101.
☎ 910 727 0008
Also in Durham.

Sam Manoogian, Ph.D.
1338 Ashley Square, Winston-Salem, North Carolina 27103.
☎ 910 765 5636
Wide range of psychological counselling.

Manoogian Psychological Associates
1338 Ashley Square, Winston-Salem, North Carolina 27103.
☎ 910 765 5636
Wide range of psychological counselling.

Organizations: AIDS: Education

AIDS Task Force of Winston-Salem
P. O. Box 20983, Winston-Salem, North Carolina 27120-0983.
☎ 910 7223 5031

Organizations: Family

Parents & Friends of Lesbians & Gays (PFLAG)—Winston-Salem
P. O. Box 15477, Winston-Salem, North Carolina 27113.
☎ 910 723 6345

NORTH DAKOTA

Area: Approximately 179,000 square kilometres
Population: Approximately 640,000
Capital City: Bismarck
Time zone: GMT minus 6 hours (CST)
Age of consent & homosexuality legislation: State has adopted the Model Penal Code or otherwise decriminalized homosexual activities.
Legal drinking age: 21

Fargo

Organizations: AIDS: Education

Dakota AIDS Project
P. O. Box 2, Fargo, North Dakota 58107.
☎ 701 287 2437

Dakota Life Foundation
P. O. Box 1773, Fargo, North Dakota 58107.
☎ 701 287 2437
Publishes *Turning Points*.

Piercers

Sterling Rose Tattooing & Piercing
1344 Main Avenue, Fargo, North Dakota 58103.
☎ 701 232 1744
By appointment only

Stores: Books: General

Food For Thought Alternative Book Store
314 10th. Street North, Fargo, North Dakota 58102.
☎ 701 239 4052

Stores: Erotica: General

☺ ■ **Adult Books & Cinema**
 ⅙ 417 Northern Pacific Avenue, Fargo, North Dakota 58102.
 ☎ 701 232 9768

Grand Forks

Organizations: Sexuality: Student

⚥▽ **University of North Dakota G&L Coalition**
 P. O. Box 8055, Grand Forks, North Dakota 58202.

Stores: Erotica: General

☺ ■ **Plain Brown Wrapper II**
 102 South 3rd. Street, Grand Forks, North Dakota 58201.
 ☎ 701 772 9021

Minot

Stores: Books: General

☺ ■ **Risque's**
 ⅙ 1514 South Broadway, Minot, North Dakota 58701.
 ☎ 701 839 9033

OHIO

Area: Approximately 106,000 square kilometres
Population: Approximately 10,900,000
Capital City: Columbus
Time zone: GMT minus 5 hours (EST)
Age of consent & homosexuality legislation: State has adopted the Model Penal Code or otherwise decriminalized homosexual activities.
Legal drinking age: 21

State Resources

Archives: Sexuality

⚥▽ **Ohio Lesbian Archives**
 ☒ c/o Crazy Ladies, 4039 Hamilton Avenue, Cincinnati, Ohio 45223.
 ☎ 513 541 1917
 ⊕ By appointment

Competitions & Conventions: Music

⚥▽ **Ohio Lesbian Festival**
 ⅙ c/o Lesbian Business Association, P. O. Box 82086, Columbus, Ohio 43202.
 ☎ 614 267 3953
 ⊕ Usually held in September
 Usually attended by many lesbians who enjoy BDSM.

Helplines: AIDS

☺ □ **Ohio AIDS Hotline**
 ⅙ c/o Columbus AIDS Task Force, Suite 329, 1500 West 3rd. Avenue, Columbus, Ohio 43212.
 ☎ 800 332 2437
 ☎ 800 332 3889
 ⊕ 09:00 - 21:00, Sat Sun - 18:00

Organizations: AIDS: Education

☺ □ **AIDS Foundation Miami Valley**
 ⅙ P. O. Box 3539, Dayton, Ohio 45401.
 ☎ 513 277 2437 ☏ 513 277 7619
 Publishes *Quest*.

☺ □ **Ohio AIDS Coalition (OAC)**
 P. O. Box 10034, Columbus, Ohio 43201.
 ☎ 614 445 8277 ☏ 614 445 8283
 Publishes *Wellness Times*.

Publishers: Newspapers: Sexuality

⚥▽ *Dinah*
 P. O. Box 1485, Cincinnati, Ohio 45201.
 Cincinnati's lesbian newsletter, published since 1975, features local & national news, opinions, poetry, reviews, etc., of interest to lesbians. Published every two months. Yearly subscription is $10.

⚥▼ *Gay People's Chronicle*
 P. O. Box 5426, Cleveland, Ohio 44101.
 ☎ 216 631 8646 ☏ 216 631 1082
 ✉ ChronOhio@aol.com
 The Chronicle is dedicated to providing Ohio's lesbian & gay community with a forum to communicate. Published every two weeks. Yearly subscription is $40.

⚥▼ *Gaybeat*
 ⅙ Suite 103, 772 North High Street, Columbus, Ohio 43215-1457.
 ☎ 614 297 1500 ☏ 614 297 1502

⚥▼ *Ohio Word*
 Word Publications, Suite 2800, Tower 1, 225 East North Street, Indianapolis, Indiana 46204-1349.

☎ 317 579 3075 ☏ 317 687 8840
⊕ 24hr. answering machine
✍ ✔
Men-oriented. 3 state editions (Indiana, Kentucky, & Ohio). No 900 phone ads, no nudity. Published every month.

Akron

Health Services

☺ □ **Akron City Hospital**
 525 East Market Street, Akron, Ohio 44304.
 ☎ 216 375 3000

Organizations: AIDS: Education

☺ □ **Northeast Ohio Task Force on AIDS**
 655 North Main Street, Akron, Ohio 443310.
 ☎ 216 375 2000

Organizations: BDSM

⚥▽ **Leather & Lace Society—Eastern Ohio**
 P. O. Box 26731, Akron, Ohio 44319.
 ✉ cz@universe.digex.net

Organizations: Body Size

⚥▽ **Girth & Mirth—Akron**
 ☎ 216 655 4259

Organizations: Family

☺ □ **Parents & Friends of Lesbians & Gays (PFLAG)—**
 ⅙ **Akron**
 3204, Cuyahoga Falls, Ohio 44223.
 ☎ 216 923 1883

Organizations: Sexuality

⚥▽ **Gay, Lesbian, & Bisexual Alliance League**
 ☒ **(GLOBAL)**
 P. O. Box 27202, Akron, Ohio 44319.
 Please address envelopes to GLOBAL, do NOT address them to Gay, Lesbian, & Bisexual Alliance League.

⚥▽ **Open Doors**
 18 North College Street, Akron, Ohio 45701.
 ☎ 61114 593 7301
 ⊕ Mon - Fri 08:00 - 16:00

Ashland

Printers: General

☺ **Bookmasters**
 P.O. Box 159, Ashland, Ohio 44805-1059.
 ☎ 419 289 6051 ☏ 419 281 1731

Athens

Organizations: AIDS: Education

☺ □ **Athens AIDS Task Force**
 ☒ 18 North College Street, Athens, Ohio 45701.
 ☎ 614 592 4397

Bowling Green

Organizations: Sexuality: Student

⚥▽ **Lesbian & Gay Alliance**
 ☒ BGSU, Box 22, University Hall, Bowling Green, Ohio 43403.
 ☎ 419 352 5242

Publishers: Magazines: Sexuality

☺ *The Journal of Sex Research*
 Bowling Green State University, Bowling Green, Ohio 43403.
 ☎ 419 372 2301

Cincinnati

Bars: BDSM

⚥▼ **The Dock**
 ⅙ 603 Pete Rose Way, Cincinnati, Ohio 45202.
 ☎ 513 241 5623

⚥▼ **Spurs**
 ⅙ 326 East 8th. Street, Cincinnati, Ohio 45202-2217.
 ☎ 513 621 2668
 ⊕ 16:00 - 02:30
 ✍ $ ⚊

Counsellors

☺ ■ **Ashland Psychological Services**
 2334 Ashland Avenue, Cincinnati, Ohio 45206.
 ☎ 513 861 8365

Health Services

☺ □ **Jewish Hospital of Cincinnati**
3200 Burnett Avenue, Cincinnati, Ohio 45229.
☎ 513 569 2000

☺ □ **STD Clinic**
⟁ 3101 Burnet Avenue, Cincinnati, Ohio 45229.
☎ 513 352 3138

☺ □ **University of Cincinnati Hospital**
234 Goodman Street, Cincinnati, Ohio 45267.
☎ 513 558 1000

☺ □ **Veterans' Affairs Medical Center**
3200 Vine Street, Cincinnati, Ohio 45220.
☎ 513 861 3100

Helplines: Sexuality

♂♀▽ **Gay & Lesbian Community Switchboard**
P. O. Box 141061, Cincinnati, Ohio 45250-1061.
☎ 513 651 0070
⏲ Mon - Fri 19:00 - 23:00

Organizations: AIDS: Education

☺ □ **AIDS Volunteers of Cincinnati**
⟁ 2183 Central Parkway, Cincinnati, Ohio 45214.
☎ 513 421 2437
Publishes *AVOC Newsletter*.

☺ □ **Greater Cincinnati AIDS Consortium**
P. O. Box 19353, Cincinnati, Ohio 45219.
☎ 513 558 4259

Organizations: BDSM

♂ **Cincinnati Chaps**
P.O. Box 3104, Cincinnati, Ohio 45201.

♂▽ **Temple of Hecate**
P. O. Box 24067, Cincinnati, Ohio 45224-0067.

Organizations: Bears

♂▽ **Cincinnati's River Bears**
P. O. Box 431, Cincinnati, Ohio 54201.
☎ 513 921 6472
Contact: Jack

♂▽ **River Bears**
P. O. Box 431, Cincinnati, Ohio 45201.

Organizations: Family

☺ □ **Parents & Friends of Lesbians & Gays (PFLAG)—**
⟁ **Greater Cincinnati**
P. O. Box 19634, Cincinnati, Ohio 45219-0634.
☎ 513 721 7900
⏲ Meets 2nd. Tue of month 19:30

Organizations: Sexuality

▽□ **Cross-Port**
P. O. Box 54657, Cincinnati, Ohio 45254-0657.
☎ 513 474 9557
✉ crossport@aol.com
Contact: Shelbi
Publishes *Cross-Port InnerView Newsletter*.

♂▽ **Greater Cincinnati Gay / Lesbian Coalition**
⟁ P. O. Box 19158, Cincinnati, Ohio 45219.
☎ 513 557 2904

Organizations: Sexuality: Student

♂▽ **Lesbian / Gay Academic Union of Greater**
⟁ **Cincinnati**
P. O. Box 19630, Cincinnati, Ohio 45219.
☎ 513 281 7496
Publishes *LGAY Newsletter*.

♂▽ **U.C. Alliance of Lesbian, Gay, & Bisexual People**
⟁ Mail Location #136, 211 Tangeman Center, Cincinnati, Ohio 45221-0136.
☎ 513 556 1449

Publishers: Newspapers: Sexuality

♂▼ *Nouveau Midwest*
P. O. Box 3176, Cincinnati, Ohio 45201.
☎ 513 621 9500

Radio: Sexuality

♂▽ *Alternating Currents*
🎧 WAIF FM 88.3, P. O. Box 6126, Cincinnati, Ohio 45206.
☎ 513 961 8900 (office)
☎ 513 749 1444 (studio during show)
⏲ Sat 15:00 - 17:00

Stores: Books: General

⚥ ▼ **Crazy Ladies Bookstore**
⟁ 4039 Hamilton Avenue, Cincinnati, Ohio 45223.
📞 513 541 4198

♂▼ **Pink Pyramid**
36A West Court Street, Cincinnati, Ohio 45202.
☎ 513 621 7465
⏲ Mon - Thu 11:00 - 21:00, Fri Sat 11:00 - 23:00

Stores: Erotica: BDSM

♂▼ **ACME Leather & Toy Co.**
326 East 8th. Street, Cincinnati, Ohio 45202-2217.
☎ 513 621 7390
⏲ Tue Thu Sun 19:00 - 01:00, Fri Sat 22:00 - 02:30
🔥 ✓ $ 💳 🏧
Catalogue available. Age statement of 21 is required.

☺ ▼ **Kinks**
⟁ 1118 Race Street, Cincinnati, Ohio 45210-1919.
☎ 513 651 2668
⏲ 14:00 - 20:00
🔥 ✓ $ 💳 🏧
Age statement of 18 is required.

Cleveland

Archives: General

⚥ □ **What She Wants Feminist Library**
⟁ P. O. Box 18465, Cleveland, Ohio 44118.
☎ 216 321 3054

Bars: BDSM

♂▼ **Leather Stallion Saloon**
2205 Saint Clair Avenue, Cleveland, Ohio 44114.
☎ 216 589 8588
⏲ 12:00 - 14:30

♂■ **Tomahawk**
11217 Detroit Avenue, Cleveland, Ohio 44102.
☎ 216 521 5443

Health Services

☺ □ **Cleveland Clinic Hospital**
9500 Euclid Avenue, Cleveland, Ohio 44195.
☎ 216 444 2200

☺ □ **Saint Luke's Medical Center**
11311 Shaker Boulevard, Cleveland, Ohio 44104.
☎ 216 368 7000

☺ □ **University Hospital of Cleveland**
2074 Abingdon Road, Cleveland, Ohio 44106.
☎ 216 844 1000
HIV & emergency departments.

☺ □ **Veterans' Affairs Medical Center**
10000 Brecksville Road, Cleveland, Ohio 44141.
☎ 216 526 3030

Helplines: Sexuality

♂▽ **Cleveland Lesbian / Gay Hotline**
⟁ P. O. Box 6177, Cleveland, Ohio 44101.
☎ 216 781 6736
⏲ 19:00 - 23:00, Sat 17:00 - 20:00, Sun 19:00 - 22:00

Manufacturers: Furniture: BDSM

☺ **VIPPS**
P. O. Box 81508, Cleveland, Ohio 44181.
☎ 216 899 1326
Portable bondage sling that comes apart in minutes.

Organizations: AIDS: Education

☺ □ **Health Issues Task Force**
⟁ 2250 Euclid Avenue, Cleveland, Ohio 44115.
☎ 216 621 0766
⏲ Mon - Fri 09:00 - 17:00
Publishes a newsletter.

Organizations: AIDS: Support

☺ □ **The Living Room**
⟁ P. O. Box 6177, Cleveland, Ohio 44101.
☎ 216 522 1998
📞 216 522 0025

Organizations: BDSM

♂ **Excalibur of Cleveland**
c/o The Leather Stallion Saloon, 2205 Saint Clair Avenue, Cleveland, Ohio 44114.

♂▽ **Ohio Broncos**
Suite 2, 6808 Detroit, Cleveland, Ohio 44102-3021.

☞▽ **Rangers**
P.O. Box 6504, Cleveland, Ohio 44101-0504.
Contact: Mr. George Roscoe

☞ **Stallions**
c/o The Leather Stallion, 2203 Saint Clair Avenue, Cleveland, Ohio 44114.

☞ **Tower City Corps**
c/o Ohio City OASIS, Attention: Club Cleveland, 2909 Detroit, Cleveland, Ohio 44113.

Organizations: Bears
☞▽ **Arktos**
P. O. Box 14838, Cleveland, Ohio 4414-0838.

Organizations: Family
☞▽ **Gay Fathers**
🕭 P. O. Box 91853, Cleveland, Ohio 44101.
☎ 216 621 0228

☺☐ **Parents & Friends of Lesbians & Gays (PFLAG)—Cleveland**
14260 Larchmere Boulevard, Cleveland, Ohio 44120.
☎ 216 321 7413

⊕ ▽ **Wives of Bisexual & Married Gay Men**
🕭 P. O. Box 770932, Lakewood, Ohio 44107.
☎ 216 529 9139

Organizations: Motorcycle
☞▽ **Trident—Cleveland**
Suite 207, 11349 Edgewater Drive, Cleveland, Ohio 44107.

☞ **Unicorn MC**
2203 Saint Clair Avenue, Cleveland, Ohio 44114.

Organizations: Sexuality
☞▽ **Bisexual & Married Gay Men**
🕭 P. O. Box 770932, Lakewood, Ohio 44107.
☎ 216 529 9139

♀ ▽ **Bisexual Women's Support Group**
🕭 P. O. Box 594, Northfield, Ohio 44067.
☎ 216 467 6442
🕘 Call 09:00 - 21:00

☞▽ **Black & White Men Together (BWMT)—Cleveland**
P. O. Box 5144, Cleveland, Ohio 44101-0144.
☎ 216 4597

☞▽ **Lesbian & Gay Community Center of Greater Cleveland**
P. O. Box 6177, Cleveland, Ohio 44101.
☎ 216 522 1999
☎ 216 781 6736 (hotline)
🕘 Hotline 15:00 - 23:00

☞▽ **Northern Ohio Coalition, Inc.**
🕭 P. O. Box 15065, Cleveland, Ohio 44115-0065.
☎ 216 771 0369

Organizations: Sexuality: Student
☞▽ **CSU Lambda Delta Lambda**
Box 79, CSU, UC 301, Cleveland, Ohio 44115.
☎ 216 261 8645

☞▽ **CWRU Gay Lesbian Bisexual Alliance**
♿ c/o Student Activities Office, Thwing SAO, 11111 Euclid Avenue, Cleveland, Ohio 44106.
☎ 216 368 2679

Piercers
☺■ **Body Work Productions**
☎ 216 421 7181
🕘 By appointment only

☺■ **Chain Link Addiction**
11623 Euclid Avenue, Cleveland, Ohio.
Some fetish clothing & other items.

Publishers: Newspapers: Sexuality
☞▼ *Cleveland For You & Akron Too!*
For You Productions, Edgewater Branch, P. O. Box 760, Lakewood, Ohio 44107.
☎ 800 560 8712
☎ 216 221 1940

⊕ *Lesbian World Newsletter*
P. O. Box 32147, Cleveland, Ohio 44132-0147.
☎ 216 289 2939 ✆ 216 289 5885
Positive, upbeat national & world news, & information for lesbians & feminists; multi-cultural, multi-ethnic. Published every month. Yearly subscription is $24.

Stores: Books: General
☺■ **Bookstore on West 25th.**
1921 West 25th. Street, Cleveland, Ohio 44113.
☎ 216 566 8897

☺■ **The Pavillion Mall Booksellers**
24031 Chagrin Boulevard, Cleveland, Ohio 44122.
☎ 216 831 5035

Stores: Erotica: General
☺■ **95th. Street News**
♿ 950 Lorain Avenue, Cleveland, Ohio 44102.
☎ 216 631 4010
🕘 07:30 - 23:00, Sun 12:00 - 21:00

☺■ **Bank News**
4025 Clark, Cleveland, Ohio 44109.
☎ 216 281 8777

☺▼ **Body Language**
♿ 3291 West 115th. Street, Cleveland, Ohio 44111.
☎ 216 251 3330 ✆ 216 476 3825
🕘 Mon - Sat 12:00 - 21:00, Sun 12:00 - 17:00
🕭 ✓ $ 💳 VISA 💳 💳 ℓ
Educational store for adults of alternative lifestyles, featuring leather, books, magazines, videos, erotic toys, etc.. Age statement of 21 is required.

☺■ **Chain Link Addiction**
11623 Euclid Avenue, Cleveland, Ohio.
Some fetish clothing & other items.

☺■ **Detroit Avenue News**
♿ 6515 Detroit Avenue, Cleveland, Ohio 44102.
☎ 216 961 3880
🕘 08:00 - 23:00, Sun 12:00 - 21:00

Columbus

Bars: BDSM
☞ **Eagle in Exile**
893 North 4th. Street, Columbus, Ohio 43201.
☎ 614 294 0069

BBSs: General
☺■ **Night Life**
✆ 614 876 2116
Cat's Lair forum for BDSM conversations.

Counsellors
☞▼ **Affirmations**
K 918 South Front Street, Columbus, Ohio 43206.
☎ 614 445 8277 ✆ 614 445 8283
☎ 614 445 8283 (TTY)
🕘 Mon - Thu 08:00 - 22:00, Fri 08:00 - 18:00, Sat varies
🕭 ✓ $ 💳 VISA 💳 💳
A center for psychotherapy & growth. A multi-disciplinary private psychotherapy practice promoting recovery, self-empowerment, positive self-esteem, & acceptance of our diversities. American Sign Language also spoken.

☺▼ **Clintonville Counseling Services**
3840 North High Street, Columbus, Ohio 43214.
☎ 614 261 1126

☺▼ **Joseph Shannon, Ph.D.**
♿ 1155 West 3rd. Avenue, Columbus, Ohio 43212.
☎ 614 297 0422
🕘 08:00 - 20:00, Sat 08:00 - 14:00

☺■ **Village Counseling, Inc.**
11 East Kossuth Street, Columbus, Ohio 43206.
☎ 614 444 7714

Health Services
☺☐ **Mount Carmel Medical Center**
793 West State Street, Columbus, Ohio 43222.
☎ 614 225 5000

☺☐ **Ohio State University Medical Center**
410 West Tenth Avenue, Columbus, Ohio 43210.
☎ 614 293 8000
HIV & emergency departments.

Helplines: Sexuality
☺▽ **North Central Mental Health Services**
1301 North High Street, Columbus, Ohio 43201.
☎ 614 299 6600
Mental helath hotline & service provider.

Organizations: AIDS: Education
☺☐ **AIDS Service Connection**

P. O. Box 16178, Columbus, Ohio 43216.
☎ 614 291 2300

☺ ☐ **Columbus AIDS Task Force**
 ⅙ Suite 329, 1500 West 3rd. Avenue, Columbus, Ohio 43212.
 ☎ 800 332 2437
 ☎ 614 488 2437
 Also deaf TTY: 800 332 3889.

☺ ☐ **Ohio State University Hospitals**
 ⅙ AIDS Clinical Trials Unit, Suite 4725, 456 West 10th. Avenue, Columbus,
 Ohio 43210.
 ☎ 614 293 8112

Organizations: AIDS: Support

☺ ☐ **Southeast Counseling Services**
 ⅊ HIV Counseling Program, 1455 South 4th. Street, Columbus, Ohio
 43207.
 ☎ 614 445 3330 ✆ 614 444 0800
 ⏰ By appointment

Organizations: BDSM

⚥ ☐ **Briar Rose**
 ⅊ P.O. Box 163143, Columbus, Ohio 43216.
 Contact: Ms. Jan Hall
 Age statement of 21 is required.

⚧▽ **Centurions of Columbus**
 P. O. Box 09208, Columbus, Ohio 43209.

⚧▽ **Dragon LC**
 P. O. Box 06417, Columbus, Ohio 43206.

☺ ▽ **The National Leather Association (NLA)—**
Columbus
 P. O. Box 2763, Columbus, Ohio 43216-2763.
 ☎ 614 470 2093
 ✉ donbear@infinet.com
 ⏰ Meets 2nd. Sun of month
 Contact: Secretary

⚧ **Vulcan LL**
 P. O. Box 18352, Columbus, Ohio 43218.

Organizations: Bears

⚧▽ **Columbus Ursine Brotherhood**
 P. O. Box 16822, Columbus, Ohio 43216.
 ✉ Chuckybear@aol.com

Organizations: Family

⚧▽ **Gay & Lesbian Parenting Group of Central Ohio**
 ⅊ P. O. Box 16235, Columbus, Ohio 43215-235.
 ☎ 614 497 8652
 Please address envelopes to GLPG/Central Ohio, do NOT address them to
 Gay & Lesbian Parenting Group of Central Ohio.

Organizations: Motorcycle

⚧▽ **Trident—Columbus**
 284 Kelton, Columbus, Ohio 43205.

Organizations: Sexuality

♂▽ **Bi-Lines**
 ⅊ P. O. Box 14773, Columbus, Ohio 43214.
 ☎ 614 341 7015

⚧▽ **Black & White Men Together (BWMT)—Columbus**
 P. O. Box 151276, Columbus, Ohio 43215.
 ☎ 614 221 2734

☒☐ **Central Ohio Gender Dysphoria Program**
 P. O. Box 82008, Columbus, Ohio 43202.
 ☎ 614 451 0111
 Contact: Mr. Meräl Crane, M.A., L.P.C.C.

⚧▽ **G/L/B Support Group**
 P. O. Box 1136, Delaware, Ohio 43015.
 ☎ 614 363 0431

⚥▽ **Momazons**
 ⅊ P. O. Box 02069, Columbus, Ohio 43202.
 ☎ 614 267 0193

Organizations: Sexuality: Student

⚧▽ **Bisexual, Gay, & Lesbian Alliance (B-GALA)**
 ⅙ 340 Ohio Union, 1739 High Street, Columbus, Ohio 43210.
 ☎ 6114 292 9212

Organizations: Sexuality: Youth

⚧▽ **Phœnix Pride Youth Group**
 ᴀⓢ Southeast Community Mental Health Center, 1455 4th. Street,
 Columbus, Ohio 43207.
 ☎ 614 445 0013 ✆ 614 445 0017
 For youth 15 - 21. Publishes *Phœnix Pride*.

Piercers

☺ ▼ **Piercology**
 874 North High Street, Columbus, Ohio 43215.
 ☎ 614 297 4743 ✆ 614 297 6855
 ⏰ Mon - Fri 12:00 - 19:00, Sat 19:00 - 24:00
 💳 ☺
 Full service body piercing salon. Please see our display advertisement.

Publishers: Books: Sexuality

☺ **Big Breakfast Publishing**
 P. O. Box 02394, Columbus, Ohio 43202.

Publishers: Directories: Sexuality

⚧▽ *Lavendar Listings*
 ⅙ P. O. Box 10814, Columbus, Ohio 43201.
 ☎ 614 299 7764 ✆ 614 299 4408
 Published once a year.

Publishers: Newspapers: Sexuality

⚥▼ *Lesbian Health News*
 P. O. Box 12121, Columbus, Ohio 43212.
 Please address envelopes to LHN, do NOT address them to *Lesbian
 Health News*.

⚧ *The News*
 P. O. Box 8296, Columbus, Ohio 43201.

⚧▼ *News of the Columbus Gay & Lesbian Community*
 P. O. Box 8296, Columbus, Ohio 43201.
 ☎ 614 263 2482
 ⏰ Call eve & WE only

⚧ *Stonewall Union Reports*
 P. O. Box 10814, Columbus, Ohio 43201-7814.

⚥▼ *The Word is Out!*
 P. O. Box 02106, Columbus, Ohio 43202.

Stores: Books: General

☺ ■ **Disco Book Store**
 973 Harrisburg Pike, Columbus, Ohio 43223.
 ☎ 614 274 9716

⚥ ▼ **Fan The Flames**

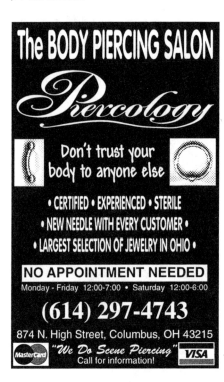

& 3387 North High Street, Columbus, Ohio 43202.
☎ 614 447 0565
🕐 Tue - Fri 11:00 - 19:00, Sat Sun 12:00 - 18:00

⚥▼ **Rainbow Bookstore**
Suite 103, 772 North High Street, Columbus, Ohio 43215.
☎ 614 297 1500

Stores: Erotica: BDSM

⚥▼ **IMRU**
235 North Lazelle, Columbus, Ohio 43215.
☎ 614 228 9660 📞 614 297 6855
☎ 614 297 8844
🕐 Wed - Sun 23:30 - 02:30

Tattooists

☺ ■ **8-Ball Tattoo**
2593 Indianola Avenue, Columbus, Ohio 43202.
☎ 614 784 8850
Body piercing also available.

Television: Sexuality

⚥▽ **Stonewall Union Lesbian / Gay Pride Report**
⚥ Cable Access Channel 21, P. O. Box 10814, Columbus, Ohio 43201-7814.
☎ 614 299 7764 📞 614 299 4408
🕐 Mon Sat 23:30

Dayton

Bars: BDSM

⚥▼ **The Edge, Inc.**
909 Patterson Road, Dayton, Ohio 45419.
☎ 513 294 0713
🕐 17:00 - 02:30
Leather shop inside.

Health Services

☺ ☐ **Combined Health District**
& Communicable Disease Clinic, 451 West 3rd. Street, Dayton, Ohio 45422-1280.
☎ 513 225 4249

☺ ☐ **Miami Valley Hospital**
One Wyoming Street, Dayton, Ohio 45409.
☎ 513 223 6192

Organizations: AIDS: Education

☺ ☐ **Community Unity Health & Wholeness Project**
& P. O. Box 4021, Dayton, Ohio 45401.
☎ 513 228 4031

Organizations: BDSM

⚥ **Gryphons**
P.O. Box 18283, Dayton, Ohio 45401-0283.

Organizations: Bears

⚥▽ **Ursus**
P. O. Box 75, Dayton, Ohio 45405.
☎ 513 643 9220
Contact: Dan or Dave

Organizations: Family

☺ ☐ **Parents & Friends of Lesbians & Gays (PFLAG)—Darke County**
1219 Northmoor Drive, Dayton, Ohio 45331.
☎ 513 547 1433

Stores: Books: General

☺ ■ **Books & Co.**
& 316A Stroop Road, Dayton, Ohio 54529.
☎ 513 298 6540

Stores: Erotica: General

☺ ■ **Exotic Bookstore**
444 East 5th. Street, Dayton, Ohio 45402.
☎ 513 228 3584

Euclid

Organizations: Bears

⚥ **Cleveland Bears**
Suite 157, 25931 Euclid Avenue, Euclid, Ohio 44132.
☎ 216 556 1570
✉ CleveBears@aol.com
🌐 http://www.skepsis.com/.gblo/bears/CLUBS/cleveland_bears.html
A social club for bears & bear admirers.

Greenville

Organizations: Family

☺ ☐ **Friends & Relatives of Gays (FROG)**
&& Great Lakes District Office, 415 Medallion Drive, Greenville, Ohio 45331.
☎ 513 548 6730

Ironton

Organizations: Bears

⚥▽ **Tri-State Bears**
P. O. Box 526, Ironton, Ohio 45638.
☎ 614 532 6307

Kent

Organizations: Sexuality: Student

⚥▽ **Lesbian, Gay, & Bisexual Union - Kent (LGBU-Kent)**
& Box 17, Student Activities, Kent State University, Kent, Ohio 44242.
🕐 Mon - Fri 09:00 - 17:00, hotline mon - Fri eve

Stores: Books: General

☺ ■ **The News & Photo Shop**
407 East Main Street, Kent, Ohio 44240.
☎ 216 678 5499

Lakewood

Organizations: Body Size

⚥▽ **Chubbies & Chasers of Cleveland**
P. O. Box 427, Lakewood, Ohio 44107.

Publishers: Newspapers: Sexuality

⚥▽ **Now Cleveland**
& P. O. Box 406, Lakewood, Ohio 44102.
☎ 216 771 0369
Published every month.

Stores: Books: General

☺ ■ **The Flying Lemur Bookstore**
P. O. Box 770222, Lakewood, Ohio 44107.
☎ 216 221 2535
🌐 http://www.apk.net/lemur/bookstr.html
🕐 Mon - Sun afternoons & early evenings. Late on weekends
Body piercing also available.

Leipsic

Suppliers: Diapers

☺ ■ **Duraline Medical Products**
P. O. Box 67, Leipsic, Ohio 45856.
☎ 800 654 3376 📞 419 943 3637
☎ 419 943 2044
Diapers & waterproof pants. Be ready to talk about your 'medical condition' when you call them. Discreet packaging upon request only.

Lima

Organizations: AIDS: Education

☺ ☐ **Lima AIDS Unit**
405 East Market, Lima, Ohio 45801.
☎ 419 228 4457

Lorain

Bars: General

⚥▼ **Nite Club**
2223 Broadway, Lorain, Ohio 44052.
☎ 216 245 6319
Some leather.

Organizations: Family

☺ ☐ **Parents & Friends of Lesbians & Gays (PFLAG)—Lorain**
P. O. Box 176, Lorain, Ohio 44052.
☎ 216 988 8215

Organizations: Sexuality

⚥▽ **Lorain Lesbian & Gay Center**
&& P. O. Box 167, Lorain, Ohio 44052.
☎ 216 960 2050
Publishes Hotlines.

Mansfield
Organizations: AIDS: Education
☺ □ **North Central Ohio AIDS Foundation**
611 Cliffside Drive, Mansfield, Ohio 44904-1501.
☎ 419 522 9357
Organizations: Sexuality
♂▽ **Lambda Support Group**
c/o 2600 Lexington Avenue, Mansfield, Ohio 44904.
☎ 419 522 0729

Marion
Organizations: Sexuality
♂▽ **Combined Forces**
P. O. Box 6132, Marion, Ohio 43302.

Mentor
Organizations: Sexuality
♂▽ **Mentor Center (HUGS East)**
P. O. Box 253, Mentor, Ohio 44061-0251.
☎ 216 974 8909

Oberlin
Organizations: Sexuality: Student
♂▽ **Oberlin College Lesbian, Gay, & Bisexual Union**
& Box 88, Wilder Hall, Oberlin, Ohio 44074.
☎ 216 775 8179
Publishes *SNAP, It's A Queer Thing.*
Publishers: Directories: Booksellers
☺ **The National Association of College Stores**
P. O. Box 58, Oberlin, Ohio 44074.
☎ 216 775 7777

Oxford
Organizations: Sexuality: Student
♂▽ **Chameleon**
& P. O. Box 382, Oxford, Ohio 45056.
☎ 614 529 3823
♂▽ **Miami University Gay, Lesbian, & Bisexual Alliance**
381 Shriver Center, Oxford, Ohio 45056.
☎ 614 529 3823

Parma
Organizations: Sexuality
▽□ **Paradise Club**
P. O. Box 29564, Parma, Ohio 44129.
☎ 216 586 9292
✉ Paradise@aol.com
Publishes *Paradise Tales.*

Reynoldsburg
Organizations: Sexuality
▽▽ **Crystal Club**
P. O. Box 287, Reynoldsburg, Ohio 43068-0287.
☎ 614 224 1165
✉ cc@stargate.com
Publishes *The Crystal Chronicle.*

Sheffield Lake
Organizations: Sexuality
▽□ **The Society for the Second Self (Tri-Ess)—Alpha Omega**
P. O. Box 2053, Sheffield Lake, Ohio 44054-0053.
Publishes *Alpha Omega Outreach.*

Springfield
Organizations: AIDS: Education
☺ □ **Clark County American Red Cross**
1830 North Limestone Street, Springfield, Ohio 45503.
☎ 513 399 3872 ✆ 513 399 6111
☺ □ **Clark County Health & Education Department**
529 East Home Road, Springfield, Ohio 45503.
☎ 513 328 2665
Piercers
☺ ■ **Piercings Unlimited**

2211 Scioto Drive, Springfield, Ohio 45506.
☎ 513 322 0877
🕐 Callofter 16:00

Steubenville
Stores: Books: General
☺ ■ **Steubenville News**
426 Market Street, Steubenville, Ohio 43952-2853.
☎ 614 282 5842

Toledo
Organizations: AIDS: Education
☺ □ **Toledo Wellness Group**
P. O. Box 391, Toledo, Ohio 43691.
☎ 419 244 6682
Organizations: Motorcycle
♂▽ **Trident—Toledo**
P. O. Box 20017, Toledo, Ohio 43620.
Organizations: Sexuality
▽▽ **Glass City Sisters**
P. O. Box 8532, Toledo, Ohio 43623.
⊕▽ **Lavendar Triangle**
& P. O. Box 178079, Toledo, Ohio 43615.
☎ 419 531 0644
Publishes *Women's Vineline.*
♂▽ **Toledo Area Gay & Lesbian Affiliation (TAGALA)**
P. O. Box 4642, Old West End Station, Toledo, Ohio 43610-0642.
☎ 419 243 9351
Publishes *TAGALA Newsletter.*
Organizations: Sexuality: Student
♂▽ **Gay & Lesbian Student Union**
& 3503-D Student Union Building, University of Toledo, Toledo, Ohio 43606-3390.
☎ 419 537 7975
Publishers: Newspapers: Sexuality
♂ **Toledo Area Gay & Lesbian Affiliation**
P. O. Box 1388, Toledo, Ohio 43603.
Publishes a newsletter.

Yellow Springs
Organizations: Sexuality: Student
♂▽ **Lesbian & Gay Rights Caucus**
& Antioch School of Law, 795 Livermore Street, Yellow Springs, Ohio 45387.
☎ 513 265 9500
Publishers: Magazines: Fetish
☺ *Batteries Not Includeed*
BNI, 130 West Limestone, Yellow Springs, Ohio 45387.
Articles, reviews, all varieties of sexual experience & fetish.

Youngstown
Organizations: Sexuality
♂▽ **Black & White Men Together (BWMT)—Youngstown**
P. O. Box 1131, Youngstown, Ohio 44501-1131.
☎ 216 782 3483
Publishers: Newspapers: Sexuality
⊕ *Life In Out*
c/o Stacy Meadows, Suite 1, 19 Illinois Avenue, Youngstown, Ohio 44505-2814.
☎ 216 782 4892
Stores: Erotica: General
☺ ■ **Uptown Bookstore**
2597 Market Street, Youngstown, Ohio 44507.
☎ 216 783 2553

OKLAHOMA

Area: Approximately 178,000 square kilometres
Population: Approximately 3,160,000
Capital City: Oklahoma City
Time zone: GMT minus 6 hours (CST)
Climate: Continental weather influenced by the Gulf of Mexico. Long, hot summers with tornadoes, & average temperatures reaching 28°C. Winters are mild, with lows averaging 2°C.

Age of consent & homosexuality legislation: Anal & oral sex is illegal in this state only between people of the same sex.
Legal drinking age: 21

State Resources

Publishers: Newspapers: Sexuality

⚥▼ **Gayly Oklahoman**
P. O. Box 60930, Oklahoma City, Oklahoma 73146.
☎ 405 528 0800
News & events publication focusing on the needs & interests of Oklahoma's gay & lesbian readership. Published twice a month. Yearly subscription is $35.

Lawton

Stores: Erotica: BDSM

☺ ■ **Things Medieval**
914 South West C Avenue, Lawton, Oklahoma 73501.
☎ 405 357 8762
Leather & chainmail clothing, BDSM toys, etc.. Also mail order.

Muskogee

Organizations: Fetish: Uniforms

⚥▽ **CHKK**
P. O. Box 1125, Muskogee, Oklahoma 74403.

Oklahoma City

Counsellors

⚥▼ **Shirley Hunter, M.Ed.**
& Suite 102, 5009 North Pennsylvania, Oklahoma City, Oklahoma 73112.
☎ 405 848 5429

☺ □ **Red Rock Mental Health Center**
440 North Lincoln Boulevard, Oklahoma City, Oklahoma 73105-5105.
☎ 405 425 0399

Health Services

☺ □ **Mercy Health Center**
4300 West Memorial Road, Oklahoma City, Oklahoma 73120.
☎ 405 755 1515

☺ ▽ **Monday Night Clinic**
& c/o HIV Prevention Services, 4400 North Lincoln Boulevard, Oklahoma City, Oklahoma 73105-5105.
☎ 405 232 5453
☎ 405 427 5812
🕐 No appointment necessary. Call only during clinic hours Mon 19:00 - 20:30
Free anonymous HIV testing. Other tests at cost.

☺ □ **Presbyterian Hospital**
700 North East 13th. Street, Oklahoma City, Oklahoma 73104.
☎ 405 271 5100

☺ □ **Saint Anthony Hospital**
1000 North Lee Street, Oklahoma City, Oklahoma 73101.
☎ 405 272 7000

⚥▽ **Testing The Limits**
& 2136 North West 39th. Street, Oklahoma City, Oklahoma 73112-8830.
☎ 405 843 8378
🕐 12:00 - 24:00
Free anonymous HIV testing.

Organizations: AIDS: Education

☺ □ **Red Rock Mental Health Center**
& AIDS Prevention Services, 440 North Lincoln Boulevard, Oklahoma City, Oklahoma 73105-5105.
☎ 405 425 0399

Organizations: AIDS: Research

☺ □ **Oklahoma City Foundation for AIDS Research**
&& 2136 North West 39th. Street, Oklahoma City, Oklahoma 73112-8830.
☎ 405 843 8378
HIV treatment. Call before visit.

Organizations: AIDS: Support

⚥▽ **AIDS Support Program**
& P. O. Box 12185, Oklahoma City, Oklahoma 73157-2185.
☎ 405 525 6277

Organizations: Bears

⚥▽ **Red Earth Bears**
P. O. Box 57561, Oklahoma City, Oklahoma 73157.
☎ 405 557 1169
📧 alanokc@aol.com or jerome@telepath. com

Organizations: Sexuality

⚥▽ **Oasis Resources Center**
&& 2135 North West 39th. Street, Oklahoma City, Oklahoma 73112.
☎ 405 525 2437
🕐 Mon - Thu 19:00 - 22:00, Fri - Sun 12:00 - 24:00

☺ □ **Red Rock Mental Health Center**
& Gay & Lesbian Outreach, 440 North Lincoln Boulevard, Oklahoma City, Oklahoma 73105-5105.
☎ 405 425 0399

⚥▽ **Sigma Beta**
P. O. Box 42122, Oklahoma City, Oklahoma 73123.

⚥▽ **The Society for the Second Self (Tri-Ess)—Sigma Beta**
P. O. Box 60354, Oklahoma City, Oklahoma 73146.

⚥▽ **Sooner Diversity**
P. O. Box 575, Norman, Oklahoma 73070.
📧 dmricks@ionet.net

Organizations: Sexuality: Student

⚥▽ **Oklahoma University Gay, Lesbian, & Bisexual Alliance**
306 Ellison Hall, 633 Elm Avenue, Norman, Oklahoma 73019-0350.
☎ 405 325 4452

Organizations: Sexuality: Youth

⚥▽ **Young Gay & Lesbian Alliance of Oklahoma City**
&& c/o Oasis Resources Center, 2135 North West 39th. Street, Oklahoma City, Oklahoma 73112.
☎ 405 525 2437
🕐 Sun 19:30
For youth up to 24 years.

Publishers: Newspapers: Sexuality

♀ ■ **Herland Voice**
& Herland Sister Resources, Inc., 2312 North West 39th. Street, Oklahoma City, Oklahoma 73112.
☎ 405 521 9696
A variety of information concerning women & lesbian issues. Published every month. Yearly subscription is free.

Stores: Books: General

♀ ■ **Herland Sister Resources, Inc.**
& 2312 North West 39th. Street, Oklahoma City, Oklahoma 73112.
☎ 405 521 9696
🕐 10:00 - 18:00, Sun 13:00 - 18:00

Stores: Erotica: General

☺ ■ **Christie's Toy Box**
6307 Southwestern, Oklahoma City, Oklahoma 73139.
☎ 405 631 1399

☺ ■ **Ingrid's Bookstore**
1124 North West Cache Road, Oklahoma City, Oklahoma 73507.
☎ 415 353 1488

☺ ■ **Naughty 'n Nice**
& 3121 South West 29th. Street, Oklahoma City, Oklahoma 73119.
☎ 405 686 1110

Tulsa

Bars: General

⚥▼ **New Age Renegade**
& 1649 South Main, Tulsa, Oklahoma 74119.
☎ 918 585 3405
Some leather.

Health Services

☺ □ **Saint John's Medical Center**
1923 South Utica Street, Tulsa, Oklahoma 74104.
☎ 918 744 2345

Helplines: Sexuality

⚥▽ **TOHR Gay / Lesbian Helpline**
P. O. Box 52729, Tulsa, Oklahoma 74152-2729.
☎ 918 743 4297
🕐 20:00 - 22:00

Organizations: AIDS: Support

☺ □ **HIV Resource Consortium**
& Suite H-1, 4154 South Harvard, Tulsa, Oklahoma 74135.
☎ 918 749 4194 📞 918 749 4213
🕐 08:30 - 17:00, support groups after hours

Organizations: Family

Organizations: Family

☺ ☐ **Parents & Friends of Lesbians & Gays (PFLAG)—** ♿ **Tulsa**
P. O. Box 52800, Tulsa, Oklahoma 74152.
☎ 918 749 4901
🕓 24hr. hotline
Publishes *FLAG of Green Country*.

Organizations: Sexual Politics

⚥ **Tulsa Oklahomans for Human Rights**
P. O. Box 52729, Tulsa, Oklahoma 74152.
☎ 918 743 4297
Publishes *Tulsa Oklahomans for Human Rights Reporter* every month.

Organizations: Sexuality

⚥▽ **Cross Dressers International (CDI)**
P. O. Box 50192, Tulsa, Oklahoma 94104.
☎ 918 582 6643
☎ 918 835 5334
🕓 Meets every other Sat
Contact: Ms. Gwen Pete

⚥▽ **Desire**
P. O. Box 50192, Tulsa, Oklahoma 74104.
Contact: Ms. Gwen Pete
For all sisters & spouses.

Publishers: Newspapers: Sexuality

⚥ *Tulsa News*
P. O. Box 4140, Tulsa, Oklahoma 74159.

Stores: Erotica: General

☺ ■ **Elite Adult Books**
814 South Sheridan, Tulsa, Oklahoma 74112.
☎ 918 838 8503

☺ ■ **Whittier Bookstore**
♿ 1 North Lewis Avenue, Tulsa, Oklahoma 74110.
☎ 918 592 0767

OREGON

Area: Approximately 249,000 square kilometres
Population: Approximately 2,850,000
Capital City: Salem
Time zone: GMT minus 7/8 hours (both Mountain Time & Pacific)
Climate: Pleasant summers, with average temperatures of approximately 15°C. Winters are rainy & mild with average lows of 3°C.
Age of consent & homosexuality legislation: State has adopted the Model Penal Code or otherwise decriminalized homosexual activities.
Legal drinking age: 21

State Resources

Organizations: Sexuality

♂ ▽ **BiNet—Oregon**
⚥ P. O. Box 8232, Portland, Oregon 97207-8232.
☎ 503 236 4941 ✆ 503 236 4941
Publishes *Northwest BiWays*.

⚥▽ **The Mpowerment Project**
♿ 775 Monroe Street, Eugene, Oregon 97402.
☎ 503 683 4303
✉ mpower@efn.org
🕓 08:00 - 17:00
Publishes *M Center Voice* every month.

⚥▽ **Oregon Gay & Lesbian Cultural Resource Center Task Force**
P. O. Box 6012, Portland, Oregon 97228.
☎ 503 295 9732

Publishers: Magazines: Sexuality

⚥▽ *Just Out*
P. O. Box 14400, Portland, Oregon 97214.
☎ 503 236 1252 ✆ 503 236 1257
Oregon's lesbian & gay news magazine. Published twice a month. Yearly subscription is $34.

Publishers: Newspapers: Sexuality

⚥▽ *Community News*
P. O. Box 663, Salem, Oregon 97308.
☎ 503 363 0006
🕓 07:00 - 17:00
Gay & lesbian news, political, & religious subjects. Accepts insolicited manuscripts. Published every month. Yearly subscription is $15.

Television: Sexuality

⚥▽ *Night Scene*

Cable Access TV, 13 North West Avenue, Portland, Oregon 97209.
☎ 503 244 6483
Call for show details.

Aloha

Organizations: Polyfidelity

☺ ☐ **The Group Marriage Alliance**
P. O. Box 5995, Aloha, Oregon 97007.
☎ 503 4525453
✉ beattie@proaxis.com

Ashland / Medford

Organizations: Family

☺ ☐ **Parents & Friends of Lesbians & Gays (PFLAG)— Rouge Valley**
P. O. Box 13, Ashland, Oregon 97520.
☎ 503 488 3436 ✆ 503 482 4017
Publishes *Jefferson Banner*.

Organizations: Sexuality

⚥▽ **Southern Oregon Lambda Association**
P. O. Box 4387, Medford, Oregon 97501.
☎ 503 773 8146

Organizations: Sexuality: Student

⚥▽ **Gay & Lesbian Alliance at Southern Oregon State College**
c/o Stevenson Union, Siskyou Boulevard, Ashland, Oregon 97550.
☎ 503 552 7702

Stores: Books: General

☺ ■ **Bloomsbury Books**
290 East Main Street, Ashland, Oregon 97520-1831.
☎ 503 488 0029

Astoria

Organizations: AIDS: Education

☺ ☐ **Clatsop County AIDS Coalition**
P. O. Box 455, Astoria, Oregon 97103.
☎ 503 338 7501

Baker City

Organizations: Sexuality

⚥▽ **Lambda Eastern Oregon Association**
P. O. Box 382, Baker City, Oregon 97814.
Publishes *LEOA Newsletter*.

Bend

Organizations: AIDS: Support

☺ ▽ **Central Oregon AIDS Support Team**
P. O. Box 9184, Bend, Oregon 97708.
☎ 503 389 4330

Organizations: Sexuality

⚥▽ **Another Side**
⚥ P. O. Box 5672, Bend, Oregon 97701.
☎ 503 388 2395
🕓 Call 24hrs.
Publishes *Another Side.*

⚥▽ **Gay & Lesbian Outreach Network (GALON)**
P. O. Box 5672, Bend, Oregon 97708-5672.
☎ 503 388 2395
🕓 Call 24hrs.
Gay & lesbian outreach network.

Central Point

Manufacturers: Piercing Jewelry

☺ ■ **Afterglow FX**
P. O. Box 3893, Central Point, Oregon 97502.
☎ 503 664 9171 ✆ 503 664 1471
Make surgical steel & Niobium jewelry. Also supply piercing supplies & publications. Catalogue, $2.

Clackamas

Organizations: BDSM

☺ ☐ **Rose City Discussion Club (RCDC)**
P. O. Box 1370, Clackamas, Oregon 97015.
☎ 503 650 7052 (voice mail)
🕓 Meets monthly
♿ ✓ $
RCDC is open to BDSM, fetishes, & orientations that are safe, sane, &

consensual. Guest speakers, socials, etc.. Publishes a newsletter every month. Yearly subscription is $36. Age statement of 21 is required.

Coos Bay

Helplines: Sexuality

☺▽ **Gay & Lesbian Outreach Network (GALON)**
P. O. Box 4212, Coos Bay, Oregon 97420.
☎ 503 269 4182
🕐 Call 24hrs.

Organizations: Sexuality

☺▽ **Gay & Lesbian Outreach Network (GALON)**
P. O. Box 4212, Coos Bay, Oregon 97420.
☎ 503 269 4182
🕐 Call 24hrs.
Publishes *GALON News*.

Corvallis

Organizations: AIDS: Education

☺☐ **Valley AIDS Information Network**
♿ 128 South West 9th. Street, Corvallis, Oregon 97333.
☎ 503 752 6322

Organizations: BDSM

☺☐ **A.S.B. Munch—Corvallis**
📧 hackbod@mail.cs.orst.edu
🕐 Tue 19:00 - 21:00
Contact: Ms. Dianne Kyra Hackborn

Organizations: Sexuality: Student

☺▽ **Lesbian, Gay, & Bisexual Alliance**
♿ Student Activities Center, Oregon State University, Corvallis, Oregon 97331.
☎ 503 737 6363

Publishers: Newspapers: Sexuality

☺▽ *Ladies Home Companion*
P. O. Box 1828, Corvallis, Oregon 97339.

Stores: Books: General

☺■ **Grass Roots**
♿ 227 South West 2nd. Street, Corvallis, Oregon 97333.
☎ 503 754 7668

☺■ **Monroe Avenue Book Bin**
2305 North West Monroe Avenue, Corvallis, Oregon 97330.
☎ 503 753 8398

Eugene

Counsellors

☺■ **Amethyst Counselling Service**
1059 Hilyard Street, Eugene, Oregon 97401.
☎ 503 484 6979
🪑 ✓
Counselling includes relationships, personal growth, & identity issues.

☺■ **Barb Ryan, M.S.**
K P. O. Box 286, Eugene, Oregon 97405.
☎ 541 345 5058
📧 barbr@efn.org
🕐 Variable, leave message on 24hr. answering machine
🪑 ✓
Feminist, wholistic counselling for individuals, couples, & groups. Specialties: abuse, intimacy, parenting, body image, & lesbian, gay & bisexual concerns.

Health Services

☺☐ **Sacred Heart General Hospital**
1255 Hilyard Street, Eugene, Oregon 97440.
☎ 503 686 7300

Organizations: AIDS: Education

☺☐ **HIV/AIDS Resources, Inc.**
P. O. Box 55113 , Eugene, Oregon 97405-0513.
☎ 503 342 5088

Organizations: Family

☺☐ **Parents & Friends of Lesbians & Gays (PFLAG)— Eugene**
♿ P. O. Box 11137, Eugene, Oregon 97440.
☎ 503 689 1630

Organizations: Polyfidelity

☺■ **Erisian Fields Cohousing**
3336 Loma Linda Drive, Eugene, Oregon 97405.
📧 shava@darkwing.uoregon.edu
🌐 http://darkwing.uoregon.edu/~shava/idyll/
A polyfidelity & pagan-friendly housing group.

Organizations: Sexuality

⊙▽ **The Lavendar Network**
P. O. Box 5263, Eugene, Oregon 97405-0263.

📰▼ **Salmacis**
P. O. Box 1604, Eugene, Oregon 97440-1604.
☎ 503 688 4282
🕐 Meets 3rd. Mon of month 20:00
Contact: Ms. Sally Ann Douglas, Social Director
The Equalitarian Feminist Social Society. Publishes *The Equalitarian Feminist* & *Femmes Together*.

Organizations: Sexuality: Student

☺▽ **Gay & Lesbian Alliance**
♿ #319 EMU, University of Oregon, Eugene, Oregon 97403.
☎ 503 686 3360

Publishers: Newspapers: Sexuality

⊕■ *Womyn's Press*
P. O. Box 562, Eugene, Oregon 97440.
Eclectic feminist newspaper; news, fiction, art, poetry, & photos - feminist expression or experience. Published every two months. Yearly subscription is $8.

Stores: Books: General

☺■ **Hungry Head Books**
♿ 1212 Williamette Street, Eugene, Oregon 97401.
☎ 503 485 0888
📧 brianw@efn.org
🕐 Mon - Sat 10:30 - 18:00, Sun 12:00 -17:00
💳 💳

☺▼ **Mother Kali's Books**
♿ Suite 102, 720 East 13th. Avenue, Eugene, Oregon 97401-3753.
☎ 503 343 4864

Stores: Military Surplus

☺■ **Action Surplus**
P. O. Box 292, Eugene, Oregon 97401.
☎ 503 746 1301

Klamath Falls

Organizations: AIDS: Education

☺☐ **Klamath County AIDS/HIV Support & Education Council**
1035 Main Street, Klamath Falls, Oregon 97601.
☎ 503 883 2437

Organizations: Sexuality

☺▽ **Klamath Area Lambda Association**
♿ P. O. Box 43, Klamath Falls, Oregon 97601.
☎ 503 883 2437
Please address envelopes to KALA, do NOT address them to Klamath Area Lambda Association.

La Grande

Organizations: Sexuality: Student

☺▽ **Gay & Lesbian Alliance of Eastern Oregon State College**
SAO, Hoke College Center, 8th. Street, La Grande, Oregon 97850.

Lake Oswego

Publishers: Directories: Sexuality

☺■ **Niche Catalog Publications**
P. O. Box 1921, Lake Oswego, Oregon 97053-3377.
☎ 503 699 5094
Publishes a "Yellow Pages" directory of the adult industry.

Newport

Stores: Books: General

☺▼ **Green Gables Bookstore**
156 South West Coast Street, Newport, Oregon 97365.
☎ 503 265 9141
🕐 Thu - Mon 10:00 - 17:00

Pacific City

Organizations: Sexuality

♂♀▽ **Tillamook County GALA**
P. O. Box 592, Pacific City, Oregon 97135.

Portland

Artists: BDSM

☺▼ **The Hun**
P. O. Box 11308, Portland, Oregon 97211.
☎ 503 285 9670 ✆ 503 285 9670

Bars: BDSM

♂♀▼ **CC Slaughter's**
1014 South West Stark Street, Portland, Oregon 97205.
☎ 503 248 9135
⏱ 17:00 - 02:30, Sun 15:00 - 02:30

BBSs: BDSM

☺■ **North Keep**
✆ 503 289 4872

Health Services

☺☐ **Good Samaritan Hospital & Medical Center**
1015 North West 22nd. Avenue, Portland, Oregon 97210.
☎ 503 229 7711
HIV & emergency departments.

☺☐ **University Hospital**
3181 South West Sam Jackson Road, Portland, Oregon 97201.
☎ 503 494 8311

☺☐ **Veterans' Affairs Medical Center**
3710 U. S. Veterans Hospital Road, Portland, Oregon 97201.
☎ 503 220 8262

Helplines: AIDS

☺☐ **Cascade AIDS Project**
♿ 620 South West 5th. Avenue, Portland, Oregon 97204-1418.
☎ 800 777 2437

Manufacturers: Clothing: Leather

☺ **Cuir Gear**
☎ 503 281 7231

Manufacturers: Erotica: Leather

☺■ **Spartacus Enterprises**
1002 South East 8th. Street, Portland, Oregon 97214.
☎ 800 666 2604 ✆ 503 239 4681
☎ 503 239 4416
⏱ Mon - Fri 08:00 - 16:30
♿ ✓ $ ⚡ 🆅🆂🅰 🅼🅲
Catalogue, $8.

Organizations: AIDS: Education

☺☐ **Cascade AIDS Project**
♿ Suite 300, 620 South West 5th. Avenue, Portland, Oregon 97204-1418.
☎ 503 223 5907
☎ 800 777 2437 (hotline)
⏱ Mon - Fri 10:00 - 21:00, Sat Sun 12:00 - 18:00
Also publishes Connections. Publishes Positive Connection.

Organizations: BDSM

♀ ▽ **B.A.D. Girls**
P. O. Box 17254, Portland, Oregon 97217-0254.

♂♀▽ **Chaps**
c/o NLA: Portland, P. O. Box 5161, Portland, Oregon 97208.
⏱ Meets monthly
Gay male education forum. Send letter for more information.

☺▽ **The National Leather Association (NLA)—Portland**
P. O. Box 5161, Portland, Oregon 97208.
☎ 503 727 3148

♂♀▽ **Oregon Guild Activists of S/M (ORGASM)**
P. O. Box 5702, Portland, Oregon 97208.
☎ 503 688 0669

♀♀▽ **Portland Power & Trust**
P. O. Box 3781, Portland, Oregon 97208.

Organizations: Body Size

♂♀▽ **Gentle Giants of Oregon**
P. O. Box 83332, Portland, Oregon 97263-0332.
☎ 503 981 4281

Organizations: Family

☺☐ **Parents & Friends of Lesbians & Gays (PFLAG)— Portland**
♿
P. O. Box 8944, Portland, Oregon 97207-8944.
☎ 503 232 7676

Organizations: Motorcycle

♂♀▽ **Harley Strokers**
P. O. Box 86686, Portland, Oregon 97286.
☎ 503 771 6136
⏱ After 17:00
♿ ✓
Free information with proof of Harley ownership.

Organizations: Sexual Politics

♂♀▽ **Right to Privacy, Inc.**
Suite 546, 921 South West Morrison, Portland, Oregon 97205.
☎ 503 228 5825 ✆ 503 228 1104
⏱ Variable.

Organizations: Sexuality

♂♀▽ **Gay Men's Community Project**
♿ P. O. Box 40741, Portland, Oregon 97240-0741.
☎ 503 331 2282

⊠☐ **Northwest Gender Alliance (NWGA)**
🜨 P. O. Box 4928, Portland, Oregon 97208.
☎ 503 646 2802
⏱ Meets monthly

♂♀▽ **Phœnix Rising**
♿ Suite 710, 620 South West 5th. Avenue, Portland, Oregon 97204-1422.
☎ 503 223 8299

⊠▽ **Trans-Port—Portland**
P. O. Box 66913, Portland, Oregon 97290-6913.
☎ 503 774 7463
⏱ Meets monthly
Publishes Trans-Port.

Organizations: Wrestling

♂♀▽ **Wrestling Club Of Portland**
P. O. Box 40066, Portland, Oregon 97240-0066.

Piercers

☺■ **Attitudes**
Studio 312, 1017 South West Morrison Street, Portland, Oregon.
☎ 503 224 0050
♿ 🆅🆂🅰 🅼🅲
Discount to RCDC members.

☺■ **Gerd**
☎ 503 253 7956

☺■ **Darryn Lagaipa**
☎ 503 284 4174

☺■ **Gary Richmond**
☎ 503 283 9571

Publishers: Magazines: Fetish

☺■ **In Uniform**
A. M. Publications, P. O. Box 3226, Portland, Oregon 97208-3226.
☎ 503 228 6935 ✆ 503 274 0038
✉ UniformMag@aol.com
Published quarterly. Yearly subscription is $24 U.S., $30 Cdn, $40 Intl.. Age statement of 21 is required.

Radio: General

♀ ☐ **Womansoul**
♿ KBOO Radio FM 90.7, 20 South East 8th., Portland, Oregon 97214.
☎ 503 231 8032

Radio: Sexuality

♀☐ **Bread & Roses**
♿ KBOO Radio FM 90.7, 20 South East 8th., Portland, Oregon 97214.
☎ 503 231 8032

Stores: Books: General

☺■ **Conant & Conant Books**
♿ P. O. Box 13104, Portland, Oregon 97213-0104.
☎ 503 241 7726

☺■ **In Other Words**
3734 South East Hawthorne Boulevard, Portland, Oregon 97214.
☎ 503 232 6003

☺■ **Laughing Horse Books**
♿ 3652 South East Division, Portland, Oregon 97202-1546.
☎ 503 236 2893

☺ ■ **Looking Glass Books**
318 South Weat Taylor Street, Portland, Oregon 97204.
☎ 503 227 4760
🕐 Mon - Fri 09:00 - 18:00, Sat 10:00 - 18:00

☺ ■ **Powell's City of Books**
1005 West Burnside, Portland, Oregon 97209.
☎ 800 228 7323 ✆ 503 228 4631
☎ 503 228 4651
🕐 Mon - Sat 09:00 - 23:00, Sun Hol 09:00 - 21:00
🍴 ✓ 💳 🔲 🔲
Large lesbian, gay, & bisexual section.

☺ ■ **Twenty-Third Avenue Book**
1015 North West 23rd. Avenue, Portland, Oregon 97210.
☎ 503 224 5097

⊕▼ **Widdershins Books**
♿ 1996 South East Ladd Avenue, Portland, Oregon 97214.
☎ 503 232 2129

Stores: Clothing: Fetish

⊕ ■ **Leather & Lace Lingerie**
8327 South East Division, Portland, Oregon 97266.
☎ 503 774 8292

Stores: Erotica: BDSM

☺ ■ **The Leatherworks, Inc.**
2908 South East Belmont, Portland, Oregon 97214-4025.
☎ 503 234 2697
📠 fip1@aol.com
🌐 http://www.lthr-pdx@europa.com
🕐 12:00 -18:00 Tue - Sat
🍴 ✓ $ 💳 🔲 🔲 Ⓓ 🔲 ℓ
Manufacturer & retailer of motorcycle & erotic leather. Established in 1975. Quality, service, & value. Also mail order through online catalogue. French & Spanish also spoken.

Stores: Erotica: General

☺ ■ **Christie's Toy Box**
8201 South East Powell Boulevard, Portland, Oregon 97266.
☎ 503 771 9979
RCDC newsletter available here. 10% discount to members.

☺ ■ **Crimson Phœnix**
♿ 1876 South West 5th. Avenue, Portland, Oregon 97201.
☎ 503 228 0129 ✆ 503 228 0129 (Call first)
🕐 Mon - Thu 10:00 - 21:00, Fri 10:00 - 23:00, Sat 11:00 - 23:00, Sun 12:00 - 16:00
🍴 💳 🔲

☺ ■ **It's My Pleasure**
4526 East Hawthorne, Portland, Oregon 97215.
☎ 503 236 0505

☺ ■ **Sin City Adult Books**
838 South West 3rd. Avenue, Portland, Oregon 97204.
☎ 503 223 6514

Roseburg

Archives: Sexuality

⊘▽ **Douglas County Gay Archives**
P. O. Box 942, Dillard, Oregon 97432-0942.
☎ 503 440 2761

Helplines: Sexuality

⊘▽ **Gay & Lesbian Switchboard**
☎ 503 672 4126

Publishers: Newspapers: Sexuality

⊘ *Gay Ol' Times*
P. O. Box 813, Roseburg, Oregon 97470.
☎ 503 679 9144
The goal of our publication is to chronicle the gay life in the rural community. We support the only rural gay & lesbian community centre in the nation. Published every two months. Yearly subscription is free.

Salem

Organizations: Sexuality

⊘▽ **Trans-Port—Capital City**
P. O. Box 3312, Salem, Oregon 97302.

Stores: Books: General

☺ ■ **Rosebud & Fish Community Bookstore**
♿ 524 State Street, Salem, Oregon 97301.
☎ 503 399 9960
🕐 10:00 - 19:00, Sun 12:00 - 17:00

Springfield

Stores: Erotica: General

☺ ■ **Exclusively Adult**
♿ 1166 South A Street, Springfield, Oregon 97477-5209.
☎ 503 726 6969
🕐 24hrs. (almost)
🍴 ✓ $ 💳 🔲 🔲
Age statement of 18 is required.

PENNSYLVANIA

Area: Approximately 116,000 square kilometres
Population: Approximately 11,900,000
Capital City: Harrisburg
Time zone: GMT minus 5 hours (EST)
Climate: Warm, humid summers with average temperatures of approximately 22°-26° (depending which part of the state you're in). Winters are cold & snowy, with average temperatures of approximately 2°. The coastal weather is moderated by the Atlantic ocean.
Age of consent & homosexuality legislation: State has adopted the Model Penal Code or otherwise decriminalized homosexual activities.
Legal drinking age: 21

State Resources

Organizations: AIDS: Education

☺ ☐ **AIDS Law Project of Pennsylvania**
♿ 5th. Floor, 924 Cherry Street, Philadelphia, Pennsylvania 19107.
☎ 215 440 8555

Organizations: AIDS: Support

☺ ☐ **Venango-Forest AIDS Support**
P. O. Box 834, Oil City, Pennsylvania 16301.
☎ 800 359 2437

Organizations: Sexuality

⊘▽ **Poconos Action Lambda Society**
P. O. Box 1375, Milford, Pennsylvania 18337.
Publishes *Spread The Word*. Please address envelopes to PALS, do NOT address them to Poconos Action Lambda Society or Spread The Word.

⊘▽ **Sesquehanna KONTACT**
♿ P. O. Box 741, Bloomsburg, Pennsylvania 17815-0741.
Publishes *Sesquehanna KONTACT*.

Publishers: Newspapers: Sexuality

⊘▼ *Au Courant*
P. O. Box 42741, Philadelphia, Pennsylvania 19101.
☎ 215 790 1179
Au Courant is a weekly newspaper serving the gay & lesbian community of the Philadelphia area, emphasizing both news & feature writing. Published every week. Yearly subscription is $98.

Allentown

Counsellors

⊠ **Patricia Klein, M.S.**
Box 3624, 1013 Brookside Road, Allentown, Pennsylvania 18106.
☎ 610 821 2955

Organizations: BDSM

☺ ■ **Leather Bondage & Whips (LBW)**
Suite 139, 3140-B Tilghman, Allentown, Pennsylvania 18104.
📠 lbw1femdom@aol.com
Contact: Mistress Lisa, Foundress & Editrix
Publishes *LBW Magazine* quarterly. Yearly subscription is $25.

Altoona

Helplines: Sexuality

⊘▽ **Gay, Lesbian, & Bisexual Helpline**
c/o Family & Childrens' Service, 2022 Broad Avenue, Altoona, Pennsylvania 16601.
☎ 814 942 8101
🕐 Thu - Sun 19:00 - 22:00

Organizations: AIDS: Education

☺ **Home Nursing Agency AIDS Intervention Project**
P. O. Box 352, Altoona, Pennsylvania 16603.

Bensalem

Organizations: Sexuality

⊠▽ **Renaissance Education Association, Inc.—Greater Philadelphia**
P. O. Box 530, Bensalem, Pennsylvania 19020.
☎ 610 957 9119
📠 bensalem@cpcn.com

Blacklick

Organizations: Body Size

⚥▽ **Girth & Mirth—Western Pennsylvania**
P. O. Box 108, Blacklick, Pennsylvania 15716.

Bryn Mawr

Organizations: Sexuality: Student

⚥▽ **Bryn Mawr / Haverford Bisexual, Gay, & Lesbian Alliance (BGALA)**
Box 1725, Brym Mawr College, Bryn Mawr, Pennsylvania 19010.

Buckingham

Organizations: AIDS: Education

☺ ☐ **F. A. C. T.**
P. O. Box 616, Buckingham, Pennsylvania 18112.
☎ 215 598 0750

Carlisle

Organizations: Sexuality: Student

⚥▽ **Dickinson College Allies**
⚧ c/o Health Education, P. O. Box 4888, Carlisle, Pennsylvania 17013.
☎ 717 240 1835

Castle Shannon

Piercers

☺ ■ **Accent In Ink**
☎ 412 563 8281

Clarion

Organizations: Sexuality: Student

⚥▽ **Gay Information & Concerns**
P. O. Box 750, Clarion, Pennsylvania 16214.
☎ 814 226 8212

Easton

Organizations: Sexuality

⚧▽ **Cross Dressers International (CDI)**
P. O. Box 61, Easton, Pennsylvania 18044.
Contact: Ms. Kristine James, Director

Edinboro

Organizations: Sexuality: Student

⚥▽ **Edinboro Gay Organization**
⚧ University Center, Edinboro University of Pennsylvania, Edinboro, Pennsylvania 16444.
☎ 814 732 2000

Erie

Health Services

☺ ☐ **Hamot Medical Center**
201 State Street, Erie, Pennsylvania 16550.
☎ 814 877 6000

Organizations: AIDS: Support

☺ ☐ **Friends From The Heart**
710 Beaumont Avenue, Erie, Pennsylvania 16505.
☎ 814 838 0123

Organizations: Sexuality

⚥▼ **Bridges**
P. O. Box 3063, Erie, Pennsylvania 16508-0063.
☎ 814 456 9833
☎ 814 453 2785
⚧ ✓
Make cheques payable to Erie Gay Community Coalition. Publishes *Erie Gay Community Newsletter* every month. Yearly subscription is $15.

⚧☐ **Erie Sisters**
Suite 261, 2115 West 8th. Street, Erie, Pennsylvania 16505.
⏲ Meets 4th. Sat, even numbered months
Publishes *Mirror Images*.

Organizations: Sexuality: Student

⚥▽ **GALA 10**
⚧ Mercy Insitute for Religious Education Lay Ministry, 501 East 38th., Erie, Pennsylvania 16546.
☎ 814 824 2572

⚥▽ **Trigon**
⚧ c/o Box 794, College Mailroom, Behrend College, Erie, Pennsylvania

16563.
☎ 814 453 6232

Stores: Erotica: General

☺ ■ **Eastern Adult Books**
1313 State Street, Erie, Pennsylvania 16501.
☎ 814 459 7014

☺ ■ **Filmore News**
2757 West 12th. Street, Erie, Pennsylvania 16505.
☎ 814 833 2667

Gettysburg

Organizations: Sexuality: Student

⚥▽ **Gettysburg College Lambda Alliance**
⚧ Box 412, Gettysburg College, Gettysburg, Pennsylvania 17325.

Harrisburg

Counsellors

☺ ■ **Bette Weinberger, ACSW**
240 Division Street, Harrisburg, Pennsylvania 17110.
☎ 717 233 7153

Health Services

☺ ☐ **Harrisburg Hospital**
111 South Front Street, Harrisburg, Pennsylvania 17101.
☎ 717 782 3131

Helplines: Sexuality

⚥▽ **Gay & Lesbian Switchboard of Harrisburg**
⚥ P. O. Box 872, Harrisburg, Pennsylvania 17108-0872.
☎ 717 234 0328
⏲ Mon - Fri 18:00 - 22:00

Organizations: BDSM

⚥▽ **Pennsmen**
P.O. Box 401, Federal Square Station, Harrisburg, Pennsylvania 17108.

Organizations: Family

☺ ☐ **Parents & Friends of Lesbians & Gays (PFLAG)—**
⚧ **Central Pennsylvania**
c/o Tressler Lutheran Social Services, P. O. Box 2001, Mechanicsburg, Pennsylvania 17055.
☎ 717 795 0330

Organizations: Sexuality

⚥▽ **Lancaster Lambda**
P. O. Box 8283, Harrisburg, Pennsylvania 17604-8283.

⚥▽ **Pink Triangle Coalition**
P. O. Box 1603, Harrisburg, Pennsylvania 17601.

⚥▽ **Renaissance Education Association, Inc.—Lower Susquehanna Valley**
P. O. Box 2122, Harrisburg, Pennsylvania 17105-2122.
☎ 717 780 1578

Organizations: Sexuality: Youth

⚥☐ **The Pink Triangle Coalition**
P. O. Box 31, Harrisburg, Pennsylvania 17603-0031.

Publishers: Newspapers: Sexuality

⚥▽ **Lavendar Letter**
P. O. Box 60184, Harrisburg, Pennsylvania 17106-0184.
☎ 717 732 8010

Stores: Erotica: General

☺ ■ **Erotic Forum**
227 North Prince Street, Harrisburg, Pennsylvania 17603.
☎ 717 393 9722

⚥▽ **V. O. I. C. E. / Den of Pleasure**
⚥ 53 North Prince Street, Harrisburg, Pennsylvania 17603.
☎ 717 299 1779

Havertown

Counsellors

⚥ ▼ **Mona Cardell, Ph.D.**
1618 Rose Glen Road, Havertown, Pennsylvania 19083.
☎ 610 446 9625

Huntington Valley

Organizations: Polyfidelity

☺ ■ **Delaware Valley Synergy**
P. O. Box 252, Huntington Valley, Pennsylvania 19006-0252.

Jenkintown

Organizations: Academic: Psychiatry

☺ ■ **American Association for Counselling & Development**
P. O. Box 216, Jenkintown, Pennsylvania 19046.
Publishes a newsletter quarterly.

King of Prussia

Publishers: Magazines: Sexuality

⚥▼ **Ladylike**
Creative Design Services, P. O. Box 61263, King of Prussia, Pennsylvania 19406.
☎ 610 640 9449 ✆ 610 648 0257
✉ info@cdspub.com
🖳 www.cdspub.com
Published quarterly. Yearly subscription is $30.

Lancaster

BBSs: BDSM

☺ ■ **The Covenant**
✆ 717 394 2819

Lansdowne

Television: Marketing

☺ **Radio & TV Interview Report**
Bradley Communications Corporation, P. O. Box 1206, 135 East Plumstead Avenue, Lansdowne, Pennsylvania 19050-8206.
☎ 800 989 1400 Ext.: 408 ✆ 610 284 3704
☎ 610 259 1070

Lehigh Valley

Counsellors

⊕ □ **Women's Counseling Services of Berk County, Inc.**
♿ 739 Washington Street, Reading, Pennsylvania 19601.
☎ 610 372 7234

Organizations: AIDS: Education

☺ □ **AIDS Services Center**
♿ P. O. Box 1800, Bethlehem, Pennsylvania 18016-1800.
☎ 610 974 8700
Publishes *Positive Plus*.

☺ □ **Fighting AIDS Continously Together (FACT)**
♿ P. O. Box 1028, Allentown, Pennsylvania 18105.
☎ 610 820 5519

Organizations: Family

⚥▽ **Gay & Lesbian Parents**
☎ 610 439 8755

☺ □ **Parents & Friends of Lesbians & Gays (PFLAG)—**
♿ **Lehigh Valley**
☎ 610 439 8755
🕒 Meets 1st. Sun of month

Organizations: Sexuality

⚥▽ **Lambda Alive**
♿ P. O. Box 4313, Reading, Pennsylvania 19606.
☎ 610 589 4854
Publishes *Lambda Alive News*.

⚥▽ **Lehigh Valley Gay & Lesbian Task Force**
P. O. Box 20253, Lehigh Valley, Pennsylvania 18002-0253.
✆ 610 250 0266

⚥▽ **Gay & Lesbian Organization of Reading & Allentown (GLORA)**
♿ P. O. Box 1952, Allentown, Pennsylvania 18105-1952.
Publishes *The Tassel*.

⚥▽ **Lehigh Valley Lesbians**
♿ ☎ 610 439 8755
🕒 Meets 1st. & 3rd. Tue of month 19:00

Organizations: Sexuality: Student

⚥▽ **Lehigh University LesBiGay Alliance**
♿ c/o Chaplain's Office, 110 Johnson Hall, 36 University Drive, Bethlehem, Pennsylvania 18015.
☎ 610 758 3877

Organizations: Sexuality: Youth

⚥▽ **Your Turf**
♿ ☎ 610 439 8755
For youth 16 - 21.

Stores: Books: General

⚥▼ **Lavendar Hearts**
♿ 13 North 9th. Street, Reading, Pennsylvania 19601.
☎ 610 372 1828

Levittown

Counsellors

⚥ **Ronald Goldstein, Ph.D.**
Suite 12, Bucks Medical Center, 1723 WoodBourne Road, Levittown, Pennsylvania 19057.
☎ 215 547 9417
🕒 By appointment

Lewisburg

Stores: Books: General

⊕ ■ **The Dwelling Place**
♿ 200 Market Street, Lewisburg, Pennsylvania 17837.
☎ 717 523 7878

Malvern

Suppliers: Miscellaneous

☺ ■ **Goodfellow Corp.**
Suite 140, 301 Lindonwood Drive, Malvern, Pennsylvania 19355.
☎ 800 821 2870 ✆ 800 283 2020
☎ 215 640 1612
Not piercing oriented, but supplies niobium wire.

Meadville

Organizations: Sexuality

⚥▽ **Oasis**
P. O. Box 622, Meadville, Pennsylvania 16335.
Publishes *Oasis Dreams* every month.

Organizations: Sexuality: Student

⚥▽ **The Committee in Support of Gay, Lesbian, & Bisexual People**
Box 186, Allegheny College, Meadville, Pennsylvania 16335.
☎ 216 371 0709

Morrisville

Organizations: BDSM

☺ □ **People Exchanging Power (PEP)—Philadelphia**
P.O. Box 812, Morrisville, Pennsylvania 19067.
☎ 215 552 8155

New Hope

Stores: Books: General

☺ ▼ **Book Gallery**
19 West Mechanic Street, New Hope, Pennsylvania 18938.
☎ 215 8622 5110

☺ ■ **Farley's Bookstore**
44 South Main Street, New Hope, Pennsylvania 18938.
☎ 215 862 2452

☺ ■ **Hemetro**
127 South Main Street, New Hope, Pennsylvania 18938.
☎ 215 862 5629

☺ ■ **Village Green Bookstore**
16 South Main Street, Doylestown, Pennsylvania 18901.
☎ 215 230 7610 ✆ 215 230 7615

Stores: Erotica: General

⚥▼ **Grownups**
2 East Mechanic Street, New Hope, Pennsylvania 18938.
☎ 215 862 9304

Norristown

Organizations: Bears

⚥▽ **Double Trouble Bears**
354 West Elm, Norristown, Pennsylvania 19401.

Philadelphia

Archives: Sexuality

⚥▼ **Gay, Lesbian, Bisexual & Transgendered Library / Archives of Philadelphia**
201 South Carmac Street, Philadelphia, Pennsylvania 19107.
☎ 215 732 2220 Ext.: Voicemail box 6
✉ lglap@aol.com

Archives: Sexuality

⬡ http://wanda.pond.com/~stevecap/la000001.htm
A project of Penguin Place (The Gay, Lesbian, Bisexual, & Transgendered Community Center of Philadelphia).

Bars: BDSM

☺▼ **Club Tyz**
1418 Rodman Street, Philadelphia, Pennsylvania 19146.
☎ 215 546 4195
🕐 Open - 03:00

Bars: General

☺■ **Bike Stop**
204 South Quince Street, Philadelphia, Pennsylvania 19107.
☎ 215 627 1662
🕐 15:00 - 02:00, Sat Sun 12:00 - 02:00
Some leather.

BBSs: BDSM

☺■ **The Digital Obsession**
✆ 610 678 4214

☺■ **Forum**
✆ 215 722 1482

☺■ **LuvCat's Lair**
✆ 215 467 7407

Counsellors

☺▽ **Gay & Lesbian Peer Counseling**
Room 4, 3601 Locust Walk, Philadelphia, Pennsylvania 19104.
☎ 215 368 6100
☎ 215 898 8888
🕐 Mon - Thu 16:00 - 22:00, Fri - 19:00

☺■ **Victor Hope, Ph.D.**
512 South 4th. Street, Philadelphia, Pennsylvania 19147.
☎ 215 925 0330

☺■ **Sidney Slutsky, Ed.D.**
Cottman Professional Building, 1936 Cottman Avenue, Philadelphia, Pennsylvania 19111.
☎ 215 722 1404

Health Services

☺□ **Graduate Hospital**
One Graduate Plaza, Philadelphia, Pennsylvania 19146.
☎ 215 893 2501
HIV & emergency departments.

☺□ **Hospital of the University of Pennsylvania**
3400 Spruce Street, Philadelphia, Pennsylvania 19104.
☎ 215 662 4000

☺□ **North Philadelphia Health System**
16th. Street & Girard Avenue, Philadelphia, Pennsylvania 19130.
☎ 215 787 9000

Helplines: Sexuality

☺▽ **Philadelphia Gay Switchboard**
P. O. Box 2091, Philadelphia, Pennsylvania 19103.
☎ 215 546 7100

⚥□ **Tell-A-Woman**
♿ Box 322, 1530 Locust Street, Philadelphia, Pennsylvania 19102.
☎ 215 564 5810
🕐 24hr. recording of local events
Publishes a newsletter.

Organizations: AIDS: Education

☺▽ **AIDS Information Network**
♿ The Safe Guards, 32 North 3rd. Street, Philadelphia, Pennsylvania 19106.
☎ 215 922 5597 ✉ 215 922 6762

☺□ **ActionAIDS, Inc.**
♿ 1216 Arch Street, Philadelphia, Pennsylvania 19107.
☎ 215 981 0088 (also TTY) ✉ 215 854 0735

☺□ **Critical Path AIDS Project**
P. O. Box 2126, Philadelphia, Pennsylvania 19103.
☎ 215 545 2212
🕐 Call 24hrs.
Publishes *Critical Path AIDS Project*.

☺□ **Philadelphia Community Health Alternatives**
Philadelphia AIDS Task Force, 1642 Pine Street, Philadelphia, Pennsylvania 19103-6711.
☎ 215 545 8686
☎ 800 732 2437 (hotline)
Also free anonymous HIV testing: call 215 735 1911.

Organizations: AIDS: Information

☺□ **AIDS Library of Philadelphia**
♿ 32 North 3rd. Street, Philadelphia, Pennsylvania 19106.

☎ 215 922 5120

Organizations: AIDS: Support

☺□ **American Civil Liberties Union**
AIDS & Civil Liberties Project, P. O. Box 1161, Philadelphia, Pennsylvania 19105.
☎ 215 592 1513

Organizations: BDSM

☺□ **A.S.B. Munch—Philadelphia**
✉ squirrel@noc.drexel.edu
🕐 Meets 3rd. Wed of month
Contact: Mr. Bob Westall

⚥▽ **Female Trouble**
P.O. Box 2284, Philadelphia, Pennsylvania 19103-0284.
☎ 215 732 6898
☎ 215 732 6869
Contact: Ms. Ketti Neil, Head Mistress

Organizations: Bears

☺▽ **Buddy Bears of Philadelphia**
2631 South Alder, Philadelphia, Pennsylvania 19148-4409.
☎ 215 467 5479
Contact: Mr. R. Smith

☺▽ **Delaware Valley Bears**
P. O. Box 1591, Philadelphia, Pennsylvania 19105-1591.
✉ dvbears@early.com
⬡ http://www.skepsis.com/.gblo/bears/CLUBS/Delaware_Valley_Bears/
🕐 Meets 2nd. Thu of month 20:00

Organizations: Bondage

☺▽ **Pittsburgh Bondage Club**
P. O. Box 8033, Philadelphia, Pennsylvania 15216-1467.

Organizations: Family

☺□ **Parents & Friends of Lesbians & Gays (PFLAG)—Philadelphia**
P. O. Box 15711, Philadelphia, Pennsylvania 19103.
☎ 215 572 1833

Organizations: Fetish: Uniforms

☺▽ **Philadelphia Uniform Patrol**
c/o The Bike Shop, 206 South Quince Street, Philadelphia, Pennsylvania 19107.

Organizations: Motorcycle

☺▽ **Philadelphians MC**
P.O. Box 3733, Philadelphia, Pennsylvania 19125.

☺▽ **Vanguards MC**
P. O. Box 2308, Philadelphia, Pennsylvania 19103.

Organizations: Sexuality

♂▽ **BiUnity**
⚥ P. O. Box 41905, Philadelphia, Pennsylvania 19101-1905.
☎ 215 724 3663

⚥▽ **Lesbian Community of Delaware County (LCDC)**
P. O. Box 193, Media, Pennsylvania 19063.

☺▽ **Philadelphia Lesbian & Gay Task Force**
♿ 1501 Cherry Street, Philadelphia, Pennsylvania 19102.
☎ 215 563 9584
☎ 215 563 4581 (hotline)

▷▽ **Philadelphia TS Support Group**
P. O. Box 15839, Philadelphia, Pennsylvania 19103.
☎ 215 975 9119
🕐 Meets monthly
Outreach & referrals.

⚥▽ **Triangle Interests**
P. O. Box 35145, Philadelphia, Pennsylvania 19128.
☎ 215 844 6348 ✉ 215 844 1506

Organizations: Sexuality: Student

☺▽ **Lesbian, Gay, & Bisexual Alliance at Penn**
♿ 243 Houston Hall, 3417 Spruce Street, Philadelphia, Pennsylvania 19104-6306.
☎ 215 898 5270

☺▽ **Penn GALA**
3rd. Floor, 3537 Locust Walk, Philadelphia, Pennsylvania 19104-6225.

☺▽ **Temple Lambda Alliance**
♿ Box 116, Room 205, Student Activities Center, 13th. Street, Philadelphia, Pennsylvania 19122.
☎ 215 232 4522

Organizations: Wrestling

♂▽ **Spartans Wrestling Club**
Drake Box 43, 1512 Spruce Street, Philadelphia, Pennsylvania 19102.
☎ 215 546 0735
⊕ Meets Wed 19:00 - 22:00

Piercers

☺■ **Inferno**
618 South Street, Philadelphia, Pennsylvania 19147.
☎ 215 627 5489

Publishers: Magazines: Sexuality

⚥□ **International Transcript / CDS**
Creative Design Services, P. O. Box 61263, King of Prussia, Pennsylvania 19406-1263.
☎ 610 640 9449 📞 610 648 0257
✉ info@cdspub.com
🖥 www.cdspub.com

Publishers: Newspapers: Sexuality

♂ **Bi Focus**
P. O. Box 30372, Philadelphia, Pennsylvania 19103.
☎ 215 726 5525
Created to inform its audience about social, political, & personal issues relevant to bisexuality, to provide a forum for exchanging opinions, & to help build a diverse, feminist, multicultural community of bisexual, bi-supportive people. Published quarterly. Yearly subscription is $12.

⊕■ **Labyrinth**
P. O. Box 59285, Philadelphia, Pennsylvania 19102.
☎ 215 546 6686 📞 215 546 1156
🖎 ✓
The monthly women's newspaper for the Philadelphia area. Book reviews, news articles, & feminist voices of all kinds. Published 10 times a year. Yearly subscription is $15.

Radio: Sexuality

⚲▽ **Amazon Country**
WXPN FM 88.5, 3905 Spruce Street, Philadelphia, Pennsylvania 19104.
☎ 215 898 6677
⊕ Sun 20:00 - 21:00

♂▽ **Gaydreams Radio**
WXPN FM 88.5, 3905 Spruce Street, Philadelphia, Pennsylvania 19104.
☎ 215 898 6677
⊕ Sun 21:00 - 22:00

Stores: Books: General

♂▼ **Book Bin East**
942 Market Street, Philadelphia, Pennsylvania 19103.
☎ 215 922 9208

☺■ **Borders Book Shop**
& 1727 Walnut Street, Philadelphia, Pennsylvania 19103.
☎ 215 568 7400
⊕ 07:00 - 22:00, Sat 09:00 - 21:00, Sun 11:00 - 19:00

☺▼ **Edward's Books**
1319 Arch Street, Philadelphia, Pennsylvania 19107.
☎ 215 563 6171

☺ **Giovanni's Room**
345 South 12th. Street, Philadelphia, Pennsylvania 19107.
☎ 215 923 2960 📞 215 923 0813
⊕ Mon Tue Thu 11:30 - 21:00, Wed - 19:00, Fri - 22:00, Sat 10:00 - 22:00, Sun 13:00 - 19:00

♂■ **Lambda Resources**
Suite 209, 7 Bala Avenue, Bala Cynwyd, Pennsylvania 19004.
☎ 215 667 9060

☺■ **Robin's Books**
1837 Chestnut Street, Philadelphia, Pennsylvania 19103.
☎ 215 567 2615

⊕□ **Women's Therapy Center**
& Suite 1703, 1930 Chestnut Street, Philadelphia, Pennsylvania 19103.
☎ 215 567 1111

Stores: Erotica: BDSM

☺■ **Leather Rose**
201 South 13th. Street, Philadelphia, Pennsylvania 19107.
☎ 215 985 2344 📞 215 985 0311
Latex fetish clothing & body piercing also available.

Stores: Erotica: General

☺▼ **Adam & Eve**
133 South 13th. Street, Philadelphia, Pennsylvania 19107.
☎ 215 925 5041 📞 215 925 8230

☺■ **Adult World**
1236 Arch Street, Philadelphia, Pennsylvania 19107.

☎ 215 972 9031

☺ **Fantasy Island**
7363 State Road, Philadelphia, Pennsylvania 19136.
☎ 215 332 5454

☺■ **Pleasure Chest**
2039 Walnut Street, Philadelphia, Pennsylvania 19103.
☎ 215 561 7480

♂■ **The Tomcat Store**
120 South 13th. Street, Philadelphia, Pennsylvania 19107.
☎ 215 985 9725

Pittsburgh

Bars: BDSM

♂▼ **Jazi's**
1241 Western Avenue, Pittsburgh, Pennsylvania 15233.
☎ 412 323 2721

Counsellors

♂▽ **Persad Center, Inc.**
& 5150 Penn Avenue, Pittsburgh, Pennsylvania 15224-1627.
☎ 412 441 9786 📞 412 363 2375
Professional mental health services.

Health Services

☺□ **Allegheny General Hospital**
320 East North Avenue, Pittsburgh, Pennsylvania 15212.
☎ 412 359 3131

☺□ **Mercy Hospital of Pittsburgh**
1400 Locust Street, Pittsburgh, Pennsylvania 15219.
☎ 412 232 7637

☺□ **Montefiore University Hospital**
3459 Fifth Avenue, Pittsburgh, Pennsylvania 15213.
☎ 412 647 8470

☺□ **Saint Francis Medical Center**
400 45th. Street, Pittsburgh, Pennsylvania 15201.
☎ 412 622 4343

☺□ **Shadyside Hospital**
5230 Centre Avenue, Pittsburgh, Pennsylvania 15232.
☎ 412 623 2121

☺□ **Veterans' Affairs Medical Center**
University Drive C, Pittsburgh, Pennsylvania 15240.
☎ 412 692 3000

Manufacturers: Piercing Jewelry

☺■ **Hellion House**
1814 Pennsylvania Avenue, Pittsburgh, Pennsylvania 15222.
☎ 412 391 1121
✉ aflu+@andrew.cmu.edu
Surgical steel rings & barbells, Niobium captive bead rings, & a wide variety of gemstone beads. Catalogue available.

Organizations: AIDS: Education

♂▽ **Persad Center, Inc.**
& 5150 Penn Avenue, Pittsburgh, Pennsylvania 15224-1627.
☎ 412 441 9786 📞 412 363 2375
Contact: Mr. Randal Forrester

☺□ **Pittsburgh AIDS Task Force**
& 4th. Floor, 905 West Street, Pittsburgh, Pennsylvania 15221.
☎ 412 624 2008
Publishes *Update*.

♂▽ **University of Pittsburgh**
Pitt Men's Study, P. O. Box 7319, Pittsburgh, Pennsylvania 15213.
☎ 412 624 2008

Organizations: BDSM

♂▽ **Three Rivers Leather Club, Inc.**
P.O. Box 5485, Pittsburgh, Pennsylvania 15206.

☺□ **Tri-State Couples Club**
P. O. Box 99626, Pittsburgh, Pennsylvania 15233.
🖎
Newsletter available to only members & other serious real people in the BDSM community. Publishes *Crackin' The Whip!* Yearly subscription is $35U.S. for U.S., $45U.S. elsewhere.

♂ **Tri-State TCC**
P.O. Box 99626, Pittsburgh, Pennsylvania 15233.

Organizations: Bears

♂ **Bears on Bikes**
P.O. Box 1451, Pittsburgh, Pennsylvania 15219.
Contact: Mr. S. Hill

Organizations: Bondage
☞ **PBC**
P.O. Box 8033, Pittsburgh, Pennsylvania 15216-1467.

Organizations: Family
☺ ☐ **Parents & Friends of Lesbians & Gays (PFLAG)—Pittsburgh**
P. O. Box 223, Monroeville, Pennsylvania 15146.
☎ 412 272 4059

Organizations: Motorcycle
☞▽ **Crucible MC**
123 Fountain Street, Pittsburgh, Pennsylvania 15212-4125.
☎ 412 322 1144
☞▽ **Pittsburgh Motorcycle Club**
P.O. Box 17198, Pittsburgh, Pennsylvania 15235.
☎ 412 795 5968
☼ Meets monthly
Contact: Mr. Peter Rapp
Age statement of 21 is required.

Organizations: Sexuality
☞▽ **Black & White Men Together (BWMT)—Pittsburgh**
1007 Franklin Avenue, Pittsburgh, Pennsylvania 15221.
☎ 412 231 3395
☼ Thu Fri 17:30 - 20:00, Sat 12:00 - 18:00, Sun 12:00 - 15:00
☞▽ **Gay & Lesbian Community Center of Pittsburgh**
P. O. Box 5441, Pittsburgh, Pennsylvania 15206.
☎ 412 422 0114
☼ Mon - Fri 18:00 - 21:30, Sat 15:00 - 18:00
Publishes *GLCC Community Newsletter*.
✉▽ **Transsexual Menace**
Suite2, 221 Morewood Avenue, Pittsburgh, Pennsylvania 15213.
✉ diana@usaor.net
⚲ http://www.echonyc.com/~degrey/Menace.html
✉▽ **Transsexual Support Group (TSG)**
P. O. Box 3214, 6020 Penn Circle South, Pittsburgh, Pennsylvania 15206.
☎ 412 661 7030
✉ tsg@usaor.net
✉☐ **Transpitt**
☞ P. O. Box 3214, Pittsburgh, Pennsylvania 15230.
☎ 412 231 1181

Organizations: Sexuality: Student
☞ **Bisexual, Gay, & Lesbian Alliance at Pitt**
University of Pittsburgh, 502 William Pitt Union, Pittsburgh, Pennsylvania 15260.
☎ 412 648 2105
Publishes a newsletter.
☞▽ **CMU-Out**
c/o Skibo Information Desk, Carnegie Mellon University, Pittsburgh, Pennsylvania 15213.
☎ 412 268 8794
☼ Meets Fri 19:30
☞▽ **Gay & Lesbian Law Caucus**
Pittsburgh School of Law, 3900 Forbes Avenue, Pittsburgh, Pennsylvania 15213.
☎ 412 648 1388

Organizations: Sexuality: Youth
☞▽ **Growing Alternative Youth**
#16-416, 4120 Brownsville Road, Pittsburgh, Pennsylvania 15227.
☎ 412 642 9099

Piercers
☺ ■ **Iron City Ink Tattoos**
328 Butler Street, Etna, Pennsylvania 15223.
☎ 412 784 9396
☼ By appointment
☺ ■ **Slacker**
1312 East Carson Street, Pittsburgh, Pennsylvania 15203.
☎ 412 381 3911
☼ By appointment

Publishers: Books: Sexuality
⚲ ▼ **Cleis Press**
P. O. Box 8933, Pittsburgh, Pennsylvania 15221.
☎ 412 937 1555 📞 412 937 1567
✉ cleis@english-server.hss.cmu.edu

☼ Mon - Fri 09:00 - 17:00
✓ 💳 💳

Publishers: Newspapers: Sexuality
☞▼ **Out**
747 South Avenue, Pittsburgh, Pennsylvania 15221.
☎ 412 243 3350 📞 412 243 4067
☼ Mon - Fri 10:00 - 16:00
⚲ ✓ 💳 💳 💳
The only gay & lesbian publication in the Pittsburgh & tri-state area (western Pennsylvania, Eastern Ohio, & West Virginia). Local & national news, opinions, health, arts, entertainment, calendar of events, & classified ads.. Published every month. Yearly subscription is $33.

Stores: Books: General
☺ ■ **Book Stall, Inc**
3604 5th. Avenue, Pittsburgh, Pennsylvania 15213.
☎ 412 683 3030
☺ ■ **Borders Book Shop**
1775 North Highland Road, Pittsburgh, Pennsylvania 15241.
☎ 412 835 5583 📞 412 835 5637
⚲ ▼ **Gertrude Stein Memorial Bookshop**
⚲ 1003 East Carson, Pittsburgh, Pennsylvania 15203.
☎ 412 481 9666
☼ Thu Fri 17:30 - 20:00, Sat 12:00 - 18:00, Sun 12:00 - 15:00
⚲ ✓ 💳 💳
☺ ▼ **Saint Elmo's Books & Music**
2214 East Carson Street, Pittsburgh, Pennsylvania 15203.
☎ 412 431 9100
☼ 10:00 - 21:00, Sun - 17:00

Stores: Erotica: General
☺ ■ **Boulevard Books**
2nd. Floor, 346 Boulevard of Allies, Pittsburgh, Pennsylvania 15222.
☎ 412 261 9119
☺ ■ **Golden Triangle News**
⚲ 816 Liberty Avenue, Pittsburgh, Pennsylvania 15222.
☎ 412 765 3790

Pocono Summit
Publishers: Magazines: BDSM
⚲ ■ **Chained**
Carter Stevens Presents, P. O. Box 727, Pocono Summit, Pennsylvania 18346.
☎ 717 839 2512
💳 💳
Age statement of 21 is required.

Publishers: Magazines: Spanking
⚲ ■ **Spanks-A-Lot**
Carter Stevens Presents, P. O. Box 727, Pocono Summit, Pennsylvania 18346.
☎ 717 839 2512
💳 💳
Age statement of 21 is required.

Publishers: Magazines: BDSM
⚲ ■ **World of Payne**
Carter Stevens Presents, P. O. Box 727, Pocono Summit, Pennsylvania 18346.
☎ 717 839 2512
💳 💳
Age statement of 21 is required.

Publishers: Newspapers: BDSM
⚲ ■ **Female Domination Forever**
Carter Stevens Presents, P. O. Box 727, Pocono Summit, Pennsylvania 18346.
☎ 717 839 2512
💳
Published every month. Yearly subscription is $45. Age statement of 21 is required.
⚲ ■ **Fetish Video Review**
Carter Stevens Presents, P. O. Box 727, Pocono Summit, Pennsylvania 18346.
☎ 717 839 2512
💳
Published every month. Yearly subscription is $45. Age statement of 21 is required.
⚲ ■ **Footprints**
Carter Stevens Presents, P. O. Box 727, Pocono Summit, Pennsylvania 18346.
☎ 717 839 2512

[VISA] [MC]
Age statement of 21 is required.
♂♀ ■ Mistress Cherie's Orchard
Carter Stevens Presents, P. O. Box 727, Pocono Summit, Pennsylvania 18346.
☎ 717 839 2512
[VISA] [MC]
Age statement of 21 is required.
♂♀ ■ S&M News
Carter Stevens Presents, P. O. Box 727, Pocono Summit, Pennsylvania 18346.
☎ 717 839 2512
[VISA] [MC]
Published every two months. Yearly subscription is $22.50. Age statement of 21 is required.

Reading
Organizations: BDSM
♂ **Reading Railmen**
P.O. Box 13124, Reading, Pennsylvania 19612.

State College
Organizations: AIDS: Education
☺ □ **The AIDS Project**
⅊ Suite 102, 301 South Allen Street, State College, Pennsylvania 16801.
☎ 800 233 2437
☎ 814 234 7087
♂♀▽ **The Page Initiative**
P. O. Box 903, State College, Pennsylvania 16804-0903.
Publishes Page One.
Organizations: Polyfidelity
☺ ■ **Loving Alternatives**
P. O. Box 10509, Calder Square, State College, Pennsylvania 16805-0509.
Organizations: Sexuality
♂ ▽ **Bisexual Women's Group (LGBSA)**
c/o Lesbian, Gay, & Bisexual Student Alliance, Penn State University, 310 Hetzel Union Building, University Park, State College, Pennsylvania 16802.
Organizations: Sexuality: Student
♂♀▽ **Lesbian, Gay, & Bisexual Student Alliance (LGBSA)**
⅊ Penn State University, 310 Hetzel Union Building, University Park, State College, Pennsylvania 16802.
☎ 814 237 1950
☎ 814 865 3327
Piercers
☺ ■ **Forbidden Fruit**
110 Hetzel Street, State College, Pennsylvania 16801.
☎ 814 234 0605

Stroudsburg / Poconos
Organizations: Sexuality: Student
♂♀▽ **East Stroudsburg University GLBSO**
⅊ Box 698 University Center ESU, East Stroudsburg, Pennsylvania 18301.
☎ 717 424 4910
Publishers: Newspapers: Sexuality
⊕ ■ **Defiance**
⅊ 400 Main Street, Stroudsburg, Pennsylvania 18360-2405.

Tionesta
Organizations: Sexuality
♂♀▽ **North West Pennsylvania G & L Task Force**
P. O. Box 213, Tionesta, Pennsylvania 16353-0213.

Wayne
Organizations: Sexuality
✉ **Renaissance Education Association, Inc.—Head Office**
Suite 719, 975 Old Eagle School Road, Wayne, Pennsylvania 19087.
☎ 610 975 9119
✉ bensalem@cpcn.com
🌐 http://www.cdspub.com/REN.html
Contact: Ms. Angela Gardiner, Co-Director of Outreach, Editor-in-Chief
Publishes Renaisance News & Views.

West Chester
Organizations: Motorcycle
♂ **Trident—Philadelphia**
307 East Minor Street, West Chester, Pennsylvania 19308.
Organizations: Sexuality: Student
♂♀▽ **Lesbian, Gay, & Bisexual Association**
⅊ Box 2331, West Chester University, West Chester, Pennsylvania 19383.
☎ 610 436 6949

West Point
Publishers: Books: Medical: General
☺ **The Merck Manual**
☎ 215 397 2340

Wilkes-Barre
Publishers: Newspapers: Sexuality
♂♀ **Spank**
P. O. Box 1092, Wilkes-Barre, Pennsylvania 18702.

Williamsport
Helplines: Sexuality
♂♀▽ **Gay & Lesbian Switchboard of Northern Pennsylvania**
P. O. Box 2510, Williamsport, Pennsylvania 17703.
☎ 717 327 1411
🕐 Mon - Fri 18:00 - 21:00
Organizations: AIDS: Education
☺ □ **AIDS Resource Alliance, Inc.**
⅊ 507 West 4th. Street, Williamsport, Pennsylvania 17701-6003.
☎ 717 322 8448
Organizations: Family
☺ □ **Parents & Friends of Lesbians & Gays (PFLAG)—Central Susquehanna**
☎ 717 742 9350
Organizations: Sexuality
♂♀▽ **Susquehanna Lambda**
P. O. Box 2510, Williamsport, Pennsylvania 17703.
☎ 717 327 1411
Publishes Susquehanna Lambda.

Willow Grove
Counsellors
✉ **Lee Etscovitz**
P. O. Box 471, Willow Grove, Pennsylvania 19090.
☎ 215 657 1560

York
Organizations: AIDS: Education
☺ □ **YHESSI**
101 East Market Street, York, Pennsylvania 17401.
☎ 717 846 6776 ✆ 717 854 0377
🕐 Mon - Fri 08:00 - 17:00 (in English & Spanish)
☺ □ **York Area AIDS Coalition**
P. O. Box 5001, York, Pennsylvania 17405.
☎ 717 846 6776
Organizations: Sexuality
♂♀▽ **York Area Lambda**
⅊ P. O. Box 2425, York, Pennsylvania 17405-2425.
☎ 717 292 1665
☎ 717 846 9636
Printers: General
☺ **Maple-Vail**
P.O. Box 2695, York, Pennsylvania 17405.
☎ 717 764 5911 ✆ 717 764 4702
Stores: Books: General
⊕ ▼ **Her Story**
⅊ 2 West Market Street, Hellam, Pennsylvania 17406.
☎ 717 757 4270
🕐 11:00 - 19:00, Sat 09:00 - 17:00, Sun 12:00 - 17:00
☺ ■ **Towne News**
1000 West Princess Street, York, Pennsylvania 17404-3521.
☎ 717 232 1100

Stores: Erotica: General

⊕▼ **Cupid's Connection**
244 North George Street, York, Pennsylvania 17401.
☎ 717 846 5029
⊕ 09:00 - 02:00, Fri Sat - 17:00

RHODE ISLAND

Area: Approximately 2,709 square kilometres
Population: Approximately 1,005,000
Capital City: Providence
Time zone: GMT minus 5 hours (EST)
Climate: Weather is moderated by the proximity of the Atlantic ocean. Summers average approximately 24°C, winters 9°C.
Age of consent & homosexuality legislation: All anal & oral sex is illegal in this state.
Legal drinking age: 21

State Resources

Health Services

☺ ☐ **Rhode Island Hospital**
593 Eddy Street, Providence, Rhode Island 02903.
☎ 401 444 4000

Helplines: Sexuality

⊕▽ **Gay & Lesbian Helpline of Rhode Island**
P. O. Box 5671, Providence, Rhode Island 02903.
☎ 401 751 3322
Publishes *Options*.

Organizations: AIDS: Education

☺ ☐ **Rhode Island Project / AIDS**
3rd. Floor, 95 Chestnut Street, Providence, Rhode Island 02903-4110.
☎ 401 831 5522
☎ 800 726 3010 (hotline)

Organizations: Sexuality

⊕▽ **Network of Rhode Island**
⅃ P. O. Box 1474, Pawtucket, Rhode Island 02862-1474.

▷⟋▽ **Silent Passage**
☎ 401 438 7477
Age statement of 21 is required.

East Greenwich

Counsellors

☺ **Summit Consulting Group, Inc**
K P. O. Box 1009, East Greenwich, Rhode Island 02818.
☎ 401 884 2778 ✆ 401 884 5068
✉ 71525.553@compuserve.com.
General counselling, sexuality issues.

East Providence

Suppliers: Electrolysis

▷⟋■ **Roxy's Electrolysis**
Suite 2, 234 Warren Avenue, East Providence, Rhode Island 02914.

Kingston

Organizations: Sexuality: Student

⊕▽ **URI Gay, Lesbian, & Bisexual Association**
⅃ c/o Student Senate, 346 Memorial Union, Kingston, Rhode Island 02881.
☎ 401 792 2097
Publishes *3 Dollar Bill*.

Providence

Bars: BDSM

⊕▼ **Yukon Trading Company**
⅃ 124 Snow Street, Providence, Rhode Island 02903.
☎ 401 274 6620
✉ mrmounty@aol.com
⊕ Sun - Thu 16:00 - 01:00 Fri Sat - 02:00
Age statement of 21 is required.

Organizations: BDSM

⊕ ☐ **Ace**
P. O. Box 261, Annex Station, Providence, Rhode Island 02901.

Organizations: Sexuality: Student

⊕▽ **Lesbian Bisexual Collective**
c/o Box 1829, Sarah Doyle, Brown University, Providence, Rhode Island 02912.
☎ 401 863 2189

⊕▽ **Lesbian, Gay, & Bisexual Alliance**
⅃ P. O. Box 1930 SAO, Brown University, Providence, Rhode Island 02912.
☎ 401 863 3062
Publishes *Not Guilty*.

⊕▽ **Rhode Island College Gay, Lesbian, or Bisexual Equality Alliance (GLOBE)**
Student Union, 600 Mount Pleasant Avenue, Providence, Rhode Island 02908.

Stores: Erotica: General

⊕■ **Upstairs Bookshop**
206 Washington Street, Providence, Rhode Island 02903.
☎ 401 272 3139

Riverside

Organizations: Bears

⊕▽ **Rhode Island Grizzlies**
P. O. Box 15373, Riverside, Rhode Island 02915.
☎ 410 727 8840

SOUTH CAROLINA

Area: Approximately 78,000 square kilometres
Population: Approximately 3,500,000
Capital City: Columbia
Time zone: GMT minus 5 hours (EST)
Climate: Warm, humid summers with an average temperature of approximately 27°C & mild winters with an average temperature of approximately 9°C. The Atlantic ocean has a moderating influence on the coastal regions.
Age of consent & homosexuality legislation: All anal & oral sex is illegal in this state.
Legal drinking age: 21

State Resources

Organizations: AIDS: Education

☺ ☐ **South Carolina AIDS Education Network, Inc.**
Suite 98, 2768 Decker Boulevard, Columbia, South Carolina 29206.
☎ 803 736 1171

Organizations: AIDS: Support

☺ ☐ **Palmetto AIDS Life Support Services of South Carolina, Inc. (PALSS)**
P. O. Box 12124, Columbia, South Carolina 29211.
☎ 800 868 7257 ✆ 803 779 7257

Organizations: Sexuality

⊕ ▽ **South Carolina Women's Consortium (SCWC)**
P. O. Box 3099, Columbia, South Carolina 29230.

Organizations: Sexuality: Student

⊕▽ **Beyond Tolerance Task Force**
c/o Student Affairs, University of South Carolina, 109 Russell House, Columbia, South Carolina 29208.
☎ 803 777 4172 ✆ 803 777 9354

Publishers: Newspapers: Sexuality

⊕▽ **Virago**
P. O. Box 11193, Columbia, South Carolina 29211.
☎ 803 246 9090

Aiken

Organizations: Sexuality

⊕▽ **Last Sunday**
284, Aiken, South Carolina 29802.

Charleston

Health Services

☺ ☐ **Naval Hospital**
☎ 803 743 7200

☺ ☐ **Veterans' Affairs Medical Center**
109 Bee Street, Charleston, South Carolina 29401.
☎ 803 577 5011

Organizations: AIDS: Support

☺ ☐ **Low Country Palmetto AIDS Support Services**
⅃ P. O. Box 207, Charleston, South Carolina 29402.
☎ 803 577 2437

Organizations: BDSM

⊕▽ **Trident Knights**
P. O. Box 31622, Charleston, South Carolina 29417.

☎ 803 769 2094
✉ Tridentkts@aol.com
🌐 http://users.aol.com/cuirlover/tks.htm
👢 ✓ $ ⚎
A levi / leather club.

Organizations: Sexuality

⚥▽ **Low Country Gay & Lesbian Information Alliance**
P. O. Box 98, Charleston, South Carolina 29401.
☎ 803 881 0129

Clemson

Organizations: Sexuality: Student

⚥▽ **Lambda Society at Clemson**
P. O. Box 5795, University Station, Clemson, South Carolina 29632.

Columbia

Bars: General

⚥■ **Lil Rascals**
1109 Assembly, Columbia, South Carolina 29201.
☎ 803 771 0121
🕐 17:00 - 06:00
Some leather.

Health Services

☺□ **Richland Memorial Hospital**
Five Richland Medical Park, Columbia, South Carolina 29203.
☎ 803 434 6512

Organizations: BDSM

⚥▽ **Levi/Leather Brigade**
P. O. Box 7214, Columbia, South Carolina 29202.
☎ 803 796 3860

Organizations: Family

☺□ **Parents & Friends of Lesbians & Gays (PFLAG)—Columbia**
493 Hickory Hill Drive, Columbia, South Carolina 29210.
☎ 803 772 7396

Organizations: Research: Sexuality

⚥ **Gay & Lesbian Advocacy Research Project**
P. O. Box 5085, Columbia, South Carolina 29250.

Organizations: Sexuality

⚥▽ **The Center**
P. O. Box 12648, Columbia, South Carolina 29211.
☎ 800 325 4297
☎ 803 771 7713
🕐 Wed 13:00 - 18:00, Fri 19:00 - 23:00, Sat 13:00 - 23:00, Sun 13:00 - 21:00

⚥▽ **Elmwood Park / Cottontown Lesbian & Gay Neighborhood Association**
☎ 803 252 2269

Publishers: Magazines: Sexuality

⚥▼ *Empathy*
Gay & Lesbian Advocacy Project, P. O. Box 5085, Columbia, South Carolina 29250.
☎ 803 791 1607
Published twice a year. Yearly subscription is $15.

Stores: Books: General

⊕▼ **Bluestocking Books**
⚬ 829 Gervais Street, Columbia, South Carolina 29201.
☎ 803 929 0114
🕐 Mon - Sat 10:00 - 18:00
Specializes in female authors.

Stores: Erotica: General

☺■ **Château IV Bookstore**
P. O. Box 23389, Columbia, South Carolina 29224-3389.
☎ 803 754 0713

☺ **Nitch Novelties**
P. O. Box 9286, Columbia, South Carolina 29290-0286.
☎ 800 445 8697

Greenville

Organizations: AIDS: Education

☺□ **AID Upstate**
P. O. Box 105, Greenville, South Carolina 29602.
☎ 803 233 8842

Organizations: Sexuality

⚥▽ **Upstate Women's Community**
⚬ P. O. Box 6652, Greenville, South Carolina 29606.
☎ 803 271 4207
Publishes a newsletter.

Greenwood

Suppliers: Diapers

☺■ **Professional Medical Products**
P. O. Box 3288, Greenwood, South Carolina 29648.
☎ 803 223 4281
☎ 800 845 4571
Disposable diaper & liners.

North Augusta

Stores: Erotica: General

☺■ **Foxes Adult Books**
111 Jefferson Davis Highway, North Augusta, South Carolina 29841.
☎ 803 279 7023

Pawleys Island

Organizations: Family

☺□ **Parents & Friends of Lesbians & Gays (PFLAG)—Pawleys Island**
P. O. Box 1761, Pawleys Island, South Carolina 29585.

Spartanburg

Organizations: Motorcycle

⚥▽ **Spartans MC**
P. O. Box 6041, Spartanburg, South Carolina 29304-6041.

West Columbia

Suppliers: Diapers

☺■ **George Disposables**
P. O. Box 5887, Old Dunbar Road, West Columbia, South Carolina 29171.
☎ 803 796 9196
Disposable diapers.

SOUTH DAKOTA

Area: Approximately 197,000 square kilometres
Population: Approximately 700,000
Capital City: Pierre
Time zone: GMT minus 6/7 hours (both CST & Mountain Time)
Age of consent & homosexuality legislation: State has adopted the Model Penal Code or otherwise decriminalized homosexual activities.

State Resources

Organizations: Sexuality

⚥▽ **The Coalition**
⚬ P. O. Box 89803, Sioux Falls, South Dakota 57105.
☎ 605 333 0603

Publishers: Newspapers: Sexuality

⚥▼ **Left of Center**
P. O. Box 88812, Sioux Falls, South Dakota 57105.
☎ 605 361 7043

⚥▼ *The Progress Tribune*
P. O. Box 88812, Columbia, South Dakota 57105.
☎ 605 361 7043

Brookings

Organizations: Sexuality

⚥▽ **Sons & Daughters**
P. O. Box 478, Brookings, South Dakota 57006.
☎ 605 692 6026
🕐 Call evenings & weekends

Hill City

Stores: Books: General

☺▼ **Oriana's Bookcafé**
P. O. Box 479, Hill City, South Dakota 57745.
☎ 800 524 4954
☎ 605 574 4878
Publishes *Bookcafé News*.

Rapid City

Stores: Erotica: General

☺■ **Monument Books**

Stores: Erotica: General

912 Main Street, Rapid City, South Dakota 57701.
☎ 605 397 9877

Sioux Falls
Bars: General
♂▼ **Club 332**
 ♿ 332 South Phillips Avenue, Sioux Falls, South Dakota 57102.
 ☎ 605 335 9874
 Some leather.

Stores: Erotica: General
☺■ **Studio One**
 311 North Dakota Avenue, Sioux Falls, South Dakota 57102.
 ☎ 605 332 9316

TENNESSEE
Area: Approximately 107,000 square kilometres
Population: Approximately 4,900,000
Capital City: Nashville
Time zone: GMT minus 5/6 hours (both EST & CST)
Climate: Inland the weather is mild with summer average highs of approximately 26˚C & winter lows of approximately 6˚C. Closer to the coast, the mountain weather is mild, but the rest of the coastal regions can experience hot, humid, & stormy summers with highs averaging approximately 27˚C, & winter lows averaging approximately 4˚C.
Age of consent & homosexuality legislation: All anal & oral sex is illegal in this state.
Legal drinking age: 21

State Resources
Publishers: Newspapers: Sexuality
♂▼ *Query*
 P. O. Box 24241, Nashville, Tennessee 37202-4241.
 ☎ 800 625 7972
 ☎ 615 327 7972
 Published every week.

Brentwood
Organizations: Sexuality
✍▽ **The Society for the Second Self (Tri-Ess)—Alpha Pi Omega**
 P. O. Box 784, Brentwood, Tennessee 37204-0784.

Chattanooga
Organizations: Family
☺□ **Parents & Friends of Lesbians & Gays (PFLAG)—Greater Chattanooga**
 P. O. Box 17252, Red Bank, Tennessee 37415.
 ☎ 615 875 5750
 ⏰ Meets 4th. Sun of month

Publishers: Books: Sexuality
🐸 **Timely Books**
 4040 Mountain Creek Road, Chattanooga, Tennessee 37415.
 ☎ 615 875 9447

Cookeville
Organizations: Sexuality
♂▽ **Middle Tennessee Gay & Lesbian Alliance**
 P. O. Box 101, Cookeville, Tennessee 38503-0101.

Publishers: Directories: Sexuality
☺ *Outposts*
 P. O. Box 1213, Cookeville, Tennessee 38503.
 Radical sexuality, art, politics, etc..

Johnson City
Counsellors
✍▼ **Mountain Home VAMC**
 ☎ 615 926 1177 Ext.: 7709

Organizations: AIDS: Education
☺□ **HIV Network, Inc.**
 P. O. Box 1512, Johnson City, Tennessee 37615-1512.
 ☎ 615 928 8888

Kingsport
Printers: General
☺■ **Donihe Graphics, Inc.**
 766 Brookside Drive, Kingsport, Tennessee 37662.
 ☎ 800 251 0337 📞 423 246 7297

☎ 423 246 2800

Knoxville
Health Services
☺○ **University of Tennessee Memorial Hospital**
 1924 Alcoa Highway, Knoxville, Tennessee 37920.
 ☎ 615 544 9000

Organizations: AIDS: Education
☺□ **AIDS Response Knoxville (ARK)**
 ♈ P. O. Box 6069, Knoxville, Tennessee 37914-6069.
 ☎ 615 523 2437 📞 615 546 2437

Organizations: Bears
♂▽ **Appalachian Bears Club of East Tennessee**
 P. O. Box 27144, Knoxville, Tennessee 37927-7144.
 ☎ 615 524 7884 (infoline)
 Contact: Mr. Casey Scott
♂▽ **Smokey Mountain Bears**
 P. O. Box 52662, Knoxville, Tennessee 37950.
 ☎ 615 531 7515

Stores: Books: General
☺■ **Chelsea Station News**
 103 West Jackson Avenue, Knoxville, Tennessee 37902.
 ☎ 615 522 6390
☺■ **Davis-Kidd Bookseller**
 113 North Peters Road, Knoxville, Tennessee 37923.
 ☎ 615 690 0136

Lavergne
Distributors: Books: General
☺ **Ingram Book**
 1125 Heil Quaker Boulevard, Lavergne, Tennessee 37086.

Liberty
Publishers: Newspapers: Sexuality
♂▼ *RFD*
 P. O. Box 68, Liberty, Tennessee 37095.
 ☎ 615 536 5176
 ⏰ 24hr. answering machine
 ✓
 A country journal for gay men everywhere. Published quarterly. Yearly subscription is $25.

Memphis
Bars: BDSM
♂▼ **Pipeline**
 ♿ 1382 Poplar, Memphis, Tennessee 38104.
 ☎ 901 726 5263
 ⏰ 14:00 - 03:00

Counsellors
☺■ **Ethelreda Collins, LCSW, BCD**
 Suite 601, 2670 Union Avenue, Memphis, Tennessee 38112.
 ☎ 901 323 6500

Health Services
☺□ **Regional Medical Center at Memphis**
 ☎ 901 575 7100
☺□ **Saint Francis Hospital**
 5959 Park Avenue, Memphis, Tennessee 38119.
 ☎ 901 765 1000

Helplines: Sexuality
♂▽ **Gay & Lesbian Switchboard**
 P. O. Box 41074, Memphis, Tennessee 38174-1074.
 ☎ 901 728 4297

Organizations: AIDS: Education
☺□ **Friends For Life**
 ♿ P. O. Box 40389, Memphis, Tennessee 38174-0389.
 ☎ 901 458 2437

Organizations: BDSM
♂▽ **Memphis Leather / Levi Alliance**
 4372 Kerwin Drive, Memphis, Tennessee 38128.
 ☎ 901 386 8625
♂▽ **Tennessee Leather Tribe**
 P. O. Box, 3293 Renners Cove, Memphis, Tennessee 38128-3436.
♂▽ **Tsarus**
 P. O. Box 41082, Memphis, Tennessee 38174-1082.

♂▽ **Wings MC**
P. O. Box 41784, Memphis, Tennessee 38174-1784.

Organizations: Family
☺□ **Parents & Friends of Lesbians & Gays (PFLAG)— Memphis**
P. O. Box 172031, Memphis, Tennessee 38187-2031.
☎ 901 761 1444

Organizations: Motorcycle
♂▽ **Riverboat Gamblers Motorcycle Club**
P. O. Box 40404, Memphis, Tennessee 38104.
☎ 901 276 9939

Organizations: Sexuality
♂▽ **Black & White Men Together (BWMT)—Memphis**
♿ P. O. Box 42157, Memphis, Tennessee 38174-2157.
☎ 901 726 1461

♂ **Memphis Bisexual Alliance**
♿ Suite 4, 1517 Court Street, Memphis, Tennessee 38104-2402.
Contact: Rev. John Prowett

♂▽ **Memphis Gay & Lesbian Center**
♿ P. O. Box 41074, Memphis, Tennessee 38174-1074.
☎ 901 276 4651

✉□ **Memphis Trans-Gender Alliance**
♿ P. O. Box 11232, Memphis, Tennessee 38111-0232.
🕐 Meets 4th. Sat of month 14:00
Publishes *Powder & Pearls* every month. Yearly subscription is $15.

✉▽ **TV/TS Support Group**
Suite 4, 1517 Court Street, Memphis, Tennessee 38104-2402.
🕐 Meets 4th. Sat of month 18:00
Contact: Rev. John Prowett

Organizations: Sexuality: Student
♂▽ **Students for Bisexual, Gay, & Lesbian Awareness (GALA)**
♿ Box 100, Office of Greek Affairs, MSU, Memphis, Tennessee 38152.
🕐 Meets Thu 19:00

Piercers
☺■ **Underground Art**
2287 Young Avenue, Memphis, Tennessee.
☎ 901 272 1864

Publishers: Newspapers: Sexuality
♂▼ *Triangle Journal News*
♿ P. O. Box 11485, Memphis, Tennessee 38111-0485.
☎ 901 454 1411
Published every month.

Radio: Sexuality
♂▽ *Gay Alternative*
♿ WEVL FM 90, P. O. Box 41773, Memphis, Tennessee 38104-1773.
🕐 Mon 18:00 - 19:00

Stores: Books: General
⊕▼ **Meristem**
♿ 930 South Cooper, Memphis, Tennessee 38104.
☎ 901 276 0282
🕐 Wed - Sat 10:00 - 18:00, Sun 13:00 - 17:00

Stores: Erotica: General
☺■ **Puss'N'Boots**
2149 Young Avenue, Memphis, Tennessee 38112.
☎ 901 276 9970
Piercing jewelry also available.

Millington
Piercers
☺■ **Ship to Shore Tattooing & Body Piercing**
4491 King Lake Land, Millington, Tennessee 38053.
☎ 901 872 0405 ✆ 901 872 0405
🕐 Every day from 15:00

Murfreesboro
Organizations: Sexuality: Student
♂▽ **MTSU Lambda Association**
♿ MTSU Box 624, Murfreesboro, Tennessee 37132.
☎ 615 780 2293
Publishes *The Pink Voice*.

Nashville
Bars: General
♂▼ **Victor / Victoria's**
♿ 111 8th. Avenue North, Nashville, Tennessee 37203.
☎ 615 244 7256
🕐 15:00 - 03:00
Some leather.

Health Services
☺□ **Metropolitan Nashville General Hospital**
72 Hermitage Avenue, Nashville, Tennessee 37210.
☎ 615 862 4490

☺□ **Veterans' Affairs Medical Center**
1310 24th. Avenue, Nashville, Tennessee 37212.
☎ 615 327 4751

Organizations: BDSM
♂▽ **Conductors L/L**
P. O. Box 40261, Nashville, Tennessee 37204.

☺□ **People Exchanging Power (PEP)—Nashville**
2426 Turner Lane, Clarksville, Tennessee 37040.

Organizations: Bears
♂▽ **Music City Bears**
P. O. Box 101592, Nashville, Tennessee 37224.

Organizations: Body Size
♂▽ **Girth & Mirth—Tennessee**
P. O. Box 121866, Nashville, Tennessee 37212.

Organizations: Sexuality
♂▽ **The Center for Lesbian & Gay Community Services**
703 Berry Road, Nashville, Tennessee 37204-2803.
☎ 615 297 0008
🕐 Call 24hrs.

✉▽ **Tennessee Vals**
♿ P. O. Box 92335, Nashville, Tennessee 37209.
☎ 615 664 6883 (voice mail)
🌐 http://www.zoom.com/tg/tvals/index.html
Publishes *Nesletter* every month.

Organizations: Sexuality: Youth
♂▽ **One-In-Teen Youth Services**
♿ 703 Berry Road, Nashville, Tennessee 37204.
☎ 615 297 0008

Publishers: Magazines: Fetish
☺■ *Get Kinky*
Modern Products, 1007 Murfreesboro Road, Nashville, Tennessee 37217-1516.

Publishers: Newspapers: Sexuality
♂ *Dore*
P. O. Box 40422, Nashville, Tennessee 37204.
☎ 615 292 9623

Stores: Books: General
☺■ **Davis-Kidd Bookseller**
♿ 4007 Hillsboro Road, Nashville, Tennessee 37215.
☎ 615 385 2645

☺■ **Dragonfly Books**
♿ 1701 Portland Avenue, Nashville, Tennessee 37212.
☎ 615 292 5699
🕐 Mon - Sat 11:00 - 19:00, Sun 13:00 - 17:00

Stores: Erotica: General
☺■ **Carousel Books**
5606 Charlotte Avenue, Nashville, Tennessee 37209.
☎ 615 352 0855

☺■ **Odyssey Book Store**
700 Division Street, Nashville, Tennessee 37203.
☎ 615 726 0243

Television: Sexuality
♂▽ *Gay Cable Nash*
Viacom Cabe, Channel 19, 703 Berry Road, Nashville, Tennessee 37204-2803.
☎ 615 297 0008
🕐 Tue Sat 21:00 - 22:00, Sat 20:00 - 21:00

Saint Bethlehem

Organizations: BDSM

People Exchanging Power (PEP)—Tennessee
P. O. Box 174, Saint Bethlehem, Tennessee 37155.
615 648 1937 615 572 9368
615 244 2438
Meet monthly
Age statement of 21 is required.

Woodlawn

Publishers: Magazines: Fetish: Foot

Pediform
Eagle Press, P. O. Box 71, Woodlawn, Tennessee 37191.
Published quarterly. Yearly subscription is $30.

TEXAS

Area: Approximately 650,000 square kilometres
Population: Approximately 117,060 ,000
Capital City: Austin
Time zone: GMT minus 6/7 hours (both CST & Mountain Time)
Climate: Hot, humid, sub-tropical weather with summer average temperatures of approximately 27°C & winter temperatures of approximately 7°C (17°C in San Antonio). Little or no snow falls in this state.
Age of consent & homosexuality legislation: Anal & oral sex is illegal in this state only between people of the same sex. It is also possible to be arrested for "trafficking in dildos" in this state. (Apparently, more having than six dildos can lead to your arrest as a trafficker!)
Legal drinking age: 21

State Resources

Organizations: AIDS: Education

AIDS Support Foundation, Inc.
Suite 41, 2610 Iowa Park Road, Wichita Falls, Texas 76305-3227.
817 691 7539
Publishes *HIV Lifeline*.

Organizations: Sexuality

Gay Service Network
585, Austin, Texas 78768.
512 445 7270

Publishers: Newspapers: Sexuality

Dimensions
P. O. Box 856, Lubbock, Texas 79408.
806 797 9647
Lesbian publication, lifestyle related, distributed in Texas, Oklahoma, New Mexico, & New Orleans bars, bookstores, etc.. Published 11 times a year. Yearly subscription is $24.

This Week in Texas (TWT)
Suite 111, 811 Westheimer Road, Houston, Texas 77006-3942.
713 527 9111
Texas' oldest gay publication, in its 20th. year. A statewide information, travel, & entertainment guide. Published every week. Yearly subscription is $69.

Abilene

Organizations: Sexuality

West Texas Gender Alliance
P. O. Box 6726, Abilene, Texas 79608.
Meets 2nd. Sat of month
Contact: Ms. Tami Maloney

Amarillo

Organizations: Sexuality

The Society for the Second Self (Tri-Ess)—Alpha Chi
P. O. Box 50266, Amarillo, Texas 79159.
806 359 7714
Meets 1st. Sat of month. Call most eve, except Wed & Sun

Arlington

Organizations: Motorcycle

Texas Cadre
P.O. Box 1041, Arlington, Texas 76010.

Organizations: Sexuality: Youth

National Youth Advocacy Alliance
P. O. Box 121690, Arlington, Texas 76012.
800 873 2820
817 535 5259
Contact: Mr. Jeff Barea
A national youth lobbying organization. Publishes *Youth Advocacy*.

Austin

Bars: BDSM

The Chain Drive
602 East 7th Street, Austin, Texas.
512 478 0295

Health Services

Saint David's Hospital
919 East 32nd. Street, Austin, Texas 78705.
512 476 7111

Seton Medical Center
1201 West 38th. Street, Austin, Texas 78705.
512 323 1000

Organizations: AIDS: Education

AIDS Services of Austin
P. O. Box 4874, 1615 West 6th. Street, Austin, Texas 78765.
512 452 2437 (info. & referral)
512 472 2273 (office)
Mon - Fri 09:00 - 18:00

Informe SIDA
P. O. Box 13501, Austin, Texas 78711.
512 472 2001
Publishes *ALLGO-PASA*.

Organizations: BDSM

Bound by Desire
P.O. Box 26583, Austin, Texas 78755.
512 473 7104
Contact: Mr. Jonnie JR

The Group with No Name (GWNN)
P. O. Box 18301, Austin, Texas 78760-9998.
gwnn@ghetto.com
http://io.com/user/crackers/GWNN.html
Meets 2nd. Sat of month
Contact: Joel
Organizes the Austin A.S.B Munch. Publishes *This Space Intentionally Left Blank*.

The National Leather Association (NLA)—Austin
P.O. Box 49801, Austin, Texas 78765-0801.
512 703 8927
Meets 3rd. Mon of month
Publishes a newsletter.

Organizations: Bears

Heart of Texas Bears
2400 Broken Oak, Austin, Texas 78745.
hotb@spdcc.com
http://spdcc.com/home/hotb/index.html

Organizations: Motorcycle

Capital City Riders MC
504 Willow, Austin, Texas 78701-4220.

Organizations: Sexuality

Austin Second Image
P. O. Box 14965, Austin, Texas 78751.
512 515 5460
Call Wed 19:00 - 21:00

Organizations: Sexuality: Student

Law Students for Gay & Lesbian Concerns
University of Texas Law School, 727 East 26th. Street, Austin, Texas 78705.
512 452 3591

Piercers

Planet K
1516 South Lamar, Austin, Texas 78704.
512 443 2292

Zoom
812 West 12th. Street, Austin, Texas 87801.
512 472 3316

Printers: General

Morgan Printing & Publishing
#135, 900 Old Koenig Lane, Austin, Texas 7856-1514.
512 459 5194 512 451 0755

Publishers: Magazines: Arts

OutArt

P. O. Box 684852, Austin, Texas 78768-4852.

Publishers: Magazines: Sexuality

⚣▼ *Fag Rag*
Snaxus Productions, P. O. Box 1034, Austin, Texas 78767.
☎ 512 416 0100 ✆ 512 416 6981
🕐 Mon - Fri 11:00 - 19:00
✓
Published twice a month. Yearly subscription is $29.

Publishers: Magazines: Shaving

⚣▼ *Smooth Buddies Bulletin*
Mercury Productions, Suite 168, 603 West 13th. Street, Austin, Texas 78701.
Published quarterly. Yearly subscription is $25.

Publishers: Miscellaneous

⚥ **Edward-William Publishing Company**
P. O. Box 332280, #292, Austin, Texas 78764.
☎ 512 288 7515

Publishers: Newspapers: Sexuality

⚣▽ *The Texas Triangle*
♿ 1615 West 6th. Street, Austin, Texas 78703.
☎ 512 476 0576 ✆ 512 472 8154
Comprehensive, professional coverage of issues & people. Published every week.

Publishers: Videos: Fetish: Mess

🕴 ■ **Messy Fun**
P. O. Box 181030, Austin, Texas 78718-1030.
Sample photos $16. Free catalogue. Age statement of 21 is required.

Stores: Books: General

⚥ ▼ **Book Woman**
♿ 918 West 12th. Street, Austin, Texas 78703.
☎ 512 472 2785
🕐 Mon - Sat 10:00 - 21:00, Sun 12:00 - 18:00
🛍 ✓ ✂ VISA MC 🔲
Women's bookstore. Also mail order.

☺ ■ **Europa Bookstore**
Dobie Mall, 2048 Guadalupe Street, Austin, Texas 78705.
☎ 512 476 0423 ✆ 512 479 0912

⚥▼ **Liberty Books**
♿ 1014-B North Lamar Boulevard, Austin, Texas 78703.
☎ 800 828 1279
☎ 512 495 9737
🕐 Mon - Sat 10:00 - 21:00, Sun 12:00 - 18:00
🛍 ✓ VISA MC

⚥▼ **Lobo Bookstore**
3204A Guadeloupe, Austin, Texas 78705.
☎ 512 454 5406
🕐 10:00 - 22:00

Stores: Erotica: General

☺ ■ **Forbidden Fruit**
♿ 512 Neches, Austin, Texas 78701.
☎ 512 478 8358 ✆ 512 478 8358
🕐 11:00 - 23:00, Sun 13:00 - 19:00
🛍 ✓ VISA MC
Also sells leather items. Age statement of 18 is required.

☺ ■ **Forbidden Fruit Uptown**
2001-A Guadalupe Street, Austin, Texas 78705.
☎ 512 478 8542
Also sells leather items.

☺ ■ **Oasis Bookstore**
♿ 9601 North Interregional Highway 35, Austin, Texas 78753.
☎ 512 835 7208

☺ ▼ **Pleasureland**
♿ 613 West 29th. Street, Austin, Texas 78705.
☎ 512 478 2339

Bellaire

Organizations: Sexuality

▷▽ **Texas Assocation of Transexuals (TATs)**
P. O. Box 142, Bellaire, Texas 88401.
☎ 713 827 5913
🕐 Meets 2nd & 4th. Sat of month

Bryan

Manufacturers: Chastity Belts

☺ ■ **Stainless Construction Company**
P. O. Box 1594, Bryan, Texas 77806.

Custom made in stainless steel.

Bulverde

Organizations: Sexuality

▷▽ **Boulton & Park Society**
P. O. Box 17, Bulverde, Texas 78163.
☎ 210 980 7788
Peer support. Publishes *Gender Euphoria*.

▷▽ **WATS**
P. O. Box 17, Bulverde, Texas 78163.
☎ 210 980 7788
🕐 Call before 21:00 Connecticut time, please
Support for women involved with transgendered men. Publishes *Partners*.

College Station

Organizations: AIDS: Education

☺ □ **Brazos Valley AIDS Foundation**
P. O. Box 9209, College Station, Texas 77842-0209.
☎ 409 260 2437

Organizations: Sexuality

⚥▽ **Brazos Valley Women's Group**
P. O. Box 133, College Station, Texas 77878.

Organizations: Sexuality: Student

⚥▽ **Gay, Lesbian, & Bisexual Aggies**
♿ #789 MSC Student Finance Center, Texas A&M University, College Station, Texas 77843-1237.
☎ 409 847 0321

Corpus Christi

Health Services

☺ □ **Memorial Medical Center**
2606 Hospital Boulevard, Corpus Christi, Texas 78405.
☎ 512 881 4000

Manufacturers: Whips

☺ ■ **Bitch Buffy**
807 Coleman Avenue, Corpus Christi, Texas 78401.
Custom whips & floggers.

Organizations: AIDS: Education

☺ □ **Coastal Bend AIDS Foundation**
♿ P. O. Box 331416, Corpus Christi, Texas 78463.
☎ 512 883 5815
☎ 512 883 2273 (hotline)
🕐 Hotline 24hrs.

Organizations: BDSM

⚥▽ **Bay Area Levi & Leather Society**
P. O. Box 33122, Corpus Christi, Texas 78463-1322.

⚥▽ **Silver Dolphins LLC**
P.O. Box 6129, Corpus Christi, Texas 78466-6129.

Organizations: Motorcycle

⚦ **Corpus Christi MC**
P.O. Box 3532, Corpus Christi, Texas 78463-3532.

⚦ **Road Riders MC**
P.O. Box 3246, Corpus Christi, Texas 78404.

Dallas / Fort Worth

Archives: Sexuality

⚥▽ **Dallas Gay & Lesbian Historic Archives**
♿ Community Center, P. O. Box 190712, Dallas, Texas 75219.
☎ 214 821 1653
☎ 214 528 4233

Bars: BDSM

⚥▼ **The Brick**
4117 Maple Street, Dallas, Texas 75219.
☎ 214 521 2024
🕐 12:00 - 02:00, Fri Sat - 04:00

☺ ▼ **The Eagle**
Suite 107, 2515 Inwood Road, Dallas, Texas 75039.
☎ 214 559 3511 ✆ 214 357 4375
🕐 Wed - Sun 16:00 - 02:00

⚥▼ **The Hidden Door**
5025 Browser Street, Dallas, Texas.
☎ 214 526 9211

Counsellors

Dennis Hartzog, M.Ed, L.P.C.
Suite B, 4235 Gilbert, Dallas, Texas 75219.
214 559 0688
Licensed professional counsellor in abuse survival, depression, grief & loss, HIV issues, relationships, working with individuals on probation for sexual offences.

Legacy Counseling Center, Inc.
Suite 212, 4054 McKinney Avenue, Dallas, Texas 75204.
214 520 6308 214 521 9172
Provides HIV/AIDS counselling for those living with or affected by HIV/AIDS. Sliding fee scale based on income. Individual & group counselling. Age statement of 18 is required. American Sign Language also spoken.

Oak Lawn Community Services
P. O. Box 191094, Dallas, Texas 75219.
214 520 8108
Mon - Fri 09:00 - 21:00
Publishes *The Vision.*

Stephen Vanek, LMSW-ACP
Suite 410, 4099 McEwen, Dallas, Texas 75244.
214 239 8775

Health Services

Dallas County Hospital
5201 Harry Hines Boulevard, Dallas, Texas 75235.
214 590 8000
HIV & emergency departments.

Nelson-Tebedo Clinic
4012 Cedar Springs, Dallas, Texas 75219.
214 528 2336 214 528 8436
Mon - Fri 09:00 - 17:00
HIV/AIDS & sexual health counselling & testing for people eleven years & up.

Saint Paul Medical Center
5909 Harry Hines Boulevard, Dallas, Texas 75235.
214 879 1000

Tarrant County Hospital
1500 South Main Street, Fort Worth, Texas 76104.
817 921 3431
HIV & emergency departments.

Veterans' Affairs Medical Center
4500 South Lancaster Road, Dallas, Texas 75216.
214 372 7001

Manufacturers: Erotica: Leather

Dungeon Enterprises, Inc.
P. O. Box 35854, Dallas, Texas 75235-0854.
214 522 2796
dungeon@ix.netcom.com
Iron shackles, collars, ball & chain, cages, & custom cells. Chain mail belts, shirts, bullwhips, jockstraps, & cats. Canvas slings.

Manufacturers: Restraints: Metal

Iron Master
Building K, 3320 Dilido Road, Dallas, Texas 75228.
214 324 4687 214 328 3425

Organizations: AIDS: Education

AIDS Arms Network
Suite 222, 2727 Oaklawn, Dallas, Texas 75219.
214 521 5191 214 528 5879

AIDS Outreach Center
1125 West Peter Smith, Fort Worth, Texas 76104.
817 335 1994

AIDS Resource Center
P. O. Box 190712, Dallas, Texas 75219.
214 521 5124
Publishes *AIDS Update.*

Organizations: AIDS: Support

AIDS Services of Dallas
P. O. Box 4338, Dallas, Texas 75208.
214 941 0523 214 941 8144

Organizations: BDSM

Branding Iron Club
P. O. Box 190471, Dallas, Texas 75219.

Cowtown Leathermen
P.O. Box 3494, Fort Worth, Texas 76113.

Dallas Area Levi / Leather Association (DALLAS)
P.O. Box 191052, Dallas, Texas 75219-8052.
214 288 9395

Disciples of de Sade
P.O. Box 190712, Dallas, Texas 75219.

The Dungeon Players
Suite 166, 2806 Reagan, Dallas, Texas 75219.

Firedancers—Dallas
P.O. Box 190712, Dallas, Texas 75219-0712.

Leather Knights
Suite 219, 4539 Cedar Springs, Dallas, Texas 75219.
214 521 3239

Leather Rose Society
P. O. Box 223971, Dallas, Texas 75222-3971.
214 289 0619
214 375 1994
leatherrose@intex.net
Meets monthly
Publishes a newsletter 10 times a year. Yearly subscription is $20U.S.. Age statement of 21 is required.

The National Leather Association (NLA)—Dallas
P.O. Box 7597, Dallas, Texas 75209-7597.
214 521 5342 Ext.: 820, press 4

Silver Spurs of Dallas
P.O. Box 111148, Carrollton, Texas 75011-1148.

Organizations: Bears

Dallas Bears
P. O. Box 190869, Dallas, Texas 75219-0869.
214 521 5342 Ext.: 880
dale@bear.net
http://www.dfw.net/~dtherio/db/

Lone Star Bears
Suite 161, 3575 North Beltline, Irving, Texas 75062-7824.
214 256 1671
tstache@computek.net
http://www.skepsis.com:80/.gblo/bears/CLUBS/Lone_Star_Bears/

T-Bear Club
9151 Boundbrook Avenue, Dallas, Texas 75243.
214 349 0815

Organizations: Family

Gay/Lesbian Parents of Dallas
P. O. Box 154031, Irving, Texas 75015-4031.
214 259 9862

Tarrant County Parents Group
P. O. Box 48382, Watauga, Texas 76148-0382.
817 656 8056

Organizations: Motorcycle

Battalion MC
P.O. Box 191227, Dallas, Texas 75129-1227.

Dallas MC
2139 West Lovers Lane, Dallas, Texas 75235.

Texas MC
P.O. Box 9188, Dallas, Texas 75219.
214 946 7089 Ext.: 4
texasmc@aol.com

Organizations: Sexuality

AGAPE
Suite 112, 1631 Dorchester, Plano, Texas 75075.
214 424 1234
Support for male-to-females & female-to-males.

BiNet—Dallas
P.O. Box 190712, Dallas, Texas 75219.
214 504 6612
Contact: Ms. Deborah Nixon

Black & White Men Together (BWMT)—Dallas
P. O. Box 190611, Dallas, Texas 75219-0611.
214 521 4765

The Center for Change, Development, & Support
7525 John T. White Road, Fort Worth, Texas 76120.
817 429 4706
Contact: Mr. George Carpenter, M.D., Director
Comprehensive professional services for the transgendered. Member HBIGDA.

Dallas Gay & Lesbian Alliance
P. O. Box 191443, Dallas, Texas 75219.
214 521 5342 Ext.: 414
Supports mainstream lesbian readers (vs. separatists or lipstick lesbians). Publishes *New Vision / Lesbian Visionaries* every two months.

⚤☐ **Delta Omega**
P. O. Box 141924, Irving, Texas 75014.
☎ 214 264 7103
🕐 Meets 2nd. Sat of month 19:30
Crossdressers & their wives. Publishes *The Texas Rose*.

▷▽ **Recast Educations & Informational Network**
P. O. Box 224001, Dallas, Texas 75222-4001.
🕐 Meets twice a month
Female-to-male support. Publishes *En*Gender*.

☺ ▽ **Significant Other Support**
c/o Recast, P. O. Box 224001, Dallas, Texas 75222-4001.
☎ 214 641 4842
Contact: Rebecca
Support for family & friends of female-to-male transsexuals.

⚥▽ **Uncut Dallas**
P. O. Box 215 163, Dallas, Texas 75221.

⚥▽ **Welcome Wagon**
P. O. Box 190132, Dallas, Texas 75219.
☎ 214 733 9644
Contact: Ms. Deb Elder
Information service for vistors & relocators to Dallas.

Organizations: Sexuality: Student

⚥ **Coalition of Lesbian/Gay Student Groups, Inc.**
P. O. Box 190712, Dallas, Texas 75219.
☎ 214 761 3802 📱 214 522 4604
Publishes *The 10th. Person*.

⚥▽ **Gay/Lesbian Association of UTA**
⚷ P. O. Box 19348-77, Arlington, Texas 76019.
☎ 817 794 5140

Organizations: Sexuality: Youth

⚥▽ **Gay & Lesbian Young Adults**
P. O. Box 190712, Dallas, Texas 75219.
☎ 214 521 5342 Ext.: 260
Publishes *Youth Street News*.

Organizations: Spirituality

⚥▽ **Shouts in the Wilderness, Leather Circle of Hope**
⚷ c/o Cathedral of Hope MCC, 5910 Cedar Springs Road, Dallas, Texas 75235.
☎ 214 351 1901 Ext.: 202
🕐 Meets bi-weekly
Contact: Mr. Jack Myars, Circle Leader
Spiritual, social, & educational support group for Christians with leather interests.

Piercers

☺ ■ **Obscurities**
4000-B Cedar Springs Road, Dallas, Texas 75219.
☎ 214 559 3706
🕐 Mon - Tue 12:00 - 20:00, Wed - Sat 12:00 - 24:00, Sun 13:00 - 18:00
⚖ ✓ VISA 💳 🏧
Age statement of 18 is required.

☺ ■ **Skin & Bones**
3603 Parry Avenue, Dallas, Texas 75226.
☎ 214 826 6647
Also make their own jewelry.

Publishers: Newspapers: Sexuality

⚥ *Alliance News*
Suite 243, 3327 Winthrop Avenue, Fort Worth, Texas 76116.

⚥▼ *Dallas Voice*
Suite 200, 300 Carlisle, Dallas, Texas 75204.
☎ 214 754 8710 📱 214 969 7271
Published every week.

Radio: Sexuality

⚥▽ *Lambda Weekly Radio*
KNON FM 89.3, P. O. Box 35031, Dallas, Texas 75235.
☎ 214 520 1375
🕐 Sun 14:00 - 16:00

Stores: Books: General

⚥▼ *Crossroads Market & Bookstore*
3930 Cedar Springs, Dallas, Texas 75219.
☎ 214 521 8919
🕐 Mon - Thu 10:00 - 22:00, Fri Sat 10:00 - 23:00, Sun 12:00 - 21:00
⚖ ✓ VISA 💳

⚥ **Curious Times**
4008D Cedar Springs, Dallas, Texas 75219.
☎ 214 522 5887

⚥▼ **Lobo After Dark**
⚷ 4008C Cedar Springs, Dallas, Texas 75219.
☎ 214 522 1132

Stores: Erotica: BDSM

☺ ▼ **Shades of Grey**
⚷ 3928 Cedar Springs Road, Dallas, Texas 75219.
☎ 214 521 4739 📱 214 526 1063
🕐 Opens 12:00, 7 days a week
⚖ $ ✓ VISA 💳 🏧 ▣
10 years in business.Leather clothing, with custom & alterations. Men's & women's wear. Largest selection of fetish boots in Texas.

Stores: Erotica: General

☺ ■ **Christie's Toy Box**
3012 Alta Mere, Fort Worth, Texas 76116.
☎ 817 244 8008

☺ ■ **Eros**
2555 Walnut Hill Lane, Dallas, Texas 75229.
☎ 214 351 3654

Stores: Military Surplus

☺ ■ **Omaha Surplus**
2600 White Settlement Road, Fort Worth, Texas 76107.

Television: Sexuality

⚥▽ *To Tell The Truth Television*
Cathedral of Hope, P. O. Box 35466, Dallas, Texas 75235-0373.
☎ 214 351 1901 Ext.: 114 📱 214 351 6099

Del Valle

Stores: Erotica: General

☺ ■ **Highway 71 News**
5246 East Highway 71, Del Valle, Texas 78617.
☎ 512 247 4070

Denton

Counsellors

⚥▽ **Harvest Counseling Associates**
⚷ 5900 South Stemmons, Denton, Texas 76205.
☎ 817 497 4020

Organizations: AIDS: Education

☺ ☐ **Harvest Ecumenical AIDS Resource Team**
⚷ 5900 South Stemmons, Denton, Texas 76205.
☎ 817 497 4020

Organizations: Sexuality: Student

⚥▽ **Courage**
⚷ c/o Student Activities Center, UNT Box 5067, Denton, Texas 76203.
☎ 817 565 6110
The lesbian, gay, & bisexual student organization at UNT.

El Paso

Helplines: Sexuality

⚥▽ **LAMBDA Services**
P. O. Box 31321, El Paso, Texas 79931-0321.
☎ 915 562 4297
📧 LAMBDAelp@aol.com
🕐 24hrs.

Organizations: AIDS: Education

☺ ☐ **Southwest AIDS Committee**
⚷ 1505 Mescalero Drive, El Paso, Texas 79925-2019.
☎ 915 533 5003
Publishes a newsletter.

Organizations: Family

☺ ☐ **Parents & Friends of Lesbians & Gays (PFLAG)— Texas**
P. O. Box 1761, El Paso, Texas 79949.
☎ 915 592 2218

Organizations: Sexuality: Youth

⚥▽ **LAMBDA Services Youth OUTreach**
⚷ P. O. Box 31321, El Paso, Texas 79931-0321.
☎ 915 562 4297

☞ LAMBDAelp@aol.com
🕐 Call 24hrs.

Printers: General
☺ **Key Press**
P.O. Box 26048, El Paso, Texas 79926.

Stores: Erotica: General
☺ ■ **Green Door**
⚥ 211 Stockyard Road, El Paso, Texas 79927.
☎ 915 858 3174
🕐 09:00 - 01:00
☺ ■ **Trixx Adult Cinema & Bookstore**
⚥ 2230 Texas, El Paso, Texas 79901.
☎ 915 532 6171

Galveston
Organizations: AIDS: Education
☺ ☐ **AIDS Coalition of Coastal Texas**
1419 Tremont Street, Galveston, Texas 77550-4519.
☎ 409 763 2437
Organizations: AIDS: Support
☺ ☐ **Community Care for AIDS-UTMB**
Route J-28, Galveston, Texas 77550.
☎ 409 938 2202
☎ 409 761 3038
Organizations: Sexuality
⚥▽ **The Rosenberg Clinic**
Gender Treatment Program, 1103 Rosenberg, Galveston, Texas 77550.
☎ 409 763 0916
Professional services organization.

Helotes
Organizations: Motorcycle
⚦ **San Antonio Rough Riders**
P.O. Box 551, Helotes, Texas 78023.

Houston
Archives: Sexuality
⚦▽ **MCC Library**
⚥ Metropolitan Community Church, 1919 Decatur, Houston, Texas 77007.
☎ 713 861 9149
Bars: BDSM
⚦▼ **Pacific Street**
710 Pacific, Houston, Texas 77006.
☎ 713 523 0213
🕐 21:00 - 02:00
Levi leather dance bar. We have the only laser light show in town with
our exclusive"Caged Heat / Men Behind Bars." Age statement of 21 is
required.
⚦▼ **Ripcord Houston**
⚥ 715 Fairview, Houston, Texas 77006.
☎ 713 521 2792
⚦▼ **Venture-N**
⚥ 2923 South Main Street, Houston, Texas 77002.
☎ 713 522 0000
🕐 12:00 - 02:00
BBSs: BDSM
☺ ■ **The Exchange**
✆ 713 521 2191
Competitions & Conventions: Sexuality
⚥▽ **ICTLEP**
5707 Firenza Street, Houston, Texas 77035-5515.
TG law conference.
Counsellors
☺ ▼ **DAPA, Family of Choice**
⚥ P.O. Box 131019, Houston, Texas 77219-1019.
☎ 800 822 2272
⚦▽ **Montrose Counseling Center**
⚥ 701 Richmond Avenue, Houston, Texas 77006-5511.
☎ 713 529 0037
🕐 08:00 - 21:00
♠ ✓ $ ⚥ 💳 💳
Non-profit out-patient mental health centre for the gay, lesbian, bisexual,
& transgendered community. Programs include HIV/AIDS, substance
abuse, & general psychotherapy. Age statement of 18 is required.

Health Services
☺ ■ **AMI Park Plaza Hospital**
1313 Hermann Drive, Houston, Texas 77004.
☎ 713 527 5000
HIV & emergency departments.
☺ ■ **AMI Twelve Oaks Hospital**
4200 Portsmouth Street, Houston, Texas 77027.
☎ 713 623 2500
HIV & emergency departments.
☺ ■ **Medical Center Hospital**
8081 Greenbriar, Houston, Texas 77054.
☎ 713 790 8100
HIV & emergency departments.
☺ ☐ **Veterans' Affairs Medical Center**
2002 Holcombe Boulevard, Houston, Texas 77030.
☎ 713 791 1414
HIV & emergency departments.
Helplines: Miscellaneous
☺ ☐ **Crisis Hotline**
P. O. Box 130866, Houston, Texas 77219-0866.
☎ 713 228 1505
Helplines: Sexuality
⚦▽ **Gay & Lesbian Switchboard of Houston**
P. O. Box 66469, Houston, Texas 77266-6469.
☎ 713 529 3211
🕐 16:30 - 24:00
Organizations: AIDS: Education
☺ ☐ **AIDS Foundation of Houston**
⚥ 3202 Weslayan Street, Houston, Texas 77027-5113.
☎ 713 623 6796
☎ 713 524 2437 (hotline)
🕐 09:00 - 21:00
Publishes Lifeline.
☺ ☐ **Department of Health & Human Services**
⚥ 5th. Floor, 800 North Stadium Drive, Houston, Texas 77054.
☎ 713 794 9020 (hotline)
Contact: AIDS Surveillance Update
Publishes Bureau of HIV/STD Prevention.
☺ ☐ **Greater Houston AIDS Alliance**
Suite 103, 811 Westheimer Road, Houston, Texas 77006.
Organizations: AIDS: Support
☺ ☐ **People With AIDS Coalition Houston, Inc.**
⚥ Suite 163, 1475 West Gray Street, Houston, Texas 77019.
☎ 713 522 5428
Organizations: BDSM
⚦ **Brotherhood of Pain**
P.O. Box 66524, Houston, Texas 77266-6524.
Age statement of 21 is required.
⚦▽ **Colt 45s**
P. O. Box 66804, Houston, Texas 77006.
☺ ☐ **The National Leather Association (NLA)—Houston**
⚦ P.O. Box 66553, Houston, Texas 77266-6553.
☎ 713 527 9666 ✆ 713 528 2850
🕐 Meets 2nd. Tue of month 19:30
⚦ **Sundance Cattle Company**
1022 Westheimer Road, Houston, Texas 77006.
☎ 713 527 9669
⚦▽ **Texas Renegade Club**
P. O. Box 131004, Houston, Texas 72219-1004.
Organizations: Bears
⚦▽ **Houston Area Bears**
P. O. box 66443, Houston, Texas 77266.
☎ 713 867 9123
☞ Bizbear@aol.com
🌐 http://www.skepsis.com:80/.gblo/bears/CLUBS/houston_area_be
ars.html
Organizations: Family
⚦▽ **Gay Fathers / Fathers First of Houston**
⚥⚥ P.O. Box 981053, Houston, Texas 77098-1053.
☺ ☐ **Parents & Friends of Lesbians & Gays (PFLAG)—**
⚥ **Houston**
P. O. Box 692444, Houston, Texas 77269-2444.
☎ 713 862 9020

Organizations: Fetish: Mess
♂▽ **SludgeMaster**
P. O. Box 541352, Houston, Texas 77254-1352.
☎ 713 552 4683

Organizations: Motorcycle
♂ **Houston Council of Clubs**
2400 Brazos Street, Houston, Texas 77006.
♂▽ **Texas Riders, Inc.**
P. O. Box 66545, Houston, Texas 77266-6545.
☎ 713 771 9726
✉ TXRiderboy@aol.com

Organizations: Sexuality
▽ **GCTC**
P. O. Box 90335, Houston, Texas 77090.
▽ **Gulf Coast Transgender Community**
P. O. Box 66643, Houston, Texas 88266.
☎ 713 780 4282
🕐 Meets 1st. Tue of month 12:00 & 3rd. Thu of month eve
Publishes *Gulf Coast Transgender Community*.
▽ **Helping CDs Anonymous (HCDA)**
Suite 334, 6904 East Highway 6 South, Houston, Texas 77083.
▽ **The Society for the Second Self (Tri-Ess)—Tau Chi**
Suite 104, 8880 Bellaire B2, Houston, Texas 77306.
☎ 713 988 8064
✉ JEFTRIS@aol.com
🖳 http://www.gomedia.com/outline/trans/sss.html
🕐 Meets 3rd. Sat of month
Contact: Ms Jane Ellen Fairfax
Publishes *The Femme Mirror* quarterly.
▽ **TS Peer Support Meetings**
Suite 560, Atrium Crest Building, 18333 Egret Bay Boulevard, Houston, Texas 77058.
☎ 713 333 2278
Contact: Ms. Alice Webb, MSW

Organizations: Sexuality: Student
♂▽ **Delta Lambda Phi Fraternity—Houston**
CA Box 219, 4800 Calhoun, Houston, Texas 77204-0001.
☎ 713 529 3211
♂▽ **Gays & Lesbians of Rice (GALOR)**
♿ P. O. Box 1892, Houston, Texas 77251.
☎ 713 527 4097

Organizations: Sexuality: Youth
♂▽ **Houston Area Teen Coalition of Homosexuals (HATCH)**
♿ P. O. Box 667053, Houston, Texas 77266-7053.
☎ 713 942 7002
♂▽ **Houston Institute for the Protection of Youth**
Suite 201, 811 Westheimer Road, Houston, Texas 77006.
☎ 713 942 9884

Organizations: Wrestling
♂▼ **Houston Wrestling Club**
♿ P. O. Box 131134, Houston, Texas 77219-1134.
☎ 713 453 7406
✓
Publishes *Take-Downs*. Yearly subscription is $25.

Publishers: Magazines: BDSM
☺■ *Villeinage*
P. O. Box 74-1193, Houston, Texas 77074.
☎ 713 778 1416
✉ fingers@phoenix.phoenix.net
BDSM, leather, fetishes, & similar topics. Published every two months.

Publishers: Magazines: Fetish
♂▼ *SludgeMaster*
P. O. Box 541352, Houston, Texas 77254-1352.
☎ 713 522 4MUD
✓
Published twice a year. Yearly subscription is $30. Age statement of 21 is required.

Publishers: Newspapers: Sexuality
☺▼ *Houston Voice*
♿ Suite 105, 811 Westheimer Road, Houston, Texas 77006. 📱 713 529 9531
☎ 800 729 8490
☎ 713 529 8490

Gay news for Texas & Louisiana. Published every week. Yearly subscription is $91.
♂ *Paz y Liberación*
P. O. Box 66450, Houston, Texas 77266.

Radio: General
🔊 *Women's Hour*
KTRU FM 91.7, P. O. Box 1892, Houston, Texas 77251-1892.
☎ 713 527 4050

Radio: Sexuality
♂▽ *After Hours*
KPFT FM 90.1, 419 Lovett, Houston, Texas 77007-4018.
☎ 713 526 4000
🕐 Sat 24:00
♂▽ *Lesbian & Gay Voices*
KPFT FM 90.1, 419 Lovett, Houston, Texas 77007-4018.
☎ 713 526 4000
🕐 Fri 18:00

Stores: Books: General
♂▼ **Crossroads Market & Bookstore**
610 West Alabama, Houston, Texas 77006.
☎ 713 942 0147
♂▼ **Inklings**
1846 Richmond Avenue, Houston, Texas 77098. 📱 713 521 3399
☎ 713 521 3369
🕐 Tue - Sat 10:30 - 18:30
♂▼ **Lobo Bookstore**
1424C Westheimer Road, Houston, Texas 77006.
☎ 713 522 5156
🕐 10:00 - 22:00

Stores: Erotica: BDSM
☺ **Leather by Boots**
P. O. Box 66307, Houston, Texas 77266. 📱 713 523 0432
☎ 713 526 2668
🕐 12:00 - 20:00 every day
Catalogue, $10.

Stores: Erotica: General
☺■ **Fountainview News**
5887 Westheimer Road, Houston, Texas 77057.
☎ 713 781 7793

Television: Sexuality
🔊 ▽ *Fem TV*
P. O. Box 66604, Houston, Texas 77266-6604.
☎ 713 755 7766
Feminist television.

Huntsville
Organizations: Sexuality: Student
♂▽ **Sam Houston GLBA**
Box 2171 SHSU, Huntsville, Texas 77341-2172.
☎ 409 291 3584

Irving
Organizations: Sexuality
▽ **The Society for the Second Self (Tri-Ess)—Delta Omega**
P. O. Box 14129, Irving, Texas 75014.

Jersey Village
BBSs: BDSM
☺■ **The Archives**
📱 713 896 1721

Lewisville
BBSs: BDSM
☺■ **Pokey's Place**
📱 214 317 7695

Longview
Stores: Erotica: General
♂■ **Newsland**
301 East Marshall, Longview, Texas 75601.
☎ 903 753 4167

Lubbock

Organizations: AIDS: Education

☺ ☐ **South Plains AIDS Resource Center**
P.O. Box 6949, Lubbock, Texas 79493.
☎ 806 796 7068 ✆ 806 796 0920
☎ 800 288 9058 (information hotline)
⏲ Mon - Fri 08:00 - 17:00
Contact: Mr. David Crader, Executive Director

Organizations: Sexuality

♂♀▽ **Lubbock Lesbian & Gay Alliance**
& P. O. Box 64746, Lubbock, Texas 79464-4746.
☎ 806 762 1019
⏲ 24hr. recording
Contact: Ms. Natalie Phillips
Publishes *Lambda Times*.

Organizations: Sexuality: Student

♂♀▽ **Gay & Lesbian Student Association**
Box 4310, SOS Office Box 8, Lubbock, Texas 79410.
☎ 806 795 8421

Stores: Books: General

♂♀▼ **Ellie's Garden**
& 2702 33rd. Street, Lubbock, Texas 79410.
☎ 806 796 0880
⏲ Mon - Sat 10:00 - 18:00, Sun 13:00 - 17:00
⬢ ✓ VISA ⬤

Manchaca

Organizations: Sexuality

♂ **Prime Timers International**
P. O. Box 436, Manchaca, Texas 78652.
☎ 512 282 2681
Contact: Mr. Woody Baldwin

Merkel

Stores: Erotica: General

☺ ■ **Adults Etc., Etc.**
Box 8, Route 1, Merkel, Texas 79536.
☎ 915 928 3894

New Waverly

Organizations: Sexuality

✉▽ **The Society for the Second Self (Tri-Ess)—Epsilon Tau**
P. O. Box 945, New Waverly, Texas 77358.

Richland Hills

Organizations: Motorcycle

♂ **Knights of Malta MC—Richland Hills**
3520 London Lane, Richland Hills, Texas 76118.

Rosebud

Organizations: Motorcycle

♂ **Heart of Texas MC**
P.O. Box 13, Rosebud, Texas 76570.

San Angelo

Organizations: AIDS: Education

☺ ☐ **San Angelo AIDS Foundation, Inc.**
& Suite 201, 3017 Knickerbocker, San Angelo, Texas 76904.
☎ 915 657 6555

San Antonio

Health Services

☺ ☐ **Audie L. Murphy Memorial Veterans' Hospital**
7400 Merton Minter Boulevard, San Antonio, Texas 78284.
☎ 210 617 5140

☺ ☐ **Santa Rosa Health Care Corporation**
519 West Houston Street, San Antonio, Texas 78207.
☎ 210 228 2011

Helplines: Sexuality

♂♀▽ **Lesbian Information San Antonio (LISA)**
P. O. Box 12327, San Antonio, Texas 78212.
☎ 210 828 5472

♂♀▽ **San Antonio Gay & Lesbian Switchboard**
P. O. Box 120402, San Antonio, Texas 78212.

☎ 210 733 7300
☎ 210 734 2833 (recorded information)
⏲ 19:00 - 23:00

Organizations: AIDS: Education

☺ ☐ **San Antonio AIDS Foundation**
⚲ 818 East Grayson Street, San Antonio, Texas 78208-1013.
☎ 210 225 4715 ✆ 210 224 7730

Organizations: AIDS: Support

☺ ☐ **PWA Coalition**
Suite 210, 12125 Jones-Maltsberger, San Antonio, Texas 78247.
☎ 210 545 4357 (hotline)

Organizations: BDSM

♂ **Chain of Command**
1032 West Woodlawn, San Antonio, Texas 78201.
☎ 210 979 7752

♂▽ **Firedancers—San Antonio**
5119 Staplehurst, San Antonio, Texas 78228.

Organizations: Family

♂♀▽ **Gay & Lesbian Parent Coalition**
& Suite 508, 2839 North West Military Drive, San Antonio, Texas 78231.
☎ 210 342 8696

Organizations: Fetish: Smoking

♂▽ **Cigar Studs**
P. O. Box 15344, San Antonio, Texas 78212.

Organizations: Fetish: Uniforms

⚣ ▼ **Patrol Uniform Club of Texas**
313 Aransas Avenue, San Antonio, Texas 78210.
☎ 210 533 6001

Organizations: Motorcycle

♂ **River City Outlaws**
P.O. Box 23548, San Antonio, Texas 78223-0548.

♂ **Tejas MC**
P.O. Box 120295, San Antonio, Texas 78212-9495.
☎ 512 223 6620

Organizations: Sexuality

♂♀▽ **The Resource Center**
121 West Woodlawn, San Antonio, Texas 78212.
☎ 210 732 0751

✉▽ **San Antonio Transexual Support Group (SATSG)**
P. O. Box 12913, San Antonio, Texas 78212.
Publishes a newsletter every month.

Organizations: Sexuality: Student

♂♀▽ **San Antonio Lambda Students Alliance (SALSA)**
& P. O. Box 12715, San Antonio, Texas 78212.
☎ 210 733 1225
Publishes a newsletter.

Piercers

☺ ■ **Planet K**
2138 Austin Highway, San Antonio, Texas.
☎ 512 654 8536

Publishers: Newspapers: Sexuality

♂▼ *The San Antonio Marquise*
P. O. Box 701204, San Antonio, Texas 78232.
☎ 210 545 3511 ✆ 210 545 3511

♂ *South Texas Voice*
P. O. Box 12023, San Antonio, Texas 78212.

♀▽ *WomanSpace*
Lesbian Information San Antonio, P. O. Box 12327, San Antonio, Texas 78212.
☎ 210 828 5472

Stores: Books: General

♂♀■ **Textures**
5309 McCullough, San Antonio, Texas 78212.
☎ 210 805 8398

Tyler

Helplines: Sexuality

♂♀▽ **Saint Ganriel Community Church**
☎ 903 581 6923

Organizations: AIDS: Education

☺ ☐ **AIDS Support Team / Dignity Foundation**

P. O. Box 74, Tyler, Texas 75710-0074.
☎ 903 566 8833

Waco

Organizations: Sexuality
⚥▽ **Gay & Lesbian Alliance of Central Texas**
 ⚘ P. O. Box 9081, Waco, Texas 76714-1428.
 ☎ 800 735 1122
 ☎ 817 741 1428
 Publishes *Central Texas Alliance News*. Please address envelopes to GLACT, do NOT address them to Gay & Lesbian Alliance of Central Texas or Central Texas Alliance News.

Wichita Falls

Organizations: Sexuality: Student
⚥▽ **Diversity**
 Suite 12764, Midwestern State University, 3410 Taft Boulevard, Wichita Falls, Texas 76308.
 ☎ 817 766 2264
 ☎ 817 692 4968

UTAH
Area: Approximately 213,000 square kilometres
Population: Approximately 1,725,000
Capital City: Salt Lake City
Time zone: GMT minus 7 hours (Mountain Time)
Age of consent & homosexuality legislation: All anal & oral sex is illegal in this state.
Legal drinking age: 21

State Resources

Organizations: AIDS: Education
☺☐ **Northern Utah AIDS Society**
 2270 Washington Boulevard, Ogden, Utah 84401. ✆ 801 778 0407
 ☎ 801 778 0379

☺☐ **Utah AIDS Foundation**
 1408 South 1100 East, Salt Lake City, Utah 84105.
 ☎ 800 366 2437
 ☎ 801 487 2323

Organizations: Sexuality
⚥▽ **Gay & Lesbian Community Council of Utah**
 ♿ 770 South 300 West, Salt Lake City, Utah 84101-2603.
 ☎ 801 539 8800

⚥▽ **Utah Stonewall Center**
 ♿ 770 South 300 West, Salt Lake City, Utah 84101.
 ☎ 801 539 8800
 Publishes *Center of Attention*.

Logan

Organizations: Sexuality
⚥▽ **Alliance of Cache Valley (GLA-CV)**
 Box 119, UMC 0100, Tagart Student Center, Logan, Utah 84322-0100.
 ☎ 801 752 1129

Midvale

Manufacturers: Furniture: BDSM
☺■ **Stocks & Bonds Ltd.**
 P. O. Box 8000-115, Midvale, Utah 84047.
 Custom made BDSM furniture. Also items from stock. Catalogue, $5.

Orem

Organizations: Sexuality
⚥▽ **The Society for the Second Self (Tri-Ess)—Alpha Rho**
 P. O. Box 1586, Orem, Utah 84059-1586.

Park City

Stores: Books: General
⚥■ **A Woman's Place**
 ♿ Park City Plaza, 1890 Bonanza Drive, Park City, Utah 84060.
 ☎ 801 649 2722
 🕐 10:00 - 21:00, Sat - 18:00, Sun 12:00 - 17:00
 No gay male material.

Pleasant Grove

Organizations: Sexuality
⚥▽ **Reflection House**
 P. O. Box 628, Pleasant Grove, Utah 84062. ✆ 801 224 4737
 ☎ 801 224 4737

Salt Lake City

Health Services
☺☐ **Holy Cross Hospital**
 1050 East South Temple, Salt Lake City, Utah 84102.
 ☎ 801 350 4111
 HIV & emergency departments.

☺☐ **Veterans' Affairs Medical Center**
 500 Foothill Drive, Salt Lake City, Utah 84148.
 ☎ 801 582 1565

Helplines: Sexuality
⚥▽ **Aardvaark Helpline**
 ☎ 801 533 0927

Organizations: BDSM
☺☐ **Power Play**
 ✉ beverly@netcom.com
 Contact: Phœnix
 Also has an e-mail list. Please send e-mail for further information.

⚥▽ **Wasatch Leathemen**
 P. O. Box 1311, Salt Lake City, Utah 84110-1311.
 ☎ 801 355 8135

Organizations: Sexuality: Student
⚥▽ **Lesbian & Gay Student Union**
 ♿ 234 Olpin Union Building, University of Utah, Salt Lake City, Utah 84112.
 ☎ 801 521 4026
 🕐 Meets Mon 19:30 - 21:00

Printers: General
☺■ **Publishers Press**
 1900 West 2300 South, Salt Lake City, Utah 84119. ✆ 801 972 6601
 ☎ 801 972 6600

Publishers: Newspapers: Sexuality
⚥▼ *Pillar of the Gay, Lesbian, & Bisexual Community*
 P. O. Box 520898, Salt Lake City, Utah 84152-0898.
 ☎ 801 328 0527 ✆ 801 466 4062
 Lesbigay community newspaper serving all of Utah, southern Idaho, & some of Nevada. Published every month. Yearly subscription is $15.

Radio: Sexuality
⚥▽ *Concerning Gay & Lesbians*
 ♿ KRCL FM 91, 208 West 800 South, Salt Lake City, Utah 84101.
 ☎ 801 363 1818
 🕐 Wed 12:30 - 13:00 (times vary)

Stores: Books: General
☺■ **Cahoots**
 878 East 900 South, Salt Lake City, Utah 84105.
 ☎ 801 538 0606

☺■ **Golden Braid Books**
 151 South 500 East, Salt Lake City, Utah 84102-1906.
 ☎ 801 322 1162

☺▼ **Hayats Magazines & Gifts**
 ♿ 228 South Main Street, Salt Lake City, Utah 84101.
 ☎ 801 531 6531
 🕐 08:00 - 23:00

☺■ **King's English Bookstore**
 ♿ 1511 South 1500 East, Salt Lake City, Utah 84105.
 ☎ 801 484 9100
 🕐 10:00 - 21:00, Sun 11:00 - 17:00

☺■ **Waking Owl**
 208 South 1300 East, Salt Lake City, Utah 84102.
 ☎ 801 582 7323

⚥■ **A Woman's Place**
 ♿ Suite 1205, 4835 South Highland Drive, Salt Lake City, Utah 84117.
 ☎ 801 278 9855
 🕐 10:00 - 21:00, Sat - 18:00, Sun 12:00 - 17:00
 No gay male material.

⚥■ **A Woman's Place**
 ♿ 1400 Foothill Drive, Salt Lake City, Utah 84108.
 ☎ 801 583 6431
 🕐 10:00 - 21:00, Sat - 18:00, Sun 12:00 - 17:00
 No gay male material.

VERMONT
Area: Approximately 24,000 square kilometres
Population: Approximately 565,000
Capital City: Montpelier
Time zone: GMT minus 5 hours (EST)

Climate: Summers are cool in the mountains. Winters are snowy & cold. Great skiing weather, but cold.
Age of consent & homosexuality legislation: State has adopted the Model Penal Code or otherwise decriminalized homosexual activities. There is legislation in place against discrimination on the basis of sexual orientation.
Legal drinking age: 18

State Resources

Organizations: AIDS: Education
☺ ⬜ **AIDS Community Resource Network (ACORN)**
⚥ P. O. Box 2057, Lebanon, New Hampshire 03766.
☎ 603 448 2220
☺ ⬜ **Lamoille County AIDS Task Force**
P. O. Box 150, Morrisville, Vermont 05661.
☎ 802 888 7153
☺ ⬜ **Vermont AIDS Council**
⚥ P. O. Box 275, Montpelier, Vermont 05601.
☎ 802 229 2557

Organizations: AIDS: Support
☺ ⬜ **Vermont Cares**
⚥ P. O. Box 5248, Burlington, Vermont 05401.
☎ 800 649 2437
☎ 802 863 2437

Organizations: Family
⚥▽ **Gay Fathers Connection**
P. O. Box 5506, Essex Junction, Vermont 05453-5506.

Organizations: Sexuality
⚥▽ **Social Alternative for Gay Men (SAM)**
⚥ P. O. Box 479, Norwich, Vermont 05055.
Publishes *SAM Newsletter*.

Organizations: Sexuality: Youth
⚥▽ **Outright Vermont**
⚥ P. O. Box 5235, Burlington, Vermont 05402-5235.
☎ 800 452 2428
☎ 802 865 9677
Youth support group with library, & education service for professional working with youth.

Bennington

Organizations: AIDS: Education
☺ ⬜ **Bennington Area AIDS Project**
P. O. Box 1066, Bennington, Vermont 05201.
☎ 800 845 2437
☎ 802 442 4481

Brattleboro

Organizations: AIDS: Education
☺ ⬜ **Brattleboro Area AIDS Project**
⚥ P. O. Box 1468, Brattleboro, Vermont 05302.
☎ 802 254 4444

Organizations: AIDS: Support
☺ ⬜ **Vermont PWA Coalition**
104 Maple Street, Brattleboro, Vermont 05301-3456.
☎ 802 257 9277

Organizations: Sexuality
⚥▽ **Brattleboro Area Gays & Lesbians (BAGAL)**
P. O. Box 875, Brattleboro, Vermont 05302-0875.
☎ 802 254 5947

Stores: Books: General
⚥ ■ **Everyone's Books**
⚥ 23 Elliott Street, Brattleboro, Vermont 05301.
☎ 802 254 8160

Burlington

Health Services
☺ ⬜ **Medical Center Hospital of Vermont**
Colchester Avenue, Burlington, Vermont 05401.
☎ 802 656 2345
⚥ ⬜ **Vermont Women's Health Center**
⚥ P. O. Box 29, Burlington, Vermont 05402.
☎ 802 863 1386 ☏ 802 863 1774

Organizations: Sexuality
⚥ ⬜ **Burlington Women's Council**
⚥ Room 14, City Hall, Burlington, Vermont 05401.

☎ 802 865 7200 ☏ 802 865 7024
🕐 Tue - Thu 09:00 - 17:00
Resource knowledgeable about most gay & lesbian activities in Burlington.

Organizations: Sexuality: Student
⚥▽ **Gay Lesbian Bisexual Alliance at UVM**
⚥ B-163 Billings, University of Vermont, Burlington, Vermont 05405.
☎ 802 656 6300

Publishers: Newspapers: Sexuality
⚥▼ **Out in the Mountains**
⚥ P. O. Box 177, Burlington, Vermont 05402.
Monthly newspaper for lesbigay readers in Vermont & west New Hampshire. The only such newspaper in this area. Published 11 times a year. Yearly subscription is $20.

Stores: Books: General
☺ ■ **Chassman & Bern Booksellers**
⚥ 81 Church Street, Burlington, Vermont 05401.
☎ 802 862 4332

Manchester Center

Stores: Books: General
☺ ■ **Northshire Bookstore**
⚥ P. O. Box 2200, Manchester Center, Vermont 05255.
☎ 802 437 3700
🕐 10:00 - 17:30, Fri - 21:00, Sat - 19:00

Montpelier

Printers: General
☺ **Capital City Press, Inc.**
P.O. Box 546, Montpelier, Vermont 05602-0546.
☎ 802 223 5207 ☏ 802 223 1194

Plainfield

Organizations: Sexuality
⚥▽ **Central Vermont Gay Liberation (CVGL)**
P. O. Box 333, Plainfield, Vermont 05667.
☎ 802 454 8078
⚥▽ **Gay, Lesbian, Bisexual Alliance of Goddard**
Goddard College, Plainfield, Vermont 05667.
☎ 802 454 8311 Ext.: 225

Rutland

Organizations: Family
☺ ⬜ **Parents & Friends of Lesbians & Gays (PFLAG)— Rutland**
11 North Street, Rutland, Vermont 05701-3011.
☎ 802 773 7601

Organizations: Sexuality
⚥▽ **Rutland Area Gay & Lesbian Connection (RAGLC)**
P. O. Box 218, Rutland, Vermont 05736.

Saint Albans

Organizations: AIDS: Education
☺ ⬜ **Franklin-Grand Isle AIDS Task Force**
P. O. Box 241, Saint Albans, Vermont 05478.
☎ 800 638 7834
☎ 802 524 7742

Saint Johnsbury

Organizations: AIDS: Education
☺ ⬜ **AIDS Community Awareness Project (ACAP)**
P. O. Box 608, Saint Johnsbury, Vermont 05819.
☎ 802 748 1149

Worcester

Organizations: Sexuality
⚥▽ **Women of the Woods (WOW)**
Box 5620, RFD 1, Worcester, Vermont 05682.
☎ 802 229 0109

VIRGINIA
Area: Approximately 103,000 square kilometres
Population: Approximately 6,220,000
Capital City: Richmond
Time zone: GMT minus 5 hours (EST)
Climate: Warm Summer with average highs of approximately 26°C & winter lows of approximately 4°C. Outside the path of most hurricanes.

Age of consent & homosexuality legislation: All anal & oral sex is illegal in this state.
Legal drinking age: 21

State Resources

Organizations: AIDS: Education

☺ ☐ **AIDS Council of Western Virginia**
 ⅊ P. O. Box 598, Roanoke, Virginia 24004.
 ☎ 800 354 3388
 ☎ 703 982 2437

☺ ☐ **Appalachian AIDS Coalition**
 ⅊ P. O. Box 513, Abingdon, Virginia 24210.
 ☎ 800 354 3388

☺ ☐ **Peninsula AIDS Foundation**
 ⅊ 326 Main Street, Newport News, Virginia 23601.
 ☎ 804 591 0971

Organizations: AIDS: Support

☺ ☐ **CARE Virginia**
 Suite 102, 3426 Washington Boulevard, Arlington, Virginia 22201-4520.

Organizations: Bears

♂♡▽ **Teddy Bear Leather Club**
 ⅊ P. O. Box 25545, Richmond, Virginia 232360.
 ☎ 804 232 0646
 Publishes *TBLC Newsletter*.

Organizations: Sexuality

♂♡▽ **Alliance of Lesbian & Gay Organizations of Western Virginia**
 P. O. Box 21111, Roanoke, Virginia 24018.

♂♡▽ **Northern Virginia Pride, Inc.**
 ⅋ P. O. Box 12404, Arlington, Virginia 22209.
 ☎ 703 528 3659
 Publishes a newsletter.

Publishers: Newspapers: Sexuality

♂♡▽ **Blue Ridge Lambda Press**
 ⅊ P. O. Box 237, Roanoke, Virginia 24002.
 ☎ 703 890 3184

♂♡▼ **Our Own Community Press**
 739 Yarmouth Street, Norfolk, Virginia 23510.
 ☎ 804 625 0700 ✆ 804 625 6024
 Serves the lesbigay community of Virginia. News & entertainment. Published every month. Yearly subscription is $14.

Alexandria

Counsellors

♀▼ **Ellen Warren, LCSW**
 Suite 1500, 1500 King Street, Alexandria, Virginia 22314.
 ☎ 703 683 0710

Organizations: Sexuality

♀▽ **Dawn**
 P. O. Box 1849, Alexandria, Virginia 22313-1849.
 Publishes *The New Dawn*. Age statement of 18 is required.

Publishers: Magazines: Sexuality

♂ **Malchus**
 Suite 301, 6036 Richmond Highway, Alexandria, Virginia 22303.
 ☎ 703 329 7896

Publishers: Miscellaneous

✉ **Reluctant Press**
 P. O. Box 11936, Alexandria, Virginia 22312.

Annandale

Organizations: Bears

♂♡▽ **Chesapeake Bay Bears**
 P. O. Box 961, Annandale, Virginia 22003-0961.

Arlington

Health Services

☺ ☐ **Arlington Hospital**
 1701 North George Mason Drive, Arlington, Virginia 22205.
 ☎ 703 558 5000

Organizations: BDSM

☺ ☐ **Black Rose**
 P.O. Box 11161, Arlington, Virginia 22210-1161.
 ☎ 301 369 7667

✉ copper@universe.digex.net
∰ http://www.br.org/
Contact: Rose
Support, educational, & social group for adults involved with dominance & submission in caring relationships. Publishes *The Petal & The Thorn* every two months. Age statement of 21 is required.

Organizations: Sexuality

♂♡▽ **Arlington Gay & Lesbian Alliance**
 ⅋ P. O. Box 324, Arlington, Virginia 22210.
 ☎ 703 522 7660
 Publishes *AGLA News*.

✉☐ **Transgender Educational Association of Greater Washington (TGEA)**
 P. O. Box 16036, Arlington, Virginia 22215.
 ☎ 301 949 3822
 ⏰ Meets 1st. Sat of month, Sep - Jun
 Publishes *The Pinnacle* every two months.

Blacksburg

Organizations: BDSM

☺ ☐ **A.S.B. Munch—Virginia**
 ✉ wombat@vt.edu
 ⏰ Meets Mon 19:00 - 21:00

Organizations: Sexuality: Student

♂♡▽ **Lambda Horizon at Virginia Tech**
 ⅊ P. O. Box 686, Blacksburg, Virginia 24063-0686.
 ☎ 703 231 3852

Charlottesville

Health Services

☺ ☐ **University of Virginia Hospital**
 2270 Ivy Road, Charlottesville, Virginia 22903.
 ☎ 804 924 9821
 HIV & emergency departments.

Helplines: Sexuality

☺ ▽ **Lesbian & Gay Student Union Helpline**
 P. O. Box 525, Newcomb Hall Station, Charlottesville, Virginia 22904.
 ☎ 804 971 4942
 ✉ lgbu@virginia.edu
 ∰ http://faraday.clas.virginia.edu/~lambda1
 ⏰ 24hrs.

Organizations: AIDS: Student

☺ **American College Health Association**
 AIDS Task Force, P. O. Box 378, University of Virginia, Charlottesville, Virginia 22908.
 ☎ 804 924 2670

Organizations: AIDS: Support

☺ ☐ **AIDS Support Group**
 P. O. Box 2322, Charlottesville, Virginia 22902.
 ☎ 804 979 7714

Organizations: Sexuality

♂♡▽ **Kindred Spirits**
 ⅊ P. O. Box 3721, Charlottesville, Virginia 22903.
 ☎ 804 971 1555
 Publishes *Kindred Spirits*.

♂♡▽ **Piedmont Triangle Society (PTS)**
 ⅊ P. O. Box 2368, Charlottesville, Virginia 22902.

Organizations: Sexuality: Student

☺ ▽ **Lesbian & Gay Student Union at the University of Virginia**
 P. O. Box 525, Newcomb Hall Station, Charlottesville, Virginia 22904.
 ☎ 804 971 4942
 ✉ lgbu@virginia.edu
 ∰ http://faraday.clas.virginia.edu/~lambda1
 Social, support, & service organization weloming University of Virginia students, faculty & staff, & others. Sponsors helpline.

Piercers

☺ ■ **G-Nation**
 P. O. Box 3401, Charlottesville, Virginia 22903.
 ☎ 804 293 4631

Stores: Books: General

☺ ■ **The Quest Bookshop**
 618 West Main Street, Charlottesville, Virginia 804 295 3377.
 ☎ 800 346 9223

Chesapeake

Stores: Erotica: BDSM

☺ ■ T.R.'s Leather Rack
P. O. Box 13307, Chesapeake, Virginia 23325-0307.
☎ 804 420 4474
🕐 09:00 - 18:00, Sun 13:00 - 17:00. Eve by appointment

Danville

Organizations: AIDS: Education

☺ ☐ Southside AIDS Venture
& 326 Taylor Drive, Danville, Virginia 24541.
☎ 804 799 5190

Denbigh

Organizations: Bears

♂▽ Tidewater Bears
P. O. Box 2241, Denbigh, Virginia 23609.

Fairfax

Organizations: Sexuality

♂▽ Fairfax Lesbian & Gay Citizens Association
& (FLGCA)
P. O. Box 2322, Fairfax, Virginia 22152.
☎ 703 451 9528

Falls Church

Archives: Sexuality

☺ ▽ Gay & Lesbian Archives of Washington, DC
P. O. Box 4218, Falls Church, Virginia 22044.
☎ 703 671 3930

Organizations: Body Size

♂▽ Girth & Mirth—Washington, D. C.
P. O. Box 4814, Falls Church, Virginia 22044.
☎ 703 461 9184

Publishers: Magazines: Sexuality

✉■ La Feminique
Suite 570, 1218 West Broad Street, Falls Church, Virginia 22046.
☎ 202 686 2992

Fredericksburg

Organizations: AIDS: Education

☺ ☐ Valley AIDS Network
College of Nursing, James Madison University, Fredericksburg, Virginia 22807.
☎ 703 564 0448

Organizations: AIDS: Support

☺ ☐ Fredericksburg Area HIV/AIDS Support Services,
& Inc.
415 Elm Street, Fredericksburg, Virginia 22401.
☎ 703 371 7532
☎ 703 371 7631

Organizations: Sexuality: Student

♂▽ Mary Washington College Gay / Lesbian /
& Bisexual Student Association
MWC Box 603, Fredericksburg, Virginia 22401-4666.

Stores: Books: General

⊕ ▼ The Purple Moon
& 810 Caroline Street, Fredericksburg, Virginia 22401.

Gloucester Point

Tattooists

☺ ■ Accent Tattoo
P. O. Box 1199, Gloucester Point, Virginia 23062.
☎ 804 642 3993
Body piercing also available.

Lynchburg

Counsellors

☺ ■ Counseling Center
415 Harrison Street, Lynchburg, Virginia 24504.
☎ 804 845 5783
🕐 Call 24hrs.

☺ ■ Jon Winder
& 2095 Langhorne Road, Lynchburg, Virginia 24501.

☎ 804 845 4927

Organizations: Sexuality: Student

⟨D⟩▽ Bridges
& Randolph-Macon Women's College, 2500 Rivermont Avenue, Lynchburg, Virginia 24503.

Newport News

Stores: Books: General

⊕ ■ Out of the Dark
530 Randolph Road, Newport News, Virginia 23601.
☎ 804 596 6220

Norfolk

BBSs: BDSM

☺ ■ Pleasure Dome
📞 804 490 LUST

Health Services

☺ ☐ Sentara Norfolk General Hospital
600 Gresham Drive, Norfolk, Virginia 23507.
☎ 804 628 3000

Helplines: Sexuality

♂▽ Gay Information Line
P. O. Box 1325, Norfolk, Virginia 23501.
☎ 804 622 4297
☎ 804 623 2277

Organizations: AIDS: Education

☺ ☐ Tidewater AIDS Crisis Task Force
& Suite 520, 740 Duke Street, Norfolk, Virginia 23510-1515.
☎ 804 626 0127
☎ 804 627 4641

Organizations: BDSM

♂▽ Knight Hawks of Virginia
P. O. Box 606, Norfolk, Virginia 23501.
☎ 804 489 8028
✉ dumusic@infi.net
Contact: Mr. Patrick Harvey

Organizations: Sexuality

⟨D⟩▽ Alternative Lifestyle Support Organization (ALSO)
& P. O. Box 891, Norfolk, Virginia 23501.
☎ 804 855 5212

✉▽ Center for Gender Reassignment
Suite 915, 142 West York Street, Norfolk, Virginia 23510-2015.
☎ 804 622 9900
Contact: Ms. Deborah Gilbert
Center for people who are seeking a permanent gender reassignment.

♂▽ The Mandamus Society
P. O. Box 1325, Norfolk, Virginia 23501.
☎ 804 625 6220

Organizations: Sexuality: Student

♂▽ Gay & Lesbian Student Union
Student Activities Office, Webb Center, Old Dominion University, Norfolk, Virginia 23508.

Publishers: Newspapers: Sexuality

♂▼ Out and About
P. O. Box 120112, Norfolk, Virginia 23502.
☎ 804 727 0037

Stores: Books: General

♂▼ Max Images
808 Spotswood Avenue, Norfolk, Virginia 23517.
☎ 804 622 3701
🕐 12:00 - 19:00, Sun - 17:00

⟨D⟩▽ Pride Bookstore
& P. O. Box 1026, Norfolk, Virginia 23501-1026.
☎ 804 855 8450
🕐 Call for hours & location
New Life MCC.

Stores: Erotica: BDSM

☺ ■ Gear, Clothing, & Accessories
733 Granby Street, Norfolk, Virginia 23510.
☎ 804 622 4438

Radford

Organizations: Sexuality: Student

☺ ▽ Radford Alternative Alliance

P. O. Box 5894, Radford University, Radford, Virginia 24142.

Richmond

Counsellors

Commonwealth Professional Services
12 South Auburn Avenue, Richmond, Virginia 23221.
804 353 1169
By appointment only
✓
Three licenced counsellors & one licenced psychologist openly serving the gay, lesbian, bisexual, transgender community with counselling, consulting, & training since 1981.

Paula Jean, Ph.D.
907 Westwood Avenue, Richmond, Virginia 23222.
804 329 3940

Health Services

Hunter Holmes McGuire Veterans' Affairs Medical Center
1201 Broad Rock Boulevard, Richmond, Virginia 23249.
804 230 0001
HIV & emergency departments.

Medical College of Virginia Hospitals
Virginia Commonwealth University, 401 North 12th. Street, Richmond, Virginia 23219.
804 786 9000

Organizations: AIDS: Education

Richmond AIDS Information Network
c/o Fan Free Clinic, P. O. Box 5669, Richmond, Virginia 23220.
804 358 2437

Richmond Street Outreach Project
1627 Monument Avenue, Richmond, Virginia 23220-2906.
804 359 4783

Organizations: AIDS: Support

Central Virginia AIDS Services & Education (CVASE)
1627 Monument Avenue, Richmond, Virginia 23220-2906.
804 359 4783

Organizations: Sexual Politics

Virginians for Justice
P. O. Box 342, Capitol Station, Richmond, Virginia 23202-0342.
Publishes *Voice of Virginians for Justice.*

Organizations: Sexuality

Richmond Area Bisexual Network (ROBIN)
c/o ICU2 Publications, Suite D, 3310 Elmwood Avenue, Richmond, Virginia 23221.
804 355 7939
Publishes *Bi Lines.*

Virginia's Secret
P. O. Box 7386, Richmond, Virginia 23221-0386.
804 222 6796
Meets monthly

Organizations: Sexuality: Student

Sexual Minority Student Alliance
Box 75, Student Activities Center, Commonwealth University, 907 Floys Avenue, Richmond, Virginia 23284-2035.
804 367 6509

Piercers

Piercing Exquisite
P. O. Box 13138, Richmond, Virginia 23225.
804 232 3096
ardvark@richmond.infi.net
By appointment only, no walk-in
✓
Age statement of 18 is required.

Publishers: Books: Erotic

The Gates of Heck
P. O. Box 15296, Richmond, Virginia 23227.
804 266 9422
804 266 9422

Publishers: Newspapers: Sexuality

Information Express
P. O. Box 14747, Richmond, Virginia 23221.

Richmond Pride
P. O. Box 14689, Richmond, Virginia 23221.

Stores: Books: General

Biff's Bookstore
2930 West Carey Street, Richmond, Virginia 23221.
804 359 4831

Phœnix Rising
19 North Belmont Avenue, Richmond, Virginia 23221.
804 355 7939
11:00 - 19:00

Roanoke

Health Services

Roanoke Memorial Hospital
Belleview at Jefferson Street, Roanoke, Virginia 24033.
703 981 7000

Organizations: AIDS: Education

Roanoke AIDS Project
P. O. Box 598, Roanoke, Virginia 24004.
703 982 2437

Organizations: AIDS: Support

Blue Ridge AIDS Support Group (BRASS)
P. O. Box 1472, Roanoke, Virginia 24007.

Organizations: BDSM

Rogues LLC
P. O. Box 12603, Roanoke, Virginia 24027-2603.
bearsday@aol.com
Meets 2nd. Sat of month

Springfield

Television: Sexuality

Gay Fairfax
P. O. Box 2322, Springfield, Virginia 22152.
703 451 9528

Staunton

Organizations: AIDS: Education

AIDS Resources of Central Shenendoah
P. O. Box 1847, Staunton, Virginia 24401.
703 886 7116

Tysons Corner

Stores: Clothing: Leather

Night Dreams
8381 Leesburg Place, Tysons Corner, Virginia.

Virginia Beach

Counsellors

Hope Damon, LCSW
Rainbow Psychotherapy, Suite 103, 5265 Providence Road, Virginia Beach, Virginia 23464.
804 495 4616
804 671 9902 (beeper)
Couples, family, groups, adult, adolescents, & children.

Bill Davis, LCSW
4616 Westgrove Court, Virginia Beach, Virginia 23455.
804 460 4655

Daniel Walter, Psy.D.
Suite 206, 5320 Providence Road, Virginia Beach, Virginia 23464.
804 424 0100

Stores: Books: General

Outright Books
Suite 111, 485 South Independence Boulevard, Virginia Beach, Virginia 23452.
804 490 6658

Williamsburg

Organizations: Sexuality: Student

Alternatives
c/o Student Activities Center, Campus Center, College of William & Mary, Williamsburg, Virginia 23185.
206 271 3309

Woodbridge
Organizations: Sexuality
ௐ▽ **Prince William Gay & Lesbian Association**
P. O. Box 4231, Woodbridge, Virginia 22194.

Woodstock
Organizations: AIDS: Support
☺ ☐ **Aid for AIDS, Inc.**
P. O. Box 147, Woodstock, Virginia 22664.
☎ 703 459 8208

WASHINGTON
Area: Approximately 172,000 square kilometres
Population: Approximately 4,890,000
Capital City: Olympia
Time zone: GMT minus 8 hours (PST)
Climate: The Pacific ocean moderates the weather on the coast. Summers are pleasant, with average highs of approximately 18°C. Winters are mild with average highs near 4°C.
Age of consent & homosexuality legislation: State has adopted the Model Penal Code or otherwise decriminalized homosexual activities.
Legal drinking age: 21

State Resources
Organizations: BDSM: Competition
⚲ **Generic Leather Productions**
Box 800, 1202 East Pike Street, Seattle, Washington 98122.
☎ 206 233 8527
✉ Scooter@stage.com
Organizes the Washington State Ms. Leather competition.
⚲ **Washington State Ms. Leather (WSMLO)**
c/o Generic Leather Productions, Box 800, 1202 East Pike Street, Seattle, Washington 98122.
☎ 206 233 8527
✉ Scooter@stage.com

Belleview
BBSs: BDSM
☺ ■ **Kinky Kumputer**
☎ 206 649 0957

Bellingham
Organizations: Sexuality: Student
ௐ▽ **Lesbian Gay Bisexual Alliance**
⛪ Viking Union Box I-1, Western Washington University, Bellingham, Washington 98225-9106.
☎ 206 650 5120
Stores: Books: General
☺ ■ **The Newsstand**
111 East Magnolia, Bellingham, Washington 98225.
Stores: Erotica: General
☺ ▼ **Great Northern Books**
1308 Railroad, Bellingham, Washington 98225.
☎ 206 733 1650

Chehalis
Distributors: Clothing: Fetish
☺ ▼ **Jim Cooke Enterprises**
276 Woodward Road, Chehalis, Washington 98532.
Black Diamond & other heavy rubber rainwear.

Everett
Organizations: AIDS: Education
☺ ☐ **North Puget Sound AIDS Foundation**
P. O. Box 526, Everett, Washington 98206.
☎ 206 659 8045

Kirkland
Manufacturers: Regalia
☺ ■ **Lannoye Emblems**
11013 Champagne Point Road, Kirkland, Washington 98034.
☎ 206 820 0955　　　　　📞 206 823 0973
🕐 Mon - Fri 09:00 - 17:00
💳 ✓
Source of club colours, patches, & pins for many motorcycle & leather clubs.

Montesano
Organizations: Sexuality
ௐ **Sonoma Bares of the Northwest**
P. O. Box 209, Montesano, Washington 98562.
☎ 360 249 6939
Social nudist group with newletter listing events, parties, things of interest to members, quotes, etc. from members. Publishes a newsletter quarterly. Yearly subscription is $10.

Mount Vernon
Organizations: Sexuality
ௐ▽ **Gay, Lesbians, & Bisexuals of Skagit (GLBS)**
♿ Suite 458, 1500A East College Way, Mount Vernon, Washington 98273.
☎ 206 428 9217
Publishes *Skagit Gay Times*. Please address envelopes to GLBS, do NOT address them to Gay, Lesbians, & Bisexuals of Skagit or Skagit Gay Times.

Olympia
Health Services
☺ ☐ **Saint Peter Hospital**
413 Lilly Road, Olympia, Washington 98506.
☎ 206 491 9480
Organizations: AIDS: Education
☺ ☐ **Olympia AIDS Task Force**
♿ Suite 1, 1408 State Avenue, Olympia, Washington 98506-4457.
☎ 206 352 2375
Publishes *Pulse*.
Organizations: BDSM
☺ ☐ **South Sound SM Leatherfolk**
1814 Amhurst Street South East, Olympia, Washington 98201-3223.
☎ 360 786 1438
Contact: Jim or Vince
Organizations: Sexuality
ௐ▽ **Lesbian Fun Society**
♿ P. O. Box 10321, Olympia, Washington 98502.
Publishes *Lesbian Fun Society News Tribute*.
Publishers: Newspapers: Sexuality
ௐ▽ *Sound Out*
P. O. Box 1844, Olympia, Washington 98507.
☎ 206 791 3355
Stores: Books: General
☺ ■ **Bulldog News**
♿ 116 East 4th. Avenue, Olympia, Washington 98501.
☎ 206 357 6397

Pullman
Organizations: Sexuality
ௐ▽ **Gay & Lesbian Association (GALA)**
♿ Suite 211, K-House, NE 720 Thatuna, Pullman, Washington 99163.
☎ 509 335 4311
Publishes *The Key*.

Seattle
Bars: BDSM
ௐ▼ **CC Slaughter's North**
1501 East Madison, Seattle, Washington 98122.
☎ 206 323 4017
ⓔ ▼ **Crescent Tavern**
1413 East Olive Way, Seattle, Washington 98122.
ௐ▼ **The Cuff**
1533 13th. Street, Seattle, Washington 98122.
☎ 206 323 1525
ௐ **The Seattle Eagle**
314 East Pike Street, Seattle, Washington 98122.
☎ 206 621 7591
Bars: Sexuality
⚧▼ **Tacky Tavern**
1706 Bellevue Avenue, Seattle, Washington 98122.
☎ 206 322 9744
🕐 12:00 - 02:00
BBSs: AIDS
☺ **Seattle AIDS Information BBS (SAIBBS)**

Box 658, 1202 East Pike Street, Seattle, Washington 98122-3934.
☎ 206 329 8617
✆ 206 323 4420
🕐 Voice line: call before 23:00. BBS 24hrs.

BBSs: BDSM

☺ ■ **#28 Barbury Lane**
✆ 206 525 2828

⚥▼ **S&M Exchange**
Box 1032, 1202 East Pike Street, Seattle, Washington 98122.
✆ 206 324 2121

Counsellors

☺▼ **Ron Anders, MSW**
♿ Suite 850, 101 Stewart Street, Seattle, Washington 98103.
☎ 206 441 1903

✍▽ **The Ingersoll Gender Center**
Suite 106, 1812 East Madison, Seattle, Washington 98122-2843.
☎ 206 329 6651
📧 ingersol@halcyon.com
🌐 http://www.halcyon.com/ingersol/iiihome.html
🕐 Mon Tue Wed Fri 18:00 - 20:00

⚥▽ **Seattle Counseling Service for Sexual Minorities**
♿ Suite 300, 200 West Mercer Street, Seattle, Washington 98119-3958.
☎ 206 282 9307

Health Services

☺ □ **45th. Street Clinic**
♿ 1629 45th. Street, Seattle, Washington 98103.
☎ 206 633 3350

☺ □ **Group Health Coöperative Central Hospital**
201 16th. Avenue, Seattle, Washington 98112.
☎ 206 326 3000
HIV & emergency departments.

☺ □ **Harborview Medical Center**
325 Ninth Avenue, Seattle, Washington 89104.
☎ 206 223 3000

☺ □ **Health Information Network**
♿ P. O. Box 30762, Seattle, Washington 98103.
☎ 206 784 5655

⚥▽ **Seattle Gay Clinic**
♿ 500 19th. Avenue East, Seattle, Washington 98112.
☎ 206 461 4540
🕐 Tue Thu 18:30 - 21:00, Sat 10:30 - 13:30

☺ □ **Swedish Medical Center**
747 Summit Avenue, Seattle, Washington 98114.
☎ 206 386 6000
HIV & emergency departments.

☺ □ **University of Washington Medical Center**
1959 North East Pacific Street, Seattle, Washington 98195.
☎ 206 548 3300

Manufacturers: Clothing: Leather

☺ **Rider Upholstery**
1116 East Pike Street, Seattle, Washington 98122.
☎ 206 323 5593
Leather wear & auto upholstery.

Organizations: Academic: Psychiatry

☺ □ **Seattle Institute for Sex Therapy Education & Research (SISTER)**
♿ 100 North East 56th. Street, Seattle, Washington 98105.
☎ 206 522 8588

Organizations: AIDS: Education

☺ □ **AIDS Prevention Project**
♿ Suite 400, 2124 4th. Avenue, Seattle, Washington 98121-2311.
☎ 206 296 4999
☎ 206 296 4843 (TDD)
🕐 Mon - Fri 08:00 - 17:00
Also anonymous HIV testing & counselling.

☺ □ **Northwest AIDS Foundation**
♿ 127 Broadway East, Seattle, Washington 98102-5711.
☎ 206 329 6923 📞 206 325 2689
☎ 206 323 2685 (TDD)
Publishes *AIDS Matters*.

☺ **People of Color Against AIDS Network**
Suite 25, 1200 South Jackson Street, Seattle, Washington 88144-2065.
☎ 206 322 7061

Organizations: AIDS: Support

☺ **American Red Cross AIDS Projects**

1900 25th. Avenue South, Seattle, Washington 98144.
☎ 206 323 2345

Organizations: BDSM

☺ □ **Alternates**
402 15th. Avenue, Seattle, Washington.
☎ 206 323 7483
🕐 Meets Thu 18:00
BDSM / leather / fetish 12-step recovery group.

⚥ ▽ **Banshees**
2716 East Marion Street, Seattle, Washington 98122.
☎ 206 329 6374

☺ □ **Collars**
Box 947, 1202 East Pike Street, Seattle, Washington 98122-3934.

Organizations: BDSM: Competition

⚥ ▼ **Washington State Mr. Leather Organization**
Box 1032, 1202 East Pike Street, Seattle, Washington 98122-3934.
☎ 206 720 4075

Organizations: BDSM

☺ ▽ **Kinky Couples**
Suite 366, 645 Southcenter Mall, Seattle, Washington 98188.

☺ ▽ **Leather Pride Project**
Box 707, 1202 East Pike Street, Seattle, Washington 98122-3934.
☎ 206 325 4275
📧 Lthrpride@aol.com
🌐 http://home.aol.com/Lthrpride
Publishes *Leather Pride!*

⚥ ■ **Northwest Leather Goddesses**
Box 687, 1202 East Pike Street, Seattle, Washington 98122-3934.
☎ 206 782 2472
Support group for dominant & switchable women.

⚥ ▽ **Outer Limits (OL)**
Box 819, 1202 East Pike Street, Seattle, Washington 98122.

☺ **Seattle Kink Information Network (SKIN)**
☎ 206 368 0384
🕐 Meets every other Sunday 19:30 - 21:30
Lectures, discussions, & workshops on BDSM & kink sensuality. Call for information & schedules. Age statement of 18 is required.

⚥▽ **Seattle Men in Leather (SML)**
Box 1199, 1202 East Pike Street, Seattle, Washington 98122-3934.
☎ 206 233 8141
📧 Scooter@stage.com
Contact: Mr. John Karr
Social club promoting Seattle's gay men's leather community, to provide cameraderie & social events. Monthly brunches, yearly BBQs, pot-lucks, etc.. Publishes a newsletter every month. Yearly subscription is $10U.S..

☺ □ **Tacoma Pride in Leather**
c/o 24th. Street Tavern, 24th. & Pacific, Seattle, Washington.
🕐 Meets last Tue of month 19:00

⚥ **Women's Welcoming Committee (WWC)**
📧 xeno@scn.org
🕐 Meets 1st. Tue of month 19:00
Assists women (only, please) of any orientation who are looking for information about BDSM & leather.

Organizations: Bears

⚥▽ **Northwest Bears**
🐾 Box 802, 1202 East Pike Street, Seattle, Washington 98122-3934.
☎ 206 233 0113
📧 bearwolf@compumedia.com
🌐 http://www.compumedia.com/~bearwolf/nwbear/

⚥▽ **Renegade Bears**
Suite 271, 9594 First Avenue North East, Seattle, Washington 98115-2012.
☎ 206 823 6639
📧 Rnegadbear@aol.com
🌐 http://www.skepsis.com:80/.gblo/bears/CLUBS/renegade_bears.html

Organizations: Body Size

⚥▽ **Girth & Mirth—Seattle**
P. O. Box 9935, Seattle, Washington 98109.
☎ 206 361 9686

Organizations: Bondage

☺ ▽ **Northwest Bondage Club**
Box 1212, 1202 East Pike Street, Seattle, Washington 98122-3934.
☎ 206 781 1575
☎ 206 824 1226
🕐 18:00 - 24:00
♿
Age statement of 18 is required.

Organizations: Family

☺ □ **Parents & Friends of Lesbians & Gays (PFLAG)—**
&. **Seattle**
1629 North 45th. Street, Seattle, Washington 98103.
☎ 206 325 7724
☎ 206 863 4206 (Tacoma)

☺ □ **Solo Parenting Alliance**
& 139 23rd. Avenue South, Seattle, Washington 98144.
☎ 206 720 1655
Publishes *Solo Connections.*

Organizations: Fisting

♂♀▽ **Cascade Handballers**
& Box 1135, 1202 East Pike Street, Seattle, Washington 98122.
☎ 206 747 5510
🕐 Meets 2nd. Fri of month 20:00 - 22:00
Contact: Gary

Organizations: Literary

☺ □ **No Safeword Writers' Group**
Box 986, 1202 East Pike Street, Seattle, Washington 98122.
✉ Danm@wolfe.net
Contact: Mr. D. C. McGlothlen

Organizations: Motorcycle

♂♀▽ **Border Riders MC**
P. O. Box 21152, Seattle, Washington 98111.
☎ 503 256 0197
☎ 206 720 4774
✉ brmc95prez@aol.com

♂♀▽ **Knights of Malta MC—Jet**
P. O. Box 21052, Seattle, Washington 98111.

Organizations: Sexual Politics

♀▽ **Lesbian Mother's Defense National Fund**
P. O. Box 21567, Seattle, Washington 98111.
☎ 206 325 2643
Publishes *Mom's Apple Pie* quarterly. Yearly subscription is $10.

☺ □ **National Campaign for Freedom of Expression**
Suite 421, 1402 3rd. Avenue, Seattle, Washington 98101-2118.
☎ 206 340 9301 ✆ 206 340 4303
🕐 Mon - Fri 09:00 - 17:00
Contact: Mr. Steven Johnson

Organizations: Sexuality

♂▽ **BiNet—Seattle**
P. O. Box 30645, Seattle, Washington 98103.
☎ 206 728 4533

♀▽ **Emerald City**
P. O. Box 31318, Seattle, Washington 98103.
☎ 206 284 1071
Publishes a newsletter.

♂ ▽ **Seattle Bisexual Men's Union**
P. O. Box 30645, Seattle, Washington 98103-0645.
☎ 206 728 4533

♀ ▽ **Seattle Bisexual Women's Network**
& P. O. Box 30645, Greenwood Station, Seattle, Washington 98103-0645.
☎ 206 783 7987
Publishes *North Bi Northwest.*

♀▽ **Transexual Lesbians & Friends**
☎ 206 292 1037
🕐 Meets Fri 18:30

Organizations: Sexuality: Student

♂♀▽ **LesBiGays, Unlimited**
& 207 HUB Box 104, FK-30, University of Washington, Seattle, Washington 98195.
☎ 206 543 6106

☺ □ **The Society for Human Sexuality**
SAO 141, Box 352238, University of Washington, Seattle, Washington 98195.
✉ sfpse@u.washington.edu
🌐 http://weber.u.washington.edu/~sfpse/
You can subscribe to our mailing list by sending an e-mail message to listproc@u.washington.edu with a body copy of: info shs.

♂♀▽ **Triangle Club**
& 1701 Broadway, Seattle, Washington 98122.
☎ 206 587 6924

Organizations: Sexuality: Youth

♂♀▽ **Gay & Lesbian Youth of Seattle**
1818 15th. Avenue, Seattle, Washington 98122.
☎ 206 322 2515

♂♀▽ **Youth Rap Group**
c/o Gay Community Social Services, Box 22228, Seattle, Washington 98122.
☎ 206 322 2873

Organizations: Watersports

♂♀▽ **Northwest Rainmakers**
Suite 150, 10115 Greenwood Avenue North, Seattle, Washington 98133.
☎ 206 292 1411
🕐 24hr. answering machine
&. ✓
Contact: Mr. Patrick Lopaka
Age statement of 18 is required.

Organizations: Wrestling

♂♀▽ **Pacific Northwest Wrestling Association**
432 Dewey Place East, Seattle, Washington 98112.

Piercers

☺ ■ **Body Circle Designs**
P. O. Box 68429, Seattle, Washington 96168.
☎ 206 244 8430 ✆ 206 244 3478
✉ bcd@bcd.seanet.com

☺ **Playspace**
616 East Pine Street, Seattle, Washington 98122.
☎ 206 329 0324 ✆ 206 727 3922
☎ 206 621 0397
🕐 12:00 - 20:00
Age statement of 18 is required. German also spoken. Please see our advertisement with SIN.

☺ ■ **WA Creations**
Suite 291, 501 North 36th. Street, Seattle, Washington.
☎ 206 632 5791
Makes gold nostril screws, fishtail labret studs, & bead rings. Also branding & cupping.

Publishers: Books: BDSM

☺ ■ **Eros Publishing**
& Box 656, 1202 East Pike Street, Seattle, Washington 98122-3934.
☎ 206 767 8269
&. ✓ VISA MC
Published *Doomed Rabbit*, a collection of recipes from members of the leather community. Only by mail order.

Publishers: Books: Erotic

☺ ■ **Artistic Licentiousness**
P. O. Box 27438, Seattle, Washington 98125.
&. ✓
A comic book that takes a humourous look at bisexuality, sexual inexperience, mysogyny, homophobia, & more. Make cheques payable to Roberta Gregory. Age statement of 18 is required.

Publishers: Books: Sexuality

☺ ■ **Infantæ Press**
P. O. Box 12466, Seattle, Washington 98111.
Publications for adult babies.

Publishers: Magazines: BDSM

♂▽ *Bitches With Whips*
DM International, P. O. Box 16188, Seattle, Washington 98116-0188.
✆ 206 937 2066
🕐 Mon - Fri 09:30 - 18:00
✓ $
Good writers, erotic non-fiction stories about female dominance, bondage, watersports, foot worship, multiple partner scenes, & much more kinky action. Published quarterly. Yearly subscription is $32U.S. for North America, $42U.S. overseas. Age statement of 21 is required. Please address envelopes to DM International, do NOT address them to Bitches With Whips. Please see our display advertisement.

♂▽ *Kinky People Places & Things*
DM International, P. O. Box 16188, Seattle, Washington 98116-0188.
✆ 206 937 2066
🕐 Mon - Fri 09:30 - 18:00
✓ $
Pansexual people who enjoy BDSM, fetish, & leather. Solid writing, erotic, tantalizing fiction, & educational, well-informed non-fiction. Published every two months. Yearly subscription is $40U.S. for North America, $54U.S. overseas. Age statement of 21 is required. Please address envelopes to DM International, do NOT address them to Kinky People Places & Things. Please see our display advertisement.

Publishers: Magazines: Sexuality

☺ ■ **Eros Comix**
P. O. Box 25070, Seattle, Washington 98125-1970.
☎ 800 657 1100 ☏ 206 524 2104
☎ 206 524 1967
⏲ Mon - Sat 10:00 - 18:00
✓ VISA MC
Sexually explicit gay & straight comic with BDSM content. Free
catalogue. Age statement of 18 is required.

⚢▽ **Teen Fag**
Chow Chow Productions, P. O. Box 20204, Seattle, Washington 98102.
☎ 206 322 6862
⚘
We're here. We're queer. Let's drink lite beer, & then go shopping. Arts,
entertainment, commentary, human interest. No subject taboo.
Published twice a year. Yearly subscription is $5 or equivalent IRCs.

⚥ **TV Connection**
DM International, P. O. Box 16188, Seattle, Washington 98116-0188.
☏ 206 937 2066
⏲ Mon - Fri 09:30 - 18:00
✓ $
For transgendered people, transvestites, & those who would like to meet
them. Everything from erotic fiction to "how to" articles. Published
quarterly. Yearly subscription is $26U.S. for North America, $36U.S.
overseas. Age statement of 21 is required. Please address envelopes to
DM International, do NOT address them to TV Connection. Please see our
display advertisement.

Publishers: Newspapers: Sexuality

⚢ **Beyond 2002**
Suite 592, 1202 East Pike Street, Seattle, Washington 98195-3934.
☎ 206 323 2332 ☏ 206 323 2170
✉ Beyond2002@eor.com

Ecce Queer
2nd. Floor, 1925 8th. Avenue, Seattle, Washington 98101.

⚲ **Lesbian Resource Center Community News**
Suite 204, 1808 Bellevue Street, Seattle, Washington 98122.
☎ 206 322 3965
Features, news, & commentary for the lesbian community, along with a
calendar of events. Published every month. Yearly subscription is $15.

⚢▼ **Seattle Gay News**
♿ P. O. Box 22007, Seattle, Washington 98122-0007.
☎ 206 324 4297 ☏ 206 322 7188
✉ sgn1@sgn.org
☒ http://www.sgn.org/sgn
⏲ Mon - Thu 09:00 - 18:00, Fri 10:00- 15:00
✓ VISA MC
News & features of interest to gay & lesbians in the northwest. Politics,
people, AIDS, films, & books. Published every week. Yearly subscription
is $45.

⚢ **Speak Out**
Hub Box 96, FK-30, Seattle, Washington 98195.

⚢▽ **TWIST**
Suite 107, 600 7th. Avenue, Seattle, Washington 98104-1902.
☎ 206 343 0311
The northwest's premier gay & lesbian newsweekly. The only paper with
two full pages of comics, compelling cover stories, & free personals.
Published every week. Yearly subscription is $25.

⚢ **Young Gay/Lesbian Life**
P. O. Box 23070, Seattle, Washington 98102-0370.

Stores: Books: General

☺ ■ **Alfi News**
113 Lake Street, Kirkland, Washington 98033.
☎ 206 827 6486

☺ ■ **Alfi News**
4427 Wallingford Avenue North, Seattle, Washington 98103.
☎ 206 632 9390

⚢▼ **Bailey/Coy Books**
♿ 414 Broadway East, Seattle, Washington 98102.
☎ 206 323 8842

⚢▼ **Beyond The Closet**
1501 Belmont Avenue, Seattle, Washington 98122.
☎ 800 238 8518
☎ 206 322 4609
⏲ 10:00 - 22:00, Fri Sat - 23:00
⚘ ✓ VISA MC AMEX

☺ ■ **Bulldog News**
♿ 401 Broadway East, Seattle, Washington 98102.
☎ 206 322 6397

☺ ■ **Bulldog News**
♿ 4208 University Way North East, Seattle, Washington 98105.

☎ 206 632 6397

☺▼ **Fremont Place Book Company**
621 North 35th., Seattle, Washington 98103.
☎ 206 547 5970

☺ ☐ **Left Bank Books**
♿ 92 Pike Street, Seattle, Washington 98101.
☎ 206 622 0195
⏲ Mon 10:00 - 18:00, Tue - Sat 10:00 - 22:00, Sun 11:00 - 17:00

☺▼ **M. Coy Books**
117 Pine Street, Seattle, Washington 98101.
☎ 206 623 5354

☺ ■ **Pistil Books & News**
1013 East Pike Street, Seattle, Washington 98122.
☎ 206 325 5401
⏲ Sun - Thu 10:00 - 22:00, Fri Sat 10:00 - 24:00
⚘ ✓ $ VISA MC
Used & new books with an emphasis on current & classic fiction, poetry,
sex / erotica, & art. Neighbourhood bookshop.

☺ ■ **Red & Black Books Collective**
♿ 432 15th. Avenue East, Seattle, Washington 98112.
☎ 206 322 7323

☺ ■ **Steve's Broadway News**
♿ 204 Broadway East, Seattle, Washington 98102.
☎ 206 324 7323

Stores: Erotica: BDSM

☺ ■ **Cramp Leather**
219 Broadway East, Seattle, Washington 98102.
☎ 206 323 9245
Part of a regular clothing store.

☺ ■ **The Crypt**
♿ 1310 East Union Street, Capitol Hill, Washington.
☎ 206 325 3882
⏲ Mon - Thu 10:00 - 24:00, Fri Sat 10:00 - 01:00, Sun 12:00 -
22:00
⚘ ✓ VISA MC AMEX

⚢■ **Seattle Leather Mercantile**
1204 East Pike Street, Seattle, Washington 98122-3909.
☎ 800 860 5847
☎ 206 860 5847
⏲ Tue - Sat 11:00 - 19:00
⚘ ✓ VISA MC
Boots, uniforms, custom leather, etc.. Also mail order.

Stores: Erotica: General

☺ ■ **Fantasy Unlimited**
P. O. Box 2602, Seattle, Washington 98101-2602.
☎ 206 682 0167 ☏ 206 328 7249
⏲ Mon - Sat 10:00 - 21:00, Sun 11:00 - 19:00
⚘ ✓ VISA MC

☺▼ **Spanky's**
♿ 3276 California Avenue, Seattle, Washington 98116.
☎ 206 938 3400

⚤▼ **Toys in Babeland**
♿ 711 East Pike Street, Seattle, Washington 98122.
☎ 206 328 2914 ☏ 206 328 2994
✉ babeland@aol.com
⏲ 12:00 - 20:00
⚘ ✓ VISA MC
Lesbian-run toy store for people of all sexualities. Large array of high-
quality dildos, harnesses, etc.. Extensive selection of sexual literature.

Suppliers: Miscellaneous

⚢▼ **Post Option Business Center**
1202 East Pike Street, Seattle, Washington 98122-3934.
☎ 206 322 2777 ☏ 206 324 8124
⚘ ✓ VISA
Mail box & voice mail services for many alternate sexuality groups.

Tattooists

☺ ■ **Dermagraphics**
94 Pike Place, Seattle, Washington.
☎ 206 622 1535
Limited body piercing also available.

☺ ■ **Tattoo You**
1017 East Pike Street, Seattle, Washington 98122.
☎ 206 324 6443
⏲ Wed - Sat 12:00 - 18:00

South Renton

Tattooists

☺ ■ **Skinprint Tattoo**

234 1/2 Wells Avenue, South Renton, Washington.
☎ 206 255 5841
Body piercing also available.

Spokane

Organizations: AIDS: Education

Spokane AIDS Network
1613 West Gardiner Avenue, Spokane, Washington 99201-1830.
☎ 509 326 6070

Spokane County Health District
AIDS Program, Suite 401, 1101 West College Avenue, Spokane, Washington 99201.
☎ 509 324 1542
Mon - Fri 08:00 - 17:00

Organizations: Family

Parents & Friends of Lesbians & Gays (PFLAG)—Spokane
P. O. Box 40122, Spokane, Washington 99202-0901.
☎ 509 624 6671

Organizations: Sexuality: Student

Gay, Lesbian, & Bisexual Alliance (GLA/EWU)
PUB-20, MS-60, Eastern Washington University, Cheney, Washington 99004.
☎ 509 359 4253
Publishes a newsletter. Please address envelopes to GLA/EWU, do NOT address them to Gay, Lesbian, & Bisexual Alliance.

Organizations: Sexuality: Youth

Odyssey
Suite 401, 1101 West College Avenue, Spokane, Washington 99201.
☎ 509 324 1547

Publishers: Newspapers: Sexuality

Stonewall News Spokane
P. O. Box 3994, Spokane, Washington 99220-3994.
☎ 509 456 8011
Serves the lesbigay community of the inland northwest. Published every month. Yearly subscription is $12.

Stores: Books: General

Auntie's Bookstore
402 West Main, Spokane, Washington 99201-0249.
☎ 509 838 0206

Tacoma

Organizations: Sexuality: Youth

Oasis
☎ 206 591 6060
Call Mon - Fri 08:00 - 16:30 for times & locations

Publishers: Newspapers: Sexuality

Tacoma Sounds
P. O. Box 110816, Tacoma, Washington 98411-0816.
☎ 206 535 4213
Local coverage of past & upcoming events, information on AIDS, items of interest to the gay community, horoscope, stories, poetry, & photos from readers. Published every month. Yearly subscription is $15.

Stores: Books: General

Imprints Bookstore
2920 Parkway, Tacoma, Washington 98466-2235.
☎ 206 383 6322
Mon - Fri 11:00 - 18:00, Sat 12:00 - 17:00

Stores: Erotica: General

Jerry's Adult Bookstore
755 Broadway, Tacoma, Washington 98402-3717.
☎ 206 272 4700

Tattooists

Skinprint Tattoo
12840 Pacific Highway South West, Tacoma, Washington.
☎ 206 582 8514
Body piercing also available.

Vancouver

Counsellors

Columbia Medical Plaza
Suite 200, 8614 East Mill Plain Boulevard, Vancouver, Washington 98664.
☎ 206 254 1814 Fax 206 254 1828
Board certified in psychiatry, adolescent, adult, & family psychiatry.

Walla Walla

Organizations: AIDS: Education

Blue Mountain Heart To Heart
P. O. Box 65, Walla Walla, Washington 99362.
☎ 509 529 4744

Wenatchee

Organizations: Sexuality

North Central Washington Gay & Lesbian Alliance (NCW GALA)
P. O. Box 234, Wenatchee, Washington 98807-0234.
☎ 509 662 8413

Yakima

Organizations: Sexuality

Together At Last Lesbians
P. O. Box 976, Yakima, Washington 98907.
☎ 509 454 4989
Please address envelopes to TALL, do NOT address them to Together At Last Lesbians.

WEST VIRGINIA

Area: Approximately 62,500 square kilometres
Population: Approximately 1,800,000
Capital City: Charleston
Time zone: GMT minus 5 hours (EST)
Age of consent & homosexuality legislation: State has adopted the Model Penal Code or otherwise decriminalized homosexual activities.
Legal drinking age: 21

State Resources

Organizations: AIDS: Education

Mountain State AIDS Network
P. O. Box 1221, Morgantown, West Virginia 26505.
☎ 800 585 4444 (in West Virginia)
☎ 304 292 9000

Organizations: AIDS: Support

HIV Care Consortium
304 South Huron Street, Wheeling, West Virginia 26003.
☎ 304 232 6295

Publishers: Newspapers: Sexuality

Out and About
P. O. Box 27, Huntington, West Virginia 25706.
☎ 304 522 9089

Berkeley Springs

Stores: Erotica: General

Action Books & Video
Box 256A, Route 522 South, Berkeley Springs, West Virginia 25411.
☎ 304 258 2529

Charleston

Health Services

Charleston Area Medical Center
3200 MacCorkle Avenue, Charleston, West Virginia 25304.
☎ 304 348 5432

Organizations: AIDS: Education

Charleston AIDS Network
P. O. Box 1024, Charleston, West Virginia 25324.
☎ 304 345 4673

Publishers: Newspapers: Sexuality

Graffitti
Suite 230, 1036 Quarrier Street, Charleston, West Virginia 25301.

Womyn's Community Newsletter
P. O. Box 5393, Charleston, West Virginia 25361-5393.

Dunbar

Organizations: Sexuality

The Valley Girls
P. O. Box 181, Dunbar, West Virginia 25064-0181.

Huntington

Health Services

Cabell Huntington Hospital
1340 Hal Greer Boulevard, Huntington, West Virginia 25701.

☎ 304 526 2000

Organizations: AIDS: Education

☺ ☐ **Huntington AIDS Force**
P. O. Box 2981, Huntington, West Virginia 25728.
☎ 304 522 4357

Organizations: Sexuality

♀♂▽ **Trans—West Virginia**
P. O. Box 2322, Huntington, West Virginia 25724.
Publishes a newsletter.

Martinsburg

Stores: Books: General

☺ ■ **Pepper's News Stand**
246 North Queen Street, Martinsburg, West Virginia 25401.
☎ 304 267 6846

Stores: Erotica: General

☺ ■ **Variety Books & Video**
255 North Queen Street, Martinsburg, West Virginia 25401.
☎ 304 263 4334

Morgantown

Helplines: AIDS

♂▽ **Gay & Lesbian Helpline**
Bisexual, Gay, & Lesbian Mountaineers (BiGLM), Student Organization
Services, P. O. Box 6444, West Virginia University, Morgantown, West
Virginia 26506-6444.
☎ 304 292 4292

Organizations: Sexuality: Student

♂▽ **Bisexual, Gay, & Lesbian Mountaineers (BiGLM)**
♿ Student Organization Services, P. O. Box 6444, West Virginia University,
Morgantown, West Virginia 26506-6444.
☎ 304 293 8200

Stores: Erotica: General

☺ ■ **Select Books & Video**
237 Walnut Street, Morgantown, West Virginia 26505.
☎ 304 292 7714

Parkersburg

Helplines: AIDS

☺ ☐ **AIDS Hotline**
P. O. Box 1274, Parkersburg, West Virginia 26102.
☎ 304 485 4803

Shepherdstown

Organizations: Sexuality

♂▽ **Lambda Panhandlers**
P. O. Box 1961, Shepherdstown, West Virginia 25443-1961.

Wheeling

Organizations: AIDS: Education

☺ ☐ **AIDS Task Force of the Upper Ohio Valley**
♿ P. O. Box 6360, Wheeling, West Virginia 26003.
☎ 304 232 6822

Stores: Erotica: General

☺ ■ **Market Street News**
♿ 1437 Market Street, Wheeling, West Virginia 26003.
☎ 304 232 2414

WISCONSIN

Area: Approximately 141,000 square kilometres
Population: Approximately 4,900,000
Capital City: Madison
Time zone: GMT minus 6 hours (CST)
Climate: Pleasant summers, with average highs near 21°C. Winters are cold
with average highs near -7°C.
Age of consent & homosexuality legislation: There is legislation in
place against discrimination on the basis of sexual orientation.
Legal drinking age: 19

State Resources

Helplines: Miscellaneous

☺ ▽ **Gay Information Services**
P. O. Box 92396, Milwaukee, Wisconsin 53202-0396.
☎ 414 444 7331
🕐 24hrs.
For 8 years, providing information to all who call. Spanish also spoken.

Organizations: AIDS: Education

☺ ☐ **AIDS Resource Center of Wisconsin, Inc.**
♿ P. O. Box 92505, Milwaukee, Wisconsin 53202.
☎ 800 359 9272 ✆ 414 273 2357
☎ 414 273 1991
Publishes *Lifelines*.

☺ ☐ **Northwest Wisconsin AIDS Project**
♿ P. O. Box 11, Eau Clair, Wisconsin 54702-0011.
☎ 800 750 2437 ✆ 715 836 9844
☎ 715 836 7710

☺ ☐ **Southeast Wisconsin AIDS Project**
♿ P. O. Box 0173, Kenosha, Wisconsin 53141-0173.
☎ 800 924 6601 ✆ 414 657 6949
☎ 414 657 6644

Organizations: AIDS: Research

☺ ☐ **Wisconsin Community-Based Research Consortium**
♿ P. O. Box 92505, Milwaukee, Wisconsin 53202.
☎ 800 359 9272 ✆ 414 273 2357
☎ 414 291 2799

Organizations: Motorcycle

♂▽ **Great Lakes Harley Owners**
P. O. Box 341611, Milwaukee, Wisconsin 53234-1611.

Publishers: Newspapers: Sexuality

♂▼ **In Step**
♿ 225 South 2nd. Street, Milwaukee, Wisconsin 53204.
☎ 414 278 7840 ✆ 414 278 5868
Statewide focus on news, organization activities, calendar of special
events, humour, variety of columns, & current listings in the guide
section. Published 25 times a year. Yearly subscription is $35. Age
statement of 21 is required.

♂▽ **Wisconsin Light**
1843 North Palmer Street, Milwaukee, Wisconsin 53212.
☎ 414 372 2773
Serving the gay & lesbian community of Wisconsin. Features local, state,
& national news, columns, opinions, reviews, & editorials. Published 25
times a year. Yearly subscription is $11.95.

Ashland

Organizations: Sexuality

♂▽ **Gay & Lesbian Support Group**
♿ Box 247A, 1411 Ellis Avenue, Ashland, Wisconsin 54806.

Beloit

Stores: Books: General

⚲ ■ **A Different World**
414 East Grand Avenue, Beloit, Wisconsin 53511.
☎ 608 365 1000

Stores: Erotica: General

☺ ■ **Naughty But Nice**
3503 East County Road, Beloit, Wisconsin 53511.
☎ 608 362 9090
🕐 Mon - Sat 08:00 - 24:00, Sun 10:00 - 23:00
Also sells BDSM items.

Cazenovia

Publishers: Magazines: Erotic

♂▼ **Steam**
PDA Press, Inc., Box 1215, Route 2, Cazenovia, Wisconsin 53924.
☎ 800 478 3268
☎ 415 243 3232
✉ steam.roller@studs.com
🕐 Mon - Fri 09:00 - 17:00
💳
Business & subscription enquiries to: PDA Press, Inc., Suite 400, 530
Howard Street, San Francisco, California 94105. Published quarterly.
Yearly subscription is $21.

Fox Valley

Organizations: AIDS: Education

☺ ☐ **Center Project, Inc.**
♿ P. O. Box 1874, Green Bay, Wisconsin 54305.
☎ 414 437 7400 ✆ 414 437 1040

☺ ☐ **Fox Valley AIDS Project**
♿ Suite 201, 120 North Morrison, Appleton, Wisconsin 54911.
☎ 414 733 2068

☺ ☐ **Winnebago Health Department**
♿ P. O. Box 68, Winnebago, Wisconsin 54985.

Organizations: AIDS: Education

☎ 414 235 5100 Ext.: 3375
Publishes *ECHO*.

Organizations: Family

☺ ☐ **Parents & Friends of Lesbians & Gays (PFLAG)— Fox Cities**
P. O. Box 75, Little Chute, Wisconsin 54140.
☎ 414 749 1629

Organizations: Sexuality: Student

♂▽ **10% Society**
& 207 Reeve Union, University of Wisconsin, Oshkosh, Wisconsin 54901.

♂▽ **Bisexual, Gay, & Lesbian Awareness**
& P. O. Box 599, Lawrence University, Appleton, Wisconsin 54912.
☎ 414 832 6600 📞 414 832 7695

Stores: Erotica: General

☺▼ **The Main Attraction**
& 1614 Main Street, Green Bay, Wisconsin 54302.
☎ 414 465 6969
🕐 24hrs.

Green Bay

Organizations: BDSM

♂▼ **Argonauts of Wisconsin**
P.O. Box 20096, Green Bay, Wisconsin 54305.

Stores: Erotica: General

☺■ **Paradise Books**
1122 Main Street, Green Bay, Wisconsin 54301.
☎ 414 432 9498

Janesville

Organizations: AIDS: Support

☺ ☐ **AIDS Support Network**
⊕ 317 Dodge Street, Janesville, Wisconsin 53545.
☎ 608 756 2550 📞 608 756 2545

La Crosse

Publishers: Newspapers: Sexuality

♀ *Leaping La Crosse News*
P. O. Box 932, La Crosse, Wisconsin 54602.

Stores: Books: General

☺▼ **Rainbow Revolution**
122 Fifth Avenue South, La Crosse, Wisconsin 54601.

Madison

Counsellors

☺■ **Harmonia Madison Center for Psychotherapy**
&5 406 North Pinckney, Madison, Wisconsin 53703.
☎ 608 255 8838

Distributors: Safer Sex Products

☺■ **Conney**
P. O. Box 44190, Madison, Wisconsin 53744-4190.
☎ 800 356 9100 📞 800 845 9095
☎ 608 271 3300
🕐 07:00 - 19:00
& ✓ $ 💳 📇 📠 🖃
Distributes N-Dex gloves, among others. Spanish also spoken.

Health Services

☺ ☐ **University Health Service**
& Blue Bus STD Clinic, 1552 University Avenue, Madison, Wisconsin 53705.
☎ 608 262 7330

☺ ☐ **University of Wisconsin Hospital & Clinics**
600 Highland Avenue, Madison, Wisconsin 53792.
☎ 608 263 6400

☺ ☐ **William S. Middleton Veterans' Hospital**
2500 Overlook Terrace, Madison, Wisconsin 53705.
☎ 608 256 1901

Manufacturers: Restraints: Medical

☺■ **Humane Restraint**
P. O. Box 16, Madison, Wisconsin 53701-0016.
☎ 800 356 7472 📞 608 849 6315
☎ 608 849 6313

Organizations: AIDS: Support

☺ ☐ **Madison AIDS Support Network**

303 Lathrop Street, Madison, Wisconsin 53705.
☎ 800 486 6276

Organizations: BDSM

♂▽ **Unicorns of Madison**
P. O. Box 536, Madison, Wisconsin 53701.

Organizations: Family

☺ ☐ **Parents & Friends of Lesbians & Gays (PFLAG)— Madison**
P. O. Box 1722, Madison, Wisconsin 53701.
☎ 608 271 0270

Organizations: Masturbation

♂▽ **Men Enjoying Mutual Masturbation & Oral Sex (MEMMOS)**
P. O. Box 3145, Madison, Wisconsin 53704-0145.
Publishes *MEMMOS Roster* quarterly. Yearly subscription is $25.

Organizations: Sexuality

♂ ▽ **Bi? Shy? Why?**
P. O. Box 321, Madison, Wisconsin 53701.
☎ 608 251 3886

♂▽ **Frontiers**
&5 Suite 103, 14 West Mifflin Street, Madison, Wisconsin 53703.
☎ 608 251 7424
Gay men's outreach. Publishes a newsletter.

♂▽ **Madison Wrestling Club**
P. O. Box 8234, Madison, Wisconsin 537008.
☎ 608 244 8675
🕐 Call evenings & WE. Meets weekly

Organizations: Sexuality: Student

♂▽ **10% Society**
& Box 614, Memorial Union, Madison, Wisconsin 53706.
☎ 608 262 7365

Printers: General

☺ **Omnipress**
P.O. Box 7214, Madison, Wisconsin 53707-7214.
☎ 608 246 2600 📞 608 246 4237

Publishers: Magazines: Sexuality

♀ *Dykes, Disability, & Stuff*
P. O. Box 8773, Madison, Wisconsin 53714-8773.

Publishers: Magazines: Spirituality

☺ *Solitary*
P. O. Box 6091, Madison, Wisconsin 53716.
☎ 608 244 0072

Publishers: Newspapers: Sexuality

⊕ ☐ *Feminist Voices*
& P. O. Box 853, Madison, Wisconsin 53701-0853.
☎ 608 241 9765
Published every month.

Stores: Books: General

☺■ **Pic-A-Book**
506 State Street, Madison, Wisconsin 53703.
☎ 608 256 1125

⊕ ▼ **A Room of One's Own**
& 317 West Johnson Street, Madison, Wisconsin 53703.
☎ 608 257 7888

Stores: Erotica: General

☺■ **State Street Arcade**
113 State Street, Madison, Wisconsin 53703-2522.
☎ 608 251 4540

Menasha

Printers: General

☺ **Banta Company**
P. O. Box, 60 Curtis Reed Plaza, Menasha, Wisconsin 54942.
☎ 414 722 7771 📞 414 722 8541

Milwaukee

Bars: BDSM

♂▼ **Boot Camp Saloon**
209 Easty National Avenue, Milwaukee, Wisconsin 53204.
☎ 414 643 6900

Health Services

♂▽ **Brady East STD Clinic**

1240 East Brady Street, Milwaukee, Wisconsin 53202-1603.
☎ 414 272 2144

☺ ☐ **Columbia Hospital**
2025 East Newport Avenue, Milwaukee, Wisconsin 53211.
☎ 414 961 3300

☺ ☐ **John L. Doyne Hospital**
8700 West Wisconsin Avenue, Milwaukee, Wisconsin 53226.
☎ 414 257 7996

☺ ☐ **Saint Luke's Medical Center**
2900 West Oklahoma Avenue, Milwaukee, Wisconsin 53215.
☎ 414 649 6000

☺ ☐ **Sinai Samaritan Medical Center**
945 North 12th. Street, Milwaukee, Wisconsin 53233.
☎ 414 345 3400

⊕ ▽ **Women's Alternative Health Clinic**
1240 East Brady Street, Milwaukee, Wisconsin 53202-1603.
☎ 414 272 2144

Organizations: Academic: Sexuality

⚥▼ **American Historical Association**
Committee on Lesbian & Gay History, c/o Jeffrey Merrick, Department of History, University of Wisconsin, P. O. Box 413, Milwaukee, Wisconsin 53201.
☎ 414 229 4924

Organizations: AIDS: Education

☺ ☐ **BESTD HIV Outreach Clinic**
1240 East Brady Street, Milwaukee, Wisconsin 53202-1603.
☎ 414 272 2144

☺ ☐ **Milwaukee AIDS Project**
🦽 P. O. Box 92505, Milwaukee, Wisconsin 53202.
☎ 800 359 9272 ✆ 414 273 2357
☎ 414 273 1991

Organizations: BDSM

⚥▽ **Beer Town Badgers**
🦽 P. O. Box 840, Milwaukee, Wisconsin 53201.

⚲▽ **Dykes Against Minority Suppression (DAMES)**
P.O. Box 1272, Milwaukee, Wisconsin 53201-1272.

☺ **Firebirds**
Suite 69, 1224 North Prospect, Milwaukee, Wisconsin 53202.

⚥▽ **Oberons**
P. O. Box 07423, Milwaukee, Wisconsin 53207.

⚥▽ **Wisconsin Leathermen's Association**
P. O. Box 897, Milwaukee, Wisconsin 53201-0897.

Organizations: Bears

⚥▽ **Brew City Bears**
P. O. Box 1252, Milwaukee, Wisconsin 53201.
📧 PoohBear8@aol.com or ChubbyCub@megaweb.com

Organizations: Body Size

⚥▽ **Girth & Mirth—Milwaukee**
P. O. Box 4203, Kenosha, Wisconsin 53143.

Organizations: Motorcycle

⚥▽ **Castaways MC**
P.O. Box 1697, Milwaukee, Wisconsin 53202-1697.

Organizations: Research: Sexuality

⚥ **New Era Institute**
3283 North 46th. Street, Milwaukee, Wisconsin 53216.
☎ 414 862 3823
Publishes *Our Causes Digest*.

Organizations: Sexuality

♂ ▽ **BiNet—Midwest**
P. O. Box 93421, Milwaukee, Wisconsin 53203-3421.

♂ ☐ **Bisexual Support Group**
⊕ P. O. Box 14081, Milwaukee, Wisconsin 53214.

⚥▽ **Black & White Men Together (BWMT)—**
⚲ **Milwaukee**
P. O. Box 12292, Milwaukee, Wisconsin 53212.
☎ 414 265 8500

▷▽ **Gemini Gender Group**
P. O. Box 44211, Milwaukee, Wisconsin 53214.
☎ 414 297 9328 (voice mail)
🕐 Meets 2nd. Sat of m onth
Publishes a newsletter.

⚲▽ **Insight**
⚲ 2038 North Bartlett, Milwaukee, Wisconsin 53202.
☎ 414 271 2565
Contact: Ms. Cheryl Orgas
Counselling for women 17 - 21.

▷▽ **Institute for Psychosexual Health**
c/o Great Lakes Gender Clinic, 3250 North Oakland Avenue, Milwaukee, Wisconsin 53211.
☎ 414 322 5407
Contact: Mr. Charles Kiley, ACSW, CICSW
Gender clinic, counselling, evaluation, support, hormone treatment, & SRS.

▷▽ **Pathways Counseling Center**
Milwaukee Transgender Program, Suite 230, First Financial Building, 2645 North Mayfair Road, Milwaukee, Wisconsin 53226-1304.
☎ 414 774 4111
Contact: Ms. Gretchen Fincke
Complete transgender program, psychotherapy, hormone therapy, & SRS.

▷▽ **Transgender Identity Group**
c/o Ivanoff & Ivanoff, Suite 1810, Clark Building, 633 West Wisconsin Avenue, Milwaukee, Wisconsin 53203-1918.
☎ 414 271 3322
Individual & group therapy.

Organizations: Sexuality: Student

⚥▽ **Gay & Lesbian Community at UWM**
⚲ Box 152, 220 East Kenwood, Milwaukee, Wisconsin 53201.
☎ 414 229 6555

⚥▽ **MGALA**
P. O. Box 92722, Milwaukee, Wisconsin 53202.

Organizations: Sexuality: Youth

⚥▽ **Gay Youth Milwaukee (GYM)**
⚲ P. O. Box 09441, Milwaukee, Wisconsin 53209.
☎ 414 265 8500

Publishers: Newspapers: Sexuality

⚥ *Hag Rag*
P. O. Box 93243, Milwaukee, Wisconsin 53203.
☎ 414 372 3330

Stores: Books: General

⚥▼ **AfterWords**
2710 North Murray, Milwaukee, Wisconsin 53211.
☎ 414 963 9089
🕐 Sun - Thu 11:00 - 22:00, Fri Sat 11:00 - 23:00

☺ ▼ **Constant Reader Bookshop**
1627 East Irving Place, Milwaukee, Wisconsin 53202.
☎ 414 291 0452

☺ ■ **Harry Schwartz Bookshop**
209 East Wisconsin, Milwaukee, Wisconsin 53202.
☎ 414 274 6400

⚥■ **People's Books**
⚲ 3512 North Oakland Avenue, Milwaukee, Wisconsin 53211.
☎ 414 962 0575 ✆ 414 962 0575
🕐 10:00 - 20:00, Sat - 18:00, Sun 12:00 - 17:00

Stores: Erotica: BDSM

☺ ■ **Tie Me Down**
1419 East Brady Street, Milwaukee, Wisconsin 53202.
☎ 414 272 3696

Television: Sexuality

⚥▽ *The Queer Program*
Warner Cable Channel 47, P. O. Box 93951, Milwaukee, Wisconsin 53203.
☎ 414 964 8423
🕐 Tue 19:00 - 20:00, repeats: Thu 16:00-17:00, Sun 11:00-12:00

⚥▽ *Yellow On Thursday*
🦽 Milwaukee Gay / Lesbian Cable Network, Tri-Cable Tonight, P. O. Box 204, Milwaukee, Wisconsin 53201.
☎ 414 265 0880

Portage

Stores: Erotica: General

☺ ■ **Naughty But Nice**
10521 Tritz Road, Portage, Wisconsin 53901.
☎ 608 742 8060
🕐 24hrs.
Also sells BDSM items.

Racine

Organizations: Sexuality

⌕▽ **Gay & Lesbian Union of Racine / Kenosha**
625 College Road, Racine, Wisconsin 53403.
☎ 414 634 0659

Organizations: Sexuality: Student

⌕▽ **UW-Parkside Gay & Lesbian Organization**
Box 200, Kenosha, Wisconsin 53141.
☎ 414 595 2244

Stores: Erotica: General

☺■ **Racine News**
316 Main Street, Racine, Wisconsin 53403.
☎ 414 634 9827

Rhinelander

Organizations: AIDS: Education

☺□ **Northern AIDS Network**
♿ P. O. Box 400, Rhinelander, Wisconsin 54501.
☎ 800 374 7678 (715 area only)
☎ 715 369 6228

Organizations: Sexuality

⌕▽ **Northern Wisconsin Lambda Society**
P. O. Box 802, Rhinelander, Wisconsin 54501.
☎ 715 362 4242

River Falls

Organizations: Sexuality: Student

⌕▽ **Gay Lesbian Bisexual Student Support**
219 East Hathorn Hall, University of Wisconsin, River Falls, Wisconsin 54022.
☎ 715 425 3530

Sheboygan

Organizations: Family

☺□ **Parents & Friends of Lesbians & Gays (PFLAG)— Lakeshore**
831 Union Avenue, Sheboygan, Wisconsin 53081-6051.
☎ 414 458 2506
☎ 414 467 0422

Stevens Point

Organizations: Sexuality: Student

⌕▽ **10% Society**
♿ Box 68, Campus Activities Office, University of Wisconsin, Stevens Point, Wisconsin 54481.
☎ 715 346 4366

Stores: Erotica: BDSM

☺■ **Eyecrusher Leather**
3304 Feltz Avenue, Stevens Point, Wisconsin 54481.
⏲ Mon - Fri 10:00 - 18:00
♣✓ $ ⚡
Wholesale. Catalogue, $15, refundable with purchase of $20 or more. Age statement of 21 is required.

Superior

Organizations: AIDS: Education

☺□ **Northern AIDS Network**
1409 Hammond Avenue, Superior, Wisconsin 54880.
☎ 800 374 7698 (715 area only)
☎ 715 394 0456

Organizations: Bears

⌕▽ **The Backwoods Bears**
P. O. Box 264, Superior, Wisconsin 54880.
✉ rstbear@primenet.com
🖥 http://www.primenet.com/~rstbear/bwbears.html

Waukesha

Stores: Erotica: General

☺■ **Holz Variety / Magazine Rack**
910 East Moreland, Waukesha, Wisconsin 53186.
☎ 414 547 9056

Wausau

Organizations: AIDS: Education

☺□ **Central Wisconsin AIDS Support Group**

P. O. Box 2071, Wausau, Wisconsin 54402.

West Allis

Stores: Erotica: General

☺■ **Naughty But Nice**
2727 South 109th. Street, West Allis, Wisconsin 53227.
☎ 414 541 7788
⏲ Mon - Sat 08:00 - 24:00, Sun 10:00 - 23:00
Also sells BDSM items.

Whitewater

Organizations: Sexuality: Student

⌕▽ **Gay Lesbian Bisexual Union**
♿ 309 McCutchen Hall, University of Wisconsin, Whitewater, Wisconsin 53190.
☎ 414 472 5738

WYOMING

Area: Approximately 252,000 square kilometres
Population: Approximately 456,000
Capital City: Cheyenne
Time zone: GMT minus 7 hours (Mountain Time)
Age of consent & homosexuality legislation: State has adopted the Model Penal Code or otherwise decriminalized homosexual activities.
Legal drinking age: 21

Casper

Organizations: Family

⌕▽ **Parents & Friends of Lesbians & Gays (PFLAG)— Casper**
♿ P. O. Box 9882, Casper, Wyoming 82609.

Organizations: Sexuality

⌕▽ **Central Wyoming Transgender Support Group**
4820 South Ash, Casper, Wyoming 82601.
☎ 307 473 2429
⏲ Meets Fri

Jackson

Organizations: Sexuality

⌕▽ **Jackson GALA**
P. O. Box 7424, Jackson, Wyoming 83001.
☎ 307 733 5349

Laramie

Organizations: Sexuality

⌕▽ **Lesbian Gay Bi Association**
P. O. Box 3625, University of Wyoming, Laramie, Wyoming 82071.
Please address envelopes to LGBA, do NOT address them to Lesbian Gay Bi Association.

Publishers: Magazines: Sexuality

⌕ **Men Into Underwear**
MJ Enterprises, P. O. Box 815, Laramie, Wyoming 82070-0815.
☎ 307 721 2027 ✆ 307 721 2027
Published every two months. Yearly subscription is $25. Age statement of 18 is required. Please address envelopes to Unique T's, do NOT address them to MJ Enterprises or Men Into Underwear.

Wales

Area: Approximately 244,490 square kilometres for whole of U.K.
Population: Approximately 57,650,000 for whole of U.K.
Capital City: London
Currency: Pound Sterling (£)
Official Language: English
Major Religions: 57% Protestant, 13% Roman Catholic
National Holiday: Queen's Birthday, early June
Time zone: GMT
Country Initials: GB
Electricity: 240 volts, 50Hz
Country Dialing Code (from elsewhere): 44
Intl. Dialing Prefix (out of the country): 0101
Long Distance Dialing Prefix (inside country): 0
Climate: Warm, dry summers, cool, wet winters.
Age of consent & homosexuality legislation: Age of consent for sexual activity is 16, but 18 for homosexual activities. Homosexual acts were decriminalized in 1967. In 1992, Homosexual acts are not permitted for the members of the military.
Legal drinking age: 18

NATIONAL RESOURCES

Mailorder: Erotica: BDSM

☺ **Simply Leather**
Corris Craft Centre, Machynlleth, Powys.
Custom heavy leather. Please mark envelopes to the attention of FRAN.

CLWYD

Wrexham

Helplines: Sexuality

⚥▽ **Wrexham Switchboard**
☎ 1248 351115
🕐 Fri 19:00 - 21:00

DYFED

Aberystwyth

Helplines: Sexuality

☺▽ **Aberystwyth Lesbian, Gay, & Bisexual Switchboard**
☎ 197 061 5076
🕐 Tue 18:00 - 20:00
Advice & information about HIV/AIDS & other sexual health & sexuality issues.

Publishers: Books: Sexuality

⚥▼ *Queer Words*
P. O. Box 23, Aberystwyth, Dyfed SY23 1AA.
☎ 1970 626503
Magazine of new lesbian & gay writing.

Carmarthen

Helplines: AIDS

☺☐ **Carmarthen AIDS Helpline**
☎ 1267 221079
🕐 Thu 18:30 - 20:30
Advice & information about HIV/AIDS & other sexual health issues.

GLAMORGAN

Cardiff

Counsellors

☺ **New Beginnings**
P. O. Box 191, Earlswood, Saint Fagans, Glamorgan CF5 4YR.

Helplines: AIDS

☺ **AIDS Helpline**
P.O. Box 304, Cardiff, Glamorgan CF1 9UD.
☎ 144 322 3443
☺☐ **Cardiff AIDS Helpline**
☎ 122 222 3443
🕐 Mon -Fri 19:00 - 22:00
Advice & information about HIV/AIDS & other sexual health issues.
☺ **Mid-Glamorgan AIDS Helpline**
P.O. Box 24, Cardiff, Glamorgan CF37 1YF.
☎ 1443 486254

Helplines: Sexuality

⚥☐ **Cardiff Friend**
☎ 1222 340101
⚥☐ **Cardiff Switchboard**
☎ 1222 374051
🕐 Thu 20:00 - 22:00

Organizations: Sexuality

⚲▽ **South Wales TV/TS Group**
56a Kinross Court, Ridgeway Road, Llan-Romney, Glamorgan VF3 9AE.

Organizations: Swingers

☺ **The Forum Society**
P. O. Box 418, Cardiff, Glamorgan CF2 4XU.
An association of approximately 50 swing clubs. Publishes a newsletter.

Swansea

Organizations: AIDS: Education

☺☐ **West Glamorgan AIDS Project**
☎ 1792 456303
🕐 Mon - Fri 10:00 - 16:00
Advice & information about HIV/AIDS & other sexual health issues.

Organizations: AIDS: Support

☺☐ **South Wales Immune Deficiency Self Help (SWISH)**
☎ 1792 722007
🕐 Wed 14:00 - 17:00
Advice & information about HIV/AIDS & other sexual health issues.

GWENT

Newport

Helplines: AIDS

☺☐ **Gwent AIDS Advice Line**
☎ 1633 422532
🕐 Mon - Fri 09:30 - 16:30
Advice & information about HIV/AIDS & other sexual health issues.

Organizations: AIDS: Support

☺☐ **Gwent AIDS Support Group**
☎ 1633 223456
🕐 Mon Wed 19:30 - 22:00
Advice & information about HIV/AIDS & other sexual health issues.

Trellech

Counsellors

⚥ **Triangle Services**
Sequola House, Trellech, Gwent NP5 4PH.
☎ 1600 860122 ✆ 1600 860122

GWYNEDD

Bangor

Helplines: Sexuality

☺▽ **Gwynedd Gay Line**
☎ 124 835 1263
🕐 Fri 19:00 - 21:00
Advice & information about HIV/AIDS & other sexual health & sexuality issues.

POWYS

Llandrindod Wells

Organizations: AIDS: Support

☺☐ **Powys AIDS Line Services (PALS)**
P.O. Box 24, Llandrindod Wells, Powys LD1 1ZZ.
☎ 1597 824200
🕐 Wed Sat 20:00 - 22:30

Welshpool

Manufacturers: Furniture: BDSM

☺ **Fesseln Fashions**
P. O. Box 27, Welshpool, Powys SY21 0ZZ.
Custom made bondage & dungeon equipment.

Publishers: Magazines: BDSM

☺■ *Fantasy of Gord*
H. G. Publications, P. O. Box 27, Welshpool, Powys SY21 0ZZ.
A bondage fantasy magazine with photos & drawings.

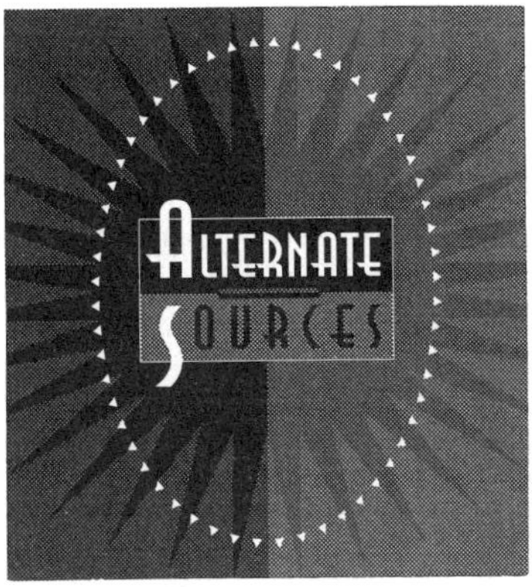

Abrasion – A term applied to any form of play that consists mainly of rubbing, stroking, pinching, or gently pricking the skin. Often referred to as an "abrasion scene."

Accessories – Items that can be used during sexual or other adult play. Can be used to refer to lubricants as well as items like handcuffs and tit-clamps.

Adult – For the purposes of this book, adult means a person of at least the age of legal majority according to the laws of the country in which he/she finds him/herself

After Hours – Operates without alcohol service after legal alcohol serving hours end.

Age Play – Play that involves taking on the rôle of someone of a different age from one's own.

AIDS – Acquired Immunodeficiency Syndrome. A common abbreviation for AIDS in most romantic languages is SIDA

Algolagnia – The dictionary definition of this is "the derivation of sexual pleasure from the giving or receipt of pain." Note that this is not necessarily BDSM, because BDSM does not necessarily include pain. It is a form of BDSM in its broadest sense.

Alternate – Within the context of this book, the term is used to indicate any major sexual orientation that is different from that of the majority, for example: homosexuality, BDSM sexuality, transsexuality, or transvestitism.

BDSM (S&M, S/M, SM) – Sado-masochism. In the context of this directory, the term is used to denote consensual adult BDSM play, not mental illness. (For a complete definition and differentiation between healthy BDSM and mental disorder, see the *Diagnostic and Statistical Manual of Mental Disorders (DSM), Revision IV (1994)* of the American Psychiatric Asscociation. You will need to look up *both* the definition of a mental disorder *and* the definition of Sexual Sadism and Sexual Masochism.) Also an abbreviation of the names Bondage and Discipline, Dominance and Submission, and Sado-masochism. This abbreviation is rapidly becoming an all-encompassing description of these communities, since it is short and sufficiently removed from "S&M" that the non-BDSM community is less likely to take a negative, prejudicial view upon hearing it.

Bondage – Catch-all phrase for restraining someone during play. Restraints could range from closing one's eyes to handcuffs to leather suits to rope to metal restraints, etc..

Bottom – The Bottom is generally the person to whom things are done during play, i.e. the person more likely to be referred to as being controlled in one manner or another. The Bottom may be able to do little but receive the ministrations of the Top.

Brown Shower – Erotic play that involves one person defecating on another. Due to the high risk of disease transmission, this practice is considered unsafe.

Bulletin Boards – Short for Computer Bulletin Boards (BBS). They are electronic means of posting mail, having conversations, advertising, etc. by computer. There are many BDSM-related boards in North America and Europe. They are often listed in the BDSM publications.

Butt Plug – A device about the size of an erect penis, designed to be inserted into the anus. Normally, these are designed with a large flange to prevent the plug from entering completely into the rectum. Used for erotic physical stimulation and as a form of mind-play. A butt plug can be left in a suitably prepared rectum for extended periods of time, e.g. during a day at the office.

Caning – Using a cane or thin rod as the main stimulus during a scene. Often during a corporal punishment scene.

Cat – Whip with many braided tails. Short for cat-o-nine tails.

Club – Club can have two meanings within the context of the BDSM/fetish and other alternate sexuality world: it can be an organization designed for players, or a bar/nightclub for them.

Cock & Ball Torture – The erotic use of pain of the male genitalia. Methods include squeezing, pinching, pulling, electricity, mild flagellation, etc..

Coming out into BDSM – The process a person goes through as he/she admits, explores, and accepts his/her BDSM sexuality.

Condom – A latex sheath used on the erect penis for the prevention of disease transmission. Available at most pharmacies. Note that lambskin condoms do not prevent the transmission of viruses such as HIV.

Consent – One of the three most important aspects of proper BDSM play. All players fully understand the potential risks of their intended play and have consented to the activities. This consent can be withdrawn or modified by any player at any time.

Counsellor – A sex or relationship therapist. May have professional psychiatry or psychology training.

Cross Dressing – As opposed to transvestitism (the use of clothes to be like the opposite sex), cross dressing is when someone gets pleasure from wearing the clothes only, not from wanting to be like the opposite sex.

Cruise – (Verb.) To seek out adult play. In particular the action of making one's intentions known to potential partners.

Cutting – A term used to describe a form a play in which one person cuts the skin of the other. It appears to be somewhat more common among women.

Depilatory – The removal of hair from the body. Usually used in reference to cold wax removal of hair.

Discipline – Play involving one person training another to obey and act in a manner that the first player wants. Also refers to the punishment given by the Top for a transgression by the Bottom.

Dominant – A person who takes the rôle of dominating another during play. It is one of many rôles one can take during a scene. The term may be somewhat more prevalent in the heterosexual community. A professional dominant will charge money for performing the rôle; reputable ones will not have sex with their clients, although they may do anything but that.

Dominatrix – A female dominant.

Fantasy – Any imagined BDSM or other event that brings pleasure to the person who thought of it.

Feminist – An advocate of women's rights and the equality of the sexes.

Fetishism – The use of objects as one of the preferred methods of producing sexual excitement.

Fisting – Inserting a hand carefully into the anus or vagina.

Flagellation – The use of a device to strike another person, often with whips, paddles, canes, rods, etc..

Flogger – This is a fairly recent term for a hitting implement that has a short handle and many, flat tails. It is usually made of leather. The effect of a flogger is due to the weight of the many strands as they land, and the texture of the material used to make it.

Gender Play – Play in which one or more of the players takes on a rôle normally associated with the opposite sex.

Golden Shower – Urinating on another person during play.

Helpline – A phone service provided (often by volunteers) to give information or counselling to anyone who requests it. Most often these are to help those concerned with their sexual identity, or families of those with alternate sexualities.

Humiliation – Fantasy play where one partner makes the other feel shame and/or embarrassment, such as making the other wet his/her pants in public.

In Rôle – The assumption of a rôle during play, often while in public, such as in a bar. While in rôle, a Top or Bottom may temporarily appear modify responses to other people.

J/O – Masturbation (also JO).

Key Word – Another word for *safeword.* Not as common as the latter.

Latex – The soft, unvulcanized sap of trees used to make condoms, dental dams, and surgical gloves.

Leather – A material often used for the manufacture of adult toys and clothing.

Lesbian – A woman who is sexually attracted to another woman.

Lingerie – Women's undergarments, usually skimpy when used in a sexual context.

Lube – Sexual lubricant.

Mail Order – Purchasing goods by mail.

Masochism – The act of enjoying, sexually or otherwise, being humiliated, beaten, bound, or otherwise made to suffer.

Master – A male dominant.

Mind Fuck – Playing a trick on someone within the context of BDSM play. (Maybe having someone believe one thing and then making another happen or putting a person in an embarrassing situation as part of a scene.)

Mistress – A female dominant.

Negotiation – The discussion and agreement, before a scene, about what the players would like to do and the limits of what they permit during the scene. Negotiation should also include discussion of any relevant medical or other physical condition that may affect play.

Network – A series of links between friends and associates.

New Guard – The "new breed" of BDSM player, armed with knowledge of safe, sane, and consensual play. Far more likely to switch from Top to Bottom (and back) than players would have been two decades ago. Also, more likely to involve spirituality in their BDSM play.

Nipple Torture – Another term for nipple play. (Also: tit torture.)

Novelties – A euphemism for adult toys and other sexual aids, such as leather clothing, whips, and vibrators.

Novice – Someone learning about BDSM play.

Old Guard – A term used to describe the way BDSM players used to define themselves. People would be Tops or Bottoms, but rarely changed or were seen to enjoy both.

Organization – A number of people brought together as a society, commercial enterprise, or charitable body.

Paddling – Play involving striking the other player with a rigid item, such as a paddle or hairbrush, usually on the buttocks.

Pain – The sensation when a stimulus is very strong and the person being stimulated would rather not be experiencing it. Hurt does *not* necessarily involve injury. (See also Injury.)

Panic Snap – A simple device used instead of a hook or eye to attach chain or rope to an anchor point or another chain or rope. It's great advantage is that it can be released without having to pull harder on the attachment. When used for suspension, it means that the suspended person does not have to be lifted further to be released. It can save time and lives. It should be used for all suspension play on each major weight bearing attachment.

Percussion Play – Any form of play involving one player striking the other, either with the hand (or other part of the body) or with an implement such as a paddle or whip. Spanking and flogging are examples of percussion play.

Phone Lines – Services, normally provided for a fee, for placing or responding to voice advertisements using a phone. Also, services to connect two or more people for the purposes of simple conversation or for sexual talk. (See also Helplines, above.)

Physical Limits – The limitations of a person's body with respect to a scene. Some people have physical conditions (such as not being able to stand in one place for too long) that stop them from enduring the physical strain put upon them during a scene.

Play – Any activity between consenting adults that produces mental, physical, and/or sexual pleasure, as in "I played with her last night."

Playroom – A place where BDSM activities can be carried out. It will often be outfitted specifically for BDSM play. Also known as a "dungeon." The term playroom is preferred, since not all BDSM play requires a dungeon atmosphere as its setting.

Pleasure/Pain – The mix of pleasurable and painful sensations, or the point at which they meet, which produce an effect where one is indistinguishable from the other. Consequently, to have more pleasure, more of what used to be painful is desired.

Predilections – Whatever turns you on.

Professional Dominant – A person who provides BDSM domination for a fee. They will not provide sexual services; the customer will have to masturbate, if required. People who provide sexual services with BDSM activities are prostitutes who also provide BDSM services.

Pushy Bottom – A term for a Bottom who deliberately, often humorously, tries to provoke his/her Top into action or further action. A term for an aggressive, dominant masochist.

Raunch – Any play that involves bodily secretions and odours as sexual turn-ons.

Reality – Cold hard fact that determines the extend to which your fantasies can be attempted safely during a BDSM scene.

Rimming – Analingus; licking of the anus.

Rubber – Vulcanized sap of trees; also a colloquialism for a condom.

Sadism – The act of enjoying, sexually or otherwise, causing someone to be humiliated, beaten, bound, or otherwise made to suffer.

Sadomasochism – A term coined be Richard von Krafft-Ebing to described both the activities of sadism and masochism.

Safe – All players have taken the necessary precautions to prevent psychological and physical damage to themselves, including the transmission of disease.

Safe, Sane, and Consensual – The reason for writing this book. If your play does not meet *all* of these criteria, you are not playing properly. This phrase has become the measure by which BDSM players judge themselves, their play, and other players. (Please see the Introduction for further information.)

Safeword – A word, preferably not the name of your partner, used to stop a BDSM scene *immediately*. Where a Bottom cannot speak, a motion of a part of the body may be substituted for the safeword. The word *safeword* is an excellent safeword.

Sane – All players are in full possession of their mental faculties and are fully aware of the risks involved in the play they intend.

Scat – Any play that involves fæces. Butyric acid can be used to simulate the smell of fæces, thereby making scat scenes safer.

Scene – A scene is any interaction between two players, be it a fleeting glance across a bar or a full weekend in the playroom.

Session – Another term for *scene*.

Slave – A rôle that may be taken up for a short scene or a prolonged relationship, where the submissive partner submits to one or more others.

S&M, S/M, SM – See BDSM.

SModdler & SMoldster – Humorous terms for *BDSM toddler* (novice) and *BDSM oldster* (experienced), respectively.

Spanking – Hitting the buttocks with a hand. When a flat, rigid implement is used, the term paddling is more appropriate.

Straight – A term used to describe heterosexual people or those who do not enjoy BDSM play, c.f. "kinky." It is used to distinguish them from homosexual or bisexual people; it is never used in this book as a pejorative term.

Submissive – A player who takes the rôle of submitting to another person. It is one of the possible rôles for a Bottom.

Support Groups – Usually, local meetings organized and chaired by volunteers as a means of providing emotional support to those having problems with their sexuality.

Suspension – Any activity in which the Bottom is suspended, upright, upside-down, or otherwise.

Switch – A person who enjoys being both the Top and the Bottom (generally at different times). Recently, switches have become more evident in the BDSM community.

Switchboard – Another term for Helpline (see above).

Tit Torture – Play primarily involving stimulation of the nipples with clamps, toothbrushes, teeth, etc..

Top – A player who takes the more controlling, perhaps dominant, rôle during play.

Torture – The use of erotic pain (without injury) during a scene. Most likely not by whipping.

Toy – Any object used during play. Most often thought of as those that can be bought in a sex store, but spatulas, toothbrushes, rubber gloves, feathers, etc., etc. can also take be used as toys. In the context of this directory, any item that is used in or to enhance adult play.

Transgender – A person who wishes to be or feels that he or she is not of the gender that his or her body would indicate. This person has yet to complete the sex change.

Transsexual – A person who has completed a sex change.

Transvestite – A person who enjoys wearing the clothes of and appearing as the opposite sex. (c.f. Cross dressing: to enjoy wearing the clothes of the opposite sex, but the clothes are not worn to allow the wearer to pass for the opposite sex.)

Vanilla – A term used to refer to non-BDSM play or players. It is never used in this book as a pejorative term.

Watersports – Any play that involves urine. Also used to refer to play involving enemas.

Whipping – Using flexible instruments, such as cat-o-nine tails and floggers, to produce erotic pain during a scene.

Workshops – Meetings for people to learn about alternate sexualities and try out aspects of them in a safe environment with knowledgeable practitioners.

Wrapping – A term that refers to the unintended wrapping of the end of a whip around the body of the Bottom and land on the side or front of the body. Often leaves marks on the Bottom. In bondage play, can refer to using strips of material (bandage, rubber, etc.) to wrap the body of the Bottom, sometimes in the style of an Egyptian mummy.

#28 Barbury Lane
Seattle 📖 351
#AIDS/HIV 📖 6
#analsex 📖 6
#anne-rice 📖 6
#bdsm 📖 6
#bdsmlounge 📖 6
#bearcave 📖 6
#bearlake 📖 6
#bearlake2 📖 6
#BiFEM!!!! 📖 6
#bifemteens 📖 6
#bisex 📖 6
#bondage 📖 6
#breasts 📖 6
#crossdres 📖 6
#d&s 📖 6
#desade 📖 6
#Dom/Sub 📖 6
#erotic 📖 6
#erotica 📖 7
#eroticsex 📖 7
#exhibitionists 📖 7
#familysex 📖 7
#femdom 📖 7
#femuscle 📖 7
#FistFuck 📖 7
#fuck 📖 7
#Gay 📖 7
#gayboysex 📖 7
#gaycouples 📖 7
#gayhelp 📖 7
#gayjackoff 📖 7
#gaynz 📖 7
#gaynz1 📖 7
#gaynzgirls 📖 7
#gaysex 📖 7
#gaySM 📖 7
#gayteenchat 📖 7
#gaytexas 📖 7
#gayuncut 📖 7
#GayWI 📖 7
#gayworld 📖 7
#gayyouth 📖 7
#goddess 📖 7
#HighHeels 📖 7
#intergen 📖 7
#jack-off 📖 7
#Jacks 📖 7
#jerk-off 📖 7
#kinkysex 📖 7
#LeChambre 📖 7
#lesbian 📖 7
#lesbians 📖 7
#lesbos 📖 7
#lezsex 📖 7
#lezsex2 📖 7
#pagan 📖 7
#pantyhose 📖 7
#peesex 📖 7
#pervert 📖 7
#polyamory 📖 7
#pornshop 📖 7
#sex 📖 7
#sex&stuff 📖 7
#spanking 📖 7
#submission 📖 7
#Swing 📖 7
#teensex 📖 7
#transgen 📖 7
#vampire 📖 7
#vampires 📖 7
#voyeurs 📖 7
#Weirdsex 📖 7
#wetstuff 📖 7
#wildsex 📖 7
#youngsex 📖 7
10 Percent
published by Browning Grace Communications 📖 217
10% Group
Minneapolis / Saint Paul, 612 363 2734 📖 280
10% Society
Fox Valley 📖 356
Madison, 608 262 7365 📖 356
Moorhead, 218 236 2227 📖 281
Stevens Point, 715 346 4366 📖 358
10% Society at NMU
Marquette 📖 277
1008 kHz
Canberra 📖 25
100th. Monkey Books
Toronto, 416 925 7633 📖 59
15 Association
San Francisco, 415 673 0452 📖 214
1st. Old Store
Provincetown, 508 487 1010 📖 272
20-20 News
Annapolis, 410 266 0514 📖 263
2NCR-FM 92.9
Lismore, 66 20 3929 📖 25
2SER FM 107.3
Sydney, 2 330 3000 (during program) 📖 27
321 News & Video
Gastonia, 704 866 0075 📖 315
3CR Community Radio, AM 855 kHz
Melbourne, 39 419 8377 📖 31
3D Radio 93.7 FM
Adelaide 📖 30
Adelaide, 8 410 0937 📖 30
3G 📖 *See* Grampian Gender Group
41 South MC
Wellington 📖 163
45th. Street Clinic
Seattle, 206 633 3350 📖 351
4ACURE-L 📖 2
4CCCC - FM 89.1
Cairns, 7 053 5866 📖 29
4TTT FM 103.9
Townsville, 7 721 1384 📖 29
519 Church Street Community Centre
Toronto, 416 392 6874 📖 57
593 Group
Atlanta, 404 853 5109 📖 245
609 Novelty
Barrie, 705 722 3244 📖 49
6RTR FM 92.1
Perth 📖 34
8-Ball Tattoo
Columbus, 614 784 8850 📖 321
93 S/M Designs
Derby 📖 22
95 BFM
Auckland, 9 366 7223 📖 161
95th. Street News
Cleveland, 216 631 4010 📖 319
99th. Floor
Chicago, 312 348 7781 📖 252
A. A. Michael Books
Evansville, 812 479 8979 📖 254
A. A. Surplus Sales, Inc.
Los Angeles, 213 680 1610 📖 206
A. D. Thompson & Co., Publishers
Santa Barbara 📖 221
A. E. L.
Albuquerque, 505 345 6484 📖 294
A. M. Publications
Portland, 503 228 6935 📖 326
A. P. M. C.
Paris 📖 20
A.S.B. Munch
Applemunch 📖 303
Atlanta 📖 244
Boston 📖 268
Chicago 📖 249
Corvallis 📖 325
Detroit 📖 275
Florida 📖 240
Huntsville 📖 191
Indianapolis 📖 255
Louisville 📖 259
Minnesota 📖 280
Palo Alto 📖 209
Philadelphia 📖 330
San Francisco Bay 📖 214
Vancouver 📖 45
Virginia 📖 347
Washington, D. C. 📖 234
AA Surplus Sales
Los Angeles, 213 526 3622 📖 206
AAA Police Supply
Boston, 617 326 8845 📖 270
AAAA 📖 *See* Alaskan AIDS Assistance Association
Aardvaark Helpline
Salt Lake City, 801 533 0927 📖 345
AASECT 📖 *See* American Association of Sex Educators, Counsellors, & Therapists
Abaton Books
Colorado Springs 📖 227
Abbey Books
Derby 📖 73
Abbott Northwestern Hospital
Minneapolis / Saint Paul, 612 863 4000 📖 279
ABC 📖 *See* Association Beaumont Continental
ABC Buchladen
Kassel, 561 77 7704 📖 123
abc Leipzig e. V.
341 719 3565 📖 125
Abco Research Associates
Monticello, 217 762 2141 📖 252
Abelman Trading Company
Hong Kong 📖 136
Aberdeen Bookshop
Dunedin 📖 162
Aberdeen HIV/AIDS Gay Support Group 📖 168
Aberdeen Lesbian, Gay, & Bisexual Switchboard
122 458 6869 📖 168
Aberdeen LesBiGay Society 📖 168
Aberystwyth Lesbian, Gay, & Bisexual Switchboard
197 061 5076 📖 359
Abigail Louise
Bristol, 117 976 0969 📖 70
ABOP Homogroep
Hendrik Ido Ambacht 📖 156
Abra Creations & Designs
Southminster 📖 68
Abrams, Steve
Chicago, 312 868 1542 📖 250
ABS 📖 *See* Nottingham AIDS Bereavement Support
Absolute Leather
Orlando, 800 447 4820 📖 241
Abundant Love Institute
Hawaii (Big Island), 808 929 9691 📖 246
Abus de Confiance
broadcast by FM 88.7 📖 99
Abusive Furniture
London 📖 81
Abva
Groningen, 50 314 1701 📖 155
ABW 📖 *See* Adult Baby World
Academic Bookbinding
Minneapolis / Saint Paul, 612 331 6381 📖 280
Academisch Ziekenhuis
Groningen, 50 361 2867 📖 155
Academisch Ziekhuis
Utrecht, 30 237 2833 📖 158
Academy
Glendale 📖 200
Academy Club
Hereford, 143 234 3241 📖 9
ACAP 📖 *See* AIDS Community Awareness Project
ACAS 📖 *See* Auckland Community AIDS Services
ACASIA 📖 *See* AIDS Care & Support In Action
Accent In Ink
Castle Shannon, 412 563 8281 📖 328
Accent Tattoo
Gloucester Point, 804 642 3993 📖 348
Access Community Radio AM 810
Auckland 📖 161
Auckland, 9 302 0238 (studio) 📖 161
Auckland, 9 525 8261 📖 161
Acceuil Rencontre Information Service (ARIS)
Lyon, 78 27 1010 📖 100, 101
ACCM 📖 *See* AIDS Community Care Montréal
Ace
Providence 📖 334
Ace Publishing, Inc,
Phœnix, 602 266 0550 📖 194
ACE Saddle Company
Woodinville 📖 182
ACESGLBI 📖 2
Aché 📖 196
ACME Leather & Toy Co.
Cincinnati, 513 621 7390 📖 318
Acme Surplus
Oakland, 415 444 9694 📖 208
Acme Toy Co.
Chicago, 312 536 1982 📖 186
Acolyte Press
Amsterdam 📖 150
ACORN 📖 *See* AIDS Community Resource Network
ACQC 📖 *See* AIDS Center of Queens County
ACRA 📖 *See* Australian Club Run Association
ACS
Bristol 📖 70
ACT-B 📖 *See* AIDS Committee of Thunder Bay
Act-HIV
Zürich, 1 291 3720 📖 179
Action Against AIDS
North Devon, 127 124 555 📖 73
Action Books & Video
Berkeley Springs, 304 258 2529 📖 354
Action Surplus
Eugene, 503 746 1301 📖 325
ActionAIDS, Inc.
Philadelphia, 215 981 0088 (also TTY) 📖 330
Actions Prévention SIDA & Aide aux Malades (APSAM - GPL)
Paris 📖 103
ACT-UP 📖 3
ACT-UP AIDS-L 📖 2
Ad Hoc
London, 171 938 1664 📖 86
Adam
Berlin, 30 292 3089 📖 109, 111
Adam & Eve
Canberra, 6 239 1121 📖 25
Carrboro, 800 274 0333 📖 187
Philadelphia, 215 925 5041 📖 331
Adam Society
Wayland 📖 273
Adam's Sensual Whips - Gillian's Toys
New York, 516 842 1711 📖 187
Adams Press
Chicago, 708 676 3426 📖 250
Adams, Roger
Brighton 📖 68
Added Dimensions Publications
Palm Springs, 619 770 9647 📖 208
ADDICT-L 📖 3
Addington Hospital
Durban, 31 35 0235 📖 171
Adelaide Bisexual Collective
8 352 5715 📖 30
Adelaide Gay Times
8 232 1544 📖 30
Adelaide GT
published by Adelaide Gay Times 📖 30
ADF Editorial Services
Lumphanan 📖 168
Adirondack GALA
Saranac Lake 📖 311
Adler & Schmitt Lederwerkstatt
Güdingen 📖 119
Adonis Atlantic Presse Editions
Nantes 📖 97
Adonis Center
Dortmund, 231 57 3619 📖 114
Adult Baby World (ABW)
Toronto 📖 40
Adult Books & Cinema
Fargo, 701 232 9768 📖 317
Adult Bookstore
Billings, 406 245 4293 📖 285
Edison, 908 985 9619 📖 290
Lewiston, 207 784 5961 📖 262
Adult Education Books
Albany 📖 296
Adult Entertainment Center
New York, 212 947 1590 📖 309
Adult Entrée
Wichita, 316 832 1816 📖 258
Adult Pursuits
Sarasota, 813 366 3501 📖 242
Sarasota, 813 923 2815 📖 242
Adult Scene Supplies
Bradford, 127 472 4726 📖 94
Adult Shop

Caldwell, 208 454 2422 🕮 247
New York, 516 472 9519 🕮 309
Adult World
Egg Harbor City, 609 965 1110 🕮 290
Philadelphia, 215 972 9031 🕮 331
Utica 🕮 312
Adults Etc., Etc.
Merkel, 915 928 3894 🕮 344
Advance Uniform Co.
Chicago, 312 922 1797 🕮 251
Adventure 1
Glasgow, 141 353 3788 🕮 170
Adventurers - Sun Coast
Saint Petersburg 🕮 241
Advocate
published by Liberation Publications Inc. 🕮 205
Advocate Men 🕮 205
AE Services
Sandbach 🕮 72
AEGIS 🕮 See American Educational Gender Information Services, Inc.
AFAN 🕮 See Aid for AIDS
AFAO 🕮 See Australian Foundation of AIDS Organizations
Affected by AIDS Support Group
Pittsfield, 413 443 7905 🕮 266
Affirmations
Columbus, 614 445 8277 🕮 319
Detroit, 313 398 4297 🕮 275
Affirmations Lesbian & Gay Community Center
Detroit, 313 398 4297 🕮 275
Affliated Big Men's Clubs
San Francisco 🕮 214
After Dark
Calgary, 403 264 7399 🕮 43
After Dark Adult Warehouse
Calgary, 403 264 7399 🕮 43
After Hours
broadcast by KPFT FM 90.1 🕮 343
After Stonewall
Ottawa, 613 567 2221 🕮 53
After Surgery Support Exchange for Transexuals (ASSET)
Greenfield 🕮 270
Afterglow FX
Central Point, 503 664 9171 🕮 324
AfterWords
Milwaukee, 414 963 9089 🕮 357
AG Leder
Hannover, 511 33 3636 🕮 121
AGALA 🕮 See Auburn Gay & Lesbian Association
AGAPE
Dallas / Fort Worth, 214 424 1234 🕮 340
AGE 🕮 See Atlanta Gender Exploration
AGEDO 🕮 See Assoziazione Genitori di Omosessuali
Agent Provocateur
London, 171 439 0229 🕮 23
AGG
Aberdeen, 122 431 7552 🕮 168
Aggressive Women Magazine
published by Swish Publications Ltd. 🕮 84
Agnes Scott Lesbian & Bisexual Alliance
Atlanta, 404 373 1632 🕮 244
AGO 🕮 See Alternative Gender-Oriented
Agora
Haarlem, 23 531 3182 🕮 155
Agora Bokhandel AB
Stockholm 🕮 176
AGT 🕮 See Associazione Gay Ticino
AHA 🕮 See Allgemeine Homosexuelle Arbeitsgemeinschaft e. V.
AHF-Switchboard (CIC)
Frankfurt am Main 🕮 117
AHO 🕮 See Aktionsgruppe Homosexualität Osnabrück e. V.
AID Atlanta
404 0600 🕮 244
Aid for AIDS
Los Angeles, 213 656 1107 🕮 203
Aid for AIDS (AFAN)
Nevada, 702 474 2437 (hotline) 🕮 286
Aid for AIDS, Inc.
Woodstock, 703 459 8208 🕮 350
AID Upstate
Greenville, 803 233 8842 🕮 335
Aide Fribourgeoise Contre le SIDA / AIDS-Hilfe
Fribourg, 37 21 9678 🕮 178
Aide Info SIDA
Bruxelles / Brussel, 2 511 4529 🕮 37
AIDES Alsace
Mulhouse, 89 60 0077 🕮 101
Strasbourg, 88 75 7363 🕮 106
AIDES Anjou
Angers, 41 87 1144 🕮 98
AIDES Aquitaine
Bordeaux, 56 52 7761 🕮 98
AIDES Armor
Brest, 98 43 1872 🕮 99
AIDES Atlantique
Nantes, 40 47 9956 🕮 102
AIDES Auvergne
Clermont-Ferrand, 73 31 3103 🕮 99
AIDES Basse-Normandie
Caen, 31 84 3663 🕮 99
AIDES Bourgogne
Dijon, 80 30 3777 🕮 99
AIDES Bretagne
Rennes, 99 79 0604 🕮 105
AIDES Champagne-Ardennes
Châlons, 26 66 8434 🕮 99
Riems, 26 49 9610 🕮 105
AIDES Côte d'Azur
Nice, 93 56 9338 🕮 102
AIDES Dauphiné-Savoie
Chambéry, 79 85 5034 🕮 99
Grenoble, 76 46 0758 🕮 100
AIDES France-Comté
Besançon, 81 81 8000 🕮 98
AIDES Haute-Normandie
Rouen, 35 69 3232 🕮 105
AIDES Languedoc-Nord
Nîmes, 66 76 2607 🕮 102
AIDES Limousin
Limoges, 55 06 1819 🕮 100
AIDES Loire & Haute-Loire
Saint Etienne, 777 80 7571 🕮 105
AIDES Lorraine-Nord
Metz, 87 36 89 63 🕮 101
AIDES Lorraine-Sud
Nancy, 83 27 9171 🕮 102
AIDES Marseille
93 33 5401 🕮 101
AIDES Monpellier Languedoc Mediterannée
Montpellier, 67 72 6303 🕮 101
AIDES Nord-Pas-de-Calais
Lille, 20 06 5959 🕮 100
AIDES Orléans Region Centre
38 53 3031 🕮 102
AIDES Pairs & Ile de France
Paris, 144 52 0000 🕮 103
AIDES Paris & Ile de France
Minitel 3615 AIDES 🕮 103
AIDES Poiteau-Charentes
Poitiers, 49 42 4545 🕮 105
AIDES Provence
Gap, 92 53 4393 🕮 99
AIDES Toulouse-Midi-Pyrénées
61 25 2571 🕮 106
AIDES—Martinique
Fort-de-France, 63 1236 🕮 149
AIDS 🕮 2
AIDS & Cancer Research Foundation
Beverly Hills, 800 373 4572 🕮 197
AIDS Action
Bridlington, 126 240 0440 🕮 77
AIDS Action Baltimore, Inc.
410 837 2437 🕮 263
AIDS Action Coalition
Huntsville, 205 533 2437 🕮 191
AIDS Action Committee
Boston, 800 235 2331 (in Massachusetts only) 🕮 266
AIDS Action Committee of Perth County
Stratford, 519 272 2437 🕮 54
AIDS Action Council
Washington, 202 293 2886 🕮 233
AIDS Action Council of the Australian Capital Territory
Canberra, 6 257 2855 🕮 25
AIDS Action Group
East London, 431 29357 🕮 171
Johannesburg, 11 642 5191 🕮 171
AIDS Action North Humberside
Hull, 1482 27060 🕮 77
AIDS Action Now!
Toronto, 416 928 2206 🕮 56
AIDS Advice
Leeds, 113 242 3204 🕮 94
AIDS Advisory Office
Stavanger, 51 56 4977 🕮 166
AIDS Alliance
Dublin, 1 733799 🕮 137
Limerick, 61 316661 🕮 138
AIDS Alliance / Cairde
Cork, 21 27 5837 (office) 🕮 137
AIDS Alliance of Greenwich
203 622 6460 🕮 230
AIDS Alliance of Howard County
Columbia, 410 313 2333 🕮 265
AIDS Alliance of Western New York
Buffalo, 716 852 6778 🕮 298
AIDS Allies
Springfield, 413 747 5144 🕮 266
AIDS Arms Network
Dallas / Fort Worth, 214 521 5191 🕮 340
AIDS Benefit Committee of New Jersey
Plainfield, 908 561 4359 🕮 289
AIDS Beratung & Betreuung
Leipzig, 341 29 5021 🕮 125
AIDS Beratung im Gesundheitsamt
Bielefeld, 521 51 3890 🕮 112
AIDS Calgary Awareness Association
800 590 8795 (information) 🕮 42
AIDS Care
Ventura, 805 683 0446 🕮 224
AIDS Care & Support In Action (ACASIA)
Birkenhead, 185 003 2925 🕮 87
AIDS Care Network
Rockford, 815 968 2437 🕮 253
AIDS Center at Hope House
Dover, 201 361 7443 (AIDS Hopeline) 🕮 290
AIDS Center of Queens County (ACQC)
New York, 718 739 2525 🕮 303
New York, 718 896 2500 🕮 303
AIDS Center of Reference
São Paulo, 11 284 4206 🕮 39
AIDS Centre
Brighton, 127 357 1660 🕮 74
Helsinki, 90 66 5081 🕮 96
AIDS Coalition of Cape Breton
Sydney, 902 567 1766 🕮 49
AIDS Coalition of Coastal Texas
Galveston, 409 763 2437 🕮 342
AIDS Coalition of North East Iowa
Waterloo, 319 234 6831 🕮 257
AIDS Coalition of Southern New Jersey
Collingswood, 800 229 2437 🕮 289
AIDS Committe of Grey-Bruce
Owen Sound, 800 331 6831 (within 519 area) 🕮 53
AIDS Committee
Santiago 🕮 64
AIDS Committee of Cambridge-Kitchener / Waterloo
519 570 3687 🕮 50
AIDS Committee of Durham
Whitby, 905 665 0051 🕮 61
AIDS Committee of Etobicoke
Toronto, 416 394 8833 (Hotline) 🕮 56
AIDS Committee of Guelph & Wellington County
519 763 2255 🕮 49
AIDS Committee of London
519 434 8160 (information) 🕮 51
AIDS Committee of North Bay & Area
705 497 3560 🕮 52
AIDS Committee of Ottawa
613 238 5014 🕮 52
AIDS Committee of Simcoe County
Barrie, 705 722 6778 🕮 49
AIDS Committee of Sudbury ACCESS
800 465 2437 (information) 🕮 54
AIDS Committee of Thunder Bay (ACT-B)
807 345 7233 (information) 🕮 54
AIDS Committee of Toronto
416 340 8844 (information) 🕮 56
AIDS Committee of Windsor
519 256 2437 (information) 🕮 61
AIDS Community Awareness Project (ACAP)
Saint Johnsbury, 802 748 1149 🕮 346
AIDS Community Care Montréal (ACCM)
5114 939 0075 (hotline) 🕮 62
AIDS Community Research Consortium
Redwood City, 415 364 6563 🕮 209
AIDS Community Resource Network (ACORN)
Lebanon, 603 448 2220 🕮 287, 346
AIDS Community Services of Western New York
Buffalo, 716 847 2441 🕮 295
AIDS Community Trust
Newcastle upon Tyne, 191 224 4848 🕮 92
AIDS Concern North Yorkshire
Harrogate, 1423 505222 🕮 88
AIDS Council of Central Australia
Alice Springs, 8 953 1118 🕮 28
AIDS Council of New South Wales
Coffs Harbour, 6 651 4056 🕮 25
Lismore, 6 622 1555 🕮 25
Newcastle, 4 929 3464 🕮 25
Sydney, 2 206 2000 🕮 26
Wollongong, 4 276 2399 🕮 27
AIDS Council of Northeastern New York
Albany, 518 434 4686 🕮 296
AIDS Council of South Australia
Adelaide, 8 362 1611 🕮 30
AIDS Council of Tasmania
Hobart, 0 224 1034 🕮 31
AIDS Council of Western Virginia
Roanoke, 800 354 3388 🕮 347
AIDS Directory
published by The Nam Charitable Trust 🕮 84
AIDS Education Project
Chicago, 312 477 4709 🕮 249
AIDS Forum
Berlin, 30 395 7505 🕮 110
AIDS Foundation Miami Valley
Dayton, 513 277 2437 🕮 317
AIDS Foundation of Chicago
312 642 5454 🕮 249
AIDS Foundation of Houston
713 623 6796 🕮 342
AIDS Foundation San Diego
619 686 5000 🕮 211
AIDS Help Line
Kolding, 75 50 5711 🕮 66
AIDS Help West
Galway, 91 252 00 🕮 137
AIDS Helpline
Belfast, 800 137 437 🕮 163
Cambridge, 122 369 765 🕮 71
Cardiff, 144 322 3443 🕮 359
Dublin, 1 724277 🕮 137
Liverpool, 151 709 9000 🕮 87
Newark, 201 877 5525 🕮 292
Norwich, 160 361 5816 🕮 88
AIDS Helpline Cork
21 27 6676 🕮 137
AIDS Hotline
Jackson, 601 371 1318 🕮 282
Parkersburg, 304 485 4803 🕮 355
AIDS Hotline - AIDS Pela Vida
Rio de Janeiro, 21 221 2221 🕮 39
AIDS Info
Århus, 86 13 6513 🕮 65
AIDS Info BBS
San Francisco, 415 626 124 🕮 212
AIDS Info Line
Helsinki, 90 66 5081 🕮 96
AIDS Infoline
Kingston, 800 565 2209 (from Kingston area) 🕮 50
AIDS Information
Dordrecht, 78 613 0284 🕮 154
AIDS Information & Counselling Service
Durban, 31 306 0758 🕮 171
Johannesburg, 11 643 2311 🕮 171
AIDS Information Collective
Amherst, 413 539 4600 🕮 266
AIDS Information Line
Winnipeg, 204 945 2437 🕮 47
AIDS Information Network
Philadelphia, 215 922 5597 🕮 330
AIDS Infostelle Winterthur
52 213 8141 🕮 179
AIDS Initiative Karlsruhe e. V.
721 1 9411 🕮 123
AIDS Law Project of Pennsylvania
Philadelphia, 215 440 8555 🕮 327
AIDS Leadership Foothills Area (ALFA)
Hickory, 704 322 1447 🕮 315

AIDS Library of Philadelphia
215 922 5120 📖 330
AIDS Lifeline
Birmingham, 121 235 3535 📖 93
AIDS Line
Melbourne, 39 347 6099 📖 32
AIDS Line West Midlands
Birmingham, 121 622 1511 📖 92
AIDS National Hotline
Auckland, 800 802 437 📖 159
AIDS Network
Hernando 📖 237
AIDS Network of Edmonton Society
403 488 5816 (information) 📖 43
AIDS New Brunswick
Fredricton, 800 561 4009 (information) 📖 48
AIDS Niagara
Saint Catharines, 905 984 8684 📖 54
AIDS Nova Scotia
Halifax, 902 425 2437 (information) 📖 48
AIDS Outreach Center
Dallas / Fort Worth, 817 335 1994 📖 340
AIDS P. E. I.
Charlottetown, 902 566 2437 📖 61
AIDS Prevention & Sexual Health Program
Toronto, 416 392 2437 📖 55
AIDS Prevention Program
Boulder, 303 441 1160 📖 226
AIDS Prevention Project
Seattle, 206 296 4999 📖 351
AIDS Project
Hawaii (Big Island), 808 969 6626 (hotline) 📖 246
Iowa City, 319 356 6040 📖 257
State College, 800 233 2437 📖 333
AIDS Project (TAP)
Portland, 800 851 2437 📖 261
AIDS Project East Bay
Oakland, 510 834 8181 📖 207
AIDS Project Hartford, Inc.
203 247 2437 📖 231
AIDS Project Hawaii
Oahu, 808 926 2122 📖 246
AIDS Project Los Angeles (APLA)
800 922 2437 (hotline) 📖 203
AIDS Project New Haven
203 624 2437 📖 231
AIDS Project of the Ozarks
Springfield, 417 881 1900 📖 282
AIDS Referral Services (ARS)
Wichita, 316 264 2437 📖 258
AIDS Regina
306 924 8420 📖 64
AIDS Relief
Crewe, 127 062 8938 📖 71
AIDS Resource Alliance, Inc.
Williamsport, 717 322 8448 📖 333
AIDS Resource Center
Dallas / Fort Worth, 214 521 5124 📖 340
Washington, 202 667 0045 📖 234
AIDS Resource Center (ARC)
New York, 212 633 2500 📖 303
AIDS Resource Center of Wisconsin, Inc.
Milwaukee, 800 359 9272 📖 355
AIDS Resource Group of Evansville, Inc.
812 421 0059 📖 254
AIDS Resources of Central Shenendoah
Staunton, 703 886 7116 📖 349
AIDS Response Knoxville (ARK)
615 523 2437 📖 336
AIDS Response of the Seacoast
Portsmouth, 603 433 5377 📖 288
AIDS Response Program
Garden Grove, 714 534 0961 📖 200
AIDS Rochester, Inc.
716 442 2220 📖 310
AIDS Saint John
506 652 2437 📖 48
AIDS Saskatoon
306 667 6876 📖 64
AIDS Service Agency
Chapel Hill, 919 990 1101 📖 313
AIDS Service Agency of Wake County
Raleigh, 919 834 2437 📖 315
AIDS Service Connection
Columbus, 614 291 2300 📖 319
AIDS Services Center
Lehigh Valley, 610 974 8700 📖 329
AIDS Services Center, Inc.
Anniston, 205 835 0923 📖 191
AIDS Services of Austin
512 452 2437 (info. & referral) 📖 338
AIDS Services of Dallas
Dallas / Fort Worth, 214 941 0523 📖 340
AIDS Services of Lower Manhattan
New York, 212 645 0875 📖 303
AIDS Services Project
Durham, 919 268 7475 📖 314
AIDS Shelter Coalition of Manitoba
Winnipeg, 204 775 9173 📖 47
AIDS Speekuur
Den Haag, 70 354 1610 📖 154
AIDS Support Foundation, Inc.
Wichita Falls, 817 691 7539 📖 338
AIDS Support Group
Charlottesville, 804 979 7714 📖 347
AIDS Support Network
Janesville, 608 756 2550 📖 356
Palmerston North 📖 162
AIDS Support Program
Oklahoma City, 405 525 6277 📖 323
AIDS Support Society
Hastings, 142 442 9901 📖 91
AIDS Support Team
Neptune, 908 776 4700 📖 291
AIDS Support Team / Dignity Foundation
Tyler, 903 566 8833 📖 344
AIDS Task Force of Alabama
Birmingham, 205 592 2437 📖 191
AIDS Task Force of Central New York
Syracuse, 315 475 2430 📖 295
AIDS Task Force of the Upper Ohio Valley
Wheeling, 304 232 6822 📖 355
AIDS Task Force of Winston-Salem
910 7223 5031 📖 316
AIDS Task Force, Inc.
Fort Wayne, 219 744 1144 📖 254
AIDS Task Group
Albury, 6 023 0340 📖 25
AIDS Telefon
Frankfurt am Main, 69 63 6036 📖 117
AIDS Telephone
Antwerpen / Anvers, 7 815 1515 📖 35
AIDS Treatment Data Network
New York, 212 268 4196 📖 295
AIDS Treatment News 📖 218
AIDS Trust of Australia
Sydney, 2 211 2044 📖 24
AIDS Unit
Hobart, 0 230 2872 📖 31
AIDS Vancouver
604 687 2437 (information) 📖 45
AIDS Vanvouver Island
Victoria, 604 384 4554 (information) 📖 47
AIDS Volunteers of Cincinnati
513 421 2437 📖 318
AIDS Wellness Program & Clinic
Santa Fe, 505 983 1822 📖 295
AIDS Yellowknife
800 661 0795 (information) 📖 48
AIDS Yukon Alliance
Whitehorse, 403 633 2437 📖 64
AIDS, A Positive Coördinated Response Society of Jasper
403 852 5274 📖 44
AIDS/AIDS Information & Ressources Québec Sud-Ouest
Athelstan, 514 264 3379 📖 61
AIDS/DTD Program
Pensacola, 904 444 8654 📖 241
AIDS/HIV Info Line
Sydney, 2 332 4268 📖 26
AIDS/HIV Nightline
San Francisco, 415 668 2437 📖 213
AIDS-Beratung
Luxembourg, 40 6251 📖 148
Neumünster, 432 1942 2837 📖 129
Westerland, 465 11 3784 📖 135
AIDS-Beratung des Gesundheitsamtes Mainz
613 122 5353 📖 126
AIDS-Beratung im Gesundheit Dresden
351 3 0126 📖 114
AIDS-Beratung im Gesundheitssamt Aachen
241 432 5326 📖 108
AIDS-Beratungsstelle des Gesundheitsamt
Köln, 221 221 4602 📖 124
AIDS-Beratungsstelle für Kölner Studierende 📖 124
AIDS-Beratungsstelle Niederbayern
Passau, 851 7 1065 📖 131
AIDS-Beratungsstelle Oberfranken
Hirschhorn, 627 28 7681 📖 122
AIDS-Beratungsstelle Unterfranken
Würzburg, 931 5 0599 📖 135
AIDS-Beratungstelle
Bamberg, 951 2 7998 📖 109
Bayreuth, 921 8 2500 📖 109
Ludwigshafen, 621 520 4440 📖 126
AIDS-Beratung-Stelle der Stadt Frankfurt
Frankfurt am Main 📖 117
AIDSBKRV 📖 2
AIDS-Hilfe
Aachen, 241 1 9411 📖 108
Aarau, 64 24 4450 📖 177
Ahlen, 238 2 4650 📖 109
Ansbach / Dinkelsbühl 📖 117
Arnstadt 📖 109
Augsburg, 821 1 9411 📖 109
Bamberg, 9551 1 9411 📖 109
Basel, 61 692 2122 📖 177
Berlin, 30 1 9411 📖 110
Bern, 31 331 3334 📖 177
Biel, 32 42 4342 (Deutsch) 📖 178
Bielefeld, 521 1 9411 📖 112
Bochum, 232 71 9411 📖 112
Bonn, 228 1 9411 📖 112
Bottrop, 204 11 9411 📖 112
Brandenburg, 338 12 3917 📖 112
Braunschweig, 531 1 9411 📖 112
Bremen, 421 1 9411 📖 113
Celle, 514 11 9411 📖 113
Chemnitz, 371 41 5223 📖 113
Dillenburg, 277 11 9411 📖 114
Dortmund, 231 52 7637 📖 114
Dresden, 351 464 0213 📖 114
Duisberg / Zweigstelle Wesel, 281 2 9980 📖 135
Duisburg, 213 41 9411 📖 114
Duisburg, 281 1 9411 📖 114
Duisburg, 284 11 9411 📖 127
Düsseldorf, 211 19411 📖 115
Eichstätt 📖 114
Eichstätt, 842 1 8488 📖 115
Essen, 201 1 9411 📖 116
Flensburg, 461 1 9411 📖 116
Frankfurt, 69 1 9411 📖 117
Freiburg, 761 1 9411 📖 117
Fulda, 661 77011 📖 118
Gelsenkircher, 209 1 9411 📖 118
Gießen, 641 1 9411 📖 118
Göttingen, 551 1 9411 📖 118
Grafschaft Bentheim, 592 1 9411 📖 129
Graubünden, 81 22 4900 📖 178
Graz, 316 81 5050 📖 34
Hagen, 233 11 9411 📖 119
Halberstadt 📖 119
Halle, 345 3 6419 📖 119
Halle, 349 32 1018 📖 112
Hamburg, 40 1 9411 📖 119
Hamm, 238 1 5575 📖 121
Hannover, 511 1 9411 📖 121
Heidelberg, 622 11 9411 📖 122
Herne, 232 36 0990 📖 122
Herzogtum Lauenburg, 454 21 9411 📖 127
Hildesheim, 512 11 9411 📖 122
Ingolstadt, 841 8 5961 📖 122
Kaiserlautern, 631 1 9411 📖 123
Kärten, 463 5 5128 📖 34
Kassel, 561 1 6801 📖 123
Kiel, 431 1 9411 📖 123
Koblenz, 261 1 9411 📖 123
Köln, 221 19411 📖 124
Konstanz, 753 11 9411 📖 125
Krefeld, 215 11 9411 📖 125
Kreis Olpe, 276 11 9411 📖 116, 130
Kreis Pinneberg / Steinfurt, 412 11 9411 📖 115
Kreis Siegen-Wittgenstein, 273 7 4253 📖 135
Kreis Unna, 230 31 9411 📖 134
Kreis Unna, 230 71 9411 📖 121
Kreis Viersen, 216 23 4987 📖 134
Kries Steinfurt, 591 5 4023 📖 131
Landau, 634 11 9411 📖 125
Leipzig, 341 232 3126 📖 125
Leverkusen 📖 125
Liechtenstein, 232 0520 📖 148
Limburg, 643 11 9411 📖 125
Lingen, 591 1 9411 📖 126
Lübeck, 451 1 9411 📖 126
Lüneburg, 413 11 9411 📖 126
Luzern, 41 51 6848 📖 178
Magdeburg 📖 126
Mainz, 613 11 9411 📖 126
Mannheim, 621 1 9411 📖 126
Marburg, 642 11 9411 📖 127
Märkischen Kreis, 235 12 3202 📖 126
Mönchengladbach / Rheydt, 216 11 9411 📖 127
Mülhausen, 360 144 6218 📖 127
München, 89 1 9411 📖 128
Münster, 251 1 9411 📖 128
Neubrandenburg, 395 44 3083 📖 129
Neumünster, 432 11 9411 📖 129
Neuss, 210 122 2925 📖 129
Nordrhein-Westfalen, 221 25 3596 📖 124
Nürnberg / Erlangen / Fürth, 911 1 9411 📖 129
Oberhausen, 208 80 6518 📖 130
Oberösterreich 📖 34
Oberwallis, 28 46 4668 📖 179
Offenbach, 69 99 3688 📖 130
Oldenburg, 441 1 9411 📖 130
Osnabrück, 541 1 9411 📖 130
Paderborn, 525 11 9411 📖 130
Pforzheim, 732 14 1110 📖 131
Potsdam 📖 131
Regensburg, 941 1 9411 📖 131
Rhein-Sieg-Kreis, 224 11 9411 📖 134
Rostock, 381 45 3156 📖 131
Saar, 681 1 9411 📖 132
Saar, 688 115 2222 📖 125
Saint Gallen, 71 23 3868 📖 179
Salzburg, 662 88 1488 📖 35
Schweiz, 1 273 4242 📖 177
Siegen-Wittgenstein, 271 2 2222 📖 132
Soest, 292 1 2888 📖 132
Solingen, 212 1 9411 📖 132
Solothurn, 65 22 9411 📖 179
Stuttgart, 711 19411 📖 132
Suhl, 368 12 0084 📖 134
Thurgau / Schaffhausen, 53 25 9338 📖 179
Thüringen, 361 731 2233 📖 116
Tirol, 512 56 3621 📖 34
Trier, 651 1 9411 📖 134
Tübingen, 707 11 9411 📖 134
Ulm, 731 3 3731 📖 134
Unterland, 713 11 9411 📖 122
Voralberg, 5574 465 26 📖 34
Wartburgkreis, 369 121 4083 📖 115
Weimar, 364 36 1451 (office) 📖 135
Westküste, 481 1 9411 📖 122
Westmünsterland, 256 1 19411 📖 109
Wien, 1 408 6186 📖 35
Wiesbaden, 611 1 9411 📖 135
Wilhelmshaven, 442 11 9411 📖 135
Wolfsburg, 536 1 9411 📖 135
Wupperthal, 202 1 9411 📖 135
Würzburg, 931 1 9411 📖 136
Zug, 42 22 4865 📖 179
Zürich, 1 461 1516 📖 179
AIDS-Hilfe (ZASA)
Zwickau, 375 78 1017 📖 136
AIDS-Info
Odense, 65 91 1119 📖 66
AIDS-Infolijn
Amsterdam, 6 022 2220 📖 152
AIDS-Informationszentrale Austria
Wien, 222 402 2353 📖 34
AIDS-Kontor
Stavanger, 51 50 8800 📖 166
AIDSLine
Birmingham, 121 622 1511 📖 93
Reading, 173 450 3377 📖 71
Southampton, 170 333 9467 📖 77
White Cross, 152 484 1011 📖 79
AIDSline Southampton
1703 339467 📖 77
AIDS-linien (AIDS Hotline)

København, 33 91 1119 66
AIDS-STAT-L 2
Aigle Noir
Montréal, 514 529 0040 61
Air Libre FM 107.6
Bruxelles / Brussel, 2 512 4587 37
Air Transilvania
Tel-Aviv 138
Aircraft News & Books
Hartford, 203 569 2324 231
Airline Books
New Orleans, 504 468 2931 261
Aiuta AIDS Ticino
91 23 1717 179
AJA Publishing Corp.
Port Chester 310
AK Schwule
Bonn, 228 21 9021 112
Akehurst Gallery
London, 181 969 0453 85
Akita, Masami
Kita-Ku 147
Akron City Hospital
216 375 3000 317
Aktionsgruppe Homosexualität Hannover (HSH)
511 66 1055 121
Aktionsgruppe Homosexualität Osnabrück e. V. (AHO)
541 2 2722 130
Alabama Adult Books
Birmingham, 205 322 7323 191
Alabama Forum 191
Alachua General Hospital
Gainesville, 904 372 4321 237
Aladdin Holdings Ltd.
Saint Thomas 183
Alameda County Leather Corps
Oakland 207
Alamo Square Distributors
San Francisco, 415 863 7410 213
Alamo Square Press
San Francisco, 415 863 7410 216, 217
Alaska Women's Bookstore
Anchorage, 907 562 4716 193
Alaskan AIDS Assistance Association (AAAA)
Anchorage, 800 478 2437 192
Alaskan Tpeople
Chugiak 193
Albany Medical Center
518 262 3125 295
Albany Trust
London, 181 675 6669 80
Albert Lea Lesbian & Gay Outreach 279
ALBGS *See* Alliance of Lesbian-Bi-Gay Students
Albino Verlag
Berlin, 30 615 0030 108
Albion Street (AIDS) Centre
Sydney, 2 332 1090 26
Ale Design
Zürich 180
Aled Richards Trust
Bath, 127 255 3355 70
Bristol, 117 955 3355 70
Alerte 97
Alexandre, Claude
Paris, 143 38 7482 104
ALFA *See* AIDS Leadership Foothills Area
Alfa Medical
Hampstead, 800 762 1586 299
Alfi News
Seattle, 206 632 9390 353
Seattle, 206 827 6486 353
Algoma AIDS Network
Sault Saint Marie, 800 361 2497 (information) 54
Algonquin College Lesbigays
Ottawa, 613 238 1717 53
ALGUQAM *See* Association des Lesbiennes & Gaies de l'Université de Québec à Montréal
Alice Kerr Sutherland Society
Hastings 91
Alice Springs Hospital
8 950 2638 28
Aliens
broadcast by Stichting M.V.S. FM 106.8, Cable 103.8 153
All Man
published by Fraction Presse SARL 97
All Out Productions
London, 171 240 2070 85
All Points North
Leeds, 113 238 0999 94
published by Silveraim Ltd. 76
All Saints AIDS Service Center
Pasadena, 818 796 5633 209
All Your Dreams Fulfilled
published by PCP 199
Allegheny General Hospital
Pittsburgh, 412 359 3131 331
Allen Wells Center for Psychotherapy & Healing
Morristown, 201 539 0301 291
Alley
Chicago, 312 883 1800 251
Alleycat Books Coöp
Newcastle upon Tyne, 191 232 5478 92
Allgemeine Homosexuelle Arbeitsgemeinschaft e. V. (AHA)
Berlin, 30 692 3600 110
Allgemeines Krankenhaus
Wien, 1 438 9510 35
Alliance
Durham, 603 862 4522 287
Alliance for Bisexual, Lesbian, & Gay Support
Kalamazoo, 616 387 2134 276
Alliance for Sexual Diversity
Portland, 207 774 4919 263
Alliance News 341
Alliance of Cache Valley (GLA-CV)
Logan, 801 752 1129 345
Alliance of Lesbian & Gay Organizations of Western Virginia
Roanoke 347
Alliance of Lesbian, Bi, & Gay Students
Wollongong, 4 221 4012 28
Alliance of Lesbian, Gay, & Bisexual Students
Atlanta, 404 605 7681 244
Alliance of Lesbian-Bi-Gay Students (ALBGS)
Lansing, 517 353 9795 277
Alliance of Massachusetts Asian Lesbians and Gay Men 269
Alliance of Professional Tattooists, Inc.
Glen Burnie, 410 768 1963 265
Allies Boulevard Bookstore Downtown
Binghamton, 607 724 8659 297
Allies Boulevard Bookstore East
Binghamton, 607 724 9749 297
Alligator News & Books
Key West, 305 294 4004 238
Allison, Judith, M.Ed., MSH
Jacksonville, 904 733 3310 238
Allmen, Robert, MS, M.Div.
New York, 516 723 0348 300
Allo SIDA
Tours 106
ALLOGAY
Bordeaux, Minitel 3615 ALLOGAY 98
Grenoble, Minitel 3615 ALLOGAY 100
Lille, Minitel 3615 ALLOGAY 100
Lyon, Minitel 3615 ALLOGAY 100
Marseille, Minitel 3615 ALLOGAY 101
Montpellier, Minitel 3615 ALLOGAY 101
Nancy, Minitel 3615 ALLOGAY 102
Nantes, Minitel 3615 ALLOGAY 102
Nice, Minitel 3615 ALLOGAY 102
Paris, Minitel 3615 ALLOGAY 103
Rennes, Minitel 3615 ALLOGAY 105
Strasbourg, Minitel 3615 ALLOGAY 106
Almont Counselling Associates
Birmingham, 205 591 5113 191
Aloft
Pasadena, 818 441 1789 209
Alper, Barbara
New York, 212 316 6518 306
ALSO *See* Alternative Lifestyle Support Organization
alt.amazon-women.admirers 4
alt.books.anne-rice 5
alt.censorship 5
alt.christnet.nudism 5
alt.christnet.sex 6
alt.clothing.lingerie 5
alt.fax.bondage 4
alt.foreplay 5
alt.homosexual 5
alt.journalism.gay-press 5
alt.lesbian.feminist.poetry 5
alt.lycra 5
alt.magazine.playboy 4
alt.magazines.pornographic 4
alt.magick.sex 5
alt.mud.sex 5
alt.nudism 5
alt.pagan 6
alt.pantyhose 5
alt.polyamory 5
alt.privacy 5
alt.recovery.addiction.sexual 6
alt.recovery.sexual-addiction 6
alt.religion.sexuality 6
alt.safe.sex 5
alt.sex 5
alt.sex.advocacy 5
alt.sex.anal 5
alt.sex.animals 5
alt.sex.asphyx 5
alt.sex.balls 5
alt.sex.bears 4
alt.sex.bestiality 5
alt.sex.bondage 4
alt.sex.boys 4
alt.sex.breast 5
alt.sex.breathless 5
alt.sex.cd-rom 6
alt.sex.cthulhu 6
alt.sex.enemas 5
alt.sex.erotica.marketplace 4
alt.sex.exhibitionism 5
alt.sex.fat 4
alt.sex.femdom 4
alt.sex.fetish.amputee 5
alt.sex.fetish.diapers 4
alt.sex.fetish.fa 4
alt.sex.fetish.fashion 5
alt.sex.fetish.feet 5
alt.sex.fetish.feet.toes 5
alt.sex.fetish.hair 5
alt.sex.fetish.motorcycles 5
alt.sex.fetish.orientals 5
alt.sex.fetish.robots 5
alt.sex.fetish.size 4
alt.sex.fetish.smoking 5
alt.sex.fetish.sportswear 5
alt.sex.fetish.tickling 5
alt.sex.fetish.waifs 4
alt.sex.fetish.watersports 6
alt.sex.fetish.wet-and-messy 5
alt.sex.fetish.wrestling 6
alt.sex.furry 4
alt.sex.girls 4
alt.sex.hello-kitty 5
alt.sex.historical 6
alt.sex.homosexual 6
alt.sex.incest 6
alt.sex.intergen 6
alt.sex.jello 5
alt.sex.jp 6
alt.sex.magazines 4
alt.sex.masturbation 5
alt.sex.motss 6
alt.sex.nasal-hair 5
alt.sex.necrophilia 5
alt.sex.orgy 6
alt.sex.pedophilia 5
alt.sex.pedophilia.boys 5
alt.sex.pedophilia.girls 5
alt.sex.preteens 5
alt.sex.reptiles 5
alt.sex.safe 6
alt.sex.sm.fig 4
alt.sex.spanking 6
alt.sex.swingers 6
alt.sex.trans 6
alt.sex.uncut 5
alt.sex.voyeurism 5
alt.sex.watersports 6
alt.sex.wizards 6
alt.sex.young 5
alt.sex.zoophile 5
alt.sex.zoophilia 5
alt.sexual.abuse.recovery 6
alt.sexual.abuse.recovery.d 6
alt.shoe.lesbians 6
alt.support.abuse-partners 6
alt.support.boy-lovers 5
alt.support.cant.urinate.in-public 6
alt.support.herpes 5
alt.support.transgendered 6
alt.transgendered 6
Alta Bates Medical Center
Berkeley, 510 204 1492 197
Alter Ego
Las Vegas, 702 796 8054 286
Stockport 68
Alternate Expressions 298
Alternate Lifestyle Alliance of Olaca
904 624 3779 240
Alternate Marketing
Palm Desert, 619 346 7374 183
Alternate Publishing Company
San Francisco, 415 864 3456 16
Alternate Sources
published by Kink, Ink 14, 15
Alternate Woman
published by Lonnie Marshall Publications 261
Alternate Woods Publishing
Boston 269
ALTERNATES 3
Seattle, 206 323 7483 351
Alternating Currents
broadcast by WAIF FM 88.3 318
Alternativa Positiva
Lisboa, 795 8296 167
Alternative Accent
broadcast by Access Community Radio AM 810 161
Alternative Access BBS
Melbourne 31
Alternative Approach Counseling & Psychotherapy Center
Montclair, 201 736 8785 291
Alternative Gender-Oriented (AGO)
Charlotte 314
Alternative Lifestyle Support Organization (ALSO)
Norfolk, 804 855 5212 348
Alternative Lifestyles Directory
published by Winter Publishing, Inc. 15
Alternative Lifestyles Fellowship
Nashua 288
Alternative Lifestyles Office
Mankato, 507 389 1455 279
Alternative Lifestyles Support Organization (ALSO)
Plymouth, 603 535 2796 288
Alternative Phone Book 251
Alternative Resources of the Triad
Greensboro, 910 274 2100 315
Alternative Sports
Glasgow, 141 423 4175 13
Alternative Youth Club - Tri State Area
Darien, 203 975 9139 230
Alternatives 205
Durham, 1209 612234 74
Williamsburg, 206 221 3309 349
Alternatives to Monogamy
Wheaton, 708 510 7027 253
Altomar Productions
Sacramento, 916 641 1930 187
Altra Faccia della Luna
broadcast by Gay Radio Sibilla FM 103 143
Altro Martedi
broadcast by Radio Popolare FM 105.5 & 107.6 143
Always On Sunday
Montclair, 201 783 1419 291
Alyson Publications, Inc.
Boston, 617 542 5679 269
Amador Communications
San Francisco, 415 431 0171 15, 20
Amalgamated American Male
New York 303
Amazon Bookstore, Inc.
Minneapolis / Saint Paul, 612 338 6560 281
Amazon Country
broadcast by WXPN FM 88.5 331
Amazon Drygoods
Davenport, 800 798 7979 183
Amazon Times 264

AMAZONS 🕮 3
Ambassador World Travel
Atlanta 🕮 245
Ambassadors
Boston 🕮 268
Amber E.
Milpitas 🕮 206
Ambitious Amazons / Lesbian Center
Lansing, 517 371 5257 🕮 277
Ambulatorio de Saude Mental SUD
São Paulo, 11 283 0005 🕮 39
Ambush 🕮 260
A-Men's Club
Århus, 86 19 1089 🕮 65
American Association for Counselling & Development
Jenkintown 🕮 329
American Association of Sex Educators, Counsellors, & Therapists (AASECT)
Chicago, 312 644 0828 🕮 188
American Bear
published by Big Bull, Inc. 🕮 228
American Book Center
Amsterdam, 20 625 5537 🕮 153
Den Haag, 70 364 2742 🕮 154
American Booksellers Association
New York, 212 463 8450 🕮 306
American Civil Liberties Union
New York, 212 944 9800 🕮 304
Philadelphia, 215 592 1513 🕮 330
American College Health Association
Charlottesville, 804 924 2670 🕮 347
American College Personnel Association
Baltimore 🕮 264
Chicago 🕮 250
American Educational Gender Information Services, Inc. (AEGIS)
Decatur, 404 939 2128 🕮 245
American Foundation for AIDS Research
Los Angeles 🕮 203
New York 🕮 303
American Group Psychotherapy Association
Boston, 617 266 1616 🕮 268
American Historical Association
Milwaukee, 414 229 4924 🕮 357
American Library Association
Chicago 🕮 250, 251
American Mental Health Counsellors Association
Phœnix 🕮 193
American Psychiatric Association
Washington 🕮 233
American Psychological Association
Washington, 202 955 7600 🕮 233
American Red Cross
Pittsfield, 800 332 2030 🕮 266
American Red Cross AIDS Projects
Seattle, 206 323 2345 🕮 351
American Social Health Association (ASHA)
Research Triangle Park, 919 361 8400 🕮 188
American Transsexual Education Center (ATEC)
Los Angeles, 213 389 6938 🕮 188
American Uniform Association (AUA)
Atlanta Brigade 🕮 244
Chicago Brigade 🕮 250
Mid-Atlantic Corps 🕮 234
New York 🕮 13
Amethyst
published by SYOL Ltd. 🕮 297
Amethyst Counselling Service
Eugene, 503 484 6979 🕮 325
AMI Park Plaza Hospital
Houston, 713 527 5000 🕮 342
AMI Twelve Oaks Hospital
Houston, 713 623 2500 🕮 342
Amigo Kerho 56
Hyvinkää, 91 453 2201 🕮 97
Amigo/CPC 🕮 36
Amitié SIDA
Nantes, 40 29 1228 🕮 102
Amok Books
Los Angeles, 213 665 0956 🕮 203
Amour
Auckland 🕮 161
Auckland, 9 379 0497 🕮 160, 161
Amour, 9 379 0497 🕮 160
Amsterdam House
20 626 2577 🕮 151
Anapol, Deborah, IRC
San Rafael 🕮 221
Anatometal
Santa Cruz, 408 462 2366 🕮 221
Anco Bar
Amsterdam, 20 624 1126 🕮 151
Andere Buchhandlung
Rostock 🕮 131
Andere Fakultät / Schwulen- & Lesbenreferat
Köln 🕮 124
Andere Kant
Bruxelles / Brussel 🕮 37
Andere Welt 🕮 108
Anders, Ron, MSW
Seattle, 206 441 1903 🕮 351
Anderschume / Kontiki 🕮 177
Anderson, Chris
London, 181 293 1947 🕮 81
Andersrum
Neustadt, 632 13 5208 🕮 129
Andreas Kneipe
Berlin, 30 218 3257 🕮 109
Androgyne
Montréal, 514 842 4765 🕮 63
Androgyny
Los Angeles, 213 467 8317 🕮 204
Androgyny Center
Durham, 919 489 8753 🕮 314
Raleigh, 919 848 0500 🕮 315
Andromeda
Bologna, 51 225976 🕮 140
Andros
San Diego 🕮 211
Androscoggin Valley AIDS Coalition (AVAC)
Lewiston, 207 786 4697 🕮 262
Angles
published by Lavendar Publishing 🕮 46
Ania Metalworks
Santa Barbara 🕮 221
Animas
Miami 🕮 239
ANKORS 🕮 *See* West Kootenay-Boundry AIDS Network, Outreach & Support Society
Ann Street Adult Entertainment Center
New York, 212 267 9760 🕮 309
Ann Summers
London, 171 437 1886 🕮 86
Anna Blaman Huis
Leeuwarden, 58 212 1829 🕮 156
Annapolis Road Books
Fort Meade, 301 674 9414 🕮 265
Annares
Leeds 🕮 94
Annette K Fashions
Düsseldorf, 211 37 4476 🕮 115
Annette's Castle
Atlanta 🕮 243
Annie's Orphans
Woodstock, 914 679 4030 🕮 183
Anonyme AIDS-Beratungsstralle des Gesundheithauses
München, 89 520 7387 🕮 128
Another Side
Bend, 503 388 2395 🕮 324
Another World
Albany 🕮 296
Brighton, 1273 675167 🕮 74
Antarius
Berlin, 30 432 8928 🕮 110
Antenne Rose
broadcast by Air Libre FM 107.6 🕮 37
Antenne SIDA du Valais Romand
Sion, 27 22 8757 🕮 179
Anthony Wojnowski's Artworks
Kitchener, 519 576 0381 🕮 23
Anthro
Glasgow 🕮 169
Antigone Books
Tucson, 602 792 3715 🕮 195
Anubis Warpus
San Francisco, 415 431 2218 🕮 216
Anvil
London, 171 407 0371 🕮 80
Anything That Moves
published by San Francisco Bay Area Bisexual Network 🕮 217
Anza Gay & Lesbian Alliance
San José, 408 534 4254 🕮 220
Aoraki Lesbian & Gay Group
Timaru, 3 615 7668 🕮 163
Apex
published by Phœnix Press 🕮 261
APG 🕮 *See* Association des Parents & Futures Parents Gais
Aphro Adult Products
Adelaide, 8 231 3632 🕮 30
Aphrodite
Toulouse, 61 62 4882 🕮 106
Aphrodite/Elle
Manchester 🕮 76
APLA 🕮 *See* AIDS Project Los Angeles
Apollo
München, 89 26 7438 🕮 128
Apollo Contakt Versand
München 🕮 107
Apolo 🕮 149
Appalachian AIDS Coalition
Abingdon, 800 354 3388 🕮 347
Appalachian Bears Club of East Tennessee
Knoxville, 615 524 7884 (infoline) 🕮 336
Applegate, Eric, PC, MS, NACA II, AAMFT, CST
Indianapolis, 317 925 1881 🕮 254
Après Noir
Sonoma, 707 935 6595 🕮 182
Trowbridge, 1225 774164 🕮 68
Aprinco Book Manufacturers
Scarborough, 416 286 6688 Ext. 22 🕮 54
APSAM - GPL 🕮 *See* Actions Prévention SIDA & Aide aux Malades
Aquala
Rie, 603 772 5529 🕮 183
Aquarius Books
Bloomington, 812 336 0988 🕮 254
Aquila MC
Agnew 🕮 196
Araba Fenice
Biella 🕮 144
Arabesque
Neuenhof, 1 242 9626 🕮 178
Zürich, 1 242 9626 🕮 180
Aradia Books
Flagstaff, 602 779 3817 🕮 193
Aragon Buchladen
Moers, 284 12 9772 🕮 127
Arbeits Gemeinschaft S/M & Öffentlichkeit
Neumünster 🕮 129
Arbeitsgemeinschaft Homosexualität Magnus
Neustrelitz 🕮 129
Arbeitsgemeinschaft Humane Sexualität
Berlin, 30 618 9039 🕮 110
Arbor Moon Alternative Bookstore
Lincoln, 402 477 5666 🕮 285
Arbuckle's Tattoo & piercing Emporium
Cedar Rapids, 319 363 1242 🕮 256
ARC 🕮 *See* AIDS Resource Center
Arc en Ciel
Montpellier, 67 60 6461 🕮 101
Arcados-Versand
Basel / Bâle, 61 681 3132 🕮 177
Arcane Bookshop
Perth, 9 328 5073 🕮 33
ARCAT 🕮 *See* Association pour la Recherche Clinique sur le SIDA & sa Thérapie
Archives
Jersey Village 🕮 343
Archives for the Protection of Gay History & Literature
Saint John 🕮 48
Archives Gaies du Québec
Montréal, 514 287 4664 🕮 61
Archives Recherches & Cultures Lesbiennes
Paris, 148 05 2589 🕮 102
Arci Gay
Antinoo, 81 552 8815 🕮 140
Arcobaleno, 40 94 1708 🕮 141
Arcobaleno, 832 30 6138 🕮 144
Bari, 80 554 3474 🕮 144
Belluno, 437 94 0209 🕮 146
Bergamo, 35 23 0959 🕮 142
Bolzano, 471 27 2165 🕮 140
Cagliari, 70 65 5998 🕮 145
Catania, 95 50 5830 🕮 145
Centaurus 🕮 146
Coccioli, 932 20471 🕮 145
Cremona, 372 20484 🕮 142
Empoli, 571 71 0301 🕮 145
Enna, 935 50 0021 🕮 145
Firenze, 55 28 8126 🕮 145
Foggia 🕮 144
Forlì, 543 34422 🕮 140
Genova, 10 247 0575 🕮 138, 142
Helios, 85 294 2221 🕮 139
Il Gabbiano, 71 203 0454 🕮 143
Legnano, 442 26053 🕮 146
Messina, 90 69 3542 🕮 145
Mestre, 41 98 3653 🕮 146
Milano, 2 839 4604 🕮 143
Nazionale, 51 644 7054 🕮 139
Nuovi Passi, 432 51 3311 🕮 141
Padova, 49 875 6326 🕮 146, 147
Pisa, 50 54 4646 🕮 146
Ragusa, 932 20471 🕮 145
Ravenna, 544 30151 🕮 141
Rieti 🕮 139
Roma, 6 446 5839 🕮 141
Rovigo 🕮 147
Sassari, 79 23 5366 🕮 145
Torino, 11 521 1116 🕮 143
Trento, 461 41 0808 🕮 146
Varese, 332 23 4055 🕮 143
Venezia, 41 72 1842 🕮 147
Vicenza, 444 50 7230 🕮 147
Arci Gay e Lesbica
Ferrara, 532 210597 🕮 140
Palermo, 91 33 5688 🕮 145
Torino, 11 521 1116 🕮 144
Arci Gayline
144 880988 🕮 138
Arcisbox
Hamburg 🕮 107
Arena 🕮 84
ARENAL
Bloomington 🕮 3
ARENAL-L 🕮 3
Argonauts of Wisconsin
Green Bay 🕮 356
Argos
Gent / Gand, 9 222 5404 🕮 38
Argos Club
Amsterdam, 20 622 6595 🕮 151
Ariel Books
Vancouver, 604 733 3511 🕮 46
ARIS 🕮 *See* Acceuil Rencontre Information Service
Aris Project
San José, 408 370 3272 🕮 219
Aristoc Distributors
Lyndhurst 🕮 183
Arizona AIDS Project
Phœnix, 602 265 3300 🕮 193
Arizona Fellowship Committee
Tucson 🕮 194
Arizona Power Exchange
Phœnix, 602 415 1123 🕮 194
Arizona Rangers MC
Phœnix 🕮 194
Arizona State Hospital
Phœnix, 602 244 1331 🕮 193
ARK 🕮 *See* AIDS Response Knoxville
Arkansas Advisor 🕮 195
Arkansas AIDS Foundation
Little Rock, 501 663 7833 🕮 195
Arkansas Gay & Lesbian Task Force Switchboard
Little Rock, 800 448 8305 (statewide) 🕮 195
Arkiv for Bøsser & Lesbiske
København, 33 11 1961 🕮 66
Arktos
Cleveland 🕮 319
Arlington Gay & Lesbian Alliance
703 522 7660 🕮 347
Arlington Hospital
703 558 5000 🕮 347
Armidale Gay Society 🕮 25
Armstrong, Paul
Toronto, 416 351 9430 🕮 55
Army & Navy Stores
Liverpool, 1928 731925 🕮 71
Macclesfield, 1625 425164 🕮 72
Stourbridge, 1384 395166 🕮 93
Walsall, 1922 725755 🕮 93
Army Classics
London, 171 247 8452 🕮 87
Army Navy Store
Saint Petersburg, 813 544 8004 🕮 241
Weymouth, 617 331 4249 🕮 273
Army Navy Stores

Birmingham, 121 744 5135 📖 93
Solihull, 121 788 3739 📖 93
Army Navy Surplus U.S.A.
Chicago, 312 348 8930 📖 252
Army Surplus Sales Inc.
Atlanta, 404 521 2227 📖 245
Army Surplus Stores
Auckland, 9 634 3792 📖 161
Army-Navy Store of Tampa, Inc.
813 229 2172 📖 243
Arocha, Jorge, ACSW
Miami, 305 285 8900 📖 238
ARS 📖 *See* AIDS Referral Services
Ars Subcutan
Mannheim, 621 318 9183 📖 127
Arsenault, Raymond, Ph.D.
Andover, 508 475 7171 📖 267
Salem, 603 898 5105 📖 288
Art & Understanding 📖 296
Art Accent Tattooing
New Orleans, 514 581 9812 📖 261
Art of Fée
Hamburg, 40 450 35353 📖 120
Artemis Creations Publishing
Brooklyn, 718 648 8215 📖 14
Arthur Hamilton, Inc.
Richmond Hill, 718 441 6066 📖 10
Artistes
Paris, 142 82 1190 📖 104
Artistic Licentiousness 📖 352
ARTpolice Agency
Minneapolis / Saint Paul, 612 291 0718 📖 281
ASA 📖 *See* Assoziazione Solidarieta AIDS
Asbl Aide Cliniques Universitaires Saint Luc
Bruxelles / Brussel, 2 764 1582 📖 36
ASBL Gai Info
Hainault, 6 828 0552 📖 38
Asgard Body Piercing
Southampton, 170 332 5059 📖 13
Asgard International
Southampton, 170 332 5059 📖 11
ASHA 📖 *See* American Social Health Association
Ashely's Boutique
Toronto, 416 767 3518 📖 40
Asheville Gay & Lesbian Information Line
704 253 2971 📖 313
Ashland Psychological Services
Cincinnati, 513 861 8365 📖 317
Ask Isadora
San Francisco, 415 386 5090 📖 212
Aslan Leathers
Toronto, 416 538 9759 📖 41
ASMF Paris 📖 103
Asnien, Carolyn, MA
New York, 212 749 4171 📖 300
Asociacion de Lucha Contra el SIDA
San José 📖 65
ASPE
Torino, 11 839 5444 📖 139
Aspen Gay & Lesbian Community
202 925 9249 📖 226
Aspinall, John, CSW
New York, 516 922 6155 📖 300
ASPYN 📖 *See* Safer Place Youth Network
ASS 📖 *See* Atlanta S&M Solidarity
Assault Hotline
800 802 437 📖 159
ASSET 📖 *See* After Surgery Support Exchange for Transexuals
Assistenza AIDS
Roma, 6 832 2315 📖 141
Associação Brasileira Interdisciplinar de AIDS
Rio de Janeiro, 21 224 1654 📖 39
Associated Counseling Professionals, Inc.
Hartford, 800 654 4320 (in Connecticut) 📖 230
Association Beaumont Continental (ABC)
Didenheim 📖 99
Association de Lutte Contre le SIDA
Lyon, 78 27 8080 📖 101
Association des Artistes Contre le SIDA
Paris, 145 00 5353 📖 103
Association des Gais & Lesbiennes de l'Université de Sherbrooke
819 564 5013 📖 63
Association des Lesbiennes & Gaies de l'Université de Québec à Montréal
514 987 3039 📖 62
Association des Parents & Futures Parents Gais (APG)
Paris, 147 36 0487 📖 103
Association Française d'Aide aux Séro-Positifs
London, 171 287 2363 📖 82
Association Gais & Lesbiennes à Liège
Liège / Luik / Luttich, 4 135 0968 📖 38
Association Ibiza
Marseille, 91 50 5012 📖 101
Association of Lesbians & Gays of Ottawa
613 233 0152 📖 52
Association of Professional Piercers
San Francisco 📖 215
Association pour la Lutte Contre le SIDA
Bruxelles / Brussel, 2 538 9192 📖 37
Association pour la Recherche Clinique sur le SIDA & sa Thérapie (ARCAT)
Paris, 149 70 8590 📖 103
Associazione Gay Ticino (AGT)
Lugano 📖 178
Assoziazione Genitori di Omosessuali (AGEDO)
Firenze, 55 28 8126 📖 145
Milano, 2 894 01749 📖 143
Torino, 11 521 1116 📖 144
Assoziazione Solidarieta AIDS (ASA)
Milano, 2 581 07084 📖 142
ASTA - Schwulen & Lesbenferat
Bamberg, 951 86 3347 📖 109
AStA-Referat Schwule & Lesben der Universität Paderborn
525 160 3174 📖 131
Astarte Shell Press
Portland, 207 828 1992 📖 263
AStA-Schwulenreferat
Düsseldorf, 211 311 5283 📖 115
Kaiserlautern, 631 205 2228 📖 123
AStA-Schwulenreferat der Uni Hamburg
40 410 3064 📖 120
At The Crossroads 📖 194
ATEC 📖 *See* American Transsexual Education Center
Atelier
Köln, 221 54 1972 📖 124
Atelier für Extravagante Mode
Berlin, 30 442 2740 📖 110
Athena Women's MC
Santa Monica, 310 458 3363 📖 222
Athens AIDS Task Force
614 592 4397 📖 317
Athlete's Bench
Glendale 📖 200
Atkol Entertainment
Plainfield, 908 756 2001 📖 187
Atlanta Eagle
404 873 2453 📖 243
Atlanta Gay Center
404 876 5372 (office) 📖 244
Atlanta Gay Center Helpline
404 892 0661 (TDD capable) 📖 244
Atlanta Gender Exploration (AGE)
404 875 9846 📖 244
Atlanta Power Exchange
Buford, 404 945 0154 📖 245
Atlanta S&M Solidarity (ASS)
404 521 3829 (voice mail) 📖 244
Atlantic City Medical Center
609 344 4081 📖 289
Atlantic First Nations AIDS Task Force
Halifax, 800 565 4255 (information) 📖 48
Atlantic Motorcycle Coördinating Council
Boston, 215 634 7156 📖 188
Atlantic News
Halifax, 902 429 5468 📖 48
Atlantic News Agency
Atlantic City, 609 344 9444 📖 289
Atlantis MC
Atlanta 📖 244
Atlas Travel East
Rockville, 800 357 4190 📖 266
Atom Age
London 📖 86
Atomage
Shinjuku-Ku 📖 148
Atomic Books
Baltimore, 410 728 5490 📖 264
Atons of Minneapolis
Minneapolis / Saint Paul, 612 333 4458 📖 280
Attic
Amsterdam, 20 638 1695 📖 151
Attika
Brindisi, 831 563051 📖 144
Attitude
London, 171 701 2175 📖 80
published by Northern & Shell 📖 85
published by The Fetish Network 📖 240
Attitudes
Portland, 503 224 0050 📖 326
Au Courant 📖 327
AUA 📖 *See* American Uniform Association
Auburn Gay & Lesbian Association (AGALA) 📖 191
Auckland Bisexual Group
9 522 1910 📖 160
Auckland Community AIDS Services (ACAS)
9 309 0156 📖 160
Auckland Gay & Lesbian Community Centre
9 378 9802 📖 159
Auckland Gay & Lesbian Trust
9 302 0590 📖 160
Auckland Hospital
9 379 7440 📖 160
Auckland University Gay Students Association 📖 160
Audie L. Murphy Memorial Veterans' Hospital
San Antonio, 210 617 5140 📖 344
Audre Lorde Clinic
London, 171 377 7311 📖 80
Auge, Rebecca, Ph.D.
Oakland, 415 426 0718 📖 207
AUGLBC-L 📖 3
Auntie's Bookstore
Spokane, 509 838 0206 📖 354
Auroboros
Toronto, 416 962 7499 📖 58
Aurora, A Northland Lesbian Center
Duluth, 218 722 4903 📖 279
aus.culture.lesbigay 📖 6
aus.sex 📖 6
aus.sex.bondage 📖 4
AUSBDSM 📖 2
AUSGBLF 📖 3
Austin Second Image
512 515 5460 📖 338
Australia TransGenerist Support Association, Inc.
New Farm, 7 236 2400 📖 29
Australian Bisexual Network
Brisbane, 7 254 0692 📖 28
Australian Club Run Association (ACRA)
Sydney 📖 26
Australian Foundation of AIDS Organizations (AFAO)
Sydney, 6 231 2111 📖 24
Australian Leather Men (ALM) 📖 24
Australian Lesbian & Gay Archives
Melbourne, 39 499 6334 📖 24
Australian National Council on AIDS
Canberra, 6 289 7186 📖 24
Autan X
Toulouse, 61 63 8790 📖 106
Author Author
Kingston, 914 339 1883 📖 299
Los Angeles, 310 798 1230 📖 205
Automatisk Telefonsvarer om AIDS
Rana, 75 13 2670 📖 165
Automones Schwulenreferat im AStA
Göttingen, 551 39 4571 📖 118
Autonomes Schwulenreferat
Mainz 📖 126
Autonomes Schwulenreferat der Uni Bielefeld
521 106 3424 📖 112
AVAC 📖 *See* Androscoggin Valley AIDS Coalition
Avalon Leather
West Hollywood 📖 225
Avalon Video International
Los Angeles, 800 222 9622 📖 23
Avatar
Los Angeles, 818 563 4626 📖 204
Avenue Services
Mountain View 📖 207
AVI Productions
Paris, 143 66 6194 📖 22
Awakenings
published by BB Publications 📖 278
Awhina 📖 163
Awhina AIDS Clinic
Wellington, 4 389 3169 📖 163
AXA
Boston 📖 268
Axfords
Brighton, 127 332 7944 📖 67
Axis
Stalybridge 📖 72
Ayr Lesbian & Gay Switchboard
1292 619000 📖 169
Ayrshire AIDS Awareness Project Support Group 📖 169
AZZLO
Shinjuku-Ku, 81 3 3225 4630 📖 148
AZZLO Discipline Co.
Shinjuku-Ku, 81 3 3225 4630 📖 148
B & D Pleasures
Long Beach, 800 827 3787 📖 202, 203
published by B & D Pleasures 📖 202
B&B Leatherworks
Calgary, 403 236 7072 📖 40, 43
B&D B&B
Laytonville, 707 984 8343 📖 202
B&D Comm
Indianapolis 📖 254
B. C. Coalition of People with Disabilities
Vancouver, 604 875 0188 📖 45
B. R. Creations
Mountain View, 415 961 5354 📖 207
B.A.D. Girls
Portland 📖 326
B-1
Breda, 76 514 5641 📖 154
Eindhoven, 40 245 1269 📖 155
Nijmegen, 80 323 7453 📖 157
Babes Silicone Dildoes
London 📖 69
Babilonia
published by Babilonia Edizione 📖 139
Babilonia Edizione
Milano, 2 569 6468 📖 139
Milano, 2 57 40 4788 📖 139
Babson Gay & Lesbian Alliance
Boston 📖 268
Babykins Products Ltd.
Richmond, 604 275 2255 Ext. 800 665 2229 📖 40
Baccus - Detroit
313 933 9344 📖 275
Back Door BBS
Mountain View, 415 756 2906 (voice, San Francisco) 📖 207
Oakland, 415 756 2906 (voice, San Francisco) 📖 207
Redwood City, 415 756 2906 (voice, San Francisco) 📖 209
San Mateo, 415 756 2906 (voice, San Francisco) 📖 220
Back Door Computing Services
San Francisco, 415 756 2906 📖 1
Backdoor
Frankfurt am Main, 69 28 4311 📖 117
Backdrop Club
Mountain View, 415 965 4499 📖 11, 206, 207
Backroom
Brooklyn, 718 951 8998 📖 297
Backroom II
Asbury Park 📖 289
Backrop
San Francisco 📖 212
Backstage
Nürnberg, 911 241 9383 📖 129
Backstairs
Hannover, 511 1 3858 📖 121
Backstreet
London, 181 980 8557 (club hours) 📖 80
Backwoods Bears
Superior 📖 358
Bad Attitude 📖 85
published by Phantasia Productions 📖 269
Badboy Books
New York, 800 458 9640 (credit card orders) 📖 306
Badlands
Washington, 202 296 0505 📖 233
Baffin Books
Helsinki, 90 694 7078 📖 96
BAGAL 📖 *See* Brattleboro Area Gays &

Lesbians
Bailey/Coy Books
Seattle, 206 323 8842 🕮 353
Baileywick Books
Danbury, 203 354 3865 🕮 230
Baker & Taylor Books
Bridgewater, 908 218 0400 🕮 290
Bakker
Hoorn, 22 921 4903 🕮 156
Baldo's Piercing Studio
Trier, 651 2 8335 🕮 134
Baldwin, Guy, MFCC
Los Angeles, 213 667 9194 🕮 203
Ball Club
Pomona, 909 622 6312 🕮 11
Baltimore Alternative 🕮 264
Baltimore Eagle
410 823 2453 🕮 263
Baltimore Gay Paper 🕮 264
Baltimore Lambda Alliance of the Deaf
410 523 8396 (TTY/TDD) 🕮 264
BAMH 🕮 *See* Bisexual & Married Homosexual Men's Support Group
Bandanna 🕮 291
Banff Regional AIDS Committee
403 762 0690 🕮 42
Bangcók, Hank
Chicago, 312 404 5838 🕮 250
Bank News
Cleveland, 216 281 8777 🕮 319
Banks, Daphnee, MSW, CSW, ACSW
Red Bank, 908 530 8483 🕮 292
Banned
London, 171 704 2766 🕮 86
Banque de Sang Cochin
Paris, 143 29 8385 🕮 103
Banshees
Seattle, 206 329 6374 🕮 351
Banta Company
Menasha, 414 722 7771 🕮 356
Bar Association for Human Rights
New York, 212 431 2156 🕮 188
Bar Mâle
Québec, 418 523 8279 🕮 63
Barbara's Bookstore
Chicago, 312 477 0411 🕮 251
Barbarella
Göteborg 🕮 173
Barbarella (Armoury)
Nottingham, 115 950 0508 🕮 89
Barbary Products
Nailsworth, 145 383 4426 🕮 75
Barbo Carlson Enterprises
Lindsborg, 913 227 3276 🕮 258
Bard Bisexual, Lesbian, & Gay Alliance
Annandale on Hudson, 914 758 6822 🕮 296
Bären Hamburg 🕮 120
Bären Stuttgart 🕮 133
Barenhohle
Sacramento, 916 488 2249 🕮 182
Barfüsser
Zürich, 1 251 4064 🕮 179
Bargain Books
Saint Charles, 800 834 4127 🕮 284
Bargain Books & News Stand
Key West, 305 294 7446 🕮 238
Barn 🕮 *See* Bisexual Atlanta Resource Center
Toronto, 416 977 4702 🕮 55
Barnes Hospital
Saint Louis, 314 362 5000 🕮 284
Barnes Memorial Library, Lambda, Inc.
Birmingham, 205 326 8600 🕮 191
Barnett's Bookstore
Athens, 706 353 0530 🕮 243
Barnett, Joyce
Toronto, 416 698 5183 🕮 55
Baron, Ronald, M.D.
Highland Park, 708 432 7007 🕮 252
Barr, Patricia, Ph.D.
Manchester, 603 647 2366 🕮 288
Bartmäner Bären Köln
221 54 2516 🕮 124
Bartmänner Schweiz, Barbus de Suisse, Barbuti Svizzeri, Barbus Svissers, Beardmen Switzerland
Zurich 🕮 177
BA-SAPPHO 🕮 3
BASIC 🕮 *See* Bay Area Services & Information Coalition
Basil's Bookstore
Cortland, 607 756 9409 🕮 298
BAST
San Francisco 🕮 2
Basta 🕮 *See* Stichting Trefcentrum HIG - COC
Hamburg, 40 24 5979 🕮 107
Basta Boots
Hamburg, 40 24 5979 🕮 107, 120
Batchelor Forum
Rochester, 716 271 6930 🕮 310
Batchelor's Library
Des Moines, 515 266 7992 🕮 256
Bates, Kirk
London, 519 679 6197 🕮 51
Bath Gay & Lesbian Switchboard
122 546 5793 🕮 70
Battalion MC
Dallas / Fort Worth 🕮 340
Batteries Not Includeed
published by BNI 🕮 322
Bawden Printing, Inc.
Eldridge, 319 285 4800 🕮 254
Baxley, Thom
Chicago, 312 275 0130 🕮 248
Bay Area AIDS Support Service
Rotorua, 7 348 1199 Ext. 8980 🕮 163
Bay Area Bisexual Network
San Francisco, 415 703 7977 🕮 215
Bay Area Boxing Club
San Francisco, 415 585 2365 🕮 216
Bay Area Levi & Leather Society
Corpus Christi 🕮 339
Bay Area Reporter 🕮 218
Bay Area Services & Information Coalition (BASIC)
Panama City, 904 785 1088 🕮 241
Bay Area Sexual Minority Youth Network
San Francisco, 415 487 6870 🕮 215
Bay Centre for Birth Control
Toronto, 416 351 3700 🕮 55
Bay Windows 🕮 269
Bayes, Marjorie, Ph.D.
Englewood, 303 377 0246 🕮 229
Bayfront Medical Center
Saint Petersburg, 813 823 1234 🕮 241
Bayley Seton Hospital
New York, 718 390 6000 🕮 302
BB Publications
Southgate 🕮 278
BBL Pony Girl Club
London 🕮 81
BBW
Mississauga 🕮 41
BC Bears
Vancouver 🕮 45
Beach Area Community Health Center
San Diego, 619 488 0644 🕮 211
Beach Board
Fort Myers, 813 278 2893 🕮 237
Beacon 🕮 203
Bear Buddies Toronto 🕮 56
Bear Club Japan
Minato-Ku 🕮 148
Bear Club U. K.
London 🕮 82
Bear Club U.K.
Beswick 🕮 75
Bear History Project
Boston, 617 262 4472 🕮 12
Bear Magazine
published by Brush Creek Media 🕮 217
Bear Man
Tequesta, 407 743 8701 🕮 183
Bear Paws of Iowa
Iowa City 🕮 257
Bear Store
San Francisco, 415 552 1506 🕮 219
BearHug - U. K.
London 🕮 82
BearHug Group
San Francisco, 415 647 9127 🕮 214
BEARS 🕮 2
Bears Down Under
Sydney, 2 550 1331 🕮 26
Bears International
New York, 212 367 7484 🕮 12
Bears LA
Valley Village, 213 850 8958 🕮 224
Bears Netherlands
Delft, 15 261 4291 🕮 154
Bears of Central Florida
Orlando, 407 240 0814 🕮 240
Bears of Mañana
Albuquerque, 505 343 0430 🕮 294
Bears of San Francisco
415 541 5000 🕮 214
Bears of Southwest Florida
Naples 🕮 239
Bears of the Old Pueblo
Tucson, 520 293 9648 🕮 194
Bears on Bikes
Pittsburgh 🕮 331
Bears San Diego
619 696 7639 🕮 211
BEARS-L 🕮 2
Beat
Brisbane, 7 252 2543 🕮 28
Melbourne, 39 827 8748 🕮 24, 32
Beate Uhse
Frankfurt am Main 🕮 117
Frankfurt am Main, 69 23 6280 🕮 117
Hannover 🕮 121
Kiel, 431 97 0833 🕮 123
Ludwigsburg, 294 190 1821 🕮 126
Nürnberg, 911 241 8915 🕮 130
Stuttgart, 771 61 3748 🕮 133
Beau Magazine
published by Sportomatic, Ltd. 🕮 19
Beauftragte für Gleigeschlechtliche Lebensweisen
Leipzig, 341 882 1189 🕮 125
Beaumont Society
London, 1582 412220 🕮 83
Beaumont Trust
London, 171 730 7453 🕮 83
Bedfordshire Lesbian & Gay Helpline
123 421 8990 🕮 70
Bee's Knees
Sydney, 2 361 4888 🕮 27
Beech, Mr. & Mrs.
Launceston 🕮 72
Beer Town Badgers
Milwaukee 🕮 357
Begegnungs- & Beratungs-Zentrum lebensart e. V.
Halle (Saale), 345 512 5103 🕮 119
Begelman, Hedda, MSW, RCSW
New York, 516 795 1320 🕮 300
Behind The Scene 🕮 196
Being Alive
Long Beach, 310 495 3422 🕮 202
Los Angeles, 213 667 3262 🕮 203
San Diego, 619 281 1400 🕮 211
Belfast Butterfly Club
158 543 0408 🕮 164
Bell Croyden, John
London, 171 935 5555 🕮 87
Bellevue Hospital Center
New York, 121 561 4141 🕮 302
Bellville Counseling Associates
Portland, 207 729 8727 🕮 262
Belmont Army Surplus
Chicago, 312 975 0626 🕮 252
Belt Up & Buckle Off
London, 171 737 6161 🕮 69
Ben's Fashion
Schiedam, 10 425 0785 🕮 150
Bendigo Gay Society, Inc.
54 270 312 🕮 31
Benedickt Taschen Verlag GmbH
Köln 🕮 124
Benjamin
Stockholm, 40 611 9923 🕮 175
Benjamin, Shiela, LCSW
Huntington Beach, 714 892 8433 🕮 201
Bennington Area AIDS Project
800 845 2437 🕮 346
Benowitz, Mindy, Ph.D.
Minneapolis / Saint Paul, 612 870 0398 🕮 279
Bent Guide to Gay/Lesbian Canada
published by ECW Press 🕮 42
Beratungsstelle
München, 89 1 9411 🕮 127
Beratungstelephon für Homosexuelle (HAZZ/SOH)
Zürich, 1 271 7011 🕮 179
Beratungstelle für Homosexuelle
Hannover, 511 36 3344 🕮 121
Berdache Books
Pittsburgh, 412 687 5563 🕮 181
Berdache Society
Anchorage 🕮 192
Bergenfield Bears
New York 🕮 304
Bergman, Tod, MSW
Hoboken, 201 795 4050 🕮 290
Berkana Press
Springfield 🕮 181
Berkeley Free Clinic
510 548 2570 🕮 197
Berkshire Alternatives 🕮 273
Berkshire Gay Switchboard
Slough, 1753 856521 🕮 71
Berlin & Brandenburg, Sachsen, Sachsen-Anhalt von Hinten
published by Bruno Gmünder Verlag 🕮 108
Berlin Jacks 🕮 110
Berliner Bären Bartmänner
30 931 6173 🕮 110
Berman Leathercraft
Boston, 617 426 0870 🕮 270
Bernet, Michael
Brooklyn, 718 284 4162 🕮 297
Bernhard Clinic
London, 181 846 1576 🕮 80
Bernstein, Gail, Ph.D.
Denver, 303 832 5123 🕮 227
Berquet, Gilles
Paris, 143 38 3343 🕮 104
Best Adult Bookstore
Irvington, 201 372 0130 🕮 290
Best Book Manufacturers
Toronto, 416 362 1872 🕮 58
Best Guide
Amsterdam, 20 600 2087 🕮 150
Best Publishing Group
49 939 1000 🕮 151
BESTD HIV Outreach Clinic
Milwaukee, 414 272 2144 🕮 357
Beth Israel Medical Center
New York, 212 420 2000 🕮 302
Beth Tyler Labs
Hartford 🕮 231
Bethany Place
Belleville, 618 234 0291 🕮 248
Better Books
Edinburgh, 131 225 1515 🕮 169
Bettinger, Michael, Ph.D., MFCC
San Francisco, 415 563 6100 🕮 213
Betty Page Social Club
Toronto, 416 972 1037 🕮 56
Vancouver, 604 688 4458 🕮 45
Between Ourselves 🕮 316
Wilmington 🕮 316
Between The Lines
published by Diva & Empress Publications, Inc. 🕮 273
Between The Sheets
Calne, 1249 822052 🕮 69
Beyond 2002 🕮 353
Beyond Monogamy, Inc.
Morley 🕮 33
Beyond The Closet
Seattle, 800 238 8518 🕮 353
Beyond Tolerance Task Force
Columbia, 803 777 4172 🕮 334
Beyond Words Bookshop
Northampton, 413 586 6304 🕮 272
BFI Productions
Orange, 714 921 1140 🕮 208
BFLO 🕮 *See* Buffalo Fetish & Leather Organization
B-GALA 🕮 *See* Bisexual, Gay, & Lesbian Alliance
BGALA 🕮 *See* Bryn Mawr / Haverford Bisexual, Gay, & Lesbian Alliance
BGALA-L 🕮 3
BGALOR 🕮 *See* Bisexuals, Gays, & Lesbians of Ryerson
B-GLAD 🕮 *See* Bisexuals, Gay Men, Lesbians, & Allies for Diversity
BGLAD 🕮 *See* Bisexual, Gays, & Lesbian Association at Dalhousie. *See also* Bisexual, Gays, & Lesbians at Davis
BHUS-Linjen

Stockholm, 20 78 3366 175
Bi Chicago
312 275 0186 250
Bi Coastal Productions (BIC)
San Diego, 407 655 0558 212
Bi Face
Vancouver, 604 688 9378 Ext. 2098 45
Bi Focus 331
Bi Line Productions
Los Angeles, 800 743 8377 205
Bi Monthly Bondage
published by Subnormal 248
Bi's R Us
Hull 61
Bi? Shy? Why?
Madison, 608 251 3886 356
BIACT-L 3
BiAtlanta
404 256 8992 244
Biblioteket
Århus, 86 13 1948 65
BIC See Bi Coastal Productions
BiCentrist Alliance
Washington 234
BIFEM-L 3
Biff's Bookstore
Richmond, 804 359 4831 349
Bifocal 281
BIG
San Francisco 188
Big & Tall
San Francisco, 415 864 3456 23
Big Ad Productions
San Francisco, 415 695 2327 217
Big Beary Bulky Boys
Edinburgh, 131 538 7775 168
Big Boys & Buddies 75
Big Breakfast Publishing
Columbus 320
Big Bull, Inc.
Denver 228
Big John's
Riverside, 714 939 0723 209
Big Men of Hawaii
Oahu 247
Big Noise
Bruxelles / Brussel, 2 512 2525 36
Big Ted & Manu 161
Big Time Publications
San Bernardino 210
BiGAYLA See Bisexual, Gay, & Lesbian Alliance at New Paltz
BiGLM See Bisexual, Gay, & Lesbian Mountaineers
Bijou Video
Chicago, 800 932 7111 187, 190
Bike Stop
Philadelphia, 215 627 1662 330
Bi-Line
Brisbane, 7 846 2770 28
Bi-Lines
Columbus, 614 341 7015 320
Bi-Link
Rotterdam 150
Billy De Frank Lesbian & Gay Community Center
San José, 408 293 4525 219
BiNet
Colorado, 303 784 5557 226
Dallas, 214 504 6612 340
Midwest 357
Oregon, 503 236 4941 324
Seattle, 206 728 4533 352
USA, 202 986 7186 265
Binghamton General Hospital
607 762 2200 296
Birmingham Adult Books
205 836 1580 191
Birmingham AIDS Outreach
205 322 4197 191
Birmingham Bi Women's Group
121 622 7351 92
Birmingham University LGB Association
121 472 1841 Ext. 254 93
BiSchoF e. V.
Fulda 118
Bisexual & Married Gay Men
Cleveland, 216 529 9139 319
Bisexual & Married Homosexual Men's Support Group (BAMH)
Adelaide, 8 362 7931 30
Bisexual Atlanta Resource Center (BARN)
404 908 3413 244
Bisexual Community Resource Center
Boston, 617 338 9595 268, 269
Bisexual Connection
Minneapolis / Saint Paul 280
Bisexual Helpline
London, 181 569 7500 79
Bisexual Information & Counseling Service
New York, 212 874 7937 300
Bisexual Phoneline (Scotland)
Edinburgh, 131 557 3620 167
Bisexual Resource Centre
Edinburgh, 131 557 3620 168
Bisexual Support Group
Milwaukee 357
San José, 408 293 2429 219
Bisexual Support Service
Long Beach, 310 597 2799 202
Bisexual Women of Color Group
New York, 212 459 4784 304
Bisexual Women's Group (LGBSA)
State College 333
Bisexual Women's Support Group
Cleveland, 216 467 6442 319
Bisexual, Gay, & Lebian Association of RIT
Rochester, 716 475 3296 311
Bisexual, Gay, & Lesbian Alliance (B-GALA)
Columbus, 6114 292 9212 320
Bisexual, Gay, & Lesbian Alliance at JHU
Baltimore, 410 516 4088 264
Bisexual, Gay, & Lesbian Alliance at New Paltz (BiGAYLA)
914 257 3097 299
Bisexual, Gay, & Lesbian Alliance at Pitt
Pittsburgh, 412 648 2105 332
Bisexual, Gay, & Lesbian Association
Stamford, 203 486 3679 232
Bisexual, Gay, & Lesbian Association, McMaster University
Hamilton, 416 525 9140 Ext. 2041 50
Bisexual, Gay, & Lesbian Awareness
Fox Valley, 414 832 6600 356
Bisexual, Gay, & Lesbian Mountaineers (BiGLM)
Morgantown, 304 293 8200 355
Bisexual, Gay, & Lesbian Youth of New York
212 620 7310 306
Bisexual, Gays, & Lesbian Association at Dalhousie (BGLAD)
Halifax, 902 494 1415 48
Bisexual, Gays, & Lesbians at Davis (BGLAD)
916 757 3848 199
Bisexual, Lesbian, & Gay Alliance at City College New York
212 650 8234 305
Bisexual, Lesbian, & Gay Alliance at York (BLGAY)
North York, 416 736 2100 Ext. 20494 52
Bisexuality & AIDS research Group
Utrecht 158
Bisexuality Newsletter
published by Gibbin Publications 202
Bisexuals in Oxford
186 520 0030 90
Bisexuals, Gay Men, Lesbians, & Allies for Diversity (B-GLAD)
Chapel Hill, 919 962 4401 313
Bisexuals, Gays, & Lesbians of Ryerson (BGALOR)
Toronto, 416 979 5000 Ext. 7527 57
Bisexuellengruppe
Bremen, 421 70 4170 113
BISEXU-L 3
bit.listserv.medforum 5
bit.listserv.medlib-l 5
bit.listserv.mednews 5
bit.med 5
Bitch Buffy
Corpus Christi 339
Bitches With Whips
published by DM International 352
Bi-The-Way
Williamstown 273
BITHRY-L 3
BiUnity
Philadelphia, 215 724 3663 330
BIVERSITY
Boston, 617 338 9595 266
BIversity Boston
617 338 9595 268
Bi-Ways
Washington 234
Bizarre
published by Spartacus 200
Bizarr-Mode
Wien 35
Bizzare Erotic Fantasies
published by B & D Pleasures 203
BJ Ventures
London, 171 734 4585 84
Black
Hamburg, 40 24 0804 119
Black & White Men Together (BWMT)
Baltimore, 410 542 6218 264
Boston 268
Charlotte, 704 563 0067 314
Chicago, 312 334 2012 250
Cleveland, 216 4597 319
Columbus, 614 221 2734 320
Dallas, 214 521 4765 340
Detroit, 313 569 8595 275
Durham 314
Greensboro 315
Indianapolis, 317 253 4297 255
Kansas City, 816 931 4470 283
Louisville, 502 637 3781 259
Louisville, 502 772 3025 259
Memphis, 901 726 1461 337
Milwaukee, 414 265 8500 357
New York, 212 330 7678 304
Pittsburgh, 412 231 3395 332
Tallahassee, 800 624 2968 (national line) 239
Youngstown, 216 782 3483 322
Black Book
published by Amador Communications 15
Black Box
Eindhoven, 40 246 4277 155
Black Box Productions Ltd.
London 84
Black Cap
London, 171 485 1742 80
Black Eagle
Toronto, 800 387 1420 55
Black Eagle Leather Co.
Mission Hills, 818 361 4674 9, 206
Black Eagle MC
Middleboro 271
Black Fire Association
Syracuse, 315 471 4563 312
Black Guard
Minneapolis / Saint Paul 280
Black Hedgehogs Rheinland
Düsseldorf 115
Black HIV/AIDS Network
London, 181 792 9223 82
Black Jack
Los Angeles, 310 338 1516 204
Black Lace
published by BLK Publishing Co. 189
Black Leather In Color (BLIC)
published by BLIC Collective 307
Black Leather Times
published by CBLT 265
Black Lesbian & Gay Centre
London, 171 732 3885 83
Black Light
Köln 108
Black Magic
London, 181 980 1365 81
Black Market
Chicago, 312 278 6780 251
Black Moon Leather
Cathedral City, 619 770 2925 198
Black On Black Leathers
El Cajon, 619 442 6614 183
Black Orchid
Fort Lauderdale, 954 437 5176 236
Black Pages International
published by Blackline Press & Services 15
Black Panther's Club
Lausanne 178
Black Rose
Arlington, 301 369 7667 347
Hobart 31
Black Sheets
published by Amador Communications 20
Black Stratsch
Berlin, 30 793 3692 111
Black Sun Studio
Montréal, 514 345 5701 62
Black Universe
København, 33 32 3113 66
Black Widow's Web
Göteborg 173
BlackFire
published by BLK Publishing Co. 189
Blackhawk MC
Rock Island, 309 788 7389 253
Blackjack Bears of Las Vegas
702 225 4513 286
Blackline Interchain
London, 171 978 4820 69
Blackline Press & Services
Berlin, 30 883 3922 15
Berlin, 30 883 7013 107
Blackliners
London, 171 738 5274 67
Blackstyle
Berlin 111
Blackthorn Books
Leicester, 116 221896 79
BLAGA See Clark University Bisexual, Lesbian, & Gay Alliane
Blair, Ralph
New York, 212 517 3171 300
Blake House Studios
Braintree 75
Blanche Baker Memorial Library & Archives
Los Angeles, 213 735 5252 203
Blasé Ltd.
London, 171 240 6525 85
Blenheim Gay / Lesbian Contact
3 578 2259 161
BLGAY See Bisexual, Lesbian, & Gay Alliance at York
BLIC Collective
New York, 212 229 2502 307
Blikk 164
Blitz
broadcast by FM 92.2, Cable 106.2 130
BLK
published by BLK Publishing Co. 189
BLK Publishing Co.
Los Angeles, 310 410 0808 189
BLMSC See Bournemouth Leather MSC
Block
London, 171 226 7453 80
Montpellier 101
BLOGS
Edinburgh 169
Bloodroot
Bridgeport, 203 576 9168 229
Bloom, Daniel, JD, CSW
New York, 212 674 0404 300
Bloomington Hospital
812 336 6821 253
Bloomsbury Books
Ashland / Medford, 503 488 0029 324
Blowfish
San Francisco, 415 864 0880 10
Blue Blood
published by CBLT 265
Blue Boy
Tilburg, 13 535 4487 158
Blue Door Bookstore
San Diego, 619 298 8610 212
Blue Haze
London 82
Blue Heron Books
Key West, 305 296 3508 238
Blue Max Cycle Club
Saint Louis 284
Blue Max MC
Los Angeles 204
Blue Moon Books
New York, 212 505 6880 181
Blue Mountain Heart To Heart
Walla Walla, 509 529 4744 354

Blue Nights
published by Pride Publishing & Typesetting, Inc. 313
Blue Ridge AIDS Support Group (BRASS)
Roanoke 349
Blue Ridge Lambda Press 347
Blue Star Publications
York, 190 462 4901 88
Blueboy Magazine 307
Bluegrass Bears
Louisville, 502 569 1889 259
Bluegrass C. O. L. T.s
Lexington 259
Bluelights Campaign
San Francisco, 415 863 3540 213
Bluemoon Films
Bromley, 181 466 8296 10
Bluestocking Books
Columbia, 803 929 0114 335
Bluestone Media
Melbourne, 39 419 9877 31
Bluff Park Rare Books
Long Beach, 310 438 9830 203
Blum, Günter
Schatthausen 132
Blume, Sue, CSW
New York, 516 379 4731 300
BMA
Ramsau 107
BMCF Antiquariat
Allmendingen 109
BNI
Yellow Springs 322
Boadecia's Books
Berkeley, 510 559 9184 197
Boalt Hall, UC Berkeley School of Law Lesbian, Gay, & Bisexual Caucus 197
Bob Miller Bookroom
Toronto, 416 922 3557 59
Bob's Rubberwear
London, 181 470 6635 68
Bobbies Bookshop
Edinburgh, 131 229 2338 169
Bobby Goldsmith Foundation
South Australia, 8 362 3106 24
Sydney, 2 360 9755 26
Bodekor, Greg, MS, CAC
Buffalo, 716 884 8670 298
Body Accents
Fishers, 317 842 0569 254
Body Armour Piercing & Tattooing
Edinburgh, 131 558 3717 169
Body Art
published by Body Art, Publications Ltd. 14
Body Art Studios
Bristol, 127 260 3923 70
Body Art, Publications Ltd.
Great Yarmouth 7, 14
Body Aware
Sonoma, 707 935 6595 188
Trowbridge, 1225 774164 68
Body Basics
Chicago, 312 404 5838 250
Body Circle Designs
Seattle, 206 244 8430 352
Body Designs
Bay Shore, 516 968 0141 296
Body Electric School
Oakland, 510 653 1594 208
Body Graphics Tattoo
Thornton, 303 254 4473 229
Body Language
Cleveland, 216 251 3330 319
Body Manipulations
Amsterdam, 20 623 3442 152
San Francisco, 415 621 0408 216
Body Modification Ezine 20
Body Piercer
Sydney, 2 360 4823 27
Body Piercing by Tee
Toronto, 416 929 7330 58
Body Play & Modern Primitives Quarterly
published by Insight Books 206
Body Politic 85
Body Positive
Bedfordshire, 1582 484499 70
Birmingham, 121 212 3636 93
Bournemouth, 1202 297386 73
Dublin, 1 671 2363 137
Grampian, 122 440 4408 168
London, 171 373 9124 67, 82
Merseyside, 151 707 2324 87
North West, 161 237 9717 76
Northern Ireland, 123 223 5515 164
Oxford, 186 520 4606 89
Shropshire, 1743 350075 90
Somerset, 1823 324417 90
Strathclyde, 141 332 5010 169
Wellington, 4 389 3169 163
West Surrey, 1483 418657 91
Body Positive Coalition of Manitoba
Winnipeg, 204 783 5848 47
Body Positive Groups
Århus, 86 18 1646 65
Body Positive Resource Center
Miami, 305 576 1111 239
Body Work Productions
Cleveland, 216 421 7181 319
Body Works Shop
Indianapolis, 317 547 9210 255
Body Worship
New York, 212 614 0124 309
Bodylink Body Piercing
Daw Park, 8 381 5093 31
Bodyshot
Port Elizabeth, 41 308016 10, 19
Bodytech
Van Nuys, 818 385 0633 224
Bodywise
Twickenham, 181 891 1485 87
Bodyworks
London, 171 721 7466 83
Boekhandel Mercurius b.v.
Amsterdam, 10 471 2313 153
Boeki, L.
Bruxelles / Brussel 37
BoisLine
Boise 247
Boîte à Films
Bordeaux, 56 44 8221 98
Boland, Jim, Ph.D.
Berkeley, 510 524 8540 196
Bold Print
Reno, 702 829 2653 287
Bold Type, Inc.
Berkeley, 800 624 8433 197
Bolt
München, 89 26 4323 127
Bolton Lesbian & Gay Switchboard
161 274 3999 78
Bon Vu Enterprises
Compton, 800 827 3787 198
Bondage Book 204
Bondage Fantasies
published by B & D Pleasures 202
Bondage Life
published by Harmony Concepts, Inc. 18
Bondage Reader
published by B & D Pleasures 202
Bondage Times
published by Tiffany Enterprises 311
Book Bin East
Philadelphia, 215 922 9208 331
Book Depot
Miami, 800 438 2750 239
Book Exchange
Birmingham 93
Darlington 73
Book Gallery
New Hope, 215 8622 5110 329
New York, 516 862 7982 308
Book Garden
Denver, 303 399 2004 228
Book Hampton
New York, 516 283 0270 308
New York, 516 324 4939 308
Book Industry Study Group
New York, 212 929 1393 304
Book Loft
Santa Cruz, 408 429 1812 222
Book Mantle
Vancouver, 604 253 1099 46
Book Marketing Council
London, 171 580 6321 83
Book Mart Press
North Bergen, 201 864 1887 292
Book Nook
Naples, 813 262 4740 239
Book Nook, Inc.
Baltimore, 410 752 5778 264
Book Sale Gallery
Ithaca, 607 272 9882 299
Book Soup
Los Angeles, 310 659 3110 205
Book Stall, Inc
Pittsburgh, 412 683 3030 332
Book Woman
Austin, 512 472 2785 339
Book-And
Buffalo, 716 856 8936 298
Bookcase
Hebden Bridge, 1422 845353 94
Bookcrafters
Chelsea, 313 475 9145 274
Bookends
Enfield, 203 745 3988 230
Bookhaven
New Haven, 203 787 2848 231
Bookie Joint
Traverse City, 616 946 8862 278
Bookland
Indianapolis, 317 639 9864 255
Bookland Of Mill Creek
Portland, 207 799 2659 263
Booklegger
Eureka, 707 445 1344 199
Bookmark
Charlottetown, 902 566 4888 61
Bookmark Bookstore
Norwich, 160 376 2855 88
Bookmarks
London, 181 802 6145 85
Bookmasters
Ashland, 419 289 6051 317
Bookpeople
Oakland, 510 632 4700 207
Books & Co.
Dayton, 513 298 6540 321
Books & Company
San Francisco, 415 441 2929 218
Books 'n' Books
Calgary, 403 228 3337 43
Books Bohemian
Los Angeles, 213 385 6761 8
Books Direct
London, 171 371 7004 67
Books In Canada
published by The Canadian Review of Books Ltd. 59
Books Upstairs
Dublin, 1 796687 137
Books, Etc.
London, 171 379 7313 85
Portland, 207 774 0626 263
San Francisco, 415 621 8631 219
Vallejo, 707 644 2935 224
Bookscene
Nottingham 89
Bookshop
Darlinghurst, 2 331 1103 27
Newtown, 2 557 4244 27
Bookshop Santa Cruz
408 423 0900 222
Books-N-Things
Saint Louis, 314 961 3755 284
Bookspeed
Edinburgh, 131 225 4950 168
Bookstore
Gloucester, 508 281 1548 270
Greenville, 601 332 2665 282
Bookstore Ltd.
Modesto, 209 521 0535 206
Bookstore Named Desire
Key West, 305 296 1000 238
Bookstore on West 25th.
Cleveland, 216 566 8897 319
Bookworld Services
Sarasota, 813 758 8094 241
Bookworm
Bridgwater, 127 842 3512 90
Derby, 150 426 1616 73
Boot Camp Saloon
Milwaukee, 414 643 6900 356
Boot Co.
Brisbane 28
Boot Factory
Helsinki, 90 148 1525 96
Boot Lovers' Digest
published by Strictly Speaking Publishing Co. 19
Bootmen Leathers
Eden, 800 216 2668 182
Boots
Antwerpen / Anvers, 3 233 2136 36
Stuttgart, 711 236 4764 132
Victoria, 604 744 5881 12
Boots & Breeches Club
Eastbourne 74
Boots & Saddle
New York, 212 929 9684 300
Border Area Lesbian & Gay Group
Cavan, 42 441 10 136
Border Riders MC
Seattle, 503 256 0197 352
Vancouver, 503 256 0197 45
Borderline Books
Tweed Heads, 7 536 4275 27
Borders Book Shop
Ann Arbor, 313 668 7652 274
Atlanta, 404 237 0707 245
Bethesda, 301 816 1067 265
Des Moines, 515 223 1620 256
Framingham, 508 875 2321 270
Indianapolis, 317 849 8660 255
Kansas City, 913 642 3642 283
Philadelphia, 215 568 7400 331
Pittsburgh, 412 835 5583 332
Borders Gay Switchboard
Hawick, 1450 370 700 167
Bordesley Army & Navy Stores
Birmingham, 121 772 5947 93
Borealis Bookstore
Ithaca, 607 272 7752 299
Borgess Medical Center
Kalamazoo, 616 383 7000 276
Born Free
Corona 198
Borras, Mildred, Ph.D.
New York, 212 505 8371 300
Borxan Publications
Vancouver, 604 264 8666 22
BoSchwul
Bochum, 232 36 8374 112
Boston AIDS Helpline
120 535 4462 79
Boston Bisexual Women's Network
617 3389595 268
Boston Book Review
617 497 0344 269
Boston City Hospital
617 534 5000 267
Boston Ducks
Boylston, 617 783 5298 270
Boston Dungeon Society
Malden 180
Boston Eagle
617 542 4494 267
Boston Gay & Lesbian Helpline
617 267 9001 (voice or TTY) 267
Boston Lesbian & Gay Community Center
617 247 2927 268
Boston Rubber Club
617 734 9582 268
Boston Unified Leather Legion (BULL)
Charlestown, 617 241 8968 270
Boston University Gay, Lesbian, & Bisexual Caucus
617 353 8974 268
Both Sides Now
Maui, 808 572 1884 246
Bottega di Monica e Patrick
Torino 144
Bottom Line 208
Bottomley, Adam
London, 181 964 5058 81
Bottomliners
London, 171 267 8882 84
Bottoms-Up
Manchester, 603 367 8304 288
Boudoir Noir 59
Boudoir Portraits
San Rafael, 415 721 5480 220
Boulder County AIDS Project
303 444 6121 226
Boulevard Books
Pittsburgh, 412 261 9119 332
Boulton & Park Society
Bulverde, 210 980 7788 339

Bound & Gagged
published by Outbound Press 📖 19
published by The Outbound Press 📖 18, 19
Bound By Design
Denver, 303 832 9741 📖 228
Bound by Desire
Austin, 512 473 7104 📖 338
Bound for Pleasure
Boston 📖 267
Bound II
Weston-Super-Mare 📖 68
Bournemouth Leather MSC (BLMSC) 📖 73
Boutique Amour
Luxembourg 📖 148
Boutique Carrefour du Sexe Inc.
Laval, 514 688 6969 📖 61
Montréal, 514 932 1311 📖 63
Boutique de Sade
Hamburg, 40 314 4119 📖 120
Boutique Demonia
Paris 📖 104
Boutique Fancy
Basel / Bâle, 61 271 4656 📖 177
Boutique Highlights
München, 89 527475 📖 128
Boutique Intim
Braunschweig, 531 4 4922 📖 113
Boutique Minuit
Bruxelles / Brussel, 2 223 0914 📖 9, 37
Boutique X
Saint Malo, 99 56 0151 📖 105
Bowerbird Designs
Sydney, 2 267 5471 📖 26
Bowers, Dan
Toronto, 416 962 6969 📖 55
Box 📖 108
Boy Toy
Denver, 303 394 4776 📖 229
Boy Trouble
broadcast by Radio Active FM 89 📖 163
Boy Zone
Wellington, 4 385 0674 📖 163
Boy's Cuir Leather Shop
Marseille 📖 101
Boy's Own
published by FTM Network 📖 85
boys & Dads Association
Toronto, 416 925 9872 Ext. 2174 📖 49
Boys From Syracuse
315 474 3616 📖 312
Boys Own
Harrogate, 1423 526467 📖 88
Boys Will Be Boys
Brisbane, 7 846 3787 📖 28
Northcote 📖 33
Sydney, 2 319 2034 📖 26
Boystown
Calgary, 403 265 2028 📖 42
Boyz
published by Silveraim Ltd. 📖 85
Bradford Friend
1274 723802 📖 94
Bradford Gay & Lesbian Switchboard
1274 722206 📖 94
Halifax, 1274 722206 📖 94
Bradley Books
Frederick, 301 662 9886 📖 265
Bradley Communications Corporation
Lansdowne, 800 989 1400 Ext. 408 📖 329
Brady East STD Clinic
Milwaukee, 414 272 2144 📖 356
Brandeis Triskelion
Boston, 617 736 4761 📖 268
Branding Iron Club
Dallas / Fort Worth 📖 340
Brandon AIDS Support, Inc.
204 726 4020 📖 47
BRASS 📖 *See* Blue Ridge AIDS Support Group
Brass Rail
Charlotte, 704 399 8413 📖 313
Brat Attack 📖 216
Brattleboro Area AIDS Project
802 254 4444 📖 346
Brattleboro Area Gays & Lesbians (BAGAL)
802 254 5947 📖 346
Braun, Etienne
Crauthem, 35 236 5102 📖 148
Braun-Brumfield
Ann Arbor, 313 662 3291 📖 274
Bravo
Tampa, 813 689 1414 📖 187, 242
Brazen Bitch Quarterly (BBQ) 📖 59
Brazos Valley AIDS Foundation
College Station, 409 260 2437 📖 339
Brazos Valley Women's Group
College Station 📖 339
Bread & Roses
broadcast by KBOO Radio FM 90.7 📖 326
Breakaway - Gay Youth Group
Perth, 9 328 9044 📖 34
Breakaway Publications Ltd.
London, 171 377 9426 📖 85
Breathing Space 📖 287
Breene Lithograph, Inc.
Van Nuys, 818 785 8500 📖 224
Brent Photographics
Burnham-on-Sea, 1278 784557 📖 90
Brew City Bears
Milwaukee 📖 357
Brewer, Sue, MSW, LCSW
Saint Petersburg, 813 347 3680 📖 241
Brian Coyle Community Center
Minneapolis / Saint Paul, 612 338 5283 📖 280
Briar Rose
Columbus 📖 320
Brick
Dallas / Fort Worth, 214 521 2024 📖 339
Bridge
Waterville, 207 872 3000 📖 263
Bridge Club
Baltimore 📖 264
Bridge, Michael, Ph.D.
Oahu, 808 526 2605 📖 246
Bridges
Erie, 814 456 9833 📖 328
Lynchburg 📖 348
New York, 516 744 2512 📖 304
Briggs Corporation
Des Moines, 800 247 2343 📖 256
Brigham Women's Hospital
Boston, 617 732 5500 📖 267
Brigid's Trove
Boston, 617 666 9390 📖 268
Brisbane Bisexual Centre
7 391 6025 📖 28
Brisbears
Nundah, 7 3226 8847 📖 29
Bristol Lesbian & Gay Switchboard
117 942 0842 📖 70
Broad Magazine 📖 75
Broadlands Medical Center
Des Moines, 515 282 2200 📖 256
Broadsheet Magazine
published by Womanlife, Inc. 📖 160
Broadway Book & Video
Minneapolis / Saint Paul, 612 338 7303 📖 281
Broadway News Center
Baltimore, 410 342 9590 📖 264
Bromfield Street Educational Foundation
Boston, 617 262 6969 📖 269
Brompton's
London, 171 370 1344 📖 80
Bronson Methodist Hospital
Kalamazoo, 616 341 6000 📖 276
Bronx
Bremen, 421 70 2404 📖 113
Bronx AIDS Services
New York, 718 295 5605 📖 303
Bronx Lebanon Hospital Center
718 590 1800 📖 297
Bronx Lesbian AIDS Task Force
New York 📖 303
Bronx Municipal Hospital Center
718 918 8141 📖 297
Brookdale Hospital Medical Center
Brooklyn, 718 240 5000 📖 297
Brookline Booksmith
Boston, 617 566 6660 📖 269
Brooklyn AIDS Task Force
718 783 0883 📖 297
Brooklyn Hospital Center
718 250 8005 📖 297
Brooklyn Lesbian Youth Sisters
718 499 0352 📖 298
BROS
Rochester, 716 323 2419 📖 12
Brother Sister 📖 32
Brother's Touch
Minneapolis / Saint Paul, 612 377 6279 📖 281
Brotherhood of Pain
Houston 📖 342
Brothers In Leather
New York 📖 303
Brothers MC, Inc.
Jacksonville, 904 353 9973 📖 238
Broward Adult Books
Fort Lauderdale, 305 792 4991 📖 237
Broward General Medical Center
Fort Lauderdale, 305 355 5610 📖 236
Brown, Ian
London, 171 916 2834 📖 80
Browning Grace Communications
San Francisco, 415 905 8590 📖 217
Brug
Gent / Gand, 9 226 3869 📖 38
Bruna
Amsterdam, 20 622 0578 📖 153
Bruno Gmünder Verlag
Berlin, 30 615 00342 📖 108
Bruno Gmünder Versand
Berlin, 30 615 00342 📖 107
Bruno's
Berlin, 30 882 4290 📖 111
Brush Away
Chislehurst, 181 467 1998 📖 78
Brush Creek Media
San Francisco, 800 234 3877 📖 217
Brush Hill Press
Boston, 800 403 4367 📖 269
Brushstrokes
Atlanta, 404 876 6567 📖 245
Bryn Mawr / Haverford Bisexual, Gay, & Lesbian Alliance (BGALA) 📖 328
BSG
Birmingham 📖 93
BS-Laden
Zürich, 1 2241 0441 📖 180
BU GLASS
Brandon, 204 727 4279 📖 47
Bücherboom
Hamburg, 40 390 5436 📖 120
Bücherkiste
Nürnberg, 911 22 2423 📖 129
Buchfink
Celle, 514 121 7420 📖 113
Buchhandlung Berliner Promenade
Saarbrücken, 681 3 2670 📖 132
Buchhandlung Decins
Hannover, 511 36 3663 📖 121
Buchladen 46
Bonn, 228 22 3608 📖 112
Buchladen am Markt
Offenbach, 69 88 3333 📖 130
Buddenbrooks
Boston, 617 536 4433 📖 269
Buddies
Denver, 303 289 9301 📖 227
Buddy
München, 89 26 8938 📖 128
Buddy Bears of Philadelphia
215 467 5479 📖 330
Buffalo
Las Vegas, 702 733 8355 📖 286
Buffalo Fetish & Leather Organization (BFLO) 📖 298
Buffalo General Hospital
716 845 5600 📖 298
Buffalo Transition Support
716 629 5421 📖 298
Bug House
São Paulo, 11 257 3131 📖 39
BULGA 📖 *See* Bulgarian Lesbian & Gay Association
Bulgarian Lesbian & Gay Association (BULGA)
Sofia, 2 58 5271 📖 40
Bulk Club U.K.
London 📖 82
Bulk Male
published by Big Bull, Inc. 📖 228
BULL 📖 *See* Boston Unified Leather Legion
Bull Durham's News
919 286 4054 📖 314
Bulldog Books
Sydney, 2 699 3507 📖 26
Bulldog News
Olympia, 206 357 6397 📖 350
Seattle, 206 322 6397 📖 353
Seattle, 206 632 6397 📖 353
Bulletin Lambda
broadcast by FM 102.3 📖 63
Bullock's Leather & Accessories
Los Angeles, 213 665 5343 📖 205
Bundaberg Gay & Lesbian Support
7 152 9999 📖 29
Bunker Hill Consultation Center
Princeton, 609 497 0899 📖 292
Bunte Tunte
Wupperthal, 202 439 2874 📖 135
Bureau 700
Gouda, 18 251 4381 📖 155
Bureau Local d'Intervention Traitant du SIDA
Victoriaville, 819 758 2662 📖 63
Bureau Régional d'Action SIDA
Gatineau, 819 568 2727 📖 61
Burgoyne, Bob, M.S.W.
Toronto, 416 463 0950 📖 55
Burlington Women's Council
802 865 7200 📖 346
Burn 📖 24
Burnet Bookstore
Syracuse, 315 471 9230 📖 312
Burnley AIDS Line
800 220 704 📖 78
Burnley Switchboard
1772 51122 📖 78
Büro für Gleichgeschlectliche Lebensfragen in Land Brandenburg
Potsdam, 331 866 5173 📖 131
Busch Counseling Center, Inc.
Tampa, 813 933 6904 📖 242
Bushido
Milano, 2 670 6420 📖 139
Butch / Femme Network
West Hollywood, 213 993 7235 📖 225
Butler's Uniforms
San Francisco, 415 863 8119 📖 219
Butte AIDS Support Services
406 494 6125 📖 285
Buzios Mode
Düsseldorf, 211 333736 📖 115
BVH - Bundesverband Homosexualität e. V.
Berlin, 30 581 8306 📖 108
BVH e. V. - Dortmund
231 28 3333 📖 114
BWMT 📖 *See* Black & White Men Together
By The Books
Russian River, 707 869 9031 📖 200
Byrum, Mildred, Ph.D.
New York, 212 674 1091 📖 300
ByteMine Adult Baby BBS
El Cajon 📖 199
C & S Constructions
Wokingham 📖 71
C. L. E. F.
Paris, 142 70 3132 📖 13
Cabell Huntington Hospital
304 526 2000 📖 354
Cable Access Channel 21
Columbus, 614 299 7764 📖 321
Cable Access TV
Portland, 503 244 6483 📖 324
Cable TV
San Francisco, 415 861 7131 📖 219
CAC 📖 *See* Cornwall AIDS Council
CADAR 📖 *See* Chester & District AIDS Relief
Café Adler
Hamburg 📖 119
Café Moustache
Paris, 146 07 7207 📖 102
Café Schwarz
Weimar, 364 3 3407 📖 135
Café Stonewall
Dortmund, 231 17 8145 📖 114
Cage
Pacific Beach, 619 531 9573 📖 208
Cahiers Gai-Kitsch-Camp (CKC)
Lille, 20 06 3391 📖 14
Cahoots
Salt Lake City, 801 538 0606 📖 345
CAIRDE

Dublin, 1 873 3799 📖 137
Caithness Gay, Bisexual, & Lesbian Connexion
Wick 📖 168
Cal State / Northridge LGBA
Los Angeles, 818 885 2393 📖 204
Calendar of Events 📖 238
Caliber
Chicago, 312 728 7228 (retail) 📖 251
California B & B Corps
Los Angeles 📖 204
California Cyclemen MC
San Diego 📖 211
California Eagles MC
San Francisco, 415 267 0560 📖 215
Callan Military Surplus
Liverpool, 151 236 8753 📖 87
Cambridge AIDS Helpline
800 697 697 📖 71
Cambridge Documentary Films, Inc.
Boston, 617 354 3677 📖 15
Cambridge Friend
122 324 6013 📖 71
Cambridge Hospital
Boston, 617 498 1000 📖 267
Camera Art
Woodland Hills, 818 766 1448 📖 23
Camouflage
Vancouver 📖 46
Camp International, Inc.
Jackson, 517 787 1600 📖 276
Campaign
published by Worlander Pty. Ltd. 📖 24
Campus Queers (GUSS)
Christchurch 📖 161
Campus Studios
Woodland Hills, 818 340 7290 📖 225
can.motss 📖 6
Canadian AIDS Society / Société Canadienne du SIDA
Ottawa, 613 230 3580 📖 41
Canadian Association of Body Arts
Toronto 📖 41
Canadian Book Marketing Centre
Toronto, 416 413 4930 📖 57
Canadian Crossdressers Club
Toronto, 416 921 6112 📖 57
Canadian Foundation for AIDS Research (CANFAR)
Toronto, 416 361 6281 📖 41
Canadian Human Rights Commission
Ottawa, 613 995 1151 📖 41
Toronto Office, 416 973 5527 📖 57
Canadian Lesbian & Gay Archives
Toronto, 416 777 2755 📖 55
Canadian Library Association
Ottawa, 613 232 9626 Ext. 301 📖 53
Canadian Review of Books Ltd.
Toronto, 416 601 9880 📖 59
Canadian Tattoo Association
Qualicum Beach 📖 41
Canadian Women's Movement Archives
Ottawa, 613 562 5910 📖 40
Canarelli, Joseph, CSW
New York, 212 529 8940 📖 300
Candle Bar
New York, 212 874 9155 📖 300
CANFAR 📖 *See* Canadian Foundation for AIDS Research
Cape Fear Valley Medical Center
Fayetteville, 910 609 4000 📖 315
Capital City Press, Inc.
Montpelier, 802 223 5207 📖 346
Capital City Riders MC
Austin 📖 338
Capital District Lesbian & Gay Community Center
Albany, 518 462 6138 📖 296
Capital Findings & Leather
Toronto, 416 363 8563 📖 60
Capital Q 📖 27
Capital Xtra!
published by Pink Triangle Press 📖 53
Capitol Men's Club
Lansing, 517 484 6342 📖 277
Capitol Tattoo
Silver Spring, 301 585 3483 📖 266
Capitulation
published by Fantastic Books Publications 📖 296
Capone, Julie, CSW
New York, 516 367 1016 📖 300
Capone, Thomas, Ph.D.
New York, 516 367 1016 📖 300
Caprice
Los Angeles 📖 182
Capson, Stephen, Psy.D.
New York, 212 769 8299 📖 300
Captial District Center for Dissociative Disorders
Albany, 518 462 0213 📖 295
CARA - Carers for People Living with AIDS
Adelaide, 8 362 3208 📖 30
Cara Friend
Belfast, 1232 238668 📖 164
Cardell, Mona, Ph.D.
Havertown, 610 446 9625 📖 328
Cardiff AIDS Helpline
122 222 3443 📖 359
Cardiff Friend
1222 340101 📖 359
Cardiff Switchboard
1222 374051 📖 359
Cardome
Brighton, 127 369 2916 📖 74
Cardozo Gay & Lesbian Law Student Alliance
New York 📖 305
CARE Virginia
Arlington 📖 347
Careline
London, 181 514 1177 📖 80
Carellas, Barbara
New York, 212 247 2354 📖 13
CARES 📖 *See* Collier AIDS Resource & Education Service, Inc.. *See also* Community AIDS Resource & Education Service
Caress Magazine
published by The Write Solution 📖 74
Caring Counseling
Reno, 702 322 7771 📖 287
Caritasverband Beratung Homosexueller Männer & AIDS Beratung
Magdeburg, 391 3 8075 📖 126
Carl Vogel Foundation, Inc.
Washington, 202 289 4898 📖 234
Carl von Ossietsky Buchhandlung
Oldenburg 📖 130
Carleton University Gay, Lesbian, & Bisexual Centre
Ottawa, 613 788 2600 Ext. 1860 📖 53
Carline Leathers
Chicago, 312 334 1444 📖 251
Carlisle Citizens Advice Bureau
122 859 1986 📖 72
Carlos Clarke, Bob
London, 171 499 9493 📖 83
Carmarthen AIDS Helpline
1267 221079 📖 359
Carmichael's Bookstore
Louisville, 502 456 6950 📖 259
Carolina Bear Lodge
Charlotte, 704 529 2891 📖 313
Carolina Trans-Sensual Alliance
Charlotte, 704 531 8838 📖 314
Carolinas Medical Center
Charlotte, 704 355 2000 📖 313
Caroline Street Books
Key West, 305 24 3931 📖 238
Carolyn's Kids
Melrose, 617 662 4432 📖 183
Carousel Books
Nashville, 615 352 0855 📖 337
Carousel Club of South Australia
Adelaide, 8 388 3644 📖 30
Carpe Diem
Torino, 11 50 0018 📖 139
Carrey Friend
Douglas, 1624 611600 📖 77
Carrousel Club, Inc.
Adelaide, 8 281 6190 📖 29
Carter Stevens Presents
Pocono Summit, 717 839 2512 📖 332, 333
Cascade AIDS Project
Portland, 503 223 5907 📖 326
Portland, 800 777 2437 📖 326
Cascade Handballers
Seattle, 206 747 5510 📖 352
CAST 📖 *See* Community AIDS Support Team
Castaways MC
Milwaukee 📖 357
Castigatio
Leiden 📖 150
Castlebar
San Francisco, 415 552 2100 📖 212
Catalog Connection
London, 171 371 7004 📖 67
Catalog X
Fort Lauderdale, 954 524 5050 📖 186, 237
Category Six Books
Denver, 303 832 6263 📖 190
Cathedral of Hope
Dallas / Fort Worth, 214 351 1901 Ext. 114 📖 341
Catholic AIDS Link
London, 171 485 7298 📖 82
Cathouse Design Studio
Liversedge, 1924 412662 📖 68
Cattlemen's Exchange Club
Phœnix, 602 266 0875 📖 193
Caught In The Act
Ottawa 📖 41
Cauldron 📖 202
CAVE 📖 *See* Centro Antivenereo
CB&V
Las Vegas 📖 286
CBLT
Gaithersburg, 301 975 7092 📖 265
CC Slaughter's
Portland, 503 248 9135 📖 326
CC Slaughter's North
Seattle, 206 323 4017 📖 350
CD Network
Rochester, 716 251 2132 📖 311
CD Research Center
Leavenworth 📖 258
CDC National AIDS Hotline
Research Triangle Park, 800 342 2437 📖 181
CDC National STD Hotline
Research Triangle Park, 800 227 8922 📖 181
CD-FORUM 📖 3
CDI 📖 *See* Cross Dressers International
CDM
Milano, 2 839 4604 📖 143
Cedars-Sinai Medical Center
Los Angeles, 310 855 5000 📖 203
Cégep de l'Outaouais
Ottawa, 613 771 4344 📖 53
CEI
Bern, 31 42 3666 📖 176
Celebrate The Self
published by Factor Press 📖 192
Celebrity Circumcision Survey Master List 📖 201
Celestial Krewe de Cuir
San Francisco, 415 255 4663 📖 214
Cell Bar
Bolton, 120 421 856 📖 78
Cell Block
Chicago, 312 665 8064 📖 248
Cellar
Bury Saint Edmund's 📖 91
Cellar Leather Club
Manchester, 161 236 8800 📖 75
Cellblock
Ottawa, 613 594 0233 📖 52
Cellblock 28
Bronx, 718 733 3144 📖 297
Centaur Magazine 📖 199
Centaur MC
Washington, 703 461 0967 📖 234
Center
Columbia, 800 325 4297 📖 335
Las Vegas, 702 733 9800 📖 286
Center for Change, Development, & Support
Dallas / Fort Worth, 817 429 4706 📖 340
Center for Contemporary Counseling
Aventura, 305 936 8000 📖 235
Center for Disease Control
Birmingham, 205 991 6920 📖 188
Center for Gender Reassignment
Norfolk, 804 622 9900 📖 348
Center For Identity Development
Montclair, 201 744 6386 📖 291
Center For Identity Development South, Ltd.
Fort Lauderdale, 305 345 5525 📖 236
Center for Lesbian & Gay Community Services
Nashville, 615 297 0008 📖 337
Center for Lesbian & Gay Studies
New York, 212 642 2924 📖 303
Center for Non-Traditional Families
New York, 212 721 1012 📖 300
Center for Research & Education in Sexuality
San Francisco, 415 338 1137 📖 215
Center News 📖 205
Center One
Fort Lauderdale, 305 537 4111 📖 236
Center Project, Inc.
Fox Valley, 414 437 7400 📖 355
Central Alberta AIDS Network Society
Red Deer, 403 346 8858 📖 44
Central Books
London, 181 986 4854 📖 80
Central City AIDS Network
Macon, 912 750 8080 📖 245
Central Illinois Gender Association (CIGA)
Washington, 309 444 9918 📖 253
Central Iowa Gender Institute
Des Moines, 515 277 7754 📖 256
Central Jersey Alliance of Gay, Lesbian, & Bisexual People
Plainfield, 908 756 4955 📖 292
Central Louisana AIDS Support Services (CLASS)
Alexandria, 800 444 7993 📖 260
Central Michigan University Lesbian & Gay Alliance
Mount Pleasant, 517 774 3822 📖 277
Central Ohio Gender Dysphoria Program
Columbus, 614 451 0111 📖 320
Central Oregon AIDS Support Team
Bend, 503 389 4330 📖 324
Central Valley AIDS Team
Fresno, 209 264 2437 📖 199, 200
Central Vermont Gay Liberation (CVGL)
Plainfield, 802 454 8078 📖 346
Central Virginia AIDS Services & Education (CVASE)
Richmond, 804 359 4783 📖 349
Central Wisconsin AIDS Support Group
Wausau 📖 358
Central Wyoming Transgender Support Group
Casper, 307 473 2429 📖 358
Centre d'Action SIDA Montréal (Femmes)
514 989 7997 📖 62
Centre de Dépistage
Mulhouse, 89 54 9033 📖 101
Centre de Prophylaxie
Lille, 20 54 5773 📖 100
Centre de Prophylaxie des MST
Dunkerque, 28 24 0400 📖 99
Centre de Prophylaxie et MST
Caen, 31 94 8422 📖 99
Centre de Santé
Aix-en-Provence, 42 23 3519 📖 97
Centre des R. O. S. É. S. de l'Abititbi-Témiscamingue
Noranda, 819 764 9111 📖 63
Centre Elisa Centrum
Bruxelles / Brussel, 2 513 2651 📖 37
Centre Figuier
Paris, 142 78 5573 📖 102
Centre for Sexuality
Vancouver 📖 45
Centre Gai & Lesbien (CGL)
Paris, 143 57 2147 📖 103
Centre Gai & Lesbien de l'UQAM
Montréal, 514 987 3039 📖 62
Centre Hospitalier
Annecy, 50 45 1649 📖 98
Argenteuil, 34 23 2620 📖 98
Bordeaux, 56 98 4607 📖 98
Meaux, 64 35 3838 📖 101
Poitiers, 49 44 3905 📖 105
Centre Hospitalier Beausecours
Metz, 87 63 1313 📖 101
Centre Hospitalier d'Alençon
33 32 3049 📖 97
Centre Hospitalier d'Amiens
22 89 0222 📖 97
Centre Hospitalier d'Angers
41 35 3419 📖 98
Centre Hospitalier d'Auxerre
86 48 4718 📖 98
Centre Hospitalier d'Epinal
29 31 3131 📖 99

Centre Hospitalier de Belfort
Beauvais, 84 28 1712 📖 98
Centre Hospitalier de Brest
98 22 3333 📖 99
Centre Hospitalier de Cahors
65 20 5050 📖 99
Centre Hospitalier de Chambéry
79 96 5050 📖 99
Centre Hospitalier de Charleville
Bordeaux, 24 56 7070 📖 98
Centre Hospitalier de Gap
92 40 6161 📖 100
Centre Hospitalier de Grenoble
76 87 6240 📖 100
Centre Hospitalier de Guéret
55 51 7000 📖 100
Centre Hospitalier de la Rochelle
46 27 3333 📖 100
Centre Hospitalier de Laval
43 66 5000 📖 100
Centre Hospitalier de Montpellier
67 33 9302 📖 101
Centre Hospitalier de Nancy
83 57 6161 📖 102
Centre Hospitalier de Nantes
40 48 3333 📖 102
Centre Hospitalier de Pau
59 84 1350 📖 104
Centre Hospitalier de Privas
Poussan, 75 64 1177 📖 105
Centre Hospitalier de Saint Denis
42 35 6067 📖 105
Centre Hospitalier de Saint Michel
45 24 4040 📖 105
Centre Hospitalier de Soissons
23 59 1102 📖 106
Centre Hospitalier de Toulouse Hôtel Dieu
61 77 8133 📖 106
Centre Hospitalier de Tours
47 34 8111 📖 106
Centre Hospitalier E. Muller
Mulhouse, 89 64 6464 📖 101
Centre Hospitalier Général
Meaux, 64 33 4935 📖 101
Centre Hospitalier Général Faconaja
Corse, 95 55 1111 📖 99
Centre Hospitalier Intercommunal
Créteil, 48 98 7758 📖 99
Centre Hospitalier la Grave
Toulouse, 61 77 7859 📖 106
Centre Hospitalier La Meynard
Fort-de-France, 50 1515 📖 149
Centre Hospitalier Laennec
Quimper, 98 90 3030 📖 105
Centre Hospitalier Louis Pasteur
Cherbourg, 33 20 7000 📖 99
Centre Hospitalier Notre Dame de la Misericorde
Corse 📖 99
Centre Hospitalier Orléans-la-Source
38 51 4361 📖 102
Centre Hospitalier R. Pontchaillou
Rennes, 99 28 4302 📖 105
Centre Hospitalier R. U. Dupuytren
Limoges, 55 06 6652 📖 100
Centre Hospitalier Regional
Nîmes, 66 27 4111 📖 102
Centre Médical
Cannes, 93 39 0636 📖 99
Centre Médico-Social
Amiens, 22 91 0770 📖 97
Boulogne-sur-Mer, 21 31 5656 📖 98
Paris, 145 43 8378 📖 103
Paris, 147 97 4049 📖 102
Saint Malo, 99 56 1156 📖 105
Centre Regional d'Information & de Prévention du SIDA (CRIPS)
Paris, 53 68 8888 📖 103
Centre SIDA Amitié
Saint Antoine des Laurentides, 514 431 7432 📖 63
Centro Antivenereo (CAVE)
Milano, 2 550 35226 📖 142
Centro d'Iniziativa Gay
Milano, 2 839 4604 📖 143
Centro de Informacion y Documentacion de las Homosexualidades en Mexico Celectivo Sol, A. C. (CIDHOM)
Mexico City 📖 149
Centro de Orientção e Aconselhamento em AIDS e Doeças Sexualmente Transmissiveis
São Paulo, 11 239 2224 📖 39
Contro do Saudo Santa Cocilia
São Paulo, 11 826 7970 📖 39
Centro Democeltico
Brescia, 30 399 4615 📖 142
Centro Dermoceltico
Venezia, 41 522 1942 📖 147
Centro Dermoceltico USL
Mestre 📖 146
Centro di Documentazione
Bologna, 51 644 6824 📖 140
Centro Epidemiologico Sardo
Cagliari 📖 145
Centro MTS
Gorizia 📖 141
Centro Ospedale di Borgo di Trento
Verona, 45 93 2647 📖 147
Centro per le Donne
Bologna, 51 233863 📖 140
Centrum Für Sexualwissenschaft e. V.
Berlin, 30 891 6046 📖 110
Centurion 📖 151
Centurions of Columbus 📖 320
Century City Hospital
Los Angeles, 310 553 6211 📖 203
Cercle Homosexuel Etudiant de l'ULB (CHE)
Bruxelles / Brussel, 2 650 2540 📖 37
Cerebus
Bournemouth, 1202 290529 📖 73
CF Publications
East Setauket, 516 689 6743 📖 299
CFLM Austria
Wien, 1 786 0835 📖 35
CFMU 93.3 FM
Hamilton, 905 525 9140 Ext. 27397 📖 50
CFRU FM 93.3
Waterloo 📖 61
CFUV FM 101.9
Victoria, 604 721 8702 📖 47
CGL 📖 *See* Centre Gai & Lesbien
Chain Drive
Austin, 512 478 0295 📖 338
Chain Gang Promotions
London, 171 284 2180 📖 84
Chain Link Addiction
Cleveland 📖 319
Chain Mail Creations
Los Angeles, 213 660 6533 📖 203
Chain Maille Fashions
Austin, 800 729 4094 📖 182
Chain of Command
San Antonio, 210 979 7752 📖 344
Chain, Steven, LCSW
Denver, 303 393 7120 📖 227
Chained
published by Carter Stevens Presents 📖 332
Chained Male
Barrie, 705 737 9791 📖 49
Chainmail 📖 238
Chains
Detroit, 313 897 3650 📖 274
Köln, 221 23 8730 📖 124
Challengers International MC
Orlando, 407 425 9836 📖 240
Chameleon
Oxford, 614 529 3823 📖 322
Chameleons
Adelaide, 8 362 3208 📖 30
Chamleon Society
Victoria Park, 15 771753 📖 34
Champagne Productions
New York, 212 982 0384 📖 19
Champaign-Urbana Bisexual Network
Champaign / Urbana 📖 248
Chandelles
Paris 📖 103
Changing Hands Bookstore
Phœnix, 602 966 0203 📖 194
Changing Men 📖 257
Changing Times Bookstore
West Palm Beach, 407 640 0496 📖 243
Channel 11
Winnipeg 📖 48
Channel Six
Bremerhaven, 471 5 6595 📖 113
Chaotic Creations
Meriden, 203 639 6105 📖 11
Chapin, Suzanne, M.A.
Danbury, 203 792 8423 📖 230
Chaps
Hamburg, 40 23 0647 📖 119
Portland 📖 326
Chapter One Books
New Brunswick, 908 828 7648 📖 291, 292
Chardmore Services
London, 181 392 9052 📖 81
Charis Books & More
Atlanta, 404 524 0304 📖 245
Charleston AIDS Network
304 345 4673 📖 354
Charleston Area Medical Center
304 348 5432 📖 354
Chart Room Saloon
Portland, 207 774 9262 📖 262
Chase Brexton Clinic
Baltimore, 410 837 2050 📖 263
Chase Products
Novi, 313 348 8191 📖 184
Chase Products & FPN6D Services
Novi, 810 348 8191 📖 183
Chassman & Bern Booksellers
Burlington, 802 862 4332 📖 346
Chastete
Lake Villa, 708 356 8300 📖 252
Château IV Bookstore
Columbia, 803 754 0713 📖 335
Chatt
published by Chatterly's 📖 59
Chatterly's
Toronto 📖 59
Chaud Business SPRL
Bruxelles / Brussel, 2 537 8404 📖 37
CHE 📖 *See* Cercle Homosexuel Etudiant de l'ULB
Checkmate & DungeonMaster
published by Telecentral Electronics 📖 15, 16
Checkpoint
Köln, 221 25 5009 📖 124
Chelmsford Lesbian & Gay Switchboard
124 542358 📖 75
Chelsea Bookstore
Long Beach, 310 434 2220 📖 203
Chelsea Psychotherapy Associates
New York, 212 206 0045 📖 300
Chelsea Station News
Knoxville, 615 522 6390 📖 336
CheLSI e. V.
Chemnitz, 371 50094 📖 113
Cherry, Roxanne, Ph.D.
Laguna Beach, 714 497 9925 📖 201
Chesapeake Bay Bears
Annandale 📖 347
Chesapeake Psychological Services
Baltimore, 410 321 1091 📖 263
Cheshire Counseling Associates
Keene, 603 357 5544 📖 287
Chest Men of America
Chicago, 312 975 9593 📖 249
Chester & District AIDS Relief (CADAR)
1244 390300 📖 71
Chester, Mark
San Francisco, 415 621 6294 📖 216
Chevalier, Remy
Weston, 203 227 2065 📖 232
Chi Town Society
Chicago 📖 250
CHIC 📖 *See* Crossdresser Heterosexual Intersocial Club
Chicago Eagle
312 728 0050 📖 248
Chicago Gender Society
312 863 7714 📖 250
Chicago Hellfire Club
312 486 2436 📖 249
Chicago Jacks 📖 250
Chicago Runaway Switchboard
800 621 3230 📖 249
Chicago Tribune 📖 251
Chicagoland Discussion Group
312 281 1097 (24hr. infoline) 📖 249
Chicos
published by Studios J. M. R. 📖 172
Children of Lesbians & Gays Everywhere (COLAGE)
Chicago, 312 583 8029 📖 250
Toronto 📖 56, 57
Children's Hospital
New Orleans, 504 8999 9511 📖 260
Chiltern Mountain Club
Boston, 617 859 2843 📖 268
ChilternAIDS
High Wycombe, 1494 444818 📖 71
Chimney Sweep Books
Santa Cruz, 408 458 1044 📖 222
Chinese HIV/AIDS Support
London, 171 287 0904 📖 82
Chiron Rising
published by Chiron Rising Publications 📖 224
Chiron Rising Publications
Victorville 📖 224
Chiron, J. P.
Angers, 41 60 3876 📖 98
CHKK
Muskogee 📖 323
Choc Monsieur
Montréal, 514 521 7558 📖 63
Chocopot
broadcast by Radio Centraal FM 101.6 📖 36
Choices Books & Music
Santa Barbara, 805 965 5477 📖 221
Choices Women's Medical Center, Inc.
Forest Hills, 718 275 6020 📖 299
Chosen Books
Royal Oak, 800 453 5758 📖 278
Chouraqui, Robert
Mons, 16 048 0917 📖 101
Chow Chow Productions
Seattle, 206 322 6862 📖 353
Chris
Chicago, 312 404 6107 📖 250
London, 181 655 2332 📖 80
Christchurch Lesbian Gay Radio Collective
3 3657 999 📖 23
Christian Hospital Northeast
Saint Louis, 314 355 2300 📖 284
Christian Hospital Northwest
Saint Louis, 314 839 3800 📖 284
Christie's Toy Box
Dallas / Fort Worth, 817 244 8008 📖 341
Oklahoma City, 405 631 1399 📖 323
Portland, 503 771 9979 📖 327
Wichita, 913 226 3004 📖 258
Christine Le Duc
Amsterdam 📖 153
Amsterdam, 20 623 1321 📖 153
Amsterdam, 20 623 8732 📖 153
Amsterdam, 20 624 8265 📖 153
Arnhem 📖 154
Breda, 76 522 5777 📖 154
Den Haag, 20 362 5295 📖 154
Eindhoven, 40 243 9081 📖 155
Groningen 📖 155
Haarlem 📖 155
Heerlen 📖 156
Hertogenbosch, 's / Den Bosch 📖 156
Nijmegen 📖 157
Rotterdam, 10 467 9527 📖 158
Utrecht, 30 242 6956 📖 158
Volendam 📖 150
Christine's Lingerie Inc.
Tampa, 813 979 0154 📖 243
Christopher Briston Enterprises
Elma 📖 182
Christopher Collection
Phœnix, 800 851 0690 📖 186
Christopher Street 📖 308
Christopher Street Bookstore
Tustin, 714 731 0224 📖 223
Christopher Street Counseling & Bookstore
Tustin, 714 731 0224 📖 223
CHRU de Nîmes
66 27 3175 📖 102
CHRW 94.7 FM
London, 519 661 3601 📖 51
Chubbies & Chasers of Cleveland
Lakewood 📖 321
Church of All Worlds
Ukiah 📖 223
Church of Epiphany
Newport Beach 📖 207

CIC See AHF-Switchboard
Cicolo Di Cultura Omosexxuale Mario Mieli
Roma, 6 541 3985 141
CIDHOM See Centro de Informacion y Documentacion de las Homosexualidades en Mexico Celectivo Sol, A. C.
CIGA See Central Illinois Gender Association
Cigar Studs
Lakewood 202
San Antonio 344
Cincinnati Chaps 318
Cincinnati's River Bears
513 921 6472 318
Cinéma Bleu Inc.
Toronto, 416 922 9112 60
Circle of Care
Fairfield, 203 255 7965 230
Circlet Press
Boston, 617 864 0492 269
Circlet Press Bookshop
Boston, 617 864 0492 8
Circumcision Resource Center
Boston, 617 523 0088 268
Circus of Books
Los Angeles, 213 666 1304 205
West Hollywood, 213 656 6533 225
Cité Sanitaire
Toulon, 94 89 9020 106
CITR FM 101.9
Vancouver, 604 685 2746 46
City Bikers MC
Denver, 303 369 0522 228
City East Adult Bookstore
Melbourne, 39 650 4763 32
City Hospital
Cape Town, 21 22 2711 170
City Lakes Crossgender Community (CLCC)
Minneapolis / Saint Paul, 612 229 3613 280
City Lights Bookstore
San Francisco, 415 362 8193 218
City Map Produkties
Amsterdam, 20 626 0702 150
City Men Shop & Video
Berlin, 30 218 2959 111
City Sex Boutique
Stuttgart, 711 24 4928 133
City Sex Shop
Kassel, 561 1 7587 123
CIUT 89.5 FM
Toronto, 416 595 0909 59
CKC See Cahiers Gai-Kitsch-Camp
CKCU FM 93.1
Ottawa 53
CKMS FM 94.5
Waterloo 61
CKWR FM 98.7
Waterloo, 519 886 9870 61
cl.freie_liebe.hetero 6
cl.freie_liebe.schwule 6
ClaireLight
Santa Rosa, 707 575 8879 222
Clan Masters
Paris 103
clari.news.crime.sex 6
clari.news.gays 6
clari.news.law.crime.sex 6
clari.news.sex 6
clari.tw.health 5
clari.tw.health.aids 5
Clark County American Red Cross
Springfield, 513 399 3872 322
Clark County Health & Education Department
Springfield, 513 328 2665 322
Clark University Bisexual, Lesbian, & Gay Alliane (BLAGA)
Worcester, 508 793 7287 273
Clark's Out of Town News
Fort Lauderdale, 305 467 1543 237
Clarke Institute of Psychiatry
Toronto, 416 979 2221 Ext. 2339 57
Clarke, Judith, MSW, ACSW, BCD
New York, 212 254 7256 300
CLASS See Central Louisana AIDS Support Services
Classic Shoe Company
Calgary, 403 938 6491 40
Clatsop County AIDS Coalition
Astoria, 503 338 7501 324
Claudia Sexshop
Würzburg, 931 1 4361 136
Claw
San Diego, 619 239 3246 211
Clay County Health Department
Moorhead, 218 299 5220 281
Claydon Hospital
Wakefield, 192 436 4144 94
CLCC See City Lakes Crossgender Community
Clean Well-Lighted Place for Books
San José, 408 255 7600 220
Cleis Press
Pittsburgh, 412 937 1555 332
Clementine's
Saint Louis, 314 664 7869 284
Cléo Dubois Academy of SM Arts
Menlo Park, 415 322 0124 206
Cleveland AIDS Support
Middlesbrough, 1642 244588 88
Cleveland Bears
Euclid, 216 556 1570 321
Cleveland Clinic Hospital
216 444 2200 318
Cleveland For You & Akron Too!
published by For You Productions 319
Cleveland Lesbian / Gay Hotline
216 781 6736 318
Cleveland Lesbian Line
Middlesbrough, 1642 217955 88
CLGSG-L 4
Clingline
Windsford 72
Clinic 275
Adelaide, 8 226 6025 30
Clinica Dermatologica
Bari 144
Clinica Dermosifilopatica
Catania, 95 32 2720 145
Firenze, 55 247 8351 145
Padova, 49 66 1011 146
Parma, 521 99 1630 141
Clinica Malatte Infettive
Napoli, 81 21095 140
Clinical Approach Counseling Center, Inc.
Coral Springs, 305 345 2292 236
Clinique Medicale de la Cité
Montréal, 514 281 1722 62
Clintonville Counseling Services
Columbus, 614 261 1126 319
Clippers
Saint Albans, 181 940 3084 77
Santa Monica 188
Clit Club
New York 303
Clone Zone
Birmingham, 121 666 6640 93
Blackpool, 125 329 4850 78
East Ancoats P. O., 161 273 5246 69
London, 171 287 3530 86
Manchester, 161 236 1398 76
Clone Zone Head Office
London, 171 737 3636 86
Clonmel Gay Group 138
Closet Case Show 309
Close-Up Productions
West Hollywood, 800 697 9009 224
Clothes For Practitioners
London, 171 820 9393 81
Clovis/Portales Common Bond
505 356 2656 294
CLSMC Eagle
Chemnitz 113
Club 119
Boston, 617 367 0713 267
Club 30
Johannesburg, 21 23 5794 171
Club 332
Sioux Falls, 605 335 9874 336
Club Australia
Sydney 26
CLUB Calgary
403 234 8973 42
Club Caprice
published by Kastley GmbH 133
Club Cuir ESMC
Marseille, 91 48 4934 101
Club de Cuir Predateurs
Outremont, 514 272 8638 63
Club des Cuirassés de Québec
418 525 8868 63
Club Domentia
San Francisco 214
Club Edelweiss
New York, 212 629 1021 300
Club für Gleichgeschlechtilch Liebende e. V. (GL)
Frankfurt am Main, 335 32 1051 117
Club Gum
Utrecht, 20 420 2117 158
Club J & G
Wilrijk 39
Club Jaecques
Amsterdam, 20 622 0323 151
Club LL
Amsterdam 152
Club MET
Montréal, 514 528 8874 62
Club Mud
Rio Nido 188
Club Neues Leben Nova
München, 89 311 3260 128
Club Sunrise
Alingsås 173
Club Travestie Extraordinaire
London, 181 788 4154 83
Club TV
published by Continental Spectator 189
Club Tyz
Philadelphia, 215 546 4195 330
Club Whiplash
London, 171 603 9654 82
Club Winnipeg 47
Club X
San Diego, 800 598 1859 211
Club X Shop 25
Perth, 9 444 5572 34
Clyde Books
Glasgow, 141 552 4699 169
CMU-Out
Pittsburgh, 412 268 8794 332
CNBC Real Personal
Fort Lee, 201 585 2622 290
Coalesce Bookstore
San Luis Obispo, 805 772 2880 220
Coalition
Sioux Falls, 605 333 0603 335
Coalition des Organismes Communautaires Québecoise de Lutte Contre le SIDA
Montréal, 5114 844 2477 61
Coalition for Bisexual, Gay, & Lesbian Youth in Peel
Mississauga, 416 925 XTRA Ext. 2142 51
Coalition for Lesbian & Gay Rights in Ontario
Toronto, 416 553 6824 49
Coalition of Lesbian/Gay Student Groups, Inc.
Dallas / Fort Worth, 214 761 3802 341
Coalition of Lesbians, Gay, & Friends
Wayne, 201 595 3427 293
Coalition of Sexuality Organizations
Middletown, 203 347 9411 Ext. 2712 231
Coalition of Ursine Brothers
Tempe, 602 730 8171 194
Coastal Bend AIDS Foundation
Corpus Christi, 512 883 5815 339
Coatney, Catherine
San Francisco, 415 431 7300 213
Cobra
Roma, 6 38 5947 142
Cobra Custom Leather Shop
Clearwater, 813 553 8884 236
COC
Alkmaar & West Friesland, 72 511 1650 151
Arnhem, 26 442 3161 154
Bergen op Zoom, 16 425 4235 154
Brabant Noordoost, 41 262 6666 157
Breda, 76 522 6662 154
Den Helder, 22 361 6807 154
Dordrecht, 78 613 1717 154
Eindhoven, 40 245 5700 155
Emmen, 59 161 1414 155
Enschede, 53 430 5177 155
Friesland, 58 212 4908 156
Gouda, 18 252 4634 155
Groningen, 50 313 2620 155
Head Office, 20 623 4596 150
Heerlen, 45 571 7387 156
Hilversum, 35 628 4789 156
Hoogeveen, 52 826 7751 156
Information Center, 20 623 4079 152
Kennemerland, 23 532 5453 155
Leiden, 71 522 0640 156
Meerlanden / Ronde Venen 151
Middleburg, 11 861 2280 156
Nijmegen, 80 323 4237 156
Roosendaal 157
Rotterdam, 10 414 1555 157
Stadtgroep Roermund, 47 532 9257 157
Tiel, 34 461 6373 158
Tilburg, 13 535 9050 158
Twente / Achterhoek 155
Uden, 41 326 5821 158
Utrecht, 30 231 8841 158
Venray, 47 851 0487 159
Vlissingen, 11 841 2248 159
Weert, 49 553 3733 159
Woerden 159
Zeeuws Vlaanderen, 11 563 0654 158
Zuid-Limburg, 43 321 8337 156
Zwolle, 38 421 0065 159
COC Magazijn
Amsterdam, 20 623 4596 152
Cockell, Denis
London, 171 437 0605 83
Cockpit
Chicago 248
Cockring
Amsterdam, 20 622 6595 151
Cocoon
Birmingham, 121 772 2800 93
Kidderminster, 156 282 9419 77
London, 171 624 1074 86
CODE See Colorado Organization of Dungeon Enthusiasts
Code-3 Supply Co.
Los Angeles, 213 617 3881 205
Cody's Books
Berkeley, 510 845 7852 197
Cogent Warriors
San Francisco 214
Cohen, Carol, M.A., LPC
Denver, 303 759 5126 227
Cohn, Beryl, RNC, MSW
Plainfield, 908 757 8981 292
COLAGE See Children of Lesbians & Gays Everywhere
Colchester Gay Switchboard
1206 767043 75
Colchester HIV/AIDS Helpline
1206 767043 75
Cold Steel
London, 171 267 7970 83
Cole, Louanne, Ph.D.
San Francisco, 415 333 9500 213
Colectivo de Lesbianas Feministas
San Juan 167
Colectivo Masiorare
Mexico City 149
Colectivo Sol
Mexico City, 5 658 3534 149
Colectivo Sol, A.C.
Mexico City 149
Coler Memorial Hospital
New York, 212 848 6000 302
Colherne
London, 181 373 9859 80
Collars
Seattle 351
College of Staten Island Lesbian, Gay, & Bisexual Alliance
New York 305
Collier AIDS Resource & Education Service, Inc. (CARES)
Naples, 813 263 2273 239
Collins, Ethelreda, LCSW, BCD
Memphis, 901 323 6500 336
Cologne Jacks
Köln, 221 54 2516 124

Colorado AIDS Project
Denver, 800 333 2437 (hotline) 📖 226
Colorado College Gay & Lesbian Alliance
Colorado Springs, 719 389 6641 📖 227
Colorado Community Directory 📖 226
Colorado Health Action Project
Denver, 303 894 8650 📖 227
Colorado Organization of Dungeon Enthusiasts (CODE)
Boulder, 303 499 6757 📖 226
Denver 📖 228
Colorado Triangle
Denver, 303 293 9009 📖 227
Colorado Woman News 📖 228
Colorlife! 📖 307
Colt 45s
Houston 📖 342
Colt Bookstore
London 📖 85
Colt Studios
Studio City, 800 445 2758 📖 186, 223
Columbia Fun Maps
New York, 212 447 7877 📖 306
Columbia Hospital
Milwaukee, 414 961 3300 📖 357
Columbia Lesbian, Bisexual, & Gay Coalition
New York, 212 854 1488 📖 305
Columbia Medical Plaza
Vancouver, 206 254 1814 📖 354
Columbia Publishing Company
Baltimore, 410 366 7070 📖 264
Columbia University
New York, 212 854 2878 📖 303
Columbus AIDS Task Force
800 332 2437 📖 320
Columbus Ursine Brotherhood 📖 320
Comba-Borel
London, 171 738 2085 📖 85
Combattre le SIDA
Paris, 146 40 0303 📖 103
Combined Forces
Marion 📖 322
Combined Health District
Dayton, 513 225 4249 📖 321
Come Again Erotic Emporium
New York, 212 308 9394 📖 190
Come Out Jungengruppe
Braunschweig, 531 391 4556 📖 112
Come Out!
published by Gay Media 📖 177
Coming Our Gruppe
Göttingen 📖 118
Coming Out
broadcast by Channel 11 📖 48
Coming Out / Being Out Group
Denver, 303 831 6268 📖 228
Coming Out Collective
Columbia, 314 442 4174 📖 283
Coming Out Group
Sydney, 2 360 2211 📖 26
Coming Out Pagan 📖 265
Coming Out Show
broadcast by Co-op Radio FM 102.7 📖 46
Comité des Personnes Atteintes du VIH
Montréal, 514 282 6673 📖 62
Comité SIDA Aide Montréal
514 282 9888 📖 62
Comité SIDA Québec
Montréal, 514 285 6471 📖 61
COMMAND
Baltimore 📖 264
Command Post, Inc.
Tampa, 813 831 9245 📖 243
Committee in Support of Gay, Lesbian, & Bisexual People
Meadville, 216 371 0709 📖 329
Committee on Homophobia
Toronto, 416 978 8087 📖 57
Committee to Preserve Sexual Liberties
San Francisco 📖 215
Common Bond 📖 294
Boston 📖 268
Common Bond Gay & Lesbian Information Line
Albuquerque, 505 266 8041 📖 294
Common Bonds
Chicago 📖 248
published by The Backdrop Club 📖 207
Common Ground 📖 295
Common Knowledge Books
Toronto, 416 539 8550 📖 59
Common Language
Ann Arbor, 313 663 0036 📖 274
Common Lives, Lesbian Lives 📖 257
Commonwealth Professional Services
Richmond, 804 353 1169 📖 349
Communidad Triangulo Rosa (CTR)
Guadalajara 📖 149
Communita Gay della Svizzera Italiana
Viganello 📖 179
Community 📖 296
Community AIDS Council
Phœnix, 602 265 2437 📖 194
Community AIDS Network
Chichester, 1243 538484 📖 91
Floral City, 904 647 6098 📖 235
Community AIDS Resource & Education Service (CARES)
Kalamazoo, 616 381 2437 📖 276
Community AIDS Support Team (CAST)
Preston, 1772 200911 📖 79
Community AIDS Treatment Information Exchange
Toronto, 800 263 1638 (information) 📖 56
Community Bookshop
Brooklyn, 718 783 3075 📖 298
Community Care for AIDS-UTMB
Galveston, 409 938 2202 📖 342
Community Center (TCC)
Boise, 208 336 3870 📖 247
Community Connections 📖 313
Community Counseling Centers of Chicago
312 769 0205 📖 248
Community Counselling & Consultation, Inc.
Palm Springs, 619 323 2118 📖 209
Community Health Project
New York, 212 675 3559 📖 303
Community Health Project Outreach to Teens
New York, 212 255 1673 📖 306
Community Health Trust, Inc.
Louisville, 502 625 5496 📖 259
Community News 📖 324
published by Queer Press, Inc. 📖 235
Community Newscenter #1
Lansing, 517 3551 7562 📖 277
Community Newscenter #4
Ann Arbor, 313 663 6168 📖 274
Community Newscenter / Webster's
Grand Rapids, 616 285 7055 📖 276
Community Outreach Program
Halifax, 902 424 6551 📖 48
Community Pride Reporter 📖 261
Community Research Initiative of South Florida
Miami, 305 667 9296 📖 239
Community Research Initiative of Toronto
416 324 9505 📖 56
Community Services Network, Inc.
Jackson, 601 373 8610 📖 282
Community Support Network of New South Wales, Inc.
Sydney, 2 283 3234 📖 26
Community Unity Health & Wholeness Project
Dayton, 513 228 4031 📖 321
Community Voice 📖 243
Community Yellow Pages 📖 204
Community-General Hospital of Greater Syracuse
315 492 5011 📖 312
Companion Publications
Laguna Hills, 714 362 4489 📖 189
Company
Amsterdam, 20 625 3028 📖 151
Company Bar
Helsinki, 90 64 4391 📖 96
Company Club
Milano, 2 282 9481 📖 142
Compass 📖 205
Compendium
London, 171 485 8944 📖 85
Complete Guide to Internet Sex Resources 📖 15
Compound
Denver, 303 722 7977 📖 227
Comprehensive AIDS Program
West Palm Beach, 407 881 9040 📖 243
Comprehensive Clinic
Fort Myers, 813 334 1448 📖 237
Conant & Conant Books
Portland, 503 241 7726 📖 326
Concept Imports
Los Angeles 📖 187
Concerning Gay & Lesbians
broadcast by KRCL FM 91 📖 345
Concord 📖 251
Concord Feminist Health Center
603 224 1737 📖 2
Concordia Queer Collective
Montréal, 514 848 7414 📖 62
Concours M. Cuir Montréal
514 933 3307 📖 62
Condom Resource Center
Oakland, 510 891 0455 📖 207
Condom Wrap
Long Beach, 310 430 3379 📖 186
Condomania
Thatcham, 1635 874393 📖 71
Condomi
Bruxelles / Brussel 📖 37
Condoms Plus
San Diego, 619 291 7400 📖 212
Conductors L/L
Nashville 📖 337
Confederate Bears
Charlotte 📖 314
Conflicto
Frederiksberg, 31 35 0380 📖 66
Congress Book Shop
Portland, 207 774 1377 📖 263
conMOCIÓN 📖 239
Connecticut Outreach Society
Farmington, 203 657 4344 📖 229
Connection Garage
Berlin, 30 218 1432 📖 111
Connexions 📖 197
Connexions Annual
published by Connexions Information Sharing Services 📖 41
Connexions Information Sharing Services
Toronto, 416 537 3949 📖 41
Conney
Madison, 800 356 9100 📖 356
Conquistadors MC
Orlando, 407 423 1546 📖 240
Constance Enterprises
Montclair, 201 746 4200 📖 182
Constant Reader Bookshop
Milwaukee, 414 291 0452 📖 357
Constantines, Inc., of the Bay Area
San Francisco 📖 215
Construction Five
Frankfurt am Main, 69 29 1356 📖 117
Construction Zone
San Francisco, 415 255 8585 📖 219
Consultorio Gay
Bologna, 51 644 6820 📖 140
Venezia, 41 524 2121 📖 147
Contact
Paris, 64 03 9794 📖 103
Contact Centre (S/M)
London 📖 12
Contact FM 89
Hamilton, 7 838 4440 📖 162
Contact S. M.
published by Chaud Business SPRL 📖 37
Contenta, Inc.
Norcross, 404 446 2235 📖 245
Continental Books
Albany 📖 296
Continental Leather Pride Committee
Denver, 303 331 2549 📖 228
Continental Spectator
New York, 800 325 4122 📖 186, 189
published by Continental Spectator 📖 189
Control-T Studios
Mission Hills, 818 898 1591 📖 206
Conversio Virium
New York, 212 316 6479 📖 304
Cook County Hospital
Chicago, 312 633 6000 📖 249
Co-op Radio FM 102.7
Vancouver, 604 684 8494 📖 46
Coordinamento Lesbische Italiano
Roma, 6 686 4201 📖 141
Copperstate Leathermen Association
Phœnix, 602 274 8194 📖 194
Cork Lesbian Line
21 27 8470 📖 136
Cornbury Society
Vancouver 📖 45
Cornelius Men
München, 89 201 4753 📖 128
Cornell Gay & Lesbian Alliance
Mount Vernon, 319 895 4224 📖 257
Cornell Lesbian, Gay, & Bisexual Alliance
Ithaca, 607 255 6482 📖 299
Cornerhouse Books
Manchester, 161 228 7621 📖 76
Cornerstone Publications
Ponsonby, 9 376 2018 📖 160
Cornhaulers L & L Club
Des Moines 📖 256
Cornwall AIDS Council (CAC)
Truro, 1872 225022 📖 72
Corporal Contacts 📖 84
Corps of Rangers
Los Angeles, 213 874 0278 📖 204
Corpus Christi MC 📖 339
Corset Digest 📖 244
COSMEP
San Francisco, 415 922 9490 📖 215
Cosmic Order of KA
Inverness, 904 726 2403 📖 188
Cosmic Wear
Köln, 221 240 1201 📖 124
Council of Southern California Motorcycle Clubs
Long Beach 📖 202
Council Physicians AIDS Office
Bodø, 75 52 4210 📖 165
Counseling Associates
Tempe, 85283 📖 194
Counseling Center
Lynchburg, 804 845 5783 📖 348
Counseling Services of Brandon
Tampa, 813 654 0166 📖 242
Countdown on Spanner
London, 171 278 3294 📖 69
Country Club
New Orleans, 504 945 0742 📖 260
Country House
Chatham, 518 392 6209 📖 298
Countrymen
Detroit, 313 836 2324 📖 275
COURAGE 📖 4
Denton, 817 565 6110 📖 341
Courageous Books
New York, 212 944 1050 📖 309
Courier Corporation
Lowell, 508 458 6351 📖 271
Courier Westford Inc.
508 692 6321 📖 273
Couto, Dan
Toronto, 171 499 9493 📖 58
Covenant
Lancaster 📖 329
Coventry Friend
1203 714199 📖 93
Cover Girl Shoes
London, 171 354 2883 📖 86
Cover Up
Nuneaton, 1203 398809 📖 68
Cowtown Leathermen
Dallas / Fort Worth 📖 340
Coyote, Ken
Santa Cruz, 408 459 8582 📖 221
Cozy Time
Calgary, 403 236 7072 📖 41
Cozy Time Adult Baby Wear
Calgary, 403 236 7072 📖 43
Cramp Leather
Seattle, 206 323 9245 📖 353
Crane Duplicating
Dennisport, 508 760 1601 📖 270
Crawford Long Hospital of Emory University
Atlanta, 404 686 4411 📖 243
Crazy Fashion
Nürnberg, 911 47 2769 📖 130
Crazy Ladies Bookstore
Cincinnati 📖 318
Crazy Sexy
Basel / Bâle, 61 271 9079 📖 177
Crazy Wisdom Bookstore
Ann Arbor, 313 665 2757 📖 274
Crazy World
Bristol 📖 70
Creative Art Collection
Luxembourg 📖 148

Creative Counseling Services
Hartford, 203 233 6962 📖 230
Creative Design Services
King of Prussia, 610 640 9449 📖 329
Philadelphia, 610 640 9449 📖 331
Creative Growth Enterprises
Concord, 510 798 0922 📖 198
Creative Imageware by J&M
Davison 📖 183
Creative Tattoo
Ann Arbor, 313 662 2520 📖 274
Crescent Tavern
Seattle 📖 350
Crewe Action for Sexual Health
127 025 1135 📖 71
Crewe L&G Switchboard
1270 250980 📖 71
Crib Sheet
published by Amber E. 📖 206
Crimson Phœnix
Portland, 503 228 0129 📖 327
CRIPS 📖 *See* Centre Regional d'Information & de Prévention du SIDA
Crisis Hotline
Houston, 713 228 1505 📖 342
Crisis Line
Alice Springs, 8 981 9227 📖 28
Crissy's Creations
San Diego 📖 183
Critical Path AIDS Project
Philadelphia, 215 545 2212 📖 330
Criticare
Billings, 406 255 7467 📖 285
Crone's Harvest
Boston, 617 983 9530 📖 269
Cronulla Gay Group
Sydney, 2 660 4615 📖 26
Croque Monsieur
broadcast by FM 89 📖 98
Cross Dressers International (CDI)
Easton 📖 328
Tulsa, 918 582 6643 📖 324
Cross Expressions
Vestal, 607 862 3203 📖 312
Cross, Clare, CSW
New York, 212 662 4609 📖 300
Crossdresser Heterosexual Intersocial Club (CHIC)
Long Beach, 714 993 7142 📖 202
Crossdressers & Friends
Overland Park, 913 791 3847 📖 258
Crossdressers InfoGuide 📖 244
Crossing Press
Freedom, 800 777 1048 📖 14
Crossings
Lexington, 606 233 7266 📖 259
Crossland Shoes
Edmonton, 403 448 0173 Ext. 5665 📖 40
Crosslynx
Glasgow, 141 332 8372 📖 169
Cross-Port
Cincinnati, 513 474 9557 📖 318
Crossroads
Royal Oak, 313 537 3267 📖 278
Crossroads Market & Bookstore
Dallas / Fort Worth, 214 521 8919 📖 341
Houston, 713 942 0147 📖 343
Crossroads of Buffalo 📖 298
Cross-Talk
Woodland Hills 📖 225
Crouch, Katherine Eustis, CSW
Albany, 518 456 5845 📖 295
Crowe, John, CRC, CAC
Albany, 518 436 1578 📖 295
Crown Books
San Francisco, 415 441 7479 📖 219
Croydon Friend
181 683 4239 📖 91
Crucible 📖 22
Crucible MC
Pittsburgh, 412 322 1144 📖 332
Cruella
published by Rogue-Hagen Publications 📖 73
Cruise Club
Bristol, 117 929 2447 📖 70
Cruise Magazine
published by Rome Enterprises, Inc. 📖 278
Cruiser 📖 177
Cruz Leather Works
København, 33 14 9017 📖 66
Crypt
Denver, 303 733 3112 📖 226
San Diego, 619 574 1579 📖 212
San Diego, 619 692 9499 📖 196
Seattle, 206 325 3882 📖 353
Crypt / North Park Adult Video
San Diego, 619 284 4724 📖 196
Crypt On Broadway
Long Beach, 310 983 6560 📖 196
Crypto Tech Corp.
San Diego, 800 331 0442 📖 211
Crystal Club
Reynoldsburg, 614 224 1165 📖 322
CS 📖 2
CS4 Media Today
broadcast by University of Birmingham 📖 93
CSU Lambda Delta Lambda
Cleveland, 216 261 8645 📖 319
CTN Magazine 📖 217
CTR 📖 *See* Communidad Triangulo Rosa
Cuckoo's Nest
Amsterdam, 20 627 1752 📖 151
Cuff
Seattle, 206 323 1525 📖 350
Cuffs
Los Angeles, 213 660 2649 📖 203
Cuir Gear
Portland, 503 281 7231 📖 326
Cuir Magazine
published by The Leather Journal 📖 225
Cuir Plus
Montréal, 514 521 7587 📖 63
Cuir Underground 📖 218
Cul D'Or
published by Omega Marketing 📖 77
Cumulative Book Index
published by H. W. Wilson Company 📖 297
Cupid's Connection
York, 717 846 5029 📖 334
Cupid's Treasures
Chicago, 800 287 4370 📖 252
Cupid's Video Boutique
Deer Park, 516 586 0066 📖 299
Curious Times
Dallas / Fort Worth, 214 522 5887 📖 341
Currie, Stuart
Christchurch, 3 3779 4601 📖 161
Curtin Stonewall Club
Bentley, 9 351 2907 📖 33
Cushing-Malloy
Ann Arbor, 313 663 8554 📖 274
Cutting Edge
Plainfield, 908 769 3250 📖 292
CVASE 📖 *See* Central Virginia AIDS Services & Education
C V G L 📖 *See* Central Vermont Gay Liberation
CWRU Gay Lesbian Bisexual Alliance
Cleveland, 216 368 2679 📖 319
Cybercore
Bologna 📖 140
Cyberoticomm
New York 📖 300
Cycle Runners MC
San Francisco 📖 215
Cycle/Wheels MC
New York 📖 304
Cycles MC
Newark 📖 292
Cypress College Lambda Union 📖 198
Czernich, Peter
Solingen, 21 258 6151 📖 132
D&S Society of Baltimore
410 385 3331 📖 264
D'Amico, Jane, MSW, CSW, CAC
New York, 516 621 3033 📖 300
D. A. B.
Louisville 📖 259
D. A. D. S.
Winfield 📖 253
D. B. Leisurewear
London 📖 68
D. S. S. G.
Tampa, 813 689 7999 📖 242
D.L.
San Francisco 📖 214
DAC Marketing, Inc.
Chicago, 800 982 4717 📖 251
Dacapo Sexladen
Stuttgart, 711 236 4734 📖 134
Daddy Magazine
published by Ganymede Press, Inc. 📖 264
Daddybear 📖 266
Dads & Sons
Laguna Beach 📖 188
Dædalus Publishing Company
San Francisco, 415 626 1867 📖 216
DAG/LC 📖 *See* Detroit Area Gay / Lesbian Council
DAGLO 📖 *See* Dartmouth Gay & Lesbian Organization
Daily Globe
Calgary 📖 43
Daily Mail 📖 85
Daily Planet News
Saint Louis, 314 367 1333 📖 284
Daisy Publications Ltd.
Bexhill-on-Sea, 142 845 018 📖 7
Dakota AIDS Project
Fargo, 701 287 2437 📖 316
Dakota Life Foundation
Fargo, 701 287 2437 📖 316
Dakota Steel, Inc.
Soquel, 800 995 0595 📖 222
DALLAS 📖 *See* Dallas Area Levi / Leather Association
Dallas Area Levi / Leather Association (DALLAS)
Dallas / Fort Worth, 214 288 9395 📖 340
Dallas Bears
Dallas / Fort Worth, 214 521 5342 Ext. 880 📖 340
Dallas County Hospital
Dallas / Fort Worth, 214 590 8000 📖 340
Dallas Gay & Lesbian Alliance
Dallas / Fort Worth, 214 521 5342 Ext. 414 📖 340
Dallas Gay & Lesbian Historic Archives
Dallas / Fort Worth, 214 821 1653 📖 339
Dallas MC
Dallas / Fort Worth 📖 340
Dallas Voice 📖 341
DAMES 📖 *See* Dykes Against Minority Suppression
Damien Center
Indianapolis, 317 632 0123 📖 254
Damon, Hope, LCSW
Virginia Beach, 804 495 4616 📖 349
Damron Address Book
published by Damron Company 📖 189
Damron Company
San Francisco, 800 462 6654 📖 189
Dana
Saint Gallen, 71 253195 📖 179
Danbury Area Gay, Lesbian, & Bisexual Youth Group
203 798 0863 📖 230
Danbury Hospital
203 797 7000 📖 230
Daniel Freeman Marina Hospital
Marina Del Rey, 310 823 8911 📖 206
Danish Book World II
Waterloo, 319 234 9340 📖 257
Danske Bjørne ApS
Padborg, 74 67 4727 📖 65
DAPA, Family of Choice
Houston, 800 822 2272 📖 342
Darakan
Bruxelles / Brussel, 2 512 2076 📖 37
Dark Alley
Blairstown, 908 362 8728 📖 289
Dark Garden Corsets
San Francisco, 415 522 9651 📖 11
Dark Side Creations
Calgary, 403 272 3134 📖 40
Dartmouth Gay & Lesbian Organization (DAGLO)
Hanover, 603 646 3636 📖 287
Daugherty & Associates
Denver, 303 266 3477 📖 227
Daughters of Aphrodite
London, 181 989 0281 📖 6
Dave's B&B on the Rio Grande
Albuquerque, 505 247 8312 📖 294
David
Sydney, 2 550 9448 📖 27
David Enterprises
Cathedral City, 619 324 4957 📖 198
David Magazine
published by David Enterprises 📖 198
David Printing
Cathedral City, 619 324 4957 📖 198
David-Versand
Saint-Gallen 📖 177
Davies Medical Center
San Francisco 📖 213
Davis Clinic
Huntsville, 205 533 2437 📖 191
Davis, Bill, LCSW
Virginia Beach, 804 460 4655 📖 349
Davis-Kidd Bookseller
Knoxville, 615 690 0136 📖 336
Nashville, 615 385 2645 📖 337
Davy's Erotheek
Utrecht, 30 243 6815 📖 158
Dawn
Alexandria 📖 347
Day Hospital
Cape Town, 21 46 1124 📖 170
DCH Regional Medical Center
Tuscaloosa, 205 759 7111 📖 192
DC-MOTSS 📖 3
DDMM-L 📖 3
De Gay Krant
published by Best Publishing Group 📖 151
De Sade's World
published by Executive Imports International 📖 307
Deaconess Medical Center
Billings, 406 657 4141 📖 285
DEAN 📖 *See* Down East AIDS Network
Dean's of Bournemouth
1202 314584 📖 73
Dean, Judith, Ed.D., M.Div., M.S.
Princeton, 609 275 6556 📖 292
Deana's Skin Art Studio
Orlando, 407 281 1228 📖 241
Decadence
Helsinki, 90 694 8898 📖 95
Decorations by SLAN
Lombard 📖 184
Dëeks
Chicago, 312 549 3335 📖 248
Defenders
Boston, 617 437 0998 📖 268
Denver, 303 322 8485 📖 228
New York, 908 324 6475 📖 303
San Francisco, 415 487 7669 📖 214
Tampa Bay, 813 996 4738 📖 238
Washington, D.C., 202 387 4516 📖 234
Défi
Perpignan, 68 52 4425 📖 105
Defiance 📖 333
Dehaan, Jan
Nieuw-Vennep 📖 156
DejaNews Partners 📖 7
Dekker / V. d. Vegt
Nijmegen, 80 322 1010 📖 157
Del Otro Lado
published by Colectivo Sol, A.C. 📖 149
Del Valle, J. L.
Paris, 143 21 8487 📖 104
Delaware Lesbian & Gay Health Advocates
Wilmington, 800 292 0429 (in Delaware only) 📖 233
Delaware Valley Bears
Philadelphia 📖 330
Delaware Valley Gay Neighbors
Yardville 📖 289
Delaware Valley Synergy
Huntington Valley 📖 328
Delectus Books
London, 181 963 0979 📖 7
Delftse Werkgroep Homosexualiteit
15 214 6893 📖 154
DELGO 📖 *See* Downeast Lesbian & Gay Organization

Delice Garden 🕮 38
Delmar Printing & Publishing
Charlotte, 704 847 9801 🕮 314
Delos
Canoga Park 🕮 197
Delta
Québec, 418 647 6808 🕮 63
Delta Boek
Ridderkerk 🕮 150
Delta Fashion
Göteborg 🕮 173
Delta International
Wilkes-Barre 🕮 12
Delta Lambda Phi Fraternity
Houston, 713 529 3211 🕮 343
Las Vegas, 702 733 9800 🕮 286
Minnesota, 612 336 4196 🕮 280
Sacramento 🕮 210
Delta Lithograph
Valencia, 805 257 0584 🕮 224
Delta Omega
Dallas / Fort Worth, 214 264 7103 🕮 341
Deluxe Book Bargains
Elmira, 607 734 9656 🕮 299
Demask
Amsterdam, 20 620 5603 🕮 8, 152, 153
Deming, Alison
Fayetteville, 315 637 8990 🕮 299
Demonia
published by Société Comedit 🕮 104
Deneuve
published by FRS Enterprises 🕮 217
Denise Robinson Body Art (DEXTRA)
Ottawa, 613 567 9033 🕮 53
Denmark Books
Aurora, 708 898 9838 🕮 248
Dental Alliance for AIDS/HIV
Chicago, 312 645 4891 🕮 249
Denver AIDS Prevention
303 893 6300 🕮 227
Denver Exchange
303 623 6665 🕮 227
Denver Leather Association
303 331 2549 🕮 228
Denver Metro Health Clinic
303 893 7296 🕮 227
Denver University Lesbian, Gay, & Bisexual Alliance (LGBA)
303 871 2321 🕮 228
Department of Health & Human Services
Anchorage, 905 343 4611 🕮 192
Houston, 713 794 9020 (hotline) 🕮 342
Derby AIDS Line
800 622738 🕮 72
Derby Friend
1332 349333 🕮 73
Derby, Phil
Oakland, 510 486 8960 🕮 208
Dermagraphics
Seattle, 206 622 1535 🕮 353
Derry Cara Friend
150 426 3120 🕮 164
Desert Adult Books
Las Vegas, 702 643 7982 🕮 286
Desert Bears
Phœnix 🕮 194
Desert Brotherhood MC
Las Vegas 🕮 286
Desert Hospital
Palm Springs, 619 323 6511 🕮 208
Desert Leathermen
Tucson 🕮 194
Desert Moon Periodicals
Santa Fe, 505 474 6311 🕮 2
Desiderio
Brescia, 30 41840 🕮 142
Desire
published by Red Sky Publishing, Limited 🕮 84
Sheffield, 114 244 2626 🕮 90
Tulsa 🕮 324
Desmodus, Inc.
San Francisco, 415 252 1195 🕮 217
Details 🕮 307
Detonator 🕮 84
Detroit Area Gay / Lesbian Council (DAG/LC)
810 853 2488 🕮 275
Detroit Avenue News
Cleveland, 216 961 3880 🕮 319
Detroit Eagle
810 873 6969 🕮 274
Deutsche AIDS-Hilfe e. V.
Berlin, 30 690 0870 🕮 108
Deutsche AIDS-Stiftung Positiv-Leben
Köln, 221 24 3535 🕮 124
DEXTRA 🕮 *See* Denise Robinson Body Art
DGSS Institut
Düsseldorf, 211 35 4591 🕮 115
Diablo Valley AIDS Center
Concord, 510 686 3822 🕮 198
Diablo Valley Girls
Concord, 510 937 8432 🕮 198
Dialogai
Genève / Genf, 22 340 0000 🕮 176
Diamond
Woodridge 🕮 253
Diamond Distribution
Southgate 🕮 278
Diaper Pail Friends (DPF)
Mill Valley 🕮 9
Dickinson College Allies
Carlisle, 717 240 1835 🕮 328
Dickinson, Pentz, McCall, Associates
Washington, 202 728 1166 🕮 233
Different Drummer Bookshop
Laguna Beach, 714 497 6699 🕮 201
Different Light
New York, 212 989 4850 🕮 308
New York, 800 343 4002 🕮 181
San Francisco, 415 431 0891 🕮 218
West Hollywood, 319 854 6601 🕮 225
Different Strokes
broadcast by Contact FM 89 🕮 162
Different Voice
broadcast by CFMU 93.3 FM 🕮 50
Different World
Beloit, 608 365 1000 🕮 355
Digital Obsession
Philadelphia 🕮 330
Digital Queers
San Francisco, 415 974 9122 🕮 215
DIGNITY 🕮 3
Dignity-Dokumentationsstelle der Diskriminierung von Menschen mit HIV/AIDS
Frankfurt am Main, 69 29 6797 🕮 108
Dimensions 🕮 338
Dinah 🕮 317
Dinos
Worms, 635 98 5200 🕮 135
Directory of Bookstores Specializing in Gay, Lesbian, & Feminist Books
published by American Library Association 🕮 251
Directory of Gay & Lesbian Community Publications in the United States & Canada
published by Redwood Empire Agency 🕮 200
Directory of Professional Groups of Gays & Lesbians
published by American Library Association 🕮 251
Dirty 🕮 307
Disability Rag 🕮 259
Disciples of de Sade
Dallas / Fort Worth 🕮 340
Disciples of Semiramis
published by Katharsis 🕮 19
Discipline Support-Line for Women
London, 181 989 0281 🕮 2
Disco Book Store
Columbus, 614 274 9716 🕮 320
Discreet Boutique
Saskatoon, 306 665 6681 🕮 64
Winnipeg, 204 947 1307 🕮 47
Dispensaire Anti-Vénérien
Béziers, 67 76 9080 🕮 98
distributors
South Bend, 219 232 8500 🕮 253
District 202
Minneapolis / Saint Paul, 612 871 5559 🕮 280
District of Columbia General Hospital
Washington, 202 675 5000 🕮 233
Disziplin
published by Vogel Verlag 🕮 110
Ditury & David
New York 🕮 308
Diva
published by Millivres Ltd. 🕮 85
Diva & Empress Publications, Inc.
Detroit, 313 961 4862 🕮 273
DivaNet 🕮 *See* Galleria Diva
Diversified Services
Brighton, 617 787 7426 🕮 184
Diversity 🕮 247
Wichita Falls, 817 766 2264 🕮 345
Diversity Magazine 🕮 44
Divine Press
Stockport, 153 274 6319 🕮 72
Divinity
published by Divine Press 🕮 72
Dixie Bears 🕮 243
DK Profashion
Silkeborg, 86 83 6470 🕮 66
DM International
Seattle 🕮 20, 21, 352, 353
Doc Roc
London, 171 916 9273 🕮 86
Doc's Leathers & Harley Davidson Gear
Toronto, 416 324 8686 🕮 60
Dock
Cincinnati, 513 241 5623 🕮 317
Docks
Paris, 143 57 3382 🕮 102
Doctor's Hospital
Little Rock, 501 661 4000 🕮 195
Dodds Bookshop
Long Beach, 310 438 9948 🕮 203
DOK 🕮 *See* Konsultatieburo voor Relaties en Seksualiteit
Dolphins Motor Club
Sydney, 2 699 6588 🕮 26
Domina 🕮 84, 307
Dominant & Submissive Pleasure
published by The Society of O 🕮 236
Dominant Domain
published by New Esoteric Press 🕮 308
Dominant Mystique
published by New Esoteric Press 🕮 308
Dominant Publications
Vancouver 🕮 46
Dominantly Yours
published by Continental Spectator 🕮 189
Domination
München, 89 930 6980 🕮 107
Orlando, 407 678 3388 🕮 240
Domination Directory International (DDI)
published by Strictly Speaking Publishing Co. 🕮 208
Dominican Santa Cruz Hospital
408 462 7700 🕮 221
Dominion News
Winnipeg, 204 942 6563 🕮 47
Dominique & Rubber Fun 🕮 70
Domino
Warwick 🕮 92
Domus
Cosenza 🕮 140
Don & Adonis
published by Foerster Verlag 🕮 108
Don-Club
Dortmund, 231 55 3221 🕮 114
Donihe Graphics, Inc.
Kingsport, 800 251 0337 🕮 336
Doorways
Saint Louis, 314 454 9599 🕮 284
Dorchester Gay & Lesbian Alliance (GALA)
Boston, 617 825 3737 🕮 268
Dore 🕮 337
Dormann, Ulf
Broenshoej, 31 60 4818 🕮 65
Dornan Uniforms
New York, 212 247 0937 🕮 309
Dornrosa - Frauenselbsthilfe e. V.
Halle (Saale), 345 202 4331 🕮 119
Dorothea Dix Hospital
Raleigh, 919 733 5324 🕮 315
Dorset Gay & Lesbian Switchboard
Bournemouth, 1202 318 822 🕮 73
Dorset Lesbian & Gay Helpline
Bournemouth, 1202 318822 🕮 73
Double Face 🕮 97
Double Trouble Bears
Norristown 🕮 329
Douglas County Gay Archives
Roseburg, 503 440 2761 🕮 327
Dove Art
San Diego, 619 270 7400 🕮 212
Down East AIDS Network (DEAN)
Ellsworth, 207 667 3506 🕮 262
Down There Press
San Francisco, 415 974 8985 🕮 14
Down Town
published by Michael Sürth Verlag 🕮 108
Down Town Redaktion Nord 🕮 121
Downeast Lesbian & Gay Organization (DELGO)
Bangor, 207 942 6503 🕮 262
Downtown Books & News
Asheville, 704 253 8654 🕮 313
DPF 🕮 *See* Diaper Pail Friends
DPF Newsletter
Mill Valley 🕮 9
Dr. Müller's Sex Shop
München 🕮 128
Stuttgart, 711 29 5561 🕮 134
Draconian Leather
Bakersfield, 805 631 8760 🕮 196
Dragazine 🕮 225
Dragon LC
Columbus 🕮 320
Dragon's Design
508 465 5185 🕮 266
Dragonfly Books
Nashville, 615 292 5699 🕮 337
Drague
Québec, 418 649 7212 🕮 63
Drake University Alternative Lifestyles
Des Moines, 515 274 4851 🕮 256
Drake's After Midnight Bookstore
Los Angeles, 213 651 5600 🕮 206
West Hollywood, 310 289 8932 🕮 225
Dream & Fantasy Fashions
Berlin, 30 792 7760 🕮 107
Dream Dresser
Beverly Hills, 213 848 3480 🕮 182
West Hollywood, 213 848 3480 🕮 225
Dream Girls
Kamloops 🕮 44
Dream Haven Books Uptown
Minneapolis / Saint Paul, 612 825 4720 🕮 281
Dream Magazine
published by Klinger Publications 🕮 211
Dream Team Productions
Spreitenbach, 77 88 9800 🕮 177
Dreams & Swords
Indianapolis, 800 937 2706 🕮 255
Dreams Adult Shop
Townsville, 7 771 4300 🕮 29
Dreamwear Club
Helsinki, 73 891396 🕮 96
dreizehn
Boston 🕮 268
Dressed To Kill
Chicago, 312 248 1860 🕮 251
Dressing For Pleasure
Montclair, 201 746 4200 🕮 291
Dressing For Pleasure Gala
Montclair, 201 746 4200 🕮 291
Dripride / Weyerhaeuser
Bowling Green, 502 843 1070 🕮 258
Driscoll, Robert, CSW
New York, 212 228 2745 🕮 300
Drolet's Army Surplus
Toronto, 416 762 6486 🕮 60
Drondale Limited
Edinburgh, 131 556 1471 🕮 169
Drummer
published by Desmodus, Inc. 🕮 217
DSA-LGB 🕮 4
DSSM
London 🕮 82
Du & Ich
published by Leine Verlag 🕮 108
Du Beffroi
Charleroi 🕮 38
Dublin Gay Switchboard
1 721 055 🕮 137
Dubuque Regional AIDS Coalition
319 589 4181 🕮 256
Dudley HIV & AIDS Support Group
Stourbridge, 1384 444300 🕮 93
Dugout Ltd.

Chicago, 312 777 1496 📖 252
Duke
Groningen, 50 313 4609 📖 155
Duke AIDS Research & Treatment Center
Durham, 919 684 5260 📖 314
Duke GALA
Washington 📖 234
Duluth Community Health Center
218 722 1479 📖 279
Dumfries & Galloway L&G Group
141 221 8372 📖 167
Greenock, 141 221 8372 📖 170
Stirling, 141 221 8372 📖 167
Dundalk News
Rochester, 716 325 2248 📖 311
Dundee LGB Switchboard Group
1382 202620 📖 170
Dungeon Club
London, 171 932 0755 📖 80
Dungeon Enterprises, Inc.
Dallas / Fort Worth, 214 522 2796 📖 340
Dungeon Players
Dallas / Fort Worth 📖 340
Duo Shop
Quimper, 98 90 7357 📖 105
Duraline Medical Products
Leipsic, 800 654 3376 📖 321
Durham Alliance Association
Oshawa, 905 434 4297 📖 52
Duro-Med Industries, Inc.
Hackensack, 201 488 5055 📖 290
Dutch Tattoo Foundation
Amsterdam 📖 152
Duval County Public Health Unit
Jacksonville, 904 633 3620 📖 238
Dwelling Place
Lewisburg, 717 523 7878 📖 329
Dyke Review 📖 217
Dyke TV
broadcast by Sang Froid 📖 310
Dykes Against Minority Suppression (DAMES)
Milwaukee 📖 357
Dykes Night Out
Edinburgh 📖 169
Dykes, Disability, & Stuff 📖 356
Dykespeak 📖 218
Dynasty
Mizuho-Ku, 52 853 1144 📖 147
EAGL 📖 *See* Einstein Association of Gays & Lesbians
Eagle
Amsterdam, 20 627 8634 📖 151
Dallas / Fort Worth, 214 559 3511 📖 339
Fort Lauderdale, 305 462 6380 📖 236
Stuttgart, 711 640 6183 📖 132
Wien, 1 587 2661 📖 35
Eagle in Exile
Columbus, 614 294 0069 📖 319
Eagle Leather
Melbourne, 39 417 2100 📖 25
Eagle Leathers
Northolt, 181 426 8047 📖 68
Eagle MC
West Palm Beach 📖 243
Eagle Press
Woodlawn 📖 338
Eagle's Nest
New York, 212 691 8451 📖 300
Earlham Lesbian, Bisexual, & Gay People's Union
Richmond, 317 983 1436 📖 255
Earth Spirit
Red Bank, 908 842 3855 📖 292
Earthling Bookstore
Santa Barbara, 805 965 1530 📖 221
Easons
Dublin, 1 73 3811 📖 137
East Anglia Bikers
London 📖 83
East Coast Bisexual Network
Boston 📖 268
East Coast Couples Network (ECCN)
Red Bank 📖 292
East Coast FTM Group
Northampton 📖 271
East Kent Friend
Canterbury, 184 358 8762 📖 78
East Lancashire Lesbian & Gay Switchboard
Burnley, 128 245 4978 📖 78
East Mercia MSC
Nottingham, 133 236 1056 📖 89
East of Eden
Garden Grove, 714 534 9811 📖 200
London, 171 251 4960 📖 86
East Side Ministry of Social Services
Detroit, 313 331 0033 📖 274
East Stroudsburg University GLBSO
Stroudsburg / Poconos, 717 424 4910 📖 333
Eastern Adult Books
Erie, 814 459 7014 📖 328
Eastern AIDS Support Triangle
King's Lynn, 1553 776655 📖 88
Eastern Currents
Santa Cruz, 800 946 9264 📖 222
Eastern Maine AIDS Network (EMAN)
Bangor, 207 990 3626 📖 262
Eastern Maine Medical Center
Bangor, 207 945 7000 📖 262
Easton, Dossie, MFCC
San Francisco, 415 488 1431 📖 213
Ebb & Flow
Scunthorpe, 1724 289292 📖 77
EBC
San Bernardino 📖 210
Ecce Queer 📖 353
Eccentric Fashion
Riken, 62 44 2221 📖 176
Rothrist 📖 178
ECCN 📖 *See* East Coast Couples Network
Echo Magazine
published by Ace Publishing, Inc, 📖 194
Eclectic Attitudes
published by The Fetish Network 📖 240
Eclectic Connection
Chicago 📖 181
Eclectic Engineering / Consensual Leather
Watertown 📖 273
Eclectics
Columbia, 314 443 0873 📖 283
Eclipse
San Mateo, 415 572 9702 📖 220
Ecoute Gai
Paris, 144 93 0102 📖 103
Ectomorph
London, 171 249 6311 📖 81
ECW Press
Toronto 📖 42
Eden Society
Pompano Beach, 305 784 9316 📖 241
Eden, Carl, CSW
New York, 212 929 7178 📖 300
Edge 📖 205
Toronto, 416 244 9117 📖 56
Edge, Inc.
Dayton, 513 294 0713 📖 321
Edinboro Gay Organization
814 732 2000 📖 328
Edinburgh Castle Hotel
Adelaide 📖 30
Edinburgh College of Art L&G Society
131 229 1442 📖 169
Edinburgh Gay Switchboard
131 556 4049 📖 168
Kirkcaldy, 131 556 4049 📖 168
Edinburgh Lesbian Line
131 557 0751 📖 168
Edinburgh LGB Centre
131 557 2625 📖 169
Edition Habit Press Ltd.
Sydney, 2 387 4339 📖 26
Edition Manfred Salzgeber Berlin
30 215 3209 📖 110
Editions Astarté
Paris, 143 38 3343 📖 104
éditions aubrey walter
London, 181 341 7818 📖 69
Editions Dominique Leroy
Paris, 146 34 6361 📖 104
Editions du Triangle Rose
Paris, 143 57 5205 📖 18
Editions Jaybird
Bruxelles / Brussel, 2 219 8007 📖 37
Editions Nitram
Montréal, 514 499 9994 📖 42
Editions SAN
Paris, 146 06 1035 📖 97
Editions Vents d'Ouest
Issy Les Moulineaux 📖 100
Editrice Cassia
Milano 📖 138
Editzioni d'Essai
Firenze, 55 717 880 📖 146
Edizione Gruppo Abele
Torino, 11 839 5444 📖 139
Edley Enterprises, Inc.
Sanbornville, 603 473 2539 📖 288
Edmonton Persons Living with HIV Society
403 488 5768 📖 43
Educational TV Channel (ETVC)
San Francisco, 510 549 2665 📖 196
Edward's Books
Philadelphia, 215 563 6171 📖 331
Edwards Brothers
Ann Arbor, 313 769 1000 📖 274
Edward-William Publishing Company
Austin, 512 288 7515 📖 339
Eerdmans Printing Company
Grand Rapids, 616 451 0763 📖 276
EFA 📖 *See* Saint Louis Effort for AIDS
Effetto Diversita
broadcast by Radio Onda Rossa FM 93.3 & 93.45 📖 141
E-Garbs
Brighton, 1273 748887 📖 74
EGG 📖 *See* English-Speaking Gay Group
Egge, Conrad, Ph.D.
Phœnix, 602 230 2025 📖 193
Ehe-Familien-Jungend & Schwulenberatung
Hohenmölsen 📖 122
Eichler, Wolfgang
Gelsenkirchen, 20 913 4794 📖 118
EIDOS Magazine
published by Brush Hill Press 📖 269
Einstein Association of Gays & Lesbians (EAGL)
New York 📖 305
Eisenberg, Edith, ACSW
New York, 718 263 0779 📖 300
Either/Or
Los Angeles, 310 374 2060 📖 205
EJB Enterprises
Fort Lauderdale, 305 563 9476 📖 237
EJINTVIO 📖 4
El Camino Hospital
Mountain View 📖 207
El Proyecto Arizona-Sonora
Tucson, 602 770 1314 📖 194
El Rubio
Groningen, 50 314 0039 📖 155
Elaine Barrie Project
Melbourne, 3 69 2613 📖 32
Electric City
broadcast by Cable TV 📖 219
Electronic Gay Community Magazine
published by Land of Awes Information Services 📖 189
ELGO 📖 *See* Emory Lesbian & Gay Organization
Elise
Eindhoven 📖 155
Elite Adult Books
Tulsa, 918 838 8503 📖 324
Elizabeth
Makamura-Ku 📖 147
Elizabeth Club
Koto-Ku, 3 3683 6092 📖 147
Nishi-Ku 📖 147
Ellaborn, Diane, LICSW, NASW
Wayland, 508 877 9671 📖 273
Elle For Leather
Manchester 📖 68
Ellen Schippers Design
Amsterdam, 20 662 3883 📖 153
Ellie's Garden
Lubbock, 806 796 0880 📖 344
Elmer, Mark, Dip. Couns.
London, 171 249 1351 📖 80
Elmhurst Hospital Center
718 334 4000 📖 299
Elmwood Park / Cottontown Lesbian & Gay Neighborhood Association
Columbia, 803 252 2269 📖 335
Eltern Schwuler Söhne & Lesbischwe Töchter
Bremen, 421 70 4170 📖 113
Eltern Telefon
Nürnberg, 911 22 2377 📖 129
E-MaleSM
San Francisco, 800 930 9366 📖 181
EMAN 📖 *See* Eastern Maine AIDS Network
Emanzipation e. V.
Frankfurt am Main, 69 297 7296 📖 117
Emerald City
Seattle, 206 284 1071 📖 352
Emerald City News 📖 258
Emission Gaie Cayenne
broadcast by FM 100 📖 106
Emission Homophobie
broadcast by Fréquence 4 FM 99.6 📖 98
Emory Lesbian & Gay Organization (ELGO)
Atlanta, 404 727 6692 📖 244
Empathy
published by Gay & Lesbian Advcacy Research Project 📖 335
Empire
München, 89 260 8403 📖 127
Empire City MC
New York 📖 304
Empire Hotel
Brisbane 📖 28
Emporio del Libro
Vicenza, 444 22 8097 📖 147
Emscher-Lipper Andersrum
broadcast by FM 96.1 or FM 104.5 📖 118
Enamored Writer 📖 238
Enchanté
Saint Petersburg, 813 972 2617 📖 241
Enclave Book Repository
Oyster Bay, 516 922 1169 📖 181
Encounter 📖 242
Endless Pain Tattoo
Hamburg 📖 121
English Palace
Hazlet, 908 739 1354 📖 180
English-Speaking Gay Group (EGG)
Bruxelles / Brussel 📖 36
Enigma
Chicago 📖 249
Roissy 📖 105
Enterprise
Boston, 617 983 3264 📖 268
Entitlement—The Book Company
Halifax, 902 420 0565 📖 48
Entraide SIDA
Namur / Namen, 8 122 2422 📖 39
Entre Nous MC
Boston 📖 268
Entre Nous Newsletter 📖 220
EON 📖 *See* Expressing Our Nature
Epidermal Intrusions 📖 194
Eppendorfer
Hamburg 📖 120
Equal Time 📖 279
Equinox
Santa Cruz, 408 457 1441 📖 221
Erex
Amsterdam 📖 153
Erie County Medical Center
Buffalo, 716 898 3000 📖 298
Erie Sisters 📖 328
Erisian Fields Cohousing
Eugene 📖 325
Erlkœnig Buchladen
Stuttgart, 711 63 9139 📖 133
Erne's Sportlade
Zürich 📖 180
Ero Box
Berlin, 30 882 1331 📖 111
Erocenter
Borås 📖 176
Halmstad 📖 173
Helsingborg 📖 174
Jönköping 📖 175
Erogenous Zone
Fullerton, 714 879 3270 📖 200
Eros
Alkmaar, 72 512 1551 📖 151
Dallas / Fort Worth, 214 351 3654 📖 341
Hartford, 203 297 2408 📖 231
Hilversum, 35 623 3588 📖 156
Rotterdam, 10 466 8805 📖 158
Tampere 📖 95
Toulouse, 61 63 4472 📖 106
Eros Boutique
Essen, 201 78 8321 📖 116

Eros Center
Riccione, 541 64 8686 141
Rimini, 541 22465 141
Eros Comix
Seattle, 800 657 1100 353
Eros Publishing
Seattle, 206 767 8269 352
EROS, The Center for Safe Sex
San Francisco, 415 255 4921 214
Erosart
Hanerau 107
Eroshop
Antibes, 93 34 09 04 98
EroSpirit Research Institute
Oakland, 800 432 3767 207
Eroteak
Lowestoft, 1502 519222 91
Erotec
Tujunga, 818 352 4344 223
Erotheek
Gouda, 18 258 2302 155
Erotic Art Museum
Hamburg 120
Erotic Corner
Hertogenbosch, 's / Den Bosch, 73 614 3436 156
Erotic Forum
Harrisburg, 717 393 9722 328
Erotic Shop
Bonn, 228 65 5041 112
München, 89 260 78709 128
Offenburg, 781 2 3553 130
Erotic Visions
New York 300
Erotic World
Münster, 251 4 7833 129
Erotica Plus
Hull, 613 777 4069 61
Las Vegas, 702 362 0079 286
Erotica Project
San Francisco, 415 558 8112 219
Erotica S. F.
San Francisco, 415 861 4101 218
Eroticism through Sensual Conduct, Attitude, & Power Exchange (Escape)
West, 702 226 5441 (voicemail) 286
Erotics Gallery
New York, 212 633 2241 308
Erotik Handlung Copenhagen
Stuttgart, 711 640 6778 134
Erotik Shop
Leipzig, 341 28 41 44 125
es.alt.sex 6
Escape See Eroticism through Sensual Conduct, Attitude, & Power Exchange
Escape Bookstore
Detroit, 313 336 6558 275
Esoterica Society
Randolph 272
Espace MAN
published by Fraction Presse SARL 97
Especially for Me
Upland, 909 946 6251 224
Essemian Press
El Cerrito, 510 232 1369 199
Essential Image
Brixham 68
Essentiel / HIV Anonyme
Montréal, 514 598 8402 62
Essex Intim
Hadleigh, 1702 555407 75
Essex Leather
Westcliff On Sea 75
Esteem
Hamilton, 7 856 1162 162
Esthesia, Anne
Calgary 41
Etc.
Auburn 191
Etcetera Magazine 244
Etcetera News
New York, 212 675 7952 309
Ethos
broadcast by 6RTR FM 92.1 34
Manchester, 161 442 3030 76
Ets Cochon
Paris 104
Etscovitz, Lee
Willow Grove, 215 657 1560 333
Ettie Rout Centre
Christchurch, 3 379 1953 161
Ettner, Randi, Ph.D.
Chicago, 708 328 3433 248
ETVC See Educational TV Channel
Eulenspiegel Society (TES)
New York, 212 388 7022 (recorded message) 303
Euro Men
Amsterdam 150
Euro X
Bruxelles / Brussel 37
Euro-Business Services Inc.
Schüpfheim, 41 485 0081 176
Eurofantasia
Sandnes, 51 662422 166
Europa 92
Leather Shop, 2 669 92448 139
Milano, 2 282 6356 139
Milano, 2 295 13708 139
Milano, 2 546 9582 139
Verona, 45 800 9714 147
Europa Bookstore
Austin, 512 476 0423 339
European Confederation of Motorcycle Clubs
Zürich 179
European Uniform Club
Schoten 39
Europost
Amsterdam 150
EURO-QUEER 3
EURO-QUEER-STUDIES 2
Euros
published by Bruno Gmünder Verlag 108
EURO-SAPPHO 3
Eurotique, Inc.
West Palm Beach, 407 624 5609 243
Evansdale Men's Support Group
319 233 4766 256
Evansville Gay & Lesbian Parents Coalition
812 422 4075 254
Eve Browne Fashions
New York 181, 182, 189
EVE Fund
San Francisco, 415 281 0292 215
Eve's Garden
New York, 800 848 3837 186, 309
Events
Birmingham 93
Evergreen Chronicles
Minneapolis / Saint Paul, 612 649 4982 281
published by The Evergreen Chronicles 281
Everlasting Tattoo
San Francisco, 415 928 6244 219
Every Woman's Coming Out Group
Denver, 303 837 1598 228
Everyone's Books
Brattleboro, 802 254 8160 346
Everywoman 84
Everywoman Books
Victoria, 604 388 9411 47
Excalibur of Cleveland 318
Excelsior MC
New York 304
Excess Motorcycle Club
Bristol 70
Exchange
Charlotte 313
Houston 342
Excite 7
Exclusively Adult
Springfield, 503 726 6969 327
Executive Express
Edmonton, 403 482 7480 43
Executive Imports International
New York 302, 307
Exeter AIDS Line
1392 411600 73
Exit 97
published by Highland Publications, c. c. 172
Exotic Body
Sacramento, 916 447 6824 210
Exotic Bookstore
Dayton, 513 228 3584 321
Exotique
Tampa, 813 889 9477 243
Expectations
Amsterdam 150, 153
London, 171 739 0292 69, 86
Exploded Views Books
North Hollywood 207
Express
published by Cornerstone Publications 160
Expressing Our Nature (EON)
Syracuse, 315 475 7013 (office) 312
Extremus Body Arts
Kansas City, 816 756 1142 283
Eyecrusher Leather
Stevens Point 358
EZS See Lesben & Schwulen Zentrum Saar
F & J Police Equipment, Inc.
Bronx, 718 665 4535 297
F Street
Chula Vista, 619 585 3314 198
El Cajon, 619 447 0381 197
Escondido, 619 480 6031 199
Gaslamp, 619 236 0841 212
Kearny Mesa, 619 292 8083 212
Mira Mesa, 619 549 8014 212
North Park, 619 298 2644 212
Pacific Beach, 619 581 0400 212
San Ysidro, 619 497 6042 212
Sports Arena, 619 221 0075 212
F. A.
Paris 104
F. A. C. T.
Buckingham, 215 598 0750 328
F2M Fraternity
New York, 908 298 8797 304
Fa. Dawi
München 107
Fab Magazine 59
Face 84
Facette 115
FACT See Fighting AIDS Continously Together
Ottawa, 819 770 1945 52
Québec 62
Factor Press
Mobile, 800 304 0077 (24hrs., orders only) 192
Mobile, 800 304 0077 (24hrs., U.S. orders only) 192
FACTS See Fife AIDS Care Through Support
London, 181 348 9195 82
Faerie Dish Rag (FDR) 205
Fag Rag 269
published by Snaxus Productions 339
Fahey / Klein Art Gallery
Los Angeles 205
Fairfax Lesbian & Gay Citizens Association (FLGCA)
703 451 9528 348
Fairy Tales
Dortmund 107
Fallen Angel
Fort Lauderdale 237
Families & Friends of Lesbians & Gays (FFLAG)
Manchester 76
Family & Children's Services
Minneapolis / Saint Paul, 612 339 9101 279
Family & Friends of PWA's Support Network
Chicago, 708 325 8488 249
Family Next Door 208
Family Planning Association
Auckland, 9 486 1014 160
Family Services Woodfield
Bridgeport, 203 368 4291 229
Family Study Institute of Fort Wayne
219 424 2455 254
Family Synergy
Culver City 198
Family Tree
Boston 268
Fan The Flames
Columbus, 614 447 0565 320, 321
Fanfare Books
Stratford, 519 273 1010 54
Fanny's
London 83
Fantasia
Orlando, 407 425 4527 240
Fantasies
Durban, 31 304 1408 171
Fantasies In Lace, Inc.
Fort Lauderdale, 305 581 8412 182
Fantasies Unlimited
Jupiter, 407 743 4244 182
Fantasmatic & Fetish Club
Namur / Namen 39
Fantastic Books Publications
Amityville, 516 753 2677 296
Fantastic!
London, 181 674 1076 83
Fantasy Erotique
London, 181 555 2996 10, 81
Fantasy Faire
Reno, 702 323 6969 287
Fantasy Fashions
Westmount 182
Woodland Hills 225
Fantasy Fayre
London 86
Fantasy for Adults Only
Missoula, 406 543 7510 285
Missoula, 406 543 7760 285
Fantasy House
Minneapolis / Saint Paul, 612 333 6313 281
Fantasy Inn
Dover 290
Fantasy Island
Philadelphia, 215 332 5454 331
Fantasy Island Innovations, Inc.
Fort Lauderdale, 800 785 9955 (orders) 184
Fantasy Isle
Danbury, 203 743 1792 230
Fantasy Leathers
Springfield 186
Fantasy Lingerie
Fountain Valley, 714 775 8356 199
Fantasy of Gord
published by H. G. Publications 359
Fantasy Unlimited
Seattle, 206 682 0167 353
Fantasy World
Hanley 91
Fantasy World Products
Webster 312
Fantasy Youth
London, 171 229 5672 82
Fantasyland Products
Owen Sound, 519 371 1215 41, 53
Farley's Bookstore
New Hope, 215 862 2452 329
Fascination
Liverpool, 151 252 2272 87
Fashion & Tools
Bremen, 421 339 8270 113
Hamburg, 40 319 2361 120
Fashion Cats
Düsseldorf, 211 787276 115
Fashion World International
Sacramento, 916 631 8777 182
Fat Girl
San Francisco, 714 550 7202 8
Fatale Video
San Francisco, 800 845 4617 187
FATE See Foundation for the Advancement of Transgendered People's Society
Faubourg-Marigny Bookstore
New Orleans, 504 943 9875 261
Faultline
Hollywood 201
Fayetteville Regional Medical Center
501 442 1000 195
Feather of Hope Aboriginal AIDS Prevention Society
Calgary, 403 488 5773 42
Febo Editores, S. A. de C. V.
Mexico City 149
Federal Bargain Stores
New York 309
Federation
Nottingham, 115 941 3435 89
Feelings
Lismore Heights 24

Felicity
London 🕮 82
Feline Films
San Francisco, 510 533 6474 🕮 216
Felise Leather
Washington, 202 342 7163 🕮 235
Felix Halle
Weimar, 364 342 0873 🕮 135
Felshin, Elaine, Ph.D.
New York, 212 533 4092 🕮 300
Fem Fashions, Inc.
New York, 212 629 5750 🕮 309
Fem TV 🕮 343
Female Domination Forever
published by Carter Stevens Presents 🕮 332
Female FYI 🕮 205
Female Mimics International
published by Leoram, Inc. 🕮 223
Female Supremacy
published by Tiffany Enterprises 🕮 311
Female Trouble
Philadelphia, 215 732 6898 🕮 330
Females Investigating Sexual Terrain (FIST)
Baltimore, 410 675 0856 🕮 264
FEMDOM-L 🕮 2
Femina Society International
Haverhill, 718 648 8215 🕮 271
Feminine Connection
Oakland, 201 337 7506 🕮 292
Feminine Disciplinary Society
London 🕮 82
Feminine Illusion
published by New Esoteric Press 🕮 308
Feminique 🕮 348
Feminist Bookstore News 🕮 217
Feminist Press at The City University of New York
212 360 5790 🕮 308
Feminist Studies 🕮 265
Feminist Voices 🕮 356
Feminists Against Censorship
London, 181 552 4405 🕮 83
Femme Erotica
Adelaide, 8 410 0636 🕮 31
FEMSUPREM 🕮 2
Fenway Community Health Center
Boston, 617 267 0900 🕮 267
Fer Rouge
published by RM Distribution, Ltd. 🕮 16
Fernando Cerqueira
Oeiras 🕮 167
Ferrari Publications
Phœnix, 602 863 2408 🕮 189
Ferron, Michael
Amsterdam 🕮 152
Fesseln Fashions
Welshpool 🕮 359
Fetasy Guide
published by Gear, Inc. 🕮 15
Feticon
Essen 🕮 116
Fetische in Leder, Latex, & Lack
Frankfurt am Main, 69 43 9187 🕮 117
Fetish
published by The Leather Journal 🕮 225
Fetish Bazaar
published by B & D Pleasures 🕮 202
Fetish Factory Ltd.
Evercreech, 1749 831397 🕮 90
Solingen, 21 258 6151 🕮 8, 11, 14, 19
Fetish Fetish
London, 171 734 8343 🕮 86
Fetish Network
North Miami Beach, 800 536 6462 🕮 184, 185, 240
Fetish Network BBS
North Miami Beach, 800 536 6462 🕮 240
Fetish Street 🕮 150
Fetish Times
published by Mang Publishing 🕮 19
Fetish Video Review
published by Carter Stevens Presents 🕮 332
Fetish World
published by New Esoteric Press 🕮 308
Fetish/SM Market
London 🕮 80
Fetters
London, 171 820 7780 🕮 81
FFA - FGC
Fort Lauderdale, 305 761 3961 🕮 236
FFA/CAC
Washington 🕮 234
FFLAG 🕮 *See* Families & Friends of Lesbians & Gays
FFT Publishing
Cairns 🕮 22
FG FM 98.2
Paris, 140 13 8800 🕮 104
fido.ger.gay 🕮 6
fido.ger.sex 🕮 6
fido7.sex 🕮 6
Fife AIDS Care Through Support (FACTS)
Buckhaven, 159 271 5200 🕮 168
Fife Friend
Kirkcaldy, 1592 266688 🕮 168
Fifth Wheel
Portsmouth, 603 436 1504 🕮 288
Fig Garden Bookstore
Fresno, 209 226 1845 🕮 200
Fight For Life
Orlando, 407 932 4482 🕮 240
Fightback Trust
East Anglia, 1284 725600 🕮 91
East Anglia, 1473 289200 🕮 91
East Anglia, 1502 501509 🕮 91
East Anglia, 1603 762656 🕮 88
Fighting AIDS Continously Together (FACT)
Lehigh Valley, 610 820 5519 🕮 329
Filia, Rich
San Diego, 619 298 1973 🕮 183
Film @ Eleven
San Francisco, 415 469 2093 🕮 215
Filmore News
Erie, 814 833 2667 🕮 328
Final Frontier
Chicago 🕮 248
Finders
Belmont Shore 🕮 184
finet.sex 🕮 6
Finnish AIDS Council
Helsinki, 90 17 5822 🕮 95
Firebirds
Milwaukee 🕮 357
Firedancers
Dallas 🕮 340
San Antonio 🕮 344
Firefly
Baltimore, 410 732 1232 🕮 264
Firekeepers of Indiana
Mishawaka 🕮 255
Fireweed 🕮 59
First 🕮 108
First Amendment
Colorado Springs, 719 630 7676 🕮 227
First City Network, Inc.
Savannah, 912 236 2489 🕮 246
First Hand 🕮 293
First In Schumode
Rosenheim, 803 11 3625 🕮 131
First Quality Products, Inc.
Great Neck, 516 829 3030 🕮 299
First Run Features
New York, 212 243 0600 🕮 302
Fischer, Ernst
Heidelberg 🕮 107
FIST 🕮 *See* Females Investigating Sexual Terrain
Fit 2 A T Leather
Denver, 303 294 9916 🕮 229
Fit To Be Tied
Seal Beach, 310 597 1234 🕮 222
Fits Like A Glove (FLAG)
North Dartmouth, 508 996 1394 🕮 13
fj.sci.medical 🕮 4
fj.sci.psychology 🕮 4
FLAG 🕮 *See* Fits Like A Glove
Flamands Roses
Lille, 20 47 6265 🕮 100
Flamingo
published by Kiss Contact 🕮 40
FLAS
Stanford-Le-Hope 🕮 75
Flash 🕮 170
Flash Video
San Francisco, 415 267 7651 🕮 218
FLC 🕮 *See* Frankfurter Lederclub e. V.
Flensburger Initiative & Treffpunkt für Schwule
461 2 5618 🕮 117
Flesh Canvas
East Molesley 🕮 91
Fleshworks
Raleigh, 919 782 5548 🕮 316
FLGCA 🕮 *See* Fairfax Lesbian & Gay Citizens Association
Fliederfunk
broadcast by FM 95.8 🕮 129
Fliederlich e. V.
Nürnberg, 911 22 2377 🕮 129
Flinders Medical Centre
Adelaide, 8 204 5192 🕮 30
Flinders University Gay Society
Adelaide, 8 201 2276 🕮 30
Flint Hills Alliance
Manhattan, 913 587 0016 🕮 258
FL-MOTSS 🕮 3
Florida Bear Hunters
Orlando 🕮 240
Florida HIV/AIDS Hotline
Tallahassee, 800 352 2437 🕮 235
Florida Keys Memorial Hospital
Key West, 305 294 5531 🕮 238
Florida Medical Center
Fort Lauderdale, 305 735 6000 🕮 236
Flying Lemur Bookstore
Lakewood, 216 221 2535 🕮 321
Flywheel, Ltd.
Egham 🕮 91
FM
San Francisco 🕮 214
FM 100
Cayenne 🕮 106
FM 100.3
Helsinki 🕮 96
FM 102.1
Brisbane, 7 252 1555 🕮 29
FM 102.3
Montréal, 514 843 4564 🕮 63
FM 103.1
Göteborg, 31 11 1430 🕮 173
FM 104.2
Düsseldorf, 211 733 6540 🕮 115
FM 104.6
Saint Louis, 89 67 6566 🕮 105
FM 105.7, Cable 83.1
Leiden, 71 512 0110 🕮 156
FM 106.7, 92.2, 89.5, & 98.7
Århus, 86 19 3222 🕮 65
FM 107.1 & 97.8
Köln, 221 13 3446 🕮 124
FM 88
Stockholm, 8 736 0216 🕮 176
FM 88.7
Caen 🕮 99
FM 89
Beauvais 🕮 98
FM 89.2
Malmö 🕮 174
FM 89.4
Alençon 🕮 97
FM 90.7
Melbourne, 39 690 0907 🕮 32
FM 91.2
Dortmund 🕮 114
FM 92.1
Hobart 🕮 31
FM 92.2, Cable 106.2
Oberhausen, 911 825 2662 🕮 130
FM 94.1
Amiens 🕮 98
FM 95.3
Örebro 🕮 174
FM 95.8
Nürnberg, 911 20 4069 🕮 129
FM 96
Béziers 🕮 98
FM 96.0, Cable 95.4
Hamburg 🕮 120
Hamburg, 40 43 6268 🕮 120
FM 96.1 or FM 104.5
Gladbeck 🕮 118
FM 96.2
Helsinki 🕮 96
FM 96.8
Biarritz 🕮 98
FM 98.9
København, 33 33 0404 🕮 66
FM 99.7
Angers 🕮 98
FM Concepts
North Hollywood 🕮 207
Focus International
Huntington, 516 549 5320 🕮 290
Focus, Inc.
Boston, 617 876 4488 🕮 267
Focused Counseling Services, Inc.
Blackwood, 609 228 8910 🕮 289
Foerster Verlag
Darmstadt, 61 513 3468 🕮 108
Frankfurt am Main, 69 297 8681 🕮 108
Foley, Lyn, ACSW
Concord, 603 224 5600 🕮 287
Folies de Sade
Bruxelles / Brussel, 2 219 7997 🕮 37
Follow Me
München, 89 202 1208 🕮 128
Fondation Nationale du Transsexualisme
Montréal, 514 526 5892 🕮 41
Fondazione Sandro Penna
Torino, 11 43 4749 🕮 138
Fondo Olivari
Milano, 2 581 00299 🕮 142
Fontanella, Robert, CSW
New York, 212 741 2739 🕮 300
Food For Thought Alternative Book Store
Fargo, 701 239 4052 🕮 316
Food For Thought Books
Amherst, 413 253 5432 🕮 267
Ottawa, 613 236 3361 🕮 53
Foot & Rope Club
Speedway 🕮 188
Foot Fraternity
Cleveland, 216 449 4114 🕮 188
Foot Friends
New York, 212 675 7352 🕮 304
Foot Guys
Lakeland 🕮 238
Foothills AIDS Awareness Association
Okotoks, 403 938 4911 🕮 44
Footmen
Saint Helens 🕮 87
Footprints
published by Carter Stevens Presents 🕮 332
Footsy
published by FLAS 🕮 75
For You 🕮 256
For You Productions
Cleveland, 800 560 8712 🕮 319
For'Hommes
Bordeaux, 56 50 6300 🕮 98
Forbidden
Portsmouth, 1705 826655 🕮 76
Forbidden Fruit
Austin, 512 478 8358 🕮 186, 339
State College, 814 234 0605 🕮 333
Forbidden Fruit Uptown
Austin, 512 478 8542 🕮 339
Föreningen BHUS
Stockholm, 8 34 1105 🕮 175
Foreskin Quarterly
published by Brush Creek Media 🕮 217
Forge Tavern
Vancouver, 604 683 2923 🕮 45
Fort Video & News
Fayetteville, 910 868 9905 🕮 315
Fort Wayne Gay & Lesbian Resource Center & Archives
Indianapolis, 219 744 1144 🕮 254
Forth Friend
Stirling, 1786 471285 🕮 167
Forum
Philadelphia 🕮 330
Forum Homosexualität und Literatur 🕮 108
Forum Society
Cardiff 🕮 359
Foundation
Bruxelles / Brussel, 2 219 3351 🕮 37
Foundation for the Advancement of Transgendered People's Society (FATE)
Vancouver, 604 254 9591 🕮 45
Fountain 🕮 236
Fountains of Pleasure
Novi, 810 348 5332 🕮 180
Fountainview News

Houston, 713 781 7793 343
Four B's Club
Edinburgh 168
Four Corner News
Buffalo, 716 877 4344 298
Four D Rubber Co. Ltd.
Heanor, 1773 763134 73
Fourth Street Bookmart
Saint Petersburg, 813 821 8824 241
Fox Studio
Venice, 310 399 4770 187
Fox Valley AIDS Project
414 733 2068 355, 356
Fox Valley Gay Association
Chicago, 708 931 1110 250
Foxes Adult Books
North Augusta, 803 279 7023 335
Foxy Lady
Malmö 174
San Francisco, 415 285 4980 219
FPE *See* Freedom of Personality Expression
FPSG
San Francisco 215
Fraction Presse SARL
Paris, 144 75 7979 97
FRAGLY *See* Framingham Regional Alliance of Gay & Lesbian Youth
Framingham Regional Alliance of Gay & Lesbian Youth (FRAGLY)
508 655 7183 270
Framingham State College Gays, Lesbians, & Friends (GLAF) 270
francom.medical 4
Franjeppot
Deurne 38
Frankel's
Toronto, 416 366 4221 60
Frankel, Susan, CSW, BCD
New York, 212 877 5114 300
Frankfurter Lederclub e. V. (FLC)
Frankfurt am Main, 69 29 3904 117
Frankfurter Schwule, Automones AStA-Schwulenreferat
Frankfurt am Main, 69 77 7575 117
Frankies Erotik Shop
Hannover, 511 262 1052 121
Franklin-Grand Isle AIDS Task Force
Saint Albans, 800 638 7834 346
Fraternity House
Washington, 202 223 4917 233
Fraternity of Enema Buddies
Chicago, 312 561 7188 12
Frederick's of Hollywood
818 993 3988 183
Fredericksburg Area HIV/AIDS Support Services, Inc.
703 371 7532 348
Frederickson & Associates
Minneapolis / Saint Paul, 612 646 8373 279
Free Clinic
Bruxelles / Brussel 36
Free Map of Amsterdam 152
Free University Hospital
Amsterdam, 20 548 9111 Ext. 199 151
Freedom Editions
London, 171 420 5555 84
Freedom FM
London, 171 916 0162 85
Freedom of Personality Expression (FPE)
Frankfurt 117
Northern Europe
Denmark, 42 13 9032 66
Norway 164
Sweden 173
Freewave Radio
broadcast by FM 105.7, Cable 83.1 156
Freie Transenstadt Hamburg
40 656 0585 120
Freies Tagungshaus Waldschlößhen
Gleichen-Reinhausen, 559 2 2382 107
Freizeitverein Priapos
Wien, 1 812 4716 35
Fremont Place Book Company
Seattle, 206 547 5970 353
French Addiction
Gainesville, 904 373 6628 237
Fréquence 4 FM 99.6
Bordeaux 98
Frequence Gaie
broadcast by FG FM 98.2 104
Frere Hospital
East London, 431 27350 171
Fresh Fruit
broadcast by KFAI FM 90.3 281
Fresno Community Hospital & Medical Center
209 442 6000 199
Friday Night Womyn's Group
Miami, 305 253 3740 239
Friedeman, Sheila, Ph.D.
Phœnix, 602 956 3006 193
Friendly Voice 241
Friends & Relatives of Gays (FROG)
Greenville, 513 548 6730 321
Friends Club
Göteborg, 31 15 5615 173
Friends For Life
Memphis, 901 458 2437 336
Friends For Life—Capital Area AIDS Services, Inc.
Baton Rouge, 504 923 2277 260
Friends From The Heart
Erie, 814 838 0123 328
Friends North
Traverse City, 616 946 1804 278
Friends of the Tattoo Archive
Berkeley 13
Frighten The Horses
published by Heat Seeking Publishing 217
Frisch, Hannah, Ph.D.
Chicago, 312 924 5057 249
Frisco
Firenze, 55 35 7351 138
FROG *See* Friends & Relatives of Gays
Front Page 316
Edmonton, 403 426 1206 43
Front Range Bears
Denver, 303 331 2705 228
Frontera Gay 212
Frontiers 225
Madison, 608 251 7424 356
Frontline
Hannover 121
Frontline Books
Manchester, 161 236 1101 23
FRS Enterprises
San Francisco, 415 863 6538 217
Fruits of Our Labors
Belfast, 207 338 2913 261
FSC
Berlin 110
FSMC
Marseille 101
FTM International
Oakland, 510 287 2646 207
FTM Network
London, 161 432 1915 85
Manchester 76
FTM Nippon
Adachi-Ku, 3 3683 6092 147
FUGS *See* Uppsala Gay Studenter
Fulham Army & Navy Store
London, 171 610 3577 87
Full Circle Books
Albuquerque, 800 951 0053 294
Full Moon Fashions
Hamburg 107
Full Moon Saloon
Orlando, 407 648 8725 240
Fuller, Cheryl, M.A., LCPC
Portland, 207 774 4436 262
Fun House
Baarle Nassau 154
Fundgeon Times
published by B & D Pleasures 202
Funny Skin
Haarlem, 23 542 1870 155
Fürsorger für Homosexuelle im Caritas Verband
Bernberg 111
Futami - Shobo Co., Ltd.
Bunkyo-Ku, 3 3942 2311 147
Future Sex
published by Kundalini Publishing, Inc. 217
Future Shock
Indianapolis, 317 251 6957 255
Fux, Andreas
Berlin, 30 442 5501 110
Fylkeslegen i Hamar
62 53 0033 165
Fylkeslegen i Ostfold
Moss, 32 25 5589 166
G & D Merchandise
New York, 212 221 8947 309
G & M Fashions Ltd.
Romford 75
G & T Breakfast Show
broadcast by Access Community Radio AM 810 161
G'Day Guide 24
G. D. C.
Amsterdam, 20 625 1301 153
G. I. Joes
Ukiah, 707 468 8834 223
G.A.Y, The Radio
broadcast by Spectrum Radio AM 558 85
G/L/B Support Group
Columbus, 614 363 0431 320
GAB *See* Gay Advice Bureau
Gabrielly, Vince
New York, 212 977 5433 (studio) 306
GACH *See* Gelders Advies Centrum Homosexualiteit
Gaeilgeori Aerach Aontaithe
Dublin 136
Gage
Paris, 146 03 2012 103
GAI *See* Gai Amitié Initiative
Gai Amitié Initiative (GAI)
Nancy 102
Gai Guide
published by The Gai Project 89
Gai Moto Club
Paris 103
Gai Project
Nottingham, 115 947 5414 89
Gaia Bookstore
Berkeley, 510 548 4172 197
Gaie France en Português 167
Gaie Livraison
Winnipeg, 204 474 0212 47
Gai-Ecoute
Montréal, 514 521 1508 62
Gaiement Vôtre
broadcast by FM 89.4 97
Gaiety Burlesk
New York, 212 221 8868 309
Gai-Kitsch-Camp (CKC)
published by Cahiers Gai-Kitsch-Camp 14
Gair, Susan, MSW, CSW
New York, 212 799 5436 300
Gais Nounours
Paris 103
GALA *See* Dorchester Gay & Lesbian Alliance. *See also* Gay & Lesbian Association. *See also* Gay & Lesbian Association of Adelaide University. *See also* Gay & Lesbian Association. *See also* Gay & Lesbian Parents Coalition. *See also* Hamilton Gay & Lesbian Alliance. *See also* Poughkeepsie Gay & Lesbian Alliance. *See also* Stichting Gay & Lesbian Association Amsterdam. *See also* Students for Bisexual, Gay, & Lesbian Awareness
GALA 10
Erie, 814 824 2572 328
GALA of CSULA
Los Angeles, 213 224 3595 204
GALA TC
Burnaby, 604 291 3182 44
Galactica
Paris, 148 74 5671 104
Galerie Janssen
Berlin 111
Galerie Leon
Phœnix, 602 263 0463 1
Galerie Michel Vidal
Paris, 143 42 2271 104
Galerie Welker
Heidelberg 122
Galesburg Adult Book & Video
309 342 7019 252
Galileo
Rockhampton 29
Galisteo News
Santa Fe, 505 984 1216 295
Gall's, Inc.
Lexington, 800 477 7766 259
Galleria Diva (DivaNet)
San Francisco, 415 285 8157 184
Galleria Erotica
Köln 124
Gallerie Reygers
München 128
Gallery Bookstore
Des Moines, 515 245 9164 256
Gallina, Raelyn
Oakland, 510 655 2855 208
GALOHI *See* Gay & Lesbians of Hawaii Island
GALON *See* Gay & Lesbian Outreach Network
GALOR *See* Gays & Lesbians of Rice
GALS *See* Gay & Lesbian Support
GaLTaS *See* Gay & Lesbian Teachers & Students Association, Inc.
GALY-NY *See* Gay & Lesbian Youth in New Jersey
GAMIT *See* Gays, Lesbians, Bisexuals, & Friends at MIT
Gamma Line
Melbourne, 39 899 0509 32
Ganymede Press, Inc.
Baltimore, 410 727 5241 264
Gaol House
Northam, 170 333 2830 76
GAPA *See* Grupo de Apoio a Pacientes de AIDS
Garcia, Dianne, MSW, Ph.D.
Brick, 908 920 8110 289
Garden Grove Hospital & Medical Center
714 537 5160 200
Garden of Eden
Garden Grove, 714 534 9805 200
GASA *See* Gay Association of South Africa
Gatehouse
Melbourne, 39 417 2182 31
Gates of Heck
Richmond, 804 266 9422 349
Gateway MC
Saint Louis 284
Gatewood, Charles
San Francisco, 415 267 7651 216
Gauntlet II
Los Angeles, 213 669 9472 203
Gauntlet, Inc.
Los Angeles, 310 657 6677 204
New York, 212 229 0180 306
Paris, 147 007360 104
San Francisco, 415 252 1404 20
San Francisco, 800 746 4728 216
Gauntlet, Inc. Mail Order & Customer Service
San Francisco, 800 746 4728 187
Gay & Lesbian & All Student Association
Syracuse 312
Gay & Lesbian Adolescent Social Services, Inc.
West Hollywood, 310 288 1757 224
Gay & Lesbian Advcacy Research Project
Columbia, 803 791 1607 335
Gay & Lesbian Advocacy Research Project
Columbia 335
Gay & Lesbian Alliance
Bloomington, 309 438 2429 248
Eugene, 503 686 3360 325
Hartford 231
New Britain 231
Portland, 207 874 6956 262
San Francisco, 415 239 3212 215
Sarasota 242
Syracuse, 315 422 5732 312
Gay & Lesbian Alliance at Brooklyn College
718 951 4234 297
Gay & Lesbian Alliance at Southern Oregon State College
Ashland / Medford, 503 552 7702 324
Gay & Lesbian Alliance at UNB/STU
Fredricton 48
Gay & Lesbian Alliance in Orange County

New York, 914 782 1525 📖 305
Gay & Lesbian Alliance of Central Texas
Waco, 800 735 1122 📖 345
Gay & Lesbian Alliance of Eastern Oregon State College
La Grande 📖 325
Gay & Lesbian Alliance of Greater Danbury
203 426 4922 📖 230
Gay & Lesbian Alliance of Syracuse (GLAS)
315 422 5732 📖 312
Gay & Lesbian Alliance of Ventura County
805 963 3636 📖 224
Gay & Lesbian Alliance San Francisco State University 📖 215
Gay & Lesbian Alliance SUC-Oswego
315 341 2955 📖 310
Gay & Lesbian Americans
Washington, 202 889 5111 📖 234
Gay & Lesbian Archives of Washington, DC
Falls Church, 703 671 3930 📖 348
Gay & Lesbian Association (GALA)
Cape Town, 21 21 5420 📖 171
Pullman, 509 335 4311 📖 350
Gay & Lesbian Association of Adelaide University (GALA)
8 362 3223 📖 30
Gay & Lesbian Association of Central Alberta
Red Deer, 403 340 2198 (recorded message) 📖 44
Gay & Lesbian Association of Durango
303 247 7778 📖 229
Gay & Lesbian Association of Simcoe County
Orillia, 613 325 0033 📖 52
Gay & Lesbian Association of Students & Staff (GLASS)
Winnipeg, 204 477 8184 📖 47
Gay & Lesbian Association of Students at SIU-E
Edwardsville, 618 692 2686 📖 252
Gay & Lesbian Association UCLA
Los Angeles, 213 825 8053 📖 204
Gay & Lesbian Association, San Joaquin County
Stockton, 209 464 5615 📖 223
Gay & Lesbian Center, Island Empire
San Bernardino, 909 884 5447 📖 210
Gay & Lesbian Centre
Montréal, 514 528 8424 📖 62
Vancouver, 604 684 6869 📖 45
Gay & Lesbian Community (GLC)
Flagstaff, 602 774 1521 📖 193
Gay & Lesbian Community Alliance
Galesburg 📖 252
Gay & Lesbian Community at UWM
Milwaukee, 414 229 6555 📖 357
Gay & Lesbian Community Center
Baltimore, 410 837 5445 📖 264
Fort Lauderdale, 305 763 1530 📖 236
New York, 212 620 7310 📖 304
Oahu, 808 951 7000 📖 247
Gay & Lesbian Community Center of Chicago
312 665 5300 📖 250
Gay & Lesbian Community Center of Colorado, Inc.
Denver, 303 831 6268 📖 227, 228
Gay & Lesbian Community Center of Pittsburgh
412 422 0114 📖 332
Gay & Lesbian Community Centre of Edmonton
403 488 3234 📖 43
Gay & Lesbian Community Council of Utah
Salt Lake City, 801 539 8800 📖 345
Gay & Lesbian Community of Howard County
Columbia 📖 265
Gay & Lesbian Community Services
Rochester, 507 281 3265 📖 281, 282
Gay & Lesbian Community Services Center
Los Angeles, 213 464 7400 📖 203, 204
Gay & Lesbian Community Services Center of Orange County
Garden Grove, 714 534 0862 📖 200
Gay & Lesbian Community Switchboard
Cincinnati, 513 651 0070 📖 318
Gay & Lesbian Counseling Center
Tustin, 714 731 0224 📖 223
Gay & Lesbian Counseling Services of the United Community Church
Jackson, 601 373 8610 📖 282
Gay & Lesbian Counselling
Johannesburg, 11 643 2311 📖 170
Gay & Lesbian Counselling & Information Service
Brisbane, 7 3839 3277 (gayline) 📖 29
Gay & Lesbian Counselling Service
Perth, 9 328 9044 📖 33
Gay & Lesbian Counselling Service of New South Wales
Sydney, 2 360 3063 (office) 📖 26
Gay & Lesbian Counselling Service of South Australia
Adelaide, 8 362 3223 📖 30
Gay & Lesbian Counselling South West
Exeter, 1392 422 016 📖 73
Gay & Lesbian Equality Network (GLEN)
Dublin, 1 872 1055 📖 136
Gay & Lesbian Guideline
Stamford, 203 327 0767 📖 232
Gay & Lesbian Health Collective, Inc.
Hartford, 203 278 4163 📖 230
Gay & Lesbian Health Service
Brisbane, 7 844 6806 📖 28
Gay & Lesbian Health Services of Saskatoon
306 665 1224 📖 64
Gay & Lesbian Helpline
Fort Wayne, 219 744 1199 📖 254
Morgantown, 304 292 4292 📖 355
Gay & Lesbian Helpline of Rhode Island
Providence, 401 751 3322 📖 334
Gay & Lesbian Helpline of Wake County
Raleigh, 919 821 0055 📖 315
Gay & Lesbian Historical Society of Northern California
San Francisco, 415 626 0980 📖 196
Gay & Lesbian Hotline
Minneapolis / Saint Paul, 612 822 8661 📖 279
New York, 914 948 4922 📖 302
Saint Louis, 314 367 0084 📖 284
Washington, 202 833 3234 📖 233
Gay & Lesbian Independent Broadcasters (GLIB)
New York, 212 473 1689 📖 308
Gay & Lesbian Info Line
Tijuana, 66 88 0267 📖 149
Gay & Lesbian Info Services
Springfield, 413 731 5403 📖 272
Gay & Lesbian Law Caucus
Pittsburgh, 412 648 1388 📖 332
Gay & Lesbian Liberation of Waterloo (GLLOW)
519 884 4569 📖 60
Gay & Lesbian Line
Sydney, 2 360 2211 📖 26
Gay & Lesbian London
broadcast by Greater London Radio 📖 85
Gay & Lesbian Network
Bangor, 207 862 5907 📖 262
Gay & Lesbian Olin Business School Alliance (GLOBAL)
Saint Louis, 314 935 6315 📖 284
Gay & Lesbian Organization of Reading & Allentown (GLORA)
Lehigh Valley 📖 329
Gay & Lesbian Outreach Network (GALON)
Bend, 503 388 2395 📖 324
Coos Bay, 503 269 4182 📖 325
Gay & Lesbian Parent Coalition
San Antonio, 210 342 8696 📖 344
Gay & Lesbian Parenting Group of Central Ohio
Columbus, 614 497 8652 📖 320
Gay & Lesbian Parents
El Toro, 714 720 9460 📖 199
Lehigh Valley, 610 439 8755 📖 329
Gay & Lesbian Parents Coalition (GALA)
Kansas City, 816 356 9589 📖 283
Gay & Lesbian Parents Coalition (GLPC—MW)
Gaithersburg, 301 762 4828 📖 265
Gay & Lesbian Parents Coalition International (GLPCI)
Florida, 407 420 2191 📖 240
Washington, D. C., 202 583 8029 📖 234
Gay & Lesbian Peer Counseling
Philadelphia, 215 368 6100 📖 330
Gay & Lesbian Peer Counselling Group
London, 519 661 3031 📖 51
Gay & Lesbian Periodicals Directory
published by New Vista Publishing 📖 15
Gay & Lesbian Phoneline
Caribou, 207 498 2088 📖 261
Gay & Lesbian Press Association
Universal City, 818 902 1476 📖 223
Gay & Lesbian Quarterly 📖 208
Gay & Lesbian Resource Center
Cedar Rapids, 319 366 2055 📖 256
Des Moines, 515 279 2110 📖 256
Santa Barbara, 805 963 3636 📖 221
Gay & Lesbian Resource Center (GLSA)
Lincoln, 402 472 5644 📖 285
Gay & Lesbian Resource Center of Ventura County
805 389 1530 📖 224
Gay & Lesbian Services Guide
published by Training By Design 📖 235
Gay & Lesbian Services Network
Kansas City, 816 374 5910 📖 283
Gay & Lesbian Student Association
Cape Girardeau, 314 651 2996 📖 282, 283
Greensboro, 910 334 5110 📖 315
Las Cruces 📖 295
Lubbock, 806 795 8421 📖 344
Gay & Lesbian Student Society (GLSS)
Durban, 31 22 3800 📖 171
Gay & Lesbian Student Union
Albuquerque, 505 277 6739 📖 294
Norfolk 📖 348
San Bernardino, 090 887 7407 📖 210
Toledo, 419 537 7975 📖 322
Gay & Lesbian Students Union
Los Angeles, 213 669 4306 📖 204
Gay & Lesbian Studies Union
Long Beach, 310 498 4181 📖 202
Gay & Lesbian Support (GALS)
Niagara Falls 📖 310
Gay & Lesbian Support Group
Ashland 📖 355
Kalamazoo 📖 276
Gay & Lesbian Switchboard
Amsterdam, 20 623 6565 📖 152
Baltimore, 410 837 8888 📖 263
Indianapolis, 317 639 5937 📖 254
Malmö, 40 11 9944 📖 173
Melbourne, 39 510 5488 📖 32
Memphis, 901 728 4297 📖 336
New York, 212 777 1800 📖 302
Roseburg, 503 672 4126 📖 327
San José, 408 293 4525 📖 219
Wilmington, 910 675 9222 📖 316
Gay & Lesbian Switchboard Cornwall
Cambourne, 120 931 4449 📖 72
Gay & Lesbian Switchboard of Charlotte
704 535 6277 (also TDD) 📖 314
Gay & Lesbian Switchboard of Harrisburg
717 234 0328 📖 328
Gay & Lesbian Switchboard of Houston
713 529 3211 📖 342
Gay & Lesbian Switchboard of Long Island (GLSB of LI)
New York, 516 737 1615 📖 302
Gay & Lesbian Switchboard of Northern Pennsylvania
Williamsport, 717 327 1411 📖 333
Gay & Lesbian Teachers & Students Association, Inc. (GaLTaS)
Sydney, 2 350 9544 📖 27
Gay & Lesbian Teen Task Force
Oahu, 808 951 7000 📖 247
Gay & Lesbian Times/Uptown 📖 196
Gay & Lesbian Union at NYU
New York, 212 998 4938 📖 305
Gay & Lesbian Union at Queens College
New York, 718 520 1866 📖 305
Gay & Lesbian Union of Racine / Kenosha
414 634 0659 📖 358
Gay & Lesbian Welfare, Auckland
9 303 3584 📖 159
Gay & Lesbian WotsOn
Sydney, 2 361 0655 📖 26
Gay & Lesbian Young Adults
Dallas / Fort Worth, 214 521 5342 Ext. 260 📖 341
Gay & Lesbian Youth in New Jersey (GALY-NY)
Convent Station, 201 285 1595 📖 289
Gay & Lesbian Youth of Hudson Valley
New York, 914 948 4922 📖 306
Gay & Lesbian Youth of Seattle
206 322 2515 📖 352
Gay & Lesbian Youth Services
Buffalo, 716 855 0221 📖 298
Gay & Lesbians of Hawaii Island (GALOHI)
Hawaii (Big Island), 808 329 0049 📖 246
Gay Academic Union
New York, 212 864 0361 📖 303
Gay Advice Bureau
East London, 431 26665 📖 171
Gay Advice Bureau (GAB)
Pretoria, 11 643 2311 📖 172
Gay Alaska 📖 192
Gay Alliance
Cape Town, 21 21 5420 📖 170
Gay Alliance, Genesee Valley
Rochester, 716 244 9030 📖 311
Gay Alternative
broadcast by WEVL FM 90 📖 337
Gay Anglia 📖 71
Gay Area Youth Switchboard
San Francisco, 415 386 4297 📖 213
Gay Association Inland Natal
Pietermaritzburg, 331 47 2109 📖 171
Gay Association of South Africa (GASA)
East Rand, 11 845 2285 📖 171
Johannesburg, 11 725 4703 📖 171
Northern Cape, 531 31393 📖 171
Northern Transvaal, 12 62 1314 📖 172
Gay Bikers (GBMCC)
Nottingham, 115 941 1454 📖 89
Gay Blade
Thornhill 📖 54
Gay Boys on Campus
Dunedin 📖 161
Gay Broadcasting Collective
Wellington, 4 385 8783 📖 163
Gay Broadcasting System
New York, 212 243 1570 📖 310
Gay Cable Nash
broadcast by Viacom Cabe, Channel 19 📖 337
Gay Cable Network
New York, 212 727 8850 📖 310
Gay Capital Events
Amsterdam, 20 689 0279 📖 152
Gay Chicago Magazine
published by Ultra Ink, Inc. 📖 251
Gay Club Hawkes Bay
Napier 📖 162
Gay Club I. L. R. E. S.
Lisboa 📖 167
Gay College Societies
Dublin, 1 872 1055 📖 137
Gay Community AIDS Project
Champaign / Urbana, 217 351 2437 📖 248
Gay Community Directory
Oahu, 808 521 6000 (24hr. tape listing) 📖 246
Gay Community News 📖 246
published by Bromfield Street Educational Foundation 📖 269
Gay Community News (GCN) 📖 136
Gay Counseling Center of Long Island
New York, 516 795 0151 📖 301
Gay Counselling
Roma, 6 702 9037 📖 141
Gay Crisis Line
Kelowna, 604 860 8486 📖 44
Gay Express
published by Verlag W.-D. Fritsch 📖 108
Gay Fairfax 📖 349
Gay Fathers
Cleveland, 216 621 0228 📖 319
Los Angeles, 310 654 0307 📖 225
Sacramento, 916 924 3237 📖 210
Sydney, 2 360 3063 📖 26
Washington, D. C., 301 9900 0638 📖 234
Gay Fathers / Fathers First of Houston 📖 342
Gay Fathers Connection
Essex Junction 📖 346
Gay Fathers Group
Rochester, 716 924 4397 📖 311
Gay Fathers I
New York, 212 874 7727 📖 304
Gay Fathers of Greater New York
212 721 4216 📖 304
Gay Fathers of Long Island
New York, 516 282 9478 📖 304

Gay Fathers of Westchester (GFW)
New York, 914 948 4922 304
Gay Film Association Lambda
Amsterdam, 20 618 5374 150
Gay FM
broadcast by 4CCCC - FM 89.1 29
Gay GAIA 291
Gay Gazette
published by Silveraim Ltd. 85
Gay Group Bloemfontein
51 30 5934 171
Gay Help Line
Galway, 91 661 34 137
Victoria, 604 383 9124 46
Gay Helpline of New Jersey
201 285 1595 289
Hackensack, 201 692 1794 289
Gay Hotline
Düsseldorf, 211 311 5283 115
Essen, 201 183 3392 116
Gay Hotline, Inc.
Tampa, 813 229 8839 242
Gay II Gay
broadcast by Wear FM 103.4FM 92
Gay Info
Montréal, 514 768 0199 62
Gay Info Line
Gent / Gand, 9 223 9399 35
Gay Info Line of New Hampshire
Concord, 603 224 1686 287
Gay Information & Concerns
Clarion, 814 226 8212 328
Gay Information Cork
21 27 1087 136
Gay Information Line
Christchurch, 3 379 3990 161
Hobart, 0 234 8179 31
Norfolk, 804 622 4297 348
Gay Information Mississauga
905 891 1716 51
Gay Information Services
Milwaukee, 414 444 7331 355
Gay International
Oslo, 22 20 3736 165
Gay Italia 139
Gay Jouren
Göteborg, 31 11 0104 173
Halmstad, 35 12 0722 173
Linköping, 13 11 0333 174
Luleå, 920 17055 174
Örebro, 19 12 2550 174
Stockholm, 8 24 7465 175
Uppsala, 18 26 0915 176
Gay Law Students at Hastings
San Francisco, 415 565 4601 215
Gay Lesbian Bisexual Alliance at UVM
Burlington, 802 656 6300 346
Gay Lesbian Bisexual Student Support
River Falls, 715 425 3530 358
Gay Lesbian Bisexual Union
Whitewater, 414 472 5738 358
Gay Liberation Forum Baden-Baden
Gaggenau 118
Gay Library
Johannesburg, 11 643 2311 171
Gay Life 108
Gay Line
Brisbane, 7 839 3277 28
Erfurt, 361 66 6764 116
Firenze, 1678 69042 (free) 145
Halifax, 902 423 7129 48
Gay Line Hagen
233 133 8833 119
Gay Lines Calgary
403 234 8973 42
Gay Male SM Activists
New York, 212 727 9878 303
Gay Married Men's Support Group
Rochester 311
Gay Media
Basel / Bâle, 61 681 3132 177
Gay Men & Lesbian Alliance
Boston, 617 573 8226 268
Gay Men of the Bronx
New York, 718 792 8078 305
Gay Men's Alliance of Hudson Valley
New York, 914 948 4922 305
Gay Men's Community Project
Portland, 503 331 2282 326
Gay Men's Health Crisis
New York, 212 807 6665 (hotline) 303
Gay Men's Health Project
Dublin, 1 602149 137
Norwich, 160 362 7514 88
Sandown 77
Santa Fe, 505 984 0911 295
Gay Men's Press
London, 181 341 7818 69
Gay Men's Psychotherapy Referral Service
New York, 212 388 2738 301
Gay Men's Support Group
Lincoln, 402 472 7450 285
University Park 295
Gay Naturists International (GNI)
Norwalk 13
Gay Network (TGT)
Stockholm 175
GAY NETWORKS MAILING LIST 3
Gay Obscessions
published by Publications Nouvelles 97
Gay Ol' Times 327
Gay Organization for Alternative Lifestyles (GOAL)
Oneonta 310
Gay Outreach Association for Lowell Students (GOALS)
508 452 3679 271
Gay People of Laurel
301 776 6891 265
Gay People Princeton 292
Gay People's Chronicle 317
Gay People's Union
Sacramento, 916 429 7381 210
Gay Phoneline of Windsor
519 973 4951 61
Gay Pleasures / Gay Treasures
New York, 212 255 5756 309
Gay Positive Buffalo
716 884 8670 298
Gay Presses of New York 308
Gay Psychological Services
New York, 212 265 1974 301
Gay Radio
broadcast by 3D Radio 93.7 FM 30
broadcast by Arci Gay 145
broadcast by FM 89.2 174
Gay Radio Information News Service (Grins)
Sydney 27
Gay Radio Programme
broadcast by 3CR Community Radio, AM 855 kHz 31
Gay Radio Sibilla FM 103
Ancona, 71 203 0454 143
Gay Raiders
Köln 124
Gay Rap Telephone Line of Topeka
913 233 6558 258
Gay Review 269
Gay Scene 308
Gay Scotland 169
Gay Service Network
Austin, 512 445 7270 338
Gay Skinhead Group
Guildford 91
Gay Spirit
broadcast by WRSU FM 88.7 291
Gay Students Alliance at Baruch College
New York 305
Gay Sunshine Press / Leyland Publications
San Francisco, 707 996 6082 216
Gay Switchboard
Gainesville, 904 332 0700 237
Trondheim, 73 52 4226 166
Wellington, 4 385 0674 163
Winterthur, 52 213 8188 179
Gay Switchboard Dublin
1 721 055 137
Gay Switchboard Johannesburg
11 643 2311 171
Gay Switchboard Limerick
61 310101 138
Gay Times
published by Millivres Ltd. 85
Gay To Z Directory
published by Gay To Z Publishing, Ltd. 84
Gay To Z Publishing, Ltd.
London, 171 793 7450 84
Gay Wave Length
broadcast by 1008 kHz 25
Gay Youth Alliance
San Diego, 619 233 9209 211
Gay Youth Calgary
403 234 9873 43
Gay Youth Milwaukee (GYM)
414 265 8500 357
Gay Youth Switchboard / Ungdomstelefonen
København, 33 13 0628 66
Gay's Innung
Jena 122
Gay's The Word
London, 171 278 7654 70
Gay, Lesbian, & Allied Student Society
Williamstown, 413 664 4511 273
Gay, Lesbian, & Bi Student Organization (GLBSO)
Hattiesburg, 601 583 7997 282
Gay, Lesbian, & Bisexual Academics, Students & Staff (GLASS)
Calgary, 403 282 8998 42
Gay, Lesbian, & Bisexual Activities
Mankato, 507 345 7799 279
Gay, Lesbian, & Bisexual Aggies
College Station, 409 847 0321 339
Gay, Lesbian, & Bisexual Alliance
Brooklyn, 718 636 3790 298
Mobile, 205 666 9824 192
Gay, Lesbian, & Bisexual Alliance (GLA/EWU)
Spokane, 509 359 4253 354
Gay, Lesbian, & Bisexual Alliance League (GLOBAL)
Akron 317
Gay, Lesbian, & Bisexual Alliance of Kingsborough
Brooklyn, 718 368 5400 298
Gay, Lesbian, & Bisexual Association of Mc Master
Hamilton, 905 525 9140 Ext. 27397 50
Gay, Lesbian, & Bisexual Community Alliance
Saint Louis, 314 935 5349 284
Gay, Lesbian, & Bisexual Community Center
Hartford, 203 724 5542 231
Gay, Lesbian, & Bisexual Community Hotline of Greater Miami
305 759 3661 239
Gay, Lesbian, & Bisexual Helpline
Altoona, 814 942 8101 327
Gay, Lesbian, & Bisexual Teens
Gainesville, 904 338 3593 237
Gay, Lesbian, & Bisexual Union
New York, 914 251 6976 305
Gay, Lesbian, & Bisexual Union (GLBSU)
Fredonia 299
Gay, Lesbian, Bisexual & Transgendered Library / Archives ofPhiladelphia 329
Gay, Lesbian, Bisexual Alliance of Goddard
Plainfield, 802 454 8311 Ext. 225 346
Gay, Lesbian, Bisexual, & Friends Association (GLBFA)
Rochester, 716 275 9379 311
Gay, Lesbian, Or Bisexual Alliance (GLOBAL)
Louisville, 502 852 4556 259
Gay, Lesbians, & Bisexuals of Skagit (GLBS)
Mount Vernon, 206 428 9217 350
Gay/Lesbian Association of UTA
Dallas / Fort Worth, 817 794 5140 341
Gay/Lesbian Information Bureau (GLIB)
Arlington 180
Gay/Lesbian Information Line
Birmingham, 205 326 8600 191
Gay/Lesbian International News Network (GLINN)
Millwaukee, 414 289 8780 180
Gay/Lesbian Parents of Dallas
Dallas / Fort Worth, 214 259 9862 340
Gaya Mater Studiorum
Bologna, 51 644 6824 140
Gaybeat 317
Gaybook 216
GayBox
Braunschweig, 531 79 6054 112
Gaydar Show
broadcast by KOPN FM 89.5 283
Gaydreams Radio
broadcast by WXPN FM 88.5 331
Gayellow Pages
published by Renaissance House 306
Gayhälsen
Göteborg, 31 60 1874 173
GayHotline
Klagenfurt, 463 50 4690 34
GAYLIB-N 3
Gayline
Adelaide, 008 11 22 33 30
Cairns, 7 051 9083 29
Canberra, 6 247 2726 25
Christchurch, 3 379 4796 161
Dunedin, 3 477 2077 161
Fredricton, 506 457 2156 48
Hamilton, 905 523 7055 50
Invercargill, 3 216 6344 162
Montréal, 514 990 1414 62
Nanaimo, 604 754 2585 44
Napier, 6 835 7190 162
Perth, 9 328 9044 33
Rotorua, 87 348 3598 163
Syracuse, 315 422 5732 312
Gayline & Lesbianline
Palmerston North, 6 358 5378 162
Gayline / Lesbianline
Auckland, 9 303 3584 160
Gayly Oklahoman 323
Gayme Magazine
published by Zymurgy 269
GAYmeinsam 135
Gaymen & Lesbians in Brookhaven (GLIB)
New York, 516 286 6867 305
GAYNET 4
Albuquerque, 505 842 5112 294
gay-net.aids 4
gay-net.coming-out 6
gay-net.diskussionen 6
gay-net.general 6
gay-net.gesundheitsecke 6
gay-net.guide.bundesweit 6
gay-net.heteros 6
gay-net.international 6
gay-net.ledérecke 4
gay-net.lesben 6
Gayphone
Syracuse, 315 443 3599 312
Gay-Plus
Freiburg, 761 7 7188 117
Gayroute
Montréal 41
Gays & Lesbians at Andover Newton Theological School (GLANTS)
Boston 268
Gays & Lesbians at Notre Dame / Saint Mary's College
Muncie 255
Gays & Lesbians at the University of Saskatoon (GLUS)
306 244 4782 64
Gays & Lesbians at U of T
Toronto, 416 971 7880 57
Gays & Lesbians Awareness Civil Rights Committee
Edmonton, 403 469 4286 43
Gays & Lesbians Everywhere in Education (GLEE)
Auckland, 9 846 1681 160
Gays & Lesbians of Humber (GLOH)
Toronto, 416 675 5051 57
Gays & Lesbians of Rice (GALOR)
Houston, 713 527 4097 343
Gays & Lesbians of Watertown (GLOW)
Boston 268
Gays & Lesbians on Campus
Edmonton, 403 403 988 4166 43
Gays South of Lake Street
Minneapolis / Saint Paul 280
Gays, Lesbian, & Bisexuals of North Bay Area (GLB NBA)
705 495 4545 52
Gays, Lesbian, & Bisexuals of UBC
Vancouver, 604 228 4638 45
Gays, Lesbians, & Bisexuals International
Toronto, 416 591 7949 57
Gays, Lesbians, & Bisexuals of Ames (GLBA)
515 233 5000 256
Gays, Lesbians, & Bisexuals United
San Luis Obispo, 805 546 8148 220
Gays, Lesbians, Bisexuals, & Friends

Carbondale, 618 453 5151 248
Gays, Lesbians, Bisexuals, & Friends at MIT (GAMIT)
Boston, 617 253 5440 268
Gaystudenterna
Lund, 46 15 7134 174
GAYTEL
Best 150
Gaytime FM
broadcast by Spectrum 162
Gaywaves
broadcast by 2NCR-FM 92.9 25
broadcast by 2SER FM 107.3 27
broadcast by FM 102.1 29
broadcast by FM 92.1 31
Gaywire
broadcast by CIUT 89.5 FM 59
Gayzette 24
Gaze Magazine 279
Gazelle
published by Les Editions Nitram 42
Gazette 236
GBMCC *See* Gay Bikers
GCTC
Houston 343
GDANC Support Group
Salisbury, 704 642 1914 316
Gear, Clothing, & Accessories
Norfolk, 804 622 4438 348
Gear, Inc.
Los Angeles, 213 683 8313 15, 205
GEC *See* Gender Education Center
Gegen den Strich Buchcafé
Düsseldorf, 211 323 7938 115
Gelders Advies Centrum Homosexualiteit (GACH)
Nijmegen 157
Gelsenkirchen Lesben- & Schwuleninitiative
209 20 1171 118
Gemini
Melbourne, 39 419 6270 33
Melbourne, 39 534 6074 33
San Diego, 619 287 1402 212
Gemini Gender Group
Milwaukee, 414 297 9328 (voice mail) 357
GENDER 3
Gender & Self Acceptance Program (GSAP)
San Francisco, 415 558 8058 213
Gender Awareness League
Los Angeles 204
Gender Centre, Inc.
Petersham, 2 569 2366 24
Gender Clinic
Brisbane, 7 839 8262 28
Gender Congruity Center
Boca Raton, 800 328 2633 235
Gender Council of Australia (W. A.), Inc.
Gosnells, 9 362 5447 33
Gender Dysphoria Program of Orange County, Inc.
San Juan Capistrano, 714 240 7020 220
Gender Dysphoria Support
Kansas City, 816 241 1411 283
Gender Education Center (GEC)
Minneapolis / Saint Paul, 612 425 5445 280
Gender Expressions
Lakewood, 310 869 4241 202
Gender Identity Center of Colorado, Inc.
Lakewood, 303 202 6466 229
Gender Identity Clinic of New England
Manchester, 203 646 8651 231
Gender Identity Project for Transsexuals
New York, 212 620 7310 305
Gender Identity Support Services for Transexuals (GISST)
Boston, 617 720 3413 266
Gender Issues Centre
Thunder Bay, 807 343 8897 54
Gender Mosaic
Ottawa, 819 770 1945 52
Gender Review 226
Gender Talk North
Keene, 603 924 8828 288
Gender Trust
London, 1305 269222 (infoline) 83
Genderstichting (Belgian Gender Foundation)
Kortrijk / Courtrai, 56 21 9541 38
General Media Inc.
New York, 212 702 6000 19, 307
Generic Leather Productions
Seattle, 206 233 8527 350
Genessee Hospital
Rochester, 716 263 6000 310
Genie Trimmers
Atlantic City 289
Genitorturers
Highland 290
Gentle Giants of Oregon
Portland, 503 981 4281 326
Gents
Greensboro, 910 855 9855 315
George Brown College Lesbian, Gay, & Bisexual Students
Toronto, 416 925 9872 Ext. 2178 57
George Disposables
West Columbia, 803 796 9196 335
Georgetown Pride
Washington, 202 687 1592 234
Georgetown University Hospital
Washington, 202 784 3000 233
Georgia Tech's Gay & Lesbian Alliance
Atlanta, 404 497 0684 244
Gerber/Hart Library & Archives
Chicago, 312 883 3003 248
Gerd
Portland, 503 253 7956 326
Gerede-Dresdener Lesben, Schwule, & Alle Anderen
351 464 0220 114
Geri-Care Products
Middlesex, 908 469 7722 291
Gerotek
Münster, 251 51 1461 129
Gertrude Stein Memorial Bookshop
Pittsburgh, 412 481 9666 332
Gesprecks- en Onthaalcentrum u. z. w. (GOC)
Antwerpen / Anvers, 3 233 1071 36
Gesundheitsamt
Eckernförde, 435 188 22567 115
Gesundheitsamt AIDS-Beratungstelle
Düsseldorf, 211 899 2663 115
Gesundheitsamt Chemnitz
371 65 4347 113
Gesundheitsamt Erfurt
361 655 1744 116
Get Booked
Las Vegas, 702 737 7780 286
Get Kinky
published by Modern Products 337
Get Wet
London, 171 627 0290 69
Getting Real
West Newton 273
Gettysburg College Lambda Alliance 328
GFMC/DC
Washington 234
G-Force
Amsterdam, 20 420 1664 151
GFW *See* Gay Fathers of Westchester
GG & GD
Amsterdam, 20 555 5822 152
Arnhem 153
Roosendaal, 16 554 1900 157
Tilburg, 13 463 1515 158
Venlo, 77 359 8822 158
Venray, 47 858 5251 158
GGALA-L 4
GGG *See* Group Gai Guyanais
GGS *See* Gisborne Gay Support
GHEM *See* Groupe Homo pour l'Expression des Minorités
GI Joe's Genuine Surplus
Malden, 617 322 8600 271
Giachetti, Diane, CSW, ACSW
Montclair, 201 998 7705 291
Gibbin Publications
Long Beach, 310 597 2799 202
Giffins MC
Newark 232
Gilson, Patrick
London, 171 371 9454 69
Giogianni, Paul, CSW
New York, 212 532 2599 301
Giovanni's Room
Philadelphia, 215 923 2960 181, 331
Girl Jock 217
Girlfriends 217
Girls CD Group
Burnwood 24
Girls Like Us, Ltd.
London, 171 359 2289 83
Girls Night Out
Brooklyn, 201 794 1665 Ext. 2021 297
Girth & Mirth
Akron, 216 655 4259 317
Alpes-Jura, 16 81 880618 98
Amsterdam, 20 625 5128 152
Belgium, 71 56 0580 12, 22
Big Dutch, 73 613 5373 156
Chicago, 312 776 9223 250
Detroit, 313 531 3907 278
Deutschland
Berlin, 30 325 5990 110
Hamburg, 40 28 0289 120
Köln, 234 925 55104 124
Mannheim / Stuttgart, 621 545 315 127
München, 89 542 0407 128
Florida, 305 791 9794 236
France, 19 47 2745 103
Italia Magnum Club, 3 531 5998 142
Los Angeles, 818 961 7900 197
Milwaukee 357
New England, 617 387 0762 268
New York, 914 699 7735 310
North Carolina, 704 274 2100 315
Rockies, 303 784 5814 228
Rotterdam, 10 414 1555 157
Saint Louis 284
San Diego, 619 685 8822 211
San Francisco, 415 552 1143 214
Seattle, 206 361 9686 351
Tennessee 337
Twin Cities, 612 938 8551 280
Washington, D. C., 703 461 9184 348
Western Pennsylvania 328
Girth & Mirth of LA
Canoga Park 197
Gisborne Gay Support (GGS)
6 867 9103 162
GISST *See* Gender Identity Support Services for Transexuals
GL *See* Club für Gleichgeschlechtilch Liebende e. V.
GL Friendly
Biloxi, 601 435 2398 282
GLA/EWU *See* Gay, Lesbian, & Bisexual Alliance
GLABA *See* Glendon Gay, Lesbian, & Bisexual Alliance
GLA-CV *See* Alliance of Cache Valley
GLAD
Dundee 170
Glad Day Books
Boston, 617 267 3010 181
Toronto, 416 961 4161 40
Glad Day Bookshop
Boston, 617 267 3010 269
Toronto, 416 961 4161 59
GLAF *See* Framingham State College Gays, Lesbians, & Friends
Glans Naked & Unashamed (GNU)
Washington 234
GLANTS *See* Gays & Lesbians at Andover Newton Theological School
GLAS *See* Gay & Lesbian Alliance of Syracuse
GL-ASB 2
Glasgow Caledonian University L&G Society
141 332 0681 169
Glasgow University L&G Society
141 334 9512 169
Glasgow University Shop 169
GLASS *See* Gay & Lesbian Association of Students & Staff. *See also* Gay, Lesbian, & Bisexual Academics, Students & Staff
Greensboro, 910 274 2100 315
Glass City Sisters
Toledo 322
GLB NBA *See* Gays, Lesbian, & Bisexuals of North Bay Area
GLB Publishers
San Francisco, 415 621 8307 13
GLBA *See* Gays, Lesbians, & Bisexuals of Ames. *See also* Wesleyan Gay, Lesbian, & Bisexual Alliance
GLBC, University of Miami
305 284 4483 239
GLBFA *See* Gay, Lesbian, Bisexual, & Friends Association
GLB-NEWS 3
GLBPOC 3
GLBS *See* Gay, Lesbians, & Bisexuals of Skagit
GLBSO *See* Gay, Lesbian, & Bi Student Organization
GLBSU *See* Gay, Lesbian, & Bisexual Union
GLC *See* Gay & Lesbian Community
GLEE *See* Gays & Lesbians Everywhere in Education
Gleebooks
Sydney, 2 660 2578 27
GLEN *See* Gay & Lesbian Equality Network
Glendale Memorial Hospital & Health Center
818 502 2201 200
Glendon Gay, Lesbian, & Bisexual Alliance (GLABA)
Toronto, 416 736 2100 Ext. 88197 57
Glendower
Independence 283
GLIB *See* Gay & Lesbian Independent Broadcasters. *See also* Gay/Lesbian Information Bureau. *See also* Gaymen & Lesbians in Brookhaven
GLINN *See* Gay/Lesbian International News Network
gLiTcH
Dunellen 290
Glittering Images
Firenze, 55 717 880 146
GLLOW *See* Gay & Lesbian Liberation of Waterloo
GLNCI / North Central Iowa
Iowa Falls 257
GLOBAL *See* Gay & Lesbian Olin Business School Alliance. *See also* Gay, Lesbian, & Bisexual Alliance League. *See also* Gay, Lesbian, Or Bisexual Alliance
Global Wrestling Alliance
Farmington, 203 524 4288 13
GLOBE *See* Rhode Island College Gay, Lesbian, or Bisexual Equality Alliance
Globe Centre
London, 171 377 2003 82
Globe Graphics Communications
Cooksville, 905 625 1010 49
Globe News
Los Angeles, 213 622 4390 205
GLOH *See* Gays & Lesbians of Humber
GLORA *See* Gay & Lesbian Organization of Reading & Allentown
Gloucester Friend
1452 306800 75
Glove Me Tender
Winnetka, 708 501 2880 253
Glover, Thomas
New York 306
GLOW *See* Gays & Lesbians of Watertown
GLPCI *See* Gay & Lesbian Parents Coalition International
GLPC—MW *See* Gay & Lesbian Parents Coalition
GLQSOC-L 3
GLR *See* Greater London Radio
GLSA *See* Gay & Lesbian Resource Center
GLSB of LI *See* Gay & Lesbian Switchboard of Long Island
GLSM *See* Gruppe Leder SM
GLSO News 259
GLSS *See* Gay & Lesbian Student Society
GLUS *See* Gays & Lesbians at the University of Saskatoon
GLWA *See* Lesbian Alliance
G-Nation
Charlottesville, 804 293 4631 347
GNI *See* Gay Naturists International

GNU 📖 *See* Glans Naked & Unashamed
GO CARE
 Monroe, 318 325 1092 📖 260
Go Info 📖 53
Go Up
 Berlin, 30 312 3045 📖 111
GOAL 📖 *See* Gay Organization for Alternative Lifestyles
 New York 📖 303
GOALS 📖 *See* Gay Outreach Association for Lowell Students
GOC 📖 *See* Gesprecks- en Onthaalcentrum u. z. w.
Goddess
 published by Rogue-Hagen Publications 📖 73
Goerings' Book Center
 Gainesville, 800 726 1487 📖 237
GOHL 📖 *See* Grupo Orgullo Homosexual de Liberación
GOLBA 📖 *See* Greeley Gay, Lesbian, & Bisexual Alliance
Gold Club
 Gent / Gand, 9 225 0353 📖 38
Gold Coast Bears
 Fort Lauderdale, 305 463 7923 📖 236
Gold'n Stream
 published by Winter Publishing, Inc. 📖 22
Goldberg, Jonathan, Ph.D.
 New York, 212 496 0535 📖 301
Golden Boy
 Lille, 20 06 3426 📖 100
Golden Braid Books
 Salt Lake City, 801 322 1162 📖 345
Golden Dawn Books
 Manchester 📖 76
Golden Gate
 Redwood City, 415 364 6913 📖 209
 San Mateo, 415 620 9639 📖 220
Golden Gate Connection
 Daly City, 415 871 7870 📖 198
Golden Gate Guards
 San Francisco, 415 431 9475 📖 214
Golden Lee Distributors
 Avon, 508 586 3900 📖 267
Golden Notebook
 Woodstock, 914 679 8000 📖 313
Golden Shower Association
 New York 📖 306
Golden Shower Buddies
 San Francisco, 415 979 0242 📖 215
Golden State Bears
 Fresno, 209 496 3875 📖 200
Golden State Peace Officers Association
 Los Angeles 📖 204
Golden Thread Booksellers
 New Haven, 203 777 7807 📖 231
Golden Triangle News
 Pittsburgh, 412 765 3790 📖 332
Goldies
 Sacramento, 916 447 5860 📖 210
 Sacramento, 916 922 0103 📖 210
Goldmine Bookshop
 Hamilton 📖 162
Goldstein Publications
 New York, 212 989 8001 📖 307
Goldstein, Ronald, Ph.D.
 Levittown, 215 547 9417 📖 329
Gonzales, Efrain
 Brooklyn 📖 298
Good Art Company
 Santa Monica, 800 345 7601 📖 222
Good Samaritan Hospital & Medical Center
 Portland, 503 229 7711 📖 326
Good Samaritan Medical Center
 West Palm Beach, 407 655 5511 📖 243
Good Samaritan Regional Medical Center
 Phœnix, 602 239 2000 📖 193
Good Sports
 South Windsor, 800 845 0084 📖 232
Good Vibrations
 Berkeley, 415 974 8980 📖 197
 San Francisco, 800 289 8423 📖 10, 219
Goodfellow Corp.
 Malvern, 800 821 2870 📖 329
Goodhew, John, M.D.
 Toronto, 416 461 2200 📖 55
Gordon, Donna, MA, NCPsyA
 Washington Township, 201 652 2957 📖 293
Görlitzer Homosexuelleninitiative 📖 118
Göteborg Gay Radio
 broadcast by FM 103.1 📖 173
Gotham Psychotherapy Associates
 New York, 212 903 4033 📖 301
Gothic Steel
 Denver, 303 837 0272 📖 227
Gottardi, Susi Medusa
 Bologna 📖 140
Gottlieb, Jody, Ph.D.
 Birmingham, 205 933 6501 📖 191
Goulburn Valley Gay Group
 Melbourne, 58 299218 📖 32
Government Sales, Inc.
 Hartford, 203 247 7787 📖 231
Government Surplus
 Glasgow, 1294 469343 📖 170
Governor's Office of Lesbian & Gay Concerns
 Albany, 518 486 3168 📖 295
Grabowski, Robert, CSW, ACSW
 New York, 718 261 1346 📖 301
Grace & Lace Letter 📖 282
Graduate Gay & Lesbian Alliance
 Buffalo, 716 645 3063 📖 298
Graduate Hospital
 Philadelphia, 215 893 2501 📖 330
Grady Memorial Hospital
 Atlanta, 404 616 4307 📖 243
Graff, Laura
 Boston 📖 269
Graffiti
 Lithonia, 404 972 9709 📖 245
Graffitti 📖 354
Graham, Sally, Ph.D.
 New York, 212 807 0543 📖 301
Grampian AIDS Line
 Aberdeen, 122 457 4000 📖 168
Grampian Gender Group (3G)
 Lumphanan, 133 988 3695 📖 168
Grand Mello
 Roma, 6 687 7309 📖 142
Grand Opening!
 Brookline, 617 731 2626 📖 190
Grand Rapids AIDS Reseource Center
 616 459 9177 📖 276
Grand Rapids Rivermen 📖 276
Grand River Books
 East Landing, 517 333 3666 📖 275
GRANITE 📖 3
Grantham HIV/AIDS Helpline
 1476 60192 📖 79
Granville Book Company
 Vancouver, 604 687 2213 📖 46
Grapevine 📖 34
Grapevine Books
 Reno, 702 786 4869 📖 287
 Timmins, 705 268 0181 📖 55
Grapik Arts Productions
 San Francisco 📖 218
Grass Roots
 Corvallis, 503 754 7668 📖 325
Grassroots Books
 Iowa City, 319 339 4678 📖 257
Graven Image
 Redwood City, 415 369 6365 📖 209
Gravesend Switchboard
 163 482695 📖 78
Gravity Plus
 La Jolla, 800 383 8056 📖 183
Great Lakes Bears
 Chicago, 312 509 5135 📖 250
 Pontiac, 313 338 1991 📖 277
Great Lakes Harley Owners
 Milwaukee 📖 355
Great Northern Books
 Bellingham, 206 733 1650 📖 350
Great Southern Tattoo Company
 College Park, 301 474 8820 📖 265
Great Triad Men
 Greensboro 📖 315
Greater Cincinnati AIDS Consortium
 513 558 4259 📖 318
Greater Cincinnati Gay / Lesbian Coalition
 513 557 2904 📖 318
Greater Houston AIDS Alliance 📖 342
Greater London Radio (GLR)
 171 224 2424 📖 85
Greater New York.Gender Alliance
 212 765 3561 📖 305
Greater Utica Lambda Fellowship 📖 312
Greeley Bears
 970 330 3732 Ext. 387 📖 229
Greeley Gay, Lesbian, & Bisexual Alliance (GOLBA)
 303 351 1484 📖 229
Green & Yellow TV 📖 281
Green Door
 El Paso, 915 858 3174 📖 342
Green Gables Bookstore
 Newport, 503 265 9141 📖 325
Greenery
 published by Lady Green 📖 217
Greenleaf Bookshop
 Bristol, 117 921 1369 📖 70
Greenwich Health Project
 London, 181 854 2966 📖 82
Greenwich Lesbian & Gay Centre
 London, 181 316 5954 📖 83
Greenwood's Bookshoppe
 Edmonton, 403 439 2005 📖 43
Griff's
 Los Angeles, 213 660 0889 📖 203
Griffin Printing & Lithograph Co.
 Glendale, 213 245 3671 📖 200
Griffin Printing/Spilman
 Sacramento, 916 649 3511 📖 210
Griffin, David Lindsey, CSW, CAC
 New York, 212 582 1881 📖 301
Griffins Motor Club
 Canberra 📖 25
Grimes, Robert
 Rockville, 301 816 3251 📖 266
Grimsby & District AIDS Line
 1472 240840 📖 77
Grins 📖 *See* Gay Radio Information News Service
GRLP
 Lisboa 📖 167
Grønn Mann
 Hønefoss 📖 165
Group
 Saint John, 709 652 2848 📖 48
Group Gai Guyanais (GGG)
 Cayenne 📖 106
Group Health Coöperative Central Hospital
 Seattle, 206 326 3000 📖 351
Group Marriage Alliance
 Aloha, 503 4525453 📖 324
Group with No Name
 Champaign / Urbana, 217 384 7333 📖 248
Group with No Name (GWNN)
 Austin 📖 338
Groupe Action Gai
 Orléans 📖 102
Groupe B. A. I., Inc.
 Montréal, 514 852 2429 📖 41
Groupe de Santé d'Antenne Rose
 Bruxelles / Brussel 📖 37
Groupe Gai de l'Université de Laval
 Québec, 418 649 9478 📖 63
Groupe Homo pour l'Expression des Minorités (GHEM)
 Lille, 20 52 1884 📖 100
Groupe SIDA Genève
 Genève / Genf, 22 700 1500 📖 178
Groupe SIDA Neuchâtel
 Neuchâtel / Neuenburg, 38 31 4924 📖 178
GROW
 Wilmington, 910 675 9222 📖 316
Growing Alternative Youth
 Pittsburgh, 412 642 9099 📖 332
Grownups
 New Hope, 215 862 9304 📖 329
Grundman, Maryann, Ph.D., LCSW
 Denver, 303 278 4392 📖 227
Grupo de Apoio a Pacientes de AIDS (GAPA)
 São Paulo 📖 40
Grupo Neuróticos Anónimos Gay
 Guadalajara 📖 149
Grupo Nueva Generación
 Guadalajara 📖 149
Grupo Orgullo Homosexual de Liberación (GOHL)
 Guadalajara 📖 149
Gruppe Leder SM (GLSM)
 Hamburg, 40 313540 📖 119
Gruppo C
 Cremona, 372 45 1755 📖 142
 Mestre, 41 98 7868 📖 146
 Verona, 45 803 0843 📖 147
Gryphons
 Dayton 📖 321
GSAP 📖 *See* Gender & Self Acceptance Program
GSN
 Guildford 📖 91
G-Spot Productions
 Brighton, 1273 676435 📖 74
Gualala Books
 707 888 4255 📖 200
Guardian 📖 85
Guelph Gay, Lesbian, & Bisexual Equality
 519 824 4120 Ext. 8575 📖 50
Guelph Gayline
 519 836 4550 📖 49
Guida Gay
 published by Babilonia Edizione 📖 139
Guide 📖 269
Guide Gai du Québec 📖 62
Gulf Area Gender Alliance
 New Orleans 📖 261
Gulf Coast Transgender Community
 Houston, 713 780 4282 📖 343
Gummi
 London 📖 69
Gundry, Nick
 London, 181 995 1590 📖 80
GUSS 📖 *See* Campus Queers
Guttman Breast Diagnostic Institute
 New York, 212 463 8733 📖 302
Guys Magazine 📖 293
GVNS
 Folkestone 📖 69
GW Miami Beach
 305 534 4763 📖 239
Gwendoline
 Bruxelles / Brussel, 2 523 3589 📖 37
Gwent AIDS Advice Line
 Newport, 1633 422532 📖 359
Gwent AIDS Support Group
 Newport, 1633 223456 📖 359
GWNN 📖 *See* Group with No Name
Gwynedd Gay Line
 Bangor, 124 835 1263 📖 359
GYM 📖 *See* Gay Youth Milwaukee
Gyncrocrat Alliance
 Saint Louis 📖 284
H.
 published by Quest Publications 📖 226
H. F. Verwoerd Hospital
 Pretoria, 12 42 3211 📖 172
H. G. Publications
 Welshpool 📖 359
H. W. Wilson Company
 Bronx, 212 588 8400 📖 297
H.E.L.P, Inc.
 Wayne, 201 666 7246 📖 293
Hag Rag 📖 357
Hahn, Louise, MA, NCC
 Winston-Salem, 910 727 0008 📖 316
HAI 📖 *See* Homosexuelle Aktion Ilmenau
Hair Club
 Bruxelles / Brussel 📖 37
Hair to Stay
 published by Winter Publishing, Inc. 📖 19
HAK - Advies Kontakt Centrum 't Koerken
 Aalst / Alost, 5 378 4279 📖 36
Halcyon 📖 88
HALO 📖 *See* Homophile Association of London Ontario Inc.
HALT 📖 *See* Homosexuelle Alternative
Halton Regional Health Department
 Burlington, 905 825 6065 📖 49
HALU 📖 *See* Homosexuelle Arbeitsgruppe Luzern
Hamburger Gay Information 📖 120
Hamilton AIDS Network
 800 563 6919 📖 50
Hamilton Book
 Poughkeepsie, 914 473 1776 📖 310
Hamilton Gay & Lesbian Alliance (GALA)
 905 523 7055 📖 50
Hamilton, China
 Woodbridge, 1728 638415 📖 91

Hamilton-Wentworth Lesbian/Gay Archives
905 528 0156 📖 50
Hamot Medical Center
Erie, 814 877 6000 📖 328
Hampshire College Gay & Bisexual Men's Alliance
Amherst, 413 549 4600 📖 267
HAND 📖 See HIV & AIDS in North Derbyshire
Handjobs
published by Avenue Services 📖 207
Hands
Köln, 221 24 3541 📖 125
Hangar
Roma, 6 488 1397 📖 141
Hanky Code
Antwerpen / Anvers, 3 226 8172 📖 36
Hannchen Mehrzweck Stiftung für Homosexuelle Selbsthilfe
Berlin, 30 391 2651 📖 108
Hans Gay-O-Theek
Rotterdam, 10 485 9079 📖 158
Hanson Percussion Instruments
Racine, 414 632 7330 📖 11
Hap's Militaria & Collectibles
Saint Petersburg, 813 527 9532 📖 241
Happy Foundation
San Antonio, 210 227 6451 📖 180
Harbor Bytes
Baltimore 📖 263
Harbor View Medical Center
San Diego, 619 235 3102 📖 211
HarborMasters
Portland 📖 262
Harborview Medical Center
Seattle, 206 223 3000 📖 351
Harbour City Bears
Sydney, 2 9904 1603 📖 26
Hard Art Design
Ulm, 731 5 6072 📖 134
Hard Candy Books
New York, 800 458 9640 (credit card orders) 📖 306
Hard Labor Leather
Los Angeles 📖 205
Hard Line
München, 89 260 6017 📖 107, 128
Hard Love Leather
Phœnix, 602 947 3520 📖 9
Hardclub 88
Paris 📖 104
Hardcore
Leipzig, 341 232126 📖 125
Hardware, Inc.
Albuquerque 📖 294
Hares & Hyenas
Melbourne, 3 9419 4445 📖 32
Melbourne, 3 9824 2839 📖 32
Haringey Lesbian & Gay Helpline
London, 181 802 0840 📖 81
Harlem Hospital Center
New York, 212 939 1340 📖 302
Harley Strokers
Portland, 503 771 6136 📖 326
Harlo Press
Detroit, 313 883 3600 📖 275
Harlow Switchboard
1279 639637 📖 75
Harm Reduction Centre
Dundee, 138 221 0919 📖 170
Harmonia Madison Center for Psychotherapy
608 255 8838 📖 356
Harmony
Manchester 📖 76
Harmony Concepts, Inc.
Los Angeles, 818 766 1448 📖 18
Harness - Sin City
Helsinki, 90 612 1513 📖 96
Harper Hospital
Detroit, 313 745 8303 📖 275
Harpies & Quines 📖 169
Harris Newsstand
Albuquerque, 505 880 8696 📖 294
Harrisburg Hospital
717 782 3131 📖 328
Harrison, James, Ph.D.
Asheville, 704 253 3055 📖 313
Harrogate Army & Navy Store
1423 504035 📖 88
Harrogate Switchboard
1423 524101 📖 88
Harry S. Truman Memorial Veterans' Hospital
Columbia, 314 443 2511 📖 283
Harry Schwartz Bookshop
Milwaukee, 414 274 6400 📖 357
Hartford Colts, MC
203 278 5616 📖 231
Hartford Health Department
203 722 6742 📖 231
Hartford Hospital
203 545 5555 📖 230
Hartman, Judith Rachael, Ph.D.
Denver, 303 722 2212 📖 227
Hartwigs Bookshop
Melbourne, 39 417 7147 📖 32
Hartzog, Dennis, M.Ed, L.P.C.
Dallas / Fort Worth, 214 559 0688 📖 340
Harvard Book Store
Boston, 617 661 1515 📖 269
Harvard Gay & Lesbian Caucus
Boston 📖 268
Harvest Counseling Associates
Denton, 817 497 4020 📖 341
Harvest Ecumenical AIDS Resource Team
Denton, 817 497 4020 📖 341
Harvey Milk AIDS Education Project
San Francisco, 415 773 9544 📖 213
Harvey Milk Archives
San Francisco, 415 824 3449 📖 212
HASG 📖 See Homosexuelle Arbeitsgruppe Saint Gallen
HASO 📖 See Homosexuelle Arbeitsgruppe
Hassle Free Clinic - Men
Toronto, 416 922 0603 📖 55
Hassle Free Clinic - Women
Toronto, 416 922 0556 📖 55
Hastings Befrienders
1424 444777 📖 91
Hastings Switchboard
1424 721394 📖 91
HATCH 📖 See Houston Area Teen Coalition of Homosexuals
Hatley, Scott, MS, CSW
New York, 212 674 4706 📖 301
Haukeland Hospital
Bergen, 55 20 0944 📖 165
Haus des Buches Carl Habel GmbH
Erfurt, 361 2 3033 📖 116
Hautnah
Berlin, 30 882 3434 📖 111
Havenzuikhuis
Rotterdam, 10 411 2800 📖 157
Hawaii Transgender Outreach
Oahu, 808 923 4270 📖 247
Hawkins, Brenda, Ed.D.
Doraville, 404 986 4247 📖 245
Hawley-Cooke
Louisville, 502 546 6660 📖 259
Louisville, 502 893 0133 📖 259
Haworth Press
Binghamton, 607 722 5857 📖 20, 22
Hayats Magazines & Gifts
Salt Lake City, 801 531 6531 📖 345
Hays & Sanders Bookstore
Fayetteville, 501 442 0832 📖 195
HAZ 📖 See Homosexuelle Arbeitsgruppen Zürich
HAZ/SOH 📖 See Schwule Ausleihbibliothek
Hazelton, Michael
Toronto, 416 604 3958 📖 55
HAZ/SOH 📖 See Beratungstelephon für Homosexuelle
HBIGDA 📖 See National Harry Benjamin Gender Dysphoria Association
HCDA 📖 See Helping CDs Anonymous
He & She
Toronto, 416 594 0171 📖 60
Headpress Magazine 📖 72
Headquarters
San Francisco, 415 626 5876 📖 212
Headquarters Military Surplus, Inc.
Tampa, 813 759 0459 📖 243
Headspace
Atlanta 📖 244
HEAL 📖 See Health Education AIDS Liason
Healing Our Spirit
Vancouver, 604 879 0906 📖 45
Health Awareness Services
Worcester, 508 756 7123 📖 273
Health Crisis Network
Miami, 800 442 5046 (in Florida) 📖 239
Health Education AIDS Liaison (HEAL)
Blackpool, 123 532 9 0052 📖 78
Health Education AIDS Liason (HEAL)
Preston, 1772 555525 📖 79
Health Education Resource Organization, Inc.
Baltimore, 410 685 1180 📖 263
Health Information Network
Seattle, 206 784 5655 📖 351
Health Issues Task Force
Cleveland, 216 621 0766 📖 318
Health Shop
Lincoln, 152 252 9222 📖 79
Health Tec, Inc.
Palmer, 413 289 1221 📖 272
Healthwise
Liverpool, 800 665544 📖 87
Heart of Texas Bears
Austin 📖 338
Heart of Texas MC
Rosebud 📖 344
Heartland AIDS Resource Council
Kansas City 📖 283
Heartland Books
East Corinth, 802 439 5655 📖 181
Hearts of the West
Santa Fe 📖 295
Heartwood Whips of Passion
Laguna Beach, 714 376 9558 📖 201
Heat Seeking Publishing
San Francisco, 415 824 0282 📖 217
Heather's Show
broadcast by CITR FM 101.9 📖 46
Heaven Sent Me
Brentwood, 516 434 4777 📖 297
Elbert, 719 495 3000 📖 186
Hedonism
Compton 📖 198
Heh! 📖 See Homosexuelle Emanzipationsgruppe
Hein & Feite Switchboard
Hamburg, 40 24 0333 📖 119
HELB 📖 See Homosexuelle Emanzipationsgruppe
Hellfire Club
New York, 212 647 0063 📖 303
Hellfire Emporium
Melbourne, 39 639 4755 📖 32
Hellion House
Pittsburgh, 412 391 1121 📖 331
Helping CDs Anonymous (HCDA)
Houston 📖 343
Helping People With AIDS
Little Rock, 501 666 6900 📖 195
Helping People With AIDS (HPA)
Rochester, 716 987 1853 📖 310
Helpline
Chemnitz, 371 1 9411 📖 113
Helseavdelingen Helsesjef Pål Gulbrandsen
Kongsberg, 32 73 1179 📖 165
Helseavdelingen Helsesjef Th. Hetland
Drammen, 32 83 8301 📖 165
Helsekontor
Fredrikstad, 33 31 7010 📖 165
Helseutvalget
Ålesund 📖 165
Helseutvalget for Homofile
Oslo, 22 33 7015 📖 164
Tromdheim, 73 52 4557 📖 166
Hemetro
New Hope, 215 862 5629 📖 329
Hencken, Joel, Ph.D.
Boston, 617 864 7711 📖 267
Henkel, Keile
Dortmund 📖 107
Henkin, William
San Francisco, 415 923 1150 📖 213, 216
Hennepin County Medical Center
Minneapolis / Saint Paul, 612 347 2121 📖 279
Henry Ford Hospital
Detroit, 313 876 2600 📖 275
Hepburn, Fran, MSW, CADC
Toms River, 908 270 2952 📖 293
Her Story
York, 717 757 4270 📖 333
Hera
published by The Women's Community Center 📖 297
Hercules Outfitters
Toronto, 416 924 7764 📖 60
Hereford & Worcester Lesbian & Gay Switchboard
1905 723097 📖 77
Herefordshire HIV/AIDS Advice Helpline
1432 278787 📖 77
Heresies 📖 307
Heriot Watt University LGB Society
Edinburgh 📖 169
Herland Book Café
Santa Cruz, 408 429 6636 📖 222
Herland Sister Resources, Inc.
Oklahoma City, 405 521 9696 📖 323
Herland Voice
published by Herland Sister Resources, Inc. 📖 323
Hermes
published by Febo Editores, S. A. de C. V. 📖 149
Herpes Association
London, 171 607 9661 📖 80
Herspectives 📖 45
Herta Gummi
London 📖 9
He-She Directory 📖 189
Het AIDS Team
Antwerpen / Anvers, 3 226 6969 📖 35
Het Jongensuur
Amsterdam, 20 622 1710 📖 152
Het Roze Haagie
Heereveen, 51 362 3293 📖 156
Hetrick-Martin Institute
New York, 212 674 2400 📖 303, 306
HIA 📖 See Homosexuelle Initiative Aalen
Hibiscus Books
Baton Rouge, 504 387 4264 📖 260
Hibiscus Coast Men's Support Group
Auckland, 9 424 8808 📖 160
Hicks, Walter Dean, Ph.D., CAS
Westmount, 609 854 3155 📖 293
Hidden Door
Dallas / Fort Worth, 214 526 9211 📖 339
Hidden Joy
Cathedral City, 619 328 1694 📖 198
Hide & Sleek
Kinghorn, 1592 891344 📖 23
Hidebound
Liverpool, 151 252 2272 📖 9
HIE 📖 See Homosexuelle Initiative Essen
Hiegel, Josef
München, 89 527132 📖 128
Higgins Collection
New Orleans, 504 949 0386 📖 184
HIGH 📖 See Homosexuelle Interessengruppe Hagen
High Heels
Stuttgart, 711 29 1676 📖 133
Highland Books
Los Angeles, 213 463 0295 📖 206
Highland General Hospital
Oakland, 510 437 4397 📖 207
Highland Publications, c. c.
Johannesburg, 11 614 9866 📖 172
Hightail Publishing
Denver, 303 458 6653 📖 228
Highway 71 News
Del Valle, 512 247 4070 📖 341
Highwaymen MC
Burnaby, 604 294 3559 📖 44
Highwaymen TNT
Washington 📖 234
Hignell Printing Limited
Winnipeg, 204 783 7237 📖 47
Hijman
Arnhem, 26 442 4938 📖 154
Hijos del Sol
Albuquerque 📖 294
Hikané 📖 270
HIL 📖 See Homosexuelle Initiative Lübeck
Hillingdon AIDS Response Trust
Uxbridge, 189 581 3874 📖 87
Hillis, Raymond, Ph.D.
Tesuque, 505 983 3549 📖 295
HIMS 📖 See Homosexuelle Initiative im Märkischen Sauerland
HIN 📖 See Homosexuelle Initiative

Neumünster
Hinnerk 📖 120
H I O B 📖 *See* Homosexuelle Informationsgruppe Ortenau / Baden
HIP 📖 *See* Homosexuelle Initiative Passau. *See also* Homosexuelles Integrationsprojekt Potsdam
Hippopotame
Münster, 251 51 8011 📖 129
Hirsute Fraternity
San Francisco 📖 214
Hirsute Pursuit
Wichita, 316 269 0913 📖 258
HIV & AIDS in North Derbyshire (HAND)
Chesterfield, 1246 550550 📖 72
HIV Care Consortium
Wheeling, 304 232 6295 📖 354
HIV Confidential Testing Service
Flemington, 908 806 4893 📖 289
HIV Education Unit
London, 181 200 0369 📖 82
HIV Groups
Århus, 86 12 4313 📖 65
HIV Network
Coventry, 1203 555616 📖 93
HIV Network, Inc.
Johnson City, 615 928 8888 📖 336
HIV Positive Peer Support Group
Christchurch, 3 379 1953 📖 161
HIV Resource Consortium
Tulsa, 918 749 4194 📖 323
HIV Support Group
Wellington, 4 389 3169 📖 163
HIV Update 📖 252
HIV/AIDS Advocacy Project
Lansing, 800 288 5923 📖 273
HIV/AIDS Gay Support Group
Aberdeen 📖 168
HIV/AIDS Resources, Inc.
Eugene, 503 342 5088 📖 325
HIV/STD Clinic
Hamilton, 7 839 9732 📖 162
HIV-Antikörpertest
Weimar, 364 36 1451 (office) 📖 134
HIV-Arbeitlung der Charité
Berlin, 30 286 4596 📖 110
HIV-Hjælpen
København 📖 66
HIV-Kontoret
Sandefjord, 33 46 5390 📖 166
HIV-Plusline
Amsterdam, 20 685 0055 📖 152
HIV-Positiven Treff
Bielefeld, 521 79 1571 📖 112
Hobson De Nero
Scarborough, 172 335 1515 📖 88
Hofstra Gay & Lesbian Student Association
New York, 516 560 6960 📖 305
Hog On Ice
San Francisco, 415 771 7909 📖 218
Hole
Hannover, 511 352 3895 📖 121
Hole In The Wall Saloon
San Francisco, 415 431 4695 📖 212
Holiday Associates
San Francisco, 415 863 7326 📖 215
Holland AIDS Resource Center
616 396 6545 📖 276
Douglas, 616 396 3538 📖 275
Hollywood Community Hospital
213 462 2271 📖 201
Holtby, Michael, LSCW
Denver, 303 722 1021 📖 227
Holy Cross Hospital
Salt Lake City, 801 350 4111 📖 345
Holy Titclamps 📖 217
Holz Variety / Magazine Rack
Waukesha, 414 547 9056 📖 358
HOME 📖 *See* Homosexuelle Emanzitpation Gruppe
Home Delivery Incontinent Supplies Co., Inc.
Ferguson, 800 538 1036 📖 283
Home Nursing Agency AIDS Intervention Project
Altoona 📖 327
HOME Zentrum
Hannover, 511 36 3633 📖 121
Hommes
published by Editions SAN 📖 97
Hommes Bookshop
New York 📖 308
Homo- en Lesbiennegroep Gehoor
Gent / Gand, 9 225 7599 📖 38
Homo laber
broadcast by FM 91.2 📖 114
Homo- Lesbiennewerking
Mechelen, 1 543 2120 📖 38
Homo Radio
broadcast by WRPI FM 91.5 📖 312
Homo- und Lesbiennejongerenkrant 📖 36
Homocentrum Laakdal en Omstreken
Veerle-Laakdal, 1 484 0455 📖 39
Homodok
Amsterdam, 20 525 2601 📖 150
Homofil Bevegelse
Indre Søre Sogn, 70 12 0915 📖 166
Nordmore & Romsdal, 70 12 0915 📖 165
Sogn og Fjordane, 70 12 0915 📖 166
Homofile Bevegelse
Head Office, 70 12 0915 📖 165
Homofile og Lesbiskes Opplysningstelefon
Oslo, 22 11 3660 📖 164
Homogezondheitzentrum
Zwolle, 38 454 6369 📖 159
Homogroep Uithoorn 📖 158
Homogroep Wageningen
31 742 2835 📖 159
Homogruppe Thürmsdorf 📖 134
Homologay
Neuchâtel / Neuenburg, 38 31 5726 📖 178
HOMologie 📖 151
Homophile Association of London Ontario Inc. (HALO)
519 433 3511 📖 51
519 433 3762 📖 51
Homophon
Bielefeld, 521 106 3424 📖 112
Homophone
Mönchengladbach, 216 14 5055 📖 127
Homophonies
broadcast by FM 94.1 📖 98
Homosaïque
Nantes 📖 102
Homosexual Information Center
Bossier City 📖 260
Universal City, 318 742 4709 📖 223
Homosexuelle Aktion Ilmenau (HAI) 📖 122
Homosexuelle Alternative (HALT)
München, 89 311 6172 📖 128
Homosexuelle Arbeitsgruppe (HASO)
Solothurn, 65 23 6620 📖 179
Homosexuelle Arbeitsgruppe Luzern (HALU)
Luzern / Lucerne, 41 51 3532 📖 178
Homosexuelle Arbeitsgruppe Saint Gallen (HASG) 📖 179
Homosexuelle Arbeitsgruppen
Basel, 61 692 6655 📖 177
Bern, 31 311 6353 📖 177
Homosexuelle Arbeitsgruppen Zürich (HAZ)
1 271 2250 📖 179, 180
1 273 1177 📖 180
Homosexuelle Emanzipationsgruppe
Hannover, 511 36 3633 📖 121
Homosexuelle Emanzipationsgruppe (Heh!)
Heilbronn, 713 18 9064 📖 122
Homosexuelle Emanzipationsgruppe (HELB)
Biberach, 735 1 8384 📖 111
Homosexuelle Emanzitpation Gruppe (HOME)
Hannover, 511 36 3633 📖 121
Homosexuelle Informationsgruppe Ortenau / Baden (HIOB)
Lahr, 782 13 8383 📖 125
Homosexuelle Initiative (HOSI)
Salzburg, 662 43 5927 📖 35
Voralberg, 557 436 8675 📖 34
Wien 📖 35
Wien, 1 216 6604 📖 35
Homosexuelle Initiative Aalen (HIA)
07361 📖 109
Homosexuelle Initiative Essen (HIE)
201 4 2924 📖 116
Homosexuelle Initiative im Märkischen Sauerland (HIMS)
Lüdenscheid, 235 13 9547 📖 126
Homosexuelle Initiative Konstanz
753 16 4535 📖 125
Homosexuelle Initiative Lübeck (HIL)
451 7 4619 📖 126
Homosexuelle Initiative Neumünster (HIN)
432 12 9097 📖 129
Homosexuelle Initiative Passau (HIP)
851 7 1973 📖 131
Homosexuelle Inititivgruppe & Freunde
Bocholt 📖 112
Homosexuelle Interessengemeinschaft Unterfranken Warum
Kitzingen, 932 12 2666 📖 123
Homosexuelle Interessengruppe Hagen (HIGH) 📖 119
Homosexuelle Kultur Duisburg 📖 115
Homosexuelle Organisation Thurgau (HOT)
Frauenfeld, 54 21 0434 📖 178
Homosexuelle Selbshilfe
Brandenburg 📖 112
Homosexuelle Selbsthilfe
Tuttlingen, 746 17 6333 📖 134
Homosexuelle Selbsthilfe e. V.
Frankfurt am Main 📖 108
Homosexuelle Selbsthilfe e. V. (HS)
Offenbach, 69 84 1933 📖 130
Homosexuellenberatung in Bartaungs- & Seelsorgenzentrum St. Petri
Hamburg, 40 33 5845 📖 120
Homosexuelles Integrationsprojekt Potsdam (HIP)
331 2 2065 📖 131
Homostudies
Nijmegen, 80 351 2938 📖 157
Tilburg, 13 466 9111 📖 158
Homostudies Utrecht
30 253 4700 📖 158
Homosum
Delfzijl, 59 661 9823 📖 154
HOMOture 📖 217
Honcho
published by Fraction Presse SARL 📖 97
published by MMG Services Inc. 📖 307
Honour
London, 171 378 8565 📖 68
London, 171 401 8219 📖 86
Hoole, Ken, MSW
Fort Collins, 303 221 0272 📖 229
Hoosier Bears of Indiana
Indianapolis, 317 293 4394 📖 253
Hope HIV Support Group
Boone, 704 264 4109 📖 313
Hope, Victor, Ph.D.
Philadelphia, 215 925 0330 📖 330
Hôpital
Carcassone, 68 25 7976 📖 99
Hôpital Antoine Beclere
Paris, 145 37 4444 📖 103
Hôpital Beauregard
Thionville, 82 55 8899 📖 106
Hôpital Boucicaut
Paris, 145 54 9292 📖 103
Hôpital Cantonal
Lausanne, 21 314 4141 📖 178
Hôpital Charles-Nicole
Rouen, 35 008 8040 📖 105
Hôpital Corantins-Celton
Issy Les Moulineaux, 45 54 9533 📖 100
Hôpital de Bellevue
Saint Etienne, 77 42 7722 📖 105
Hôpital de la Fontaine
Paris, 142 35 6808 📖 103
Saint Denis, 42 35 6808 📖 105
Hôpital Edouard Herriot
Lyon, 72 34 4689 📖 100
Hôpital Henri Mondor
Créteil, 49 81 2295 📖 99
Hôpital Jean Martial
Cayenne, 885 📖 106
Hôpital Lariboisère
Paris, 149 95 6565 Ext. 2120 📖 103
Hôpital Pellegrin
Bordeaux, 56 98 4607 📖 98
Hôpital Saint Antoine
Paris, 143 44 3333 📖 103
Hôpital Saint Charles
Montpellier, 67 33 6490 📖 101
Hôpital Saint Louis
Paris, 142 49 9924 📖 103
Hôpital Saint-André
Bordeaux, 56 91 4424 📖 98
Hôpital Tarnier
Paris, 143 29 1289 📖 103
Horizon Bookstore
Champaign / Urbana, 217 328 2988 📖 248
Horizons Community Services, Inc.
Chicago, 312 472 6469 📖 250
Hors Château
Liège / Luik / Luttich, 4 123 5588 📖 38
Horstman, William, Ph.D.
San Francisco, 415 431 1790 📖 213
Horsts Laden
Berlin, 30 881 3929 📖 111
Horwitz, Richard, CSW, CAC
New York, 212 780 9400 📖 301
HOSI 📖 *See* Homosexuelle Initiative
Hospices Civils de Strasbourg
88 16 1718 📖 106
Hospital das Clinicas da Faculdade de Medicina
São Paulo, 11 282 2811 📖 39
Hospital Emilio Ribas
São Paulo, 11 881 2433 📖 39
Hospital of the University of Pennsylvania
Philadelphia, 215 662 4000 📖 330
Hospital São Paulo
11 549 8777 📖 39
HOT 📖 *See* Homosexuelle Organisation Thurgau
Hot & Bothered
published by USECA Communications Inc. 📖 53
Hot Ash
New York, 718 789 6147 📖 12
Hot Leather Versand
Hannover, 511 57 4251 📖 107
Hot Love
Helsinki, 90 773 3004 📖 97
Hot Pockets BBS
Portland, 503 232 2803 📖 1
Hot Rubber Company
Berlin 📖 108
Zürich 📖 177
Hot Shop
München, 89 487 214 📖 128
Hotel Adler
Hamburg, 40 24 5640 📖 119
Hôtel Dieu
Lyon, 78 42 2926 📖 100
Hotflash
Saint Louis 📖 284
Hothead Paisan 📖 231
Hots Spots 📖 236
Hotshots
published by Sunshine Publishing Co. 📖 211
House of David
Leicester 📖 79
House of Harlot
London, 171 706 2315 📖 68
House of Whacks
Chicago, 312 761 6969 📖 250, 251
Houseman's
London, 171 837 4473 📖 85
Housk, Randall
London, 181 764 8248 📖 83
Houston Area Bears
713 867 9123 📖 342
Houston Area Teen Coalition of Homosexuals (HATCH)
713 942 7002 📖 343
Houston Council of Clubs 📖 343
Houston Institute for the Protection of Youth
713 942 9884 📖 343
Houston Voice 📖 343
Houston Wrestling Club
713 453 7406 📖 343
Howard Brown Health Center
Chicago, 312 871 5777 📖 249
Howell Adult Book Store
908 363 9680 📖 290
Howick Gay Youth Group
Auckland, 9 534 2643 📖 160
HPA 📖 *See* Helping People With AIDS
Hraca, Kim, M.A., MFCC
Berkeley, 510 601 1859 📖 196, 197
HS 📖 *See* Homosexuelle Selbsthilfe e. V.
HSH 📖 *See* Aktionsgruppe Homosexualität Hannover
HTC
Phœnix, 602 278 1037 📖 193
HTC Body Adornment Studio
Phœnix, 602 278 1037 📖 194

Hubba Hubba
Boston, 617 492 9082 📖 270
Huch! Schwulen- & Lesben-Zentrum
Kiel, 431 17090 📖 123
Hudson Video & News
Rochester, 716 342 8310 📖 311
Hugendubel
Frankfurt am Main, 69 29 9820 📖 117
HUGS East 📖 *See* Mentor Center
Hull Lesbian Line
1482 214331 📖 77
Hulptelefoon
Doetinchem, 31 434 5884 📖 154
Humane Restraint
Madison, 800 356 7472 📖 356
Humanicare International, Inc.
North Brunswick, 201 214 0660 📖 292
Human-Nature & Postorder AEV
Hoorn, 22 923 2994 📖 156
Humberside Friend
Hull, 1482 443333 📖 77
Humboldt Buchhandlung
Bremen, 421 7 7721 📖 113
Hun
Portland, 503 285 9670 📖 326
Hung Jury
Los Angeles, 213 850 3618 📖 204
Hungry Head Books
Eugene, 503 485 0888 📖 325
Hunter Holmes McGuire Veterans' Affairs Medical Center
Richmond, 804 230 0001 📖 349
Hunter, Shirley, M.Ed.
Oklahoma City, 405 848 5429 📖 323
Huntington AIDS Force
304 522 4357 📖 355
Huntington Memorial Hospital
Pasadena, 818 397 5000 📖 209
Huntsville Hospital
205 533 8020 📖 191
Hurley Medical Center
Flint, 810 257 9000 📖 275
Hurricane Alice 📖 281
Hus 1 'Huset
Stockholm, 8 30 8338 📖 175
Hush-A-Bye Baby Club
Gravesend, 163 457 1396 📖 78
Husky Magazine 📖 217
HX (Homo Xtra) 📖 307
Hyacinth AIDS Foundation
New Brunswick, 800 433 0254 (in New Jersey) 📖 289
Hyatt, Diane, MSW, CISW
Stamford, 203 964 1847 📖 232
Hyde Park News
Perth, 9 328 5265 📖 34
Hygia-Versand
Pforzheim 📖 107
Hyssna
København, 35 37 7700 📖 66
H•M - Lederwerk
Bremen, 421 37 1430 📖 108
I, I & E Group
Twickenham, 181 894 2835 📖 87
Ian King Engineering Designs Ltd.
Near Marden 📖 78
Ian's
New York, 212 420 1857 📖 309
New York, 212 838 3969 📖 309
Ibiza
published by Association Ibiza 📖 101
ICARE 📖 *See* Iowa Center AIDS Resources & Education
Icebreakers
Auckland, 9 376 6633 (Youthline) 📖 160
Dunedin, 3 477 2077 📖 162
Hamilton, 7 856 3161 📖 162
Napier, 6 835 7190 📖 162
Wellington, 4 385 0674 📖 163
Icon 📖 59
Icon Detroit
Berkeley, 313 831 1852 📖 274
ICTLEP
Houston 📖 342
Idaho AIDS Foundation
Boise, 800 677 2437 📖 247
Idaho Women's Network
Boise, 208 344 5738 📖 247
Identity
London, 171 487 3797 📖 82
Identity Newspaper
published by Identity, Inc. 📖 192
Identity, Inc.
Anchorage, 907 258 4777 📖 192
IDPA 📖 *See* International Dungeon & Playroom Association
IEM 📖 *See* International Estetic Men
IFGE 📖 *See* International Foundation for Gender Education
IGLAB 📖 *See* Ithaca Gay & Lesbian Activities Board
IGLHRC 📖 *See* International Gay & Lesbian Human Rights Commission
IGTA 📖 *See* International Gender Transient Affinity
IHBa 📖 *See* Initiative Homosexualität Bamberg
IHS 📖 *See* Initiativgruppe Homosexualität Stuttgart e. V.
IHT 📖 *See* Innitiativgruppe Homosexualität Tübingen
IIAV
Amsterdam, 20 665 0820 📖 151
Il Bolero
Montréal, 514 270 6065 📖 63
Il Seme
Cosenza 📖 140
ILGA 📖 *See* International Lesbian & Gay Association
Illico 📖 97
Illinois Masonic Medical Center
Chicago, 312 975 1600 📖 249
Illusions Social Club
Calgary, 403 236 7072 📖 42
Illusions Social Club II
Edmonton 📖 43
Illustrated Men
Sylmar, 818 367 3938 📖 223
Image Leather
San Francisco, 415 621 7551 📖 218
Images
Thompson, 203 779 9708 📖 232
Images in Ink
Howell, 908 901 6205 📖 290
IMAX International
Riccione, 541 642160 📖 141
IMC 📖 *See* Italia Motor Club Milano
IME of Western Michigan
Grand Rapids 📖 276
Impact 📖 260
Imperia Press
London, 181 989 0281 📖 15
Imperial Books
Burnaby, 604 432 9940 📖 44
Imperial Point Medical Center
Fort Lauderdale, 305 776 8500 📖 236
Imperial Queens of New York & Long Island
212 580 9862 (New York City) 📖 305
Imprints - Booksellers
Adelaide, 8 231 4454 📖 30
Imprints Bookstore
Tacoma, 206 383 6322 📖 354
IMRU
Columbus, 614 228 9660 📖 321
IMRU of Gloucester County College
Sewell, 609 468 5000 Ext. 750 📖 293
In Distress
Birmingham, 121 428 3192 📖 93
In Line Diffusion
Bologna, 51 22 5976 📖 140
Milano, 2 20 1894 📖 143
Torino, 11 38 6512 📖 144
IN Newsweekly
published by IN Publications 📖 269
In Other Words
Portland, 503 232 6003 📖 326
In Other Words, Ltd.
Plymouth, 1752 663 889 📖 73
IN Publications
Boston, 617 292 0212 📖 269
In Step 📖 224, 355
In Step Magazine 📖 282
In The Flesh
published by OB Enterprises 📖 307
In The Life 📖 295
In The Pink, The Girls Own Show
broadcast by 95 BFM 📖 161
In Touch 📖 207
In Touch Hotline
Chicago, 312 996 5535 📖 249
In Uniform
published by A. M. Publications 📖 326
In Your Face 📖 308
Inciting Desire 📖 221
Inclinations
Nonantum, 617 893 4597 📖 271
INCON
Columbia 📖 183
Indecent Exposure
Laurel, 301 725 5683 📖 265
Independence News
Charlotte, 704 332 8430 📖 314
Independent Bookshop
Sheffield, 114 273 7722 📖 90
Independent Publishers Group (IPG)
Chicago, 312 337 0747 📖 249
Independent Review 📖 25
Indiana AIDS Hotline
Indianapolis, 317 257 4673 📖 254
Indiana CARES, Inc.
Indianapolis, 317 630 9075 📖 253
Indiana Crossdressers Society (IXE)
Indianapolis, 317 781 0834 📖 253
Indiana University Medical Center
Indianapolis, 317 274 5000 📖 254
Indiana Word
published by Word Publications 📖 253
Indianapolis Youth Group
317 541 8726 📖 255
Infantæ Press
Seattle 📖 352
Infectious Diseases Clinic
Indianapolis, 317 635 8378 📖 254
Inferno
Philadelphia, 215 627 5489 📖 331
Wildwood 📖 293
Info SIDA
Montréal, 514 521 7432 (SIDA) 📖 62
Infofoon Amsterdam
20 675 3026 📖 150
Infogai
published by Publicació Degana del Moviment Gai a Catalunya 📖 172
Infoline
Paris, 136 65 5678 📖 103
Infoline of Eastern Connecticut
Norwich, 203 886 0516 📖 232
Infor Homo
Bruxelles / Brussel, 2 733 1024 📖 36, 37
Informagay
Torino, 11 436 5000 📖 144
Information Express 📖 349
Informationszentrum für Männer
Frankfurt am Main, 69 597 0959 📖 117
Informazioni AIDS
Bologna, 51 624 0644 📖 140
Informazioni Gay
Bologna, 51 624 7054 📖 140
Informe SIDA
Austin, 512 472 2001 📖 338
Informher
published by Friday Night Womyn's Group 📖 239
Ingersoll Gender Center
Seattle, 206 329 6651 📖 351
Ingram Book
Lavergne 📖 336
Ingrid's Bookstore
Oklahoma City, 415 353 1488 📖 323
Iniquity 📖 307
Initiative Homosexualität Bamberg (IHBa)
951 2 4729 📖 109
Initiativgruppe Homosexualität Stuttgart e. V. (IHS)
711 62 4870 📖 133
Inklings
Houston, 713 521 3369 📖 343
Inland Northwest Gay People's Alliance
Moscow, 208 882 8034 📖 247
Inner Bookshop
Oxford, 186 524 5301 📖 90
Inner Circle
Bristol, 117 929 3754 📖 70
Innitiativgruppe Homosexualität Tübingen (IHT)
707 14 2763 📖 134
Innovations
Boston 📖 270
Raleigh, 919 833 4833 📖 316
Innvestments
Orleans 📖 272
INSA 📖 *See* Intersex Society of North America
Insel
268 5 7612 📖 122
Insight
Milwaukee, 414 271 2565 📖 357
Insight Books
Menlo Park, 415 324 0543 📖 206
Insitute for Personal Growth
New Brunswick, 908 246 8439 📖 291
Institut Prophylactique
Paris, 145 55 3894 📖 103
Institute for Gender Study & Treatment
Arvada, 303 423 9885 📖 226
Institute for Human Identity
New York, 212 799 9432 📖 301
Institute for Psychosexual Health
Milwaukee, 414 322 5407 📖 357
Institute of Gay & Lesbian Education
West Hollywood, 310 652 1786 📖 225
Institute of Lesbian Studies
Chicago 📖 249
Institute of Psychiatry
London, 171 703 5411 📖 81
Institute of Psycho-Analysis
London, 171 580 4952 📖 81
Institute of Psychosexual Medicine
London, 171 580 0631 📖 81
Institute of Psycho-Synthesis
London, 181 959 2330 📖 81
Institute of Psychotherapy & Social Studies
London, 171 284 4762 📖 82
Instituto de SIDA de San Juan
809 723 2424 📖 167
Instituto Lambda
Barcelona 📖 172
Intabooks
London 📖 85
Integrity Indexing
Charlotte, 704 335 9936 📖 314
Inter-Bike Denmark
København 📖 13
Interchange
San Anselmo 📖 210
Intermale
Amsterdam, 20 625 0009 📖 8
Intermale Gay Bookstore
Amsterdam, 20 625 0009 📖 153
International Gay & Lesbian Human Rights Commission (IGLHRC)
San Francisco, 415 255 8680 📖 215
International Directory of Bisexual Groups
published by Bisexual Community Resource Center 📖 269
International Dungeon & Playroom Association (IDPA)
Pasadena 📖 12
International Estetic Men (IEM)
Paris, 142 96 0574 📖 104
International Estetic Men (IEM)
Paris, 142 41 2141 📖 97, 104
Paris, 145 22 6901 📖 104
International Foundation for Gender Education (IFGE)
Boston, 617 899 2212 📖 268
International Gay & Lesbian Archives
Los Angeles, 213 662 9444 📖 1
International Gay & Lesbian Association (ILGA)
Köln, 221 52 0206 📖 108
International Gender Transient Affinity (IGTA)
Freshwater 📖 77
International Leatherman
published by Brush Creek Media 📖 217
International Lesbian & Gay Association (ILGA)
Utrecht, 30 234 0912 📖 158
International Mackintosh Society
Folkestone 📖 78
International Male Mail
Schüpfheim, 41 485 0081 📖 8
International Mr. Fantasy
Omaha 📖 285
International Mr. Leather, Inc.
Chicago, 800 545 6753 (in U.S.A.) 📖 1
International Ms Leather
Omaha, 402 451 7987 📖 1
International Roadmasters

Ferndale 📖 275
International Sexual Minorities Information Resource (ISMIR)
Pittsburgh, 412 422 3060 📖 13, 15
International Transcript / CDS
published by Creative Design Services 📖 331
International Wavelength, Inc.
San Francisco, 415 749 1100 📖 215
Internationalist Books
Chapel Hill, 919 942 1740 📖 313
Intersex Society of North America (INSA)
Canada 📖 50
Intervention Régionale & Information sur le SIDA (IRIS)
Sherbrooke, 800 567 391 (information) 📖 63
Intim Boutique
Rendsburg 📖 131
Rottweil, 741 1 2714 📖 131
Intim Shop
Donaueschingen 📖 114
Intimate Treasures
San Francisco, 415 863 5002 📖 186
Intimshop
Oldenburg, 441 2 7291 📖 130
Into You
London, 171 253 5085 📖 87
Invincible
London, 171 237 4017 📖 68, 86
Iowa Artistry
Cedar Rapids 📖 256
Iowa Center AIDS Resources & Education (ICARE)
Iowa City, 319 338 2135 📖 257
Iowa Woman Endeavors, Inc.
Iowa City 📖 255
Iowa Woman Magazine
published by Iowa Woman Endeavors, Inc. 📖 255
IPG 📖 *See* Independent Publishers Group
IPS
Stockholm, 8 747 1493 📖 175
Ipswich AIDS Helpline
1473 232007 📖 91
IQ Magazine 📖 85
Ireland, Chris
Sydney, 2 331 2689 📖 27
IRIS 📖 *See* Intervention Régionale & Information sur le SIDA
Iris Books
Gainesville, 904 375 7477 📖 237
Iron City Ink Tattoos
Pittsburgh, 412 784 9396 📖 332
Iron Cross MC
Montréal, 514 931 2202 📖 62
Iron Eagles MC
Dorchester 📖 270
Iron Guard BC NYC
New York, 908 245 5323 📖 304
Iron Master
Dallas / Fort Worth, 214 324 4687 📖 340
Isaacs, Robert, CSW
New York, 212 229 0090 📖 301
ISBN Agency
New York, 212 337 6975 📖 304
Island Gay Community Centre
Victoria, 604 383 9124 📖 47
Island Lesbian & Gay Association
Vineyard Haven, 508 693 3563 📖 272
Island Lesbian Connection 📖 246
Island Lifestyle Magazine
published by Lifestyle Publishing Inc. 📖 246
Isle of Wight Switchboard
Ryde, 1983 525123 📖 77
Islington Army & Navy Store
London, 171 833 4805 📖 87
ISMIR 📖 *See* International Sexual Minorities Information Resource
ISMIR Events Calendar
published by International Sexual Minorities Information Resource 📖 15
Istar, Arlene, CSW, CAC
Albany, 518 439 9270 📖 295
Istituti Ospedale
Cremona, 372 40 5518 📖 142
Istituto Dermopatico dell'Immacolata
Roma 📖 141
Istituto Malattie Infettive
Sassari, 79 231 1659 📖 145
Istvan, John Emery, M.S., MSW, LCSW
Trumbull, 203 268 8858 Ext. 304 📖 232
It's My Pleasure
Portland, 503 236 0505 📖 327
It's Okay!
published by Phœnix Counsel, Inc. 📖 54
Italia Motor Club Milano (IMC)
2 0250 4889 📖 143
Ithaca Gay & Lesbian Activities Board (IGLAB) 📖 299
Ithaca Lesbian, Gay, & Bisexual Task Force
607 347 4605 📖 299
IUPUI Advocate
Indianapolis, 317 274 0079 📖 255
Ivy's Bookshop
Victoria, 604 598 2713 📖 47
IXE 📖 *See* Indiana Crossdressers Society
J & S Sports Products
Warren, 810 754 6971 📖 278
J Barnicoat Ltd.
Penryn, 132 637 2628 📖 72
J's Hangout
New York, 212 242 9292 📖 304
J. B. Productions
Santa Clara 📖 221
J. G. Strydom Hospital
Johannesburg, 11 726 5128 📖 171
J. Whitaker & Sons
London, 171 836 8911 📖 84
J/O Enthusiasts
Washington, 202 452 5906 📖 234
J/OE
Baltimore 📖 264
Jack's Number Two
Houston 📖 188
Jack, Sarah
London, 181 509 9751 📖 80
Jackaroos MC
Melbourne, 39 885 1612 📖 32
Jackhammer
San Francisco, 415 252 0290 📖 212
Jackson GALA
307 733 5349 📖 358
Jackson Hospital & Clinic
Montgomery, 205 293 8000 📖 192
Jackson Memorial Hospital
Miami, 305 324 8111 📖 239
Jacobs, Mindy, Ph.D.
Washington, 202 543 0303 📖 233
Jacques, Trevor
Toronto, 416 962 1040 📖 13
Jacqui
San Francisco, 415 626 6551 📖 213
Jaguar
San Francisco, 415 863 4777 📖 219
Jahn, Harald
Wien, 1 505 5490 📖 35
Jail
Mannheim, 621 85 9626 📖 126
James Adult Centre
Mansfield, 1623 420425 📖 89
James Bondage
Tampa 📖 242
James Publishing Group, Inc.
Chicago 📖 251
James Whale Show
broadcast by Mike Mansfield TV 📖 87
James White Review 📖 281
James, George, Ph.D.
Birmingham 📖 191
Janssen Verlag
Berlin 📖 110
Janus
London, 171 437 1741 📖 85
JARG 📖 *See* Jersey AIDS Relief Group
Jarratt, Kent, ACSW
New York, 212 674 7370 📖 301
Jay Fashions
Stanford-Le-Hope 📖 68
Jaybird's Toybox
Fort Lauderdale 📖 184
Jazi's
Pittsburgh, 412 323 2721 📖 331
JDL
Stoke-on-Trent, 1782 518564 📖 68
Jean Paul
published by Editions SAN 📖 97
Jean, Paula, Ph.D.
Richmond, 804 329 3940 📖 349
Jeans Mode Trends
Berlin, 30 881 4157 📖 111
Jennifer & Friends
Sparks 📖 287
Jensen & Morrow
London, 171 729 1115 📖 81
Jerry's Adult Bookstore
Tacoma, 206 272 4700 📖 354
Jerry's Army & Navy Store
Malden, 617 324 6990 📖 271
Jerry's Misc. Services
Fairview Heights, 618 397 2709 📖 183
Jersey AIDS Relief Group (JARG)
Saint Helier, 1534 58886 📖 64
Jersey Shore Gay & Lesbian Community Center
Asbury Park, 908 493 0730 📖 289
Jeunes & Etudiant(e)s Homosexuel(le)s de Tour (JEHT)
Paris, 47 20 5530 📖 103
Jewish AIDS Trust
London, 181 200 0369 📖 67, 82
Jewish Hospital of Cincinnati
513 569 2000 📖 318
Jewish Lesbian & Gay Helpline
London, 171 706 3123 📖 67
JG Leathers
Delta 📖 41
JH Press
New York 📖 306
Jim Bridges' Boutique
Studio City, 818 761 6650 📖 223
Jim Cooke Enterprises
Chehalis 📖 350
Jim Johnson Surplus
Garden Grove, 714 534 2973 📖 200
JK Perfect Personal Products
Phœnix 📖 183
JMPG
Burbank 📖 197
Jock 📖 307
John Coutts Library Services, Ltd.
Niagara Falls, 905 356 6382 📖 51
John Floyd Video
West Hollywood, 800 697 9009 📖 224
John L. Doyne Hospital
Milwaukee, 414 257 7996 📖 357
John Smith
Glasgow, 141 221 7472 📖 169
Glasgow, 141 334 2769 📖 169
Johns Hopkins Hospital
Baltimore, 410 955 5000 📖 263
Jones, Jeanette
Chigwell 📖 75
Jones, Linda, CSW, ACSW
New York, 212 982 9232 📖 301
Jones, Mark
Phœnix, 602 265 4435 📖 193, 194
Joseph-Beth Booksellers
Lexington, 606 273 2911 📖 259
Jostens Printing & Publishing
Visalia, 209 651 3300 📖 224
Journal
Koblenz, 261 30 9768 📖 123
Journal Gaie Presence 📖 97
Journal of Gay & Lesbian Psychotherapy
published by Haworth Press 📖 20
Journal of Gay & Lesbian Social Services
published by Haworth Press 📖 20
Journal of Homosexuality
published by Haworth Press 📖 22
Journal of Sex Research 📖 317
Jox
Berlin 📖 111
Joy Melbourne
broadcast by FM 90.7 📖 32
JP L'Agora
Bruxelles / Brussel, 2 511 1220 📖 37
JS Leather
Salisbury, 1722 328588 📖 94
JUB 📖 *See* Jungendberatung Düsseldorf
Judith's Room
New York, 212 727 7330 📖 308
Jugendgruppe Jackpoint
Saint Gallen 📖 179
Jugendgruppe Rose
Basel / Bâle, 61 692 6655 📖 177
Jugendgruppe Space
Bern 📖 178
Jugendgruppe WIGWAM
Saint Moritz 📖 179
June Addams Book Shop
Champaign / Urbana, 217 356 2555 📖 248
June Mazer Collection & Archive
West Hollywood, 310 659 2478 📖 224
Junge Lesben & Schwule im Thurgau (LuST)
Mammern, 71 72 3413 📖 178
Jungendberatung Düsseldorf (JUB)
211 67 3058 📖 115
Jungendnetwerk Lambda e. V.
Berlin 📖 110
Jungendnetzwerk Lambda Niedersachsen e. V.
Braunschweig 📖 112
Jungle Vine 📖 246
Juran, Shelley, Ph.D.
Brooklyn, 718 625 6526 📖 297
JuRonCo
Peoria, 309 673 8724 📖 10
Just Books
Belfast, 123 232 5426 📖 164
Just For The Record
broadcast by Public Access Television 📖 261
Just Leathers
Caldmore 📖 68
Just Out 📖 324
K. A. B. Kühn / Clabes Versandhandel GbR
Duisberg, 203 33 4482 📖 107
K. G. Saur Publishing Company
New York, 212 751 3033 📖 306
K. L. Graphics
Hawaii (Big Island), 808 325 3157 📖 181
K. O. X.
Montréal, 514 523 0064 📖 61
Kâa, Heïdi
Bruxelles / Brussel, 2 223 0914 📖 36
Kacmer Publishing Co.
Alton, 618 465 9370 📖 247
KAE BokImport
Oslo 📖 164
Kaiser Foundation Hospital
Oahu, 808 834 5333 📖 246
San Francisco, 415 202 2000 📖 213
Kalake Kaptive Bead
Sacramento, 914 447 9443 📖 209
Kalamazoo Gay / Lesbian Center
616 345 7878 📖 276
Kalani Honua, Inc.
Hawaii (Big Island), 808 965 7828 📖 246
Kali-Shiva Society
Winnipeg, 204 477 9506 📖 47
Kanal Gay
broadcast by FM 95.3 📖 174
Kansas City Cave Bears
816 986 9696 📖 283
Kansas City Free Health Clinic
816 753 5144 📖 283
Kansas City Pioneers 📖 283
Kantonspital
Baden, 56 84 2111 📖 177
Liestal, 61 91 9111 📖 178
Kantonsspital Basel
Basel / Bâle, 61 265 4161 📖 177
KARES 📖 *See* Kelowna & Area AIDS Resources, Education, & Support
Karmen, Mel, Ph.D.
San Diego, 619 296 9442 📖 211
Karo Design
Hamburg, 40 279 6121 📖 119, 120
Kassan, Lee, MA
New York, 212 989 3613 📖 301
Kastley
Darwen, 125 487 3247 📖 78
Kastley GmbH
Stuttgart, 711 76 9074 📖 107, 133
Katacombes
Montréal, 514 523 0064 📖 62
Katharsis
Bunnell, 904 437 2642 📖 16, 18, 19, 20
published by Katharsis 📖 16
published by Katharsis 📖 16, 20
Kayser Novelty Co.
Austal, 2 606 0002 📖 24
KBDI-TV, Channel 12

Denver, 303 446 2518 📖 229
KBOO Radio FM 90.7
Portland, 503 231 8032 📖 326
KCM 📖 *See* Schwulen- & Lesbenzentrum Münster
Keeffe, Corky, M.A.
Colorado Springs, 719 578 9730 📖 226
Keith, III, Paul, M.D.
Los Angeles, 213 964 1440 📖 203
Keller's
Paris, 143 55 1152 📖 102
Kellner, Bernhard
Hannover 📖 121
Kelowna & Area AIDS Resources, Education, & Support (KARES)
604 862 2437 📖 44
Kelso, Betsy, Psy.D.
Denver, 303 757 6969 📖 227
Ken Marcus Studio
Hollywood, 213 937 7214 📖 201
Kennestone Hospital
Marietta, 404 793 5000 📖 245
Kent County Council
Folkestone, 1303 248 177 📖 78
Kentuckiana People With AIDS Coalition (KIPWAC)
Louisville, 502 574 5493 📖 258
Owensboro, 502 683 2438 📖 260
Kentucky Gay & Lesbian Educational Center
Louisville, 502 636 0935 📖 258
Kentucky Woman
Brighton, 1273 674631 📖 23
Kentucky Word
published by Word Publications 📖 258
Kepler's Books
Palo Alto, 415 324 4321 📖 209
Kerner, Bruce, Psy.D.
New York, 212 682 1288 📖 301
Kert, Kelvin
Paris, 148 03 2885 📖 104
Key
published by Sussex Mailbox 📖 70
Key Largo
London, 171 ?49 7599 📖 86
Key Press
El Paso 📖 342
Key West Island Bookstore
305 294 2904 📖 238
Key West Wreckers LLC
305 296 3338 📖 238
Keyhole Bookshop
Tweed Heads, 7 536 3197 📖 27
KFAI FM 90.3
Minneapolis / Saint Paul, 612 341 3144 📖 281
Kick Publishing Company
Detroit, 313 438 0704 📖 275
Kick! Magazine
published by Kick Publishing Company 📖 275
Kießling Handelsagentur
München, 89 35 65 1745 📖 128
Kill City
Melbourne 📖 33
Kimberly Press
Santa Barbara, 805 964 6469 📖 221
Kindred Spirits
Charlottesville, 804 971 1555 📖 347
Kinesis 📖 46
King Edward VIII Hospital
Durban, 31 35 0235 📖 171
King's English Bookstore
Salt Lake City, 801 484 9100 📖 345
King's Leathers
Bradenton, 813 751 2167 📖 236
Kingfisher
Inverness, 146 379 1681 📖 168
Kings County Hospital Center
Brooklyn, 718 245 3131 📖 297
Kingston AIDS Project
800 565 2209 (information) 📖 50
Kingston Lesbian, Gay, & Bisexual Association
613 545 2960 📖 50
Kink
published by Dominant Publications 📖 46
Kink Distributors
Petaluma, 800 805 4657 📖 209
Kink Video
Brooklyn, 718 832 3952 📖 187
Kink, Ink
Toronto, 416 962 1040 📖 14, 15
Kinks
Cincinnati, 513 651 2668 📖 318
Kinky Bar
Stockholm, 8 653 5739 📖 175
Kinky Club
Amsterdam, 20 620 5603 📖 151
Helsinki 📖 95
Kinky Couples
Seattle 📖 351
Kinky Kumputer
Belleview 📖 350
Kinky People Places & Things
published by DM International 📖 352
Kinsel, Kevin, MSW, CSW, PC
Detroit, 810 541 6830 📖 274
Kinsey Institute
Bloomington, 812 855 7686 📖 253
KIPWAC 📖 *See* Kentuckiana People With AIDS Coalition
Kirkenes Sykehus Sjefslege Arnt Uchtermann
78 99 1701 📖 165
Kirklees AIDS Response
Huddersfield, 1484 432433 📖 94
Kirklees Lesbian & Gay Switchboard
Huddersfield, 1484 538070 📖 94
Kiss Contact
Sofia, 2 22 5607 📖 40
Kitchen Table, Women of Color Press
Brooklyn, 718 935 1082 📖 14
Kitchener / Waterloo Sexual Assault Support Centre
519 741 8633 (Hotline) 📖 50
Kitsch
Pau, 59 27 6867 📖 105
Kiwi Bears
Auckland 📖 160
Klamath Area Lambda Association
Klamath Falls, 503 883 2437 📖 325
Klamath County AIDS/HIV Support & Education Council
Klamath Falls, 503 883 2437 📖 325
Klein Enterprises
Johannesburg, 11 642 8989 📖 170
Klein, Patricia, M.S.
Allentown, 610 821 2955 📖 327
Klick, Schwulengruppe Zürich Oberland
Hinwil, 55 48 4753 📖 178
Klinger Publications
San Diego 📖 211
Klinik HIV Station
Dortmund, 231 4 5090 📖 114
Klinikken for Kønssygdomme
Ålborg 📖 65
Klinikum an Küchwald Infectktionsklinik
Chemnitz, 371 33 2644 📖 113
Klinikum der Johan-Gutenburg Universit_at
Mainz, 613 11 7197 📖 126
Klix Leather Products
Bury, 161 763 7488 📖 11
Klondyke Kontact 📖 193
Kloster, Doris
New York, 212 614 6621 📖 306
Klub A-3 e. V. - Anders als Andere
Magdeburg 📖 126
Klub Einblick e. V.
Schwerin, 385 764 9720 📖 132
Klystra
Hawaii (Big Island), 808 325 3157 📖 186
Knast
Berlin, 30 219 1026 📖 110
Knickers & Upskirts 📖 70
Knight Cruisers
Lexington, 606 225 4315 📖 259
Knight Hawks of Virginia
Norfolk, 804 489 8028 📖 348
Knight Publishing
Los Angeles 📖 204
Knights d'Orleans
New Orleans 📖 261
Knights of Leather
Minneapolis / Saint Paul, 612 870 7473 (answering machine) 📖 280
Knights of Malta MC
Dogwood 📖 45
Jet 📖 352
Richland Hills 📖 344
Western 📖 287
Knights of Malta of California Clubs, Inc.
Cable Car Chapter 📖 215
Motherlode Chapter 📖 206
Knights on Iron MC
San Diego 📖 211
Knights Wrestling Club
New York, 718 639 5141 📖 306
KNON FM 89.3
Dallas / Fort Worth, 214 520 1375 📖 341
Knopf, Norton, Ph.D.
Chicago, 312 363 5011 📖 249
Know How
Milano, 2 66 98 7065 📖 143
Koen Book Distributors
Moorestown, 609 235 4444 📖 291
Köln Oliv
228 234451 📖 124
Kommuneoverlegen
Gjøvik, 61 17 5600 Ext. 235 📖 165
Konsultatieburo voor Relaties en Seksualiteit (DOK)
Antwerpen / Anvers, 3 234 0848 📖 36
Kooky Shop
Brighton 📖 74
Kools
Hannover, 511 262 1540 📖 121
Kopacsi, Rosemarie, Ph.D., ACSW
Montclair, 201 338 4834 📖 291
Koplin, James, M.Ed., MSW
Hartford, 203 724 4204 📖 230
KOPN FM 89.5
Columbia, 314 874 5676 📖 283
Koppel, Mark, Ph.D.
New York, 212 362 7027 📖 301
KPFT FM 90.1
Houston, 713 526 4000 📖 343
Kramer Books & Afterwords
Washington, 202 387 1400 📖 235
Kraus Eule, Norma, LCSW
Auburn, 207 784 8747 📖 262
Kraze
Hockley 📖 93
KRCL FM 91
Salt Lake City, 801 363 1818 📖 345
Kreger, Kenneth, MA, CSW, LPC
Flint, 810 234 3658 📖 275
Krewe of Apollo de Lafayette 📖 260
Krieger, Irwin, LCSW
New Haven, 203 776 2966 📖 231
Kringen
Eindhoven 📖 155
Nijmegen, 80 344 0030 📖 157
Rotterdam, 10 419 8310 📖 157
Kringen, Regio Amerfoort
Hoogland, 33 456 1509 📖 156
Kristiansan Helserâd
Kristiansand, 38 02 9755 📖 166
Kroll, Eric
New York, 212 684 2465 📖 306
Kromar Printing
Winnipeg, 204 775 8721 📖 47
KTRU FM 91.7
Houston, 713 527 4050 📖 343
Kubs/Kiwi United Bear Social
Auckland 📖 160
Kumpel
published by Vogel Verlag 📖 110
Kundalini Publishing, Inc.
San Francisco, 415 541 7725 📖 217
Kunomeiden GMBH
Frankfurt am Main 📖 117
Kunstbanett
Köln 📖 124
Kunsthaus Fischinger
Stuttgart 📖 133
Kunzmann
Ispringen 📖 122
Pforzheim, 7231 89774 📖 131
Kuopion AIDS-Tukikeskus
971 281 1959 📖 96
Kurbash
Toronto, 416 921 0665 📖 55
Kuumba
published by BLK Publishing Co. 📖 189
KW Enterprises
New York, 212 727 1973 📖 10
L & L Society
Bay City, 517 982 8054 📖 274
L'Hermite, Christian
Sydney, 2 212 2088 📖 27
L. C. Fantasia
Lindsay, 705 328 3998 📖 51
L. U. R. E.
New York, 212 741 3919 📖 300
L.U.U. Bookshop
Leeds, 113 244 4974 📖 94
L/SM Round-Up
San Francisco, 415 754 2990 📖 214
La Ampurdanesa
Barcelona, 3 301 8879 📖 172
La Carnivale
Rego Park, 212 689 6397 📖 310
La Conchiglia
Capri, 81 837 6577 📖 140
La Fourmi Ailée
Paris, 143 29 4099 📖 104
La Librairie des Femmes
Paris 📖 104
La Loge de Thalie
Bruxelles / Brussel, 2 734 5705 📖 37
La Luz de Jesus
Los Angeles, 213 651 5875 📖 205
La Madrona
San Francisco 📖 215
La Sex Shoppe
Anchorage, 907 522 1987 📖 193
Labyrinth 📖 331
Toronto, 416 417 6583 📖 60
Läderverkstan
Stockholm, 8 668 5869 📖 175
Ladies After Dark
Fort Wayne 📖 254
Ladies Home Companion 📖 325
Lady Elizabeth
Ellesmere Port, 151 353 0126 📖 68
Lady Green
San Francisco 📖 217
Lady Iris
Portsmouth, 603 436 3634 📖 288
Lady Midnight
Berkeley, 510 845 3823 📖 183
Lady O Society
London 📖 82
Ladylike
published by Creative Design Services 📖 329
Lafayette CARES
318 233 2437 📖 260
Lafferty, Norma, MSW
Denville, 201 586 3694 📖 290
Lagaipa, Darryn
Portland, 503 284 4174 📖 326
LAGC 📖 *See* Los Angeles Gender Center
Laguna Honda Hospital
San Francisco, 415 664 1580 📖 213
Lake, Moira
London, 181 943 5507 📖 80
Lakeland Elements
Morecombe, 152 441 3607 📖 69
Lakes - Mountains Coinnection
Campton, 603 726 3667 📖 287
LAMBDA
Lexington 📖 4
Saint Cloud, 612 654 5166 📖 282
Lambda Alive
Lehigh Valley, 610 589 4854 📖 329
Lambda Alliance of Gay Men & Lesbians
Bozeman, 406 994 3836 📖 285
Lambda Association of Fayetteville
910 484 7337 📖 315
Lambda Association of Staten Island
New York, 718 979 8890 📖 305
Lambda Book Report
published by Lambda Rising, Inc. 📖 235
Lambda Club, University of Victoria 📖 47
Lambda Community Center
Fort Collins, 303 224 3247 📖 229
Sacramento, 916 447 5755 📖 210
Lambda Counseling Services
Kansas City, 816 531 7133 📖 283
Lambda Delta Lambda Sorority
Los Angeles, 213 825 6322 📖 204
Lambda Eastern Oregon Association
Baker City 📖 324
Lambda Edition 📖 108
Lambda Group
Terre Haute 📖 255
Lambda Horizon at Virginia Tech
Blacksburg, 703 231 3852 📖 347

Lambda Lesbian & Gay Student Association
New York, 212 237 8738 📖 305
Lambda Line
Ottawa, 613 233 8212 📖 52
Lambda of Northeast Louisiana
Monroe, 318 387 0442 📖 260
Lambda Panhandlers
Shepherdstown 📖 355
Lambda Passages
Miami, 305 754 6900 📖 239
Lambda Press
Ottawa 📖 53
Lambda Publications
Chicago, 312 871 7610 📖 251
Lambda Report
broadcast by KBDI-TV, Channel 12 📖 229
Lambda Resourcer Center
Birmingham, 205 326 8600 📖 191
Lambda Resources
Philadelphia, 215 667 9060 📖 331
Lambda Rising
Baltimore, 410 234 0069 📖 264
Rehoboth Beach, 302 227 6969 📖 233
Washington, 202 462 6969 📖 235
Washington, 800 621 6969 📖 8
Lambda Rising Online
Washington, 800 621 6969 📖 8
Lambda Rising, Inc.
Washington, 202 462 7924 📖 235
LAMBDA Services
El Paso, 915 562 4297 📖 341
LAMBDA Services Youth OUTreach
El Paso, 915 562 4297 📖 341
Lambda Society at Clemson 📖 335
Lambda Support Group
Mansfield, 419 522 0729 📖 322
Lambda Weekly Radio
broadcast by KNON FM 89.3 📖 341
Lambda Youth & Family Empowerment
San Francisco, 415 565 7681 📖 215
Lambda Youth Network
Culver City 📖 198
Lambda Youth Services
Syracuse, 315 422 9741 📖 312
Lambda-Junge Lesben & Schwule im Freistaat Sachsen e. V.
Dresden 📖 114
Lambda-Nachrichten
published by Homosexuelle Initiative 📖 35
Lammas Women's Books & More
Baltimore, 410 752 1001 📖 264
Lamoille County AIDS Task Force
Morrisville, 802 888 7153 📖 346
Lamothe, Denise, Psy.D.
Manchester, 603 627 3739 📖 288
LA-MOTSS
Los Angeles 📖 3
LA-MOTSS-ANNOUNCE
Los Angeles 📖 3
Lamp Bookshop
Wigan 📖 76
Lampe
Hamburg 📖 107
Lancashire Family & Partners Support
Leyland, 1772 621111 📖 79
Lancaster Lambda
Harrisburg 📖 328
Lancaster Lesbian & Gay Switchboard
1524 847437 📖 78
Kendal, 1524 847437 📖 72
Penrith, 1524 847437 📖 72
Lance Publications
London 📖 85
Land Beyond
Sydney 📖 27
Land in Sight
Frankfurt am Main, 69 44 3095 📖 117
Land of Awes Information Services
Wichita, 316 269 0913 📖 189
Landeskrankenhaus Innsbruck / Department of Dermatology & Venerology
512 2 8711 Ext. 448 📖 34
Landeskrankenhaus Salzburg, Dept. Dermatologie
662 3 1581 📖 34
Landforeningen mot AIDS
Oslo, 22 17 0700 📖 164
Landry, Patricia, CSW, BCD
New York, 516 794 2626 📖 301
Landsforeningen for Bøsser og Lesbiske (LBL)
Afdeling Sudjylland, 75 54 1948 📖 66
Århus, 86 12 1948 📖 65
Head Office, 33 13 1948 📖 65
København, 33 13 1948 📖 66
Odense, 66 17 7692 📖 66
Rådgivning, 98 16 4507 📖 65
Landsforeningen for Lesbisk og Homofil Frigjøring (LLH)
Akershus 📖 164
Bodø, 75 52 2775 📖 165
Kristiansand, 38 02 0048 📖 166
Kristiansund 📖 165
Mjøsa, 61 19 5152 📖 165
Mo 📖 165
Oslo, 22 36 1948 📖 164
Stavanger, 51 53 1446 📖 166
Tromsø, 77 68 5643 📖 166
Trondheim, 73 52 4226 📖 166
Lanem Fashions
Chesham 📖 68
Langley Outreach
604 534 7921 📖 44
Lannoye Emblems
Kirkland, 206 820 0955 📖 350
Lansing General Hospital
517 372 8220 📖 277
Larmes D'Eros
Paris, 143 38 3343 📖 104
Larmes D'Hollywood
Liège / Luik / Luttich, 4 122 0472 📖 38
Larry's Guide to the Ghetto 📖 58
Larvik Helserâd
33 18 6372 📖 166
Sandefjord, 33 48 6372 📖 166
Las Vegas Bears
702 658 7548 📖 286
Las Vegas Bugle 📖 286
Lashes by Sarah
San Francisco, 415 621 6048 📖 187
LASS 📖 *See* Leicestershire AIDS Support Services
Last Frontier
Anchorage 📖 192
Last Gasp of San Francisco
415 824 6636 📖 213
Last Sunday
Aiken 📖 334
Last Word Newsstand
Forestville, 707 869 0571 📖 199
Lasting Impressions
Ames, 515 233 2819 📖 256
Latest Isssue 📖 210
Latex America
Miami 📖 183
Latex Seduction
Nantes 📖 97
Latexa
Praestoe 📖 65
Lathrop, Brian, NCPsy.A.
New York, 212 727 9797 📖 301
Latina Lesbian History Project
Binghamton 📖 296
Laughing Horse Books
Portland, 503 236 2893 📖 326
Laughing Moon Bookstore
Damariscotta, 207 563 5537 📖 262
Laura's Lair
Ava 📖 282
Laurel News Agency
301 725 9671 📖 265
Laurie Lane's Leather World
Melbourne, 3 9827 9974 📖 32
Lavendar & Lace
New York, 212 255 6758 📖 305
Lavendar Books
Los Angeles, 213 464 7400 Ext. 204 📖 205
Lavendar Circle Press
Red Bank 📖 292
Lavendar Enterprises
Binghamton, 607 771 1986 📖 189
Lavendar Express 📖 289
Lavendar Hearts
Lehigh Valley, 610 372 1828 📖 329
Lavendar Heights
New York, 212 569 2023 📖 305
Lavendar Jade's
Clifton Park, 518 798 3304 📖 181
Lavendar Letter 📖 328
Lavendar Life
published by Lavendar Enterprises 📖 189
Lavendar Listings 📖 320
Lavendar Morning 📖 276
Lavendar Network
Eugene 📖 325
Lavendar Pages 📖 218
Lavendar Prairie News 📖 248
Lavendar Publishing
Vancouver, 604 688 0265 📖 46
Lavendar Reader 📖 222
Lavendar Triangle
Toledo, 419 531 0644 📖 322
Lavendar Wimmin
broadcast by WUSB FM 90.1 📖 308
Lavendelschwert Buchladen
Köln, 221 23 2626 📖 124
Lavender's
Naples, 941 594 9499 📖 240
LAVG 📖 *See* Lincolnshire AIDS Voluntary Group
Law Students for Gay & Lesbian Concerns
Austin, 512 452 3591 📖 338
Lawrence Corner
London 📖 87
Lawrence Publishing Company (NZ) Ltd.
Auckland, 9 377 9031 📖 160
Lawrence, Robert
London, 181 472 2430 📖 80
Laws Leather
Cleveland, 216 961 0939 📖 184
Lazy J Leather
Kansas City, 913 287 7432 📖 257
LBGA 📖 *See* Lesbian, Bisexual, Gay Alliance
LBL 📖 *See* Landsforeningen for Bøsser og Lesbiske
LBW 📖 *See* Leather Bondage & Whips
LC Nordwest
Bremen 📖 113
LC Saar
Saarbrücken 📖 132
LC Stuttgart e. V.
711 640 6138 (Eagle bar) 📖 132
LCATF 📖 *See* Lee County AIDS Task Force
LCDC 📖 *See* Lesbian Community of Delaware County
LCH 📖 *See* Lederclub Hamburg
Leader Ship
Paris 📖 104
Leaping La Crosse News 📖 356
Leather & Lace
Denver, 800 441 4695 📖 229
Leather & Lace Society
Eastern Ohio 📖 317
Leather & Lace Lingerie
Portland, 503 774 8292 📖 327
Leather & Lace WMC, Inc.
Sacramento, 916 452 7469 📖 210
Leather & Lust
Linden, 908 925 7110 📖 182
Leather / SM / Fetish Community Outreach
New York 📖 12
Leather Archives & Museum
Chicago, 312 878 6360 📖 1
Leather Bar
Johannesburg 📖 171
Madrid, 91 308 1462 📖 172
Leather Bondage & Whips (LBW)
Allentown 📖 327
Leather by Boots
Houston, 713 526 2668 📖 343
Leather by Danny (& Cohorts)
617 288 2203 📖 266
Leather Caucus of Toronto
416 962 1040 📖 56
Leather Closet
Orlando, 407 649 2011 📖 241
Leather Corps
Los Angeles 📖 204
Leather Creations
Hartford, 203 742 0157 📖 230
Leather Etc.
San Francisco, 415 864 7558 📖 219
Leather Factory
El Paso, 800 433 3201 📖 190
Leather First
Sacramento 📖 209
Leather Group
Edinburgh, 131 558 1270 📖 168
Leather Harvest
East Hartford, 203 290 8981 📖 230
Leather Journal
published by Leather Journal 📖 17
published by The Leather Journal 📖 16
West Hollywood, 213 656 5073 📖 16, 17, 225
Leather Knights
Boston 📖 268
Dallas / Fort Worth, 214 521 3239 📖 340
Leather Links
published by B & D Pleasures 📖 203
Leather Maker
Los Angeles, 213 461 1095 📖 205
Leather Man, Inc.
New York, 800 243 5330 📖 184, 309
Leather Master
Key West, 305 292 5051 📖 238
Leather Masters
San José, 800 417 2636 (outside California) 📖 220
Leather Men Düsseldorf 📖 115
Leather Motor Club Torino
11 669 2599 📖 144
Leather Post / Taz Men
Atlanta, 404 873 5080 📖 245
Leather Pride Project
Seattle, 206 325 4275 📖 351
Leather Rack
Washington, 202 797 7401 📖 235
Leather Rose
Philadelphia, 215 985 2344 📖 331
Leather Rose Society
Dallas / Fort Worth, 214 289 0619 📖 340
Leather Scribes
Los Angeles, 213 665 5343 📖 12
Leather Shop
Shawnee Mission, 913 268 3652 📖 258
Leather Shoppe
Albuquerque, 505 266 6690 📖 294
Leather Stallion Saloon
Cleveland, 216 589 8588 📖 318
Leather Stitches
San Francisco, 415 546 4075 📖 213
Leather Tiger
Fort Myers, 813 334 4084 📖 237
Orlando, 407 839 0710 📖 240
Tampa, 813 248 8814 📖 242
Leather Underground
Baltimore, 410 528 0991 📖 264
Leather Underground, Inc.
Fort Lauderdale, 305 561 3977 📖 9, 237
Leather United - Chicago 📖 249
Leather WISDOM 📖 *See* Leather Women Into Sadism Dominance Obedience & Masochism
Leather Women Into Sadism Dominance Obedience & Masochism (Leather WISDOM)
Santa Clara 📖 221
Leather Workshop
Brighton, 1273 600427 📖 74
Leathercraft
Toronto, 416 924 5018 📖 60
Leatherhead Shop
Louisville 📖 259
Leatherhood
Sacramento, 916 456 8649 📖 184
Leatherline
Loughborough 📖 69
Leathermasters International
Los Angeles, 213 664 6422 📖 12
Leathermen
Atlanta 📖 244
Leathermen Yearning for Northern eXcitement (LYNX)
Bonfield, 705 776 2638 📖 49
Leatherworks Ltd.
London, 171 359 9778 📖 81
Leatherworks, Inc.
Portland, 503 234 2697 📖 327
Lebensart e. V.
Cottbus, 355 48 8156 📖 114
Lebensberatung Für Transsexuelle Menschem Im Saarland
Saarbrücken, 681 583912 📖 132

Leda
San Marcos 📖 181
Leder- & Motorradclub Zürich (LMZ) 📖 179
Leder Art & Design
Hannover, 511 350 5633 📖 121
Leder Beratungstelefon
Stuttgart, 711 61 7318 📖 132
Leder Boutique bei Günther
Berlin, 30 302 8494 📖 111
Leder Jeans Club Ost (LJC Ost)
Nürnberg, 911 24 1471 📖 129
Leder Spezial
Hertogenbosch, 's / Den Bosch, 73 612 8849 📖 156
Lederclub Dresden 📖 114
Lederclub Hamburg (LCH) 📖 119
Lederclub HH
Hamburg, 40 24 0804 📖 119
Lederclub Leipzig 📖 125
Lederfreunde Rhein-Ruhr Essen (LFRR)
201 236161 📖 116
Leder-Gummistudio
Gelsenkirchen, 209 22214 📖 118
Lederklub SAM
Praha 📖 65
Lee County AIDS Outreach
Auburn, 205 887 5244 📖 191
Lee County AIDS Task Force (LCATF)
Sanford 📖 316
Lee Memorial Hospital
Fort Myers, 813 332 1111 📖 237
Lee's Mardi Gras Boutique
New York, 212 645 1888 📖 309
New York, 212 947 7773 📖 308
Leeds Gay Switchboard
113 245 3588 📖 94
Leeds Lesbian Line
113 245 3588 📖 94
Leeds Parent's Friend
113 267 4627 📖 94
Leeds University Lesbian, Gay, & Bisexual Society 📖 94
Leffler's
Melbourne, 3 9690 3577 📖 33
Left Bank Books
Saint Louis, 314 367 6731 📖 284
Seattle, 206 622 0195 📖 353
Left Bank Bookstall
Chicago, 708 383 4700 📖 251
Left of Center 📖 335
Leg Tease
published by Rem-mer Ltd. 📖 296
Lega Volontari Anti-HIV
Ravenna, 544 40 9625 📖 141
Legacy Counseling Center, Inc.
Dallas / Fort Worth, 214 520 6308 📖 340
Lehigh University LesBiGay Alliance
Lehigh Valley, 610 758 3877 📖 329
Lehigh Valley Gay & Lesbian Task Force 📖 329
Lehigh Valley Lesbians
610 439 8755 📖 329
Lehne, Gregory, Ph.D.
Baltimore, 410 366 0642 📖 263
Leicester Lesbian & Gay Communities' Resource Centre
116 255 0667 📖 79
Leicester Lesbian & Gayline
116 255 0667 📖 79
Leicestershire AIDS Support Services (LASS)
116 255 9995 📖 79
Leine Verlag
Hannover, 511 31 1619 📖 108
Leisure Look
Hailsham 📖 74
Lemaire, Guy
Liège / Luik / Luttich 📖 38
Lenny's News
New Orleans, 504 866 5127 📖 261
New Orleans, 504 897 0005 📖 261
Lenox Hill Hospital
New York, 212 434 2000 📖 302
Leon County Health Department
Tallahassee, 904 487 3155 📖 242
Leoram, Inc.
Studio City, 818 898 1591 📖 223
Lesben- & Schwuengruppe Emden
49 212 6501 📖 116
Lesben & Schwulen Zentrum Saar (EZS)
Saarbrücken, 681 37 4055 📖 132
Lesbewell
Birmingham, 121 442 4481 📖 93
Lesbian & Gay Advisory Commission
San Francisco 📖 215
Lesbian & Gay Alliance
Bowling Green, 419 352 5242 📖 317
Lesbian & Gay Archives of New Zealand
Wellington, 4 474 3000 Ext. 8663 📖 159
Lesbian & Gay Bashing Reporting & Information Line
Toronto, 416 392 6877 (Hotline) 📖 56
Lesbian & Gay Bereavement Project
London, 181 455 8894 📖 81
Lesbian & Gay Campus Organization
Saint Louis, 314 553 5380 📖 284
Lesbian & Gay Collective of Mount Royal College
Calgary 📖 43
Lesbian & Gay Community Center of Greater Cleveland
216 522 1999 📖 319
Lesbian & Gay Community Center of New Orleans
504 522 1103 📖 261
Lesbian & Gay Community Library
Adelaide, 8 362 3106 📖 30
Lesbian & Gay Community Network of Western Michigan
Grand Rapids, 616 458 3511 📖 276
Lesbian & Gay Community Switchboard
Phœnix, 602 234 2762 📖 193
Lesbian & Gay Concerns Network (LGCN)
Oneonta, 607 432 1289 📖 310
Lesbian & Gay Convenors
Callaghan, 49 68 1281 📖 25
Lesbian & Gay Counselling & Consulting Services
Vancouver, 604 222 7807 📖 45
Lesbian & Gay Film Festival
Cork, 21 27 8470 📖 136
Lesbian & Gay Freedom Movement
London, 181 552 4405 📖 83
Lesbian & Gay Health Project
Durham, 919 286 4107 📖 314
Lesbian & Gay Helpline
Chicago, 312 929 4357 📖 249
Columbia, 314 449 4477 📖 283
Lesbian & Gay Historical Society of San Diego
619 260 1522 📖 210
Lesbian & Gay Law Student at NYU
New York 📖 305
Lesbian & Gay Male Advocates
Ann Arbor, 313 763 4186 📖 274
Lesbian & Gay Men's Community Center
San Diego, 619 692 4297 📖 211
San Diego, 619 692 4297 (information) 📖 211
Lesbian & Gay Pink Pages, Chicago
published by DAC Marketing, Inc. 📖 251
Lesbian & Gay Pride 📖 22
Lesbian & Gay Resource Center
Denver, 303 629 3317 📖 228
Lesbian & Gay Rights Caucus
Yellow Springs, 513 265 9500 📖 322
Lesbian & Gay Rights Resource Centre
Wellington 📖 159
Lesbian & Gay Student Association
Muncie 📖 255
Lesbian & Gay Student Group
Wellington 📖 163
Lesbian & Gay Student Union
Salt Lake City, 801 521 4026 📖 345
Lesbian & Gay Student Union at the University of Virginia
Charlottesville, 804 971 4942 📖 347
Lesbian & Gay Student Union Helpline
Charlottesville, 804 971 4942 📖 347
Lesbian & Gay Students Association
New York, 212 431 2100 📖 305
Lesbian & Gay Students of the Toronto Board of Education
416 397 3755 📖 57
Lesbian & Gay Studies
London, 171 420 5555 📖 84
Lesbian & Gay Support Group, Fordham University
New York 📖 305
Lesbian & Gay Voices
broadcast by KPFT FM 90.1 📖 343
Lesbian & Gay Youth Group
Albany, 518 462 6138 📖 296
Lesbian & Gay Youth of Rochester
716 251 9604 📖 311
Lesbian & Gay Youth Ottawa Hull
613 729 1000 📖 53
Lesbian & Gay Youth/Calgary
403 262 1626 📖 43
Lesbian / Gay Academic Union of Greater Cincinnati
513 281 7496 📖 318
Lesbian / Gay Resource Line
Kalamazoo, 616 345 7878 📖 276
Lesbian Alliance (GLWA)
Lansing, 517 394 1454 (TDD available) 📖 277
Lesbian Bisexual Collective
Providence, 401 863 2189 📖 334
Lesbian Bisexual Gay Alliance
Keene, 603 352 1909 📖 288
Lesbian Calendar
published by TLC Productions 📖 189
Lesbian Centre
Vancouver, 604 254 8458 📖 45
Lesbian Coalition
Auckland 📖 160
Lesbian Community of Delaware County (LCDC)
Philadelphia 📖 330
Lesbian Connection 📖 277
Boulder, 303 443 1105 📖 226
Lesbian Contradiction 📖 218
Lesbian Ethics 📖 294
Lesbian Fun Society
Olympia 📖 350
Lesbian Gay Bi Association
Laramie 📖 358
Lesbian Gay Bi Youth Line
Toronto, 800 268 9688 📖 56
Lesbian Gay Bisexual Alliance
Bellingham, 206 650 5120 📖 350
Lesbian Health News 📖 320
Lesbian Health Project
West Hollywood, 213 650 1508 📖 225
Lesbian Herstory Webweaving Collective
New York, 718 768 3953 📖 300
Lesbian Information Line 📖 62
Lesbian Information Line/Womyn's Collective of Calgary
403 265 9458 📖 42
Lesbian Information San Antonio (LISA)
210 828 5472 📖 344
Lesbian Interest Press (LIP) 📖 312
Lesbian Line
Brisbane, 7 839 3288 📖 28
Invercargill, 3 218 3877 📖 162
Limerick, 61 310101 📖 138
Wellington, 4 389 8082 📖 163
Lesbian Mother's Defense National Fund
Seattle, 206 325 2643 📖 352
Lesbian Network 📖 25
Adelaide, 8 341 6964 📖 30
Lesbian News 📖 196, 222
Lesbian Radio
broadcast by Plains FM 96.9 📖 161
Lesbian Resource Center Community News 📖 353
Lesbian Sex Mafia
New York, 212 222 9299 📖 303
Lesbian Show
broadcast by Co-op Radio FM 102.7 📖 46
Lesbian Sisters
broadcast by Overnight Productions FM 90.7 📖 207
Lesbian Support
Auckland, 8 846 7441 📖 160
Lesbian Support Group
Christchurch 📖 161
Oahu, 808 951 7000 📖 247
Lesbian Support Rap Group
Albuquerque, 505 266 0022 📖 294
Lesbian Switchboard
New York, 212 741 2610 📖 302
Lesbian Voices 📖 287
Lesbian World Newsletter 📖 319
Lesbian, Bisexual, & Gay Alliance
Boulder, 303 492 8567 📖 226
Lesbian, Bisexual, & Gay Men's Counseling Collective
Amherst, 413 545 2645 📖 266
Lesbian, Bisexual, Gay Alliance (LBGA)
Amherst, 413 545 0154 📖 267
Lesbian, Gay, & Bi Youth
Vancouver, 604 688 9378 Ext. 2067 📖 46
Lesbian, Gay, & Bisexual Aliance
College Park, 301 314 8467 📖 265
Lesbian, Gay, & Bisexual Alliance
Ames, 515 294 2104 📖 256
Buffalo, 716 645 3063 📖 298
Corvallis, 503 737 6363 📖 325
New York, 516 632 6469 📖 305
Princeton, 609 258 4522 📖 292
Providence, 401 863 3062 📖 334
Santa Barbara, 805 893 4578 📖 221
Lesbian, Gay, & Bisexual Alliance at Penn
Philadelphia, 215 898 5270 📖 330
Lesbian, Gay, & Bisexual Alliance at Plattsburgh
518 564 3200 📖 310
Lesbian, Gay, & Bisexual Alliance of UMBC
Baltimore, 410 788 8765 📖 264
Lesbian, Gay, & Bisexual Alliance SUNY Albany (LGBA)
518 442 5672 📖 296
Lesbian, Gay, & Bisexual Association
West Chester, 610 436 6949 📖 333
Lesbian, Gay, & Bisexual Association at SUNY Postsdam
Potsdam, 315 267 2184 📖 310
Lesbian, Gay, & Bisexual Caucus
Albany, 518 465 2406 📖 296
Boston 📖 269
Lesbian, Gay, & Bisexual Center
Boston, 617 287 7983 📖 269
Lesbian, Gay, & Bisexual Coalition
De Kalb, 815 753 0584 📖 252
Lesbian, Gay, & Bisexual Collective of Douglas College
New Westminster, 604 527 5111 📖 44
Lesbian, Gay, & Bisexual Community at Boston College
617 552 2979 📖 269
Lesbian, Gay, & Bisexual Community Center
Miami, 305 531 3666 📖 239
Lesbian, Gay, & Bisexual Community, Carleton College
Northfield, 507 663 4154 📖 281
Lesbian, Gay, & Bisexual Coöperative at Yale
New Haven, 203 432 1585 📖 231
Lesbian, Gay, & Bisexual Issues Committee (LGBIC)
Kingston, 613 545 4816 📖 50
Lesbian, Gay, & Bisexual Organization
San Diego, 619 534 4297 📖 211
Lesbian, Gay, & Bisexual Resource Center (LGBRC)
Minneapolis / Saint Paul, 612 654 5166 📖 280
Lesbian, Gay, & Bisexual Student Alliance
Hartford, 203 523 4841 Ext. 267 📖 231
Lesbian, Gay, & Bisexual Student Alliance (LGBSA)
State College, 814 237 1950 📖 333
Lesbian, Gay, & Bisexual Student Association (LGBSA)
Ypsilanti 📖 278
Lesbian, Gay, & Bisexual Student Union
Newark, 302 451 8066 📖 233
San Diego, 619 594 2737 📖 211
Tallahassee, 904 644 8804 📖 242
Lesbian, Gay, & Bisexual Student Union of the University of Florida
Gainesville, 904 332 0700 📖 237
Lesbian, Gay, & Bisexual Students' Association
Vancouver, 604 324 3881 📖 45
Lesbian, Gay, & Bisexual Support Group
Springfield, 413 458 4273 📖 272
Lesbian, Gay, & Bisexual Switchboard
Champaign / Urbana, 217 384 8040 📖 248
Lesbian, Gay, & Bisexual Teen Support Group
Kalamazoo, 616 327 8107 📖 276
Lesbian, Gay, & Bisexual Union - Kent (LGBU-Kent)
216 672 2068 📖 321
Lesbian, Gay, & Bisexual Union SUNY (LGBU)

Binghamton, 607 777 2202 📖 297
Lesbian, Gay, & Bisexual Youth of Toronto
416 925 XTRA Ext. 2880 📖 57
Lesbian, Gay, Bisexual Association
Fullerton, 714 773 2067 📖 200
Lesbian/Gay Film Festival
New York, 212 966 5656 📖 302
Lesbian/Gay Phoneline
Hamilton, 905 523 7055 📖 50
Lesbians & Gay MEn of New Brunswick
908 247 0515 📖 291
Lesbians at Queens College
New York, 718 263 5668 📖 305
Lesbians in Colorado 📖 228
Lesbians In Law (LIL)
San Francisco 📖 215
Lesbians, Bisexuals, & Gays of McGill
Montréal, 514 398 6822 📖 62
Lesbigais de l'Université de Québec à Hull 📖 61
LesBiGay Services of Kansas
Lawrence, 913 864 3091 📖 257
LesBiGayline
Iowa City, 319 335 3215 📖 257
Lesbigays Cité Collégiale
Ottawa 📖 53
LesBiGays, Unlimited
Seattle, 206 543 6106 📖 352
Lesbisch Archief
Amsterdam, 20 618 5879 📖 151
Lesbische & Schwule Aktiongemeinschaft
Linz, 732 274 7382 📖 34
Leschemins de Trans
Kortrijk / Courtrai 📖 38
Lesch-Selbsthilfegruppe Lesben & Schwule
Duisburg 📖 115
Lesko, Kathryn, Ph.D.
New York, 212 598 4090 📖 301
Leslie Shoe Company 📖 *See* Sexy Shoes
Leslie, David
London, 181 857 7146 📖 83
Lestalk
published by Rose Publications 📖 284
Lethbridge AIDS Connection Society
403 328 8186 📖 44
Letter
published by The Letterhead 📖 258
Letterhead
Louisville, 502 772 7570 📖 258
Leurquin, Jacques
Namur / Namen, 81 22 7502 📖 39
Levi/Leather Brigade
Columbia, 803 796 3860 📖 335
Levi/Leather Plainsmen
Saskatoon 📖 64
Levin, Betty, MA
Millburn, 201 763 1035 📖 291
Lewinter, Beth, MSW, CSW
Montclair, 201 783 6351 📖 291
Lewisham Friend
London, 181 690 6195 📖 81
Lexicon 📖 217
Lexington Gay & Lesbian Services Organization
606 231 0335 📖 259
Leydig Trust
London, 171 739 0388 📖 15
Leyland Publications
San Francisco, 707 996 6082 📖 216
LFRR 📖 *See* Lederfreunde Rhein-Ruhr Essen
LGB 📖 *See* London Bisexual Group
LGB Awareness League
Birmingham 📖 191
LGB Guide to Great Britain 📖 22
LGBA 📖 *See* Denver University Lesbian, Gay, & Bisexual Alliance. *See also* Lesbian, Gay, & Bisexual Alliance SUNY Albany
LGBIC 📖 *See* Lesbian, Gay, & Bisexual Issues Committee
LGBPSYCH
Montréal 📖 2
LGBRC 📖 *See* Lesbian, Gay, & Bisexual Resource Center
LGBSA 📖 *See* Bisexual Women's Group. *See also* Lesbian, Gay, & Bisexual Student Alliance. *See also* Lesbian, Gay, & Bisexual Student Association
LGBU 📖 *See* Lesbian, Gay, & Bisexual Union SUNY
LGBU-Kent 📖 *See* Lesbian, Gay, & Bisexual Union - Kent
LGCN 📖 *See* Lesbian & Gay Concerns Network
LGS 📖 *See* Saint Louis Gender Foundation
LIAAC 📖 *See* Long Island Association for AIDS Care, Inc.
Liberation 📖 30
Liberation Publications Inc.
Los Angeles, 213 871 1225 📖 205
Liberation Publishers
Johannesburg, 11 648 5032 📖 172
Libertarian Alliance
London, 171 821 5502 📖 83
Libertarians for Gay & Lesbian Concerns Newsletter 📖 274
Liberty
London, 171 403 3888 📖 83
Liberty Books
Austin, 800 828 1279 📖 339
Modesto, 209 524 7603 📖 206
Libidex
London, 171 613 3329 📖 68
Libido
London, 171 916 0180 📖 86
published by Libido, Inc. 📖 19
Libido, Inc.
Chicago, 312 275 0842 📖 19
Libidos-Erotheek
Aalst / Alost, 5 370 6428 📖 36
Antwerpen / Anvers, 3 226 0245 📖 36
Antwerpen / Anvers, 3 233 1001 📖 36
Gent / Gand, 9 223 9388 📖 38
Kortrijk / Courtrai, 5 625 7601 📖 38
Mechelen / Malines, 1 555 6845 📖 38
Librairie d'Albret
Bordeaux, 56 52 2929 📖 98
Librairie du Bon Secours
Bruxelles / Brussel, 2 512 2303 📖 37
Librairie Erotique
Dijon, 80 30 7409 📖 99
Librarie La Scarabée D'or
Paris, 146 34 6361 📖 104
Library Corporation
Washington, 800 624 0559 📖 234
Library Journal 📖 307
Library of Congress
Washington, 202 707 6372 📖 234
Libreria Babele
Milano, 2 669 2986 📖 139
Roma, 6 687 6628 📖 142
Libreria Gruppo Abele
Torino, 11 54 5420 📖 138
Libreria Internazionale Luxemburg
Torino, 11 561 3896 📖 144
Lidec
Montréal, 514 843 5991 📖 62
Lidéfix
Bruxelles / Brussel, 2 241 1804 📖 37
Liechenstein, Joyce, Ph.D.
New York, 212 673 4427 📖 301
LIFE 📖 *See* Long Island Femme Expression
Life In Out 📖 322
Lifesigns
Colorado Springs, 719 634 2488 📖 226
Lifestyle
Holsworthy 📖 68
Lifestyle Books
Albany, 518 433 1290 📖 296
Lifestyle Explorers Club
Land 'O Lakes 📖 238
LifeStyle Leather & Wood
Gillsville, 706 869 9606 📖 187
Lifestyle Online 📖 1
Lifestyle Publishing Inc.
Oahu, 808 737 6400 📖 246
Lifestyles
Buena Park, 714 821 9953 📖 197
Lifestyles for the 90's
Boston, 617 891 6060 📖 270
Lifestyles Organization
Anaheim, 714 821 9953 📖 187
Lighthouse Center
Phœnix, 602 451 0819 📖 193
Ligne 2
Paris, 143 20 9132 📖 104
LIL 📖 *See* Lesbians In Law
Lil Rascals
Columbia, 803 771 0121 📖 335
Lila Archiv e. V.
Berlin, 30 448 5713 📖 109
Lillehammer Helseråd
61 25 3540 📖 165
Lima AIDS Unit
419 228 4457 📖 321
Limburg Motorclub
Roermund, 47 533 3119 📖 157
Lincoln Gay & Lesbian Switchboard
152 253 5553 📖 79
Lincoln Medical & Mental Health Center
Bronx, 718 579 5700 📖 297
Lincolnshire AIDS Voluntary Group (LAVG)
1522 513999 📖 79
Line
Saint Petersburg, 813 586 4297 📖 241
Lingerie by Barbie
Calgary, 403 236 7072 📖 43
LINK
Toronto, 416 466 7198 📖 57
LINKS
San Francisco, 415 695 7955 📖 214
Lion Regiment
Boise, 208 322 8174 📖 247
Lion's Roar
San Francisco, 415 588 1850 📖 214
Lioness Books
Sacramento, 916 442 4657 📖 210
Lippman, Susan, CSW
New York, 718 639 5969 📖 301
LIS 📖 3
LISA 📖 *See* Lesbian Information San Antonio
Lite & Lively 📖 53
Literary Market Place
New York, 212 645 9700 📖 306
Literatussi 📖 120
Litfass
Halle (Saale), 345 2 4263 📖 119
LITFASS Der Buchladen
Dortmund, 231 83 4724 📖 114
Little Denmarks Books
South Bend, 219 233 9538 📖 255
Little Shoe Box
London, 171 607 1247 📖 86
Little Sister's Book & Art Emporium
Vancouver, 800 567 1662 📖 40, 46
Little Store
Provincetown, 508 487 0208 📖 272
Live The Dream
Van Nuys, 818 361 6737 📖 224
Liverbirds
Liverpool, 151 709 3181 📖 87
Liverpool Bisexual & Married Gays Group
161 708 9552 📖 87
Lives of the Secular Saints
London 📖 79
Living Art Association
Sacramento, 916 339 0331 📖 209
Living Batch Bookstore
Albuquerque, 505 262 1619 📖 294
Living Colour Tattoo
Ottawa, 613 789 7187 📖 53
Living Pens
Avoca 📖 195
Living Room
Cleveland, 216 522 1998 📖 318
Liz Lewitt - Wholesale
Bristol, 117 929 3754 📖 11
LJC Ost 📖 *See* Leder Jeans Club Ost
LL&SS
Vaasa, 962 42123 📖 97
LLH 📖 *See* Landsforeningen for Lesbisk og Homofil Frigjøring
LMC Vienna
Wien, 1 798 5484 📖 35
LMT 94.4 FM
Paris 📖 104
LMZ 📖 *See* Leder- & Motorradclub Zürich
LNBi 📖 *See* Vereniging Landelijk Netwerk voor Bisexualiteit
Lobo After Dark
Dallas / Fort Worth, 214 522 1132 📖 341
Lobo Bookstore
Austin, 512 454 5406 📖 339
Houston, 713 522 5156 📖 343
LOBOCS MC
Long Beach 📖 202
Lock, Stock, & Leather
Las Vegas, 702 796 9801 📖 286
Locker Jocks
Piscataway 📖 292
Loco
Stoneleigh, 181 786 7347 📖 68
Lodestar Books
Birmingham, 205 939 3356 📖 191
Lodge
Royal Leamington Spa 📖 92
Loft Lesbian & Gay Community Services Center, Inc.
New York, 914 948 4922 📖 305
Logden House
Washington, 202 726 5159 📖 1
Loge 70 (Schweitz)
Zürich 📖 177
Login Publishers Consortium
Chicago, 312 733 8228 📖 249
Logos
Siena 📖 146
London Apprentice
171 739 5949 📖 80
London Bisexual Group (LGB) 📖 83
London Blues
181 940 3084 📖 83
London East AIDS Network
181 519 9545 📖 82
London Friend
171 837 3337 (men) 📖 81
London Leather Cave
181 875 1607 📖 86
London Lesbian & Gay Switchboard
171 837 7324 📖 67
London Lesbian Line
171 251 6911 📖 79
London Lighthouse
171 792 1200 📖 82
London Piercing Clinic
181 656 7180 📖 83
London Pink Pathways 📖 54
Lone Star Bears
Dallas / Fort Worth, 214 256 1671 📖 340
Long Beach Community Hospital
310 498 1000 📖 202
Long Beach Directory
published by Turkey Media Services 📖 202
Long Island Association for AIDS Care, Inc. (LIAAC)
New York, 516 385 2437 📖 303
Long Island Connection
East Meadow 📖 299
Nassau 📖 299
Long Island Crisis Center
New York, 516 679 1111 (hotline) 📖 302
Long Island Eagle
Bay Shore, 516 968 2750 📖 296
Long Island Femme Expression (LIFE)
Ronkonkoma, 516 283 1333 📖 311
Long Island Gay & Lesbian Youth, Inc.
New York, 516 627 3340 📖 306
Long Island Gay Men's Group
New York, 516 694 2407 📖 305
Long Island Gay Men's Social Group
New York, 516 334 2773 📖 305
Long Island Ravens
Bay Shore, 516 666 6091 📖 296
Lonnie Marshall Publications
Thibodaux, 504 369 6976 📖 261
Looking Glass Books
Portland, 503 227 4760 📖 327
Loop 📖 46
Lorain Lesbian & Gay Center
216 960 2050 📖 321
Lords of Leather
New Orleans, 602 233 9042 Ext. 270 📖 261
Lormer Military Shop
Saint Petersburg, 813 527 2721 📖 241
Los Angeles Gender Center (LAGC)
Santa Monica 📖 222
Los Angeles Times Book Review 📖 205
Lothian LGYM
Edinburgh 📖 169
Lotus Foot Love Club
Coram 📖 298
Loud & Queer
broadcast by RDU FM 98.3 📖 161
Louisville Gender Society

812 944 5570 259
Louisville Nightwings 259
Love & Flash
Hameln, 51 51 28769 121
Love Boutique
Los Angeles, 310 453 3459 206
Tarzana, 818 342 2400 223
Love Toy Books
Boston, 617 451 2168 270
Lovecraft
London 86
Mississauga, 416 276 5772 51
Toronto, 416 923 7331 60
Lovejoy, Gary, Ph.D.
Phœnix, 602 957 2368 193
Lovejoys
London, 171 437 0811 85
Loveland
Bern, 31 311 4533 178
Løvetann 164
Loveworks
Lafayette, 318 988 5000 260
Loving Alternatives
Greenwood 254
published by Omnific Designs West 212
State College 333
Loving Brotherhood
Sussex, 201 875 4710 293
Low Country Gay & Lesbian Information Alliance
Charleston, 803 881 0129 335
Low Country Palmetto AIDS Support Services
Charleston, 803 577 2437 334
Löwengrube
München, 89 26 5750 127
Lowson's Army & Navy Store
Glasgow, 141 427 0961 170
LSMA Köln
221 54 2516 124
Lubbock Lesbian & Gay Alliance
806 762 1019 344
Lucerne Medical Center
Orlando, 407 649 6111 240
Lucifer's Armory
New York 186
Lucrezia & De Sade
Melbourne, 3 9416 3826 32
Luna Books
Washington, 202 332 2543 235
Lunaria Feminist Bookstore
Northampton, 413 586 7851 (voice & TDD) 272
Lüneburger Schwulengruppe & Rosa Telefon
Lüneburg, 413 11 9411 126
Lush
London, 171 253 2975 81
Lust See Junge Lesben & Schwule im Thurgau
published by Nummer Verlag 135
Luton Switchboard
1234 218990 70
LuvCat's Lair
Philadelphia 330
Lycos Incorporated
Marlborough, 508 229 0717 7
Lyndon Distributors Limited
Van Nuys, 818 988 0228 224
Lynn, Rusty, BD, MSW, LCSW
Bethesda, 301 652 6448 265
LYNX See Leathermen Yearning for Northern eXcitement
Lyon-Martin Women's Health Services
San Francisco, 415 565 7674 213
M & J Army Surplus
Toronto, 416 253 0827 60
M & M Productions
San Francisco, 510 533 6474 218
M & S Connexion
Mannheim, 621 85 8374 127
M. Coy Books
Seattle, 206 623 5354 353
M. E. C. See Mecs En Caoutchouc
M. J. Production
Rotterdam 157
Mac Leather
Toronto, 416 469 3459 (Brian) 56
Mac Mac
Stoke Abbot, 1308 68227 73
Macalester Gays, Lesbians, & Bisexuals United
Minneapolis / Saint Paul, 612 696 6248 280
MacAuley, Donna
Toronto, 416 925 9497 55
Mach
published by Desmodus, Inc. 217
Machismo 307
Macho City Shop
Zürich, 1 251 1222 180
Macho Men's Shop
Zürich, 1 241 3215 180
Macho-Versand
Zürich, 1 241 3215 177
Mack's Leathers
Vancouver, 604 688 6225 41, 46
MacNeill Library Service
Vancouver, 604 732 1335 45
Macquarie University Gay & Lesbian Association
Sydney 27
MACT See Men of All Colors Together
Madison AIDS Support Network
800 486 6276 356
Madison Wrestling Club
608 244 8675 356
MAFIA See Mid-America Fists In Action
MAG Jeunes Gais
Paris, 143 70 5009 103
Magayzine
published by Bodyshot 19
Magazine
San Francisco, 415 441 7737 218
Magazine Fugues 62
Magazine Rack
Ypsilanti, 313 482 6944 278
Magazine RG 63
MAGGIE See Mid-America Gender Group Information Exchange
Magic America
Bologna, 51 235882 140
Firenze, 55 21 2840 146
Genova, 10 31 6783 142
Milano, 2 29 52 4386 143
Milano, 2 349 4118 143
Milano, 2 423 9980 143
Milano, 2 546 5679 143
Milano, 2 688 1057 143
Milano, 2 761 0083 143
Modena, 59 21 6774 140
Parma, 521 20 6273 141
Rimini, 541 39 1977 141
Roma, 6 769 02211 142
Torino, 11 817 7007 144
Udine, 432 29 7345 141
Verona, 45 800 5234 147
Magic Color Photo Lab
Oceanside, 619 967 6014 23
Magic Moments
Hastings, 1424 853366 74
Magic Shoe Company
London, 171 791 3331 68
Magic Top Video Club
Padova, 49 807 2414 147
Magick & Fetish Shop
Los Angeles, 213 660 1575 205
Magni
Braunschweig, 531 4 2429 113
Magnum Club
Milano, 2 536273 138
Magnus
published by Magnus Verlag 108
Magnus Hirschfeld Centrum
Hamburg, 40 279 0060 120
Magnus Hirschfeld Zentrum
Erlangen, 913 18 0050 116
Magnus Verlag
Berlin, 30 787 93431 108, 111
Mags 'R' Us
New York, 212 627 2245 308
Mail & Female
Amsterdam, 20 693 6074 150, 153
Mail2Male
published by FFT Publishing 22
Mailshoppe Inc.
Toronto, 416 921 6960 59
Main Attraction
Fox Valley, 414 465 6969 356
Main Street Clinic
Jacksonville, 904 358 3386 238
Maine Gay & Lesbian Film Festival
Portland 261
Maine Gender Resource & Support Service
Bangor 262
Maine Medical Center
Portland, 207 871 0111 262
Maine Progressive 262
Mainliners
London, 171 737 3141 67
Maison des Homosexualités
Paris, 142 77 7277 104
Maitresse
Fairport, 800 456 8464 183
Maize 281, 295
MALAGA See Mobile Area Lesbian & Gay Assembly
Malaprop's Bookstore
Asheville, 704 254 6734 313
Malchus 347
Male Box
Colorado Springs 226
Male Hide Leathers
Chicago, 312 929 0069 252
Male Image
London, 181 885 5488 67
Male Xpress Ltd.
London, 181 340 8644 67
Malebox
published by Pink Triangle Press 42
Malebox Direct Mail Service
Ottawa, 613 237 7133 42
Malebox Warehouse
Ottawa, 613 237 7133 41
Male-order Leather
Danbury 186
Malestop
New York 300
Malibu Sales
Los Angeles, 213 871 1225 186
Malin, Martin, Ph.D.
Baltimore, 410 528 1638 263
Malkin, Joyce, LCSW-C, LICSW
Washington, 202 363 8119 233
Mall City Cruisers
Kalamazoo 276
Mallon, David, MSW
Long Beach, 310 434 8236 202
Malloy Lithographing
Ann Arbor, 313 665 6113 274
Mama Bears
Oakland, 510 428 9684 208
Mama Raga 235
Man Bag
published by The ARTpolice Agency 281
Man Fashion
Oslo, 22 36 0603 164
Man Leder Shop
Köln 125
Man Shop
Duisburg, 203 2 3300 115
Man To Man
Bruxelles / Brussel 37
Man's BCN
Barcelona, 93 301 5419 172
Man's Hand Films
San Francisco, 415 771 3918 187
Man's Pleasurechest
Berlin 111
Man's World
Köln, 221 25 2423 125
Manawatu Gay Rights Association Inc.
Palmerston North 163
Manchester Gay Parents Group 75
Manchester Lesbian & Gay Switchboard
161 274 3999 75
Manchester Superchain MSC 76
Manchester Transvestite / Transgender Hotline
161 274 3705 75
Mandamus Society
Norfolk, 804 625 6220 348
Mandate
published by MMG Services Inc. 307
Mang Publishing
London, 171 436 0385 19
Manhandler Saloon
Chicago, 312 871 3339 248
Manhattan
Paris, 143 54 9886 102
Manhattan Psychotherapy
New York, 212 724 8767 301
Manhole
Chicago, 312 975 9244 248
Maniac
published by Editions Astarté 104
Manifest
Leiden, 71 512 5691 156
Manifest Reader
published by Alternate Publishing Company 16
Männer Aktuell
published by Bruno Gmünder Verlag 108
Männerschwarm Buchladen
Hamburg, 40 43 6093 120
Männertreu
Nürnberg, 911 26 2676 129
Mann-O-Meter e. V.
Berlin, 30 216 8008 107
Manoogian Psychological Associates
Winston-Salem, 910 765 5636 316
Manoogian, Sam, Ph.D.
Winston-Salem, 910 765 5636 316
Manphone-Schwulenberatung
Nordhorn, 592 17 6590 129
Manpower Network
Johannesburg 171
Manscape 312
Manshots 312
Manson, Susan, MS, MFCC
Los Angeles, 213 280 9925 203
Man-to-Man Gay Information Centre
Amsterdam, 20 625 8797 152
Maple-Vail
York, 717 764 5911 333
MAPP See Midwest AIDS Prevention Project
Maracle Press
Oshawa, 905 723 3438 52
Marathon Films
Toluca Lake, 800 426 4207 22
Marc Sanders Mail Order
Oakland, 510 444 3204 186
Marc's Smokeshop
Ottawa, 613 789 8886 53
Marci & Friends 295
Marco 139
Marginal Distribution
Peterborough, 705 745 2326 54
Maricopa Medical Center
Phœnix, 602 267 5011 193
Mariner Wear
Barrington 183
Mariposa Education & Research Foundation
Topanga, 818 704 4812 223
Mark Allen Productions
Las Vegas, 800 858 5568 286
Marked Men
Petersham 25
Market Street News
Wheeling, 304 232 2414 355
Market Tavern
London, 171 622 5655 80
Marks, Al, Ph.D.
San Diego, 619 296 6134 211
Marlow Heights Periodicals
Temple Hills, 301 899 6458 266
Marquette County Health Department
906 475 7651 277
Marquis de Sade
Boston, 617 426 2120 270
Marquis Magazine
published by The Fetish Factory Ltd. 14, 19, 90
Marquis Masquerade 89
Nottingham, 115 981 9113 89
Married Men's Group
Charlotte 314
Marschall, Rick, CSW, CAC
New York, 212 620 7155 301
Marshall, John
Teddington, 181 977 6180 87
Martifoto
Den Haag, 70 368 1865 13
Martijn
Amsterdam, 20 693 4793 150
Mary Washington College Gay / Lesbian / Bisexual Student Association
Fredericksburg 348
Masco Communication
Philadelphia, 215 625 8501 190

MASG 📖 *See* Merseyside AIDS Support Group
Masquerade Books
New York, 800 458 9640 (credit card orders) 📖 306, 307
Masquerade Erotic Newsletter
published by Masquerade Books 📖 307
Mass Bay Counseling Associates
Boston, 617 739 7832 📖 267
Massachusetts Army Navy Store
Boston, 617 267 1559 📖 270
Massachusetts General Hospital
Boston, 617 726 2000 📖 267
Massad
Rotterdam, 10 466 4368 📖 157
Massad Mailorder
Rotterdam, 10 466 4368 📖 9
Masta Entertainment
San Francisco, 800 996 2782 📖 187
Master Leather
Oslo 📖 165
Master Leathers
Amsterdam, 20 624 5573 📖 153
Tucson 📖 186
Master's Toychest
Roselle, 908 245 5223 📖 292
Master's Way
published by Church of Epiphany 📖 207
Masters & Slaves Together
San Francisco 📖 12
West Hollywood 📖 12
MASTER-SLAVE 📖 2
Mastery Magazine
published by Alternate Woods Publishing 📖 269
Mates
Provincetown, 508 487 3732 📖 272
Matlovich Society
Portland, 203 773 1209 📖 262
Matrix 📖 295
Matt
New Orleans 📖 260
Matthews, Ingham, & Lake Inc.
Don Mills, 416 445 8800 📖 49
Maui Lesbian/Gay Youth Project
808 575 2681 (Karen) 📖 246
Mavericks 📖 293
Santa Fe 📖 188
MAW 📖 *See* Monadnock Area Womyn
Max & Million
München, 89 52 7452 📖 128
Max & Moritz Jugendgruppe
Stuttgart, 711 297936 📖 133
Max Images
Norfolk, 804 622 3701 📖 348
Max Wonder
Silver Spring, 301 585 3333 📖 266
Maxitosh
Bristol 📖 70
Mayer Laboratories
Oakland, 510 452 5555 📖 208
Mayers, Terry, M.Ed., BCSW, ACSW
New Orleans, 504 524 5973 📖 260
Mayesm, John
Wellington, 4 384 5549 📖 163
Maynooth Gay & Lesbian Society
1 628 6035 📖 138
Mayor's Office for the Lesbian & Gay Community
New York, 212 788 2706 📖 305, 306
Maze
New York 📖 300
Mazurkewicz, Terry
New Preston, 203 639 2345 📖 229
MC Faucon, Inc.
Montréal 📖 62
MC Nordlicht Hamburg 📖 120
MCC Library
Houston, 713 861 9149 📖 342
McCarthy, Mark, M.S., LPC
Kansas City, 816 931 0011 📖 283
McClemens, Mary Anne, M.A., LPCMH
Willmington, 302 475 3359 📖 233
McConnell, John, Ph.D.
San Diego, 619 296 1216 📖 211
McEwen, Chase, ACSW, LCSW
Tampa, 813 932 9300 📖 242
MCF Leather Motor Club Firenze 📖 145
McGinley, Robert, Ph.D.
Buena Park, 714 821 9939 📖 197
McGovern, Maureen, MSW
New York, 212 929 1498 📖 301
McIntyre Media
Toronto, 416 245 7800 📖 58
McKayne, Stella
Chicago, 312 905 1941 📖 249
McLaren Morris & Todd Ltd.
Mississauga, 905 677 3592 📖 51
McLaren Regional Medical Center
Flint, 810 762 2000 📖 275
MCLB 📖 *See* Motorradclub LederBären Berlin
M-Club
Baden 📖 177
McNally Robinson Booksellers
Winnipeg, 204 452 2644 📖 47
McNaughton & Gunn
Saline, 313 429 5411 Ext. 265 📖 278
MCRA 📖 *See* MSC Rhône-Alpes
Mebray Ltd
Romford 📖 75
Mec Zone
Paris, 140 82 9418 📖 102
Mecs en Caoutchouc
Dammarie les Lys 📖 99
Mecs En Caoutchouc (M. E. C.)
Dammarie Les Lys 📖 12
Médecins du Monde
Lyon, 78 60 2384 📖 100
MEDGAY-L 📖 2
Medical Center Hospital
Houston, 713 790 8100 📖 342
Medical Center Hospital of Vermont
Burlington, 802 656 2345 📖 346
Medical Center of Delaware
Wilmington, 302 733 1000 📖 233
Medical Center of Louisiana at New Orleans
504 568 3201 📖 260
Medical Center of North Hollywood
818 980 9200 📖 207
Medical Centre
Nelson, 3 546 8881 📖 162
Medical College of Virginia Hospitals
Richmond, 804 786 9000 📖 349
Medical Disposables Company
Marietta, 404 422 3036 📖 245
Mediquip
Okehampton, 1837 53710 📖 11
Medway & Maidstone Lesbian & Gay Switchboard
Chatham, 1634 826925 📖 78
Meester Terry's SM Society & School
Amsterdam, 20 671 0682 📖 153
MEGA Scene 📖 208
Megalesia
Montréal 📖 62
Meikänainen
Helsinki 📖 96
Meisner, Judith, Ph.D., LCSW, LMFT
Saint Petersburg, 813 327 1672 📖 241
Melbourne Leather Men, Inc.
39 645 3747 📖 32
Melbourne Leather Pride Association
9 530 2244 📖 32
Melbourne Sexual Health Centre
39 347 0244 (& TTY) 📖 32
Melbourne Star Observer
published by Bluestone Media 📖 31
Melbourne University Gay Society 📖 32
Melbourne Wankers 📖 32
Melrose Army Navy Store
Boston, 617 665 9729 📖 270
MEMMOS 📖 *See* Men Enjoying Mutual Masturbation & Oral Sex
Memorial Hospital of South Bend
219 234 9041 📖 255
Memorial Hospital of Tampa
813 873 6400 📖 242
Memorial Medical Center
Corpus Christi, 512 881 4000 📖 339
Memphis Bisexual Alliance 📖 337
Memphis Gay & Lesbian Center
901 276 4651 📖 337
Memphis Leather / Levi Alliance
901 386 8625 📖 336
Memphis Trans-Gender Alliance 📖 337
Men Enjoying Mutual Masturbation & Oral Sex (MEMMOS)
Madison 📖 356
Men Into Underwear
published by MJ Enterprises 📖 358
Men of All Colors Together (MACT)
West Hollywood 📖 225
Men of Discipline
New York, 212 366 0861 📖 303
Men on Men Project
Halifax, 1422 366298 📖 94
Men Only Selbsthilfzentrum
Hoyerswerda 📖 122
Men Shaving Men
Vancouver 📖 46
Men Under Control
published by CF Publications 📖 299
Men's Bar
København, 33 12 7303 📖 66
Men's Center
Minneapolis / Saint Paul, 612 822 5892 📖 280
Men's Coming Out Group
Denver, 303 831 6238 📖 228
Men's Gay & Bisexual Coming Out Group
Wollongong, 4 221 4012 📖 28
Men's Rap Group
Albuquerque, 505 266 8041 📖 294
Men's Support Group
Saint Louis, 314 231 9100 📖 284
Menamore Levi / Leather Club
Wilmington, 910 675 9222 Ext. 534 📖 316
Menfriends
Christchurch, 3 377 1701 📖 161
Menkes, David
New York, 212 989 3706 📖 303
Mentor Center (HUGS East)
216 974 8909 📖 322
Mephisto Leather
Sydney, 2 332 3218 📖 27
Merck Manual
published by Merck Research Laboratories 📖 333
Merck Research Laboratories
West Point, 215 397 2340 📖 333
Mercury Mail Order
San Francisco, 415 621 1188 📖 186
Mercury Morocycle Club
Auckland 📖 159
Mercury Productions
Austin 📖 339
Mercy
New York 📖 300
Mercy Health Center
Oklahoma City, 405 755 1515 📖 323
Mercy Hospital
Iowa City, 319 339 0300 📖 256
Miami, 305 854 4400 📖 239
Mercy Hospital of Pittsburgh
412 232 7637 📖 331
Meristem
Memphis, 901 276 0282 📖 337
Merlins Ear & Body Piercing Jewelry
Eastbourne, 132 343 0595 📖 74
Merril Company
Los Angeles, 213 231 4133 📖 204
Merrimack Valley Counseling
Lowell, 508 687 4383 📖 271
Merrimack Valley Lesbians
Newburyport, 508 521 2239 📖 271
Merrimack Valley Youth Group
603 424 7759 📖 288
Merrymeeting AIDS Support Services
Brunswick, 207 725 4955 📖 262
Merseyside AIDS Support Group (MASG)
Liverpool, 151 709 9000 (also TTY) 📖 87
Merseyside Friend
Liverpool, 151 708 9552 (men) 📖 87
Messy Fun
Austin 📖 339
Metal Morphosis
London, 171 434 4554 📖 84
Metamorphosis
New York, 718 728 4615 📖 301
Methodist Hospital of Indiana
Indianapolis, 317 929 2000 📖 254
Metra 📖 277
Metro
London, 181 316 5954 📖 81
Metro Area Committee on AIDS
Halifax, 902 425 4882 📖 48
Metro Gay Wrestling Alliance, Inc. (MGWA)
New York, 212 563 7066 📖 306
Metro Leather Society
Royal Oak, 313 547 8919 📖 278
Metro Line 📖 231
Metro News
Cape Giradeau, 314 335 8633 📖 283
Metro Place de Clichy
København 📖 66
Metrolina AIDS Project
Charlotte, 800 289 2437 📖 314
Metrolina Community Service Project
Charlotte, 704 535 6277 (also TDD) 📖 314
Metropole Lithographers
Toronto, 416 538 4511 📖 58
Metropolitan Gender Network
New York, 201 794 1665 Ext. 332 📖 305
Metropolitan Hospital
Grand Rapids, 616 247 7200 📖 276
Metropolitan Hospital Center
New York, 212 230 6262 📖 302
Metropolitan Nashville General Hospital
615 862 4490 📖 337
Metropolitan Slave
published by Selective Publishing, Inc. 📖 16
Metropolitan Slave Online
Oakbrook, 708 986 8550 📖 1
Metrosource 📖 307
Metrowest Medical Center
Framingham, 508 383 1020 📖 270
Mexicanos Contre el SIDA
Mexico City, 5 530 2771 📖 149
Meyerson, Adam
Northampton, 413 582 0424 📖 272
MFGE 📖 *See* Minnesota Freedom of Gender Expression
MGALA
Milwaukee 📖 357
MGL Sexy Lingerie
Paris, 142 21 3334 📖 104
MGLTF 📖 *See* Mississipi Gay & Lesbian Task Force
MGM 📖 *See* Monadnock Gay Men. *See also* Mutal Gay Mens' Support Group
MGWA 📖 *See* Metro Gay Wrestling Alliance, Inc.
Miami University Gay, Lesbian, & Bisexual Alliance
Oxford, 614 529 3823 📖 322
Miami Valley Hospital
Dayton, 513 223 6192 📖 321
Michael Sürth Verlag
Köln, 220 38 5767 📖 108
Michael's Thing Magazine 📖 307
Michelle Fashions
Buckhurst Hill, 181 504 0418 📖 75
Michiana AIDS Support Group
South Bend, 219 232 6930 📖 255
Michigan Society for Domination & Submission (MSDS) 📖 273
Mic-Man
Paris, 142 74 3980 📖 102
Mid-America Fists In Action (MAFIA)
Chicago, 312 539 1669 📖 249
Mid-America Gender Group Information Exchange (MAGGIE)
Saint Louis, 314 997 9897 📖 284
Middle Tennessee Gay & Lesbian Alliance
Cookeville 📖 336
Mid-Glamorgan AIDS Helpline
Cardiff, 1443 486254 📖 359
Midi Gai Loisirs 📖 101
Midian Books
Tamworth, 1827 281391 📖 67
Midland Book Centre
Birmingham 📖 93
Midland Link MSC
Birmingham 📖 93
Midlands Communication Network
Council Bluffs 📖 256
Mid-Michigan Bears
Mount Morris, 810 687 5927 📖 277
Mid-Missouri AIDS Project
Columbia, 413 875 2437 📖 282
Mid-New York AIDS Coalition
Utica 📖 312
Midnight Adult Book & Video
San Diego, 619 222 9973 📖 212

San Diego, 619 299 7186 212
Midnight Blue
Atlanta, 404 766 6288 245
Midnight Iguana Tattoing, Inc.
Athens, 706 549 0190 243
Midnight Lady
Luton, 158 239 1854 68
Midnight Special Books
Santa Monica, 310 393 2923 222
Midnight Sun Rainwear
Soldotna 183
Midway Family Services
Minneapolis / Saint Paul, 612 222 0311 279
Midway Hospital Medical Center
Los Angeles, 213 938 3161 203
Midwest Adult Bookstore
Columbia, 314 442 6622 283
Midwest AIDS Prevention Project (MAPP)
Detroit, 313 545 1435 275
Midwest Men's Center, Chicago
312 348 3254 250
MIELS *See* Mouvement d'Information & d'Entraide dans la Lutte Contre Le SIDA à Québec
MIENS *See* Mouvement d'Information, d'Education, & d'Entraide dans la Lutte Contre Le SIDA
Mike Arlen's Guys
published by Wetherby Studios 84
Mike Mansfield TV
London, 171 494 3061 87
Mike's
Ludwigshafen 126
Mike's Custom Leathers
Charlestown, 617 241 8968 265
Mike's Men
Charlestown, 617 241 8968 270
Mikes Läder
Stockholm, 8 644 0466 176
Military & Police Club International
San Diego 13
Military & Police Uniform Association
West Hollywood, 213 650 5112 225
Military & Police Uniform Association Newsletter
published by Military & Police Uniform Association 225
Miller, Niela, M.S. Ed., LCSW, LMHC
Nagog Woods, 508 264 4565 180, 189
Miller, Wynn, MSW, CSW
New York, 212 989 4641 301
Miller-Dawn Medical Center
Duluth, 218 727 8762 279
Millivres Ltd.
London 85
London, 171 267 0021 67
London, 171 482 2576 85
Milton Keynes Lesbian & Gay Switchboard
1908 666266 71
High Wycombe, 1908 666266 71
Milwaukee AIDS Project
800 359 9272 357
Milwaukee Gay / Lesbian Cable Network
414 265 0880 357
Mind Candy Emporium
Hollywood, 818 907 3199 184
Mindanao Printing Company
Minneapolis / Saint Paul, 612 774 3768 280
Mineshaft
Manchester, 161 237 9937 75
Minnesota AIDS Project
Duluth, 218 727 2437 279
Marsall, 507 532 3825 279
Minneapolis / Saint Paul, 612 341 2060 278
Rochester, 507 282 8771 281
Minnesota Freedom of Gender Expression (MFGE)
Minneapolis / Saint Paul, 612 220 9027 (voice mail) 280
Minnesota Leather Den
Brooklyn Center, 612 292 0542 279
Brooklyn Center, 612 561 6526 279
Minnesota Leather Encounter, Inc.
Minneapolis / Saint Paul 280
Minnesota Underground
Waseca 282
Minnesota Womens' Press 281
Minstry of Health AIDS Hotline
Toronto, 800 668 AIDS (English) 56
Miroir des Hommes
Tours, 47 37 4646 106
Mirrored Dragon's Dream
Omaha 285
Mirza, Inc.
Roselle, 908 245 5323 292
misc.education.medical 5
misc.health.aids 5
Mischief Moon
Sydney, 2 361 3332 27
Miss Prim's Muir Reform Academy
Hereford, 143 234 3241 24
Miss Tresse's Finishing Academy
Toronto, 416 622 2485 24
Mississipi Gay & Lesbian Task Force (MGLTF)
Biloxi, 601 435 2398 282
Mississipi Phœnix Coalition, Inc.
Jackson, 601 373 8610 282
Mississipi Voice 282
Mister B
Amsterdam, 20 422 0003 23
Mister Mosse's Boy Shop
Helsinki 97
Mistress
published by Olympia Publishing (UK) Ltd. 16
Mistress Cherie's Orchard
published by Carter Stevens Presents 333
Mistress Jacqueline Magazine
published by Pacific Force 201
Mitchell Press Ltd.
Vancouver, 604 731 5211 46
MJ Enterprises
Laramie, 307 721 2027 358
MLC *See* Montana Lesbian Coalition. *See also* Münchner-Löwen Club e. V.
MLCV *See* Moto Leather Club Veneto
MMG Services Inc.
New York, 212 966 8400 307
MMV Erotic Shop
Celle 113
MnBears
Minneapolis / Saint Paul, 612 220 1382 280
Mobile AIDS Support Services
205 433 6277 192
Mobile Area Lesbian & Gay Assembly (MALAGA)
205 450 0501 192
Mobile Infirmary Medical Center
205 431 2408 192
Mobiles Team AIDS des Landes Brandenburg
Cottbus, 355 48 8156 114
Moda Moda
Bruxelles / Brussel, 2 537 6919 36
Modern Armour
Letchworth, 1462 483458 77
Modern Products
Nashville 337
Modern Style
Köln, 221 121 1080 124
Modern Times Bookstore
San Francisco, 415 282 9246 218
Modernway Books
Dunedin, 3 477 6636 162
Mohawk Leather
Atlanta, 404 874 4732 245
Molotov
Hamburg, 40 319 2633 119
Molvig, Karen, Psy.D.
Gardiner, 207 582 1559 262
Mom Guess What! 210
Momazons
Columbus, 614 267 0193 320
Mon Cherie's The Chamber
Atlanta, 404 248 1612 243
Monadnock Area Lesbian / Gay Parents
Keene, 603 352 6741 288
Monadnock Area Womyn (MAW)
Keene, 603 352 6741 288
Monadnock Gay Men (MGM)
Keene, 603 357 5544 288
Monadnock Outright
Francestown, 603 547 2545 287
Monarch Social Club
Mississauga, 416 949 6602 51
Monash University Gay Collective
Melbourne, 39 565 4195 32
Monash University Gayline
Melbourne, 39 565 4195 32
Monday Night Clinic
Oklahoma City, 405 232 5453 323
Monique
Ferndown 69
Monique of Hollywood
Los Angeles 183
Monmouth Ocean Transgender Group (MOTG)
Red Bank 292
Monroe Avenue Book Bin
Corvallis, 503 753 8398 325
Montague, John
Toronto, 416 463 6097 55
Montana American West Company
Bozeman, 800 262 9269 187
Montana Lesbian Coalition (MLC)
Helena 285
Montanus Aktuell
Bremen, 421 17 1077 113
Bremerhaven 113
Göttingen 118
Hagen 119
Hamburg 120
Hildesheim 122
Karlsruhe 123
Lübeck 126
Mönchengladbach, 216 11 5527 127
München, 89 59 4377 128
Nürnberg, 911 23 2803 130
Oldenburg 130
Osnabrück, 541 2 2787 130
Solingen 132
Montclair State College
201 893 5271 291
Montefiore Medical Center
Bronx, 718 920 4321 297
Montefiore University Hospital
Pittsburgh, 412 647 8470 331
Montgomery AIDS Outreach
205 269 1002 192
Montgomery Medical & Psychological Institute
Alabama, 205 244 9613 192
Florida, 904 462 4826 235
Georgia, 404 321 9343 188
Montgomery, Roy
Toronto 56
Montreal's Electronic Dungeon
Montréal 62
Montrose Counseling Center
Houston, 713 529 0037 342
Monument Books
Rapid City, 605 397 9877 335
Moon Dog
New York 300
Moon Mystique
Iowa City, 319 338 5752 257
Mooncussers MC
Provincetown 272
Moonglow Dining Club
London 82
Moonlight Fashion
Bielefeld 107
Moonlight Leather Association of the Deaf
San Diego 211
Mooring & Mooring
Los Angeles 186
Moose Leather
San Diego, 619 297 6935 212
Moray House College L&G Society
Edinburgh, 131 556 5184 169
More Than You Can Count
New Brunswick, 908 819 0601 291
More! Productions
Berkeley, 510 845 5457 197
Morena & Orta Gender Issues Specialists
Puebla, 22 44 3826 149
Morey, Craig
Emeryville, 510 601 0606 199
Morgan J. Cowin Photography
San Rafael, 415 459 7722 221
Morgan Printing & Publishing
Austin, 512 459 5194 338
Morgan's Toybox
Pasadena 184
Morgan, Luke
London, 171 790 1346 81
Morrison, Craig
London, 171 278 5367 81
Morrow, David
New York, 212 645 6797 306
Mosaic Books
New York, 212 475 8623 309
Moser, Charles, Ph.D, M.D.
San Francisco, 415 621 4369 213
Moses H. Cone Memorial Hospital
Greensboro, 910 574 7000 315
Motail
Pangbourne 67
MOTG *See* Monmouth Ocean Transgender Group
Mother Kali's Books
Eugene, 503 343 4864 325
Mother's Little Helper Diaper Service
San José, 800 394 9727 220
Moto Leather Club Veneto (MLCV)
Vicenza, 444 32 1290 138
Motor City Bears
Royal Oak, 810 988 0227 278
Motorcity Men of Leather
Pontiac, 313 352 0182 277
Motorcycle Men of Alberta
Red Deer, 403 346 8927 44
Motorcycle Sports Club
Johannesburg, 11 726 1552 171
Motorcyclemen of New Mexico
Albuquerque, 505 247 8312 294
Motorradclub LederBären Berlin (MCLB)
30 215 1458 110
Mots à la Bouche
Paris, 142 78 8830 104
Mount Carmel Medical Center
Columbus, 614 225 5000 319
Mount Diablo Medical Center
Compton, 510 682 8200 198
Mount Lawley Medical Centre
Perth, 9 227 2455 33
Mount Royal College Bookstore
Calgary, 403 240 6300 43
Mount Sinai Medical Center
Miami Beach, 305 674 2121 239
New York, 212 241 6500 302
Mountain AIDS Coalition
Asheville, 704 253 4647 313
Mountain Home VAMC
Johnson City, 615 926 1177 Ext. 7709 336
Mountain Men of Leather
Denver 228
Mountain State AIDS Network
Morgantown, 800 585 4444 (in West Virginia) 354
Mountain Top Publishing
Denver, 303 985 3034 228
Mountain Valley Men
Conway, 207 925 1034 287
Mountaintop Design & Typography
Lakewood, 303 985 0202 229
Mourthé, Christophe
Paris, 142 82 1054 104
Moustache
Berlin, 30 281 7277 109, 110
Mouvement d'Information & d'Entraide dans la Lutte Contre Le SIDA à Québec (MIELS)
418 649 0788 (information) 63
Mouvement d'Information, d'Education, & d'Entraide dans la Lutte Contre Le SIDA (MIENS)
Chicoutimi, 418 693 8983 61
Mouvement SIDA Québec
418 649 1720 63
Moving Violations
Boston, 617 695 8093 268
Moyes, Jan
Livermore 202
Mozes, David, Ph.D.
Wilmington, 302 658 3067 233
Mpowerment Project
Eugene, 503 683 4303 324
Mr Surplus Army Navy Stores
Toronto, 416 977 2769 60
Mr. & Ms. Olympus
West Hollywood, 213 656 5073 224
Mr. Chaps Leatherworks
Hamburg, 40 24 3109 120
Mr. Deaf International Leather
Dallas / Fort Worth, 214 540 6439 TDD

📖 1
Mr. Drummer
San Francisco, 415 974 1156 📖 214
Mr. S – Fetters, U.S.A.
San Francisco, 800 746 7677 📖 184, 219
Mr. SM
published by Orange Press ApS 📖 66
MS Panther Köln e. V.
221 73 9483 📖 124
MS Rotterdam 📖 157
Ms. Charade
Vancouver, 604 669 2195 📖 46
Ms. Kitty's Adult Shop
Bozeman, 406 586 6989 📖 285
Ms. Leather Sacramento
916 921 1466 📖 209
Ms. San Francisco Leather 📖 212
MSC Amsterdam 📖 152
MSC Barcelona 📖 172
MSC Belgium
Bruxelles / Brussel, 2 479 9692 📖 37
MSC Berlin e.V.
30 861 8847 📖 110
MSC Black Angels Köln
Aachen 📖 108
MSC Finland
Helsinki, 0 680 2948 📖 95
MSC Hamburg e. V. 📖 120
MSC Hannover
511 66 8557 📖 121
MSC Iceland
Reykjavik, 1 17101 📖 136
MSC London
181 840 4041 📖 83
MSC Madrid
Barcelona 📖 172
MSC Rhein-Main, Frankfurt
Wiesbaden 📖 135
MSC Rhône-Alpes (MCRA)
Lyon, 72 33 0339 📖 101
MSC Rote Erde Dortmund 📖 114
MSC Scotland
Edinburgh 📖 168
MSC Südwest
Freiburg 📖 117
MSC Suisse Romande
Lausanne 📖 178
MSC Viking
Köln 📖 124
M S D S 📖 *See* Michigan Society for Domination & Submission
MTSU Lambda Association
Murfreesboro, 615 780 2293 📖 337
Mud Buddies
San Diego 📖 211
Mud Honey
New York, 212 995 5593 📖 309
Mud Maniacs
Seascale 📖 72
Mueller, Richard
Las Vegas, 702 796 9592 📖 286
MUGALS 📖 *See* Murdoch University Gay & Lesbian Society
Muir Cap & Regalia
Scarborough, 416 757 2815 📖 54
Mulé, Nick, M.S.W.
Toronto, 416 926 9135 📖 49
Multi Sexy Boutique
Mexico City, 5 264 4195 📖 149
Multicom4
Buffalo, 716 442 1669 📖 298
Rochester, 716 442 1669 📖 310
Multiprint, Inc.
Chatham, 201 635 6400 📖 290
Multitek Services
London, 181 960 5759 📖 84
Mum'sTattoo
Vancouver, 614 984 7831 📖 46
Mummy Hazel High Heels - H. B. Enterprises
Gravesend, 163 457 1396 📖 9
Münchner Hochschwule - Schwulenreferat der LMU
München, 89 2180 2072 📖 128
Münchner-Löwen Club e. V. (MLC)
München 📖 128
Municipality of Anchorage
907 343 4611 📖 192
Munro's Bookstore
Victoria, 604 382 2464 📖 47
Murdoch University Gay & Lesbian Society (MUGALS)
9 332 6335 📖 33
Murray & Vern
Manchester, 161 236 7440 📖 75
Murray Street STD Clinic
Perth, 9 270 1122 📖 33
Murrell, Pat, MSW, LCSW
Saint Louis, 314 569 5795 📖 282
Musafar, Fakir
Menlo Park, 415 324 0543 📖 206
Museum für Angewandte Kunst
Gera 📖 118
Museum of Sex
Amsterdam 📖 151
Mushroom Bookshop
Nottingham, 115 958 2506 📖 89
Music City Bears
Nashville 📖 337
Musk
Düsseldorf, 211 35 2154 📖 115
Muskegon Area AIDS Resource Services
616 722 2437 📖 277
Musson, Victoria
Tamworth, 1827 281391 📖 13
Mustang Books & Videos
Upland, 909 981 0227 📖 224
Musy, Gerard
Paris 📖 104
Mutal Gay Mens' Support Group (MGM)
Auckland, 9 534 2643 📖 160
Muther's
Toronto, 416 466 8616 📖 55
MVS
Herne, 23 231 8028 📖 122
MX
published by Out of London Limited 📖 85
My Comrade 📖 307
My Sin
Rotterdam, 10 404 6568 📖 157
My Sisters' Words
Syracuse, 315 428 0227 📖 312
Myriad Network
Williamstown 📖 273
Myrtle Bookstore
Worcester, 508 755 7541 📖 273
Mystery Loves Company
Baltimore, 410 276 6708 📖 264
Mystic Bookshop
London, 519 673 5440 📖 51
Mystic Rose Books
Fairfield, 203 371 6912 📖 230
N. M. A.
Darlington, 132 548 1631 📖 74
N. S. P.
Paris, 140 09 6969 📖 18
N. Y. C.
Toulouse, 61 59 4645 📖 106
Na Und e. V.
Oldenburg, 441 777 5923 📖 130
Nahani
Saratoga Springs, 518 587 4322 📖 311
Naiad Press, Inc.
Tallahassee, 904 539 5965 📖 242
Nam Charitable Trust
London, 171 737 1846 📖 84
NAMBLA 📖 *See* North American Man Boy Love Association
NAMES Project Foundation
San Francisco, 415 882 5500 📖 213
Namibian Leather Corps
Swakopmund, 641 4979 📖 149
Napa Valley AIDS Project
707 258 2437 📖 207
Natal Gay Community
Durban 📖 171
National AIDS Hotline
London, 800 567 123 📖 67
National Association of College Stores
Oberlin, 216 775 7777 📖 322
National Association of People With AIDS
Chicago 📖 249
National Book Network
Lanham, 301 459 8696 📖 265
National Campaign for Freedom of Expression
Seattle, 206 340 9301 📖 352
National Campaign for Reform of the Obscene Publications Acts
London 📖 83
National Center for Lesbian Rights
New York, 212 343 9589 📖 188
San Francisco, 415 392 6257 📖 188
National Coalition for Gay, Lesbian, & Bisexual Youth
San José, 408 269 6125 📖 220
National Coming Out Day
Washington, 800 866 6263 📖 234
National Council for Research on Women
New York, 212 274 0730 📖 304
National Dildo Club
Los Angeles 📖 188
National Foot Network (NFN)
Brooklyn, 718 832 3952 📖 188
National Friend
London 📖 81
National Gay & Lesbian Domestic Violence Victims' Network
Aurora, 303 266 3477 📖 226
National Gay & Lesbian Task Force
Washington, 202 332 6483 📖 234
National Gay & Lesbian Task Force Campus Project
Washington, 202 332 6483 📖 234
National Gay Rights Coalition (NGRC)
Auckland 📖 159
National Gay Youth Network
San Francisco 📖 215
National Gender Dysphoria Organization & Support Group (NGDO)
Detroit, 313 842 5228 📖 275
National Harry Benjamin Gender Dysphoria Association (HBIGDA)
Sonoma, 707 938 2871 📖 181
National Health AIDS-line
050 03 4000 📖 164
National Herpes Hotline
Research Triangle Park, 800 230 6039 📖 181
National Hospital
Bloemfontein, 51 70411 📖 171
National Institutes of Health
Bethesda, 301 496 3227 📖 265
National Leather Association (NLA)
Arkansas 📖 196
Atlanta, 404 624 1676 (24hr. recording) 📖 244
Austin, 512 703 8927 📖 338
British Columbia, 604 945 3668 📖 44
Central Arizona 📖 194
Columbus, 614 470 2093 📖 320
Dallas, 214 521 5342 Ext. 820, press 4 📖 340
Deaf International 📖 12
Detroit, 810 354 5841 📖 278
Florida 📖 236
Houston, 713 527 9666 📖 342
Indianapolis, 317 634 4272 📖 255
International Headquarters, 614 899 4406 (information/message line) 📖 12
Kansas City 📖 283
Los Angeles, 213 856 5643 📖 225
Metro New York, 212 802 9295 📖 303
New England 📖 271
New Orleans 📖 261
New South Wales 📖 26
Portland, 503 727 3148 📖 326
Russian River 📖 200
Toronto, 416 925 9872 Ext. 2089 📖 56
National Lesbian & Gay Federation
Dublin, 1 671 0939 📖 136
National Lesbian & Gay Health Association
Washington, 202 939 7880 📖 188
National Minority AIDS Council
Washington, 202 544 1076 📖 234
National Native American AIDS Prevention Center
Oakland, 800 283 2437 (AIDS line) 📖 207
National Organization for Women, Inc.
Washington, 202 331 0066 📖 234
National Organization of Circumcision Information Resource Centers (NOCIRC)
San Anselmo, 415 488 9883 📖 210
National Organization of Restoring Men (NORM)
Concord, 510 827 4077 📖 198
National Organization of Sexual Enthusiasts (NOSE)
Atlanta, 404 377 5760 📖 244
National Organization to Halt the Abuse & Routine Mutilation of Males (NOHARMM)
San Francisco, 415 826 9351 📖 215
National People Living with AIDS Union
Wellington, 4 382 8791 📖 159
National Reproductions Corporation
Madison Heights, 313 298 7900 📖 277
National Runaway Switchboard
800 621 4000 📖 181
National Shemale Directory
published by Salishon Society 📖 189
National Task Force on AIDS Prevention
San Francisco, 415 749 6700 📖 213
National Tattoo Association
New Hyde Park 📖 188
National Transvestite Line
Dublin, 1 671 0939 📖 136
National Women's Mailing List
Jenner, 707 632 5763 📖 201
National Youth Advocacy Alliance
Arlington, 800 873 2820 📖 338
Natkiel, Dan
New York 📖 303
Naughty 'n Nice
Oklahoma City, 405 686 1110 📖 323
Naughty But Nice
Beloit, 608 362 9090 📖 355
Michigan City, 219 879 6363 📖 255
Oshawa, 416 576 5826 📖 52
Portage, 608 742 8060 📖 357
West Allis, 414 541 7788 📖 358
Naughty Nancy
Seattle, 206 547 7042 📖 183
Naughty Victorian
Annapolis, 410 626 1879 📖 263
Nauti Nik Naks
Tauranga 📖 163
Naval Hospital
Charleston, 803 743 7200 📖 334
Oakland 📖 207
NAZ Project
London, 181 536 0208 📖 67
London, 181 563 0205 📖 67
NBM Publishing
New York, 800 886 1223 📖 306
NCW GALA 📖 *See* North Central Washington Gay & Lesbian Alliance
NCWC 📖 *See* Northern California Wrestling Club
ne.motss 📖 6
Nebraska AIDS Project
Omaha, 800 782 2437 📖 285
Necronomicon 📖 73
Nederbears
Amsterdam 📖 152
Nederlandse Vereniging Humanits
Amsterdam, 20 626 2445 📖 152
Utrecht, 54 727 2048 📖 158
Nederlandse Vereniging voor Sexuele Hervorming (NVSH)
Amsterdam, 20 623 9359 📖 152
Utrecht 📖 150
Needleworks
Birmingham, 121 622 6602 📖 93
Neikrug Photographica, Ltd.
New York, 212 288 7741 📖 308
Nelson HIV/AIDS Support Network
3 546 1540 📖 162
Nelson, Joan, M.A., Ed.D.
San Anselmo, 415 453 6221 📖 210
Nelson-Tebedo Clinic
Dallas / Fort Worth, 214 528 2336 📖 340
NE-SOCIAL-MOTSS 📖 3
NESS 📖 *See* Northeast Erotic Spanking Society
Network
Lafayette 📖 255
Network for the 10% Plus 📖 289
Network of Rhode Island
Pawtucket 📖 334
Neue Regel
Jacksonville 📖 238
Neuens Co-Op
Paris 📖 104
Neuer Freundeskreis Homosexueller

Kitzingen 🕮 123
Neuer Weg
Würzburg, 931 35 5910 🕮 136
Neutral Corner
San Diego, 619 685 3696 🕮 211
New Action
Berlin, 30 211 8256 🕮 110
New Age
London, 181 809 6119 🕮 67
New Age Renegade
Tulsa, 918 585 3405 🕮 323
New Beginnings
Cardiff 🕮 359
New Clinton Book Mart
Rochester, 716 325 9322 🕮 311
New Cross Army Surplus
Manchester, 161 832 9683 🕮 76
Oldham, 161 633 6967 🕮 76
New England Bears
Boston, 617 762 7821 Ext. 4 🕮 268
New England Deaconess Hospital
Boston, 6177 632 2000 🕮 267
New England Medical Center
Boston, 617 956 5000 🕮 267
New Era Institute
Milwaukee, 414 862 3823 🕮 357
New Esoteric Press
New York, 718 846 1140 🕮 308
New Hampshire Gay Parents
Manchester, 603 527 1082 🕮 287
New Hampshire Hospital
Concord, 603 271 5200 🕮 287
New Hanover Regional Medical Center
Wilmington, 910 343 7000 🕮 316
New Jersey AIDS Connection
Montclair, 201 481 1412 🕮 291
New Jersey Lesbian & Gay Coalition
New Brunswick, 201 763 0668 🕮 289
New Jersey Lesbian & Gay Film Festival
Montclair 🕮 288
New Man im WOS
Nürnberg, 911 20 3443 🕮 130
New Men & Women of Minnesota
Minneapolis / Saint Paul, 612 220 1920 🕮 280
New Mexico AIDS Services
Albuquerque, 505 266 0911 🕮 293
New Mexico Association of People Living With AIDS (NMPLA)
Albuquerque, 505 266 0342 🕮 293
Santa Fe, 505 982 5995 🕮 293
New Orleans Bondage Club 🕮 261
New Orleans PWA Coalition
504 944 3663 🕮 261
New Phazes Newsletter 🕮 227
New School Gay, Lesbian, Bisexual Collective
New York 🕮 305
New Vista Publishing
619 727 8718 🕮 15
New Voice 🕮 285
New Words
Boston, 617 876 5310 🕮 269
New World Rubber Men
Port Townsend, 206 385 3811 🕮 12
New York
München, 89 59 1056 🕮 127
New York Bears
212 367 7484 🕮 304
New York Bisexual Network
212 459 4784 🕮 305
New York Bondage Club
212 315 0040 🕮 304
New York Boys & Dads 🕮 304
New York City Department of Health
212 788 4315 🕮 302
212 788 4399 🕮 302
New York City Gender Alliance (NYCGA)
212 570 7389 🕮 305
New York Downtown Hospital
212 312 5000 🕮 302
New York Femmes
212 388 2736 🕮 305
New York Girl & Partner
Centereach 🕮 298
New York Hospital
212 746 5454 🕮 302
New York Metro D&S Singles
Brooklyn, 718 648 8215 🕮 297
New York Native
published by That New Magazine 🕮 308
New York Review of Books 🕮 307
New York State Division of Human Rights
212 870 8604 🕮 295
800 532 2437 🕮 295
New York Strap & Paddle Association
718 367 7484 🕮 304
New Zealand AIDS Foundation
Auckland, 9 309 5560 🕮 160
Auckland, 9 378 9802 🕮 159
Christchurch, 3 379 3353 🕮 161
Dunedin, 3 474 7732 🕮 161
Hawkes Bay, 6 835 5554 🕮 162
Head Office, 4 303 3124 🕮 159
Waikato, 7 838 557 🕮 162
Wellington, 4 389 3169 🕮 163
New Zealand Gender Dysphoria Foundation (NZGDF)
Auckland 🕮 160
New Zealand Prostitutes Collective
Auckland, 9 366 6106 🕮 160
Wellington, 4 382 8791 🕮 163
New Zealand Swing Club
Wellington, 4 384 8214 🕮 163
Newark Beth Israel Medical Center
201 926 7000 🕮 292
Newark Community Health Centers, Inc.
201 565 0355 🕮 292
Newcastle AIDS Hotline
4 926 6866 🕮 25
Newcastle Friend
Newcastle upon Tyne, 191 261 8555 🕮 92
Newcastle Gay & Lesbian Information Service
4 929 6733 🕮 25
Newcastle Gay Youthline
Newcastle upon Tyne, 191 233 1551 🕮 92
Newcastle Lesbian Line
Newcastle upon Tyne, 191 261 2277 🕮 92
Newfoundland & Labrador AIDS Committee Inc.
Saint John's, 709 579 8656 🕮 48
News 🕮 320
News - Books - Cards
Fort Lauderdale, 305 726 5544 🕮 237
News & Photo Shop
Kent, 216 678 5499 🕮 321
News from Nowhere
Liverpool, 151 708 7270 🕮 87
News of the Columbus Gay & Lesbian Community 🕮 320
News Stand
Winnipeg, 204 453 2644 🕮 47
Newsbreak
Swansea, 508 675 9380 🕮 272
Newsland
Longview, 903 753 4167 🕮 343
Newsland Bookstore
Albuquerque, 505 242 0694 🕮 294
Newsstand
Bellingham 🕮 350
Newsstand Adult Bookshop
Boulder, 303 442 9515 🕮 226
News-Telegraph
published by Piasa Publishing Company 🕮 282, 283
Next! Body Piercing
Vancouver, 604 684 6398 🕮 46
Nexus
London 🕮 84
NFN 🕮 *See* National Foot Network
NGDO 🕮 *See* National Gender Dysphoria Organization & Support Group
NGRC 🕮 *See* National Gay Rights Coalition
NH Lambda
Concord, 603 627 8675 🕮 287
Nice 'n' Naughty
Cape Town, 21 434 3585 🕮 170
Niche Catalog Publications
Lake Oswego, 503 699 5094 🕮 325
Nichols, Margaret, Ph.D.
Jersey City, 201 798 5926 🕮 290
Night Dreams
Tysons Corner 🕮 349
Night Life
Columbus 🕮 319
Night Scene
broadcast by Cable Access TV 🕮 324
Nightlife
Burlington, 508 658 4421 🕮 270
Nightlines
published by Lambda Publications 🕮 251
Nightshift
Wien, 1 586 2337 🕮 35
Nightstick
New York 🕮 300
Nightstyle Designs
Runcorn 🕮 72
Nikky / Natural Baby Co., Inc.
Titusville, 609 737 2895 🕮 293
Nima
Köln, 22 123 6328 🕮 125
Nimbus
Grand Rapids 🕮 276
Nine & A Half Weeks
Atlanta, 404 815 9622 🕮 245
Nine Plus Club, Inc.
New York 🕮 304
Nirvana
Glasgow, 141 552 5706 🕮 169
Nitch Novelties
Columbia, 800 445 8697 🕮 335
Nite Club
Lorain, 216 245 6319 🕮 321
NK Products
Teaneck 🕮 183
NLA 🕮 *See* National Leather Association
NLA-FRIENDS 🕮 2
NMPLA 🕮 *See* New Mexico Association of People Living With AIDS
No Hope * No Fear
Chicago, 312 772 1960 🕮 252
No Safeword Writers' Group
Seattle 🕮 352
NO/AIDS Task Force
New Orleans, 800 992 4379 (hotline) 🕮 260
Noah's Ark
Karlstad, 570 11222 🕮 176
Linköping, 13 19 1000 🕮 174
Stockholm, 8 23 5060 🕮 175
Växjö, 470 77 0966 🕮 175
Visby, 498 21 6850 🕮 173
Noahs Ark
Malmö, 40 11 5215 🕮 174
Noble Distributors
New York, 800 662 5372 🕮 302
NOCIRC 🕮 *See* National Organization of Circumcision Information Resource Centers
Nocturne Productions
Ferndale, 810 542 7980 🕮 275
Noelle Nielson Softwear
West Hollywood 🕮 183
NOHARMM 🕮 *See* National Organization to Halt the Abuse & Routine Mutilation of Males
Noir
Windsor, 519 252 3653 🕮 61
Noir Leather
Royal Oak, 810 541 3979 🕮 278
Nomad
Northcote 🕮 33
San Francisco, 415 563 7771 🕮 216
Noone, Kenneth, CSW, CAC
New York, 718 820 39700 🕮 301
Noose
New York, 212 807 1789 🕮 309
Noose II
New York, 212 807 1789 🕮 309
Noose Letter
published by Winter Publishing, Inc. 🕮 19
Norcal Printing
San Francisco, 415 282 8856 🕮 216
Norfolk Friend
Norwich, 1603 628055 🕮 88
Nørhaven A/S
Viborg 🕮 67
NORM 🕮 *See* National Organization of Restoring Men
Normandale Community College Lesbian & Gay Network
Minneapolis / Saint Paul, 612 832 6544 🕮 280
Norsemen
Manchester, 603 641 3450 🕮 287
North American Man Boy Love Association
San Francisco, 415 564 2602 🕮 215
North American Man Boy Love Association (NAMBLA)
New York, 212 807 8578 🕮 305
North Carolina State Lesbian / Gay Student Union
Raleigh, 929 829 9553 🕮 316
North Central Bronx Hospital
718 519 3500 🕮 297
North Central Mental Health Services
Columbus, 614 299 6600 🕮 319
North Central Ohio AIDS Foundation
Mansfield, 419 522 9357 🕮 322
North Central Washington Gay & Lesbian Alliance (NCW GALA)
Wenatchee, 509 662 8413 🕮 354
North Colorado Medical Center
Greeley, 303 352 4121 🕮 229
North Country Bears
Minneapolis / Saint Paul, 612 588 2506 🕮 279
North Devon Lesbian & Gay Switchboard
Barnstaple, 1271 321111 🕮 73
North East Bi Group
Gateshead 🕮 92
North End News
Rochester, 716 271 1426 🕮 311
North Florida Regional Medical Center
Gainesville, 904 333 4000 🕮 237
North General Hospital
New York, 212 424 4000 🕮 302
North Idaho AIDS Coalition
Coeur D'Alene, 800 677 2437 🕮 247
North Iowa AIDS Project
Mason City, 515 423 0025 🕮 257
North Keep
Portland 🕮 326
North of Scotland NUS
Dundee 🕮 170
North Park Review 🕮 212
North Philadelphia Health System
215 787 9000 🕮 330
North Puget Sound AIDS Foundation
Everett, 206 659 8045 🕮 350
North Shore Gay & Lesbian Alliance
Marblehead, 617 745 3848 🕮 271
North Staffordshire Lesbian & Gay Switchboard
Sandbach, 1782 266998 🕮 72
Stoke-on-Trent, 1782 266998 🕮 91
North Street Bookshop
Binghamton, 607 785 9606 🕮 297
North Suburban Gay Association
Chicago, 708 251 8853 🕮 250
North West Gay Support
Wivenhoe 🕮 31
North West Pennsylvania G & L Task Force
Tionesta 🕮 333
North Woods Radical Faerie Circle
Minneapolis / Saint Paul, 612 334 1948 🕮 280
Northampton AIDS Information Line
1604 28999 🕮 89
Northampton Lesbian & Gayline
1604 39722 (men) 🕮 88
Northamptonshire Gayline
Wellingborough, 1933 223591 🕮 89
Northbound Leather Ltd.
Toronto, 416 972 1037 🕮 41, 56, 60
Northeast Erotic Spanking Society (NESS)
Waltham 🕮 273
Northeast Ohio Task Force on AIDS
Akron, 216 375 2000 🕮 317
Northeast Ursamen
New Preston, 203 639 2345 🕮 232
Northern & Shell
London, 171 987 5090 🕮 85
Northern AIDS Network
Rhinelander, 800 374 7678 (715 area only) 🕮 358
Superior, 800 374 7698 (715 area only) 🕮 358
Northern Association of Fantasy Fetishists
Leeds 🕮 94
Northern California Leather Association of the Deaf
San Francisco 🕮 214
Northern California Wrestling Club (NCWC)
San Francisco 🕮 216
Northern Colorado AIDS Project
Fort Collins, 303 223 6227 🕮 229

Northern Concord
Manchester, 161 274 3705 📖 76
Northern Kentucky AIDS Consortium
Covington, 606 291 0770 📖 258
Northern Ohio Coalition, Inc.
Cleveland, 216 771 0369 📖 319
Northern Territory AIDS Council, Inc.
Darwin, 8 41 3288 📖 28
Northern Utah AIDS Society
Ogden, 801 778 0379 📖 345
Northern Virginia Pride, Inc.
Arlington, 703 528 3659 📖 347
Northern Voice
Bartlet, 603 374 1833 📖 287
Northern Wisconsin Lambda Society
Rhinelander, 715 362 4242 📖 358
Northland Gay Men's Center
Minneapolis / Saint Paul, 218 722 8585 📖 280
Northshire Bookstore
Manchester Center, 802 437 3700 📖 346
Northtown Books
Arcata, 707 822 2834 📖 196
Northwest AIDS Foundation
Seattle, 206 329 6923 📖 351
Northwest Bears
Seattle, 206 233 0113 📖 351
Northwest Bondage Club
Seattle, 206 781 1575 📖 351
Northwest Gender Alliance (NWGA)
Portland, 503 646 2802 📖 326
Northwest Leather Goddesses
Seattle, 206 782 2472 📖 351
Northwest Louisiana AIDS Task Force
New Orleans, 318 221 8219 📖 260
Northwest Michigan Gender Society
Petosky 📖 277
Northwest Rainmakers
Seattle, 206 292 1411 📖 352
Northwest Wisconsin AIDS Project
Eau Clair, 800 750 2437 📖 355
Northwestern Connecticut AIDS Project
Torrington, 203 482 1596 📖 232
Northwestern Memorial Hospital
Chicago, 312 908 2000 📖 249
Northwestern University Bisexual, Gay, & Lesbian Alliance
Chicago, 708 491 2375 📖 250
Northwind
Vancouver, 604 253 1258 📖 46
Norwich AIDS Helpline
1603 615816 📖 88
Norwich Gay Men's Health Project
1603 62514 📖 88
Norwich Lesbian & Gayline
1603 592505 📖 88
Great Yarmouth, 1603 592505 📖 88
NOSE 📖 *See* National Organization of Sexual Enthusiasts
NOSS 📖 *See* Núdeo de Orientção em Saude Social
Nostro Mondo
São Paulo, 11 257 4481 📖 39
Northern Kentucky AIDS Task Force
Newport, 606 491 6611 📖 259
Nottingham AIDS Bereavement Support (ABS)
115 962 0920 📖 89
Nottingham AIDS Information Project
115 941 1989 📖 89
Nottingham Friend
115 947 4717 📖 89
Nottingham Lesbian & Gay Switchboard
115 941 1454 📖 89
Nottingham Women's Bi Group 📖 89
Nouveau Midwest 📖 318
Nouvelle
Charleroi, 7 131 8133 📖 38
Nova Radio FM 101.5
Firenze, 55 30 8461 📖 146
Nova Scotia PWA Coalition
Halifax, 902 429 7922 📖 48
Now Cleveland 📖 321
Now Voyager
Provincetown, 508 487 0848 📖 272
Nowhere To Hide
broadcast by CKMS FM 94.5 📖 61
NSS Seminars, Inc.
Ben Lomand, 408 336 9281 📖 181, 196
Nu Haven Books & Video
New Haven, 203 562 5867 📖 231
Núdeo de Orientção em Saude Social (NOSS)
Rio de Janeiro, 21 262 6362 📖 39
Nugget's Bar
Melbourne, 39 417 2832 📖 31
Nuit du Desir
Bruxelles / Brussel 📖 37
Number One
Essen, 201 23 6682 📖 116
Numbers 📖 307
Sydney, 2 361 6099 📖 27
Numbers Pub
Pensacola, 904 438 9004 📖 241
Nummer
published by Nummer Verlag 📖 135
Nummer Verlag
Wiesbaden, 611 37 7765 📖 135
Nürnberger Schwulenpost 📖 129
NUS East of Scotland Area LGB Network
Edinburgh, 131 558 1541 📖 169
Nussdorf, Gerrie, Ph.D.
New York, 212 691 1818 📖 301
Nu-West Productions
San Marcos, 619 630 9979 📖 220
nv.bi 📖 6
nv.motss 📖 6
NVSH 📖 *See* Nederlandse Vereniging voor Sexuele Hervorming
NW Thames HIV Project
London, 171 724 7443 📖 82
NWGA 📖 *See* Northwest Gender Alliance
NYCGA 📖 *See* New York City Gender Alliance
Nylon Club
Courcouronnes, 164 97 0506 📖 99
NYPT
New York 📖 13
NZGBLF 📖 3
NZGDF 📖 *See* New Zealand Gender Dysphoria Foundation
«O» Magazine
published by RM Distribution, Ltd. 📖 19
O Productions
New York, 212 243 3700 Ext. 412 📖 308
O'Brien, Maureen, CSW, ACSW
Albany, 518 462 0213 📖 295
O'Brien, Terence
Sacramento, 916 979 3515 📖 209
O'Connor, A Gallery
Toronto, 416 921 7149 📖 59
O'Donnell, Elke, Ph.D.
Boston 📖 267
OAC 📖 *See* Ohio AIDS Coalition
Oak Lawn Community Services
Dallas / Fort Worth, 214 520 8108 📖 340
Oakhaus
Bloomington, 309 454 2128 📖 248
Oaklawn
Goshen, 219 533 1234 📖 254
Oasis
Meadville 📖 329
Tacoma, 206 591 6060 📖 354
Oasis AIDS Care Centre
London, 181 874 3230 📖 82
Oasis Bookstore
Austin, 512 835 7208 📖 339
Oasis Resources Center
Oklahoma City, 405 525 2437 📖 323
OB Enterprises
New York 📖 307
Obelisk The Bookstore
San Diego, 619 297 4171 📖 212
Oberlin College Lesbian, Gay, & Bisexual Union
216 775 8179 📖 322
Oberons
Milwaukee 📖 357
Obscurities
Dallas / Fort Worth, 214 559 3706 📖 341
Observer 📖 121, 195
Obsession 📖 307
Occhiolino
Torino, 11 54 9440 📖 144
Ocean (County) Lesbian-Gay Alliance, Inc.
Seaside Park, 908 793 3603 📖 289
Ochsengarten
München, 89 26 6446 📖 127
OCLA 📖 *See* Orange Coast Leather Assembly
October Books
Southampton, 1703 224489 📖 77
Octopus Books
Ottawa, 613 236 2589 📖 53
Vancouver, 604 253 0013 📖 46
odd isn't. it?
Toronto, 416 515 0009 📖 60
Odysseus
published by Odysseus International Ltd. 📖 189
Odysseus International Ltd.
Port Washington, 516 944 5330 📖 189
Odyssey
Spokane, 509 324 1547 📖 354
Odyssey Book Store
Nashville, 615 726 0243 📖 337
Odyssey Magazine 📖 218
Œdipus MC
Hollywood 📖 201
Off Broadway Emporium
Council Bluffs, 712 328 2673 📖 256
off our backs 📖 235
Off The Beaten Path
Tempe, 602 839 4771 📖 194
Offbeat
broadcast by CFUV FM 101.9 📖 47
Officers Club
North Little Rock 📖 196
Offrande
published by A. P. M. C. 📖 20
Ohio AIDS Coalition (OAC)
Columbus, 614 445 8277 📖 317
Ohio AIDS Hotline
Columbus, 800 332 2437 📖 317
Ohio Broncos
Cleveland 📖 318
Ohio Lesbian Archives
Cincinnati, 513 541 1917 📖 317
Ohio Lesbian Festival
Columbus, 614 267 3953 📖 317
Ohio State University Hospitals
Columbus, 614 293 8112 📖 320
Ohio State University Medical Center
Columbus, 614 293 8000 📖 319
Ohio Word
published by Word Publications 📖 317
OH-MOTSS 📖 3
OHO
Helsinki 📖 96
OISE
Toronto 📖 59
OK To Be Us
Toronto, 416 397 3755 📖 57
Oklahoma City Foundation for AIDS Research
405 843 8378 📖 323
Oklahoma University Gay, Lesbian, & Bisexual Alliance
Oklahoma City, 405 325 4452 📖 323
Ökumenischer Arbeitskreis AIDS
Hamburg, 40 43 4696 📖 119
OL 📖 *See* Outer Limits
Olaf Lesbian & Gay Alliance (OLAGA)
Northfield, 507 663 2305 📖 281
OLAGA 📖 *See* Olaf Lesbian & Gay Alliance
Old Fort Bears
Fort Wayne 📖 254
Old Reliable
Los Angeles 📖 187
Old Wives Tales
San Francisco, 415 821 4675 📖 218
OLGSR 📖 *See* Organization for Lesbian & Gay Student Rights
OLLIE of ORLANDO
407 843 5621 📖 187
Olympia AIDS Task Force
206 352 2375 📖 350
Olympia Publishing (UK) Ltd.
Ryde, 1983 811783 📖 16, 18, 19
Omaha Players Club
402 451 7987 📖 285
Omaha Surplus
Dallas / Fort Worth 📖 341
Omega Centre Bookstore
Toronto, 416 975 9086 📖 40
Omega Literary Arts Magazine 📖 208
Omega Marketing
Southampton 📖 77
OMEN
Omaha 📖 285
Omikron
Indianapolis 📖 255
Omni Adult Bookstore
Fort Lauderdale, 305 584 6825 📖 237
Omnific Designs West
San Dimas, 909 592 5217 📖 212
Omnipress
Madison, 608 246 2600 📖 356
OMPO 📖 22
Ompos's Gay House
Roma, 6 93 54 7567 📖 141
On Our Backs 📖 217
On The Issues
published by Choices Women's Medical Center, Inc. 📖 299
On The Wilde Side 📖 308
On Your Knees
Southfield 📖 278
Once Upon a Time (OUT)
Bloomington, 309 828 3998 📖 248
Onda Gay
broadcast by Radio Città Aperta FM 99.8 & 100.1 📖 146
One Way
Paris, 148 87 4610 📖 102
One-In-Teen Youth Services
Nashville, 615 297 0008 📖 337
Ontario AIDS Network
Ottawa, 613 230 3580 📖 49
OPC Supply
Omaha, 402 451 7987 📖 187
Open Arms
South Bend 📖 255
Open Doors
Akron, 61114 593 7301 📖 317
Open Enterprises, Inc.
San Francisco 📖 219
Open Hands 📖 235, 251
Open Road Riders of Chicagoland
708 795 1803 📖 250
Opening Books
Huntsville, 205 536 5880 📖 192
Opera
Berne, 31 228458 📖 178
Opplysnigstelefon om AIDS
Kongsberg, 32 83 3070 📖 165
Optic Verve
Toronto, 416 515 7260 📖 58
Options Bisexual Group
Vancouver, 604 688 9378 Ext. 2097 📖 45
Options Clinic
London, 519 673 4427 📖 51
Options Magazine
published by AJA Publishing Corp. 📖 310
Options Nightclub
Brisbane, 7 831 4214 📖 28
Oracle
North Hollywood 📖 207
Oral Majority
published by Winter Publishing, Inc. 📖 22
Orange Coast Leather Assembly (OCLA)
Garden Grove, 714 534 0862 📖 200
Orange County Blade 📖 201
Orange County Directory
published by Turkey Media Services 📖 202
Orange Press ApS
Holbæck 📖 66
Orb & Scepter
Las Vegas, 702 251 7201 📖 286
Orbita Gay Macho
published by Gay Club I. L. R. E. S. 📖 167
Order of the Marquis & Chevalier
Novi, 810 348 5332 📖 277
Oregon Gay & Lesbian Cultural Resource Center Task Force
Portland, 503 295 9732 📖 324
Oregon Guild Activists of S/M (ORGASM)
Portland, 503 688 0669 📖 326
Organization for Gay Awareness
Montclair, 201 746 6196 📖 289
Organization for Lesbian & Gay Student Rights (OLGSR)
Washington, 202 635 5291 📖 234
ORGASM 📖 *See* Oregon Guild Activists of

S/M
  Edinburgh 🕮 168
Oriana's Bookcafé
  Hill City, 800 524 4954 🕮 335
Original Bookstore
  Orlando, 407 648 4546 🕮 241
Orion
  Braunschweig, 531 4 3283 🕮 113
Orlando Eagle
  407 843 6334 🕮 240
Orlando Regional Medical Center
  407 841 5111 🕮 240
Orsi Italiani Girth & Mirth
  Milano, 2 481 8685 🕮 138
Orsiciliani
  Masalucia 🕮 145
Oscar Wilde Buchladen
  Frankfurt am Main, 69 28 1260 🕮 117
Oscar Wilde Memorial Bookstore
  New York, 212 255 8097 🕮 182, 309
Oslo Piercing Studio
  22 19 9265 🕮 164
Ospedale
  Pordenone, 434 65 2512 🕮 141
Ospedale A Cardanelli
  Campobasso, 874 99791 🕮 143
Ospedale Amedeo di Savoia
  Torino, 11 771 0514 AIDS information 🕮 144
Ospedale Civico
  Palermo, 91 48 9004 🕮 145
Ospedale Civile
  Alghero, 79 95 0235 🕮 145
  Aosta, 165 3041 🕮 146
  Asti, 141 3941 🕮 144
  Avellino 🕮 140
  Biella, 15 35031 🕮 144
  Caserta, 81 23 1111 🕮 140
  Catanzaro, 961 42613 🕮 139
  Cuneo, 171 44182 Ext. 441 🕮 144
  Pescara, 85 37 3111 Ext. 406 🕮 139
  Sondrio, 342 81 3470 🕮 143
  Teramo, 861 4291 🕮 139
Ospedale Civile dell'Annunziata
  Cosenza, 984 7291 🕮 139
Ospedale Civile Ruiniti
  Venezia, 41 78 4304 🕮 147
Ospedale Civile S. Chiara
  Trento, 461 92 5125 🕮 146
Ospedale Cotugno
  Napoli, 81 25 7033 🕮 140
Ospedale Di Cattinara
  Trieste, 40 79 5338 🕮 141
Ospedale di Summa
  Brindisi, 831 2042 🕮 144
Ospedale di Venere
  Bari, 80 35 0731 🕮 144
Ospedale Gen. Reg. S. M. Battuti
  Treviso, 422 58 2625 🕮 147
Ospedale Generale Provinciale
  Macerata, 733 2571 🕮 143
  Terni, 744 57141 🕮 146
Ospedale Guadagna
  Palermo, 91 39 7111 🕮 145
Ospedale Macchi
  Varese, 332 27 8234 🕮 143
Ospedale Madonna dei Cieli
  Catanzaro, 961 41921 🕮 139
Ospedale Malacrino
  Crotone, 965 34711 🕮 140
Ospedale Mauriziano
  Torino, 11 50801 🕮 144
Ospedale Maurizio Ascoli
  Catania, 95 759 1111 🕮 145
Ospedale Molinette
  Torino 🕮 144
Ospedale Morgagni
  Forli, 545 73 1717 🕮 140
Ospedale Pascale
  Napoli, 81 25 7300 🕮 140
Ospedale Pellegrini Nuovo
  Napoli, 81 780 1122 🕮 140
Ospedale Policlinico Monteluce
  Perugia, 75 66118 🕮 146
Ospedale Provinciale
  Matera, 835 2431 🕮 139
Ospedale Provinciale San Francesco di Paola (Pescopagano)
  Potenza, 971 26929 🕮 139
Ospedale Regina Marherita
  Messina, 90 292 6284 🕮 145
Ospedale S. Camillo de Lellis
  Chieti, 871 64141 🕮 139
Ospedale S. Chiara
  Pisa, 50 59 2111 🕮 146
Ospedale S. Gallicano
  Roma 🕮 141
Ospedale S. Salvatore di Muraglia
  Pesaro, 721 36 4052 🕮 143
Ospedale San Antonio
  Alessandria, 131 3061 🕮 144
Ospedale San Carlo
  Potenza, 971 3595 🕮 139
Ospedale San Lazzaro
  Torino, 11 66251 🕮 144
Ospedale San Martino
  Genova, 10 35351 🕮 142
Ospedale San Matteo
  Pavia, 382 39 0660 Ext. 3881 🕮 143
Ospedale San Salvatore
  L'Aquila, 862 7781 🕮 139
Ospedale Santa Anna
  Brescia, 301 58 5329 🕮 142
Ospedale Spallanzani
  Roma, 6 55 4021 🕮 141
Ospedale SS. Annunziata
  Taranto 🕮 145
Ospedale SS. Trinita
  Cagliari, 70 285 2294 🕮 145
Ospedale Umberto I
  Ancona, 71 5961 3270 🕮 143
Ospedale V. Emanuele
  Caltanissetta, 934 32611 🕮 145
Ospedali Riuniti
  Bergamo, 35 26 9111 🕮 142
Ostfreisische Schwulen- & Lesbeninitiative
  Emden, 492 12 9522 🕮 116
Other Place
  Cork, 21 27 8470 🕮 137
Other Pony Club
  Hereford, 143 234 3241 🕮 9, 11
Other Side Bookshop
  Cork, 21 27 8470 🕮 137
Other Way Press
  London, 181 998 1519 🕮 84
Ottawa Gayline / Télégai Ottawa
  613 238 1717 🕮 52
Ottawa Knights
  613 237 9072 Ext. 2038 🕮 52
Ottawa Physicians for Lesbian & Gay Health
  613 563 3331 🕮 52
Ottawa Women's Bookstore
  613 230 1156 🕮 53
Oude Mol
  Nijmegen, 80 322 1734 🕮 157
Oulu AIDS-Tukikeskes
  98 137 9398 🕮 95
Our Kids
  Detroit, 616 388 5656 🕮 275
Our Own Community Press 🕮 347
Our Paper 🕮 220
Our Place
  Raleigh, 919 833 8968 🕮 316
Our Print Shop
  San José, 408 452 0570 🕮 220
Our Times 🕮 78
Our World Television 🕮 212
Our World Too
  Saint Louis, 314 533 5322 🕮 182
OUT 🕮 332. *See also* Once Upon a Time
  Bloomington, 812 855 5688 🕮 253
  published by Out Publishing, Inc. 🕮 307
  South Bend, 219 237 4125 🕮 255
Out & About 🕮 217
  Inverness 🕮 168
  Plympton, 8 302 3212 🕮 31
  Portsmouth, 603 659 2139 🕮 288
  published by Out & About, Inc. 🕮 307
Out & About - The Gay Radio Show
  broadcast by CKWR FM 98.7 🕮 61
Out & About Books
  Orlando, 407 896 0204 🕮 241
Out & About Indiana
  Indianapolis, 317 925 9126 🕮 253
Out & About, Inc.
  New York, 800 929 2268 🕮 307
Out & Out
  broadcast by 2SER FM 107.3 🕮 27
Out Among Friends
  Biddleford, 207 799 0297 🕮 262
Out and About 🕮 348, 354
Out For Good
  East Waterboro, 207 247 3461 🕮 262
Out Front 🕮 228
Out in the Mountains 🕮 346
Out In The Nineties
  broadcast by Gay Broadcasting System 🕮 310
Out Loud
  broadcast by 3D Radio 93.7 FM 🕮 30
Out Magazine 🕮 308
Out of London Limited
  171 581 1521 🕮 85
Out of the Dark
  Newport News, 804 596 6220 🕮 348
Out On Campus
  Vancouver, 604 688 9378 Ext. 2064 🕮 45
  Windsor, 519 971 7617 🕮 61
Out On The Shelves
  Vancouver, 604 684 5307 🕮 45
Out Pages 🕮 236
Out Publishing, Inc.
  New York, 212 334 9119 🕮 307
Out Reach
  Albuquerque, 505 255 3552 🕮 294
Out This Week
  broadcast by All Out Productions 🕮 85
Out!
  published by Lawrence Publishing Company (NZ) Ltd. 🕮 160
Out! Books
  Brighton, 1273 623356 🕮 74
Out! Bookshop
  Auckland, 9 377 7770 🕮 160
  Christchurch, 3 366 7352 🕮 161
  Wellington, 4 385 4400 🕮 163
Out! Looks
  Brighton, 1273 623356 🕮 74
Out! Magazine 🕮 294
Out! Mailorder
  Auckland, 900 51993 🕮 159
OUT! Resource Guide
  published by Lambda Publications 🕮 251
OutArt 🕮 338
OUTawa Magazine 🕮 53
Outbound Press
  New York, 212 727 2751 🕮 18, 19
Outcasts
  San Francisco, 415 668 4622 🕮 214
Outcomers
  Drogheda, 1 872 1055 🕮 138
Outer Limits
  Chicago, 708 259 0410 🕮 248
Outer Limits (OL)
  Seattle 🕮 351
OutFit
  Asheville, 704 277 7815 🕮 313
Out-In-Africa
  Cape Town, 21 24 1532 🕮 170
Outlines
  published by Lambda Publications 🕮 251
Outlooks Magazine 🕮 279
OutNow 🕮 196
Outposts 🕮 336
OutProud!
  San José 🕮 189
Outrage 🕮 24
Outreach Institute of Gender Studies
  Augusta, 207 621 0858 🕮 13
Outreach of Daytona Beach
  904 672 6069 🕮 236
Outreach Rand
  Johannesburg, 11 643 2311 🕮 171
Outreach UFS
  Charlotte, 704 332 9034 🕮 314
Outright
  Durham, 800 879 2300 (within NC) 🕮 314
  Portland, 207 774 4357 🕮 263
  published by Liberation Publishers 🕮 172
Outright Books
  Virginia Beach, 804 490 6658 🕮 349
Outright Vermont
  Burlington, 800 452 2428 🕮 346
Outright Youth in Kingston (OYINK)
  613 545 2960 🕮 50
Outright! 🕮 89
Outsiders
  London, 171 739 0388 🕮 13
Outspace Schwul-Lesbische Jungendgruppe
  Hannover, 511 36 3633 🕮 121
Outspoken
  published by Kalani Honua, Inc. 🕮 246
Outspoken Productions
  Manchester, 161 228 6228 🕮 76
Outwaves
  broadcast by Christchurch Lesbian Gay Radio Collective 🕮 23
Outwords 🕮 298
Outwrite Bookstore & Coffeehouse
  Atlanta, 404 607 0082 🕮 245
Overlooked Opinions, Inc.
  Chicago 🕮 252
Overnight Productions
  Los Angeles, 213 874 0874 🕮 205
Overnight Productions FM 90.7
  North Hollywood, 818 833 0283 🕮 207
OxAIDS
  Oxford, 800 393999 🕮 89
Oxenbury, Jane, M. Ed., C. Psyc.
  Calgary, 403 240 2501 🕮 42
Oxford Books
  Atlanta, 404 262 3332 🕮 245
Oxford Friend
  1865 726 893 🕮 89
Oxford Gay & Lesbian Centre
  186 520 0030 🕮 90
Oxford Lesbian & Gay Switchboard
  1865 793 999 🕮 89
OYINK 🕮 *See* Outright Youth in Kingston
Oz
  Fayetteville, 910 485 2037 🕮 315
Ozark Feminist Review 🕮 195
Ozark Mountain Bears
  Avoca 🕮 195
Ozbears Australia Inc.
  Sydney, 2 550 1331 🕮 26
Ozbears of South Australia
  Lobethal, 8 389 4292 🕮 31
P+E
  Rotterdam, 10 474 8360 🕮 150
P. A. U. K.
  Nuneaton 🕮 92
P. E. S., Inc.
  Las Vegas, 702 474 2991 🕮 181
P. I. Group
  Haddam 🕮 230
P. M. Club
  Tampa 🕮 242
P. M. Productions
  West New York, 800 336 9696 🕮 187
P. T. Max
  Baltimore, 410 539 6965 🕮 263
pa.motss 🕮 6
PACE
  London, 171 700 1323 🕮 82
Pacific Bears California LMC
  Russian River, 707 869 3783 🕮 200
  San Francisco, 415 905 9575 🕮 215
Pacific Book House
  Oahu 🕮 247
Pacific Center
  Head Office, 510 841 6224 🕮 197
Pacific Center for Human Growth
  Walnut Creek, 510 939 7711 🕮 224
Pacific Coast MC
  Los Angeles 🕮 204
Pacific Force
  Hollywood 🕮 201
Pacific Island AIDS Trust
  Wellington, 4 473 4493 🕮 159
Pacific Northwest Wrestling Association
  Seattle 🕮 352
Pacific Street
  Houston, 713 523 0213 🕮 342
PACK 🕮 *See* Positive Action Coalition of Kansas, Inc.
PACT 🕮 *See* People With AIDS Coalition of Tucson
Paddles 🕮 25
  New York, 212 463 8599 🕮 300
Padula, Lee, Ph.D.
  Livonia, 313 953 3333 🕮 277
Pagan Metal
  London, 171 287 3830 🕮 84, 86
Pagan Press
  New York, 212 674 3321 🕮 308
Page Initiative
  State College 🕮 333

Page One
Pasadena, 818 798 8418 📖 209
Page One Books
Hull, 148 241 925 📖 77
Page, Ken, CSW
New York, 212 420 0394 📖 301
Pageprint Limited
Edinburgh, 131 539 0666 📖 169
Pages
published by Lifestyle Publishing Inc. 📖 246
Toronto, 416 598 1447 📖 59
Pages Video & More
Saint Louis, 314 361 3420 📖 284
Paips Essonne
Palaiseau, 42 61 1522 📖 102
Paisano Publications
Agoura Hills, 818 889 8740 📖 196
PAL 📖 *See* Project AIDS Lafayette
Palette Hamburg e. V. im Schantezhof
40 430 2777 📖 119
Palm Beach County AIDS Clinic
West Palm Beach, 407 845 4444 📖 243
Palm Beach County Health Department
West Palm Beach, 407 837 3090 📖 243
Palm Beaches Medical Center
West Palm Beach, 407 842 6141 📖 243
Palm Springs Directory
published by Turkey Media Services 📖 202
Palm Springs Leather Order of the Desert
619 770 3192 📖 208
Palmetto AIDS Life Support Services of South Carolina, Inc. (PALSS)
Columbia, 800 868 7257 📖 334
PALS 📖 *See* Powys AIDS Line Services. *See also* People of Alternate Lifestyles
PALSS 📖 *See* Palmetto AIDS Life Support Services of South Carolina, Inc.
Pan Biblioteket
København, 33 11 1961 📖 66
Pan Information
København, 33 13 0112 📖 2
Panasewicz, T. Roman
Las Vegas 📖 286
Panda Bear
New Orleans, 504 529 3593 📖 261
Pandora Book Peddlars
North Haledon, 201 427 5733 📖 292
Pandora Books for Open Minds
Kalamazoo, 616 388 5656 📖 276
Panos Institute
Washington, 202 483 0044 📖 233
Panozzo, David, CSW
Woodcliff Lake 📖 293
Pantaleo, Michael, CSW, CAC
New York, 212 691 2312 📖 301
Pantheon of Leather
West Hollywood, 213 656 5073 📖 224
Panther LL, Inc.
Atlanta 📖 244
Paper Shop
Chelmsford 📖 75
Paper Skyscraper
Charlotte, 704 333 7130 📖 314
Pappy's
Lake Charles, 318 436 2819 📖 260
Para Publishing
Santa Barbara, 805 968 7277 📖 221
Parachute 📖 257
Paradis
Frederiksberg, 31 12 6017 📖 66
Paradise 📖 307
Oostende / Ostende, 5 951 3672 📖 39
Paradise Books
Green Bay, 414 432 9498 📖 356
Paradise Club
Parma, 216 586 9292 📖 322
Paradise Sexy Shop
Perugia, 75 527 0121 📖 146
Paradiso Bodyworks
London, 171 287 2487 📖 86
Paragon
Amsterdam 📖 2, 8, 153
Paramour Magazine 📖 269
Paraphernalia from Beyond Planet X
Columbus, 614 272 8984 📖 186
Parent's Enquiry
Dublin, 1 872 1055 📖 136
Edinburgh 📖 168
London, 181 698 1815 📖 82
Parents & Friends of Lesbians & Gays (PFLAG)
Akron, 216 923 1883 📖 317
Ann Arbor, 313 769 1684 📖 274
Annapolis, 410 849 3524 📖 263
Atlanta, 404 691 4729 📖 244
Baltimore, 410 433 3524 📖 264
Bendigo, 53 483 033 📖 31
Berkshire, 413 243 2382 📖 272
Boone, 704 264 4109 📖 313
Boston, 617 547 2440 📖 268
Brampton, 905 457 4570 📖 57
Calgary, 403 282 6592 📖 42
Casper 📖 358
Castle Hill 📖 25
Central Pennsylvania, 717 795 0330 📖 328
Central Susquehanna, 717 742 9350 📖 333
Charlotte, 704 364 1474 📖 314
Chicago, 312 472 3079 📖 250
Chico, 916 891 5718 📖 198
Cleveland, 216 321 7413 📖 319
Cloverdale 📖 33
Colorado Springs, 719 634 2488 📖 227
Columbia, 803 772 7396 📖 335
Connecticut, 203 544 8724 📖 229
Darke County, 513 547 1433 📖 321
Denver, 303 333 0286 📖 228
Des Moines, 515 274 4851 📖 256
Detroit, 810 478 8408 📖 275
Eugene, 503 689 1630 📖 325
Flat Rock, 704 696 8250 📖 315
Flint, 313 631 4910 📖 275
Fox Cities, 414 749 1629 📖 356
Fredericton 📖 48
Gainesville, 904 377 8131 📖 237
Grand Junction, 303 242 2966 📖 229
Grand Rapids, 616 285 9133 📖 276
Greater Chattanooga, 615 875 5750 📖 336
Greater Cincinnati, 513 721 7900 📖 318
Greensboro, 910 274 2100 📖 315
Guelph & Kitchener / Waterloo, 519 623 0492 (Hotline) 📖 49
Hallowell, 207 623 2349 📖 262
Hamilton-Wentworth, 905 528 0854 📖 50
Hartford, 203 633 7184 📖 231
Healdsburg, 707 431 8364 📖 201
Hinsdale, 708 325 8488 📖 250
Houston, 713 862 9020 📖 342
Kalamazoo, 616 327 8107 📖 277
Lafayette, 318 984 2216 📖 260
Lakeshore, 414 458 2506 📖 358
Lansing, 517 349 3612 📖 277
Las Vegas, 702 369 8700 📖 286
Lehigh Valley, 610 439 8755 📖 329
Lincoln, 402 467 4599 📖 285
Long Beach, 310 984 8335 📖 202
Long Island, 516 938 8913 📖 304
Lorain, 216 988 8215 📖 321
Los Angeles, 310 472 8952 📖 204
Louisville, 502 589 3316 📖 259
Madison, 608 271 0270 📖 356
Marin County, 415 479 3535 📖 206
Melbourne, 39 700 7190 📖 32
Memphis, 901 761 1444 📖 337
Mid-Hudson, 914 221 9559 📖 310
Mid-Peninsula, 415 857 1058 📖 222
Minnesota, 612 458 3240 📖 278
Monmouth / Ocean Counties, 908 905 6823 📖 289
National Office, 800 432 6459 📖 188
New Hampshire, 603 623 6023 📖 287
New Orleans, 504 895 3936 📖 261
New York City, 212 463 0629 📖 304
North Jersey, 201 267 8414 📖 289
Norwich, 203 822 9216 📖 232
Omaha, 402 291 6781 📖 285, 286
Orange County, 714 997 8047 📖 221
Orlando, 407 896 0689 📖 240
Pawleys Island 📖 335
Pensacola 📖 241
Philadelphia, 215 572 1833 📖 330
Pioneer Valley, 413 532 4883 📖 266
Pittsburgh, 412 272 4059 📖 332
Portage 📖 277
Portland, 207 766 5158 📖 262
Portland, 503 232 7676 📖 326
Queens, 718 460 4064 📖 304
Raleigh, 919 380 9325 📖 315, 316
Rochester, 716 436 7051 📖 311
Rouge Valley, 503 488 3436 📖 324
Rutland, 802 773 7601 📖 346
Sacramento, 916 444 9510 📖 210
Saint Catharines, 905 934 9933 📖 54
Saint Cloud, 612 259 4238 📖 280
Saint Louis, 314 821 3524 📖 284
San Diego, 619 579 7640 📖 211
San Francisco, 415 921 8850 📖 214
San Juan, 809 726 2888 📖 167
Seattle, 206 325 7724 📖 352
South Australia, 8 837 7108 📖 29
South Bay, 408 270 8182 📖 223
Southeast Region, 704 922 9273 📖 314
Southern Minnesota, 507 282 0484 📖 279
Spokane, 509 624 6671 📖 354
Texas, 915 592 2218 📖 341
Thunder Bay, 807 345 1516 📖 54
Toronto, 416 322 0600 📖 57
Tucson 📖 195
Tulsa, 918 749 4901 📖 324
Tuscaloosa, 205 348 7210 📖 192
Vancouver, 604 688 9378 Ext. 2060 📖 45
Ventura County, 805 644 5863 📖 224
Victoria, 604 688 9378 Ext. 2091 📖 47
Washington Metropolitan Area, 301 439 3524 📖 234
Waterloo, 319 234 6531 📖 257
Westchester, 914 698 3619 📖 304
Western New York, 716 883 0384 📖 298
Western North Carolina, 704 277 7815 📖 313
Wilmington, 910 392 6475 📖 316
Winnipeg, 204 284 5208 📖 47
Winston-Salem, 910 723 6345 📖 316
Parents d'Enfants Homosexuels
Liège / Luik / Luttich, 4 180 3491 📖 38
Parents of Lesbian & Gay Children
Adelaide, 8 267 5366 📖 30
Parents of Lesbians & Gays
Auckland, 9 846 7889 📖 160
Paris Adult Bookstore
Lewiston, 207 784 6551 📖 262
Park Central Counselling
Phœnix, 602 274 0327 📖 193
Parkinson, Phil
London, 181 767 7464 📖 80
Parkview Memorial Hospital
Fort Wayne, 219 484 6636 📖 254
Parkway Books & Videos
Travis, 707 437 9969 📖 223
Parlee Plus/ Equal Time the News 📖 296
Parry Sound - Muskoka AIDS Committee
MacTier, 800 267 2437 (Hotline) 📖 51
Partages
Paris 📖 103
PARTNERS 📖 3
Partners Task Force for Gay & Lesbian Couples
Seattle, 206 955 1206 📖 188
Passages Counseling Center
New York, 516 698 9222 📖 301
Passion
Silkeborg, 86 81 3370 📖 65
Passion Flower
Oakland, 510 601 7750 📖 208
Passion, Our Leather Soul
published by Diamond 📖 253
PASTELS
Leeds, 113 267 4627 📖 94
Pat's Tats
Woodstock, 914 679 4429 📖 312
Paths Untrodden Book Service
New York, 212 661 5997 📖 182
Pathways Counseling Center
Milwaukee, 414 774 4111 📖 357
Patrioli, Tony
Milano 📖 143
Patrol Uniform Club of Texas
San Antonio, 210 533 6001 📖 344
Patterson Printing
Benton Harbor, 616 925 2177 📖 274
Patti, Vincent-John, ACSW
New York, 212 473 3623 📖 301
Paul C Leather
Chicago, 312 508 0848 📖 182, 249
Pavillion Mall Booksellers
Cleveland, 216 831 5035 📖 319
Paws Magazine 📖 307
PAWS Social Club
Johannesburg, 11 794 3620 📖 171
PAYSO 📖 *See* Positivity About Youth Sexual Orientation
Paz y Liberación 📖 343
PBC
Pittsburgh 📖 332
PC Bear Lair
San Mateo 📖 220
PCP
Danville 📖 199
PDA Press, Inc.
Cazenovia, 800 478 3268 📖 355
San Francisco, 800 478 3268 📖 218
PDS 📖 *See* Publishers Distribution Service
PDX-MOTSS 📖 3
Pearls Booksellers
Long Beach, 310 438 8875 📖 203
Pearne, Dennis, Ed.D.
Belmont Center, 617 484 0013 📖 267
Peck, Janet, M.S.
Colchester, 203 537 3977 📖 230
Pediform
published by Eagle Press 📖 338
Peel Health Department - Sexual Health Info-Line
Toronto, 905 840 1333 📖 57
Peel HIV/AIDS Network (PHAN)
Mississauga, 905 890 8770 📖 51
Peer Education Project
London, 181 955 4366 Ext. 4383 📖 83
Peer Support Program
Denver, 303 831 6268 📖 228
PEG 📖 *See* Plymouth Eddystone Group
Pegasus
Raleigh, 919 782 2481 📖 316
Pegasus Leatherworks
Marietta 📖 245
Pegasus Motorcycle Owners Club
San Francisco, 415 334 1166 📖 215
Pegasus Unusual Books
Pocatello, 208 232 6493 📖 247
PEI Gay Phoneline
Charlottetown, 902 566 9733 📖 61
Pendragons of Birminham
Hoover 📖 191
Peninsula AIDS Foundation
Newport News, 804 591 0971 📖 347
Penis Power Quarterly
published by Added Dimensions Publications 📖 208
Penn GALA
Philadelphia 📖 330
Pennine AIDS Link
Bradford, 127 439 5815 📖 94
Pennsmen
Harrisburg 📖 328
Penrose Hospital
Colorado Springs, 719 630 5000 📖 226
Penthouse
published by Penthouse International, Ltd. 📖 307
Penthouse Forum
published by General Media Inc. 📖 307
Penthouse International, Ltd.
New York, 212 496 6100 📖 307
Penthouse Variations
published by General Media Inc. 📖 19
Pentonville Rubber Company
London, 171 837 0283 📖 81
Penzance Lesbian Line
1736 62869 📖 72
People Exchanging Power
Central Florida, 407 678 3388 📖 240
People Exchanging Power (PEP)
Atlanta, 404 621 7961 (voice mail) 📖 244
Nashville 📖 337
Paradise 📖 247
Philadelphia, 215 552 8155 📖 329
Tennessee, 615 648 1937 📖 338
People for Lesbian, Gay, & Bisexual Concerns

Champaign / Urbana, 217 333 1187 248
People In The North
Elizabeth Vale, 8 282 1206 31
People Like Us
Chicago, 312 248 6363 182, 251
People Like You
broadcast by CKCU FM 93.1 53
People Living with AIDS
Perth, 9 221 3002 33
People Living With AIDS (PLWA)
South Australia, 8 362 2799 30
People of Alternate Lifestyles (PALS)
Little Rock, 501 374 3605 195
Owen Sound, 519 371 8707 53
People of Color Against AIDS Network
Seattle, 206 322 7061 351
People With AIDS Coalition
Baltimore, 410 625 1677 263
People With AIDS Coalition Houston, Inc.
713 522 5428 342
People With AIDS Coalition of Long Island, Inc.
New York, 516 225 5797 303
People With AIDS Coalition of Tucson (PACT)
602 770 1710 194
People With HIV/AIDS
Los Angeles, 213 667 3262 203
People With HIV/AIDS Support Group
Durham, 919 286 4107 314
People's Books
Milwaukee, 414 962 0575 357
Peoria City County Health Department
309 679 6028 252
PEP See People Exchanging Power
Pepper's News Stand
Martinsburg, 304 267 6846 355
Pepperland
Bruxelles / Brussel, 2 513 5751 37
Perceptions 64
Perez Books
Cathedral City, 619 321 5597 198
Perforations
Brighton, 127 332 6577 74
Perforations Piercing Studio
Washington, 202 289 8863 234
Perlman, Graham
London, 171 274 2754 80
Perlswig, Ellis, M.D.
New Haven, 203 777 1876 231
Perrin & Treggett Booksellers
Denville, 800 770 8811 290
Perry, Michael, Ph.D.
Encino, 818 784 9199 199
Persad Center, Inc.
Pittsburgh, 412 441 9786 331
Personally Speaking 258
Persons with AIDS Society of British Columbia
Vancouver, 604 681 2122 45
Perth Lesbian & Gay Group
1738 23917 (men) 170
Perth Switchboard
1738 828840 170
Pervert Scouts
San Francisco, 415 285 7985 214
PET See Prevention, Education, & Treatment Center
Peter's Palace
Portsmouth, 603 436 9622 288
Peterborough AIDS Helpline
1733 62334 71
Peterborough AIDS Resource Network
800 361 2895 (information) 54
Peterborough Friend
1733 61499 71
Peterson, Ronald, Ph.D.
Phœnix, 602 234 3500 193
Petruchio
Berkeley 197
PFLAG See Parents & Friends of Lesbians & Gays
PFLAG-TALK 2
pgh.motss 6
PG-Jouren
Stockholm, 20 78 4414 175
Phambili Books
Johannesburg, 11 29 4944 172
PHAN See Peel HIV/AIDS Network
Phantasia Productions
Boston 269
Phase
published by Blasé Ltd. 85
Phi Pi Epsilon
Sverige 175
Phi, Alpha, Gamma
Tucson, 916 753 2090 223
Philadelphia Center
Shreveport, 318 222 6633 261
Philadelphia Community Health Alternatives
215 545 8686 330
Philadelphia Gay News (PGN)
published by Masco Communication 190
Philadelphia Gay Switchboard
215 546 7100 330
Philadelphia Lesbian & Gay Task Force
215 563 9584 330
Philadelphia TS Support Group
215 975 9119 330
Philadelphia Uniform Patrol 330
Philadelphians MC 330
Philippe Moda Pelle
Herentals, 1 421 9103 38
Philly Hair Razors
Atlanta, 215 784 7140 244
Phœnix
Zürich, 1 734 2469 179
Phœnix Books
Kansas City, 816 931 5794 283
Phœnix Bookstore
Lexington, 606 255 9881 259
Phœnix Centre
London 83
Phœnix Counsel, Inc.
Saint Catharines, 905 685 0496 54
Phœnix Men's Room
New Orleans, 504 945 9264 260
Phœnix Press
Portland, 207 282 8091 261
Phœnix Pride Youth Group
Columbus, 614 445 0013 320
Phœnix Project
Aurora 226
Phœnix Resource 193
Phœnix Rising 218
Portland, 503 223 8299 326
Richmond, 804 355 7939 349
San Diego 211
Phœnix Society
Parow East 170
Phœnix Transgender Support
Asheville, 704 259 9428 313
Phœnix Uniform Club
San Francisco, 415 863 3127 214
Phönix
Berlin, 30 213 8580 110
Phun Ink Press
Boulder, 303 575 5652 226
Phylea
Paris, 142 76 0190 104
Physicians Association for AIDS Care
Chicago, 312 222 1326 249
PI Versand
Kirchlinteln, 42 36 1058 107
Pianeta Viola
Brescia, 30 242 1840 142
Piasa Publishing Company
Kansas City, 800 303 5468 283
Saint Louis, 800 301 5468 282
Pic-A-Book
Madison, 608 256 1125 356
Picador, Div. of Pan Macmillan
London 84
Pictou County AIDS Coalition
New Glasgow, 902 755 4647 48
Piedmont Hospital
Atlanta, 404 605 5000 243
Piedmont Triangle Society (PTS)
Charlottesville 347
Piercing Experience
Atlanta, 800 646 0393 244
Piercing Exquisite
Richmond, 804 232 3096 349
Piercing Fans International Quarterly (PFIQ)
published by Gauntlet, Inc. 20
Piercing Urge
Melbourne, 3 9530 2244 24
Sydney, 2 360 3179 27
Piercing World
published by P. A. U. K. 92
Piercings Unlimited
Springfield, 513 322 0877 322
Piercology
Columbus, 614 297 4743 320
Pig Pen
Ottawa 52
Pike's Peak Tattoo
Colorado Springs, 719 632 6141 227
Pike, Ben
Monrovia, 818 358 9582 206
Pikes Peak Gay & Lesbian Community Center Help Line
Colorado Springs, 719 471 4429 227
Pillar of the Gay, Lesbian, & Bisexual Community 345
Pillow Talk
Croydon, 181 688 8197 91
Maidstone, 1622 661504 78
Margate, 1843 294069 78
Pink & Purple
Darmstadt 114
Pink Antenna 59
Pink Channel
broadcast by FM 96.0, Cable 95.4 120
Pink Cross
Bern, 31 372 3300 177
Pink Elephant
broadcast by Dream Team Productions 177
Pink Express 162
Pink Homo
Duisburg, 203 87 1083 115
Pink List
London, 181 964 4523 85
Pink Pages 49
Pink Panther
Villingen-Schwenningen, 772 05 9088 134
Pink Paper 312
published by Silveraim Ltd. 85
Pink Power 111
Pink Practice
London, 181 809 7218 80
Pink Pussy
Adelaide, 8 271 5975 31
Pink Pussycat Boutique
Fort Lauderdale, 305 563 4445 237
Miami, 305 448 7656 239
New York, 212 243 0077 309
Pink Pyramid
Cincinnati, 513 621 7465 318
Pink Shop
Lausanne, 21 311 6969 178
Pink Times 90
Pink Triangle Coalition
Harrisburg 328
Pink Triangle Group
Kuala Lumpur, 3 981 2863 148
Pink Triangle Press
Ottawa, 613 237 7133 42, 53
Toronto, 800 268 9872 59
Vancouver, 604 684 9696 46
Pink Triangle Services Library
Ottawa, 613 563 4818 52
Pink Triangle Youth of Edmonton
403 488 1754 43
Pinkboard
Sydney 26
Pinkpot
Birmingham, 121 476 4627 93
Pipeline
Memphis, 901 726 5263 336
Pipeline Books
London, 171 729 3491 80
Pipeline Bookshop
London, 171 240 3319 85
Pistil Books & News
Seattle, 206 325 5401 353
Pitié-Salpêtrière
Paris, 145 70 2172 103
Pittsburgh AIDS Task Force
412 624 2008 331
Pittsburgh Bondage Club
Philadelphia 330
Pittsburgh Motorcycle Club
412 795 5968 332
Places of Interest
published by Ferrari Publications 189
Plain Brown Wrapper II
Grand Forks, 701 772 9021 317
Plains FM 96.9
Christchurch 161
Plakidas, Nicolas
München, 89 314 3540 128
Planet 23 Productions
Boston 269
Planet Alice
Grenoble, 76 42 7032 100
Planet Homo 225, 239
Planet K
Austin, 512 443 2292 338
San Antonio, 512 654 8536 344
Planet Sex Ball
London, 171 739 0388 80
Planet Sex The Handbook
published by The Leydig Trust 15
Planning Familial
Luxembourg, 48 5976 148
Plastic Cow Productions
Danville, 510 736 2153 198
Platinum Video
Sherman Oaks, 818 503 0280 187
Plato's Bookstore
Wichita, 316 269 9036 258
Platt, Keith Allen, LCSW
West Palm Beach, 407 835 3934 243
Platzjabbeck
Köln, 221 21 8173 124
Playboy 251
PLAYBOY MAILING LIST 3
Playgirl 307
Playguy
published by MMG Services Inc. 307
Playland Magazine 220
Playmates
Hollywood, 213 464 7636 201
Playspace
Seattle, 206 329 0324 352
Pleasurable Alternatives
Hawthorne, 201 238 0305 290
Pleasurable Piercings, Inc.
Hawthorne, 201 238 0305 290
Pleasure
Hannover 122
Kassel, 561 77 4437 123
Pleasure Bound
published by Olympia Publishing (UK) Ltd. 19
Pleasure Chest
Chicago, 312 525 7151 252
Miami, 305 448 2214 239
New York, 212 242 2158 309
Philadelphia, 215 561 7480 331
West Hollywood, 800 753 4536 (orders) 225
Pleasure Dome
Norfolk 348
Pleasure Palace
New York, 212 265 5213 309
Pleasure Palace I
Iowa City, 319 351 9444 257
Pleasure Palace II
Ames, 515 232 7717 256
Pleasure Place
Washington, 202 333 8570 235
Washington, 202 483 3297 235
Washington, 800 386 2386 10
Pleasure Spot
Sydney, 2 361 0433 24
Pleasure Zone
Atlanta, 404 414 1137 245
Pleasureland
Austin, 512 478 2339 339
San Diego, 619 237 9056 212
Pleasures Entertainment Centers, Inc.
Denver, 303 722 5892 229
Plus Voice 251
PLUSS
Oslo, 22 11 4900 164
Plusvoice
Chicago, 312 929 9761 249
PLWA See People Living With AIDS
Plymouth Eddystone Group (PEG)
1752 251666 73
PMC Transgender Counseling & Consultation
Coralville, 319 354 3189 1
pnw.motss 6
Poach Gay Guide 189
Pocket Guide to Hawaii 247

Pocono Warriors
Woodbridge 📖 293
Poconos Action Lambda Society
Milford 📖 327
Point Gai
Paris, 47 20 5530 📖 103
Pointer to Sex Information on the Net (PtSlotN) 📖 15
Pokey's Place
Lewisville 📖 343
POLEN
Mexico City 📖 149
Policlinico
Bari, 80 27 1111 📖 144
Napoli, 81 45 5365 📖 140
Policlinico di Careggi
Firenze, 55 439 9620 📖 145
Policlinico Gemelli
Roma, 6 330527 📖 141
Polished Knob
published by Planet 23 Productions 📖 269
Polk Gay & Lesbian Alliance
Lakeland, 813 644 0085 📖 238
POLY 📖 4
POLY-BOSTON 📖 267
Polyester Books
Melbourne, 3 9419 5223 📖 33
POLYFIDELITY 📖 4
Polymorph Body Art Gallery
Sydney, 2 519 8923 📖 27
Pop As
München, 89 260 9191 📖 127
Porcupine's Quill Inc.
Erin, 519 833 9158 📖 49
Porno Pen
published by Amador Communications 📖 20
Port City Press, Inc.
New York, 212 921 9166 📖 306
Port Kar BBS
Toronto 📖 55
Porter Memorial Hospital
Denver, 303 778 1955 📖 227
Porter, Theresa, Psy.D.
Meriden, 203 237 8978 📖 231
Portland Power & Trust 📖 326
Portsmouth Lesbian & Gay Switchboard
1705 655 077 📖 76
Positif
Roma, 6 488 1859 📖 141
Positiivi-yhdistys
Helsinki, 90 685 1846 📖 96
Positiva Gruppen
Stockholm, 8 720 1960 📖 175
Positive Action
Camberley, 127 668 6377 📖 91
Positive Action Coalition of Kansas, Inc. (PACK)
Topeka 📖 257
Positive Action for HIV
Lancaster, 800 220704 📖 78
Positive Advocacy
York, 13774 229133 📖 88
Positive Friends
Melbourne, 39 481 3413 📖 32
Positive Image
Pomona, 909 622 6312 📖 11
Positive People Portsmouth
1705 816429 📖 76
Positive Place
London, 181 694 9988 📖 82
Positive Straight Men
Toronto, 416 923 3253 📖 56
Positive Support
Nottingham, 115 942 5133 📖 89
Positive Times
published by Silveraim Ltd. 📖 69
Positive Women's Network
Vancouver, 604 681 2122 📖 45
Positive Youth Outreach
Toronto, 416 506 1400 📖 56
Positively East
London 📖 82
Positively Friends 📖 226
Positively Irish Action on AIDS
London, 181 983 4293 📖 82
Positively Women
London, 171 490 2327 📖 67
Positivgruppen
Frederiksberg, 38 33 3244 📖 66
Positivia Gruppen-Väst
Göteborg, 70 760 7092 📖 173
Positivity About Youth Sexual Orientation (PAYSO)
London, 519 434 1604 📖 51
Post
Vancouver 📖 45
Post Option Business Center
Seattle, 206 322 2777 📖 353
Poster Hut
Atlanta, 404 633 7491 📖 245
Potomac Area Lifestyles
Baltimore 📖 264
Potomac Area Polyamory Network
Silver Spring, 301 587 1193 📖 266
Potomac MC
Washington 📖 234
Poughkeepsie Gay & Lesbian Alliance (GALA)
914 473 1500 📖 310
Pourquoi Pas?
Saarbrücken, 681 417018 📖 132
Powder Puffs of California (PPOC)
Yorba Linda, 714 779 9013 📖 226
Powell's City of Books
Portland, 800 228 7323 📖 327
Power Circle
Santa Cruz 📖 221
Power Exchange
Walkersville 📖 266
Power of Passion
Oldenburg 📖 130
Power Play
Salt Lake City 📖 345
Power Xchange
published by Pacific Force 📖 201
Power, John, MSW
Chicago, 312 327 9886 📖 249
POWERarts Presence Provider
Toronto, 416 962 9696 📖 55
PowerPlay
published by Brush Creek Media 📖 217
Powys AIDS Line Services (PALS)
Llandrindod Wells, 1597 824200 📖 359
POZ 📖 307
PPOC 📖 *See* Powder Puffs of California
PPS. Gallery
Berlin 📖 111
Prairie Lights Bookstore
Iowa City, 319 337 2681 📖 257
Prairie Moon
Arlington Heights, 708 342 9608 📖 247
Prairie Rose Gender Club
Dugald, 204 257 2759 📖 47
Precision Body Piercing
Oakland, 510 547 7751 📖 208
Precision Metal
Sunnyvale 📖 223
Preferred Stock 📖 228
Prenzelberger AIDS Projekt 📖 110
Presbyterian Hospital
Charlotte, 704 384 4942 📖 313
Oklahoma City, 405 271 5100 📖 323
Presbyterian Hospital in the City of New York
212 305 2500 📖 302
President News
Fayetteville 📖 315
Prestige Periodical Distributors
Port Chester, 914 939 2362 📖 2
Preston Bisexual Group 📖 79
Preston Gay Information Service
1772 51122 📖 79
Preston Graphics
Sunrise 📖 242
Prevention Auckland
9 357 0415 📖 160
Prevention, Education, & Treatment Center (PET)
Miami, 305 538 0525 📖 239
Priape
Montréal, 800 461 6969 📖 41, 63
Toronto, 800 461 6969 📖 60
Priarie Lesbian & Gay Community
Moorhead, 701 237 0556 📖 281
Pride & Unity for Male Prostitutes (PUMP)
Auckland 📖 159
Christchurch 📖 161
Dunedin 📖 161
Wellington, 4 382 8791 📖 163
Pride Agenda Bookshop
Chicago, 708 524 8429 📖 251
Pride at UIC
Chicago, 312 996 4424 📖 250
Pride Bookstore
Norfolk, 804 855 8450 📖 348
Pride FM
broadcast by G-Spot Productions 📖 74
Pride in Life, Gays & Lesbians of Southeastern New Brunswick
Riverview, 506 855 8064 📖 48
Pride Leathers
Rochester, 716 242 7840 📖 311
Pride Path Magazine 📖 298
Pride Publishing & Typesetting, Inc.
Charlotte, 704 531 9988 📖 313
Pride Publishing & Typsetting, Inc.
Charlotte, 704 531 9988 📖 314
Pride S. I. S.
Kapiti / Horowhenua, 6 368 1195 📖 162
Pride, Inc.
Helena, 406 549 4466 📖 285
PRIDENET
published by PRIDENET, Incorporated 📖 59
PRIDENET, Incorporated
Toronto, 416 955 9050 📖 59
Prime
published by Virtual Universe Publications Ltd. 📖 85
Prime Timers International
Manchaca, 512 282 2681 📖 344
Primeval Body
Los Angeles, 213 666 9601 📖 204
Primitive Leather
Northampton 📖 272
Prince George AIDS Society
604 562 1172 📖 44
Prince Institute
Palm Springs 📖 208
Prince William Gay & Lesbian Association
Woodbridge 📖 350
Princeton Hospital
Orlando, 407 295 5151 📖 240
Prinz Eisenherz Buchladen
Berlin, 30 313 9936 📖 111
Priscilla's
Waterville, 207 873 2774 📖 263
Prism 📖 46
Private Case
Royston 📖 67
Private Pleasures
Toronto, 416 237 0626 📖 60
Private Tymes
published by Phun Ink Press 📖 226
Privaty Shop
La Spezia, 187 52 4268 📖 142
Pro Familia Homosexuellenberatung
Duisburg, 203 35 0700 📖 115
Hannover, 511 36 3606 📖 121
Professional Body Piercing by Jack
Santa Barbara, 805 962 0296 📖 221
Professional Medical Products
Greenwood, 803 223 4281 📖 335
Professional Press
Chapel Hill, 919 942 8020 📖 313
Pro-Fun
Frankfurt am Main, 69 59 3590 📖 107
Program for Gay, Lesbian, & Bisexual Concerns
Amherst, 413 545 4824 📖 267
Progress Tribune 📖 335
Project 10
Montréal, 514 989 4585 📖 62
Project AIDS Lafayette (PAL)
800 524 3229 (in state) 📖 255
Project Inform
San Francisco, 800 822 7422 📖 213, 214
Project Lazarus
New Orleans, 504 949 3609 📖 261
Project Sigma
London 📖 83
Project X 📖 307
Projet X
published by Editions du Triangle Rose 📖 18
Prostitutes for Safer Sex Project
Toronto, 416 964 0150 📖 56
Proteus
Halle (Saale), 345 50 3649 📖 119
Proud Out Loud 📖 294
Provenant Saint Anthony Hospital
Denver, 303 629 3511 📖 227
Providence Hospital
Anchorage, 907 562 2211 📖 192
Washington, 202 269 7000 📖 233
Provincetown Advocate 📖 272
Provincetown Bookshop
508 487 0964 📖 272
Provincetown Magazine 📖 272
Provincetown Positive PWA Coalition
508 487 3998 📖 272
Provincetown Purchase Company
508 487 3232 📖 272
Prowler Press Ltd.
London, 181 348 9963 📖 67
PSGV Transgendered Group
Pomona, 909 620 8987 📖 209
Psychology & Counselling Associates
San Francisco, 415 863 9559 📖 213
Psychotherapeutische Beratungsstelle
Bielefeld, 521 12 3216 📖 111
Psychotherapy Center
Little Rock, 501 374 3605 📖 195
Psychotherapy Institute
Toronto, 416 968 0640 📖 55
PTS 📖 *See* Piedmont Triangle Society
PtSlotN 📖 *See* Pointer to Sex Information on the Net
Public Access Television
New Orleans, 214 351 1901 📖 261
Public Eye
London, 181 840 4027 📖 79
Public Health Clinic
Miami, 305 324 2434 📖 239
Public Health STD Centre
Palmerston North, 6 350 8602 📖 162
Public House Bookshop
Brighton, 127 328 357 📖 74
Publicació Degana del Moviment Gai a Catalunya
Barcelona, 93 318 1666 📖 172
Publications Nouvelles
Paris, 148 24 3955 📖 97
Publishers Distribution Service (PDS)
Traverse City, 616 929 0733 📖 278
Publishers Group West
Emeryville, 510 658 3453 📖 199
Publishers Press
Salt Lake City, 801 972 6600 📖 345
Publishers Weekly 📖 307
Pulse Magazine 📖 170
PUMP 📖 *See* Pride & Unity for Male Prostitutes
Pump It Up!
published by Mirza, Inc. 📖 292
Purdue Gay Alliance
Lafayette, 812 497 2712 📖 255
Pure
London, 171 394 1717 📖 81
Pure Imagination
Marietta, 770 424 5151 📖 14
Purple Moon
Fredericksburg 📖 348
Purple Passion
New York, 212 807 0486 📖 309
Purple Stone Press & Productions
Malden, 617 321 3569 📖 271
Purr...effect
Sydney, 2 332 1370 📖 27
Puss'N'Boots
Memphis, 901 276 9970 📖 337
Pussy Cat
published by Black Box Productions Ltd. 📖 84
Pussywhipped!
published by Six of the Best Publishing 📖 18
PW Multitek Services
London, 181 960 5759 📖 81
PWA Coalition
Broward County, 3305 565 9119 📖 236
Hawaii, 808 948 4792 📖 246
San Antonio, 210 545 4357 (hotline) 📖 344
PWA Coalition Colorado
Denver, 303 837 8214 📖 228
PWA Coalition of Dade County

Miami, 305 576 1111 📖 239
PWA Coalition of Maine
Portland, 207 773 8500 📖 261
PWA Coalition of New York, Inc.
800 828 3280 (hotline) 📖 303
PWA Coalition of Palm Beach
West Palm Beach, 407 697 8033 📖 243
PWA Coalition of Tampa Bay
813 238 2887 📖 242
PWA Support Groups
Asheville, 704 277 7815 📖 313
PWAlive Publications, Inc.
Minneapolis / Saint Paul, 612 640 7927 📖 281
Px3
Chicago, 312 854 6172 📖 252
Q & M Stores
Birmingham, 121 458 4614 📖 93
Birmingham, 121 771 3134 📖 93
Q Community Events Calendar 📖 163
Q Notes
published by Pride Publishing & Typsetting, Inc. 📖 314
Q Things
London, 171 384 2129 📖 10
Q. W. Hq. P.
Boston 📖 267
qc Magazine
Calgary, 403 630 2061 📖 42
published by qc Magazine 📖 42
QG
Paris, 148 87 7418 📖 102
Q-GLU 📖 *See* Queens Gay & Lesbians United
QN 📖 3
QNA 📖 4
Qpido
Malmö 📖 174
QRC 📖 *See* Queer Resource Center
QSA 📖 2
QSM
San Francisco, 800 537 5815 📖 7
QSTUDY-L 📖 2
QuAC Voice
broadcast by 4TTT FM 103.9 📖 29
Quad Cities AIDS Coalition
Davenport, 319 324 8638 📖 256
Quad-City Society for Sexuality Education
Davenport, 319 324 6941 📖 256
Quadland, Michael, Ph.D.
New York, 212 691 1617 📖 301
Quälgeister - FSG Berlin e.V.
30 694 7829 📖 110
Quality Books
Lake Bluff, 708 295 2010 📖 252
Quality Control
Birmingham 📖 93
Quality Paperback Book Club
New York, 212 522 4200 📖 181
Quartet Books Limited
London 📖 84
Quasimode
Hannover 📖 122
Quebecor America Book Group
New York, 212 827 2700 📖 306
Queen Margaret College L&G Society
Edinburgh, 131 339 3961 📖 169
Queen's Medical Center
Oahu, 808 538 9011 📖 247
Queen, Carol
San Francisco, 415 978 0891 📖 216
Queens Gay & Lesbians United (Q-GLU)
New York, 718 639 4951 📖 305
Queens Hospital Center
New York, 718 883 3000 📖 302
Queensboro Community College Lesbian & Gay Male Alliance
New York, 718 631 6212 📖 305
Queensland AIDS Committee
Gold Coast, 7 538 4611 📖 29
Townsville, 7 721 1384 📖 28
Queensland AIDS Council
Brisbane, 7 844 1990 📖 28
Cairns, 7 051 1028 📖 29
Noosa, 7 443 7702 📖 29
Surfer's Paradise, 7 532 2673 📖 29
Toowooba, 7 639 1820 📖 29
Townsville, 7 721 1384 📖 29
Queensland Bisexual Network
Brisbane 📖 29
Queensland Positive People
Brisbane, 7 846 3939 📖 28
Queensland Pride 📖 29
Queer Biz Oy
Helsinki, 0 7002 8710 📖 96
Queer Community
Grinnell 📖 256
Queer Guide - Brighton 📖 74
Queer Press
Toronto, 416 978 8201 📖 58
Queer Press, Inc.
Tallahassee, 904 671 7982 📖 235
Queer Program
broadcast by Warner Cable Channel 47 📖 357
Queer Resource Center (QRC)
Berkeley, 510 643 8929 📖 197
Queer Talk
broadcast by WFTL Radio 📖 237
Queer TV 📖 27
Queer Words 📖 359
QueerAmerica
published by OutProud! 📖 189
QUEERCAMPUS 📖 4
Queer-e 📖 22
Querelle
Milano, 2 68 3900 📖 142
Query 📖 336
Quest Bookshop
Charlottesville, 800 346 9223 📖 347
Quest Magazine
published by Quest Publications 📖 226
Quest Publications
Denver, 303 722 5965 📖 226
Question de Genre
Lille, 20 06 3391 📖 2
QUIM 📖 84
Quimby's Queer Store
Chicago, 312 342 0910 📖 252
Quintessential Transfigurations
Calgary, 403 270 7550 📖 43
QUT Campus Queers
Brisbane 📖 29
QX 📖 85
R B Books
Slough, 175 353 9565 📖 71
R. K. Unlimited
Milwaukee, 414 342 1411 📖 186
R. L.
Bristol 📖 230
R. O. S. PO.
Milano 📖 143
R. R. Bowker
New Providence, 908 665 2883 📖 292
R. R. Donnelly & Sons
Chicago, 312 326 8000 📖 250
R2B2 Books
Vancouver, 604 732 5087 📖 46
Racine News
414 634 9827 📖 358
Racine, Christianne
Ottawa, 613. 562 0523 📖 52
Rack
Lexington, 606 233 7266 📖 259
Radford Alternative Alliance 📖 348, 349
Rådgivningskontoret mot AIDS
Tønsberg, 33 31 6840 📖 167
Rådgivningstjenesten for Homofile
Trondheim, 73 52 3330 📖 166
Rådgivningstjenesten for Homofile og Lesbiske i Tromsø
77 68 5643 📖 166
Radiance, The Magazine For Large Women 📖 22
Radical Chick 📖 308
Radical Faerie Circle
Chicago, 312 235 8315 📖 250
Russian River, 707 887 9851 📖 199
Radical Leather
Sydney, 2 331 7544 📖 27
Radio & TV Interview Report
broadcast by Bradley Communications Corporation 📖 329
Radio Active FM 89
Wellington 📖 163
Radio Bigoudi
broadcast by Radio Campus FM 91.4 📖 100
Radio Campus FM 91.4
Lille 📖 100
Radio Centraal FM 101.6
Antwerpen / Anvers, 3 236 5076 📖 36
Radio Città Aperta FM 99.8 & 100.1
Mestre 📖 146
Radio Dreyekland
broadcast by FM 104.6 📖 105
Radio Filzlaus
broadcast by Wiener Warmenradio FM 107.3 📖 35
Radio Gribouille
broadcast by FM 99.7 📖 98
Radio Lightfire
broadcast by FM 96.0, Cable 95.4 📖 120
Radio Onda Rossa FM 93.3 & 93.45
Roma, 6 491750 📖 141
Radio One FM 91
Blenheim 📖 161
Radio Popolare FM 105.5 & 107.6
Milano, 2 80 8249 📖 143
Radio Punto Stereo FM 88.5, 103.5
Pesaro 📖 143
Radio Rosa
broadcast by FM 106.7, 92.2, 89.5, & 98.7 📖 65
broadcast by FM 98.9 📖 66
Radio SETA
broadcast by FM 100.3 📖 96
Radio Studio Aperto FM 88.25
Torino 📖 139
Radio Tilla
broadcast by FM 107.1 & 97.8 📖 124
Radio Toinen linja
broadcast by FM 96.2 📖 96
RAGE 📖 *See* Rosa Aktionsgruppe Essen
Rage Fashions
Birmingham, 121 233 4488 📖 93
Raging Rhino Productions
Hollywood 📖 238
RAGLC 📖 *See* Rutland Area Gay & Lesbian Connection
Railey, Julie, ACSW
Lansing, 517 332 1449 📖 277
Raiments
Pasadena 📖 182
Rainbow Books
Thunder Bay, 807 345 6272 📖 55
Rainbow Bookshop
Winterthur, 52 213 8188 📖 179
Rainbow Bookstore
Columbus, 614 297 1500 📖 321
Rainbow Center
Macon, 912 750 8080 📖 245
Rainbow Clinic
London, 171 346 3488 📖 80
Rainbow Gender Alliance (RGA)
San José, 408 984 4044 (recording) 📖 219
Rainbow MC
San Francisco 📖 215
Rainbow People
Tucson 📖 195
Rainbow Radio Network
broadcast by CHRW 94.7 FM 📖 51
Rainbow Revolution
La Crosse 📖 356
Rainbow Youth Trust
Auckland, 9 376 4155 📖 160
Rainbows Ltd.
Huntsville, 205 722 9220 📖 192
Rainmakers Club
New York 📖 306
Rainvain
Bothell 📖 183
Ram Bookstore
Chicago, 312 525 9528 📖 252
Ram Leathers
Brighton, 127 350 8272 📖 69
Ramrod
Boston, 617 266 2986 📖 267
Rana Helseråd
5 15 2500 📖 165
Ranch & Cuffs
Albuquerque, 505 275 1616 📖 294
Rand Gay Organization (RGO)
Johannesburg, 11 932 2713 📖 171
Rangers
Cleveland 📖 319
Rangers MC
Brisbane 📖 28
RAP
Los Angeles, 213 964 1637 📖 204
Raphael, Jerry, Ph.D.
New York, 212 982 6135 📖 301
Rapids AIDS Project
Cedar Rapids, 319 393 9579 📖 256
Rapture
Santa Rosa 📖 222
Rat & Tat
Rostock 📖 131
Rat & Tat Rosa Telefon
Saarbrücken, 681 37 4650 📖 132
Rat & Tat Zentrum
Bremen, 421 70 4170 📖 113
Ratgeber Schwul Darmstadt
615 16 5384 📖 114
Raunch
published by Tom's Ranch 📖 194
Raven in the Grove
Pacific Grove, 408 649 6057 📖 208
Rawhide
New Orleans, 504 525 8106 📖 260
New York, 212 242 9332 📖 300
RAWhips
Eugene 📖 187
Ray's Playpen
Kansas City, 816 753 7692 📖 283
RBW Graphics
Mississauga, 905 677 7468 📖 51
RCDC 📖 *See* Rose City Discussion Club
RCGA 📖 *See* River City Gender Alliance
RDU FM 98.3
Christchurch 📖 161
Re/Search Publications
San Francisco, 415 362 1465 📖 15
Reach HIV Support Group
Wolverhampton, 1902 25702 📖 94
Reachout of Saint Lawrence County, Inc.
Potsdam, 315 265 2422 📖 310
Reactive Metals Studio, Inc.
Clarkdale, 602 634 3434 📖 193
Read All About It
Brighton, 127 320 5824 📖 74
Read All Over
Sarasota, 813 923 1340 📖 242
Reader's Feast
Hartford, 203 232 2710 📖 231
Reading Lesbian & Gay Helpline
1734 597269 📖 71
Reading Railmen 📖 333
Real World Emporium
Lansing, 517 487 6495 📖 182
rec.arts.bodyart 📖 5
rec.arts.erotica 📖 4
Recast Educations & Informational Network
Dallas / Fort Worth 📖 341
Record 📖 308
RECOVERY 📖 4
Red & Black Books Collective
Seattle, 206 322 7323 📖 353
Red Admiral Project
London 📖 67
Red Barn Adult Bookstore
Berlin, 609 767 1525 📖 289
Red Devil Studios
West Hollywood, 213 851 0445 📖 225
Red Door Clinic
Minneapolis / Saint Paul, 612 348 6363 📖 279
Red Earth Bears
Oklahoma City, 405 557 1169 📖 323
Red Hankies of San Diego
619 688 8668 📖 211
Red Herring Coöp Books
Halifax, 902 422 5087 📖 48
Red Lantern Books
Hartford, 203 289 5000 📖 231
Red Lights Sex Center
Tampere 📖 95
Red Plaid
published by The James Publishing Group, Inc. 📖 251
Red Ring Studios
Richmond, 317 966 4667 📖 255
Red River Books
Cambourne, 1209 714805 📖 72
Red Rock Mental Health Center
Oklahoma City, 405 425 0399 📖 323
Red Sky Publishing, Limited

London, 171 627 5155 84
Redboard Video
San Francisco, 415 296 8712 218
Redbook
Boston, 617 522 1464 269, 270
Redeemer
published by Redemption Films 84
Redemption
published by Borxan Publications 22
Redemption Films
London 84
Redwood Empire Agency
Guernville, 707 869 1146 200
Re-Enchantment for Women
London 82
Referat für Schwule & Lesben
Rostock, 381 379 2481 131
Reflection House
Pleasant Grove, 801 224 4737 345
Reflections
East Dedham 270
Refuge
Charlotte, 704 372 5499 314
Regal Mag & Toy Shop
Nelson 162
Regalia
Schenectady, 518 374 1900 311
Regard
published by Infor Homo 36
Regenbogen Buchhandlung
Nürnberg, 911 33 7785 130
Regensburger Schwulen & Lesben Initiative (RESI)
941 5 1441 131
Regiment of the Black & Tans
Los Angeles, 818 893 1966 204
Regina Gayline
306 569 0125 64
Regina Students Homophile Society, Inc.
306 522 7343 64
Regional Hospital
Limerick, 61 281 11 138
Regional Medical Center at Memphis
901 575 7100 336
Registrar of Copyrights
Washington, 202 707 6372 234
Regulation
London, 171 226 0665 86
Regulator Bookshop
Durham, 919 286 2700 315
Rekroom
Calgary, 403 265 4749 42
Relais d'Espérance
Québec, 418 522 3301 63
Relatives Group
Århus 65
relcom.sci.libraries 5
Religion
Bristol, 117 929 3754 70
Reluctant Press
Alexandria 347
Remawear
Todmorden 68
Remedy Versand
Hamburg, 40 24 5979 10, 120
Rem-mer Ltd.
Amityville, 516 753 2677 296
Renaissance Books
Springfield, 417 883 5161 284
Renaissance Education Association, Inc.
Baltimore 264
Delaware, 302 995 1396 233
Greater Philadelphia, 610 957 9119 327
Head Office, 610 975 9119 333
Lower Susquehanna Valley, 717 780 1578 328
Northern New Jersey, 201 663 0772 291
Renaissance House
New York, 212 674 0120 306, 308
Renas Boutique
Seymor, 203 888 5164 183
Renate Buccone
København, 31 22 1041 66
Rendel, Brian, M.A, NCC
Dowagiac, 616 782 9811 275
Rendez-Vous
published by Chaud Business SPRL 37
Rendezvous Lounge
Atlantic City, 609 347 8539 289
Renegade Bears
Seattle, 206 823 6639 351
Renegades
New York, 201 217 1646 (recorded message) 304
Rennaissance
South Jersey, 609 435 5401 291
Reno Informer 287
Reno's Leather Underground
Sparks 287
Rensselaer Gay, Lesbian, & Bisexual Alliance
Albany, 518 271 2655 296
Repentence
London 82
Report
published by ST Publishing 85
Reporter 176
Research Medical Center
Kansas City, 816 276 4000 283
RESI *See* Regensburger Schwulen & Lesben Initiative
Resource Center
San Antonio, 210 732 0751 344
Resources for Feminist Research
published by OISE 59
Resources Mailing Lists
Boston, 617 825 8895 269
Respect
Hamilton 162
Response of Suffolk County
New York, 516 751 7500 302
Restrictive Practice
Newport Pagnell 69
RETHINKING AIDS 2
Retro Systems
San Francisco 18
Return to Sender
Vancouver, 604 683 6363 46
Review
Villa Park, 708 620 6946 253
Revolt Shop
Hamburg, 40 31 2848 121
REW Video
San José, 800 528 1942 181
Rex Hospital
Raleigh, 919 783 3100 315
Reynolds, Jan, M.A., MFCC
Los Angeles, 213 937 3787 203
RFD 336
RFSL *See* Riksförbundet för Sexuellt Likaberättigande
RGA *See* Rainbow Gender Alliance
RGL Designs
Nelson, 1282 697866 9
RGN
Frattochie, 6 93 54 7567 22
RGO *See* Rand Gay Organization
Rhinocerous Books
New York, 800 458 9640 (credit card orders) 306
Rhode Island College Gay, Lesbian, or Bisexual Equality Alliance (GLOBE)
Providence 334
Rhode Island Grizzlies
Riverside, 410 727 8840 334
Rhode Island Hospital
Providence, 401 444 4000 334
Rhode Island Project / AIDS
Providence, 401 831 5522 334
Ribakoff, Robin, M.F.C.T.
Encino, 818 957 4065 199
Richard Kasak Books
New York, 800 458 9640 (credit card orders) 306
Richard Roudebush Veterans' Affairs Medical Center
Indianapolis, 317 635 7401 254
Richards, Janet
Toronto, 416 588 2030 55
Richland Memorial Hospital
Columbia, 803 434 6512 335
Richmond AIDS Information Network
804 358 2437 349
Richmond Area Bisexual Network (ROBIN)
804 355 7939 349
Richmond Pride 349
Richmond Street Outreach Project
804 359 4783 349
Richmond, Gary
Portland, 503 283 9571 326
Rider Upholstery
Seattle, 206 323 5593 351
Riders MC
Boston 268
Riemer Foundation
Chicago, 312 935 7233 249
Riga
San Francisco, 415 552 1525 218
Right Hand Productions
Bussum, 21 591 4288 154
Right to Privacy, Inc.
Portland, 503 228 5825 326
Rik Production
Hamburg, 40 24 5979 119, 120
Riksförbundet för Sexuellt Likaberättigande (RFSL)
Borås, 33 10 6970 176
Eskilstuna 175
Falun, 23 28485 173
Gävle, 26 18 0967 173
Göteborg, 31 11 0133 173
Göteborg, 31 11 6151 173
Halland, 35 21 4800 173
Helsingborg, 42 12 3532 174
Karlstad, 54 15 2090 176
Kristianstad, 54 10 6590 174
Linköping, 13 13 2022 174
Luleå, 920 17055 174
Lund, 46 15 7134 174, 175
Malmö, 40 11 9962 174
Norrköping, 11 23 8250 174
Nyköping, 155 21 0229 175
Örebro, 19 14 4232 174
Östersund, 63 10 0668 173
Piteå älvdal & norra Västerbotten, 910 22222 174
Piteå älvdal & norra Västerbotten, 911 14440 174
Rådgivningen, 40 611 9950 173
Rådgivningen, 8 736 0210 175
Stockholm, 8 736 0213 175
Sundsvall, 60 17 1330 174
Trollhätan, 520 11766 176
Umeå, 90 11 4710 176
Uppsala, 18 23 4750 176
Väterås, 21 11 8041 176
Vätterstad, 36 18 8360 175
Växjö, 470 20808 175
Rila, Margo
San Francisco, 415 861 4551 213
Riley Snow, Wynelle, M.D.
Bristol, 860 582 1178 229
Rimba
Prinsenbeek, 76 541 4484 150
Ring
Hayward, 415 522 9697 201
Ringed Men
Rozelle 25
Ringmasters
Sun Valley 187
Rings & Things
Brighton, 127 367 0619 74
Montclair, 201 783 9633 291
Rings of Desire
New Orleans, 504 524 6147 261
Rip Off Press, Inc.
Auburn, 800 468 2669 196
Ripcord Houston
713 521 2792 342
Ripplesmooth
Birmingham, 121 515 1994 11
Rising Moon Books & Beyond
Charlotte, 704 332 7473 314
Rising Tide Press
Huntington Station, 516 427 1289 299
Risque's
Minot, 701 839 9033 317
Rita Dean Gallery
San Diego, 619 338 8153 212
Rites of Passage
Allston, 617 783 1918 266
Ritual
Albuquerque, 505 255 1549 294
Ritual Magazine
published by Ritual World 84
Ritual Shoes
London, 171 287 2096 86
Ritual World
London, 171 287 1025 84
Rivendell Marketing Company
Westfield, 908 232 2021 190
River Bears
Cincinnati 318
River Bend Vision 256
River City Gender Alliance (RCGA)
Council Bluffs 256
River City Outlaws
San Antonio 344
Riverboat Gamblers Motorcycle Club
Memphis, 901 276 9939 337
RLGA *See* Rockland Lesbian Gay Alliance
RM Distribution, Ltd.
Kirkland, 514 851 0264 16
Venice, 310 289 1412 19
Roach, Barbara, L.C.S.W.
Long Beach, 310 424 1755 202
Road Riders MC
Corpus Christi 339
Roads Less Travelled
Boise, 208 375 9090 182
Roanoke AIDS Project
703 982 2437 349
Roanoke Memorial Hospital
703 981 7000 349
RoB
Amsterdam, 20 625 4686 153
London, 171 735 7893 86
San Francisco, 415 252 1198 219
Robert Gordon University LGB Society
Aberdeen 168
Roberts, Lynne, CSW, ACSW
New York, 212 749 1596 301
ROBIN *See* Richmond Area Bisexual Network
Robin & Rik Leathermakers
Amsterdam, 20 627 8924 153
Robin's Books
Philadelphia, 215 567 2615 331
Rochdale Lesbian & Gay Switchboard
1706 59964 76
Rochester Custom Leathers
800 836 9047 311
Rochester General Hospital
716 338 4000 310
Rochester Rams MC
716 244 9812 311
Rock Valley Bears
Rockford, 815 963 7962 253
Rockland Lesbian Gay Alliance (RLGA)
New York, 914 353 6925 305
Rocky Mountain Lambda Lions
Denver 228
Rocky Mountain Oyster
published by Mountain Top Publishing 228
Rocky Mountaineers MC
Denver, 303 733 7047 228
Rocquet, Olivier
Montréal La Cluse 101
Rodeo Riders
Chicago 250
Rodgers, Luanna, M.A., MFCC
San Francisco, 415 641 8890 213
Rogers, Linda, Ph.D.
Saint Louis, 314 727 1907 284
Rogue-Hagen Publications
Derby 73
Rogues LLC
Roanoke 349
Romano, Nino, CSW, MSW
New York, 212 242 2896 301
Romantasy
San Francisco, 415 673 3137 Ext. 03 23
Rome Enterprises, Inc.
Royal Oak, 810 545 9040 278
Rome Gay News
published by RGN 22
Romeo & Julius
Ingolstadt 122
Romeo Trading Co. Ltd.
London, 171 607 7212 87
Rondelle, Gordon
London, 171 485 0134 83
Roode Hand
Den Haag, 70 364 8861 154
Roodhorst
Amsterdam, 20 624 5181 153

Rooie Rat
Utrecht, 30 231 7189 🕮 151
Room of One's Own
Madison, 608 257 7888 🕮 356
Roosevelt Hospital
New York, 212 523 4000 🕮 302
Rosa Aktionsgruppe Essen (RAGE)
201 23 6096 🕮 116
Rosa Blum
Gelnhausen, 605 11 2561 🕮 118
Rosa Engel-SchwulLesbische Aktion Hamm
Hamburg, 238 1 5575 🕮 120
Rosa Greif-Schwul-Lesbischer AK im Vorpommern e. V.
Greifswald, 383 4 3463 🕮 118
Rosa Gruppe Arnsberg
293 1 3670 🕮 109
Rosa Hilfe
Dortmund, 231 83 1919 🕮 114
Frankfurt am Main, 69 28 8080 🕮 117
Freiburg, 761 2 5161 🕮 117
Hannover, 511 458 1624 🕮 121
Magdeburg, 391 34 3364 🕮 126
Mannheim, 621 31 8594 🕮 126
Nürnberg, 911 1 9446 🕮 129
Würzburg, 931 1 9446 🕮 135
Rosa Hilfe im KCM
Münster, 251 6 0440 🕮 128
Rosa Hilfe Schwalm-Alsfed
Schwalmstadt, 669 2 7085 (helpline) 🕮 132
Rosa Linse Leipzig 🕮 125
Rosa Lüste
Wiesbaden, 611 37 7765 🕮 135
Rosa Mickrowelle
broadcast by FM 104.2 🕮 115
Rosa Rummet
Göteborg, 31 11 6151 🕮 173
Stockholm, 8 736 0215 🕮 176
Rosa Strippe e. V.
Bochum, 232 71 9411 🕮 112
Rosa Telefon
Aachen, 241 3 4633 🕮 108
Augsburg, 821 15 9242 🕮 109
Bamberg, 951 2 4729 🕮 109
Bayreuth, 921 85 2928 🕮 109
Bonn, 228 63 00339 🕮 112
Braunschweig, 531 1 9411 🕮 112
Bremerhaven, 471 4 4010 🕮 113
Chur, 81 21 6766 🕮 178
Dornbirn, 557 436 8675 🕮 34
Duisburg, 203 66 3383 🕮 114
Elmshorn, 412 16 5058 🕮 115
Erfurt, 361 731 2458 🕮 116
Flensburg, 461 2 1347 🕮 116
Freiburg, 761 2 5161 🕮 117
Gera, 365 710 6303 🕮 118
Gießen, 641 38 9294 🕮 118
Heidelberg, 622 118 3770 🕮 122
Ingolstadt, 841 30 5608 🕮 122
Karlsruhe, 721 37 9352 🕮 123
Kassel, 561 2 7413 🕮 123
Kiel, 431 1 7099 🕮 123
Koblenz, 261 6 3557 🕮 123
Köln, 753 16 4535 🕮 124
Krefeld, 215 177 0643 🕮 125
Landau, 634 18 8688 🕮 125
Limburg, 643 12 3711 🕮 125
Lingen, 591 1 9411 🕮 125
Lübeck, 451 7 4619 🕮 126
Minden, 571 88 0038 🕮 127
Passau, 851 7 1973 🕮 131
Putbus, 291 498 🕮 131
Salzburg, 662 43 5927 🕮 35
Siegen, 271 5 3297 🕮 132
Stuttgart, 711 1 9446 🕮 132
Trier, 651 1 9411 🕮 134
Tübingen, 707 14 4843 🕮 134
Ulm, 731 3 7332 🕮 134
Weimar, 364 3 3407 🕮 135
Wien, 1 26 6604 🕮 35
Wiesbaden, 611 1 9446 🕮 135
Wupperthal, 202 45 0004 🕮 135
Rosa Telefon der Pro Familia
Marburg, 642 12 2800 🕮 127
Rosa Telefon Hinterland
Biederkopf, 735 1 5055 🕮 111
Rosa Zone 🕮 112
Rosa, Lydia, ACSW
New York, 914 834 2128 🕮 301
RosaLinde
Menden, 237 390 3455 🕮 127
Rosarote Panthe-Schwul-Lesbische Aktion-gemeinschaft Steiermark
Graz 🕮 34
Rose
Phœnix 🕮 194
Rose City Discussion Club (RCDC)
Clackamas, 503 650 7052 (voice mail) 🕮 324
Rose Drempel
Leuven / Louvain, 1 620 0606 🕮 38
Rose Printing
Tallahassee, 904 576 4151 🕮 242
Rose Publications
Saint Louis, 314 773 3220 🕮 284
Rose's Club
Sheffield, 114 261 9444 🕮 90
Rosebud & Fish Community Bookstore
Salem, 503 399 9960 🕮 327
Rosebud Productions
Woodland Hills, 818 702 8040 🕮 225
Rosenberg Clinic
Galveston, 409 763 0916 🕮 342
Rosenberg, Miriam, M.D., Ph.D.
Boston, 508 358 7512 🕮 267
Ross, Dale
Berkeley, 313 544 7041 🕮 274
Ross, Joellyn, Ph.D.
Cherry Hill, 609 424 1065 🕮 290
Rouge Magazine
published by Breakaway Publications Ltd. 🕮 85
Routledge Press
Andover, 1264 342923 🕮 76
New York 🕮 306
Roxy's Electrolysis
East Providence 🕮 334
Royal Darwin Hospital
8 720 8007 🕮 28
Roze Waas
Sint Niklaas, 3 776 7270 🕮 39
rpi.libraries 🕮 5
Rubber & Rivets
Fullerton, 714 671 1402 🕮 200
Rubber Ball
London, 181 968 0234 🕮 80
Rubber Corps
San Francisco, 415 267 7604 🕮 214
Rubber Design Modevertriebsgesellschaft
Kaarst 🕮 123
Rubber Lady
Barnet 🕮 68
Rubber Mask & Costume Company
Telford, 1952 883994 🕮 90
Rubber Men's Club
London 🕮 83
Rubber Nipple Club
London 🕮 83
Rubber Plantation
Manchester, 161 839 5920 🕮 76
Rubber Rebel
published by Gear, Inc. 🕮 205
Rubber Sex Groep
Amsterdam 🕮 152
Rubber Tree
Seattle, 206 633 4750 🕮 191
Rubberotica
San Rafael 🕮 220
Rubberstuffers
London, 171 278 0508 🕮 87
Rubbertree Rainwear
Vancouver, 604 885 1282 🕮 40
Rubberworks
Boston, 617 734 9582 🕮 267
Rubenstein, Maggi, R.N., MFCC, Ph.D.
San Francisco, 415 584 0172 🕮 213
Rubyfruit Books
Tallahassee, 904 222 2627 🕮 242
Rubyfruit Erotica
Toronto 🕮 41
Ruderman, Jerome, JD, MS
New York, 212 877 7344 🕮 301
Rurals MC
Roermund 🕮 157
Rush-Presbyterian-Saint Luke's Medical Center
Chicago, 312 942 5000 🕮 249
Rutgers University Press
New Brunswick 🕮 291
Ruth, Richard, Ph.D.
Wheaton, 301 933 3072 🕮 266
Rutland Area Gay & Lesbian Connection (RAGLC) 🕮 346
Ruward
Den Haag, 70 363 0879 🕮 154
RVG-Import Oy
Helsinki, 90 719781 🕮 97
Ryan, Barb, M.S.
Eugene, 541 345 5058 🕮 325
Ryan, Janet
Kansas City 🕮 283
Rycroft Gallery
San José 🕮 220
Ryder Publishing
London 🕮 67
S & L Sales Company
Los Angeles 🕮 205
S & M Club
San Francisco, 415 552 7339 🕮 214
S O S Army Surplus Ltd.
Edmonton, 403 422 3348 🕮 44
S&M Exchange
Seattle 🕮 351
S&M Fabrications
Hollinswood, 195 229 9978 🕮 90
S&M News
published by Carter Stevens Presents 🕮 333
S. A. D. E.
Barcelona, 3 450 4816 🕮 172
published by S. A. D. E. 🕮 172
S. A. M. Co.
Brooklyn, 718 748 7593 🕮 298
S. E. London's Lesbian, Gay, & Bisexual Helpline
181 316 5954 🕮 79
S. H. S. Services
Winnipeg, 204 694 3164 🕮 10
S. W. 3
Hannover, 511 131 7279 🕮 121
S. Wolbrecht
Göteborg, 31 83 3910 🕮 173
S3C3 🕮 *See* Sober, Safe, Sane, Consensual Club - Chicago
SAAFE 🕮 *See* Southern Alberta Association for Fetish / Fantasy Education / Exploration
Sabazio 🕮 22
Saber MC
Hollywood 🕮 237
Sabra Lesbian Coalition
Las Cruces 🕮 294
Sachs
Albuquerque, 505 266 1661 🕮 294
Sacramento AIDS Foundation
916 448 2437 🕮 209
Sacramento Gender Association
916 482 7742 🕮 210
Sacramento Leather Association
916 863 3398 (voice mail) 🕮 209
Sacred Heart General Hospital
Eugene, 503 686 7300 🕮 325
Sacred Heart Tattoos
Atlanta, 404 222 0393 🕮 245
SAD
Amsterdam, 20 662 4206 🕮 152
Sade
Weston-Super-Mare 🕮 70
Sadean
published by Katharsis 🕮 18
Saegert, Linda
New York, 516 825 2289 🕮 301
SAFE 🕮 *See* South Australia Fetish / Fantasy Enthusiasts
broadcast by Access Community Radio AM 810 🕮 161
Safe Afro-Arab Health & AIDS Respite Action (SAHARA)
London, 181 795 3317 🕮 82
Safe Way / Verien für Prävention für Schwule und Bisexuelle Männer
Wien 🕮 35
Safer Place Youth Network
Raleigh, 929 851 9544 🕮 316
SAG 🕮 *See* Seacoast Gay Men
SAGA 🕮 *See* Sudbury All Gay Alliance
Boone 🕮 313
Sage 🕮 244
Saginaw Valley State College Gay & Lesbian Alliance 🕮 278
SAHARA 🕮 *See* Safe Afro-Arab Health & AIDS Respite Action
SAIBBS 🕮 *See* Seattle AIDS Information BBS
SAIM 🕮 *See* Sufficient As I Am
Saint Alphonsus Regional Medical Center
Boise, 208 378 2121 🕮 247
Saint Andrew's University GaySoc
Saint Andew's 🕮 168
Saint Anthony Hospital
Oklahoma City, 405 272 7000 🕮 323
Saint Anthony's Hospital
Saint Petersburg, 813 825 1100 🕮 241
Saint Austell Switchboard
1726 69111 🕮 72
Saint Clare's Hospital & Health Center
New York, 212 586 1500 🕮 302
Saint Crispin L/L Fraternity
Orlando, 407 843 5621 🕮 240
Saint David's Hospital
Austin, 512 476 7111 🕮 338
Saint Elizabeth's Medical Center of Boston
617 789 3000 🕮 267
Saint Elmo's Books & Music
Pittsburgh, 412 431 9100 🕮 332
Saint Francis Hospital
Memphis, 901 765 1000 🕮 336
Saint Francis Hospital & Medical Center
Hartford, 203 286 4600 🕮 230
Saint Francis Medical Center
Oahu, 808 547 6011 🕮 247
Pittsburgh, 412 622 4343 🕮 331
Saint Francis Regional Medical Center
Wichita, 316 268 5000 🕮 258
Saint Ganriel Community Church
Tyler, 903 581 6923 🕮 344
Saint Helens Lesbian & Gay Helpline
1744 454823 🕮 87
Saint John's Episcopal Hospital - South Shore
Far Rockaway, 718 868 7000 🕮 299
Saint John's Medical Center
Tulsa, 918 744 2345 🕮 323
Saint John's University Lesbian, Gay, & Bisexual Alliance
New York, 718 390 8829 🕮 305
Saint Joseph County Health Department
South Bend, 219 284 9725 🕮 255
Saint Joseph Hospital
Denver, 202 837 7111 🕮 227
Saint Joseph Hospital & Medical Center
Chicago, 312 665 3000 🕮 249
Saint Joseph Medical Center
Albuquerque, 505 848 8000 🕮 294
Fort Wayne, 219 425 3000 🕮 254
Saint Joseph's Hospital
Lexington, 606 278 3436 🕮 259
Tampa, 813 870 4000 🕮 242
Saint Joseph's Hospital of Atlanta
404 851 7001 🕮 244
Saint Joseph's Medical Center
Bloomington, 309 622 3311 🕮 248
South Bend, 219 237 7111 🕮 255
Saint Louis Effort for AIDS (EFA)
314 367 2382 🕮 284
Saint Louis Gender Foundation (LGS)
314 997 9897 (voice mail) 🕮 284
Saint Louis Lifestyles 🕮 284
Saint Luke's Hospital
Tempe, 602 968 9411 🕮 194
Saint Luke's Hospital Center
New York, 212 523 4000 🕮 302
Saint Luke's Medical Center
Cleveland, 216 368 7000 🕮 318
Denver, 303 839 6100 🕮 227
Milwaukee, 414 649 6000 🕮 357
Saint Marks Bookshop
New York, 212 260 7853 🕮 309
Saint Marks Women's Health Collective
New York, 212 228 7482 🕮 302
Saint Mary Medical Center
Long Beach, 310 491 9000 🕮 202
Saint Mary's Health Services
Grand Rapids, 616 774 6399 🕮 276
Saint Mary's Hospital
West Palm Beach, 407 844 6300 🕮 243
Saint Mary's Hospital & Medical Center
San Francisco, 415 668 1000 🕮 213
Saint Mary's Medical Center
Duluth, 218 726 4000 🕮 279

Saint Mary's Medical Center of Evansville
812 479 4000 📖 254
Saint Mary's Regional Medical Center
Reno, 702 323 2041 📖 287
Saint Michael's Emporium
New York, 212 995 8359 📖 9
Saint Paul Medical Center
Dallas / Fort Worth, 214 879 1000 📖 340
Saint Peter Hospital
Olympia, 206 491 9480 📖 350
Saint Vincent Hospital
Santa Fe, 505 983 3361 📖 295
Saint Vincent Hospital & Health Care Center
Indianapolis, 317 338 2345 📖 254
Saint Vincent Infirmary Medical Center
Little Rock, 501 660 3000 📖 195
Saint Vincents' Medical Center of Richmond
New York, 718 876 1234 📖 302
SAK Publishing
Novi 📖 277
SALGA 📖 *See* Southern Appalachian Lesbian & Gay Alliance
Salisbury Lesbian & Gay Switchboard
1722 415051 📖 94
Salisbury News Agency
410 543 4469 📖 266
Salishon Society
Eugene, 503 688 4282 📖 180, 189
Sally's II
New York, 212 944 6000 Ext. 212 📖 300
Salmacis
Eugene, 503 688 4282 📖 325
SALO 📖 *See* Springfield Area Lesbian Outreach
Salon
San Francisco, 415 552 4213 📖 219
San Francisco, 415 673 4492 📖 219
SALSA 📖 *See* San Antonio Lambda Students Alliance
Salt City Book & Video
Mattydale, 315 454 0629 📖 299
SAM 📖 *See* Scottish AIDS Monitor. *See also* Social Alternative for Gay Men
Sam Houston GLBA
Huntsville, 409 291 3584 📖 343
Sam's Tiffany's on the Park
Detroit 📖 274
Samanta
Hamm, 2381 402586 📖 107
Samons, Sandra, ACSW
Ann Arbor, 313 663 7871 📖 274
Samotowka, Ted
Mississauga, 905 760 3390 📖 51
SAMPA 📖 *See* Solidariedade, Apoio Moral e Psicologico Aplicados a AIDS
San Angelo AIDS Foundation, Inc.
915 657 6555 📖 344
San Antonio AIDS Foundation
210 225 4715 📖 344
San Antonio Gay & Lesbian Switchboard
210 733 7300 📖 344
San Antonio Lambda Students Alliance (SALSA)
210 733 1225 📖 344
San Antonio Marquise 📖 344
San Antonio Rough Riders
Helotes 📖 342
San Antonio Transexual Support Group (SATSG) 📖 344
San Bernadino County Medical Center
San Bernardino, 909 387 8111 📖 210
San Diego Community Research Group
619 291 2437 📖 211
San Diego North County Gay & Lesbian Association
619 945 2478 📖 211
San Francisco AIDS Foundation
415 864 5855 📖 214
San Francisco Bay Area Bisexual Network
415 703 7977 📖 217
San Francisco Bay Times 📖 218
San Francisco Bondage Club 📖 214
San Francisco Dungeon 📖 184
San Francisco Gender Information 📖 215
San Francisco General Hospital Medical Center
415 206 8000 📖 213
San Francisco God-Damned Independents
415 431 7645 📖 214
San Francisco Leather Bears 📖 214
San Francisco Leather Works
415 566 7376 📖 213
San Francisco Sentinel 📖 218
San Francisco Sex Information
415 989 7374 📖 213
San Francisco Whip Company
415 804 7676 📖 187
San Joaquin AIDS Foundation
Stockton, 800 367 2437 (hotline) 📖 222
San José Medical Center
408 998 3212 📖 219
San Mateo County AIDS Program
415 573 2588 📖 220
Sandia Leathermen
Albuquerque 📖 294
Sandler, Karen, D.O.
Los Angeles, 213 931 1463 📖 203
SandMen
San Diego 📖 211
Sandmutopia Guardian
published by The Utopian Network 📖 307
Sandmutopia Supply Company
San Francisco, 415 252 1195 📖 184
Sanford Video & News
919 774 9124 📖 316
Sang Froid
New York, 212 343 9335 📖 310
Santa Barbara Cottage Hospital
805 682 7111 📖 221
Santa Barbara Paddle Company
800 569 0971 📖 221
Santa Clara County Health Department
San José, 408 299 4151 📖 219
Santa Clara Valley Medical Center
San José, 408 299 5100 📖 219
Santa Cruz AIDS Project
408 427 4999 (hotline) 📖 221
Santa Cruz Lesbian, Gay, & Bisexual Community Center
408 425 5422 📖 221
Santa Rosa Adult Books & Video
707 542 8248 📖 222
Santa Rosa Health Care Corporation
San Antonio, 210 228 2011 📖 344
Santa Rosa Memorial Hospital
707 546 3210 📖 222
Santé & Plaisir Gai (SPG)
Marseille, 142 72 7386 📖 101
Santerineross, John
Newark, 201 743 6290 📖 292
Sapphex Learn
Tampa, 813 961 6064 📖 235
Sapphire 📖 73
SAPPHO 📖 4
Sappho & Apoll Schwulen & Lesben-Jungendgruppe
Bremen, 421 70 4170 📖 113
Sappho's Isle 📖 295
Sarah's Bare Necessities
Concord, 510 680 8445 📖 198
Sarasota Memorial Hospital
813 955 1111 📖 241
SARCH 📖 *See* Schwullesbisches Archiv Hannover
SAS 📖 *See* Schwule Aktion Südwest
Saskatoon Gayline
306 665 1224 📖 64
SATRU
Johannesburg 📖 172
SATSG 📖 *See* San Antonio Transexual Support Group
Satyricons MC
Las Vegas, 702 733 8355 📖 286
Satyrs MC
Los Angeles, 213 257 0624 📖 204
Savage
published by Paisano Publications 📖 196
Savage Gifts & Leather
Albany, 518 434 2324 📖 296
Save-More Sport Store
Toronto, 416 368 3536 📖 60
Savoy
Manchester 📖 76
Sax Leather
Sydney, 1800 674 340 (order line) 📖 24, 27
SB Publishing, Ltd.
Stockton-on-Tees 📖 92
SBD
Barcelona, 93 451 7564 📖 172
SBSN 📖 *See* Sydney Bisexual Support Network
Scala B. V.
Amsterdam 📖 152
Scandinavian Leather Men (SLM)
Göteborg, 31 833910 📖 173
København, 33 32 0601 📖 66
Malmö, 40 30 1893 📖 174
Oslo, 22 20 2095 📖 164
Stockholm, 8 643 3100 📖 175
Scarecrow Press
Metuchen, 201 548 8600 📖 291
Scargall, Peter
Toronto, 416 486 0014 📖 55
Scat Times
published by Winter Publishing, Inc. 📖 20
Scenario 📖 91
Scene
published by F. A. 📖 104
Scene 22
Brighton, 127 362 6682 📖 74
Scene Gear
Hoboken 📖 184
Scene One
Bradford 📖 94
published by Shadow Lane 📖 223
SchAM 📖 *See* Schwule Aktion Mannheim e. V.
Schau Mode
Rodgau, 610 61 8379 📖 107
SCHE 📖 *See* Society of Cross-Dressing Hardware Engineers
Schein, Michael
Cockeysville 📖 11
Scherma, Robert, Psy.D.
New York, 212 969 0988 📖 301
Schernoff, Michael, CSW, ACSW
New York, 212 675 9563 📖 301
Schlagzeilen 📖 120
Schlesinger, Jay, Ph.D.
New York, 516 582 2188 📖 301
SchLUB 📖 *See* Schwule-Lesbische Unigruppe
Schmidt, Beverly, RCSW
New York, 516 329 0474 📖 301
SchMIT-Z
Trier, 561 14 1416 📖 134
Schneiderei Ottokar Fischer
Düsseldorf, 211 35 9486 📖 115
Schochet, Rachel, Ph.D., MFCC
San Francisco, 415 641 1292 📖 213
Scholtens
Groningen, 50 313 9788 📖 155
School of Professional Body Piercing
Bay Shore, 516 968 0141 📖 296
Schooler, C.
New York, 212 243 1224 📖 301
SchuLZ 📖 *See* Schwulen- & Lesben-Zentrum
SCHWARM 📖 *See* Schwule Arbeitsgruppe Minden
Schwarz Bar
Brighton, 1273 624462 📖 74
Schwarze Mode
Berlin, 30 784 5922 (shop) 📖 107, 110, 111
SchwBile Referat
Duisburg, 203 37 0047 📖 115
Schweizerische Organisation Homosexuellen (SOH)
Zürich, 1 271 7011 📖 180
SchwIM 📖 *See* Schwule Initiative Minden
Schwugs! 📖 *See* Schwulengruppe Suhl
Schwuguntia - Verein zur Förderung Sozialer & Kulturelle Interessen e. V.
Mainz 📖 126
SchwUL 📖 *See* Schwule an der Univesität Leipzig
Schwul & Lesben in Plauen (SLiP) 📖 131
Schwul in Eisenach
Wartburgkreis, 369 121 4083 📖 115
Schwul in Paderborn
525 12 1959 📖 131
Schwule Aktion Bremerhaven
471 4 4010 📖 113
Schwule Aktion Lübeck 📖 126
Schwule Aktion Mannheim e. V. (SchAM)
621 31 8594 📖 127
Schwule Aktion Südwest (SAS)
Stuttgart, 711 52 5341 📖 133
Schwule Akzeptanz Gera (SIAG) 📖 118
Schwule an der Christian Albrecht Universität
Kiel 📖 123
Schwule an der Univesität Leipzig (SchwUL)
341 719 2261 📖 125
Schwule Arbeitsgruppe Minden (SCHWARM) 📖 127
Schwule Ausleihbibliothek (HAZ/SOH)
Zürich, 1 271 2250 📖 179
Schwule Beratung
Fulda, 661 19446 📖 117
Schwule Coming Out Gruppe
Osnabrück, 541 2 2722 📖 130
Schwule Gruppe Germersheim
727 4 4089 📖 118
Schwule Gruppe Oberberg
Gummersbach, 226 59152 📖 119
Schwule Gruppe Witten 📖 135
Schwule Gruppe Wupperthal 📖 135
Schwule Hannöversche Studenten (SHS)
Hannover, 511 49 4575 📖 121
Schwule Hilfe Göttingen
551 8 3355 📖 118
Schwule im Westerwald (SIW)
Altenkirchen 📖 109
Schwule in der AIDS-Hilfe (SidAH)
Aachen, 241 52 2558 📖 109
Schwule Initiativ Gruppe Mülheim And der Ruhr (SIGMAR)
208 806516 📖 127
Schwule Initiative
Clausthal-Zellerfeld, 532 3 4794 📖 113
Schwule Initiative Gladbeck
204 32 5412 📖 118
Schwule Initiative Minden (SchwIM)
571 88 0038 📖 127
Schwule Initiative Rheingau (SIR)
Wiesbaden, 611 7 5141 📖 135
Schwule Initiative Siegen (SIS-ters) 📖 132
Schwule Internationale Berlin e. V.
30 315 2615 📖 110
Schwule Jungendclique Frankfurt
Frankfurt am Main, 69 28 3535 📖 117
Schwule Jungendgruppe Koblenz (SJK) 📖 123
Schwule Männer
published by Bruno Gmünder Verlag 📖 108
Schwule Pressearchiv Bonn
228 21 6587 📖 107
Schwule Uni Gruppe (SchWUnG)
Karlsruhe, 721 69 1041 📖 123
Schwule Väter
Münster, 251 3 4969 📖 128
Stuttgart 📖 133
Schwüle Väter
Erfurt, 361 731 2233 📖 116
Schwule Väter & Ehemänner
Bremen, 421 70 4170 📖 113
Schwule Väter Köln
221 23 2626 📖 124
Schwule-Lesbische Unigruppe (SchLUB)
Bern 📖 178
Schwule-Lesbische Unigruppe (SLUG)
Basel / Bâle, 61 692 6655 📖 177
Schwulen & Lesben Zentrum
Bonn, 228 63 0029 📖 112
Schwulen- & Lesben-Initiative der Universität Dortmund 📖 114
Schwulen- & Lesben-Zentrum (SchuLZ)
Köln, 221 52 0206 📖 124
Schwulen- & Lesbenzentrum Münster (KCM)
251 66 56886 📖 128
Schwulen-Archiv Köln
221 44 2757 📖 124
Schwulen Selbsthilfegruppe
Olpe 📖 130
Schwulenforum Trier
651 14 1461 📖 134
Schwulengruppe Biedenkopf
Marburg, 642 11 9411 📖 127
Schwulengruppe Darmstadt
615 14 5691 📖 114
Schwulengruppe Düsseldorf
211 36 4260 📖 115
Schwulengruppe Elmshorn
412 18 8943 📖 116

Schwulengruppe Freudstadt

Schwulengruppe Freudstadt 117
Schwulengruppe HX/HOL
Holzminden, 553 11 0807 122
Schwulengruppe Limburg / Weilburg
643 12 3711 125
Schwulengruppe Marburg
642 12 6001 127
Schwulengruppe Suhl (Schwugs!) 134
Schwulengruppen
Erfurt, 361 731 2233 116
Schwulengruppen Biedenkopf 111
Schwulenreferat
Trier, 651 201 2117 134
Schwulenreferat an den Aachener Hochschulen
241 3 4633 109
Schwulenreferat AStа in der FH Fulda
661 60 2162 118
Schwulenreferat beim AStа der TU
Braunschweig, 531 391 4555 112
Schwulenreferat beim AStA der WW-Uni
Münster, 251 83 3057 129
Schwulenreferat der Bochumer Ruhr-Universität
232 700 2226 112
Schwulenreferat Fachhochschule Neiderrhein
Krefeld, 215 177 6878 125
Schwulenreferat im AStA der Carl von Ossietsky Universität Oldenburg
441 798 2578 130
Schwulenreferat im AStA der Christian Albrecht Universität
Kiel, 431 880 2647 123
Schwulenreferat im AStA der Fachhochschule
Münster, 251 8 2001 129
Schwulenreferat im AStA der GH Essen
201 183 3392 116
Schwulenreferat im SprecherInnenrat der Friedrich-Alexander Universität Erlangen Nürnberg
913 185 6695 116
Schwulenzentrum Bochum
232 758 3858 112
Schwuler Väter
Weimar, 364 36 1451 (office) 135
Schwules Archiv
Frankfurt am Main, 69 29 6797 117
Schwules Pressearchiv Berlin
30 694 1077 109
Schwules Überfalltelefon
Köln, 221 1 9228 124
Schwul-lesbische Filmtage
Halle (Saale), 345 512 5103 119
Schwul-Lesbische Initiative Preetz
434 2 4566 131
Schwul-lesbische Jungendegruppe
Uelzen, 581 7007 134
Schwül-lesbischer Stammtisch
Geldern, 2831 89233 118
Schwullesbisches Archiv Hannover (SARCH)
511 66 1055 121
Schwul-Lesbisches Presse-Archiv
Köln, 221 81 0451 124
SchwUlm
731 3 7332 134
SchWUnG *See* Schwule Uni Gruppe
Schwusos
Tübingen 134
SchwuZ-Schwules Zentrum
Karlsruhe, 721 37 9352 123
sci.anthropology 4
sci.med.aids 5
sci.med.diseases.hepatitis 5
sci.psychology 4
sci.psychology.journals.psyche 4
sci.psychology.research 4
sci.psychology.research.psychotherapy 4
SCL «O» Fashion
Didenheim, 89 06 1040 99
SCMA
Laguna Beach 201
Scoop 236
Scorpion 73
Scots Scene 169
Scotsgay
published by Pageprint Limited 169
Scottish AIDS Monitor
Dundee, 138 246 1167 170
Edinburgh, 131 555 4850 168
Glasgow, 141 353 3133 169
Scottish AIDS Monitor (SAM)
Inverness, 146 324 1000 168
Scottsdale Memorial Hospital
Phœnix, 602 481 4000 193
Scoville, Rob
Albuquerque, 505 843 7435 294
Screaming Leather
San Francisco 213
Screw Magazine
published by Goldstein Publications 307
Scunthorpe Gay Helpline
1724 271661 77
SCWC *See* South Carolina Women's Consortium
sdnet.motss 6
Seacoast Gay Men (SAG)
Portsmouth, 603 898 1115 288
Seacoast Outright
Portsmouth, 800 639 6095 (teenline) 288
Seahorse Society
London 83
New South Wales, 2 569 6239 26
Queensland 28
Victoria 32
Sealwear
Bournemouth, 1202 290675 73
Seattle AIDS Information BBS (SAIBBS)
206 329 8617 350
Seattle Bisexual Men's Union
206 728 4533 352
Seattle Bisexual Women's Network
206 783 7987 352
Seattle Counseling Service for Sexual Minorities
206 282 9307 351
Seattle Eagle
206 621 7591 350
Seattle Gay Clinic
206 461 4540 351
Seattle Gay News 353
Seattle Institute for Sex Therapy Education & Research (SISTER)
206 522 8588 351
Seattle Kink Information Network (SKIN)
206 368 0384 351
Seattle Leather Mercantile
800 860 5847 353
Seattle Men in Leather (SML)
206 233 8141 351
Sec 52 Buchladen & Galerie
Zürich, 1 271 1818 177
Second Skin
New Orleans, 504 561 8167 261
Secret Magazine 36
Secrets Boutique
Köln, 221 24 4100 125
Séduction
Laval 41
Montréal, 514 876 3636 63
Seksuaalinen Tasavertaisuus ry (SETA)
Head Office, 3580 135 8302 95
Helsingin Seudun, 3580 135 8302 95
Joensuun, 9 732 6033 96
Jyrässendun, 941 310 0660 95
Kokkola, 96 831 0469 97
Kuopio, 971 261 9566 96
Lahti, 918 781 8954 95
Oulu, 98 137 6932 96
Rovaniemi, 96 031 0141 96
Tampere, 93 114 8721 95
Turku, 921 250 0695 96
Selbsthilfegruppe
Stuttgart, 7143 33502 133
Selbsthilfegruppe Gießen
641 38 9294 118
Select Books & Video
Morgantown, 304 292 7714 355
Selective Publishing, Inc.
Oakbrook, 708 986 8550 16
Senior Action in a Gay Environment (S. A. G. E.) 308
Sentara Norfolk General Hospital
804 628 3000 348
Sentrum Legekontor
Tromsø, 77 68 2549 166
Sentry Box
London, 171 735 1116 81
Sentury Publications
Chicago, 312 935 1790 251
Sept
Bruxelles / Brussel, 2 513 1414 36
Sequoia Hospital
Redwood City, 415 369 5811 209
Serenity
Hollywood, 305 436 9477 238
Serhume
Mexico City 149
Serieys, Philippe
Rosny sous Bois, 145 28 2157 105
Sernier, Conrad, ACSW, CSW
New York, 212 260 2590 301
Séro-Zéro
Montréal, 514 286 0439 62
Serri di Piazza, Arcobaleno
Trieste 141
Servant's Quarters
published by Six of the Best Publishing 18
Service aux Séro-Positifs
Bruxelles / Brussel, 2 219 6795 37
Service of Mankind Church
East 230
El Cerrito, 510 874 4974 (hotline) 199
Service Spécialisé SIDA Québec
Laval, 514 668 1230 61
Services Départmental de Vénérologie
Amiens, 22 89 4630 97
Services for Men (& Their Families)
West Medford, 617 395 2450 273
Sesquehanna KONTACT
Bloomsburg 327
Sestienda
Barcelona, 93 318 8676 172
SETA *See* Seksuaalinen Tasavertaisuus ry
SETA Information Service
Helsinki, 90 135 8302 95
SETA Library
Helsinki, 90 135 8302 96
Seton Medical Center
Austin, 512 323 1000 338
Severin's Kiss
London, 181 342 9136 83
Severn Links
Bristol 90
Sex & Gay Shop
Hamm 121
Sex 10
Helsinki, 90 60 2368 97
Sex 42
Helsinki 97
Sex Bazar
Braunschweig, 531 4 0440 113
Sex Center
Lille, 20 51 0891 100
Sex Imtim
Braunschweig, 531 4 3541 113
Sex Information & Education Council (SIECCAN)
Toronto, 416 466 5304 41
Sex Information & Education Council (SIECUS)
New York, 212 819 9770 304
Sex Institute
New York, 212 674 7111 303
Sex Magik Faeries Circle
San Francisco 214
Sex Market
Oulu 97
Sex Pool
Berlin, 30 214 1989 111
Sex Shop
Heidelberg, 622 12 9899 122
Karlsruhe, 721 2 9185 123
Le Mans, 43 28 5139 100
Rochefort, 46 99 9363 105
Saintes, 46 74 5172 106
Stuttgart, 711 62 5340 134
Tampere 95
Sex Shop Erotik Kaufhaus
Schwerin 132
Sex World
Minneapolis / Saint Paul, 612 672 0556 281
Sexashop
Grenoble, 76 46 7086 100
Marseille, 91 33 7191 101
Sexbox
Berlin, 30 233 3953 111
SEX-L 4
Sexotica
Zürich, 1 273 0179 180
SEXTALK 4
Sexual Assault Centre - Hamilton & Area
905 525 4162 (24 hrs.) 50
Sexual Assault Centre for Quinte & District
Belleville, 800 909 7007 (24hrs.) 49
Sexual Assault Centre of Brantford
Toronto, 519 751 3471 (24 hrs.) 57
Sexual Assault Support Centre - Ottawa
613 234 2266 (24 hrs.) 52
Sexual Assault/Rape Crisis Centre of Peel
Mississauga, 905 273 3337 51
Sexual Identity Center (SIC)
Oahu, 808 926 1000 246
Sexual Minorities Alligned for Community, Education, & Support (SM Aces)
Annandale on Hudson 296
Sexual Minority Student Alliance
Richmond, 804 367 6509 349
Sexual Minority Youth Assistance League
Washington, 202 546 5911 233
Sexual Minority Youth Assistance League
Washington, 202 546 5940 234
Sexual Reality
broadcast by TOPS FM 104.1 28
Sexuallberatungsstelle der Abteilung für Sexualforschung
Hamburg 120
Sexy Cats
Düsseldorf 115
Sexy Shoes (Leslie Shoe Company)
Rogers City, 517 734 4030 183
Sexy Shop
Konstanz, 752 1220 2526 125
Toulon, 94 62 6393 106
Sexyland
Bochum 112
Ludwigshafen 126
Zürich, 1 242 7989 180
Sezione Malattie Infettive dell'Ospedale
La Spezia, 187 53 5111 142
SFHR
Jönköping, 36 11 4751 175
sfnet.keskustelu.psykologia 4
SGBB Mailbox
Hamburg 107
Sh!
London, 171 613 5458 68, 86
Shades of Grey
Dallas / Fort Worth, 214 521 4739 341
Shades of Lavendar
Brooklyn, 718 499 0352 297
Shadow Lane
Studio City, 818 985 9151 223
Shadowfax Leathercraft
Sarasota, 941 371 5242 241
Shadyside Hospital
Pittsburgh, 412 623 2121 331
Shaft
Rotterdam, 10 414 1486 157
Shakespeare & Co.
New York, 212 529 1330 309
Shakti *See* South Asian Lesbian & Gay Network
Shamakami
published by Shamakami, Incorporated 22
Shamakami, Incorporated
San Francisco, 415 442 7958 22
Shaman Body Piercing
New York, 212 505 8488 306
Shand Hospital at the University of Florida
Gainesville, 904 395 0111 237
Shannon, Joseph, Ph.D.
Columbus, 614 297 0422 319
Shared Times
Lowell, 508 441 9081 271
Shaw, Nanette, Ph.D.
New York, 212 505 7869 301
Shaynew Press
San Francisco, 415 391 9525 182
She Bang 85
She'an'Me Fun Fashions
London, 171 603 2402 86
Uxbridge, 1895 271668 87
Shear-Davis
Ann Arbor, 313 741 0123 274

Sheeba
Beaconsfield 61
Sheela-Na-Gig
Galway, 91 668 49 137
Sheenan Memorial Hospital
Buffalo, 716 848 2000 298
Sheffield Bisexual Women's Group 90
Sheffield Friend
114 275 8880 90
Sheffield Gayphone
114 258 8199 90
Sheffield Lesbian Line
114 258 1238 90
Shelix
Northampton 271
Shell, John, Ph.D.
Denver, 303 377 6169 227
Shiny
published by G & M Fashions Ltd. 75
Shiny Fashion
Ittingen, 7266 3595 122
Salzwedel, 3901 33927 132
Shiny Things
Montréal, 514 284 0868 63
Ship to Shore Tattooing & Body Piercing
Millington, 901 872 0405 337
Shipmates of Baltimore, Inc. 264
Shiwa
Aschaffenberg 109
Shock
Malmö, 40 11 1080 174
Shoe Express
Lafayette, 800 874 0469 (orders) 183
Shoecraft
Melbourne, 5 221 4802 24
Shomer-Tec
Bellingham, 206 733 6214 187
Shop 28
Oldenburg 130
Shotgun Video
San Francisco, 415 626 5070 218
Shouts in the Wilderness, Leather Circle of Hope
Dallas / Fort Worth, 214 351 1901 Ext. 202 341
Show Me Bears
Saint Louis, 314 995 2690 284
Showgrade Ltd.
Stockport 68
Shrewsbury AIDS Helpline
1743 261113 90
Shropshire Lesbian & Gay Switchboard
Telford, 1743 232393 90
SHS *See* Schwule Hannöversche Studenten
Shunga Comix
Keego Harbor 276
SIAG *See* Schwule Akzeptanz Gera
SIC *See* Sexual Identity Center
SID'Aventure
Rennes, 99 78 2132 105
SIDA Centre
Newcastle upon Tyne, 191 232 2855 92
SIDA MST Info
Charleroi, 7 156 0580 38
SIDA-AIDS Moncton
506 859 9616 48
Sidaction Trois-Rivières
819 374 5740 63
SidAH *See* Schwule in der AIDS-Hilfe
Sidney's Newstand
New Orleans, 504 524 6872 261
SIECCAN *See* Sex Information & Education Council
SIECUS *See* Sex Information & Education Council
Siegessäule
published by Magnus Verlag 111
Sierra AIDS Council
Sonora, 209 533 2873 222
Sierra Pacific Productions
Marina Del Rey, 800 828 4336 181
Sierra Voice 281
SigMa
Washington, 202 728 7589 234
Sigma Beta
Oklahoma City 323
SIGMAR *See* Schwule Initiativ Gruppe Mülheim And der Ruhr
Sign of the Times
London, 171 938 4744 86
Sign Of The Wolf Tattoo
Weirs Beach, 603 366 2557 288
Signals 293
Significant Other Support
Dallas / Fort Worth, 214 641 4842 341
Silent Passage
401 438 7417 334
Silkwood Books, Inc.
Rochester, 716 473 8110 311
Silver Anchor Enterprises
Crystal Springs, 800 848 7464 (800 Tit Ring) 236
Silver Dolphins LLC
Corpus Christi 339
Silver Fox
Pocatello, 208 234 2477 247
Silver Moon
London, 171 836 7906 85
Silver News
Hyattsville, 301 779 1024 265
Silver Smoke
Bloomington, 708 653 1287 248
Silver Spurs of Dallas
Dallas / Fort Worth 340
Silver State Leather Association
Sparks, 702 331 7059 287
Silveraim Ltd.
London, 171 296 6000 69, 85
Manchester, 161 236 4999 76
Silverlake Leather
Los Angeles, 213 665 5326 206
Silverman, Philip, Ph.D.
Washington, 202 822 0078 233
Silvermans Ltd.
London, 171 790 5257 87
Silverstein, Charles, Ph.D.
New York, 212 799 8574 301
Simon, Liz, BCSW
New Orleans, 504 899 6024 260
Simply Leather
Machynlleth 359
Simpson, Gary
Luton, 1582 505839 71
SIN
Seattle, 206 329 0324 190
Sin City Adult Books
Portland, 503 223 6514 327
Sinai Hospital of Baltimore
410 578 5678 263
Sinai Samaritan Medical Center
Milwaukee, 414 345 3400 357
Sin-A-Matic
Fürth, 911 709 017 118
Sin-A-Matique
Brighton, 1273 329154 69
Since May Productions
Union City, 201 864 7837 293
(sin)ch
Oakland, 510 451 7716 207
Sine Qua Non
Albuquerque 294
Sing Heavenly Muse! 281
Single Step Co-op
Lancaster, 1524 63021 78
Sinister Wisdom
published by Sinister Wisdom, Inc. 197
Sinister Wisdom, Inc.
Berkeley 197
SIR *See* Schwule Initiative Rheingau
Sir Steve's Leather
Guelph 41
Sir!
published by ST Publishing 84
Sirens MC
New York, 212 807 8211 304
Sirens MC San Francisco
415 530 9328 215
SIS *See* Swan's Inner Sorority
SISA Intervention Prévention Ecoute
Joliette, 514 752 4004 61
Sissy Exposé
published by Leoram, Inc. 223
SISTER *See* Seattle Institute for Sex Therapy Education & Research
Sisterhood Bookstore
Los Angeles, 310 477 7300 181
SIS-ters *See* Schwule Initiative Siegen
Sisters' & Brothers' Bookstore
Albuquerque, 505 266 7317 294
Sisterspirit Bookstore
San José, 408 293 9372 220
SISTI *See* Society for Initiatives & Services in Transgender Issues
SIW *See* Schwule im Westerwald
Six of the Best Publishing
Berkeley, 510 208 2835 18
Sjinderhannes
Roermund, 47 533 3119 157
SJK *See* Schwule Jungendgruppe Koblenz
Skarupe
Hamburg, 40 701 7388 120
SKIN *See* Seattle Kink Information Network
Skin & Bones
Dallas / Fort Worth, 214 826 6647 341
Skin Deep Tattoo
Maui, 808 661 8531 246
Skin Parlor
Hollywood 201
Skin Tight
Ottawa, 613 523 2708 53
Rotterdam, 10 436 3756 151
Skin To Skin
Ramsgate 69
Skin Two
London, 181 968 0234 86
published by Tim Woodward Publishing Ltd. 84
Skinner Jack's Bath House
North Hollywood 207
Skinnydippers
Woodside, 718 651 4689 312
Skinprint Tattoo
South Renton, 206 255 5841 353
Tacoma, 206 582 8514 354
Skint
Norwich 68
SKVdC Sekretariat
Berlin 110
Skyclad Publishing
Kansas City, 816 753 7816 22
Skye
New Baltimore 277
Slacker
Pittsburgh, 412 381 3911 332
Slant 218
Slawson Communications
San Marcos, 619 744 2299 220
Slimwear Of America
Eastsound, 360 376 5213 183
Sling
Boston, 617 742 4084 267
SLiP *See* Schwul & Lesben in Plauen
Slippery When Wet
published by More! Productions 197
SLM *See* Scandinavian Leather Men
SLMA *See* Solano Lambda Men's Association
SLMC *See* Sylter Männer Leder Club
slo.sex 6
SLOSH *See* Society for Lovers Of Slapstick Happenings
SludgeMaster 343
Houston, 713 552 4683 343
SLUG *See* Schwule-Lesbische Unigruppe. *See also* South Bay Leather Uniform Group
Slutsky, Sidney, Ed.D.
Philadelphia, 215 722 1404 330
SM / Leather / Fetish Community Outreach Project (SM-COP)
New York 12
SM Aces *See* Sexual Minorities Alligned for Community, Education, & Support
SM Bisexuals
London, 171 278 3294 69
SM Bladet / SM Shop
København, 33 32 3303 66
SM Board
Wyoming, 717 655 2880 1
SM Gays
London 69
SM Group
Thornton Heath 75
SM Toy Hamburg 107
SM Versand
Oldenburg, 441 72340 107
Small Etc.
Bayside 296
Small Gazette
published by Small Etc. 296
Small Press Traffic
San Francisco, 415 285 8394 218
Smart Alternative
London, 181 840 6431 81
SMC *See* Zentralschweizer Schwulen-Motorrad-Club
SMC Dresden 114
SM-COP *See* SM / Leather / Fetish Community Outreach Project
Smedley's Bookshop
Ithaca, 607 273 2325 299
SMia
Oslo, 92 42 0878 164
SMiL Denmark
København, 1 81 05 50 66
SMil Norge
Oslo, 22 17 0501 164
Smith College Lesbian, Gay, & Bisexual Alliance
Northampton, 413 585 4907 272
Smith, Ira
New York, 212 260 6396 300
Smith, Marilee, Psy.D.
Greeley, 303 351 6688 229
Smith, Richard
Miami, 809 541 4500 238
SML *See* Seattle Men in Leather
Smoke Exchange
New York 12
Smoke Shop
Wilmington, 302 655 2861 233
Smokey Mountain Bears
Knoxville, 615 531 7515 336
Smooth Buddies Bulletin
published by Mercury Productions 339
sm-org 4
Smorgasmatron!
London 87
SNAP *See* Southern Nevada Association of Pride
Snax Club
Berlin 110
Snaxus Productions
Austin, 512 416 0100 339
SNC London 82
SNHAGLY *See* Southern New Hampshire Gay & Lesbian Youth
Snyder, Robert, Ph.D.
Saint Louis, 314 727 9088 284
Sober, Safe, Sane, Consensual Club - Chicago (S3C3) 249
soc.bi 6
soc.gender.issues 6
soc.libraries.talk 5
soc.motss 6
soc.support.transgendered 6
soc.support.youth.gay-lesbian-bi 5
Social Alternative for Gay Men (SAM)
Norwich 346
Société Comedit
Paris, 143 57 09 93 104
Society
Chicopee, 413 592 7239 265
Unionville, 413 592 7239 232
Society for Human Sexuality
Seattle 352
Society for Initiatives & Services in Transgender Issues (SISTI)
Oakland, 510 601 7975 207, 208
Society for Lesbian & Gay Philosophy
Moorhead, 218 236 4087 281
Society for Lovers Of Slapstick Happenings (SLOSH)
Harrogate 69
Society for Scientific Study of Sex
Mount Vernon, 319 895 8407 257
Society for the Psychological Study of Lesbian & Gay Issues
Washington, 202 366 6037 233
Society for the Second Self (Tri-Ess)
Alpha Chi, 806 359 7714 338
Alpha Omega 322

Alpha Pi Omega 📖 336
Alpha Rho 📖 345
Alpha Zeta 📖 194
Alpha, 213 876 6141 📖 204
Beta Chi, 601 982 7678 📖 282
Beta Gamma 📖 280
Chi Delta Mu, 201 663 0772 📖 292, 297
Chi, 708 364 9514 📖 253
Delta Omega 📖 343
Delta, 303 595 5875 📖 228
Epsilon Tau 📖 344
Kappa Beta 📖 314
Lambda Chi Lambda, 607 547 4118 📖 310
Mu Sigma, 501 227 8798 📖 195
Nu Phi Chi 📖 312
Phi 📖 294
Phi Epsilon Mu 📖 243
Phi Sigma 📖 42
Sigma Beta 📖 323
Sigma Epsilon, 404 552 4415 (helpline) 📖 246
Sigma Nu Rho, 609 586 1351 📖 293
Sigma Rho Gamma 📖 191, 192
Sigma Sigma Beta 📖 202
Tau Chi, 713 988 8064 📖 343
Tau Lambda 📖 242
Theta Upsilon Gamma 📖 286
Tulare, 209 688 9246 📖 223
Society of Cross-Dressing Hardware Engineers (SCHE)
Boston 📖 268
Society of Janus
San Francisco, 415 985 7117 📖 214
Society of O
Clearwater 📖 236
Society of Spankers
Toronto, 416 925 9872 Ext. 2102 📖 58
Sociologisch Instituut
Amsterdam, 20 525 2226 📖 152
Socket Science Labs
San Francisco, 415 334 1828 📖 213
Sodomite Invasion Review 📖 46
SOH 📖 *See* Schweizerische Organisation Homosexuellen
Soho Books
Nottingham, 115 978 3567 📖 89
Sojourner - The Women's Forum 📖 269
Solano Country Gay & Lesbian Information Line
Fairfield, 7007 448 1010 (recorded message) 📖 199
Solano Lambda Men's Association (SLMA)
Fairfield, 707 449 1010 (tape recording) 📖 199
SOLAS
Edinburgh, 131 659 5116 📖 168
Solent Gay Switchboard & AIDSline
1703 637363 📖 64
Southampton, 1703 637363 📖 77
Solent Lesbian Line
1703 405111 📖 64
Southampton, 1703 405111 📖 77
Solidariedade, Apoio Moral e Psicologico Aplicados a AIDS (SAMPA)
São Paulo, 11 571 7396 📖 39
Solitary 📖 356
Solo Parenting Alliance
Seattle, 206 720 1655 📖 352
Soma Studios
Santa Barbara 📖 221
Somandros
Los Angeles, 213 465 7589 📖 204
Some Bizarre
published by SB Publishing, Ltd. 📖 92
Somerset AIDS Advice
Taunton, 1823 332727 📖 90
Sonoma Bares of the Northwest
Montesano, 360 249 6939 📖 350
Sonoma County Women's Voices 📖 222
Sons & Daughters
Brookings, 605 692 6026 📖 335
Grand Rapids, 616 459 8877 📖 276
Sons of Capone
Bonfield 📖 49
Sons of Satan
San Francisco, 415 695 2913 📖 214
Sooner Diversity
Oklahoma City 📖 323
Sorgentelefon HALU
Luzern / Lucerne, 41 51 3532 📖 178
Sorodz
Oakland, 510 839 2588 📖 207
Sorority Magazine 📖 59
Sortilège 📖 104
SOS Gay
Milano, 2 832 2762 📖 142
Sound Out 📖 350
Source Bookstore
Southington, 203 621 6255 📖 232
Source Leather Shop
Forestville 📖 199
Sources 📖 42
South Arkansas Fight AIDS
El Dorado 📖 195
South Asian Lesbian & Gay Network (Shakti)
London, 171 837 2782 📖 79
South Australia Bisexual Network
Adelaide, 8 344 6146 📖 30
South Australia Fetish / Fantasy Enthusiasts (SAFE)
Adelaide 📖 30
South Australia Transexual Support
Adelaide, 1800 182 233 📖 30
South Bay Intinet
Sunnyvale, 408 730 9622 📖 223
South Bay Leather Uniform Group (SLUG)
San José, 408 929 7584 📖 219
South Bay Lesbian & Gay Community Center
Los Angeles, 310 379 2850 📖 204
South Bay Times 📖 220
South Bucks Rainwear
Didcot, 1235 811666 📖 68
South Carolina AIDS Education Network, Inc.
Columbia, 803 736 1171 📖 334
South Carolina Women's Consortium (SCWC)
Columbia 📖 334
South East Alaska Gay & Lesbian Alliance
Juneau, 907 586 4297 📖 193
South Florida Bears
Miami, 305 685 1841 📖 12
South Florida Polyamorists 📖 235
South Goes Mad
Roermund 📖 157
South Jersey AIDS Alliance
Atlantic City, 800 281 2437 (in New Jersey) 📖 289
South Miami Hospital
305 661 4611 📖 239
South Mississipi AIDS Task Force
Biloxi, 601 435 1234 📖 282
South Pacific MC
Sydney 📖 26
South Peace AIDS Council
Grande Prairie, 403 538 3388 📖 44
South Plains AIDS Resource Center
Lubbock, 806 796 7068 📖 344
South Shore Gay & Lesbian Alliance
Bridgewater, 508 293 5183 📖 270
South Shore Hospital & Medical Center
Miami Beach, 305 672 2100 📖 239
South Sound SM Leatherfolk
Olympia, 360 786 1438 📖 350
South Texas Voice 📖 344
South Wales Immune Deficiency Self Help (SWISH)
Swansea, 1792 722007 📖 359
South Wales TV/TS Group
Cardiff 📖 359
South Yorkshire AIDSline
Sheffield, 800 844334 📖 90
South Yorkshire Connections
Barnsley, 122 673 0703 📖 90
Southeast Counseling Services
Columbus, 614 445 3330 📖 320
Southeast Wisconsin AIDS Project
Kenosha, 800 924 6601 📖 355
Southeastern Connecticut AIDS Project
New London, 203 447 0884 📖 231
Southend Lesbian & Gay Switchboard
1702 480344 📖 75
Southern Alberta Association for Fetish / Fantasy Education / Exploration (SAAFE)
Calgary 📖 42
Southern Appalachian Lesbian & Gay Alliance (SALGA)
Asheville, 704 645 5908 📖 313
Southern Bears
Atlanta, 404 908 3381 📖 244
Southern Books
Dunedin 📖 162
Southern Colorado AIDS Poject
Colorado Springs, 719 578 9092 📖 227
Southern Gay Dreams
broadcast by WRFG 📖 245
Southern Gay Health Project
Cork, 21 27 8470 📖 137
Southern Health Board
Wilton, 21 96 6844 📖 137
Southern Nevada Association of Pride (SNAP)
Las Vegas, 702 798 9455 📖 286
Southern New Hampshire Gay & Lesbian Youth (SNHAGLY)
Nashua, 603 672 0792 📖 288
Southern Ontario Bears
Toronto 📖 56
Southern Oregon Lambda Association
Ashland / Medford, 503 773 8146 📖 324
Southern Region Motor Club (SRMC)
Adelaide, 8 266 3268 📖 30
Southern Sisters
Chapel Hill, 919 682 0739 📖 313
Southern Tier AIDS Program, Inc.
Johnson City, 800 333 0892 📖 295
Southern Voice 📖 244
Southland Social Group
Invercargill 📖 162
Southside AIDS Venture
Danville, 804 799 5190 📖 348
Southside Hospital
Bay Shore, 516 968 3000 📖 296
Southwest AIDS Committee
El Paso, 915 533 5003 📖 341
Southwest Louisiana AIDS Council
Lake Charles, 318 439 5145 📖 260
Southwest Men At Large
Tempe, 602 730 8171 📖 194
Soyez, Jean-François
Bruxelles / Brussel 📖 37
SPACE 📖 *See* Swindon Project for AIDS Counselling & Education
Spadola, Madeline, Ms.Ed, CADAC
Boston, 617 625 0761 📖 267
Spandex from the Imagination of Mark I. Chester
San Francisco, 415 621 6294 📖 186
Spank 📖 333
Spank Promotions
Bristol, 117 929 3754 📖 70
Spankclub
Bruxelles / Brussel, 2 523 6878 📖 36
Spanking Times
published by Tiffany Enterprises 📖 311
SPANK-L 📖 4
Spanks-A-Lot
published by Carter Stevens Presents 📖 332
Spanky's
Seattle, 206 938 3400 📖 353
Spanner Trust
London 📖 13
Sparrow Hospital
Lansing, 517 482 2700 📖 277
Spartacus
Garden Grove, 714 971 1113 📖 200
Liège / Luik / Luttich, 4 123 1259 📖 38
Los Angeles, 213 654 8108 📖 206
published by Bruno Gmünder Verlag 📖 108
Toulouse, 61 62 6145 📖 106
Spartacus Books
Vancouver, 604 688 6138 📖 46
Spartacus Centurion
Garden Grove, 714 971 1113 📖 200
Spartacus Enterprises
Portland, 800 666 2604 📖 326
Spartan MC
Alexandria 📖 263
Spartans MC
Spartanburg 📖 335
Spartans Wrestling Club
Philadelphia, 215 546 0735 📖 331
Sparta-Shop
Lübeck, 451 7 2453 📖 126
Speak Out 📖 353
Speaking Out 📖 54
Spearhead
Toronto 📖 56
Special Clothes
Alexandria, 703 683 7343 📖 182
Speckert, Josefina, M.Ed.
Pittsfield 📖 272
Spectator Magazine 📖 199
Spectrum
Iowa City, 319 354 1703 📖 257
Nelson, 3 525 9781 📖 162
Nelson, 3 547 2827 📖 162
San Anselmo, 415 457 1115 📖 210
Spectrum Radio AM 558
London, 181 905 5000 📖 85
Spellbound Limited
London 📖 69
Spencer Gifts
Atlantic City 📖 289
Spezial Schuversand
Recklinghausen 📖 131
SPG 📖 *See* Santé & Plaisir Gai
SPICE 📖 *See* Wives'/Partners' Concerns
Spijker
Amsterdam, 20 620 5919 📖 151
Spike
New York, 212 243 9688 📖 300
West Hollywood, 213 656 9343 📖 224
Spinsters Ink
Minneapolis / Saint Paul, 612 558 9655 📖 281
Splash 📖 74
Spokane AIDS Network
509 326 6070 📖 354
Spokane County Health District
509 324 1542 📖 354
Sportomatic, Ltd.
Port Chester, 914 939 2362 📖 19
Sports Locker
London, 171 221 9166 📖 86
Sportsheets
Huntington Beach, 800 484 9954 Ext. 7962 📖 196
Sportsman Hotel
Brisbane, 7 831 2892 📖 28
Springfield Area Lesbian Outreach (SALO)
217 525 4297 📖 253
Springfield Books & Video
413 781 6833 📖 272
Sprinkle, Annie
East Hampton, 516 329 9020 📖 299
Spunk 📖 205
published by Studio Iguana 📖 216
Spurs
Cincinnati, 513 621 2668 📖 317
Squish
published by Big Time Publications 📖 210
SRMC 📖 *See* Southern Region Motor Club
SSSH
West Haddon 📖 89
ST Publishing
London 📖 84, 85
St. Martin's Press
New York 📖 306
Stablemaster Bar
Amsterdam, 20 625 0148 📖 151
Stablemaster Hotel
Amsterdam, 20 625 0148 📖 151
Stacey's Bookshop
San Francisco, 415 421 4687 📖 218
Städtiches Gesundheitsamt-Beratungstelle für Geschlechtskrankheiten
Stuttgart 📖 132
Städtische Poliklinik für Haut- & Geschlechtskrankheiten
Zürich, 1241 8900 📖 179
Städtisches Gesundheitsamt AIDS Beratungstelle
Stuttgart, 711 216 6292 📖 132
Stainless Construction Company
Bryan 📖 339
Stainless Steel Ball
Brighton, 1273 323758 📖 13
Stainless Steel Body Art
Toronto, 416 504 1433 📖 58
Staircase Tattoos
Santa Cruz, 408 425 7644 📖 221
Stairwell Leathers
Calgary, 403 276 2471 📖 43
Stall

Frankfurt am Main, 69 29 1880 📖 117
Stallion Book & Video Centre
Manchester, 161 237 3401 📖 76
Stallions
Cleveland 📖 319
Stamford Health Department
203 967 2437 📖 232
Stamford Hospital
203 325 7000 📖 232
Stamp Out AIDS
New York, 212 354 8899 📖 303
Stanford Hygenic Corp.
Long Island City, 718 389 6433 📖 182
Stanford Lesbian, Gay, & Bisexual Community Center
415 725 4222 (office) 📖 222
Star Magazine 📖 208
Star Maker Video
New York, 212 541 6877 📖 308
Starbright Productions
San Francisco 📖 218
Starburst
Lithis, 813 633 9653 📖 238
Starlight
Buckhurst Hill, 181 559 2369 📖 69
Stars 📖 307
STARS MC
Albany 📖 296
State Street Arcade
Madison, 608 251 4540 📖 356
State Street Bookstore
Rochester, 716 263 9919 📖 311
State University Association of Lesbians & Gays
Grand Rapids 📖 276
Staten Island AIDS Task Force
New York, 718 981 3366 📖 303
Station House
San Francisco 📖 212
STD Clinic
Cincinnati, 513 352 3138 📖 318
Fort Lauderdale, 305 797 6900 📖 236
Fort Wayne, 219 428 7504 📖 254
Galway, 91 460 00 📖 137
Ottawa, 613 234 0747 📖 52
Steam
published by PDA Press, Inc. 📖 355
Steel City Centurions
Pelham, 205 664 0609 📖 192
Stein, Virginia, MA
Somerville, 908 722 6343 📖 293
Steinhorn, Audrey
Poughkeepsie, 914 452 0374 📖 310
Steinmeier Photography
Chicago, 312 642 4707 📖 250
S-TEK
Montréal 📖 62
Stephan Richter Photography
Reutlingen, 71 212 2525 📖 131
Stepping Stones
Palo Alto, 415 583 9685 📖 209
Sterling
Needham Heights, 508 586 4442 📖 271
Sterling Rose Tattooing & Piercing
Fargo, 701 232 1744 📖 316
Steubenville News
614 282 5842 📖 322
Steve's Broadway News
Seattle, 206 324 7323 📖 353
Stewart's Army Surplus
Glasgow, 141 337 2550 📖 170
Stichting Bisexualiteit Nederland
Amsterdam, 20 664 2337 📖 152
Stichting Ede
Renkum, 31 731 8890 📖 157
Stichting Gay & Lesbian Association Amsterdam (GALA)
20 616 1979 📖 152
Stichting Gay Association
Roermund, 47 533 3119 📖 157
Stichting Homo Groep Gemert
49 236 6894 📖 155
Stichting M.V.S. FM 106.8, Cable 103.8
Amsterdam, 20 620 8866 📖 153
Stichting Nederlands Gender Centrum
Amstelveen, 20 612 4099 📖 151
Stichting Omd
Terheijden 📖 158
Stichting Reborn
Capelle a/d Ijssel, 10 458 3469 📖 154
Stichting SMet...!
Amsterdam 📖 152
Stichting Trefcentrum HIG - COC (Basta)
Den Haag, 70 365 9090 📖 154
Stichting Urania
Hilversum 📖 151
Stichting Werkgroep Biseksualiteit
Amsterdam, 20 634 0065 📖 152
Den Haag, 70 346 4767 📖 154
Stiefel 📖 108
Stiefelknecht
Köln, 221 21 3001 📖 124
Wien, 1 545 2301 📖 35
Stiletto Shoes AB
Stockholm, 750 53237 📖 176
Still Smokin'
Vancouver 📖 45
Stilletto
New York 📖 309
Stimulation
Hull, 1482 218068 📖 77
Stirling University LGB Society
178 646 7166 📖 167
Stockholm Gay Center
8 736 0212 📖 175
Stockholm Gay Radio
broadcast by FM 88 📖 176
Stockholm Rubber Men's Club
8 643 3100 📖 175
Stockroom
Los Angeles, 800 755 8697 📖 186, 206
Stocks & Bonds
Baltimore, 410 426 8158 📖 263
Stocks & Bonds Ltd.
Midvale 📖 345
Stonewall Alliance of Chico
916 893 3336 📖 198
Stonewall Library & Archives
Fort Lauderdale, 954 522 2317 📖 236
Stonewall News
published by That New Magazine 📖 308
Stonewall News Spokane 📖 354
Stonewall Union Lesbian / Gay Pride Report
broadcast by Cable Access Channel 21 📖 321
Stonewall Union of Students
Northbridge 📖 33
Stonewall Union Reports 📖 320
Stonewall Youth Group
Edinburgh, 131 556 4040 📖 169
Stop AIDS
Los Angeles, 310 659 4778 📖 204
Stop AIDS Byelarus
Minsk 📖 40
Stop AIDS Chicago
312 871 3300 📖 249
Stop AIDS Projekt Berlin
30 218 2011 📖 110
STOPRAPE 📖 3
Stormy Leather
San Francisco, 415 626 1672 📖 219
Stortford Lodge Bookshop
Hastings 📖 162
Stoughton Army Navy Center
Boston, 617 341 0769 📖 270
Straight to Hell (The Manhattan Review of Unnatural Acts) 📖 307
Strangeblades & More
Manchester, 203 645 9394 📖 187
Strapko, Nasncy, Ph.D.
Plymouth, 603 536 1306 📖 288
Stratègie
Paris, 145 32 1820 📖 102
Strathclyde Lesbian & Gay Switchboard
Glasgow, 141 332 8372 📖 169
Strathclyde University Union Shop
Glasgow 📖 169
Stretch
Amsterdam, 20 627 4305 📖 153
Strictly Speaking Publishing Co.
Palm Springs 📖 19, 208
Strictly Stories
Toronto, 416 622 2485 📖 10, 18
Strong Memorial Hospital of the University of Rochester
716 275 2100 📖 310
Stronghold at the Clock Hotel
Sydney, 2 360 4373 📖 26
Strout, David, LSMW
San Francisco 📖 213
Strubco, Inc.
New York, 212 242 1900 📖 308
Stud
Fort Lauderdale, 305 525 7883 📖 236
Students for Bisexual, Gay, & Lesbian Awareness (GALA)
Memphis 📖 337
Studio 2
Manchester, 1475 837930 📖 76
Studio Blu
Firenze, 55 422 3767 📖 146
Studio Iguana
San Francisco 📖 216
Studio One
Sioux Falls, 605 332 9316 📖 336
Studio Strak
Melbourne, 3 809 2632 📖 31, 32
Studio-7
El Cajon, 619 440 1020 📖 199
Studios J. M. R.
Barcelona, 93 239 6105 📖 172
Studs
San Francisco, 415 495 1811 📖 212
STUDS-30, Inc.
Novi, 810 348 5332 📖 277
Stuurgroep AIDS Preventie Homo's
Amsterdam, 20 671 2815 📖 150
su.gay 📖 6
Subculture
published by Strictly Stories 📖 18
Sublime
published by M. J. Production 📖 157
Submission
London, 171 284 2180 📖 80
Oahu, 808 942 0670 📖 247
Submissive Females
Maidenhead 📖 71
Subnormal
Bloomington 📖 248
Suburban Network 📖 252
Subwave Design
København, 33 12 1452 📖 66
Sudbury All Gay Alliance (SAGA)
705 670 2262 📖 54
Sudbury Sexual Assault Crisis Centre
705 675 1323 (24 hrs.) 📖 54
Sufficient As I Am (SAIM)
Baltimore, 410 837 5445 📖 264
Suffolk Lesbian & Gay Switchboard
Ipswich, 1473 232212 📖 91
Summit Consulting Group, Inc
East Greenwich, 401 884 2778 📖 334
Sun Leather & Lace
Louisville, 502 634 4705 📖 259
Suncoast Leather Club
Miami 📖 239
Sundance
Springfield, 217 788 5243 📖 253
Sundance Cattle Company
Houston, 713 527 9669 📖 342
Sunday Society
Chicago, 312 486 3126 📖 250
Sunderland Lesbian & Gay Young Peoples Group
191 565 7905 📖 92
SunMaster
Toronto, 416 763 5830 📖 24
Sunnypatch Works
Oshawa, 905 571 3896 📖 52
Sunrays MC
Hollywood 📖 237
Sunrise Center
Corte Madera, 415 924 5483 📖 198
Sunshine Club
Hadley 📖 270
Sunshine Gifts
Palmdale, 805 265 0652 📖 209
Sunshine News
Springfield, 417 831 2298 📖 284
Sunshine Publishing Co.
San Diego, 619 278 9080 📖 211
Superia Supplies
Hove, 127 377 8816 📖 69
Support Line 📖 237
Support Plus
Medfield, 800 229 2910 📖 271
Supporters of Worcester Area Gay & Lesbian Youth
508 755 0005 📖 273
Surrey & East Hants AIDSlink Ltd.
Guildford, 1483 300150 📖 91
Survivors
London, 171 833 3737 📖 82
Survivors of Transexuality Anonymous
New York, 212 969 0888 (voice mail) 📖 305
Susquehanna Lambda
Williamsport, 717 327 1411 📖 333
Sussex AIDS Helpline
Brighton, 127 357 1660 📖 74
Sussex County AIDS Committee
Rehoboth Beach, 302 945 3205 📖 233
Sussex Lancers MSC
Brighton 📖 74
Sussex Mailbox
Haywards Heath, 1444 482443 📖 70
Sussex Safer Sex Supplies Ltd.
Brighton, 1273 625222 📖 74
Sutherland's Books
Regina, 306 565 2808 📖 64
Sutter General Hospital
Sacramento, 916 454 2222 📖 209
Suzie Q Pleasure & Pain
Esslingen 📖 116
SVG
Hertogenbosch, 's / Den Bosch, 73 641 4141 📖 156
Hilversum, 35 629 2475 📖 156
Nijmegen, 80 322 6141 📖 156
Oss, 41 263 4245 📖 157
Roermund, 47 532 8112 📖 157
Valkenswaard, 40 204 0505 📖 158
Veghel, 41 336 7915 📖 158
Venlo, 77 354 0404 📖 158
SVGD
Haarlem, 23 531 9026 📖 155
Swan's Inner Sorority (SIS)
San José, 408 297 1423 📖 220
Swedish Medical Center
Seattle, 206 386 6000 📖 351
Sweet Sixties
Rotterdam, 10 213 2032 📖 157
Sweethearts Adult Bookshop
Townsville, 7 251 1431 📖 29
Swindon Project for AIDS Counselling & Education (SPACE)
1793 420620 📖 94
Swingers Bookstore
Anchorage, 907 561 5039 📖 193
SWISH 📖 *See* South Wales Immune Deficiency Self Help
Swish Publications Ltd.
London 📖 84
Switchboard
Frankfurt am Main, 69 28 3535 📖 117
Hannover, 511 41 3932 📖 121
Skellefteå, 910 22222 📖 176
Switchboard of Miami, Inc.
305 358 4357 📖 239
Sydney Bisexual Support Network (SBSN)
2 310 2798 📖 26
Sydney Bondage Club 📖 26
Sydney Leather Pride Association 📖 26
Sydney Star Observer 📖 27
Sylter Männer Leder Club (SLMC)
Westerland, 465 1 7849 📖 135
Syndicat PTT de la Manche CFDT
Saint Lô, 33 57 0697 📖 105
Synergy Book Service
Flemington, 908 782 101 📖 182
SYOL Ltd.
Binghamton, 607 723 5790 📖 297
Syracuse University Gay, Lesbian, Bisexual Student Association
315 443 3599 📖 312
Syren
Los Angeles, 213 936 6693 📖 205
T & P Men
Fruemsen, 81 757 1144 📖 13
T. B.'s Camelot
Wichita, 316 688 5343 📖 258
T. S. C.
Worthing 📖 92
T.O.M.
Rochester 📖 311
T.R.'s Leather Rack
Chesapeake, 804 420 4474 📖 348
Tab International

published by Mailshoppe Inc. 📖 59
Tabasco
Firenze, 55 21 3000 📖 146
Tabby
Westcliff On Sea 📖 69
Taboo Center
Malmö, 40 97 6410 📖 174
Taboo Tabou
Chicago, 312 548 2266 📖 252
Tacky Tavern
Seattle, 206 322 9744 📖 350
Tacoma Pride in Leather
Seattle 📖 351
Tacoma Sounds 📖 354
Tad's Total Adult Discount Store
Calgary, 403 237 8237 📖 43
Calgary, 403 244 8239 📖 43
Taffeta 📖 70
TAGALA 📖 *See* Toledo Area Gay & Lesbian Affiliation
TAGL 📖 *See* Toronto Area Gay/Lesbian Phoneline & Crisis Counselling
TAGS 📖 *See* Torquay AIDS Support Group
Tailors Unlimited
Wien, 1 505 4941 📖 35
Takoma Park Lesbians & Gays (TPLAG)
Baltimore, 301 891 3953 📖 264
TAKOTS 📖 *See* Teenage Kids of Ts
Talana Gamah & leish
London, 181 979 2429 📖 11
talk.rape 📖 6
Talking Leaves... Books
Buffalo, 716 837 8554 📖 298
Tallahassee Memorial Regional Medical Center
904 681 1155 📖 242
TAM Design
Salem, 603 898 0316 📖 183
Tamaki Makaurau 📖 161
Tamara Bane Gallery
Los Angeles, 213 651 1400 📖 205
Tampa AIDS Network
813 978 8683 📖 242
Tampa Bay Bondage Club
Largo, 813 832 2999 📖 238
Tampa Bay Trailblazers 📖 242
Tampa Bay Wrestling Club
Saint Petersburg 📖 241
Tampa General Healthcare
813 251 7000 📖 242
Tampere AIDS-Tukikeskus
93 113 3307 📖 95
TAMUGLB 📖 4
Tan Ya Hide Ltd.
Auckland, 9 623 0397 📖 161
Tandy Leather Co.
817 244 6404 📖 190
Tanner, Mark, M.D.
Atlanta, 404 355 2000 📖 244
Tannery Row
San Anselmo 📖 210
Tantra Magazine 📖 294
Taos Book Shop
505 758 3733 📖 295
TAP 📖 *See* AIDS Project. *See also* Tucson AIDS Project, Inc.
TAPE 📖 *See* Triangle Area Power Exchange
Tarheel Leather Club
Greensboro, 910 288 4709 📖 315
Tarrant County Hospital
Dallas / Fort Worth, 817 921 3431 📖 340
Tarrant County Parents Group
Dallas / Fort Worth, 817 656 8056 📖 340
Tartan Skirt
published by ADF Editorial Services 📖 168
Tartarus
Saint Louis 📖 284
Task Force Surplus Supplies
Stirling, 1786 451136 📖 167
Tass Surtur
Stockholm 📖 176
Taste of Latex
published by DM International 📖 20, 21
Taste of Leather
San Francisco, 800 367 0786 📖 219
Tatau Obscur
Berlin 📖 110
TATs 📖 *See* Texas Assocation of Transexuals
Tattered Cover Book Store
Denver, 800 833 9327 📖 228
Tattler 📖 260
Tattoo Club of Great Britain
Oxford, 186 571 6877 📖 69
Tattoo Connection
Berlin 📖 111
Tattoo Directory 📖 207
Tattoo Factory
Butler, 201 838 7828 📖 290
Tattoo Santa Barbara
805 962 7552 📖 221
Tattoo World
Fort Pierce, 407 465 6255 📖 237
Tattoo You
Seattle, 206 324 6443 📖 353
Tattooing & Piercing Studio
Amsterdam, 20 625 7812 📖 152
Tauranga Gay Support Group 📖 163
Tavistock Centre
London, 171 435 7111 📖 81
Tayfriend
Dundee 📖 170
Tayland House
Shawseen 📖 272
Taylor, Brad, M.A.
Los Angeles, 310 576 5455 📖 203
T-Bear Club
Dallas / Fort Worth, 214 349 0815 📖 340
T-Bears of Boston
Millis, 508 376 5892 📖 271
TCBA 📖 *See* Twin Cities Bondage Association
TCC 📖 *See* Community Center
TCNE 📖 *See* Tiffany Club of New England, Inc.
TDA - Atlanta 📖 244
Te Roopu Tatautoko
Wellington, 4 389 9676 📖 159
Tea With The Boys
broadcast by Radio One FM 91 📖 161
Tease!
published by Pure Imagination 📖 14
Teddy Bear Leather Club
Richmond, 804 232 0646 📖 347
Teen Fag
published by Chow Chow Productions 📖 353
Teen Options Clinic
Manchester, 603 429 1616 📖 288
Teenage Kids of Ts (TAKOTS)
Aurora 📖 226
Teeside Friend
Middlesbrough, 1642 248888 📖 88
Teestube Schwuler Treff
Kleve, 282 12 3157 📖 123
Tejas MC
San Antonio, 512 223 6620 📖 344
Telecentral Electronics
Wyoming, 717 655 2880 📖 15, 16
Telefon des Vertrauens
Neustrelitz, 398 1 4995 📖 129
Rostock, 381 45 3156 📖 131
Schwerin, 385 80 0618 📖 132
Telefonberatung Homosexualität
Göttingen, 551 4 3438 📖 118
Telefono AIDS
Perugia, 75 63942 📖 146
Telefono Amica
Milano, 1678 27182 📖 142
Telefono Amico Gay
Milano, 1678 27182 📖 142
Telefono Gay
Milano, 2 581 00299 📖 142
Telephono Rosa
Barcelona, 93 237 7070 📖 172
Telephono Viola
Forli, 543 34422 📖 140
Tell-A-Woman
Philadelphia, 215 564 5810 📖 330
Tels Quels 📖 36
Tels Quels Meeting Point
Bruxelles / Brussel, 2 512 4587 📖 37
Temple Lambda Alliance
Philadelphia, 215 232 4522 📖 330
Temple of Hecate
Cincinnati 📖 318
Ten Percent 📖 205
Ten Percent of U
Allendale, 616 895 6611 📖 274
Tenbusch, Lynne, Ph.D.
Ann Arbor, 313 973 3232 📖 274
Tendences Gaies
broadcast by FM 96 📖 98
Tender Loving Couples
Claymont 📖 232
Tender Moments / The Other You
Fort Myers, 813 945 1448 📖 237
Tennessee Leather Tribe
Memphis 📖 336
Tennessee Vals
Nashville, 615 664 6883 (voice mail) 📖 337
Tennklubben
Bergen 📖 165
Tentacle
Grantham, 1572 768440 📖 11
Terrace Gay Connection
604 638 1632 📖 45
Terrence Higgins Trust
London, 171 242 1010 📖 67
London, 171 831 0330 📖 82
Territory University Gay Society (TUGS)
Darwin, 8 941 1711 📖 28
Terry Mangan Library
Denver, 303 831 6268 📖 227
TES 📖 *See* Eulenspiegel Society
Testing The Limits
Oklahoma City, 405 843 8378 📖 323
TEWAHO 📖 *See* Transgender Education, Welfare, & Health Organization
Texarkana AIDS Project, Inc.
501 773 1994 📖 194
Texas Assocation of Transexuals (TATs)
Bellaire, 713 827 5913 📖 339
Texas Cadre
Arlington 📖 338
Texas MC
Dallas / Fort Worth, 214 946 7089 Ext. 4 📖 340
Texas Renegade Club
Houston 📖 342
Texas Riders, Inc.
Houston, 713 771 9726 📖 343
Texas Triangle 📖 339
Textures
San Antonio, 210 805 8398 📖 344
TFM Co.
Tiverton, 1884 34958 📖 11
TGEA 📖 *See* Transgender Educational Association of Greater Washington
TGIC 📖 *See* Transgenderists' Independence Club
TGT 📖 *See* Gay Network
Thames Valley Positive Support (TVPS)
Slough, 1628 603 400 📖 71
Thamesdown Lesbian & Gay Line
Swindon, 1793 644585 📖 94
That New Magazine
New York, 212 627 2120 📖 308
Theseus Counseling Services
Augusta, 207 621 0858 📖 262
Boston, 617 868 3157 📖 267
Things
Zaragoza, 76 44 6362 📖 172
Things Medieval
Lawton, 405 357 8762 📖 323
Third Eye Centre
Glasgow 📖 170
This Ain't The Rosedale Library
Toronto, 416 929 9912 📖 59
This Month in Mississipi 📖 282
This Way Out
broadcast by Access Community Radio AM 810 📖 161
broadcast by Overnight Productions 📖 205
This Week Guide 📖 261
This Week in Saint Louis (TWISL)
published by Kacmer Publishing Co. 📖 247
This Week in Texas (TWT) 📖 338
Thompson, Deb-Ann, Ph.D, NCACII, CACIII
Denver, 303 758 6634 📖 227
Thomson, Deb-Ann
Denver, 303 433 3001 📖 227
Thomson-Shore, Inc.
Dexter, 313 426 3939 📖 275
Thor Publications
Bronx 📖 297
Thrasher, Bob, M.A.
Long Beach, 310 435 1749 📖 202
Thread City Book & Novelty
Willimantic, 203 456 8131 📖 232
Three Birds Bookstore
Tampa, 813 247 7041 📖 243
Three Lives & Co., Ltd.
New York, 212 741 2069 📖 309
Three Rivers Leather Club, Inc.
Pittsburgh 📖 331
Three Worlds
London, 181 767 7464 📖 80
Threshold
Marina Del Rey, 213 845 0889 📖 206
Throb
Atlanta, 404 522 0355 📖 245
Throbbs
Claremont San Dimas 📖 198
Throbnet
Wentzville 📖 285
Thud 📖 85
Thunder Bay District Health Unit
807 625 5981 📖 54
Thunder Bay Physical & Sexual Assault Centre
807 344 4502 (24 Hrs.) 📖 54
Thunderbolt Book Club
London 📖 82
Thüringer Lederclub (TLC)
Erfurt, 361 731 2233 📖 116
Tiberius ASC
Wien, 1 55 8319 📖 35
Tidewater AIDS Crisis Task Force
Norfolk, 804 626 0127 📖 348
Tidewater Bears
Denbigh 📖 348
Tie Me Down
Milwaukee, 414 272 3696 📖 357
Tiffany Club of New England, Inc. (TCNE)
Woburn, 617 891 8325 📖 273
Tiffany Club Wives' Support Group
Woburn, 617 891 9325 📖 273
Tiffany Enterprises
Ronkonkoma, 516 467 0480 📖 311
Tight Situation
London, 181 857 7146 📖 68
Tightropes
Halifax 📖 48
Tijuana AIDS / SIDA Organization
Mexico City, 66 80 9963 📖 149
Tillamook County GALA
Pacific City 📖 326
Tim Swig Associates Group
Stone Harbor, 609 368 2482 📖 293
Tim Woodward Publishing Ltd.
London, 181 968 0234 📖 84
Time Out 📖 84
Portland, 207 871 9940 📖 262
Time Out Youth
Charlotte, 704 377 3399 📖 314
Timely Books
Chattanooga, 615 875 9447 📖 336
Times 📖 85
Times of the Heartland 📖 285
Times Square Books
Rochester, 716 325 9570 📖 311
Tina
Barcelona 📖 172
Tinkerbell's Treasures
London 📖 68
Tino Trevino's Leather Den
New York, 212 620 0828 📖 309
Tir-State Gay / Lesbian Awareness Dialogue Group
Amherst, 603 673 5391 📖 287
Titan
Pensacola 📖 241
TLC 📖 *See* Transgender Liberation Coalition. *See also* Thüringer Lederclub.
TLC Productions
Northampton, 413 586 5514 📖 189
To Tell The Truth Television
broadcast by Cathedral of Hope 📖 341
Todd Friedman Photography
Beverly Hills, 310 239 4818 📖 197
Todd Kaplan Gallery
Santa Monica, 310 659 5075 📖 222
Together At Last Lesbians
Yakima, 509 454 4989 📖 354

TOHR Gay / Lesbian Helpline
Tulsa, 918 743 4297 323
Toko Koschnick, Peter
Hamburg, 40 439 1847 120
Tokyo Boeki Shokai Ltd.
Shinjuku-Ku 148
Toledo Area Gay & Lesbian Affiliation 322
Toledo Area Gay & Lesbian Affiliation (TAGALA)
419 243 9351 322
Toledo Wellness Group
419 244 6682 322
Tollyboy Products
Sheffield, 1742 890575 90
Tom of Finland Company Inc.
Los Angeles, 800 334 6526 10, 206
Tom of Finland Foundation
Los Angeles, 213 250 1685 1
Tom's Bar
Berlin, 30 213 4570 110
Tom's Boutic
Lyon, 78 30 1984 101
Tom's House
Berlin, 30 218 5544 109
Tom's Ranch
Phœnix, 602 241 1604 194
Tom's Saloon
Hamburg, 40 280 3056 119
Tom's Toybox
New Orleans, 504 523 7827 261
Tomahawk
Cleveland, 216 521 5443 318
Tomcat Store
Philadelphia, 215 985 9725 331
Tomes & Treasures
Tampa, 813 251 9368 182, 243
Tool Shed
Sydney, 2 565 1599 27
Toolbox
Toronto, 416 466 8616 55
Topeka AIDS Project
913 232 3100 258
TopHat's Calendar of Erotica
published by Champagne Productions 19
TOPPS *See* Transexual Outreach
TOPS FM 104.1
Darwin, 8 941 1711 28
Torbay AIDS Group Supporters
Torquay, 180 329 9266 73
Toronto Area Gay/Lesbian Phoneline & Crisis Counselling (TAGL)
416 964 6600 56
Toronto Bisexual Network
416 925 XTRA Ext. 2015 57
Toronto Centre for Lesbian & Gay Studies 56
Toronto People With AIDS Foundation
416 506 1400 56
Toronto Women's Bookstore
416 922 8744 59
Torquay AIDS Support Group (TAGS)
1803 299266 73
Torrington Video Books
860 496 7747 232
Torso
published by MMG Services Inc. 307
Torture Garden
London, 171 490 0379 82
Toucan Productions
Cape Coral, 813 945 3007 236
Touch
Apeldoorn 153
Touché
Chicago, 312 465 7400 248
Touchpoint 193
Touchpoint Network for the Non-Monogamous
Chloride 193
Tours Elisa 2000
47 20 000899 106
Tower Books
Sacramento, 916 444 6688 210
Tower City Corps
Cleveland 319
Tower Newsstand
Lowell, 508 452 8693 271
Towne News
York, 717 232 1100 333
Townsend, Larry
Beverly Hills, 213 463 2333 184
Townsville Gay & Lesbian Resource & Information Network
7 772 6446 29
Townsville Gayline
7 772 6622 29
Townsville General Hospital
7 781 9369 29
Towson State University Gay & Lesbian Outreach
Baltimore, 410 830 4007 264
Toy Box
Upland, 909 982 9407 224
Toys For Tops
Long Beach, 310 425 1070 202
Toys in Babeland
Seattle, 206 328 2914 353
Seattle, 800 658 9119 186
Toy-Versand
Zürich 177
TPA Network
Chicago, 312 404 8726 188
TPLAG *See* Takoma Park Lesbians & Gays
Track
Montréal, 514 521 1419 62
Trader
New York 309
Trader Tom's Fantasy Depot
Fort Lauderdale, 305 524 4759 237
Tradesmen, Inc.
Charlotte 314
Trail Books
Miami, 305 262 4776 239
Training By Design
Washington, 202 546 1549 235
Trangender Forum
Pacifica 208
Trans
West Virginia 355
Trans Post-Op Recovery Residence (TransPORRS)
Montréal 62
Trans Reality
Nürnberg, 911 22 2377 129
Trans Support
Portland 263
Transequal
Saint Catharines, 905 688 0276 49
TransEssex
Basildon, 1268 583761 74
Transexual Lesbians & Friends
Seattle, 206 292 1037 352
Transexual Menace
Pittsburgh 332
Transexual Organization Self Help
Toms River 293
Transexual Outreach (TOPPS)
Auckland, 9 366 6106 160
Transexual Support Group (TSG)
Pittsburgh, 412 661 7030 332
Transfert
Paris, 142 60 4842 102
Transformatie
Den Haag 154
Transformation
published by Spartacus 200
Transformation Ltd.
Birmingham, 121 554 2429 93
Bristol, 117 959 3413 70
London, 171 388 0627 86
Newcastle upon Tyne, 191 230 1105 92
Prestwich, 161 773 2572 76
Prestwich, 161 773 4477 76
TRANSGEN 4
Transgender Education, Welfare, & Health Organization (TEWAHO)
Wellington, 4 479 2610 159
Transgender Educational Association of Greater Washington (TGEA)
Arlington, 301 949 3822 347
Transgender Identity Group
Milwaukee, 414 271 3322 357
Transgender Liberation Coalition (TLC)
Sydney, 2 358 5664 26
Transgender Network
Poughkeepsie 310
Transgender Rights
New York, 212 979 8547 304
Transgender Support Group of Baltimore
410 837 5445 264
Transgendered Alliance
Boston 268
Transgendered Magazine 271
Transgenderists' Independence Club (TGIC)
Albany, 518 436 4513 296
Transidentitas
Offenbach, 69 800 1008 130
TRANSITAS
Erfurt, 361 731 2233 116
Transition Support
Toronto 57
Translucere
Chicago, 312 477 6006 251
Trans-Net
Chesterfield, 1246 275799 72
Transpitt
Pittsburgh, 412 231 1181 332
TransPORRS *See* Trans Post-Op Recovery Residence
Trans-Port
Capital City 327
Portland, 503 774 7463 326
Transsexual Voice 244
Transsexuals In Prison
Montréal 62
Transsisters, The Journal of Transsexual Feminism
published by Skyclad Publishing 22
Trans-Trap
Edinburgh, 131 555 6416 169
Trans-tukipiste
Helsinki, 90 41 1135 96
Transupport
Portland 263
TransVamp
published by TransVamp Publications, Ltd. 22
TransVamp Publications, Ltd.
Philadelphia, 215 898 4714 22
Transvestite's Guide
published by The WayOut Publishing Company 84
Transvestites Transexuals Group Minorities Trust
Wellington, 4 844 764 160
Transvision
København 66
Trap
Paris, 143 54 5353 102
Trasek
Helsinki, 90 241 1135 95
TRASH 290
Trashy Lingerie
Los Angeles, 310 652 4543 205
Travel Keys Tours
Sacramento, 916 452 5200 210
Travesty/Transsexualle
Istanbul, 1 578925 180
Trax
Calgary, 403 265 8477 42
Treasure Box Video & News
Greensboro, 910 373 9849 315
Treasure Chest
Portland, 207 772 2225 263
Treare Chest II
Waterville, 207 873 7411 263
Treffpunkt Regenbogen
Düsseldorf, 221 72 0186 115
Treville Edition, Ltd.
Shibuya-Ku, 3 3481 5611 148
Triad Gender Association
Greensboro 315
Triad Health Project
Greensboro, 910 275 1654 315
Triangle 240
Triangle Area Power Exchange (TAPE)
Raleigh 315
Triangle Club
Seattle, 206 587 6924 352
Triangle Coalition
Columbia, 314 882 4427 283
Triangle Express Productions
Long Beach, 310 491 1046 203
Triangle Foundation
Detroit, 313 537 3323 275
Triangle Interests
Philadelphia, 215 844 6348 330
Triangle Journal News 337
Triangle Lesbian & Gay Alliance
Durham, 919 929 4053 314
Triangle Rising 195
Triangle Rose
broadcast by FM 96.8 98
Triangle Services
Trellech, 1600 860122 359
Triangle Television, Inc.
Auckland, 9 376 7385 (Jim Blackman, President) 160, 161
Triangle World & Leather Palace
Kalamazoo, 616 373 4005 276
triangle.motss 6
Tribe
published by Columbia Publishing Company 264
Triborough Triangles
Attleboro Falls, 508 223 4636 267
Tribune
Maastricht, 43 325 1978 156
Tri-Cities Gay & Lesbian Alliance
Bay City, 517 799 2583 274
Trident
Baltimore 264
Cleveland 319
Columbus 320
Detroit 275
Fort Lauderdale 236
Kingston 50
Los Angeles, 213 383 4866 204
Michigan, 313 271 4901 273
New York, #2 304
Philadelphia 333
Rochester 311
Toledo 322
Washington, D.C., 301 297 7539 265
Windy City 252
Trident International DC Hall, Inc.
Greenbelt 265
Trident Knights
Charleston, 803 769 2094 334
Tri-Ess *See* Society for the Second Self
Trigon
Erie, 814 453 6232 328
Tri-Graphic Printing (Ottawa) Ltd.
613 731 7441 53
Tri-State Alliance
Evansville, 812 484 4853 253
Tri-State Bears
Ironton, 614 532 6307 321
Tri-State Couples Club
Pittsburgh 331
Tri-State Polyamory
New Providence 292
Tri-State TCC
Pittsburgh 331
Tri-State Transgendered Club
Deer Park, 301 453 3538 265
Trivia 267
Trixx Adult Cinema & Bookstore
El Paso, 915 532 6171 342
Tromsø Komm. Helsekontor
77 62 0485 166
Trondeheim Rode Kors
Trondheim, 73 52 8810 166
Trondheim AIDS og Infeksjonshelsetjenesten
73 99 7990 166
Trondheim Helseråd
Trondheim, 73 59 7740 166
Trongate Books
Glasgow, 141 552 1545 170
Tronsmo Bokhandel
Oslo, 22 20 2509 164
True Colors
San Antonio, 800 745 0555 182
True Grace Corsets
Wokingham, 1734 785577 71
Truman Medical Center
Kansas City, 816 556 3000 283
TRUST (FF National Network)
San Francisco 188
TRUST, The Handballing Newsletter
published by Alamo Square Press 218
Trusted Servants
San Francisco, 415 552 0301 214
TS Gesellschaft Hamburg e.V.
40 7549 5910 120
TS Peer Support Meetings
Houston, 713 333 2278 343
Tsarus

Memphis 📖 336
Tschul's
Berlin, 30 612 5143 📖 111
TSG 📖 *See* Transexual Support Group
TSH
Essen, 201 78 6999 📖 116
Münster, 251 43240 📖 128
TS-Selbsthilfe Gruppe
Saint Gallen 📖 179
TSSG
Minneapolis / Saint Paul, 612 653 7936 📖 280
TTBM
Paris, 148 04 8088 📖 104
Tucholsky Buchladen
Offenbach, 69 99 7090 📖 130
Tucson AIDS Project, Inc. (TAP)
602 326 2437 📖 194
Tucson Arizona Levi/Leathermen 📖 194
Tucson Knight Owls 📖 194
Tucson Medical Center
602 327 5461 📖 194
Tuff Stuff
Phœnix, 602 254 9561 📖 184
TUGS 📖 *See* Territory University Gay Society
Tulane University Hospital & Clinincs
New Orleans, 504 588 5263 📖 260
Tullous, Don
Sacramento, 916 485 5033 📖 210
Tulsa News 📖 324
Tulsa Oklahomans for Human Rights
918 743 4297 📖 324
Tunbridge Wells Switchboard
Royal Tunbridge Wells, 1892 535876 📖 78
Turk Street News & Video
San Francisco, 415 885 2040 📖 219
Turkey Media Services
Long Beach, 310 434 7129 📖 202
Turnaround
London, 171 609 7836 📖 80
Turun AIDS-Tukikeskus
Turku, 921 253 4746 📖 96
Tuscaloosa Lesbian Coalition
205 333 8227 📖 192
TV Connection
published by DM International 📖 353
TV Selbsthilfegruppe
Münster 📖 129
TV Self Help Group
London, 171 289 5240 📖 83
TV/TS Support Group
Memphis 📖 337
TVPS 📖 *See* Thames Valley Positive Support
TVS Verein Transvestitin & Arbeitsgruppe TS
Wien 📖 35
TV-TS Confidential
published by Writer's Etc. 📖 288
TVV
Hattersheim 📖 122
tw.bbs.rec.motorcycle 📖 5
tw.bbs.sci.medicine 📖 5
tw.bbs.sci.psychology 📖 4
tw.bbs.sci.sex 📖 4
Twenty Club (XX)
Hartford 📖 231
Twentysomething
New York, 212 967 7711 Ext. 3163 📖 306
Twenty-Third Avenue Book
Portland, 503 224 5097 📖 327
Twilight 📖 110
Twilight Zone
Berlin, 30 218 1432 📖 110
Twin Cities Bondage Association (TCBA)
Minneapolis / Saint Paul 📖 280
TWIST 📖 353
Twitchell, Carol, Psy.D.
Sarasota, 941 365 9424 📖 241
Two Sisters Bookshop
San Mateo, 415 323 4778 📖 220
Two Wheelers Auxiliary Troop
Omaha 📖 286
Two-Spirited People of the First Nations Native Awareness Project
Toronto, 416 944 9300 📖 56
TWS Ent.
Florence 📖 191
Tyger Tyger
London, 171 622 5655 📖 83
U.C. Alliance of Lesbian, Gay, & Bisexual People
Cincinnati, 513 556 1449 📖 318
U.S. Conference of Mayors
Washington, 202 293 7330 📖 234
UAB G/L Student Union
Birmingham 📖 191
Überfalltelefon
München, 89 1 9411 📖 128
Ubiquity Distributors
Brooklyn, 718 875 5491 📖 181
UC Irvine GLBSU
714 856 4260 📖 201
uc.motss 📖 6
UCHSC
Denver, 303 270 8870 📖 227
UCSD Medical Center
San Diego, 619 294 6222 📖 211
Uglesett
Bergen 📖 165
UGON 📖 *See* United Gay Organization of Namibia
Uitkomst
published by Gesprecks- en Onthaalcentrum u. z. w. 📖 36
uiuc.soc.bisexuals 📖 6
uiuc.soc.gay-men 📖 6
UK Lambda
Lexington 📖 259
uk.gay-lesbian-bi 📖 6
UK-MOTSS 📖 4
UK-MOTSS-WOMEN 📖 4
Ultimate Productions
Santa Clara 📖 221
Ultra Ink, Inc.
Chicago, 312 327 7271 📖 251
Ultra-Sex Alliance
Ann Arbor 📖 274
Un Mercoledi da Leone
broadcast by Nova Radio FM 101.5 📖 146
Una Deva
Shepton Mallet, 174 983 1397 📖 69
Unabridged Books
Chicago, 312 883 9119 📖 251
Uncirc South Australia
Adelaide 📖 30
Uncircumcised Society of America (USA)
San Francisco 📖 214
Uncut
San Francisco 📖 214
Uncut Club
Los Angeles 📖 204
Uncut Dallas
Dallas / Fort Worth 📖 341
Underground
Fort Lauderdale 📖 236
London, 181 875 1607 📖 80
Vancouver 📖 45
Underground Art
Memphis, 901 272 1864 📖 337
Unforgettable Fire 📖 291
Ungdomsgruppen for Bøsser og Lesbiske i Sønderjylland
Sønderborg, 74 62 1148 📖 67
Unicorn Books
Boston, 617 646 3680 📖 270
Unicorn Bookstore
West Hollywood, 310 652 6253 📖 225
Unicorn MC
Cleveland 📖 319
Unicorns of Madison 📖 356
Uniforms, Inc.
Los Angeles, 213 383 1395 📖 205
Santa Ana, 714 541 3546 📖 221
Unigaie
Genève / Genf 📖 178
UNIGLOW 📖 *See* University of Northern Iowa Gay & Lesbian Outreach
Union of Lesbians, Gays. & Bisexuals
Riverside, 909 787 3337 📖 209
Unique Creations
Las Vegas, 702 365 1818 📖 184
Unique News
Niagara Falls, 716 282 9282 📖 310
Unique Quality Products, Inc.
New York, 212 580 4335 📖 309
Unisex Adult Bookstore
Brick Town, 908 295 0166 📖 289
Unita Sanitaria Locale (USL)
Aosta, 165 55 2675 📖 146
Lecce, 832 6851 📖 144
Unitec Gay & Lesbian Support Association
Auckland, 9 815 0440 📖 160
United Army Surplus
Chicago, 312 671 8610 📖 252
United Book
Worcester, 508 752 9293 📖 273
United Gay Organization of Namibia (UGON)
Windhoek 📖 149
United Hospitals Medical Center
Newark, 201 268 8000 📖 292
United Leatherfolk of Connecticut
East Hartford 📖 230
United Services
Dayville, 203 774 2020 📖 230
United Theological Seminary Lesbian & Gay Caucus
Minneapolis / Saint Paul, 612 633 8703 📖 280
Universal Brotherhood of Leatherlords
Phœnix 📖 194
Universal News Agency
Los Angeles, 213 467 3850 📖 205
Universitätshautklinik
Jena, 364 1 822 2048 📖 122
University & Childrens' Hospital
Columbia, 314 882 8000 📖 283
University Bi Community
Minneapolis / Saint Paul, 612 626 2344 📖 280
University Bookstore
Iowa City, 319 335 3179 📖 257
University Center Bookstore
Missoula, 406 4921 📖 285
University College London 📖 81
University Health Service
Madison, 608 262 7330 📖 356
University Hospital
Albuquerque, 505 843 2121 📖 294
Newark, 201 982 4300 📖 292
Portland, 503 494 8311 📖 326
Syracuse, 315 464 5540 📖 312
University Hospital of Cleveland
216 844 1000 📖 318
University Hospital of Zürich
1 255 2306 📖 179
University Hospitals & Clinics
Jackson, 610 984 1000 📖 282
University Lesbian, Gay, & Bisexual Alliance
Duluth 📖 279
University Lesbians
Minneapolis / Saint Paul, 612 625 1611 📖 280
University Medical Center
Jacksonville, 904 549 5000 📖 238
Las Vegas, 702 383 2000 📖 286
Tucson, 602 694 0111 📖 194
University of Alabama Gay & Lesbian Alliance
Tuscaloosa, 205 348 7120 📖 192
University of Alabama Hospital
Birmingham, 205 975 7545 📖 191
University of Birmingham
121 414 6060 📖 93
University of California - Davis Medical Center
Sacramento, 916 734 3096 📖 209
University of California Irvine Medical Center
Orange, 714 456 5678 📖 208
University of Chicago Gay & Lesbian Alliance
312 702 9734 📖 250
University of Cincinnati Hospital
513 558 1000 📖 318
University of County Cork Gay Society
21 27 6871 📖 137
University of Kansas Hospital
Kansas City, 913 588 1270 📖 257
University of Manitoba
Winnipeg, 204 474 8411 📖 47
University of Maryland Medical System
Baltimore, 410 328 8667 📖 263
University of Massachusetts Medical Center
Worcester, 508 856 0011 📖 273
University of Michigan
Ann Arbor, 313 763 4186 📖 274
University of Michigan Hospitals
Ann Arbor, 313 936 4000 📖 274
University of Minnesota
Minneapolis / Saint Paul, 612 625 1500 📖 280
Minneapolis / Saint Paul, 612 626 9765 📖 280
University of Minnesota Hospital
Minneapolis / Saint Paul, 612 626 3000 📖 279
University of Minnesota Lesbian & Gay Law Students Association
Minneapolis / Saint Paul, 612 625 1000 📖 280
University of Nebraska Medical Center
Omaha, 402 559 7400 📖 285
University of New South Wales Gay & Lesbian Department
Sydney, 2 663 0461 📖 27
University of North Carolina - Wilmington
910 395 3119 📖 316
University of North Dakota G&L Coalition
Grand Forks 📖 317
University of Northern Iowa Gay & Lesbian Outreach (UNIGLOW)
Waterloo, 319 273 2676 📖 257
University of Ottawa Lesbigays
613 230 3076 📖 53
University of Pittsburgh
412 624 2008 📖 331
University of South Alabama Medical Center
Mobile, 205 471 7000 📖 192
University of South Australia Gay, Lesbian, & Bisexual Association
Ingle Farm, 8 302 3212 📖 31
University of South Florida Gay, Lesbian, & Bisexual Coalition
Tampa, 813 974 4297 📖 242
University of Southern California Medical Center
Los Angeles, 213 226 2622 📖 203
University of Sunderland LGB Group 📖 92
University of Teeside LGB Group
Middlesbrough, 164 234 2234 📖 88
University of Tennessee Memorial Hospital
Knoxville, 615 544 9000 📖 336
University of Toronto Bookstore
416 978 7918 📖 59, 60
University of Toronto Sexual Education & Peer Counselling Centre
416 591 7949 📖 57
University of Virginia Hospital
Charlottesville, 804 924 9821 📖 347
University of Washington Medical Center
Seattle, 206 548 3300 📖 351
University of Wisconsin Hospital & Clinics
Madison, 608 263 6400 📖 356
University Students' Council - GLBi Commissioner
London, 519 661 3574 📖 51
Unleashed
published by Unlimited 📖 94
Unlimited
Leeds 📖 94
Up The Stairs Community Center
Fort Wayne, 219 744 1144 📖 254
Update 📖 201, 212
Upper Manhattan Task Force on AIDS
New York, 212 870 3352 📖 303
Uppsala Gay Studenter (FUGS) 📖 176
Upstairs Bookshop
Providence, 401 272 3139 📖 334
Upstate Women's Community
Greenville, 803 271 4207 📖 335
Uptown Bookstore
Youngstown, 216 783 2553 📖 322
Uptown Novelties
Atlanta, 404 875 9210 📖 245
Urania Books
Jacksonville, 904 744 7879 📖 238
Urban Fitness
published by Urban Publishing, Inc. 📖 201
Urban Primitive
Toronto, 416 966 9155 📖 60
Urban Publishing, Inc.
Laguna Beach 📖 201
Urban Tribe
Atlanta, 404 365 2407 📖 244
URI Gay, Lesbian, & Bisexual Association
Kingston, 401 792 2097 📖 334
Ursine Group
Iowa City 📖 257
Ursus

Dayton, 513 643 9220 321
Ursus Club
Bern, 31 311 7406 177
USA *See* Uncircumcised Society of America
USECA Communications Inc.
Ottawa, 613 241 9499 53
USL *See* Unita Sanitaria Locale
USUA Bisexual, Gay, & Lesbian Association
Tucson, 602 621 7585 195
Utah AIDS Foundation
Salt Lake City, 800 366 2437 345
Utah Stonewall Center
Salt Lake City, 801 539 8800 345
Utica Tri's, MC 312
Utopian Network
New York, 516 842 1711 307
uw.alt.sex.beastiality 6
uw.alt.sex.bondage 4
UWOUT
London, 519 432 3078 51
UW-Parkside Gay & Lesbian Organization
Racine, 414 595 2244 358
UZI
Denver, 303 832 4870 229
V. I. D. A.
Phœnix, 602 938 3932 194
V. I. Products, Inc.
Three Oaks, 616 756 3561 183
V. Jensen
Whittier, 310 943 8139 225
V. O. I. C. E. / Den of Pleasure
Harrisburg, 717 299 1779 328
V. V. S. M.
Lovendegem 38
Vaar
Dordrecht 154
Vacaville Book Co.
Fairfield, 707 449 0550 199
Vagevuur
Eindhoven, 40 244 2744 12
Vaincre le SIDA (VLS)
Paris, 144 78 7550 103
Valdosta State College Gay & Lesbian Association
912 247 0181 246
Valentine & Son, Inc.
Chicago, 312 939 3221 251
Valentine Products
Feltham 87
Valhalla
London, 181 674 9002 81
Valkyrie
Leighton Buzzard 70
Valley AIDS Information Network
Corvallis, 503 752 6322 325
Valley AIDS Network
Fredericksburg, 703 564 0448 348
Valley Bears
Sacramento, 916 484 7840 209
Valley Gay Alliance
Springfield, 413 736 2324 272
Valley Girls
Dunbar 354
Valley Hospital Medical Center
Las Vegas, 702 388 4000 286
Valley Medical Center of Fresno
209 453 4000 199
Valley Woman Books & Gifts
Fresno, 209 233 3600 200
Valley Women's Voice 267
Van Velsor, Gary
San Francisco, 415 558 9977 23
Van Volumes Limited
Thorndike, 413 283 8556 272
Vancouver Activists in SM (VASM)
604 434 1369 45
Vancouver General Hospital
604 536 2053 45
Vancouver Jacks
604 688 9378 Ext. 2034 45
Vancouver Leather Alliance
604 688 9378 Ext. 2035 45
Vanek, Stephen, LMSW-ACP
Dallas / Fort Worth, 214 239 8775 340
Vanguards MC
Philadelphia 330
Variety Books & Video
Martinsburg, 304 263 4334 355
VASM *See* Vancouver Activists in SM
Vassar Brothers Hospital
Poughkeepsie, 914 454 8500 310
Vassar Gay People's Alliance
Poughkeepsie, 914 437 7203 310
Vault
New York, 212 255 6758 300
vegas.bi 6
vegas.motss 6
VEHN *See* Verein zur Erforschung der Geschichte der Homosexuellen in Niedersachsen
Venango-Forest AIDS Support
Oil City, 800 359 2437 327
Venhälsan
Stockholm, 8 616 2500 175
Växjö, 470 88205 175
Venture-N
Houston, 713 522 0000 342
Tucson, 602 882 8224 194
Venue Services Limited
London, 171 916 0162 80
Vénus
Le Mans, 43 23 0615 100
Venus Adult Book Shop
Wollongong, 4 275 2121 28
Venus Infers 217
Venus Modern Body Arts, Inc.
New York, 212 473 1954 303, 306
Venus Photography
Minneapolis / Saint Paul, 612 338 1302 281
Venus Versand
Paderborn 107
Verdantmom
Camarillo, 805 987 3162 197
Verein für Lesben & Schwule
Greifswald 119
Verein für Sexuelle Emanzipation e. V. (VSE)
Braunschweig, 531 33 2423 112
Stuttgart 133
Verein für Sexuelle Gleichberechtigung e. V.
München, 89 260 3056 128
Verein Schwulenkultur e. V.
Hamburg, 40 430 0695 119
Verein zur Erforschung der Geschichte der Homosexuellen in Niedersachsen (VEHN)
Hannover, 511 66 1055 121
Verein zur Förderung der Erforschung der Geschichte der Homosexuellen in Nordrhein-Westfalen
Köln 124
Verein zur Verbesserung der Lebenssituation Homosexueller Frauen & Männer e. V.
Offenbach, 69 87 2700 130
Vereinigung Homosexualität & Gesellschaft e. V. (VHG)
Bayreuth, 921 85 2928 109
Vereniging Landelijk Netwerk voor Bisexualiteit (LNBi)
Amsterdam, 77 354 9776 150
Vereniging LKGT&T
Amsterdam, 76 593 3901 150
Vereniging Studiegroep Sado-Masochisme (VSSM)
Almelo, 20 420 2117 151
Amsterdam, 20 420 2117 150, 152
Arnhem, 20 420 2117 153
Eindhoven, 20 420 2117 155
Groningen, 20 420 2117 155
Rotterdam, 20 420 2117 157
Utrecht, 20 420 2117 158
Verhey, Gregory, MSW, CSW
New York, 212 447 3473 301
Verkeerd Geparkeerd Homojongeren
Gent / Gand 38
Verlag Rosa Winkel
Berlin, 30 853 4042 108
Verlag W.-D. Fritsch
Hamburg, 40 220 4001 108
Vermont AIDS Council
Montpelier, 802 229 2557 346
Vermont Cares
Burlington, 800 649 2437 346
Vermont PWA Coalition
Brattleboro, 802 257 9277 346
Vermont Women's Health Center
Burlington, 802 863 1386 346
Vernon's Specialties, Inc.
Nonantum, 617 894 1744 271
Versatile Fashions
Orange, 800 546 2902 208
Tustin, 800 546 2902 186
Vertigo Books
Washington, 202 429 9272 235
Very Special Clothes
Marathon 182
Vesta, Dianna
North Miami Beach, 800 433 8474 240
Vest-Agder Sentralsykehus
Kristiansand, 38 02 9080 166
Veterans Leather
Brooklyn, 718 768 0300 298
Veterans' Affairs Medical Center
Albany, 518 462 3311 296
Albuquerque, 505 265 1711 294
Ann Arbor, 313 761 5458 274
Baltimore, 410 605 7001 263
Biloxi, 601 388 5541 282
Boston, 617 232 9500 267
Bronx, 718 584 9000 297
Brooklyn, 718 630 3500 297
Charleston, 803 577 5011 334
Cincinnati, 513 861 3100 318
Cleveland, 216 526 3030 318
Dallas / Fort Worth, 214 372 7001 340
Fort Wayne, 219 426 5431 254
Houston, 713 791 1414 342
Jackson, 610 362 4471 282
Kansas City, 816 861 4700 283
Lexington, 502 895 3401 259
Lexington, 606 233 4511 259
Los Angeles, 310 478 3711 203
Manchester, 603 624 4366 288
Miami, 305 324 4455 239
Minneapolis / Saint Paul, 612 725 2000 279
Nashville, 615 327 4751 337
New Orleans, 504 568 0811 260
New York, 212 686 7500 302
Northampton, 413 584 4040 271
Pittsburgh, 412 692 3000 331
Portland, 503 220 8262 326
Saint Louis, 314 984 6661 284
Salt Lake City, 801 582 1565 345
Syracuse, 315 476 7461 312
Washington, 202 745 8000 233
VGC Uniforms
Chicago, 312 545 3676 251
Chicago, 312 779 6121 251
VHG *See* Vereinigung Homosexualität & Gesellschaft e. V.
Viacom Cabe, Channel 19
Nashville, 615 297 0008 337
Vibration
Perth, 9 242 4501 34
Vice
Los Angeles 203
Victor / Victoria's
Nashville, 615 244 7256 337
Victoria AIDS Respite Care Society
Vancouver, 604 388 6220 45
Victoria Persons with AIDS Society
604 383 7494 47
Victoria Regine
Wolverhampton, 1902 336191 68
Victorian AIDS Council
Melbourne, 39 483 6700 32
Melbourne, 39 483 6777 32
Melbourne, 39 483 6788 32
Video Book & News
Waterbury, 203 573 1066 232
Videomag Plus
Montréal, 514 871 1653 63
Viking Bears
Stockholm 175
Viking Press/Banta
Eden Prairie, 612 941 8780 279
Vikings MC
Boston, 617 451 5377 268
Village
Pittsburgh, 412 422 3060 1
Village Book & News
Buffalo, 716 887 5027 298
Village Bookshop
Manchester, 161 236 6441 76
Village Clinic
Winnipeg, 204 453 2144 (information) 47
Village Club
Brighton, 127 367 4816 74
Village Counseling, Inc.
Columbus, 614 444 7714 319
Village Green Bookstore
Buffalo, 716 827 5895 298
Buffalo, 716 884 1200 298
Fairport, 716 425 7950 299
New Hope, 215 230 7610 329
Rochester, 716 442 1151 311
Rochester, 716 723 1600 311
Village Voice
New York, 212 475 3300 308
Villeinage 343
Vimpex GmbH
Bad Bramstedt, 419 25 0010 107
VIPPS
Cleveland, 216 899 1326 318
Virago 334
Virginia's Secret
Richmond, 804 222 6796 349
Virginia's Sectret
Richmond 349
Virginians for Justice
Richmond 349
Virtjack Studios
Genève / Genf 14
Virtual Universe Publications Ltd.
London, 171 240 9156 85
Visibilia
Bologna, 51 263592 140
Vision SM Club
Melbourne 32
Visions & Dreams
Wichita, 316 942 6333 258
Visitors Guide to Gay Britain
published by Gay To Z Publishing, Ltd. 84
Vitale, Anne, Ph.D.
San Rafael, 415 456 4452 220
Vitaletti, Robert, Ph.D.
Denver, 303 628 5425 227
Viva TS - Selbsthilfe München e. V.
89 13481 128
Viveros, Brian
Corona 198
Vivre Autrement en Aquitaine
Blanquefort, 56 81 8062 98
VLS *See* Vaincre le SIDA
Vogel Verlag
Berlin 110, 111
Voice & Vision Productions
Royal Oak 278
Voice Literary Supplement
published by The Village Voice 308
Voice Magazine 196
Voices Magazine 260
Voices of Positive Women
Toronto, 416 324 8703 56
Voksne Babyers Verden
Langeskov, 65 38 3413 65
Volanti, Ron
Riverside, 708 484 8412 252
Voller's
Portsmouth, 1705 660 740 76
Volumé 298
Volumes
Toronto, 416 366 9522 60
Volumes of Pleasure
San Luis Obispo, 805 528 5565 220
Voyages
San Francisco, 415 495 4937 (service) 182
Vrije Boekhandel
Tilburg, 13 543 5944 158
Vrolijk Boekhandel
Amsterdam, 20 623 5142 153
VSE *See* Verein für Sexuelle Emanzipation e. V..
VSSM *See* Vereniging Studiegroep Sado-Masochisme
Vulcan America Southern California
Los Angeles 204
Vulcan LL
Columbus 320
Vyxyn's Leatherworks & Urbane Armory
Madisonville 186
W. & G. Foyles

London 📖 85
W. H. Smith
London, 171 237 5235 📖 85
London, 171 730 1200 📖 85
WA Creations
Seattle, 206 632 5791 📖 352
Wagga Wagga AIDS Task Force
6 923 4811 📖 27
Wagner, Dick, MSW, ACSW
Saint Louis, 314 965 1942 📖 284
WAIF FM 88.3
Cincinnati, 513 961 8900 (office) 📖 318
Waiheke Island Gay Support Group
Auckland, 9 372 7972 📖 160
Wairau Hospital
Blenheim, 3 577 1914 📖 161
Wake County Department of Health
Raleigh, 919 250 3950 (counslling & testing) 📖 315
Waking Owl
Salt Lake City, 801 582 7323 📖 345
Walden Books
Oahu, 808 922 4154 📖 247
Waldo-Knox AIDS Coalition
Belfast, 207 338 1427 📖 261
Walford, Virginia, Ph.D.
Ladner, 604 940 2838 📖 44
Walhalla
Antwerpen / Anvers, 3 233 6291 📖 36
Oostende / Ostende 📖 39
Walker, Sylvia, MSW, ACSW
Plainfield, 908 561 6073 📖 292
Wall
New York 📖 300
Wallace, Timothy, Ph.D.
Hartford, 203 233 6229 📖 230
Wally World
San Mateo 📖 220
Walsh, Eileen, M.S.
Pawling, 914 855 5306 📖 295
Walsworth Publishing Company
Marceline, 816 376 3543 📖 284
Walter's Leder Boutique
Berlin, 30 211 1897 📖 111
Walter, Daniel, Psy.D.
Virginia Beach, 804 424 0100 📖 349
Walthamweston Hospital & Medical Center
617 647 6000 📖 273
Wanda
published by N. S. P. 📖 18
Wanda's Wenches
Charlestown 📖 270
War & Peace
Glasgow, 141 334 9129 📖 170
Glasgow, 141 552 1101 📖 170
Glasgow, 141 552 2240 📖 170
Wardrobes by Carolyn
Melrose, 617 662 4432 📖 182
Warehouse
Antwerpen / Anvers, 3 225 2376 📖 36
Warlocks MC
San Francisco 📖 215
Warlords, Inc.
Atlanta, 404 315 9000 📖 245
Warner Cable Channel 47
Milwaukee, 414 964 8423 📖 357
Warren, Ellen, LCSW
Alexandria, 703 683 0710 📖 347
Warrington AIDSline
1925 417134 📖 72
Warrington Switchboard
1925 59572 📖 72
Warriors MC
Los Angeles 📖 204
Wasatch Leathemen
Salt Lake City, 801 355 8135 📖 345
Washington - Baltimore Alliance
301 277 5475 📖 234
Washington Blade 📖 235
Washington County AIDS Task Force
Fayetteville, 501 443 2437 📖 195
Washington State Mr. Leather Organization
Seattle, 206 720 4075 📖 351
Washington State Ms. Leather (WSMLO)
Seattle, 206 233 8527 📖 350
Washoe Medical Center
Reno, 702 328 4100 📖 287
Water Boys of San Diego
619 525 7755 📖 188
Water Hole Custom Leather, Inc.
East Hartford, 800 390 6674 📖 230
Waterstones
Cork, 21 27 6002 📖 137
Dublin, 1 679 1415 📖 137
London, 171 284 4948 📖 86
London, 171 434 4291 📖 86
Manchester 📖 76
WATS
Bulverde, 210 980 7788 📖 339
WATS Support, Unity, & Pride (WATSUP)
Doublview 📖 33
Watson, Jacob, M.A., L.C.P.C.
Portland, 207 870 8656 📖 262
Watson, Trevor
London, 181 749 2881 📖 83
WATSUP 📖 *See* WATS Support, Unity, & Pride
WAVES 📖 232
Way Out West Bookshop
Penrith, 4 731 3094 📖 25
Wayne's LeatheRack
Los Angeles, 213 655 1016 📖 206
Wayout Club
London 📖 80
WayOut Publishing Company
London 📖 84
Wayout Wine Bar
London, 181 363 0948 📖 80
Wayves 📖 48
We Are Everywhere
broadcast by CFRU FM 93.3 📖 61
We Are Visible 📖 206
We Enjoy Shaving
Reno 📖 188
We The People 📖 222
Wear FM 103.4FM
Sunderland, 191 515 2103 📖 92
WearHouse Uniforms
Glendale, 818 243 4440 📖 200
Hawthorne, 310 676 9180 📖 200
Weathervain
Kew Gardens, 181 940 0156 📖 91
Web
Amsterdam, 20 623 6758 📖 151
Webeverlag
Mülheim 📖 127
Wedda, Susan, MSW, ACSW, BCD
Flint, 810 234 3658 📖 275
Wedge Bookshop
Coventry 📖 93
Weekly News 📖 235
Weeks, Alan
London, 171 284 2621 📖 80
Weene, Kenneth, Ph.D.
New York, 516 496 8023 📖 302
Weinberger, Bette, ACSW
Harrisburg, 717 233 7153 📖 328
Welcome Wagon
Dallas / Fort Worth, 214 733 9644 📖 341
Wellington, Susan, MC
Wilmington, 302 658 8808 📖 233
Wendell's Leather Shop
San Francisco, 415 474 4104 📖 219
Wendell's Magazines
New York, 212 645 1197 📖 309
Wendy's
Los Angeles 📖 183
Werkgroep Facet
Eindhoven, 40 241 5475 📖 155
Werkgroep Gehuwde Homo's Lesbiennes en Partners
Wondelgem, 9 153 8065 📖 39
Werkgroep Homofile Achterhoek
Doetinchem, 31 436 0811 📖 154
Wesley Medical Center
Wichita, 316 688 2468 📖 258
Wesleyan Gay, Lesbian, & Bisexual Alliance (GLBA)
Manchester, 203 347 9411 Ext. 2712 📖 231
West & Wilde Bookshop
Edinburgh, 131 556 0079 📖 169
West Alabama AIDS Outreach
Tuscaloosa, 205 758 2437 📖 192
West College Gay & Lesbian Student Union
San José, 408 867 2200 Ext. 358 📖 220
West Florida Growlers
Tampa, 813 821 1075 📖 242
West Florida Regional Medical Center
Pensacola, 904 494 5000 📖 241
West Glamorgan AIDS Project
Swansea, 1792 456303 📖 359
West Kootenay-Boundry AIDS Network, Outreach & Support Society (ANKORS)
Grand Forks, 800 421 2437 (information) 📖 44
West Kootenays Gays & Lesbians
Kootnays, 604 325 3504 📖 44
West Lynn Military Surplus
Vancouver 📖 46
West Midlands Friend
Birmingham, 121 622 7351 📖 92
West Midlands Lesbian & Gay Switchboard
Birmingham, 121 622 6589 📖 92
Coventry, 121 622 6589 📖 93
Kenilworth, 121 622 6589 📖 92
Royal Leamington Spa, 121 622 6589 📖 92
Stratford-upon-Avon, 121 622 6589 📖 92
West Norfolk Gay & Lesbian Helpline
King's Lynn, 1553 630012 📖 88
West of Boston Lesbians (Wobbles)
Marlborough, 508 386 7737 📖 271
West of Scotland Area NUS
Glasgow, 141 636 6477 📖 169
West Oz Marsupial Bears And Their Supporters (Wombats)
Perth, 9 279 7949 📖 33
West Paces Medical Center
Atlanta, 404 351 0351 📖 244
West Suburban Gay Association
Glen Ellyn, 708 790 9742 (info hotline) 📖 252
West Texas Gender Alliance
Abilene 📖 338
West Video
Voorburg, 79 351 3193 📖 159
West, Jeanne
Palo Alto, 415 494 2952 📖 209
West, Kim
London, 171 729 6960 📖 68
Westchester News
Miami, 305 264 6210 📖 239
Western AIDS Alliance/Cairde
Galway, 91 66266 📖 137
Western Australian AIDS Council
Perth, 9 227 8619 📖 33
Perth, 9 429 9900 📖 33
Western Canada Leather / Fetish Clans Council
Calgary, 403 273 1765 📖 42
Western Express 📖 194
Western Kentucky University Lambda
Bowling Green 📖 258
Western New York Sentinel 📖 298
Western North Carolina AIDS Project
Asheville, 704 252 7489 📖 313
Westgate Industrial Rubber
Newcastle upon Tyne, 1632 654858 📖 92
Westminster Books
Fredricton, 506 454 1442 📖 48
Westside Publishing
Perth, 9 242 2146 📖 33
Westward Bound
Launceston, 1566 776907 📖 67
Wetherby Studios
London, 171 373 1107 📖 84
Wetlook Unlimited
Leeds 📖 69
WEVL FM 90
Memphis 📖 337
WFHB
Bloomington, 812 323 1200 📖 254
WFTL Radio
Fort Lauderdale, 800 874 3454 📖 237
Whangarei Health HIV/AIDS Coördinator
9 438 2070 Ext. 3543 📖 163
Whangarei STD Clinic
9 438 2079 📖 163
What She Wants Feminist Library
Cleveland, 216 321 3054 📖 318
Wheeler, Joe
Chicago, 312 835 3468 📖 249
Wheels MC
New York 📖 304
Whip Me Raw
Albuquerque, 505 873 4981 📖 186
Whipping Post
published by La Carnivale 📖 310
Whips
published by Thor Publications 📖 297
White Crane Newsletter 📖 218
White Rabbit Books
Charlotte, 704 377 4067 📖 314
White Rabbit Books & Things
Greensboro, 910 272 7604 📖 315
Whitehall Company
Naples, 800 321 9290 📖 239
Whitesox
Wettingen 📖 177
Whiting, Joyce, ACSW
Manchester, 603 666 4299 📖 288
Whitman-Walker Clinic
Washington, 202 797 3500 📖 233
Whittier Bookstore
Tulsa, 918 592 0767 📖 324
Wholesale Boot Supply
Eagan, 612 452 4695 📖 279
WholeSM Publishing Corporation
Toronto, 416 962 1040 📖 58
Whorezine 📖 217
WHP
Pijnakker, 15 369 7765 📖 157
Why Not
Bruxelles / Brussel, 2 512 7587 📖 36
WHZ
Zoetermeer, 79 321 0128 📖 159
Wichita Gay & Lesbian Alliance
316 267 1852 📖 258
Wichita Gay Info Line
316 269 0913 📖 258
Wichita Transgender Alliance
Kechi 📖 257
Wicked Ways
Alexandria, 703 379 4735 📖 182
Wicked Women
published by Wicked Women 📖 22
Sydney, 2 517 2163 📖 22
Widdershins Books
Portland, 503 232 2129 📖 327
Wiener Warmenradio FM 107.3
1 332 1096 📖 35
Wig Service Shop
Cherry Hill, 609 428 8448 📖 290
WIHG
Gorinchem, 18 363 6710 📖 155
Wilbro
Lincoln 📖 79
Wild Designs
London, 181 766 7550 📖 68, 70
Wild G.A.L.S.
Sydney, 2 550 9552 📖 27
Wild One
Sydney, 2 557 1550 📖 26
Wild Side
published by TWS Ent. 📖 191
Wild Times
published by S & L Sales Company 📖 205
Wildcat Books
Fresno, 209 237 4525 📖 200
Wildcat Collection
Brighton, 1273 323758 📖 11
wilde
published by PDA Press, Inc. 📖 218
Wilde Alliance
Perth 📖 34
Wilde's
Ottawa, 613 567 4858 📖 53
Wilder, Vic
London, 181 871 2443 📖 81
Wildfire Club
London, 181 989 0281 📖 15
Willems, Dany
Bruxelles / Brussel, 2 218 5126 📖 37
William Beaumont Hospital
Royal Oak, 810 551 5000 📖 278
William Mitchell College of Law Gay & Lesbian Association
Minneapolis / Saint Paul, 612 646 3966 📖 280
William S. Middleton Veterans' Hospital
Madison, 608 256 1901 📖 356
William Wishard Memorial Hospital
Indianapolis, 317 639 6671 📖 254
Williams Bisexual, Gay, & Lesbian Union

Williamstown, 413 597 2413 📖 273
Williams, Mark, Ph.D.
New York, 212 254 0529 📖 302
Willowood Press
Minot, 701 838 0579 📖 189
Wilson Barber's Quarterly
published by Oakhaus 📖 248
Wilton, Jim, MSW, CSW
Ann Arbor, 313 663 5021 📖 274
Wind, Mark, MA, CAC, NCAC II
New York, 212 929 4390 📖 302
Winder, Jon
Lynchburg, 804 845 4927 📖 348
Windfaire Exxxotic Gifts
Atlanta, 404 634 9463 📖 186
Windfire
Grand Rapids, 616 459 5900 📖 276
Kalamazoo 📖 276
Traverse City, 616 922 4800 📖 278
Windsong Books & Records
Fort Bragg, 707 964 2050 📖 199
Windy City Times
published by Sentury Publications 📖 251
Wings MC
Memphis 📖 337
Wingspan
Tucson, 602 624 1779 📖 195
Winnebago Health Department
Fox Valley, 414 235 5100 Ext. 3375 📖 355
Winnipeg Gay / Lesbian Resource Centre
204 284 5208 📖 47
Winnipeg Leather/Levi Club 📖 47
Winter Publishing, Inc.
South Dartmouth, 508 999 0078 📖 15, 19, 20, 22
Winterthur Schwule (WISCH)
52 213 8188 📖 179
Winthrop Army Navy Store
Boston, 617 539 0617 📖 270
Wire 📖 242
WISCH 📖 *See* Winterthur Schwule
Wisconsin Community-Based Research Consortium
Milwaukee, 800 359 9272 📖 355
Wisconsin Leathermen's Association
Milwaukee 📖 357
Wisconsin Light 📖 355
Wiseman, Jay
Berkeley 📖 197
Wishing Well
Santee 📖 222
Witchel, Joy, CSW, CAC
New York, 212 477 8258 📖 302
With The Times
Calgary, 403 244 8020 📖 43
Witte Raven
Antwerpen / Anvers, 3 828 6900 📖 35
Gent / Gand, 9 220 4197 📖 38
Leuven / Louvain, 1 620 0906 📖 38
Oostende / Ostende, 5 950 2882 📖 39
Wives of Bisexual & Married Gay Men
Cleveland, 216 529 9139 📖 319
Wives'/Partners' Concerns ((SPICE))
Little Rock 📖 195
WIWA International
Köln, 221 25 3115 📖 125
WMUA
Amherst, 413 545 2876 📖 267
Wobbles 📖 *See* West of Boston Lesbians
WOBS 📖 *See* Women of the Beaumont Society
Wohlthat'sche Buchhandlung
Bremen, 421 1 4320 📖 113
Mainz, 613 122 2353 📖 126
Wolech, Helmut
Wien, 222 30 6988 📖 35
Wolf Pack S&M
Dearborn 📖 274
Wolfmark Woodworks
Grand Rapids, 616 774 9518 📖 276
Wolfs
Long Beach, 310 433 9251 📖 202
Los Angeles 📖 203
San Diego, 619 291 3730 📖 210
Wolverton, Gwen, Psy.D.
Montclair, 201 746 1414 📖 291
Woman To Woman 📖 195
Woman to Womon Books
Edmonton, 403 454 8031 📖 43
Woman's Place
Park City, 801 649 2722 📖 345
Salt Lake City, 801 278 9855 📖 345
Salt Lake City, 801 583 6431 📖 345
Woman's Place Bookstore
Calgary, 403 263 5256 📖 43
Woman's Prerogative
Ferndale, 810 545 5702 📖 275
Woman's Touch
Linden, 908 486 8022 📖 291
Womanist 📖 53
Womankind Books Inc.
Huntington Station, 516 427 1289 📖 181
Womanlife, Inc.
Auckland, 9 376 4587 📖 160
Womanline
Auckland, 9 376 5173 📖 160
Womanlink
Berkeley 📖 15
published by Womanlink 📖 15
Womansline Books
London, 519 679 3416 📖 51
Womansoul
broadcast by KBOO Radio FM 90.7 📖 326
WomanSpace
published by Lesbian Information San Antonio 📖 344
Wombats 📖 *See* West Oz Marsupial Bears And Their Supporters
Women & AIDS Resource Network
Brooklyn, 718 596 6007 📖 297
Women Centered News 📖 296
Women In Print
Vancouver 📖 46
Women of Power Magazine 📖 272
Women of the Beaumont Society (WOBS)
London, 1223 441246 (South) 📖 83
Women of the Woods (WOW)
Worcester, 802 229 0109 📖 346
Women United of Nevada
Las Vegas, 702 366 8421 📖 286
Women who Administer Punishment (WhAP)
published by Retro Systems 📖 18
Women's Alternative Health Clinic
Milwaukee, 414 272 2144 📖 357
Women's Book Club
London, 171 437 1019 📖 86
Women's Book Store
Vancouver, 604 684 0523 📖 46
Women's Bookshop
Hamilton, 905 525 2970 📖 50
Women's Community Center
Binghamton, 607 724 3462 📖 297
Women's Counseling Services of Berk County, Inc.
Lehigh Valley, 610 372 7234 📖 329
Women's Hour
broadcast by KTRU FM 91.7 📖 343
Women's Leather Network
West Hollywood, 213 993 7235 📖 225
Women's Library
Fayetteville, 501 582 4636 📖 195
Women's Media Project
broadcast by WMUA 📖 267
Women's Motorcycle Contingent
San Francisco, 415 395 8318 📖 215
Women's Press
Toronto, 416 921 2425 📖 58
Women's Project
Little Rock, 501 372 5113 📖 196
Women's Review of Books 📖 16
Women's SM Group
London, 171 833 8554 📖 82
Women's Studies
Minneapolis / Saint Paul, 612 624 9326 📖 280
Women's Studies Quarterly
published by Feminist Press at The City University of New York 📖 308
Women's Therapy Center
Philadelphia, 215 567 1111 📖 331
Women's Times 📖 212
Women's Welcoming Committee (WWC)
Seattle 📖 351
Women's Word Books
Springfield 📖 181
Women's Words Books
Hopkinton, 603 228 8000 📖 181
Womenspace 📖 286
WomenWise 📖 279
WomenWorks 📖 279
Womonspace / Lesbian Lifeline
Edmonton, 403 425 0511 📖 43
Womontyme Distribution Company
Long Beach, 800 247 8903 📖 181
Womyn's Braille Press, Inc.
Minneapolis / Saint Paul, 612 872 4352 📖 281
Womyn's Community Newsletter 📖 354
Womyn's Press 📖 325
Womyn's Ware
Vancouver, 604 254 2543 📖 46
Womyn's Words 📖 241
Woodbury Products, Inc.
Island Park, 516 431 4242 📖 299
Woodhouse, Alan
Wolverhampton, 1902 331413 📖 94
Woodworks
Middleton 📖 73
Worcester County Lesbian & Gay Alliance
508 829 9898 📖 273
Word is OUT! 📖 320
broadcast by WUSB FM 📖 311
Word Publications
Indianapolis, 317 579 3075 📖 253, 258, 317
Wordplay
Saint John's, 709 726 9193 📖 48
Wordsworth
Boston, 617 354 5201 📖 270
Worlander Pty. Ltd.
Sydney, 2 332 3620 📖 24
World Book & News
Los Angeles, 213 465 4352 📖 205
World Development Centre
Waterford 📖 138
World Domination
New York 📖 183
World Eye Bookshop
Greenfield, 413 772 2186 📖 270
World of Payne
published by Carter Stevens Presents 📖 332
World's Biggest Bookstore
Toronto, 416 977 7009 📖 60
Worldwide Adult Bookstore
Cathedral City, 619 321 1313 📖 198
Worldwide Magazines
Detroit, 313 866 6020 📖 275
Worldwide News
Rochester, 716 546 7140 📖 311
Worn Out West
San Francisco, 415 431 6020 📖 218
Worn To Be Wild
Louisville 📖 259
Wos Markt
Kiel 📖 123
WOW 📖 *See* Women of the Woods
WOW!
Charlotte, 704 364 5435 📖 314
WPC 📖 8
Toronto, 416 962 1040 📖 7
Wrapaway
Sydney, 2 550 1622 📖 26
Wrapped
Amsterdam, 20 420 4022 📖 153
Wrasslin' Bears
San Francisco, 415 673 6434 📖 216
Wrestling Club Of Portland 📖 326
Wrexham Switchboard
1248 351115 📖 359
WRFG
Atlanta, 404 523 3471 📖 245
Write Solution
Hove, 1273 726281 📖 74
Writer's Etc.
West Franklin, 603 934 3379 📖 288
WRPI FM 91.5
Troy, 518 276 6248 📖 312
WRSU FM 88.7
New Brunswick, 908 932 8800 📖 291
WSMLO 📖 *See* Washington State Ms. Leather
WSO - Westside Observer
published by Westside Publishing 📖 33
WüHST 📖 *See* Würzburger Schwulengruppe
Würzburger Schwulengruppe (WüHST)
931 41 2646 📖 136
WUSB FM
Stony Brook, 516 632 6500 📖 311
WUSB FM 90.1
New York, 516 632 6901 📖 308
W W C 📖 *See* Women's Welcoming Committee
WXPN FM 88.5
Philadelphia, 215 898 6677 📖 331
Wyle, Stephen
Fenton, Stoke-On-Trent 📖 69
X Factor
Bristol, 203 583 6284 📖 230
X!
Santa Monica 📖 222
Xandria Collection
San Francisco, 415 468 3812 📖 10
Xantippe
Amsterdam, 20 623 5854 📖 153
Xclusiv Distributors, Inc.
Brooklyn, 718 439 1271 📖 297
X-Corrigia
Toronto 📖 56
X-Large
Bern, 31 352 7886 📖 177
Xpressions
Toronto, 416 812 6879 📖 57
Xtasy Down Under Male Emporium
New York, 212 262 0178 📖 309
XTC Leather of New York
Hazlet, 908 739 1354 📖 186
Xtra! 📖 35
published by Pink Triangle Press 📖 59
Xtra! West
published by Pink Triangle Press 📖 46
X-Treme Designs Ltd
Calgary 📖 40
XX 📖 *See* Twenty Club
XXXLNT
Miami 📖 239
X-zess
Bergkirchen, 8131 78941 📖 109
¡Y Que! 📖 149
Yager Kupferman, Roz, BS, MA, Psy.A.
Teaneck, 201 837 6381 📖 293
Yago Holdings Ltd.
Birmingham, 1675 464834 📖 68
Yahoo Corporation
Mountain View, 415 934 3230 📖 7
Yale GALA, DC
Washington 📖 234
Yale- New Haven Hospital
203 785 7200 📖 231
Yalesbians
New Haven, 203 432 0388 📖 231
Yamazaki, Shinji
Shinjuku-Ku, 81 3 3225 4630 📖 148
Yanko
Paris, 142 60 5528 📖 104
Paris, 145 26 1841 📖 104
Ye CG Brits
Rocky Hill 📖 232
Yellow On Thursday
broadcast by Milwaukee Gay / Lesbian Cable Network 📖 357
Yellowstone AIDS Project
Billings, 406 252 1212 📖 285
Yelsky, Miriam, Ph.D.
New York, 212 243 0261 📖 302
YHESSI
York, 717 846 6776 📖 333
YMCA
Dundee, 138 220 0352 📖 170
York AIDS Action Ltd.
1904 639595 📖 88
York Area AIDS Coalition
717 846 6776 📖 333
York Area Lambda
717 292 1665 📖 333
York Gay Line
1904 612828 📖 88
York Lesbian Line
1904 646812 📖 88
Yorkshire Mesmac
Bradford, 127 439 5815 📖 94
Young & Gay
Melbourne, 39 865 6700 📖 32
Young & Welshans Books
Flint, 800 366 8290 📖 276
Young Gay & Lesbian Alliance of Oklahoma City

Young Gay/Lesbian Life

405 525 2437 📖 323
Young Gay/Lesbian Life 📖 353
Young Gays
Adelaide, 8 362 3223 📖 30
Young Gays Club (YGC) 📖 22
Yount, Jack
Zephyrs Hills, 813 783 7377 📖 243
Your Ass & My Face 📖 281
Your Turf
Lehigh Valley, 610 439 8755 📖 329
Youth Health Services
New York, 212 230 7408 📖 302
Youth Magazine 📖 235
Youth Outreach Program
Los Angeles, 213 464 7400 Ext. 1702 📖 204
Youth Rap Group
Seattle, 206 322 2873 📖 352
Youthlink - Inner City
Toronto, 416 922 3335 📖 58
Yukon Trading Company
Providence, 401 274 6620 📖 334
YWCA AIDS Minority Outreach
Shreveport, 504 226 8717 📖 261
Z&O
published by Vogel Verlag 📖 111
Zack White Leather
Ramseur, 800 633 0396 📖 316
Zak Designs
Indiana, 814 446 5319 📖 186
Zapata
Kiel, 431 73 8323 📖 123
Kiel, 431 9 3639 📖 123
Zardoz
Hannover 📖 122
Zart & Heftig
Zürich 📖 180
ZASA 📖 *See* AIDS-Hilfe
Zauberflöte 📖 129
ZEH 📖 *See* Zentrale Erfassung Homosexuellendiskriminierung
Zeiger, Robyn, Ph.D., CPC
Silver Spring, 301 445 7333 📖 266
Zeitgeist
published by Zeitgeist International 📖 84
Zeitgeist International
London, 171 607 2977 📖 84
Zelterman, Irene, CSW
New York, 718 832 3739 📖 302
Zenana
Wolverhampton 📖 68
Zenith Foundation
Vancouver 📖 45
Zentrale Erfassung Homosexuellendiskriminierung (ZEH)
Hannover 📖 108
Zentralschweizer Schwulen-Motorrad-Club (SMC)
Luzern / Lucerne 📖 178
zer.t-netz.sex 📖 6
zer.z-netz.gesundheit.diskussion 📖 5
zer.z-netz.gesundheit.drogen 📖 5
zer.z-netz.gesundheit.krankheiten 📖 5
zer.z-netz.wissenschaft.psychologie 📖 4
Zeus
Los Angeles 📖 205
Zipper Mail Order
London, 171 267 0021 📖 9
Zipper Store
London, 171 284 0537 📖 86
Zip-Up Leathers
Denver, 303 733 7442 📖 227
Zizo
Gent / Gand, 9 223 6929 📖 36
published by Zizo 📖 36
Zoo
Chicago 📖 248
Zoom
Austin, 512 472 3316 📖 338
Zoomorph 📖 22
Zwart Op Wit
Amsterdam, 20 622 8174 📖 153
Zweite Haut
Berlin, 30 821 8603 📖 111
Zymurgy
Boston, 617 695 8015 📖 269

Index by Organization Type

ACCOMMODATION
BDSM
All Sexes & Sexualities

Backdrop Club 📖 206
Castlebar 📖 212
Country House 📖 298
Domino 📖 92
Fantasy Inn 📖 290
Lodge 📖 92
Logden House 📖 1
Westward Bound 📖 67

Female

B&D B&B 📖 202

Gay

Amsterdam House 📖 151
Dave's B&B on the Rio Grande 📖 294
Gatehouse 📖 31
Hotel Adler 📖 119
Moustache 📖 109
Muther's 📖 55
Stablemaster Hotel 📖 151
Tom's House 📖 109

ARCHIVES
BDSM
All Sexes & Sexualities

Leather Archives & Museum 📖 1
Lives of the Secular Saints 📖 79
Tom of Finland Foundation 📖 1

GENERAL
All Sexes & Sexualities

Museum of Sex 📖 151

Female

Canadian Women's Movement Archives 📖 40
IIAV 📖 151
What She Wants Feminist Library 📖 318
Women's Library 📖 195

SEXUALITY
All Sexes & Sexualities

Gay & Lesbian Archives of Washington, DC 📖 348
Happy Foundation 📖 180
Homosexual Information Center 📖 223, 260

Female

Centro per le Donne 📖 140

Lesbian

Archives Recherches & Cultures Lesbiennes 📖 102
June Mazer Collection & Archive 📖 224
Latina Lesbian History Project 📖 296
Lesbian Herstory Webweaving Collective 📖 300
Lesbisch Archief 📖 151
Ohio Lesbian Archives 📖 317

Lesbian, Gay, Bi, & Transgendered

Anna Blaman Huis 📖 156
Archives for the Protection of Gay History & Literature 📖 48
Archives Gaies du Québec 📖 61
Arci Gay 📖 143
Arkiv for Bøsser & Lesbiske 📖 66
Australian Lesbian & Gay Archives 📖 24
Barnes Memorial Library, Lambda, Inc. 📖 191
Biblioteket 📖 65
Blanche Baker Memorial Library & Archives 📖 203
Canadian Lesbian & Gay Archives 📖 55
Centro di Documentazione 📖 140
Colectivo Sol 📖 149
Dallas Gay & Lesbian Historic Archives 📖 339
Douglas County Gay Archives 📖 327
Fondazione Sandro Penna 📖 138
Fondo Olivari 📖 142
Fort Wayne Gay & Lesbian Resource Center & Archives 📖 254
Gay & Lesbian Historical Society of Northern California 📖 196
Gay Library 📖 171
Gay, Lesbian, Bisexual & Transgendered Library / Archives of Philadelphia 📖 329
Gerber/Hart Library & Archives 📖 248
Hamilton-Wentworth Lesbian/Gay Archives 📖 50
Harvey Milk Archives 📖 212
HAZ/SOH 📖 *See* Schwule Ausleihbibliothek
Homodok 📖 150
International Gay & Lesbian Archives 📖 1
Lesbian & Gay Archives of New Zealand 📖 159
Lesbian & Gay Community Library 📖 30
Lesbian & Gay Historical Society of San Diego 📖 210
Libreria Gruppo Abele 📖 138
Lila Archiv e. V. 📖 109
MCC Library 📖 342
National Gay Rights Coalition 📖 159
NGRC 📖 *See* National Gay Rights Coalition
Ompos's Gay House 📖 141
Out On The Shelves 📖 45
Pan Biblioteket 📖 66
Pink Triangle Services Library 📖 52
SARCH 📖 *See* Schwullesbisches Archiv Hannover
Schwule Ausleihbibliothek 📖 179
Schwule Pressearchiv Bonn 📖 107
Schwulen-Archiv Köln 📖 124
Schwules Archiv 📖 117
Schwules Pressearchiv Berlin 📖 109
Schwullesbisches Archiv Hannover 📖 121
Schwul-Lesbisches Presse-Archiv 📖 124
SETA Library 📖 96
Stonewall Library & Archives 📖 236
Terry Mangan Library 📖 227
Verein Schwulenkultur e. V. 📖 119

ARTISTS
BDSM
All Sexes & Sexualities

Anthro 📖 169
Bowers, Dan 📖 55
Gottardi, Susi Medusa 📖 140
Hun 📖 326
Matt 📖 260
Mercy 📖 300
Panasewicz, T. Roman 📖 286
Preston Graphics 📖 242
Sheeba 📖 61
Smith, Ira 📖 300

Heterosexual

Viveros, Brian 📖 198

Heterosexual, Male

Moyes, Jan 📖 202

EROTIC
All Sexes & Sexualities

Q. W. Hq. P. 📖 267
Smith, Richard 📖 238

Gay

Galerie Leon 📖 1

FETISH
All Sexes & Sexualities

Chris 📖 80

BARS
BDSM
All Sexes & Sexualities

Black Eagle 📖 55
Dungeon Club 📖 80
Eagle 📖 339
Hus 1 'Huset 📖 175
Inner Circle 📖 70
Kinky Bar 📖 175
Maze 📖 300
Moda Moda 📖 36
Paddles 📖 300
Sade 📖 70
Skin Parlor 📖 201
Sling 📖 267
Spank Promotions 📖 70

Gay

Aigle Noir 📖 61
Anco Bar 📖 151
Andreas Kneipe 📖 109
Anvil 📖 80
Argos Club 📖 151
Attic 📖 151
Attitude 📖 80
Backstage 📖 129
Backstairs 📖 121
Backstreet 📖 80
Badlands 📖 233
Baltimore Eagle 📖 263
Bar Mâle 📖 63
Barfüsser 📖 179
Barn 📖 55
Batchelor Forum 📖 310
Big Noise 📖 36
Black 📖 119
Block 📖 80, 101
Bolt 📖 127
Boot Camp Saloon 📖 356
Boots 📖 36, 132
Boots & Saddle 📖 300
Boston Eagle 📖 267
Boystown 📖 42
Brass Rail 📖 313
Brick 📖 339
Brompton's 📖 80
Bronx 📖 113
Buddies 📖 227
Buffalo 📖 286
Café Adler 📖 119
Café Moustache 📖 102
Candle Bar 📖 300
Cattlemen's Exchange Club 📖 193
CC Slaughter's 📖 326
CC Slaughter's North 📖 350
Cell Bar 📖 78
Cell Block 📖 248
Cellar Leather Club 📖 75
Cellblock 📖 52
Cellblock 28 📖 297
Chain Drive 📖 338
Chains 📖 124, 274
Chaps 📖 119
Chart Room Saloon 📖 262
Chicago Eagle 📖 248
Club 119 📖 267
Club Jacques 📖 151
Cockring 📖 151
Colherne 📖 80
Colorado Triangle 📖 227
Company 📖 151
Company Bar 📖 96
Company Club 📖 142
Compound 📖 227
Construction Five 📖 117
Crossings 📖 259
Cuckoo's Nest 📖 151
Cuff 📖 350
Cuffs 📖 203
Dëeks 📖 248
Detroit Eagle 📖 274
Dock 📖 317
Docks 📖 102
Don-Club 📖 114
Eagle 📖 35, 132, 151, 236
Eagle in Exile 📖 319
Eagle's Nest 📖 300
Fascination 📖 87
Faultline 📖 201
Forge Tavern 📖 45
Fraternity House 📖 233
Gaol House 📖 76
Gauntlet II 📖 203
G-Force 📖 151
Griff's 📖 203
Hangar 📖 141
Hanky Code 📖 36
Headquarters 📖 212
Hidden Door 📖 339
Hole 📖 121
Hole In The Wall Saloon 📖 212
Jackhammer 📖 212

Jail 🕮 126
Jazi's 🕮 331
K. O. X. 🕮 61
Katacombes 🕮 62
Keller's 🕮 102
Knast 🕮 110
Kurbash 🕮 55
L. U. R. E. 🕮 300
Leather Bar 🕮 171, 172
Leather Stallion Saloon 🕮 318
Lederklub SAM 🕮 65
London Apprentice 🕮 80
Long Island Eagle 🕮 296
Löwengrube 🕮 127
Manhandler Saloon 🕮 248
Manhattan 🕮 102
Market Tavern 🕮 80
Mec Zone 🕮 102
Men's Bar 🕮 66
Metro Place de Clichy 🕮 66
Mic-Man 🕮 102
Mineshaft 🕮 75
Moustache 🕮 110
Musk 🕮 115
N. Y. C. 🕮 106
New Action 🕮 110
New York 🕮 127
Nightshift 🕮 35
Nugget's Bar 🕮 31
Number One 🕮 116
Numbers Pub 🕮 241
Ochsengarten 🕮 127
One Way 🕮 102
Orlando Eagle 🕮 240
P. T. Max 🕮 263
Pacific Street 🕮 342
Phœnix 🕮 179
Phœnix Men's Room 🕮 260
Phönix 🕮 110
Platzjabbeck 🕮 124
Pop As 🕮 127
QG 🕮 102
Ramrod 🕮 267
Ranch & Cuffs 🕮 294
Rawhide 🕮 260, 300
Rekroom 🕮 42
Rendezvous Lounge 🕮 289
Ripcord Houston 🕮 342
Sam's Tiffany's on the Park 🕮 274
Schwarz Bar 🕮 74
Seattle Eagle 🕮 350
Sept 🕮 36
Shaft 🕮 157
Sjinderhannes 🕮 157
Snax Club 🕮 110
Spartacus 🕮 38
Spijker 🕮 151
Spike 🕮 224, 300
Sportsman Hotel 🕮 28
Spurs 🕮 317
Stablemaster Bar 🕮 151
Stall 🕮 117
Stiefelknecht 🕮 35, 124
Stratègie 🕮 102
Stronghold at the Clock Hotel 🕮 26
Stud 🕮 236
Sweet Sixties 🕮 157
Tom's Bar 🕮 110
Tom's Saloon 🕮 119
Tomahawk 🕮 318
Toolbox 🕮 55
Touché 🕮 248
Track 🕮 62
Transfert 🕮 102
Trap 🕮 102
Trax 🕮 42
Twilight Zone 🕮 110
Underground 🕮 45, 80
Ursus Club 🕮 177
Venture-N 🕮 194
Web 🕮 151
Why Not 🕮 36
Wolfs 🕮 202, 203, 210

Heterosexual

Vault 🕮 300

Lesbian, Gay, Bi, & Transgendered

Adam 🕮 109
Atlanta Eagle 🕮 243
Clementine's 🕮 284
Club Tyz 🕮 330
Country Club 🕮 260
Drague 🕮 63
Edge, Inc. 🕮 321
Edinburgh Castle Hotel 🕮 30
Empire 🕮 127
Manhole 🕮 248
Oz 🕮 315
Pipeline 🕮 336
Querelle 🕮 142
Venture-N 🕮 342
Village Club 🕮 74

Male

Crescent Tavern 🕮 350
Full Moon Saloon 🕮 240
Yukon Trading Company 🕮 334

FETISH

All Sexes & Sexualities

Kinky Club 🕮 151
Stimulation 🕮 77
Submission 🕮 80
Vice 🕮 203

GENERAL

All Sexes & Sexualities

Mon Cherie's The Chamber 🕮 243

Gay

Bike Stop 🕮 330
New Age Renegade 🕮 323
Nite Club 🕮 321

Lesbian, Gay, Bi, & Transgendered

Club 332 🕮 336
Lil Rascals 🕮 335
Victor / Victoria's 🕮 337

SEXUALITY

Transgender

Club Edelweiss 🕮 300
Sally's II 🕮 300

Transvestite

Beat 🕮 28
Black Cap 🕮 80
Blue Boy 🕮 158
Bug House 🕮 39
Duke 🕮 155
El Rubio 🕮 155
Empire Hotel 🕮 28
Gold Club 🕮 38
Nostro Mondo 🕮 39
Options Nightclub 🕮 28
Tacky Tavern 🕮 350
Wayout Club 🕮 80
Wayout Wine Bar 🕮 80

BBSS

ADULT BABY

All Sexes & Sexualities

ByteMine Adult Baby BBS 🕮 199

AIDS

All Sexes & Sexualities

AIDS Info BBS 🕮 212
SAIBBS 🕮 *See* Seattle AIDS Information BBS
Seattle AIDS Information BBS 🕮 350

BDSM

All Sexes & Sexualities

#28 Barbury Lane 🕮 351
Academy 🕮 200
Andros 🕮 211
Annette's Castle 🕮 243
Archives 🕮 343
Athlete's Bench 🕮 200
B&D Comm 🕮 254
Backrop 🕮 212
Boston Dungeon Society 🕮 180
Bound for Pleasure 🕮 267
Common Bonds 🕮 248
Covenant 🕮 329
Cyberoticomm 🕮 300
Delos 🕮 197
Denver Exchange 🕮 227
Digital Obsession 🕮 330
Exchange 🕮 313, 342
Fetish Network BBS 🕮 240
Final Frontier 🕮 248
Forum 🕮 330
gLiTcH 🕮 290
Harbor Bytes 🕮 263
Hedonism 🕮 198
Hotflash 🕮 284
Inferno 🕮 293
Kinky Kumputer 🕮 350
Laura's Lair 🕮 282
Leather First 🕮 209
Long Island Connection 🕮 299
LuvCat's Lair 🕮 330
Minnesota Underground 🕮 282
Mirrored Dragon's Dream 🕮 285
Montreal's Electronic Dungeon 🕮 62
Moon Dog 🕮 300
Multicom4 🕮 298, 310
North Keep 🕮 326
Oracle 🕮 207
Outer Limits 🕮 248
Pig Pen 🕮 52
Pleasure Dome 🕮 348
Pokey's Place 🕮 343
Port Kar BBS 🕮 55
Power Exchange 🕮 266
Rapture 🕮 222
SM Board 🕮 1
Station House 🕮 212
Throbbs 🕮 198
Throbnet 🕮 285
Titan 🕮 241
Underground 🕮 236
Wall 🕮 300
Wally World 🕮 220
X! 🕮 222
Zoo 🕮 248

Gay

Backroom II 🕮 289
Cockpit 🕮 248
Fountains of Pleasure 🕮 180
Hot Pockets BBS 🕮 1
Male Box 🕮 226
Metropolitan Slave Online 🕮 1
Nightstick 🕮 300
Skinner Jack's Bath House 🕮 207
Studs 🕮 212

Heterosexual

English Palace 🕮 180

Lesbian, Gay, Bi, & Transgendered

S&M Exchange 🕮 351

BEARS

Gay

PC Bear Lair 🕮 220

GENERAL

All Sexes & Sexualities

Beach Board 🕮 237
Erotic Visions 🕮 300
Night Life 🕮 319
POWERarts Presence Provider 🕮 55

SEXUALITY

All Sexes & Sexualities

Graffiti 🕮 245
Lifestyle Online 🕮 1
Village 🕮 1

Bisexual

Bi-Link 🕮 150

Gay

Back Door BBS 🕮 207, 209, 220
Back Door Computing Services 🕮 1
Gay Blade 🕮 54
Malestop 🕮 300

Lesbian, Gay, Bi, & Transgendered

Alternative Access BBS 🕮 31
Arcisbox 🕮 107
Backroom 🕮 297
Gay Network 🕮 175
Gay/Lesbian Information Bureau 🕮 180
Gay/Lesbian International News Network 🕮 180
GayBox 🕮 112
GAYTEL 🕮 150
GLIB 🕮 *See* Gay/Lesbian Information Bureau
GLINN 🕮 *See* Gay/Lesbian International News Network
Pinkboard 🕮 26
SGBB Mailbox 🕮 107
S-TEK 🕮 62
TGT 🕮 *See* Gay Network

COMPETITIONS & CONVENTIONS (SEE ALSO ORGANIZATIONS: BDSM: COMPETITIONS)

BDSM

All Sexes & Sexualities

Fetish/SM Market 🕮 80
Mr. & Ms. Olympus 🕮 224
Pantheon of Leather 🕮 224

Female

International Ms Leather 🕮 1
Ms. Leather Sacramento 🕮 209
Ms. San Francisco Leather 🕮 212

Gay

Concours M. Cuir Montréal 🕮 62
International Mr. Leather, Inc. 🕮 1

Heterosexual

Domination 🕮 240

Male

Mr. Deaf International Leather 🕮 1

FETISH

Clothing

All Sexes & Sexualities

Dressing For Pleasure Gala 🕮 291
Feticon 🕮 116
Planet Sex Ball 🕮 80
Rubber Ball 🕮 80

MUSIC

Lesbian

Ohio Lesbian Festival 🕮 317

SEXUALITY

All Sexes & Sexualities

Lifestyles 🕮 197

Transgender

ICTLEP 🕮 342
Salishan Society 🕮 180
Sexual Identity Center 🕮 246
SIC 🕮 *See* Sexual Identity Center

COUNSELLORS

All Sexes & Sexualities

Albany Trust 🕮 80
Allen Wells Center for Psychotherapy & Healing 🕮 291
Allison, Judith, M.Ed., MSH 🕮 238
Almont Counselling Associates 🕮 191
Aloft 🕮 209
Alternative Approach Counseling & Psychotherapy Center 🕮 291
Amethyst Counselling Service 🕮 325
Anders, Ron, MSW 🕮 351
Applegate, Eric, PC, MS, NACA II, AAMFT, CST 🕮 254
Arsenault, Raymond, Ph.D. 🕮 267, 288
Ashland Psychological Services 🕮 317
Ask Isadora 🕮 212
Asnien, Carolyn, MA 🕮 300
Aspinall, John, CSW 🕮 300
Associated Counseling Professionals, Inc. 🕮 230
Baldwin, Guy, MFCC 🕮 203
Banks, Daphnee, MSW, CSW, ACSW 🕮 292
Baxley, Thom 🕮 248
Bayes, Marjorie, Ph.D. 🕮 229
Benowitz, Mindy, Ph.D. 🕮 279
Bernet, Michael 🕮 297
Bernstein, Gail, Ph.D. 🕮 227
Bettinger, Michael, Ph.D., MFCC 🕮 213
Bisexual Information & Counseling Service 🕮 300
Blair, Ralph 🕮 300
Bloom, Daniel, JD, CSW 🕮 300
Blume, Sue, CSW 🕮 300
Brown, Ian 🕮 80
Burgoyne, Bob, M.S.W. 🕮 55
Busch Counseling Center, Inc. 🕮 242
Byrum, Mildred, Ph.D. 🕮 300
Canarelli, Joseph, CSW 🕮 300
Capone, Julie, CSW 🕮 300
Capone, Thomas, Ph.D. 🕮 300

Counsellors

Center For Identity Development 291
Center For Identity Development South, Ltd. 236
Center for Non-Traditional Families 300
Centrum Für Sexualwissenschaft e. V. 110
Chiron, J. P. 98
Clintonville Counseling Services 319
Cohen, Carol, M.A., LPC 227
Cohn, Beryl, RNC, MSW 292
Cole, Louanne, Ph.D. 213
Collins, Ethelreda, LCSW, BCD 336
Columbia Medical Plaza 354
Commonwealth Professional Services 349
Community Counseling Centers of Chicago 248
Counseling Center 348
Counseling Services of Brandon 242
Creative Counseling Services 230
Cross, Clare, CSW 300
Crouch, Katherine Eustis, CSW 295
Crowe, John, CRC, CAC 295
DAPA, Family of Choice 342
Daugherty & Associates 227
Davis, Bill, LCSW 349
Deming, Alison 299
Dickinson, Pentz, McCall, Associates 233
Easton, Dossie, MFCC 213
Eden, Carl, CSW 300
Eisenberg, Edith, ACSW 300
Elmer, Mark, Dip. Couns. 80
Family Study Institute of Fort Wayne 254
Focus, Inc. 267
Focused Counseling Services, Inc. 289
Foley, Lyn, ACSW 287
Fontanella, Robert, CSW 300
Frederickson & Associates 279
Fuller, Cheryl, M.A., LCPC 262
Gair, Susan, MSW, CSW 300
Garcia, Dianne, MSW, Ph.D. 289
Goldberg, Jonathan, Ph.D. 301
Gordon, Donna, MA, NCPsyA 293
Gottlieb, Jody, Ph.D. 191
Grabowski, Robert, CSW, ACSW 301
Graham, Sally, Ph.D. 301
Grundman, Maryann, Ph.D., LCSW 227
Gundry, Nick 80
H.E.L.P, Inc. 293
Harmonia Madison Center for Psychotherapy 356
Hartman, Judith Rachael, Ph.D. 227
Hartzog, Dennis, M.Ed, L.P.C. 340
Hatley, Scott, MS, CSW 301
Hawkins, Brenda, Ed.D. 245
Henkin, William 213
Hepburn, Fran, MSW, CADC 293
Hillis, Raymond, Ph.D. 295
Hoole, Ken, MSW 229
Hope, Victor, Ph.D. 330
Horstman, William, Ph.D. 213
Hraca, Kim, M.A., MFCC 196, 197
In Distress 93
Isaacs, Robert, CSW 301
Istar, Arlene, CSW, CAC 295
Istvan, John Emery, M.S., MSW, LCSW 232
Jack, Sarah 80
James, George, Ph.D. 191
Jarratt, Kent, ACSW 301
Juran, Shelley, Ph.D. 297
Kassan, Lee, MA 301
Keeffe, Corky, M.A. 226
Kinsel, Kevin, MSW, CSW, PC 274
Knopf, Norton, Ph.D. 249
Koppel, Mark, Ph.D. 301
Kraus Eule, Norma, LCSW 262
Kreger, Kenneth, MA, CSW, LPC 275
Krieger, Irwin, LCSW 231
Lafferty, Norma, MSW 290
Lake, Moira 80
Landry, Patricia, CSW, BCD 301
Lathrop, Brian, NCPsy.A. 301
Lawrence, Robert 80
Legacy Counseling Center, Inc. 340
Lehne, Gregory, Ph.D. 263
Lifesigns 226
Lighthouse Center 193
Lippman, Susan, CSW 301
Lovejoy, Gary, Ph.D. 193
Malkin, Joyce, LCSW-C, LICSW 233
Mallon, David, MSW 202
Manhattan Psychotherapy 301
Manoogian Psychological Associates 316
Manoogian, Sam, Ph.D. 316
Manson, Susan, MS, MFCC 203
Marks, Al, Ph.D. 211
Marschall, Rick, CSW, CAC 301
Mayesm, John 163
McCarthy, Mark, M.S., LPC 283
McClemens, Mary Anne, M.A., LPCMH 233
McConnell, John, Ph.D. 211
McEwen, Chase, ACSW, LCSW 242
McGovern, Maureen, MSW 301
Merrimack Valley Counseling 271
Miller, Wynn, MSW, CSW 301
Molvig, Karen, Psy.D. 262
Montclair State College 291
Mozes, David, Ph.D. 233
Murrell, Pat, MSW, LCSW 282
Nelson, Joan, M.A., Ed.D. 210
New Beginnings 359
Noone, Kenneth, CSW, CAC 301
O'Brien, Terence 209
Oxenbury, Jane, M. Ed., C. Psyc. 42
Panozzo, David, CSW 293
Park Central Counselling 193
Parkinson, Phil 80
Perlman, Graham 80
Perlswig, Ellis, M.D. 231
Perry, Michael, Ph.D. 199
Peterson, Ronald, Ph.D. 193
Pinkpot 93
PMC Transgender Counseling & Consultation 1
Porter, Theresa, Psy.D. 231
Power, John, MSW 249
Quadland, Michael, Ph.D. 301
Railey, Julie, ACSW 277
Red Admiral Project 67
Red Rock Mental Health Center 323
Rendel, Brian, M.A, NCC 275
Ribakoff, Robin, M.F.C.T. 199
Rila, Margo 213
Riley Snow, Wynelle, M.D. 229
Roach, Barbara, L.C.S.W. 202
Rodgers, Luanna, M.A., MFCC 213
Rogers, Linda, Ph.D. 284
Romano, Nino, CSW, MSW 301
Ross, Dale 274
Ross, Joellyn, Ph.D. 290
Rubenstein, Maggi, R.N., MFCC, Ph.D. 213
Ruderman, Jerome, JD, MS 301
Ruth, Richard, Ph.D. 266
Ryan, Barb, M.S. 325
Saegert, Linda 301
Schlesinger, Jay, Ph.D. 301
Schmidt, Beverly, RCSW 301
Schochet, Rachel, Ph.D., MFCC 213
Sernier, Conrad, ACSW, CSW 301
Shannon, Joseph, Ph.D. 319
Simon, Liz, BCSW 260
Slutsky, Sidney, Ed.D. 330
Smith, Marilee, Psy.D. 229
Snyder, Robert, Ph.D. 284
Spadola, Madeline, Ms.Ed, CADAC 267
Steinhorn, Audrey 310
Summit Consulting Group, Inc 334
Tenbusch, Lynne, Ph.D. 274
Three Worlds 80
Twitchell, Carol, Psy.D. 241
United Services 230
Vanek, Stephen, LMSW-ACP 340
Verdantmom 197
Village Counseling, Inc. 319
Vitaletti, Robert, Ph.D. 227
Wagner, Dick, MSW, ACSW 284
Walker, Sylvia, MSW, ACSW 292
Wallace, Timothy, Ph.D. 230
Walter, Daniel, Psy.D. 349
Watson, Jacob, M.A., L.C.P.C. 262
Wedda, Susan, MSW, ACSW, BCD 275
Weeks, Alan 80
Weene, Kenneth, Ph.D. 302
Weinberger, Bette, ACSW 328
Wilton, Jim, MSW, CSW 274
Winder, Jon 348
Witchel, Joy, CSW, CAC 302
Wolverton, Gwen, Psy.D. 291
Woodhouse, Alan 94
Zelterman, Irene, CSW 302

Female

Benjamin, Shiela, LCSW 201
Brewer, Sue, MSW, LCSW 241
Captial District Center for Dissociative Disorders 295
Cardell, Mona, Ph.D. 328
Jean, Paula, Ph.D. 349
O'Brien, Maureen, CSW, ACSW 295
Women's Counseling Services of Berk County, Inc. 329
Zeiger, Robyn, Ph.D., CPC 266

Gay

Bellville Counseling Associates 262
Egge, Conrad, Ph.D. 193
Gay Men's Psychotherapy Referral Service 301
Holtby, Michael, LSCW 227
Kerner, Bruce, Psy.D. 301

Lesbian

Levin, Betty, MA 291
Rosa, Lydia, ACSW 301
Stein, Virginia, MA 293

Lesbian, Gay, Bi, & Transgendered

Affirmations 319
Allmen, Robert, MS, M.Div. 300
Alternative Lifestyles Office 279
Androgyny Center 314, 315
Armstrong, Paul 55
Arocha, Jorge, ACSW 238
Barnett, Joyce 55
Barr, Patricia, Ph.D. 288
Bates, Kirk 51
Begelman, Hedda, MSW, RCSW 300
Bergman, Tod, MSW 290
Bodekor, Greg, MS, CAC 298
Boland, Jim, Ph.D. 196
Borras, Mildred, Ph.D. 300
Bridge, Michael, Ph.D. 246
Bunker Hill Consultation Center 292
Capson, Stephen, Psy.D. 300
Careline 80
Chain, Steven, LCSW 227
Chapin, Suzanne, M.A. 230
Chelsea Psychotherapy Associates 300
Chesapeake Psychological Services 263
Christopher Street Counseling & Bookstore 223
Clarke, Judith, MSW, ACSW, BCD 300
Currie, Stuart 161
D'Amico, Jane, MSW, CSW, CAC 300
Damon, Hope, LCSW 349
Driscoll, Robert, CSW 300
East Side Ministry of Social Services 274
Family & Children's Services 279
Felshin, Elaine, Ph.D. 300
Frankel, Susan, CSW, BCD 300
Frisch, Hannah, Ph.D. 249
Gay & Lesbian Adolescent Social Services, Inc. 224
Gay & Lesbian Counseling Center 223
Gay & Lesbian Counseling Services of the United Community Church 282
Gay & Lesbian Peer Counseling 330
Gay Counseling Center of Long Island 301
Gay Psychological Services 301
Giachetti, Diane, CSW, ACSW 291
Giogianni, Paul, CSW 301
Gotham Psychotherapy Associates 301
Griffin, David Lindsey, CSW, CAC 301
Harrison, James, Ph.D. 313
Harvest Counseling Associates 341
Hazelton, Michael 55
Hencken, Joel, Ph.D. 267
Hicks, Walter Dean, Ph.D., CAS 293
Horwitz, Richard, CSW, CAC 301
Hunter, Shirley, M.Ed. 323
Hyatt, Diane, MSW, CISW 232
Insitute for Personal Growth 291
Institute for Human Identity 301
Jacobs, Mindy, Ph.D. 233
Jones, Linda, CSW, ACSW 301
Karmen, Mel, Ph.D. 211
Kelso, Betsy, Psy.D. 227
Kopacsi, Rosemarie, Ph.D., ACSW 291
Koplin, James, M.Ed., MSW 230
Lambda Counseling Services 283
Lamothe, Denise, Psy.D. 288
Lesbian & Gay Counselling & Consulting Services 45
Lesbian & Gay Male Advocates 274
Lesbian, Bisexual, & Gay Men's Counseling Collective 266
Lesko, Kathryn, Ph.D. 301
Lewinter, Beth, MSW, CSW 291
Liechenstein, Joyce, Ph.D. 301
MacAuley, Donna 55
Mass Bay Counseling Associates 267
Mayers, Terry, M.Ed., BCSW, ACSW 260
Midway Family Services 279
Montague, John 55
Montrose Counseling Center 342
Mulé, Nick, M.S.W. 49
Nichols, Margaret, Ph.D. 290
Nussdorf, Gerrie, Ph.D. 301
Oak Lawn Community Services 340
Page, Ken, CSW 301
Pantaleo, Michael, CSW, CAC 301
Passages Counseling Center 301
Patti, Vincent-John, ACSW 301
Peck, Janet, M.S. 230
Persad Center, Inc. 331
Pink Practice 80
Platt, Keith Allen, LCSW 243
Psychology & Counselling Associates 213
Psychotherapeutische Beratungsstelle 111
Psychotherapy Center 195
Psychotherapy Institute 55
Racine, Christianne 52
Raphael, Jerry, Ph.D. 301
Reynolds, Jan, M.A., MFCC 203
Richards, Janet 55
Roberts, Lynne, CSW, ACSW 301
Rosenberg, Miriam, M.D., Ph.D. 267
Scargall, Peter 55
Scherma, Robert, Psy.D. 301
Schernoff, Michael, CSW, ACSW 301
Seattle Counseling Service for Sexual Minorities 351
Shaw, Nanette, Ph.D. 301
Shell, John, Ph.D. 227
Silverman, Philip, Ph.D. 233
Silverstein, Charles, Ph.D. 301
Strout, David, LSMW 213
Thomson, Deb-Ann 227
Thrasher, Bob, M.A. 202
Triangle Services 359
Verhey, Gregory, MSW, CSW 301
Walford, Virginia, Ph.D. 44
Walsh, Eileen, M.S. 295
Wellington, Susan, MC 233
Whiting, Joyce, ACSW 288
Whitman-Walker Clinic 233
Williams, Mark, Ph.D. 302
Wind, Mark, MA, CAC, NCAC II 302
Yager Kupferman, Roz, BS, MA, Psy.A. 293

Transgender

Auge, Rebecca, Ph.D. 207
Baron, Ronald, M.D. 252
Caring Counseling 287
Center for Contemporary Counseling 235
Central Iowa Gender Institute 256
Cherry, Roxanne, Ph.D. 201
Cheshire Counseling Associates 287
Clinical Approach Counseling Center, Inc. 236
Counseling Associates 194
Dean, Judith, Ed.D., M.Div., M.S. 292
Ellaborn, Diane, LICSW, NASW 273
Etscovitz, Lee 333
Ettner, Randi, Ph.D. 248
Free University Hospital 151
Friedeman, Sheila, Ph.D. 193
Gender & Self Acceptance Program 213
Gender Clinic 28
Goldstein, Ronald, Ph.D. 329
GSAP *See* Gender & Self Acceptance Program
Hahn, Louise, MA, NCC 316

HBIGDA See National Harry Benjamin Gender Dysphoria Association
Ingersoll Gender Center 351
Institute for Gender Study & Treatment 226
Klein, Patricia, M.S. 327
LAGC See Los Angeles Gender Center
Los Angeles Gender Center 222
Lynn, Rusty, BD, MSW, LCSW 265
Malin, Martin, Ph.D. 263
Meisner, Judith, Ph.D., LCSW, LMFT 241
Metamorphosis 301
Miller, Niela, M.S. Ed., LCSW, LMHC 180
Morena & Orta Gender Issues Specialists 149
Mountain Home VAMC 336
National Harry Benjamin Gender Dysphoria Association 181
O'Donnell, Elke, Ph.D. 267
Ospedale Mauriziano 144
Padula, Lee, Ph.D. 277
Pearne, Dennis, Ed.D. 267
Prince Institute 208
Samons, Sandra, ACSW 274
Schooler, C. 301
Services for Men (& Their Families) 273
Speckert, Josefina, M.Ed. 272
Strapko, Nasncy, Ph.D. 288
Theseus Counseling Services 262, 267
Thompson, Deb-Ann, Ph.D, NCACII, CACIII 227
Vitale, Anne, Ph.D. 220
Warren, Ellen, LCSW 347
West, Jeanne 209
Yelsky, Miriam, Ph.D. 302

Transvestite

Taylor, Brad, M.A. 203

DISTRIBUTORS

BOOKS

Erotic

All Sexes & Sexualities

Eve Browne Fashions 181
Prestige Periodical Distributors 2

Fetish

All Sexes & Sexualities

Flywheel, Ltd. 91

General

All Sexes & Sexualities

Alamo Square Distributors 213
Amok Books 203
Baker & Taylor Books 290
Bookpeople 207
Bookspeed 168
Bookworld Services 241
Bulldog Books 26
Central Books 80
distributors 253
Edition Habit Press Ltd. 26
Golden Lee Distributors 267
Independent Publishers Group 249
Ingram Book 336
IPG See Independent Publishers Group
J Barnicoat Ltd. 72
John Coutts Library Services, Ltd. 51
KAE BokImport 164
Koen Book Distributors 291
Last Gasp of San Francisco 213
Login Publishers Consortium 249
MacNeill Library Service 45
Marginal Distribution 54
National Book Network 265
PDS See Publishers Distribution Service
Pipeline Books 80
Publishers Distribution Service 278
Publishers Group West 199
Quality Books 252
Slawson Communications 220
Turnaround 80

Lesbian, Gay, Bi, & Transgendered

Venue Services Limited 80

CLOTHING

Fetish

All Sexes & Sexualities

Basta 107

Jim Cooke Enterprises 350

EROTICA

BDSM

All Sexes & Sexualities

Screaming Leather 213

Chastity Belts

All Sexes & Sexualities

Tim Swig Associates Group 293

General

All Sexes & Sexualities

Cybercore 140
Kink Distributors 209
Right Hand Productions 154
Scala B. V. 152
Studio Strak 31
Tokyo Boeki Shokai Ltd. 148
Xclusiv Distributors, Inc. 297

Gay

Paragon 2

Lesbian, Gay, Bi, & Transgendered

Executive Imports International 302

MAGAZINES

General

All Sexes & Sexualities

Desert Moon Periodicals 2
Ubiquity Distributors 181
Wrapaway 26

PIERCING JEWELRY

All Sexes & Sexualities

IMAX International 141

SAFER SEX PRODUCTS

All Sexes & Sexualities

Conney 356

VIDEOS

BDSM

All Sexes & Sexualities

Lyndon Distributors Limited 224

Gay

Close-Up Productions 224

Erotic

All Sexes & Sexualities

First Run Features 302
Noble Distributors 302

Gay

Edition Manfred Salzgeber Berlin 110
Sierra Pacific Productions 181

Heterosexual

John Floyd Video 224

Political

Lesbian, Gay, Bi, & Transgendered

Gay Film Association Lambda 150

Safer Sex

All Sexes & Sexualities

REW Video 181

FILM FESTIVALS

SEXUALITY

Lesbian, Gay, Bi, & Transgendered

Lesbian & Gay Film Festival 136
Lesbian/Gay Film Festival 302
Maine Gay & Lesbian Film Festival 261
New Jersey Lesbian & Gay Film Festival 288
Out-In-Africa 170
Question de Genre 2
SchwuHesbische Filmtage 119

HEALTH SERVICES

All Sexes & Sexualities

45th. Street Clinic 351
Abbott Northwestern Hospital 279
Academisch Ziekenhuis 155
Academisch Ziekhuis 158
Addington Hospital 171
AIDES Atlantique 102
AIDES Haute-Normandie 105
AIDES Lorraine-Sud 102
AIDES Poiteau-Charentes 105
AIDES Provence 99
AIDS Prevention & Sexual Health Program 55
AIDS Unit 31
Akron City Hospital 317
Alachua General Hospital 237
Albany Medical Center 295
Alice Springs Hospital 28
Allegheny General Hospital 331
Allgemeines Krankenhaus 35
Alta Bates Medical Center 197
AMI Park Plaza Hospital 342
AMI Twelve Oaks Hospital 342
Araba Fenice 144
Arizona State Hospital 193
Arlington Hospital 347
Asbl Aide Cliniques Universitaires Saint Luc 36
Atlantic City Medical Center 289
Auckland Hospital 160
Audie L. Murphy Memorial Veterans' Hospital 344
Audre Lorde Clinic 80
Barnes Hospital 284
Bay Centre for Birth Control 55
Bayfront Medical Center 241
Bayley Seton Hospital 302
Beach Area Community Health Center 211
Bellevue Hospital Center 302
Berkeley Free Clinic 197
Bernhard Clinic 80
Beth Israel Medical Center 302
Binghamton General Hospital 296
Bloomington Hospital 253
Borgess Medical Center 276
Boston City Hospital 267
Broadlands Medical Center 256
Bronson Methodist Hospital 276
Bronx Lebanon Hospital Center 297
Bronx Municipal Hospital Center 297
Brookdale Hospital Medical Center 297
Brooklyn Hospital Center 297
Broward General Medical Center 236
Buffalo General Hospital 298
Cabell Huntington Hospital 354
Cambridge Hospital 267
Cape Fear Valley Medical Center 315
Carolinas Medical Center 313
CAVE See Centro Antivenereo
Cedars-Sinai Medical Center 203
Centre de Dépistage 101
Centre de Prophylaxie 100
Centre de Prophylaxie des MST 99
Centre de Prophylaxie et MST 99
Centre de Santé 97
Centre Figuier 102
Centre Hospitalier 98, 101, 105
Centre Hospitalier Beausecours 101
Centre Hospitalier d'Alençon 97
Centre Hospitalier d'Amiens 97
Centre Hospitalier d'Angers 98
Centre Hospitalier d'Auxerre 98
Centre Hospitalier d'Epinal 99
Centre Hospitalier de Belfort 98
Centre Hospitalier de Brest 99
Centre Hospitalier de Cahors 99
Centre Hospitalier de Chambéry 99
Centre Hospitalier de Charleville 98
Centre Hospitalier de Gap 100
Centre Hospitalier de Grenoble 100
Centre Hospitalier de Guéret 100
Centre Hospitalier de la Rochelle 100
Centre Hospitalier de Laval 100
Centre Hospitalier de Montpellier 101
Centre Hospitalier de Nancy 102
Centre Hospitalier de Nantes 102
Centre Hospitalier de Pau 104
Centre Hospitalier de Privas 105
Centre Hospitalier de Saint Denis 105
Centre Hospitalier de Saint Michel 105
Centre Hospitalier de Soissons 106
Centre Hospitalier de Toulouse Hôtel Dieu 106
Centre Hospitalier de Tours 106
Centre Hospitalier E. Muller 101
Centre Hospitalier Général 101
Centre Hospitalier Général Faconaja 99
Centre Hospitalier Intercommunal 99
Centre Hospitalier la Grave 106
Centre Hospitalier Laennec 105
Centre Hospitalier Louis Pasteur 99
Centre Hospitalier Notre Dame de la Misericorde 99
Centre Hospitalier Orléans-la-Source 102
Centre Hospitalier R. Pontchaillou 105
Centre Hospitalier R. U. Dupuytren 100
Centre Hospitalier Regional 102
Centre Médical 99
Centre Médico-Social 97, 98, 102, 103, 105
Centro Antivenereo 142
Centro de Orientção e Aconselhamento em AIDS e Doeças Sexualmente Transmissiveis 39
Centro de Saude Santa Cecilia 39
Centro Democeltico 142
Centro Dermoceltico 147
Centro Dermoceltico USL 146
Centro Epidemiologico Sardo 145
Centro MTS 141
Centro Ospedale di Borgo di Trento 147
Century City Hospital 203
Charleston Area Medical Center 354
Children's Hospital 260
Christian Hospital Northeast 284
Christian Hospital Northwest 284
Cité Sanitaire 106
City Hospital 170
Claydon Hospital 94
Cleveland Clinic Hospital 318
Clinic 275 30
Clinica Dermatologica 144
Clinica Dermosifilopatica 141, 145, 146
Clinica Malatte Infettive 140
Clinique Medicale de la Cité 62
Coler Memorial Hospital 302
Colorado Health Action Project 227
Columbia Hospital 357
Combined Health District 321
Community-General Hospital of Greater Syracuse 312
Comprehensive Clinic 237
Cook County Hospital 249
Crawford Long Hospital of Emory University 243
Dallas County Hospital 340
Danbury Hospital 230
Daniel Freeman Marina Hospital 206
Davies Medical Center 213
Day Hospital 170
DCH Regional Medical Center 192
Deaconess Medical Center 285
Delaware Lesbian & Gay Health Advocates 233
Denver Metro Health Clinic 227
Department of Health & Human Services 192
Desert Hospital 208
Dispensaire Anti-Vénérien 98
District of Columbia General Hospital 233
Doctor's Hospital 195
Dominican Santa Cruz Hospital 221
Dorothea Dix Hospital 315
Duluth Community Health Center 279
Duval County Public Health Unit 238
Eastern Maine Medical Center 262
Ebb & Flow 77
El Camino Hospital 207
Elmhurst Hospital Center 299
Erie County Medical Center 298
Fayetteville Regional Medical Center 195
Flinders Medical Centre 30
Florida Keys Memorial Hospital 238
Florida Medical Center 236
Free Clinic 36
Frere Hospital 171
Fresno Community Hospital & Medical Center 199
Fylkeslegen i Hamar 165
Fylkeslegen i Ostfold 166
Garden Grove Hospital & Medical Center 200
Genessee Hospital 310
Georgetown University Hospital 233
Gesundheitsamt 115
Gesundheitsamt Chemnitz 113
Gesundheitsamt Erfurt 116
GG & GD 152, 157, 158

Health Services

Glendale Memorial Hospital & Health Center 🕮 200
Good Samaritan Hospital & Medical Center 🕮 326
Good Samaritan Medical Center 🕮 243
Good Samaritan Regional Medical Center 🕮 193
Goodhew, John, M.D. 🕮 55
Graduate Hospital 🕮 330
Grady Memorial Hospital 🕮 243
Group Health Coöperative Central Hospital 🕮 351
Gruppo C 🕮 142, 146, 147
H. F. Verwoerd Hospital 🕮 172
Hamot Medical Center 🕮 328
Harbor View Medical Center 🕮 211
Harborview Medical Center 🕮 351
Harlem Hospital Center 🕮 302
Harper Hospital 🕮 275
Harrisburg Hospital 🕮 328
Harry S. Truman Memorial Veterans' Hospital 🕮 283
Hartford Hospital 🕮 230
Haukeland Hospital 🕮 165
Havenzuikhuis 🕮 157
Health Awareness Services 🕮 273
Health Information Network 🕮 351
Healthwise 🕮 87
Helseavdelingen Helsesjef Pål Gulbrandsen 🕮 165
Helsekontor 🕮 165
Helseutvalget 🕮 165
Hennepin County Medical Center 🕮 279
Henry Ford Hospital 🕮 275
Herpes Association 🕮 80
Highland General Hospital 🕮 207
HIV Confidential Testing Service 🕮 289
HIV/STD Clinic 🕮 162
HIV-Antikörpertest 🕮 134
Hollywood Community Hospital 🕮 201
Holy Cross Hospital 🕮 345
Hôpital 🕮 99
Hôpital Antoine Beclere 🕮 103
Hôpital Beauregard 🕮 106
Hôpital Boucicaut 🕮 103
Hôpital Cantonal 🕮 178
Hôpital Charles-Nicole 🕮 105
Hôpital Corantins-Celton 🕮 100
Hôpital de Bellevue 🕮 105
Hôpital de la Fontaine 🕮 103, 105
Hôpital Edouard Herriot 🕮 100
Hôpital Jean Martial 🕮 106
Hôpital Lariboisère 🕮 103
Hôpital Pellegrin 🕮 98
Hôpital Saint Antoine 🕮 103
Hôpital Saint Charles 🕮 101
Hôpital Saint Louis 🕮 103
Hôpital Saint-André 🕮 98
Hôpital Tarnier 🕮 103
Hospices Civils de Strasbourg 🕮 106
Hospital das Clinicas da Faculdade de Medicina 🕮 39
Hospital Emilio Ribas 🕮 39
Hospital of the University of Pennsylvania 🕮 330
Hospital São Paulo 🕮 39
Hôtel Dieu 🕮 100
Hunter Holmes McGuire Veterans' Affairs Medical Center 🕮 349
Huntington Memorial Hospital 🕮 209
Huntsville Hospital 🕮 191
Hurley Medical Center 🕮 275
Illinois Masonic Medical Center 🕮 249
Imperial Point Medical Center 🕮 236
Indiana University Medical Center 🕮 254
Infectious Diseases Clinic 🕮 254
Institut Prophylactique 🕮 103
Istituti Ospedale 🕮 142
Istituto Dermopatico dell'Immacolata 🕮 141
Istituto Malattie Infettive 🕮 145
J. G. Strydom Hospital 🕮 171
Jackson Hospital & Clinic 🕮 192
Jackson Memorial Hospital 🕮 239
Jewish Hospital of Cincinnati 🕮 318
John L. Doyne Hospital 🕮 357
Johns Hopkins Hospital 🕮 263
Kaiser Foundation Hospital 🕮 213, 246
Kansas City Free Health Clinic 🕮 283
Kantonspital 🕮 177, 178
Kantonsspital Basel 🕮 177
Keith, III, Paul, M.D. 🕮 203
Kennestone Hospital 🕮 245
King Edward VIII Hospital 🕮 171
Kings County Hospital Center 🕮 297
Kirkenes Sykehus Sjefslege Arnt Uchtermann 🕮 165
Klinikken for Kønssygdomme 🕮 65
Klinikum an Küchwald Infectktionsklinik 🕮 113
Kommuneoverlegen 🕮 165
Kristiansan Helseråd 🕮 166
Laguna Honda Hospital 🕮 213
Landeskrankenhaus Innsbruck / Department of Dermatology & Venerology 🕮 34
Landeskrankenhaus Salzburg, Dept. Dermatologie 🕮 34
Lansing General Hospital 🕮 277
Larvik Helseråd 🕮 166
Lee Memorial Hospital 🕮 237
Lega Volontari Anti-HIV 🕮 141
Lenox Hill Hospital 🕮 302
Leon County Health Department 🕮 242
Lillehammer Helseråd 🕮 165
Lincoln Medical & Mental Health Center 🕮 297
Long Beach Community Hospital 🕮 202
Lucerne Medical Center 🕮 240
Main Street Clinic 🕮 238
Maine Medical Center 🕮 262
Maricopa Medical Center 🕮 193
Marquette County Health Department 🕮 277
Massachusetts General Hospital 🕮 267
McLaren Regional Medical Center 🕮 275
Médecins du Monde 🕮 100
Medical Center Hospital 🕮 342
Medical Center Hospital of Vermont 🕮 346
Medical Center of Delaware 🕮 233
Medical Center of Louisiana at New Orleans 🕮 260
Medical Center of North Hollywood 🕮 207
Medical Centre 🕮 162
Medical College of Virginia Hospitals 🕮 349
Melbourne Sexual Health Centre 🕮 32
Memorial Hospital of South Bend 🕮 255
Memorial Hospital of Tampa 🕮 242
Memorial Medical Center 🕮 339
Mercy Health Center 🕮 323
Mercy Hospital 🕮 239, 256
Mercy Hospital of Pittsburgh 🕮 331
Methodist Hospital of Indiana 🕮 254
Metropolitan Hospital 🕮 276
Metropolitan Hospital Center 🕮 302
Metropolitan Nashville General Hospital 🕮 337
Metrowest Medical Center 🕮 270
Miami Valley Hospital 🕮 321
Midway Hospital Medical Center 🕮 203
Miller-Dawn Medical Center 🕮 279
Mobile Infirmary Medical Center 🕮 192
Monday Night Clinic 🕮 323
Montefiore Medical Center 🕮 297
Montefiore University Hospital 🕮 331
Moser, Charles, Ph.D, M.D. 🕮 213
Moses H. Cone Memorial Hospital 🕮 315
Mount Carmel Medical Center 🕮 319
Mount Diablo Medical Center 🕮 198
Mount Lawley Medical Centre 🕮 33
Mount Sinai Medical Center 🕮 239, 302
Murray Street STD Clinic 🕮 33
National Hospital 🕮 171
National Institutes of Health 🕮 265
Naval Hospital 🕮 207, 334
Nelson-Tebedo Clinic 🕮 340
New England Deaconess Hospital 🕮 267
New England Medical Center 🕮 267
New Hampshire Hospital 🕮 287
New Hanover Regional Medical Center 🕮 316
New York City Department of Health 🕮 302
New York Downtown Hospital 🕮 302
New York Hospital 🕮 302
Newark Beth Israel Medical Center 🕮 292
North Central Bronx Hospital 🕮 297
North Colorado Medical Center 🕮 229
North Florida Regional Medical Center 🕮 237
North General Hospital 🕮 302
North Philadelphia Health System 🕮 330
Northwestern Memorial Hospital 🕮 249
Ohio State University Medical Center 🕮 319
Orlando Regional Medical Center 🕮 240
Ospedale 🕮 141
Ospedale A Cardanelli 🕮 143
Ospedale Amedeo di Savoia 🕮 144
Ospedale Civico 🕮 145
Ospedale Civile 🕮 139, 140, 143, 144, 145, 146
Ospedale Civile dell'Annunziata 🕮 139
Ospedale Civile Ruiniti 🕮 147
Ospedale Civile S. Chiara 🕮 146
Ospedale Cotugno 🕮 140
Ospedale Di Cattinara 🕮 141
Ospedale di Summa 🕮 144
Ospedale di Venere 🕮 144
Ospedale Gen. Reg. S. M. Battuti 🕮 147
Ospedale Generale Provinciale 🕮 146
Ospedale Guadagna 🕮 145
Ospedale Macchi 🕮 143
Ospedale Madonna dei Cieli 🕮 139
Ospedale Malacrino 🕮 140
Ospedale Maurizio Ascoli 🕮 145
Ospedale Molinette 🕮 144
Ospedale Morgagni 🕮 140
Ospedale Pascale 🕮 140
Ospedale Pellegrini Nuovo 🕮 140
Ospedale Policlinico Monteluce 🕮 146
Ospedale Provinciale 🕮 139
Ospedale Provinciale San Francesco di Paola (Pescopagano) 🕮 139
Ospedale Regina Marherita 🕮 145
Ospedale S. Camillo de Lellis 🕮 139
Ospedale S. Chiara 🕮 146
Ospedale S. Gallicano 🕮 141
Ospedale S. Salvatore di Muraglia 🕮 143
Ospedale San Antonio 🕮 144
Ospedale San Carlo 🕮 139
Ospedale San Lazzaro 🕮 144
Ospedale San Martino 🕮 142
Ospedale San Matteo 🕮 143
Ospedale San Salvatore 🕮 139
Ospedale Santa Anna 🕮 142
Ospedale Spallanzani 🕮 141
Ospedale SS. Annunziata 🕮 145
Ospedale SS. Trinita 🕮 145
Ospedale Umberto I 🕮 143
Ospedale V. Emanuele 🕮 145
Ospedali Riuniti 🕮 142
Palm Beach County AIDS Clinic 🕮 243
Palm Beach County Health Department 🕮 243
Palm Beaches Medical Center 🕮 243
Parkview Memorial Hospital 🕮 254
Penrose Hospital 🕮 226
People In The North 🕮 31
Peoria City County Health Department 🕮 252
Piedmont Hospital 🕮 243
Pitié-Salpêtrière 🕮 103
Policlinico 🕮 140, 144
Policlinico di Careggi 🕮 145
Policlinico Gemelli 🕮 141
Porter Memorial Hospital 🕮 227
Presbyterian Hospital 🕮 313, 323
Presbyterian Hospital in the City of New York 🕮 302
Princeton Hospital 🕮 240
Provenant Saint Anthony Hospital 🕮 227
Providence Hospital 🕮 192, 233
Public Health Clinic 🕮 239
Public Health STD Centre 🕮 162
Queen's Medical Center 🕮 247
Queens Hospital Center 🕮 302
Rana Helseråd 🕮 165
Red Door Clinic 🕮 279
Regional Medical Center at Memphis 🕮 336
Research Medical Center 🕮 283
Rex Hospital 🕮 315
Rhode Island Hospital 🕮 334
Richard Roudebush Veterans' Affairs Medical Center 🕮 254
Richland Memorial Hospital 🕮 335
Roanoke Memorial Hospital 🕮 349
Rochester General Hospital 🕮 310
Roosevelt Hospital 🕮 302
Royal Darwin Hospital 🕮 28
Rush-Presbyterian-Saint Luke's Medical Center 🕮 249
Sacred Heart General Hospital 🕮 325
Saint Alphonsus Regional Medical Center 🕮 247
Saint Anthony Hospital 🕮 323
Saint Anthony's Hospital 🕮 241
Saint Clare's Hospital & Health Center 🕮 302
Saint David's Hospital 🕮 338
Saint Elizabeth's Medical Center of Boston 🕮 267
Saint Francis Hospital 🕮 336
Saint Francis Hospital & Medical Center 🕮 230
Saint Francis Medical Center 🕮 247, 331
Saint Francis Regional Medical Center 🕮 258
Saint John's Episcopal Hospital - South Shore 🕮 299
Saint John's Medical Center 🕮 323
Saint Joseph County Health Department 🕮 255
Saint Joseph Hospital 🕮 227
Saint Joseph Hospital & Medical Center 🕮 249
Saint Joseph Medical Center 🕮 254, 294
Saint Joseph's Hospital 🕮 242, 259
Saint Joseph's Hospital of Atlanta 🕮 244
Saint Joseph's Medical Center 🕮 248, 255
Saint Luke's Hospital 🕮 194
Saint Luke's Hospital Center 🕮 302
Saint Luke's Medical Center 🕮 227, 318, 357
Saint Mary Medical Center 🕮 202
Saint Mary's Health Services 🕮 276
Saint Mary's Hospital 🕮 243
Saint Mary's Hospital & Medical Center 🕮 213
Saint Mary's Medical Center 🕮 279
Saint Mary's Medical Center of Evansville 🕮 254
Saint Mary's Regional Medical Center 🕮 287
Saint Paul Medical Center 🕮 340
Saint Peter Hospital 🕮 350
Saint Vincent Hospital 🕮 295
Saint Vincent Hospital & Health Care Center 🕮 254
Saint Vincent Infirmary Medical Center 🕮 195
Saint Vincents' Medical Center of Richmond 🕮 302
SAMPA 🕮 *See* Solidariedade, Apoio Moral e Psicologico Aplicados a AIDS
San Bernadino County Medical Center 🕮 210
San Francisco General Hospital Medical Center 🕮 213
San José Medical Center 🕮 219
Sandler, Karen, D.O. 🕮 203
Santa Barbara Cottage Hospital 🕮 221
Santa Clara Valley Medical Center 🕮 219
Santa Rosa Health Care Corporation 🕮 344
Santa Rosa Memorial Hospital 🕮 222
Sarasota Memorial Hospital 🕮 241
Scottsdale Memorial Hospital 🕮 193
Sentara Norfolk General Hospital 🕮 348
Sentrum Legekontor 🕮 166
Sequoia Hospital 🕮 209
Services Départmental de Vénérologie 🕮 97
Seton Medical Center 🕮 338
Sezione Malattie Infettive dell'Ospedale 🕮 142
Shadyside Hospital 🕮 331
Shand Hospital at the University of Florida 🕮 237
Sheenan Memorial Hospital 🕮 298
Sinai Hospital of Baltimore 🕮 263
Sinai Samaritan Medical Center 🕮 357
Solidariedade, Apoio Moral e Psicologico Aplicados a AIDS 🕮 39
South Miami Hospital 🕮 239
South Shore Hospital & Medical Center 🕮 239
Southside Hospital 🕮 296
Sparrow Hospital 🕮 277
Städtiches Gesundheitsamt-Beratungstelle für Geschlechtskrankheiten 🕮 132

Städtische Poliklinik für Haut- & Geschlechtskrankheiten 179
Stamford Hospital 232
STD Clinic 52, 137, 236, 254, 318
Strong Memorial Hospital of the University of Rochester 310
Sutter General Hospital 209
SVG 156, 157, 158
SVGD 155
Swedish Medical Center 351
Tallahassee Memorial Regional Medical Center 242
Tampa General Healthcare 242
Tanner, Mark, M.D. 244
Tarrant County Hospital 340
Townsville General Hospital 29
Tromsø Komm. Helsekontor 166
Truman Medical Center 283
Tucson Medical Center 194
Tulane University Hospital & Clinincs 260
UCHSC 227
UCSD Medical Center 211
Unita Sanitaria Locale 144, 146
United Hospitals Medical Center 292
Universitätshautklinik 122
University & Childrens' Hospital 283
University Health Service 356
University Hospital 292, 294, 312, 326
University Hospital of Cleveland 318
University Hospital of Zürich 179
University Hospitals & Clinics 282
University Medical Center 194, 238, 286
University of Alabama Hospital 191
University of California - Davis Medical Center 209
University of California Irvine Medical Center 208
University of Cincinnati Hospital 318
University of Kansas Hospital 257
University of Maryland Medical System 263
University of Massachusetts Medical Center 273
University of Michigan Hospitals 274
University of Minnesota Hospital 279
University of Nebraska Medical Center 285
University of South Alabama Medical Center 192
University of Southern California Medical Center 203
University of Tennessee Memorial Hospital 336
University of Virginia Hospital 347
University of Washington Medical Center 351
University of Wisconsin Hospital & Clinics 356
USL *See* Unita Sanitaria Locale
Valley Hospital Medical Center 286
Valley Medical Center of Fresno 199
Vassar Brothers Hospital 310
Venhälsan 175
Vest-Agder Sentralsykehus 166
Veterans' Affairs Medical Center 203, 233, 239, 254, 259, 260, 263, 267, 271, 274, 279, 282, 283, 284, 288, 294, 296, 297, 302, 312, 318, 326, 331, 334, 337, 340, 342, 345
Village Clinic 47
Wairau Hospital 161
Walthamweston Hospital & Medical Center 273
Washoe Medical Center 287
Wesley Medical Center 258
West Florida Regional Medical Center 241
West Paces Medical Center 244
Whangarei STD Clinic 163
William Beaumont Hospital 278
William S. Middleton Veterans' Hospital 356
William Wishard Memorial Hospital 254
Yale- New Haven Hospital 231
Youth Health Services 302

Female

Brigham Women's Hospital 267
Concord Feminist Health Center 2
Guttman Breast Diagnostic Institute 302
Hassle Free Clinic - Women 55
Lesbian Health Project 225
Lyon-Martin Women's Health Services 213
Saint Marks Women's Health Collective 302
Vermont Women's Health Center 346
Women's Alternative Health Clinic 357

Lesbian

New York City Department of Health 302

Lesbian, Gay, Bi, & Transgendered

Arci Gay 143
Brady East STD Clinic 356
Chase Brexton Clinic 263
DOK *See* Konsultatieburo voor Relaties en Seksualiteit
Fenway Community Health Center 267
Gay & Lesbian Health Collective, Inc. 230
Gay & Lesbian Health Service 28
Gay & Lesbian Health Services of Saskatoon 64
Helseavdelingen Helsesjef Th. Hetland 165
Helseutvalget for Homofile 166
Homogezondheitzentrum 159
Howard Brown Health Center 249
Konsultatieburo voor Relaties en Seksualiteit 36
Lesbian & Gay Health Project 314
New York City Department of Health 302
Ospedale Generale Provinciale 143
Rådgivningstjenesten for Homofile og Lesbiske i Tromsø 166
Rainbow Clinic 80
Seattle Gay Clinic 351
Testing The Limits 323

Male

Family Planning Association 160
Hassle Free Clinic - Men 55

Transgender

Centre for Sexuality 45

HELPLINES

AIDS

All Sexes & Sexualities

ACASIA *See* AIDS Care & Support In Action
AIDES Paris & Ile de France 103
AIDS Care & Support In Action 87
AIDS Concern North Yorkshire 88
AIDS Help Line 66
AIDS Helpline 71, 87, 88, 137, 163, 292, 359
AIDS Hotline 282, 355
AIDS Hotline - AIDS Pela Vida 39
AIDS Info Line 96
AIDS Infoline 50
AIDS Lifeline 93
AIDS Line West Midlands 92
AIDS National Hotline 159
AIDS Telefon 117
AIDS Telephone 35
AIDS/HIV Info Line 26
AIDS/HIV Nightline 213
AIDS-Hilfe 148
AIDS-Infolijn 152
AIDSLine 71, 77, 79, 93
AIDSline Southampton 77
AIDS-linien (AIDS Hotline) 66
Allo SIDA 106
Assistenza AIDS 141
Automatisk Telefonsvarer om AIDS 165
Blackliners 67
Body Positive 67, 169
Boston AIDS Helpline 79
Burnley AIDS Line 78
Cambridge AIDS Helpline 71
Cardiff AIDS Helpline 359
Carlisle Citizens Advice Bureau 72
Carmarthen AIDS Helpline 359
Cascade AIDS Project 326
CDC National AIDS Hotline 181
ChilternAIDS 71
Colchester HIV/AIDS Helpline 75
Derby AIDS Line 72
Eastern AIDS Support Triangle 88
Exeter AIDS Line 73
Florida HIV/AIDS Hotline 235
Grampian AIDS Line 168
Grantham HIV/AIDS Helpline 79
Grimsby & District AIDS Line 77
Gwent AIDS Advice Line 359
Health Crisis Network 239
Herefordshire HIV/AIDS Advice Helpline 77
Idaho AIDS Foundation 247
Indiana AIDS Hotline 254
Info SIDA 62
Informazioni AIDS 140
Ipswich AIDS Helpline 91
Jewish AIDS Trust 67
Kent County Council 78
Lesbian & Gay Bereavement Project 81
Mainliners 67
Metro 81
Mid-Glamorgan AIDS Helpline 359
Minstry of Health AIDS Hotline 56
National AIDS Hotline 67
National Health AIDS-line 164
NAZ Project 67
Newcastle AIDS Hotline 25
Northampton AIDS Information Line 89
Norwich AIDS Helpline 88
Ohio AIDS Hotline 317
Opplysnigstelefon om AIDS 165
Peterborough AIDS Helpline 71
Positive Action for HIV 78
Rosa Hilfe 121
SAM *See* Scottish AIDS Monitor
Santa Cruz AIDS Project 221
Scottish AIDS Monitor 168
Shrewsbury AIDS Helpline 90
SISA Intervention Prévention Ecoute 61
South Yorkshire AIDSline 90
Surrey & East Hants AIDSlink Ltd. 91
Sussex AIDS Helpline 74
Telefono AIDS 146
Terrence Higgins Trust 67
Trondeheim Rode Kors 166
Warrington AIDSline 72
Western Australian AIDS Council 33

Female

Positively Women 67

Lesbian, Gay, Bi, & Transgendered

AHA *See* Allgemeine Homosexuelle Arbeitsgemeinschaft e. V.
AIDS Helpline Cork 137
Allgemeine Homosexuelle Arbeitsgemeinschaft e. V. 110
Ecoute Gai 103
Gay & Lesbian Helpline 355
Gay Helpline of New Jersey 289
Helpline 113

MISCELLANEOUS

All Sexes & Sexualities

Crisis Hotline 342
Gay Information Services 355
In Touch Hotline 249
Reachout of Saint Lawrence County, Inc. 310
Response of Suffolk County 302

Female

Discipline Support-Line for Women 2

SEXUAL HEALTH

All Sexes & Sexualities

San Francisco Sex Information 213

SEXUALITY

All Sexes & Sexualities

Aberystwyth Lesbian, Gay, & Bisexual Switchboard 359
Bedfordshire Lesbian & Gay Helpline 70
Bradford Friend 94
Bradford Gay & Lesbian Switchboard 94
Bristol Lesbian & Gay Switchboard 70
Burnley Switchboard 78
Centre Hospitalier La Meynard 149
Colchester Gay Switchboard 75
Dorset Lesbian & Gay Helpline 73
East Lancashire Lesbian & Gay Switchboard 78
Gay & Lesbian Switchboard 219
Gay & Lesbian Switchboard Cornwall 72
Gwynedd Gay Line 359
Hastings Befrienders 91
Hastings Switchboard 91
Infoline of Eastern Connecticut 232
Jewish Lesbian & Gay Helpline 67
Leder Beratungstelefon 132
Lesbian & Gay Student Union Helpline 347
London Lesbian & Gay Switchboard 67
Medway & Maidstone Lesbian & Gay Switchboard 78
Merseyside Friend 87
North Central Mental Health Services 319
Parent's Enquiry 136
Planning Familial 148
Regional Hospital 138
South Yorkshire Connections 90
Southern Health Board 137
West Midlands Friend 92
West Midlands Lesbian & Gay Switchboard 92, 93

Bisexual

Bi-Line 28
Bisexual Helpline 79
Bisexual Phoneline (Scotland) 167

Female

Tell-A-Woman 330
Womanline 160
Womonspace / Lesbian Lifeline 43

Gay

Gay Helpline of New Jersey 289
Gay Information Cork 136
Gay Lines Calgary 42
Gayline 162
Hein & Feite Switchboard 119
Mann-O-Meter e. V. 107
Men on Men Project 94
Sheffield Gayphone 90
Solent Gay Switchboard & AIDSline 64, 77

Lesbian

Cleveland Lesbian Line 88
Cork Lesbian Line 136
Edinburgh Lesbian Line 168
Hull Lesbian Line 77
Leeds Lesbian Line 94
Lesbian Information Line/Womyn's Collective of Calgary 42
Lesbian Information San Antonio 344
Lesbian Line 28, 138, 162
Lesbian Switchboard 302
LISA *See* Lesbian Information San Antonio
London Lesbian Line 79
Newcastle Lesbian Line 92
Penzance Lesbian Line 72
Sheffield Lesbian Line 90
Solent Lesbian Line 64, 77
Telefono Amica 142
York Lesbian Line 88

Lesbian, Gay, Bi, & Transgendered

Aardvaark Helpline 345
Aberdeen Lesbian, Gay, & Bisexual Switchboard 168
Acceuil Rencontre Information Service 100
Affirmations 275
ALLOGAY 98, 100, 101, 102, 103, 105, 106
Alternative Resources of the Triad 315
Arci Gay 139, 141, 142, 143, 146
Arci Gayline 138
ARIS *See* Acceuil Rencontre Information Service
Arkansas Gay & Lesbian Task Force Switchboard 195
ASBL Gai Info 38
Asheville Gay & Lesbian Information Line 313
Assault Hotline 159
Atlanta Gay Center Helpline 244

Helplines: Sexuality

Ayr Lesbian & Gay Switchboard 🕮 169
Bath Gay & Lesbian Switchboard 🕮 70
Beauftragte für Gleigeschlechtliche Lebensweisen 🕮 125
Beratungsstelle 🕮 127
Beratungstelephon für Homosexuelle 🕮 179
Beratungstelle für Homosexuelle 🕮 121
Berkshire Gay Switchboard 🕮 71
BHUS-Linjen 🕮 175
Billy De Frank Lesbian & Gay Community Center 🕮 219
Bolton Lesbian & Gay Switchboard 🕮 78
Borders Gay Switchboard 🕮 167
Boston Gay & Lesbian Helpline 🕮 267
Café Stonewall 🕮 114
Cambridge Friend 🕮 71
Cara Friend 🕮 164
Cardiff Friend 🕮 359
Cardiff Switchboard 🕮 359
Carrey Friend 🕮 77
Chelmsford Lesbian & Gay Switchboard 🕮 75
CheLSI e. V. 🕮 113
Cleveland Lesbian / Gay Hotline 🕮 318
Common Bond Gay & Lesbian Information Line 🕮 294
Community Services Network, Inc. 🕮 282
Consultorio Gay 🕮 140, 147
Coventry Friend 🕮 93
Crewe L&G Switchboard 🕮 71
Crisis Line 🕮 28
Croydon Friend 🕮 91
Derby Friend 🕮 73
Derry Cara Friend 🕮 164
Dialogai 🕮 176
Dorset Gay & Lesbian Switchboard 🕮 73
Dublin Gay Switchboard 🕮 137
Dumfries & Galloway L&G Group 🕮 167, 170
Dundee LGB Switchboard Group 🕮 170
East Kent Friend 🕮 78
Edinburgh Gay Switchboard 🕮 168
Fife Friend 🕮 168
Flint Hills Alliance 🕮 258
Forth Friend 🕮 167
Freies Tagungshaus Waldschlößhen 🕮 107
Gai-Ecoute 🕮 62
GALON 🕮 *See* Gay & Lesbian Outreach Network
Gay & Lesbian Center, Island Empire 🕮 210
Gay & Lesbian Community Center of Colorado, Inc. 🕮 227
Gay & Lesbian Community Services Center 🕮 203
Gay & Lesbian Community Switchboard 🕮 318
Gay & Lesbian Counselling 🕮 170
Gay & Lesbian Counselling Service 🕮 33
Gay & Lesbian Counselling South West 🕮 73
Gay & Lesbian Guideline 🕮 232
Gay & Lesbian Helpline 🕮 254
Gay & Lesbian Helpline of Rhode Island 🕮 334
Gay & Lesbian Helpline of Wake County 🕮 315
Gay & Lesbian Hotline 🕮 233, 279, 284, 302
Gay & Lesbian Info Line 🕮 149
Gay & Lesbian Info Services 🕮 272
Gay & Lesbian Line 🕮 26
Gay & Lesbian Outreach Network 🕮 325
Gay & Lesbian Phoneline 🕮 261
Gay & Lesbian Switchboard 🕮 32, 152, 173, 254, 263, 302, 316, 327, 336
Gay & Lesbian Switchboard of Charlotte 🕮 314
Gay & Lesbian Switchboard of Harrisburg 🕮 328
Gay & Lesbian Switchboard of Houston 🕮 342
Gay & Lesbian Switchboard of Long Island 🕮 302
Gay & Lesbian Switchboard of Northern Pennsylvania 🕮 333
Gay & Lesbian WotsOn 🕮 26
Gay Area Youth Switchboard 🕮 213
Gay Community Directory 🕮 246
Gay Counselling 🕮 141
Gay Crisis Line 🕮 44
Gay Help Line 🕮 46, 137
Gay Hotline 🕮 115, 116
Gay Hotline, Inc. 🕮 242
Gay Info 🕮 62
Gay Info Line 🕮 35
Gay Info Line of New Hampshire 🕮 287
Gay Information Line 🕮 31, 161, 348
Gay Jouren 🕮 173, 174, 175, 176
Gay Line 🕮 28, 48, 116, 145
Gay Line Hagen 🕮 119
Gay Phoneline of Windsor 🕮 61
Gay Rap Telephone Line of Topeka 🕮 258
Gay Switchboard 🕮 163, 166, 179, 237
Gay Switchboard Johannesburg 🕮 171
Gay Switchboard Limerick 🕮 138
Gay Youth Switchboard / Ungdomstelefonen 🕮 66
Gay, Lesbian, & Bisexual Community Hotline of Greater Miami 🕮 239
Gay, Lesbian, & Bisexual Helpline 🕮 327
Gay/Lesbian Information Line 🕮 191
GayHotline 🕮 34
Gayline 🕮 25, 30, 33, 44, 48, 50, 62, 161, 162, 163, 312
Gayline & Lesbianline 🕮 162
Gayline / Lesbianline 🕮 160
Gayphone 🕮 312
Gays, Lesbian, & Bisexuals of North Bay Area 🕮 52
Gerede-Dresdener Lesben, Schwule, & Alle Anderen 🕮 114
GLB NBA 🕮 *See* Gays, Lesbian, & Bisexuals of North Bay Area
Gloucester Friend 🕮 75
GLSB of LI 🕮 *See* Gay & Lesbian Switchboard of Long Island
Gravesend Switchboard 🕮 78
Group 🕮 48
Guelph Gayline 🕮 49
HAK - Advies Kontakt Centrum 't Koerken 🕮 36
HALO 🕮 *See* Homophile Association of London Ontario Inc.
Haringey Lesbian & Gay Helpline 🕮 81
Harlow Switchboard 🕮 75
Harrogate Switchboard 🕮 88
HAZ 🕮 *See* Homosexuelle Arbeitsgruppen Zürich
HAZ/SOH 🕮 *See* Beratungstelephon für Homosexuelle
Hereford & Worcester Lesbian & Gay Switchboard 🕮 77
Homofile og Lesbiskes Opplysningstelefon 🕮 164
Homophile Association of London Ontario Inc. 🕮 51
Homophon 🕮 112
Homophone 🕮 127
Homosexuelle Arbeitsgruppen Zürich 🕮 179
Homosexuelle Selbsthilfe e. V. 🕮 130
HS 🕮 *See* Homosexuelle Selbsthilfe e. V.
Hulptelefoon 🕮 154
Humberside Friend 🕮 77
Infofoon Amsterdam 🕮 150
Infoline 🕮 103
Infor Homo 🕮 36
Informagay 🕮 144
Informazioni Gay 🕮 140
Isle of Wight Switchboard 🕮 77
Kirklees Lesbian & Gay Switchboard 🕮 94
Lambda Line 🕮 52
LAMBDA Services 🕮 341
Lancaster Lesbian & Gay Switchboard 🕮 72, 78
Landsforeningen for Bøsser og Lesbiske 🕮 66
Landsforeningen for Lesbisk og Homofil Frigjøring 🕮 166
LBL 🕮 *See* Landsforeningen for Bøsser og Lesbiske
Leeds Gay Switchboard 🕮 94
Leicester Lesbian & Gayline 🕮 79
Lesbian & Gay Bashing Reporting & Information Line 🕮 56
Lesbian & Gay Community Switchboard 🕮 193
Lesbian & Gay Health Project 🕮 314
Lesbian & Gay Helpline 🕮 249, 283
Lesbian & Gay Men's Community Center 🕮 211
Lesbian / Gay Resource Line 🕮 276
Lesbian Gay Bi Youth Line 🕮 56
Lesbian, Gay, & Bisexual Alliance 🕮 256
Lesbian, Gay, & Bisexual Switchboard 🕮 248
Lesbian/Gay Phoneline 🕮 50
LesBiGayline 🕮 257
Lewisham Friend 🕮 81
Lincoln Gay & Lesbian Switchboard 🕮 79
Line 🕮 241
LLH 🕮 *See* Landsforeningen for Lesbisk og Homofil Frigjøring
London Friend 🕮 81
Long Island Crisis Center 🕮 302
Luton Switchboard 🕮 70
Manchester Lesbian & Gay Switchboard 🕮 75
Manphone-Schwulenberatung 🕮 129
Milton Keynes Lesbian & Gay Switchboard 🕮 71
Monash University Gayline 🕮 32
National Friend 🕮 81
Newcastle Friend 🕮 92
Newcastle Gay & Lesbian Information Service 🕮 25
Newcastle Gay Youthline 🕮 92
Norfolk Friend 🕮 88
North Devon Lesbian & Gay Switchboard 🕮 73
North Staffordshire Lesbian & Gay Switchboard 🕮 72, 91
Northampton Lesbian & Gayline 🕮 88
Northamptonshire Gayline 🕮 89
Norwich Lesbian & Gayline 🕮 88
Nottingham Friend 🕮 89
Nottingham Lesbian & Gay Switchboard 🕮 89
Ottawa Gayline / Télégai Ottawa 🕮 52
Oxford Friend 🕮 89
Oxford Lesbian & Gay Switchboard 🕮 89
Pan Information 🕮 2
PEI Gay Phoneline 🕮 61
Perth Switchboard 🕮 170
Peterborough Friend 🕮 71
PG-Jouren 🕮 175
Philadelphia Gay Switchboard 🕮 330
Pikes Peak Gay & Lesbian Community Center Help Line 🕮 227
Portsmouth Lesbian & Gay Switchboard 🕮 76
Preston Gay Information Service 🕮 79
Pride S. I. S. 🕮 162
Rat & Tat Rosa Telefon 🕮 132
Ratgeber Schwul Darmstadt 🕮 114
Reading Lesbian & Gay Helpline 🕮 71
Regina Gayline 🕮 64
Relais d'Espérance 🕮 63
RFSL 🕮 *See* Riksförbundet för Sexuellt Likaberättigande
Riksförbundet för Sexuellt Likaberättigande 🕮 173, 174, 175
Rochdale Lesbian & Gay Switchboard 🕮 76
Rosa Hilfe 🕮 114, 117, 126, 129, 135
Rosa Hilfe im KCM 🕮 128
Rosa Telefon 🕮 34, 35, 108, 109, 112, 113, 114, 115, 116, 117, 118, 122, 123, 124, 125, 126, 127, 131, 132, 134, 135, 178
Rosa Telefon der Pro Familia 🕮 127
Rosa Telefon Hinterland 🕮 111
Rose Drempel 🕮 38
S. E. London's Lesbian, Gay, & Bisexual Helpline 🕮 79
Saint Austell Switchboard 🕮 72
Saint Ganriel Community Church 🕮 344
Saint Helens Lesbian & Gay Helpline 🕮 87
Salisbury Lesbian & Gay Switchboard 🕮 94
San Antonio Gay & Lesbian Switchboard 🕮 344
Saskatoon Gayline 🕮 64
Schwule Aktion Bremerhaven 🕮 113
Schwule Beratung 🕮 117
Schwules Überfalltelefon 🕮 124
Scunthorpe Gay Helpline 🕮 77
Seksuaalinen Tasavertaisuus ry 🕮 95
SETA 🕮 *See* Seksuaalinen Tasavertaisuus ry
SETA Information Service 🕮 95
Sexual Minority Youth Assistance League 🕮 233
Shakti 🕮 *See* South Asian Lesbian & Gay Network
Sheffield Friend 🕮 90
Shropshire Lesbian & Gay Switchboard 🕮 90
Solano Country Gay & Lesbian Information Line 🕮 199
Sorgentelefon HALU 🕮 178
SOS Gay 🕮 142
South Asian Lesbian & Gay Network 🕮 79
Southend Lesbian & Gay Switchboard 🕮 75
Strathclyde Lesbian & Gay Switchboard 🕮 169
Suffolk Lesbian & Gay Switchboard 🕮 91
Sunderland Lesbian & Gay Young Peoples Group 🕮 92
Switchboard 🕮 117, 121, 176
Switchboard of Miami, Inc. 🕮 239
TAGL 🕮 *See* Toronto Area Gay/Lesbian Phoneline & Crisis Counselling
Teeside Friend 🕮 88
Telefon des Vertrauens 🕮 129, 131, 132
Telefonberatung Homosexualität 🕮 118
Telefono Amico Gay 🕮 142
Telefono Gay 🕮 142
Telephono Rosa 🕮 172
Telephono Viola 🕮 140
Tels Quels Meeting Point 🕮 37
Thamesdown Lesbian & Gay Line 🕮 94
TOHR Gay / Lesbian Helpline 🕮 323
Toronto Area Gay/Lesbian Phoneline & Crisis Counselling 🕮 56
Townsville Gayline 🕮 29
Tunbridge Wells Switchboard 🕮 78
Überfalltelefon 🕮 128
Vivre Autrement en Aquitaine 🕮 98
Warrington Switchboard 🕮 72
West Kootenays Gays & Lesbians 🕮 44
West Norfolk Gay & Lesbian Helpline 🕮 88
Wichita Gay Info Line 🕮 258
Wrexham Switchboard 🕮 359
York Gay Line 🕮 88

Transgender

AEGIS 🕮 *See* American Educational Gender Information Services, Inc.
American Educational Gender Information Services, Inc. 🕮 245

Transvestite

Manchester Transvestite / Transgender Hotline 🕮 75
National Transvestite Line 🕮 136

STDS

All Sexes & Sexualities

CDC National STD Hotline 🕮 181
National Herpes Hotline 🕮 181

YOUTH

All Sexes & Sexualities

Chicago Runaway Switchboard 🕮 249
National Runaway Switchboard 🕮 181

INTERNET MAILING LISTS

ACADEMIC

All Sexes & Sexualities

ACESGLBI 🕮 2

Lesbian, Gay, Bi, & Transgendered

EURO-QUEER-STUDIES 🕮 2
LGBPSYCH 🕮 2
MEDGAY-L 🕮 2
QSA 🕮 2
QSTUDY-L 🕮 2

AIDS

All Sexes & Sexualities

4ACURE-L 🕮 2
AIDS 🕮 2
AIDSBKRV 🕮 2
AIDS-STAT-L 🕮 2
RETHINKING AIDS 🕮 2

Lesbian, Gay, Bi, & Transgendered

ACT-UP AIDS-L 🕮 2

BDSM

All Sexes & Sexualities

AUSBDSM 2
BAST 2
MASTER-SLAVE 2
NLA-FRIENDS 2
Heterosexual, Male
FEMDOM-L 2
FEMSUPREM 2
Lesbian, Gay, Bi, & Transgendered
GL-ASB 2
BEARS
Gay
BEARS 2
BEARS-L 2
FAMILY
All Sexes & Sexualities
PFLAG-TALK 2
FETISH
Cigars
Gay
CS 2
LIBRARY
Lesbian, Gay, Bi, & Transgendered
GAYLIB-N 3
SEXUAL POLITICS
All Sexes & Sexualities
STOPRAPE 3
Bisexual
BIACT-L 3
Lesbian, Gay, Bi, & Transgendered
ACT-UP 3
QN 3
SEXUALITY
All Sexes & Sexualities
ALTERNATES 3
ARENAL 3
GENDER 3
SEX-L 4
SEXTALK 4
Bisexual
ARENAL-L 3
BISEXU-L 3
BITHRY-L 3
BIVERSITY 266
Female
BIFEM-L 3
PARTNERS 3
SAPPHO 4
Heterosexual
POLY 4
POLY-BOSTON 267
POLYFIDELITY 4
Heterosexual, Male
AMAZONS 3
PLAYBOY MAILING LIST 3
Lesbian
BA-SAPPHO 3
EURO-QUEER 3
EURO-SAPPHO 3
LIS 3
UK-MOTSS-WOMEN 4
Lesbian, Gay, Bi, & Transgendered
ADDICT-L 3
AUGLBC-L 3
AUSGBLF 3
BGALA-L 3
DC-MOTSS 3
DDMM-L 3
DIGNITY 3
FL-MOTSS 3
GAY NETWORKS MAILING LIST 3
GLB-NEWS 3
GLBPOC 3
GLQSOC-L 3
GRANITE 3
LA-MOTSS 3
LA-MOTSS-ANNOUNCE 3
NE-SOCIAL-MOTSS 3
NZGBLF 3
OH-MOTSS 3
PDX-MOTSS 3
QNA 4
QUEERCAMPUS 4
UK-MOTSS 4
Transgender
TRANSGEN 4
Transvestite
CD-FORUM 3
SPANKING
Gay
SPANK-L 4
STUDENT
Lesbian, Gay, Bi, & Transgendered
CLGSG-L 4
DSA-LGB 4
GAYNET 4
GGALA-L 4
LAMBDA 4
TAMUGLB 4
SUPPORT
All Sexes & Sexualities
COURAGE 4
RECOVERY 4
Lesbian, Gay, Bi, & Transgendered
EJINTVIO 4

INTERNET NEWSGROUPS
ACADEMIC
Anthropology
All Sexes & Sexualities
sci.anthropology 4
Psychiatry
All Sexes & Sexualities
fj.sci.medical 4
fj.sci.psychology 4
francom.medical 4
sci.psychology 4
sci.psychology.journals.psyche 4
sci.psychology.research 4
sci.psychology.research.psychotherapy 4
sfnet.keskustelu.psykologia 4
tw.bbs.sci.psychology 4
zer.z-netz.wissenschaft.psychologie 4
Sexuality
All Sexes & Sexualities
tw.bbs.sci.sex 4
AIDS
Lesbian, Gay, Bi, & Transgendered
gay-net.aids 4
BDSM
All Sexes & Sexualities
alt.sex.bondage 4
alt.sex.femdom 4
alt.sex.sm.fig 4
aus.sex.bondage 4
sm-org 4
uw.alt.sex.bondage 4
Lesbian, Gay, Bi, & Transgendered
gay-net.lederecke 4
BEARS
Gay
alt.sex.bears 4
BODY SIZE
All Sexes & Sexualities
alt.sex.fat 4
alt.sex.fetish.fa 4
alt.sex.fetish.size 4
alt.sex.fetish.waifs 4
BODY TYPE
All Sexes & Sexualities
alt.sex.furry 4
Heterosexual, Male
alt.amazon-women.admirers 4
BONDAGE
All Sexes & Sexualities
alt.fax.bondage 4
EROTICA
All Sexes & Sexualities
alt.magazine.playboy 4
alt.magazines.pornographic 4
alt.sex.erotica.marketplace 4
alt.sex.magazines 4
rec.arts.erotica 4
FETISH
Adult Baby
All Sexes & Sexualities
alt.sex.fetish.diapers 4
Age
All Sexes & Sexualities
alt.sex.boys 4
alt.sex.girls 4
alt.sex.pedophilia 5
alt.sex.pedophilia.boys 5
alt.sex.pedophilia.girls 5
alt.sex.preteens 5
alt.sex.young 5
alt.support.boy-lovers 5
Amputee
All Sexes & Sexualities
alt.sex.fetish.amputee 5
Animal
All Sexes & Sexualities
alt.sex.animals 5
alt.sex.bestiality 5
alt.sex.hello-kitty 5
alt.sex.reptiles 5
alt.sex.zoophile 5
alt.sex.zoophilia 5
Balls
All Sexes & Sexualities
alt.sex.balls 5
Breasts
All Sexes & Sexualities
alt.sex.breast 5
Breathing
All Sexes & Sexualities
alt.sex.asphyx 5
alt.sex.breathless 5
Clothing
All Sexes & Sexualities
alt.clothing.lingerie 5
alt.lycra 5
alt.pantyhose 5
alt.sex.fetish.fashion 5
alt.sex.fetish.sportswear 5
Enemas
All Sexes & Sexualities
alt.sex.enemas 5
Exhibitionism
All Sexes & Sexualities
alt.sex.exhibitionism 5
Foot
All Sexes & Sexualities
alt.sex.fetish.feet 5
alt.sex.fetish.feet.toes 5
Foreskin
Gay
alt.sex.uncut 5
Hair
All Sexes & Sexualities
alt.sex.fetish.hair 5
Mess
All Sexes & Sexualities
alt.mud.sex 5
alt.sex.fetish.wet-and-messy 5
alt.sex.jello 5
Miscellaneous
All Sexes & Sexualities
alt.sex.fetish.orientals 5
alt.sex.nasal-hair 5
Transgender
alt.sex.fetish.robots 5
Motorcycle
All Sexes & Sexualities
alt.sex.fetish.motorcycles 5
Necrophilia
All Sexes & Sexualities
alt.sex.necrophilia 5
Smoking
All Sexes & Sexualities
alt.sex.fetish.smoking 5
Tickling
All Sexes & Sexualities
alt.sex.fetish.tickling 5
Voyeurism
All Sexes & Sexualities
alt.sex.voyeurism 5
LIBRARY
All Sexes & Sexualities
relcom.sci.libraries 5
rpi.libraries 5
soc.libraries.talk 5
LITERATURE
All Sexes & Sexualities
alt.censorship 5
Sexuality
alt.lesbian.feminist.poetry 5
MASTURBATION
All Sexes & Sexualities
alt.sex.masturbation 5
MEDICAL
AIDS
All Sexes & Sexualities
clari.tw.health.aids 5
misc.health.aids 5
sci.med.aids 5
Drugs
All Sexes & Sexualities
zer.z-netz.gesundheit.drogen 5
General
All Sexes & Sexualities
alt.support.herpes 5
bit.listserv.medforum 5
bit.listserv.medlib-l 5
bit.listserv.mednews 5
bit.med 5
clari.tw.health 5
misc.education.medical 5
sci.med.diseases.hepatitis 5
tw.bbs.sci.medicine 5
zer.z-netz.gesundheit.diskussion 5
zer.z-netz.gesundheit.krankheiten 5
MISCELLANEOUS
All Sexes & Sexualities
alt.nudism 5
MOTORCYCLE
All Sexes & Sexualities
tw.bbs.rec.motorcycle 5
PIERCING
All Sexes & Sexualities
rec.arts.bodyart 5
POLYFIDELITY
Heterosexual
alt.polyamory 5
SEXUAL POLITICS
All Sexes & Sexualities
alt.privacy 5
alt.sex.advocacy 5
SEXUALITY
All Sexes & Sexualities
alt.books.anne-rice 5
alt.christnet.nudism 5
alt.foreplay 5
alt.magick.sex 5
alt.safe.sex 5
alt.sex 5
alt.sex.anal 5
alt.sex.cd-rom 6
alt.sex.historical 6
alt.sex.incest 6
alt.sex.intergen 6

Internet Newsgroups: Sexuality

alt.sex.jp 6
alt.sex.orgy 6
alt.sex.safe 6
aus.sex 6
cl.freie_liebe.hetero 6
clari.news.crime.sex 6
clari.news.law.crime.sex 6
clari.news.sex 6
es.alt.sex 6
fido.ger.sex 6
fido7.sex 6
finet.sex 6
slo.sex 6
uw.alt.sex.beastiality 6
zer.t-netz.sex 6

Bisexual

nv.bi 6
soc.bi 6
uiuc.soc.bisexuals 6
vegas.bi 6

Gay

uiuc.soc.gay-men 6

Lesbian

alt.shoe.lesbians 6
gay-net.lesben 6

Lesbian, Gay, Bi, & Transgendered

alt.homosexual 5
alt.journalism.gay-press 5
alt.sex.homosexual 6
alt.sex.motss 6
aus.culture.lesbigay 6
can.motss 6
cl.freie_liebe.schwule 6
clari.news.gays 6
fido.ger.gay 6
gay-net.diskussionen 6
gay-net.general 6
gay-net.gesundheitsecke 6
gay-net.guide.bundesweit 6
gay-net.heteros 6
gay-net.international 6
ne.motss 6
nv.motss 6
pa.motss 6
pgh.motss 6
pnw.motss 6
sdnet.motss 6
soc.gender.issues 6
soc.motss 6
su.gay 6
triangle.motss 6
uc.motss 6
uk.gay-lesbian-bi 6
vegas.motss 6

Transgender

alt.support.transgendered 6
alt.transgendered 6
soc.support.transgendered 6

Transvestite

alt.sex.trans 6

Youth

Lesbian, Gay, Bi, & Transgendered

soc.support.youth.gay-lesbian-bi 5

SPANKING

All Sexes & Sexualities

alt.sex.spanking 6

SPIRITUALITY

All Sexes & Sexualities

alt.christnet.sex 6
alt.pagan 6
alt.religion.sexuality 6
alt.sex.cthulhu 6
alt.sex.wizards 6

SUPPORT

All Sexes & Sexualities

alt.recovery.addiction.sexual 6
alt.recovery.sexual-addiction 6
alt.sexual.abuse.recovery 6
alt.sexual.abuse.recovery.d 6
alt.support.abuse-partners 6
talk.rape 6

Lesbian, Gay, Bi, & Transgendered

gay-net.coming-out 6

Male

alt.support.cant.urinate.in-public 6

SWINGERS

Heterosexual

alt.sex.swingers 6

WATERSPORTS

All Sexes & Sexualities

alt.sex.fetish.watersports 6
alt.sex.watersports 6

WRESTLING

All Sexes & Sexualities

alt.sex.fetish.wrestling 6

INTERNET ORGANIZATIONS

SEXUALITY

Lesbian

Daughters of Aphrodite 6

INTERNET RELAY CHAT (IRC) CHANNELS

All Sexes & Sexualities

#AIDS/HIV 6
#analsex 6
#anne-rice 6
#bdsm 6
#bdsmlounge 6
#bondage 6
#breasts 6
#d&s 6
#desade 6
#Dom/Sub 6
#erotic 6
#erotica 7
#eroticsex 7
#exhibitionists 7
#familysex 7
#femdom 7
#femuscle 7
#FistFuck 7
#fuck 7
#goddess 7
#HighHeels 7
#intergen 7
#kinkysex 7
#LeChambre 7
#pagan 7
#pantyhose 7
#peesex 7
#pervert 7
#pornshop 7
#sex 7
#sex&stuff 7
#spanking 7
#submission 7
#teensex 7
#vampire 7
#vampires 7
#voyeurs 7
#Weirdsex 7
#wetstuff 7
#wildsex 7
#youngsex 7

Bisexual

#bisex 6

Female

#BiFEM!!!! 6
#bifemteens 6

Gay

#bearcave 6
#bearlake 6
#bearlake2 6
#Gay 7
#gayboysex 7
#gaycouples 7
#gayhelp 7
#gayjackoff 7
#gaynz 7
#gaynz1 7
#gaysex 7
#gaySM 7
#gayteenchat 7
#gaytexas 7
#gayuncut 7
#GayWI 7
#gayworld 7
#gayyouth 7
#Jack-off 7
#Jacks 7
#jerk-off 7

Heterosexual

#polyamory 7
#Swing 7

Lesbian

#gaynzgirls 7
#lesbian 7
#lesbians 7
#lesbos 7
#lezsex 7
#lezsex2 7

Transgender

#transgen 7

Transvestite

#crossdres 6

INTERNET SEARCH ENGINES

GENERAL

All Sexes & Sexualities

DejaNews Partners 7
Excite 7
Lycos Incorporated 7
Yahoo Corporation 7

MAILORDER

ADULT TOYS

Electrical

All Sexes & Sexualities

P. E. S., Inc. 181

Miscellaneous

All Sexes & Sexualities

Motail 67
New Age 67

BOOKS

BDSM

All Sexes & Sexualities

Blue Moon Books 181
Fernando Cerqueira 167
QSM 7
Ryder Publishing 67
WPC 7, 8

Gay

E-MaleSM 181

Heterosexual

Leda 181

Erotic

All Sexes & Sexualities

Black Widow's Web 173
Daisy Publications Ltd. 7
Delectus Books 7
K. L. Graphics 181
Midian Books 67

General

All Sexes & Sexualities

Body Art, Publications Ltd. 7
Books Direct 67
Eclectic Connection 181
Enclave Book Repository 181
Omega Centre Bookstore 40
Private Case 67
Prowler Press Ltd. 67
Quality Paperback Book Club 181
Womankind Books Inc. 181

Female

Berkana Press 181
Sisterhood Bookstore 181
Women's Word Books 181
Women's Words Books 181
Womontyme Distribution Company 181

Sexuality

All Sexes & Sexualities

Circlet Press Bookshop 8
Gaie Livraison 47
NSS Seminars, Inc. 181
Shaynew Press 182
Synergy Book Service 182

Gay

Intermale 8
Paragon 8
Paths Untrodden Book Service 182

Lesbian

Fat Girl 8
Heartland Books 181

Lesbian, Gay, Bi, & Transgendered

Berdache Books 181
Books Bohemian 8
Bruno Gmünder Versand 107
Delta Boek 150
Different Light 181
Giovanni's Room 181
Glad Day Books 40, 181
Lambda Rising 8
Lambda Rising Online 8
Lavendar Jade's 181
Little Sister's Book & Art Emporium 40
Male Image 67
Male Xpress Ltd. 67
Millivres Ltd. 67
Oscar Wilde Memorial Bookstore 182
Our World Too 182
People Like Us 182
Real World Emporium 182
Roads Less Travelled 182
Tomes & Treasures 182
True Colors 182

CATALOGUES

General

All Sexes & Sexualities

Catalog Connection 67

CLOTHING

Adult Baby

All Sexes & Sexualities

Special Clothes 182
Very Special Clothes 182

Chainmail

All Sexes & Sexualities

Barenhohle 182
Chain Maille Fashions 182

Gay

Chained Male 49

Corsets

All Sexes & Sexualities

Axfords 67

Fetish

All Sexes & Sexualities

ACE Saddle Company 182
Alter Ego 68
Après Noir 182
B&B Leatherworks 40
BMA 107
Bootmen Leathers 182
Caprice 182
Classic Shoe Company 40
Constance Enterprises 182
Crossland Shoes 40
Decadence 95
Demask 8
Dream Dresser 182
Eccentric Fashion 176
Fairy Tales 107
Fantasy Fashions 182
Fashion World International 182
Fetish Factory Ltd. 8
Honour 68
House of Harlot 68
Lanem Fashions 68
Latexa 65
Leather & Lust 182
Lifestyle 68
Passion 65
Paul C Leather 182
Raiments 182
Rimba 150
Samanta 107
Schau Mode 107
Schwarze Mode 107
Showgrade Ltd. 68
Skint 68
Stanford Hygenic Corp. 182
Things 172
Tight Situation 68
Victoria Regine 68

Voyages 182
Wicked Ways 182
X-Treme Designs Ltd 40
Yago Holdings Ltd. 68

Female

Cathouse Design Studio 68
Jay Fashions 68
Sh! 68

Gay

Apollo Contakt Versand 107
IEM *See* International Estetic Men
International Estetic Men 97
International Male Mail 8

Heterosexual, Male

Fantasies Unlimited 182

Lesbian, Gay, Bi, & Transgendered

Zipper Mail Order 9

Male

Après Noir 68
Christopher Briston Enterprises 182
D. B. Leisurewear 68

Transgender

Wardrobes by Carolyn 182

Transvestite

Fantasies In Lace, Inc. 182

Footwear

All Sexes & Sexualities

Adams, Roger 68
Lady Elizabeth 68
Leslie Shoe Company *See* Sexy Shoes
Magic Shoe Company 68
Sexy Shoes 183
Shoecraft 24
Zenana 68

Female

Aristoc Distributors 183
Shoe Express 183

Male

Filia, Rich 183

General

All Sexes & Sexualities

Amazon Drygoods 183
Maitresse 183
Midnight Lady 68
Noelle Nielson Softwear 183

Transvestite

Eve Browne Fashions 182

Industrial

All Sexes & Sexualities

Cover Up 68

Leather

All Sexes & Sexualities

Black Eagle Leather Co. 9
Black On Black Leathers 183
Saint Michael's Emporium 9
World Domination 183

Female

Elle For Leather 68

Gay

Bear Man 183
JDL 68

Lingerie

All Sexes & Sexualities

Frederick's of Hollywood 183
Lady Midnight 183
Monique of Hollywood 183

Transvestite

Body Aware 68

Miscellaneous

All Sexes & Sexualities

Gravity Plus 183

Rubber

All Sexes & Sexualities

Abra Creations & Designs 68
Aquala 183
Basta Boots 107
Creative Imageware by J&M 183
Essential Image 68
Herta Gummi 9
Invincible 68
Jerry's Misc. Services 183
Lampe 107
Latex America 183
Latex Seduction 97
Libidex 68
Loco 68
Mariner Wear 183
Midnight Sun Rainwear 183
Naughty Nancy 183
Rainvain 183
Remawear 68
Rubber Lady 68
Rubbertree Rainwear 40
South Bucks Rainwear 68
Wendy's 183
West, Kim 68
Wild Designs 68

Female

Full Moon Fashions 107

Gay

Dark Side Creations 40
Fa. Dawi 107

Male

Bob's Rubberwear 68

EROTICA

All Sexes & Sexualities

Aladdin Holdings Ltd. 183
Between The Sheets 69
Christopher Collection 186
Condom Wrap 186
Fantasyland Products 41
Fischer, Ernst 107
Forbidden Fruit 186
Get Wet 69
Gilson, Patrick 69
Good Vibrations 10
Groupe B. A. I., Inc. 41
Intimate Treasures 186
Klystra 186
Marc Sanders Mail Order 186
Montana American West Company 187
S. H. H. Services 10
Sin-A-Matique 69
Spellbound Limited 69
Tabby 69
Una Deva 69
Wyle, Stephen 69

Female

Pleasure Spot 24

Gay

Bodyshot 10
Colt Studios 186
David-Versand 177
Editrice Cassia 138
Heaven Sent Me 186
Henkel, Keile 107
Malebox Warehouse 41
Malibu Sales 186
M-Club 177
Mercury Mail Order 186
Toy-Versand 177

Lesbian, Gay, Bi, & Transgendered

Beat 24
CEI 176
Danske Bjørne ApS 65
Europost 150
Fantasy Erotique 10
Frisco 138
Klein Enterprises 170
Nice 'n' Naughty 170
Out! Mailorder 159

Adult Baby

All Sexes & Sexualities

ABW *See* Adult Baby World
Adult Baby World 40
Carolyn's Kids 183
Cozy Time 41
Diaper Pail Friends 9
DPF *See* Diaper Pail Friends

Heterosexual

Annie's Orphans 183
Ashely's Boutique 40
Babykins Products Ltd. 40
BBW 41
Crissy's Creations 183
Hygia-Versand 107
INCON 183
JK Perfect Personal Products 183
NK Products 183
Renas Boutique 183
Slimwear Of America 183
TAM Design 183
Tinkerbell's Treasures 68
V. I. Products, Inc. 183
Voksne Babyers Verden 65

Male

Mummy Hazel High Heels - H. B. Enterprises 9

BDSM

All Sexes & Sexualities

Academy Club 9
Ben's Fashion 150
Bound II 68
Boutique Minuit 9
Chase Products 184
Decorations by SLAN 184
Diversified Services 184
Domination 107
Dream & Fantasy Fashions 107
Esthesia, Anne 41
Fantasy Island Innovations, Inc. 184
Feelings 24
Fetish Network 184, 185
Finders 184
Hard Line 107
Hard Love Leather 9
Hidebound 9
Just Leathers 68
Kastley GmbH 107
Laws Leather 184
Leather Man, Inc. 184
Leather Underground, Inc. 9
Leatherhood 184
Leatherline 69
Massad Mailorder 9
Mind Candy Emporium 184
Monique 69
Moonlight Fashion 107
Morgan's Toybox 184
Northbound Leather Ltd. 41
Other Pony Club 9
Ram Leathers 69
RGL Designs 9
S. A. D. E. 172
Simply Leather 359
SM Toy Hamburg 107
SM Versand 107
Strictly Stories 10
Tuff Stuff 184
Unique Creations 184
Venus Versand 107
Whip Me Raw 186
Zak Designs 186

Female

Mail & Female 150

Gay

Alternate Marketing 183
Chase Products & FPN6D Services 183
Euro-Business Services Inc. 176
Higgins Collection 184
Jaybird's Toybox 184
K. A. B. Kühn / Clabes Versandhandel GbR 107
Sandmutopia Supply Company 184
Tom of Finland Company Inc. 10
Townsend, Larry 184

Heterosexual

San Francisco Dungeon 184

Heterosexual, Female

DivaNet *See* Galleria Diva
Galleria Diva 184

Lesbian

Aslan Leathers 41
Scene Gear 184

Male

Eagle Leathers 68
Mr. S – Fetters, U.S.A. 184

Bondage

All Sexes & Sexualities

JuRonCo 10
Lucifer's Armory 186
Male-order Leather 186
Mooring & Mooring 186
Paraphernalia from Beyond Planet X 186
Spandex from the Imagination of Mark I. Chester 186

Male

KW Enterprises 10

Dildos

All Sexes & Sexualities

Babes Silicone Dildoes 69

Enemas

All Sexes & Sexualities

Arthur Hamilton, Inc. 10

Gas Masks

All Sexes & Sexualities

Restrictive Practice 69

General

All Sexes & Sexualities

Blowfish 10
Christine Le Duc 150
Continental Spectator 186
Erosart 107
Séduction 41
Superia Supplies 69
Toys in Babeland 186
Versatile Fashions 186
Windfaire Exxxotic Gifts 186
Xandria Collection 10

Female

Eve's Garden 186

Gay

Caught In The Act 41
Clone Zone 69
Pro-Fun 107

Lesbian, Gay, Bi, & Transgendered

Catalog X 186
Gayroute 41
Priape 41
Q Things 10
Rubyfruit Erotica 41

Leather

All Sexes & Sexualities

Acme Toy Co. 186
Belt Up & Buckle Off 69
Fantasy Leathers 186
Master Leathers 186
Pleasure Place 10
R. K. Unlimited 186
Sax Leather 24
Sir Steve's Leather 41
Skin To Skin 69
Stockroom 186
Vyxyn's Leatherworks & Urbane Armory 186

Gay

Blackline Press & Services 107
PI Versand 107
Remedy Versand 10
Vimpex GmbH 107

Heterosexual

XTC Leather of New York 186

Lesbian, Gay, Bi, & Transgendered

Expectations 69, 150
Hot Leather Versand 107
Macho-Versand 177
Mack's Leathers 41
P+E 150

Pony

All Sexes & Sexualities

JG Leathers 41

Rubber

All Sexes & Sexualities

Lakeland Elements 69
Wetlook Unlimited 69

Gay

Black Light 108

MILITARY SURPLUS

All Sexes & Sexualities

Shomer-Tec 187

PIERCING JEWELRY

All Sexes & Sexualities

Bravo 187
Gauntlet, Inc. Mail Order & Customer Service 187
Ringmasters 187

SAFER SEX PRODUCTS

All Sexes & Sexualities

Adam & Eve 187
Hot Rubber Company 108, 177
OPC Supply 187
Starlight 69

VIDEOS

BDSM

All Sexes & Sexualities

GVNS 69
Kayser Novelty Co. 24

Gay

Masta Entertainment 187
P. M. Productions 187

Body Type

Gay

Altomar Productions 187

Erotic

Gay

Atkol Entertainment 187
Bijou Video 187
Euro Men 150
Fox Studio 187
Old Reliable 187

Male

Man's Hand Films 187

Fetish

All Sexes & Sexualities

Concept Imports 187

Gay

Kink Video 187

Heterosexual

Platinum Video 187

Sexuality

All Sexes & Sexualities

Bluemoon Films 10
Lifestyles Organization 187

Female

Fatale Video 187

Watersports

All Sexes & Sexualities

Schein, Michael 11

MANUFACTURERS

ADULT TOYS

BDSM

All Sexes & Sexualities

LifeStyle Leather & Wood 187
Silver Smoke 248
Sportsheets 196

Electrical

All Sexes & Sexualities

Erotec 223

Masturbation

All Sexes & Sexualities

Abco Research Associates 252

Percussion

All Sexes & Sexualities

Hanson Percussion Instruments 11
Santa Barbara Paddle Company 221

CHASTITY BELTS

All Sexes & Sexualities

Chastete 252
Stainless Construction Company 339
Tollyboy Products 90

CLOTHING

Chainmail

All Sexes & Sexualities

Strangeblades & More 187

Lesbian, Gay, Bi, & Transgendered

Chain Mail Creations 203

Corsets

All Sexes & Sexualities

(sin)ch 207
B. R. Creations 207
C & S Constructions 71
Dark Garden Corsets 11
Paul C Leather 249
Talana Gamah & leish 11
True Grace Corsets 71
Voller's 76
Wilbro 79

Fetish

All Sexes & Sexualities

Black Magic 81
Demask 152
Fantasyland Products 53
Lush 81
Pure 81
Schwarze Mode 110
Valhalla 81
Wild One 26

Female

Karo Design 119

Footwear

All Sexes & Sexualities

Abelman Trading Company 136
Coatney, Catherine 213

General

All Sexes & Sexualities

Kingfisher 168

Leather

All Sexes & Sexualities

Black Eagle Leather Co. 206
Cuir Gear 326
Jacqui 213
Leather Creations 230
Liz Lewitt - Wholesale 11
Rider Upholstery 351
Wilder, Vic 81

Lesbian, Gay, Bi, & Transgendered

San Francisco Leather Works 213

Rubber

All Sexes & Sexualities

Amour 160
Atelier für Extravagante Mode 110
Clothes For Practitioners 81
Ectomorph 81
Fetish Factory Ltd. 11
I, I & E Group 87
Jensen & Morrow 81
Kastley 78
Kunzmann 131
Maxitosh 70
Murray & Vern 75
Rik Production 119
Ripplesmooth 11
Rubber Mask & Costume Company 90
Tentacle 11
Westgate Industrial Rubber 92

Gay

Rubberworks 267

ENEMA EQUIPMENT

All Sexes & Sexualities

Mediquip 11

EROTICA

BDSM

All Sexes & Sexualities

Brigid's Trove 268
Crypto Tech Corp. 211
Eclectic Engineering / Consensual Leather 273
Hard Line 128
James Bondage 242
Leather by Danny (& Cohorts) 266
Zip-Up Leathers 227

Lesbian, Gay, Bi, & Transgendered

Fantasy Erotique 81

General

Female

Socket Science Labs 213

Leather

All Sexes & Sexualities

Dungeon Enterprises, Inc. 340
Federation 89
Grimes, Robert 266
Klix Leather Products 11
Leather Stitches 213
Leatherworks Ltd. 81
Mac Leather 56
Northbound Leather Ltd. 56
Paul C Leather 249
Shadowfax Leathercraft 241
Smart Alternative 81
Spartacus Centurion 200
Spartacus Enterprises 326
Wolfmark Woodworks 276

Gay

L. C. Fantasia 51
Menkes, David 303

Pony

All Sexes & Sexualities

BBL Pony Girl Club 81

Rubber

All Sexes & Sexualities

Anderson, Chris 81
Morrison, Craig 81
Rubberotica 220

Gay

Sentry Box 81

FURNITURE

BDSM

All Sexes & Sexualities

Abusive Furniture 81
Beech, Mr. & Mrs. 72
Bottomley, Adam 81
Domino 92
Dragon's Design 266
Eroteak 91
Fesseln Fashions 359
Mazurkewicz, Terry 229
Nocturne Productions 275
Pegasus Leatherworks 245
S&M Fabrications 90
Stocks & Bonds 263
Stocks & Bonds Ltd. 345
TFM Co. 11
Toys For Tops 202
VIPPS 318
Woodworks 73
X-zess 109

Bondage

All Sexes & Sexualities

Ian King Engineering Designs Ltd. 78

PIERCING JEWELRY

All Sexes & Sexualities

Afterglow FX 324
Anatometal 221
Asgard International 11
Barbarella 173
Barbary Products 75
Body Designs 296
Bowerbird Designs 26
Chaotic Creations 11
Dakota Steel, Inc. 222
Good Art Company 222
Gothic Steel 227
Hellion House 331
HTC 193
Jones, Mark 193
Kalake Kaptive Bead 209
Merlins Ear & Body Piercing Jewelry 74
Natkiel, Dan 303
P. A. U. K. 92
Precision Metal 223
PW Multitek Services 81
Reactive Metals Studio, Inc. 193
Rings & Things 291
Silver Anchor Enterprises 236
Toucan Productions 236
Venus Modern Body Arts, Inc. 303
Wildcat Collection 11

PROSTHETICS

All Sexes & Sexualities

Bodytech 224

REGALIA

All Sexes & Sexualities

Lannoye Emblems 350
Muir Cap & Regalia 54
OLLIE of ORLANDO 187

RESTRAINTS

BDSM

All Sexes & Sexualities

Fantasy World Products 312

Gay

Fetters 81

Leather

All Sexes & Sexualities

Dean's of Bournemouth 73

Medical

All Sexes & Sexualities

Humane Restraint 356

Metal

All Sexes & Sexualities

Morgan, Luke 81

Lesbian, Gay, Bi, & Transgendered

Iron Master 340

RUBBER SHEETING

All Sexes & Sexualities

Four D Rubber Co. Ltd. 73
Pentonville Rubber Company 81

SAFE SEX PRODUCTS

All Sexes & Sexualities

Bodywise 87

SLINGS

All Sexes & Sexualities

Chardmore Services 81

WHIPS

All Sexes & Sexualities

Adam's Sensual Whips - Gillian's Toys 187
AE Services 72
Bitch Buffy 339
Draconian Leather 196
Heartwood Whips of Passion 201
Lashes by Sarah 187
Mark Allen Productions 286
McKayne, Stella 249
Montgomery, Roy 56
Quality Control 93
RAWhips 187
San Francisco Whip Company 187
Sorodz 207
Sunnypatch Works 52
Wheeler, Joe 249

ORGANIZATIONS

ACADEMIC

AIDS

All Sexes & Sexualities

Bisexuality & AIDS research Group 158

Gay

ICARE *See* Iowa Center AIDS Resources & Education
Iowa Center AIDS Resources & Education 257

Psychiatry

All Sexes & Sexualities

AASECT *See* American Association of Sex Educators, Counsellors, & Therapists
American Association for Counselling & Development 329
American Association of Sex Educators, Counsellors, & Therapists 188
American Mental Health Counsellors Association 193
American Psychiatric Association 233
American Psychological Association 233
Institute of Psychiatry 81
Institute of Psycho-Analysis 81
Institute of Psychosexual Medicine 81
Institute of Psycho-Synthesis 81
Institute of Psychotherapy & Social Studies 82
Seattle Institute for Sex Therapy Education & Research 351

SISTER 📖 *See* Seattle Institute for Sex Therapy Education & Research
Tavistock Centre 📖 81
University College London 📖 81

Lesbian, Gay, Bi, & Transgendered

American Group Psychotherapy Association 📖 268
Society for the Psychological Study of Lesbian & Gay Issues 📖 233

Sexology

All Sexes & Sexualities

Sex Institute 📖 303

Sexuality

All Sexes & Sexualities

Society for Scientific Study of Sex 📖 257

Lesbian

Institute of Lesbian Studies 📖 249

Lesbian, Gay, Bi, & Transgendered

American Historical Association 📖 357
Arbeitsgemeinschaft Humane Sexualität 📖 110
Center for Lesbian & Gay Studies 📖 303
Gay Academic Union 📖 303
Institute of Gay & Lesbian Education 📖 225
Society for Lesbian & Gay Philosophy 📖 281
Sociologisch Instituut 📖 152
Toronto Centre for Lesbian & Gay Studies 📖 56

AIDS

Chinese

All Sexes & Sexualities

Chinese HIV/AIDS Support 📖 82

Education

All Sexes & Sexualities

ACAP 📖 *See* AIDS Community Awareness Project
ACAS 📖 *See* Auckland Community AIDS Services
ACORN 📖 *See* AIDS Community Resource Network
ACQC 📖 *See* AIDS Center of Queens County
Action Against AIDS 📖 73
ActionAIDS, Inc. 📖 330
AFAN 📖 *See* Aid for AIDS
AFAO 📖 *See* Australian Foundation of AIDS Organizations
AID Atlanta 📖 244
Aid for AIDS 📖 286
AID Upstate 📖 335
AIDS Action 📖 77
AIDS Action Coalition 📖 191
AIDS Action Committee 📖 266
AIDS Action Council 📖 233
AIDS Action Group 📖 171
AIDS Action North Humberside 📖 77
AIDS Alliance 📖 137
AIDS Alliance / Cairde 📖 137
AIDS Alliance of Greenwich 📖 230
AIDS Alliance of Howard County 📖 265
AIDS Alliance of Western New York 📖 298
AIDS Allies 📖 266
AIDS Arms Network 📖 340
AIDS Calgary Awareness Association 📖 42
AIDS Care Network 📖 253
AIDS Center at Hope House 📖 290
AIDS Center of Queens County 📖 303
AIDS Center of Reference 📖 39
AIDS Coalition of Cape Breton 📖 49
AIDS Coalition of Coastal Texas 📖 342
AIDS Coalition of North East Iowa 📖 257
AIDS Coalition of Southern New Jersey 📖 289
AIDS Committee of Durham 📖 61
AIDS Committee of London 📖 51
AIDS Committee of North Bay & Area 📖 52
AIDS Committee of Ottawa 📖 52
AIDS Committee of Sudbury ACCESS 📖 54
AIDS Committee of Toronto 📖 56
AIDS Community Awareness Project 📖 346
AIDS Community Resource Network 📖 287, 346
AIDS Community Services of Western New York 📖 295
AIDS Community Trust 📖 92
AIDS Council of Central Australia 📖 28
AIDS Council of New South Wales 📖 25, 26, 27
AIDS Council of Northeastern New York 📖 296
AIDS Council of Western Virginia 📖 347
AIDS Education Project 📖 249
AIDS Foundation Miami Valley 📖 317
AIDS Foundation of Chicago 📖 249
AIDS Foundation of Houston 📖 342
AIDS Foundation San Diego 📖 211
AIDS Information Collective 📖 266
AIDS Initiative Karlsruhe e. V. 📖 123
AIDS Law Project of Pennsylvania 📖 327
AIDS Leadership Foothills Area 📖 315
AIDS New Brunswick 📖 48
AIDS Nova Scotia 📖 48
AIDS Outreach Center 📖 340
AIDS Prevention Program 📖 226
AIDS Prevention Project 📖 351
AIDS Project 📖 246, 257, 261, 333
AIDS Project East Bay 📖 207
AIDS Project Hartford, Inc. 📖 231
AIDS Project Hawaii 📖 246
AIDS Project New Haven 📖 231
AIDS Project of the Ozarks 📖 282
AIDS Referral Services 📖 258
AIDS Resource Alliance, Inc. 📖 333
AIDS Resource Center 📖 303, 340
AIDS Resource Center of Wisconsin, Inc. 📖 355
AIDS Resource Group of Evansville, Inc. 📖 254
AIDS Resources of Central Shenendoah 📖 349
AIDS Response Knoxville 📖 336
AIDS Rochester, Inc. 📖 310
AIDS Saint John 📖 48
AIDS Service Agency 📖 313
AIDS Service Agency of Wake County 📖 315
AIDS Service Connection 📖 319
AIDS Services Center 📖 329
AIDS Services of Austin 📖 338
AIDS Services of Lower Manhattan 📖 303
AIDS Services Project 📖 314
AIDS Support Foundation, Inc. 📖 338
AIDS Support Team 📖 291
AIDS Support Team / Dignity Foundation 📖 344
AIDS Task Force of Central New York 📖 295
AIDS Task Force of the Upper Ohio Valley 📖 355
AIDS Task Force of Winston-Salem 📖 316
AIDS Task Force, Inc. 📖 254
AIDS Treatment Data Network 📖 295
AIDS Trust of Australia 📖 24
AIDS Vancouver 📖 45
AIDS Vanvouver Island 📖 47
AIDS Volunteers of Cincinnati 📖 318
AIDS Wellness Program & Clinic 📖 295
AIDS Yellowknife 📖 48
AIDS, A Positive Coördinated Response Society of Jasper 📖 44
AIDS/AIDS Information & Ressources Québec Sud-Ouest 📖 61
AIDS/DTD Program 📖 241
AIDS-Informationszentrale Austria 📖 34
Aled Richards Trust 📖 70
ALFA 📖 *See* AIDS Leadership Foothills Area
American Red Cross 📖 266
Androscoggin Valley AIDS Coalition 📖 262
Appalachian AIDS Coalition 📖 347
ARC 📖 *See* AIDS Resource Center
ARCAT 📖 *See* Association pour la Recherche Clinique sur le SIDA & sa Thérapie
Aris Project 📖 219
ARK 📖 *See* AIDS Response Knoxville
ARS 📖 *See* AIDS Referral Services
ASA 📖 *See* Assoziazione Solidarieta AIDS
Associação Brasileira Interdisciplinar de AIDS 📖 39
Association de Lutte Contre le SIDA 📖 101
Association des Artistes Contre le SIDA 📖 103
Association pour la Lutte Contre le SIDA 📖 37
Association pour la Recherche Clinique sur le SIDA & sa Thérapie 📖 103
Assoziazione Solidarieta AIDS 📖 142
Athens AIDS Task Force 📖 317
Atlantic First Nations AIDS Task Force 📖 48
Auckland Community AIDS Services 📖 160
Australian Foundation of AIDS Organizations 📖 24
Australian National Council on AIDS 📖 24
AVAC 📖 *See* Androscoggin Valley AIDS Coalition
Banff Regional AIDS Committee 📖 42
BASIC 📖 *See* Bay Area Services & Information Coalition
Bay Area Services & Information Coalition 📖 241
Bennington Area AIDS Project 📖 346
BESTD HIV Outreach Clinic 📖 357
Bethany Place 📖 248
Birmingham AIDS Outreach 📖 191
Black HIV/AIDS Network 📖 82
Blue Mountain Heart To Heart 📖 354
Bluelights Campaign 📖 213
Boulder County AIDS Project 📖 226
Boys From Syracuse 📖 312
Brattleboro Area AIDS Project 📖 346
Brazos Valley AIDS Foundation 📖 339
Bronx AIDS Services 📖 303
Brooklyn AIDS Task Force 📖 297
Butte AIDS Support Services 📖 285
CARES 📖 *See* Collier AIDS Resource & Education Service, Inc.. *See also* Community AIDS Resource & Education Service
Carl Vogel Foundation, Inc. 📖 234
Cascade AIDS Project 📖 326
Center Project, Inc. 📖 355
Central City AIDS Network 📖 245
Central Louisana AIDS Support Services 📖 260
Central Wisconsin AIDS Support Group 📖 358
Charleston AIDS Network 📖 354
Clark County American Red Cross 📖 322
Clark County Health & Education Department 📖 322
CLASS 📖 *See* Central Louisana AIDS Support Services
Clatsop County AIDS Coalition 📖 324
Clay County Health Department 📖 281
Coalition des Organismes Communautaires Québecoise de Lutte Contre le SIDA 📖 61
Coastal Bend AIDS Foundation 📖 339
Collier AIDS Resource & Education Service, Inc. 📖 239
Colorado AIDS Project 📖 226
Columbia University 📖 303
Columbus AIDS Task Force 📖 320
Combattre le SIDA 📖 103
Comité SIDA Québec 📖 61
Community AIDS Network 📖 235
Community AIDS Resource & Education Service 📖 276
Community AIDS Treatment Information Exchange 📖 56
Community Health Trust, Inc. 📖 259
Community Unity Health & Wholeness Project 📖 321
Comprehensive AIDS Program 📖 243
Crewe Action for Sexual Health 📖 71
Critical Path AIDS Project 📖 330
Dakota AIDS Project 📖 316
Dakota Life Foundation 📖 316
Damien Center 📖 254
DEAN 📖 *See* Down East AIDS Network
Dental Alliance for AIDS/HIV 📖 249
Denver AIDS Prevention 📖 227
Department of Health & Human Services 📖 342
Deutsche AIDS-Hilfe e. V. 📖 108
Deutsche AIDS-Stiftung Positiv-Leben 📖 124
Dignity-Dokumentationsstelle der Diskriminierung von Menschen mit HIV/AIDS 📖 108
Doorways 📖 284
Down East AIDS Network 📖 262
Dubuque Regional AIDS Coalition 📖 256
Eastern Maine AIDS Network 📖 262
EFA 📖 *See* Saint Louis Effort for AIDS
EMAN 📖 *See* Eastern Maine AIDS Network
F. A. C. T. 📖 328
FACT 📖 *See* Fighting AIDS Continously Together
FACTS 📖 82
Feather of Hope Aboriginal AIDS Prevention Society 📖 42
Fighting AIDS Continously Together 📖 329
Finnish AIDS Council 📖 95
Foothills AIDS Awareness Association 📖 44
Fox Valley AIDS Project 📖 355, 356
Franklin-Grand Isle AIDS Task Force 📖 346
Friends For Life 📖 336
Friends For Life—Capital Area AIDS Services, Inc. 📖 260
Gay Community AIDS Project 📖 248
GO CARE 📖 260
Grand Rapids AIDS Reseource Center 📖 276
Greater Cincinnati AIDS Consortium 📖 318
Greater Houston AIDS Alliance 📖 342
Greenwich Health Project 📖 82
GROW 📖 316
HAND 📖 *See* HIV & AIDS in North Derbyshire
Harm Reduction Centre 📖 170
Hartford Health Department 📖 231
Harvest Ecumenical AIDS Resource Team 📖 341
Harvey Milk AIDS Education Project 📖 213
HEAL 📖 *See* Health Education AIDS Liason
Health Education AIDS Liaison 📖 78
Health Education AIDS Liason 📖 79
Health Issues Task Force 📖 318
Heartland AIDS Resource Council 📖 283
HIV & AIDS in North Derbyshire 📖 72
HIV Education Unit 📖 82
HIV Network, Inc. 📖 336
HIV/AIDS Advocacy Project 📖 273
HIV/AIDS Resources, Inc. 📖 325
Holland AIDS Resource Center 📖 275, 276
Home Nursing Agency AIDS Intervention Project 📖 327
Huntington AIDS Force 📖 355
Hyacinth AIDS Foundation 📖 289
Idaho AIDS Foundation 📖 247
Indiana CARES, Inc. 📖 253
Informe SIDA 📖 338
Instituto de SIDA de San Juan 📖 167
Intervention Régionale & Information sur le SIDA 📖 63
IRIS 📖 *See* Intervention Régionale & Information sur le SIDA
Kirklees AIDS Response 📖 94
Klamath County AIDS/HIV Support & Education Council 📖 325
Lafayette CARES 📖 260
Lamoille County AIDS Task Force 📖 346
Landforeningen mot AIDS 📖 164
LCATF 📖 *See* Lee County AIDS Task Force
Lee County AIDS Task Force 📖 316
LIAAC 📖 *See* Long Island Association for AIDS Care, Inc.
Lima AIDS Unit 📖 321
Long Island Association for AIDS Care, Inc. 📖 303
MAPP 📖 *See* Midwest AIDS Prevention Project
Merrymeeting AIDS Support Services 📖 262
Metro Area Committee on AIDS 📖 48
Metrolina AIDS Project 📖 314
Mexicanos Contre el SIDA 📖 149
Michiana AIDS Support Group 📖 255
Mid-Missouri AIDS Project 📖 282
Mid-New York AIDS Coalition 📖 312
Midwest AIDS Prevention Project 📖 275
MIELS 📖 *See* Mouvement d'Information & d'Entraide dans la Lutte Contre Le SIDA à Québec
Milwaukee AIDS Project 📖 357
Minnesota AIDS Project 📖 278, 279, 281
Mobiles Team AIDS des Landes Brandenburg 📖 114
Montgomery AIDS Outreach 📖 192
Mountain AIDS Coalition 📖 313
Mountain State AIDS Network 📖 354
Mouvement d'Information & d'Entraide dans la Lutte Contre Le SIDA à Québec 📖

63
Mouvement SIDA Québec 🕮 63
Municipality of Anchorage 🕮 192
Muskegon Area AIDS Resource Services 🕮 277
NAMES Project Foundation 🕮 213
Napa Valley AIDS Project 🕮 207
National Minority AIDS Council 🕮 234
National Native American AIDS Prevention Center 🕮 207
National People Living with AIDS Union 🕮 159
Nebraska AIDS Project 🕮 285
New Jersey AIDS Connection 🕮 291
New Mexico AIDS Services 🕮 293
New York State Division of Human Rights 🕮 295
New Zealand AIDS Foundation 🕮 159, 161, 162, 163
Newark Community Health Centers, Inc. 🕮 292
Newfoundland & Labrador AIDS Committee Inc. 🕮 48
NO/AIDS Task Force 🕮 260
North Central Ohio AIDS Foundation 🕮 322
North Idaho AIDS Coalition 🕮 247
North Iowa AIDS Project 🕮 257
North Puget Sound AIDS Foundation 🕮 350
Northeast Ohio Task Force on AIDS 🕮 317
Northern AIDS Network 🕮 358
Northern Colorado AIDS Project 🕮 229
Northern Kentucky AIDS Consortium 🕮 258
Northern Territory AIDS Council, Inc. 🕮 28
Northern Utah AIDS Society 🕮 345
Northwest AIDS Foundation 🕮 351
Northwest Louisiana AIDS Task Force 🕮 260
Northwest Wisconsin AIDS Project 🕮 355
Northwestern Connecticut AIDS Project 🕮 232
Northern Kentucky AIDS Task Force 🕮 259
Nottingham AIDS Information Project 🕮 89
NW Thames HIV Project 🕮 82
OAC 🕮 *See* Ohio AIDS Coalition
Oaklawn 🕮 254
Ohio AIDS Coalition 🕮 317
Ohio State University Hospitals 🕮 320
Olympia AIDS Task Force 🕮 350
Ontario AIDS Network 🕮 49
Outreach UFS 🕮 314
OxAIDS 🕮 89
PACE 🕮 82
Pacific Island AIDS Trust 🕮 159
PACK 🕮 *See* Positive Action Coalition of Kansas, Inc.
PAL 🕮 *See* Project AIDS Lafayette
Panos Institute 🕮 233
Peninsula AIDS Foundation 🕮 347
Pennine AIDS Link 🕮 94
People of Color Against AIDS Network 🕮 351
People With HIV/AIDS 🕮 203
PET 🕮 *See* Prevention, Education, & Treatment Center
Philadelphia Center 🕮 261
Philadelphia Community Health Alternatives 🕮 330
Physicians Association for AIDS Care 🕮 249
Pictou County AIDS Coalition 🕮 48
Pittsburgh AIDS Task Force 🕮 331
Plusvoice 🕮 249
Positive Action 🕮 91
Positive Action Coalition of Kansas, Inc. 🕮 257
Positive Youth Outreach 🕮 56
Positively East 🕮 82
Positively Irish Action on AIDS 🕮 82
Prevention, Education, & Treatment Center 🕮 239
Project AIDS Lafayette 🕮 255
Project Inform 🕮 213, 214
Prostitutes for Safer Sex Project 🕮 56
PWA Coalition 🕮 236
Quad Cities AIDS Coalition 🕮 256
Queensland AIDS Committee 🕮 29
Queensland AIDS Council 🕮 29
Rapids AIDS Project 🕮 256
Red Rock Mental Health Center 🕮 323
Rhode Island Project / AIDS 🕮 334
Richmond AIDS Information Network 🕮 349
Richmond Street Outreach Project 🕮 349
Riemer Foundation 🕮 249
Roanoke AIDS Project 🕮 349
Sacramento AIDS Foundation 🕮 209
Safe Afro-Arab Health & AIDS Respite Action 🕮 82
SAHARA 🕮 *See* Safe Afro-Arab Health & AIDS Respite Action
Saint Louis Effort for AIDS 🕮 284
San Angelo AIDS Foundation, Inc. 🕮 344
San Antonio AIDS Foundation 🕮 344
San Francisco AIDS Foundation 🕮 214
San Joaquin AIDS Foundation 🕮 222
San Mateo County AIDS Program 🕮 220
Santa Clara County Health Department 🕮 219
Scottish AIDS Monitor 🕮 168, 170
Séro-Zéro 🕮 62
SIDA MST Info 🕮 38
SIDA-AIDS Moncton 🕮 48
Sidaction Trois-Rivières 🕮 63
Sierra AIDS Council 🕮 222
South Arkansas Fight AIDS 🕮 195
South Carolina AIDS Education Network, Inc. 🕮 334
South Jersey AIDS Alliance 🕮 289
South Mississipi AIDS Task Force 🕮 282
South Peace AIDS Council 🕮 44
South Plains AIDS Resource Center 🕮 344
Southeast Wisconsin AIDS Project 🕮 355
Southeastern Connecticut AIDS Project 🕮 231
Southern Colorado AIDS Poject 🕮 227
Southern Tier AIDS Program, Inc. 🕮 295
Southside AIDS Venture 🕮 348
Southwest AIDS Committee 🕮 341
Southwest Louisiana AIDS Council 🕮 260
SPACE 🕮 *See* Swindon Project for AIDS Counselling & Education
Spokane AIDS Network 🕮 354
Spokane County Health District 🕮 354
Stamford Health Department 🕮 232
Stamp Out AIDS 🕮 303
Staten Island AIDS Task Force 🕮 303
Stop AIDS Byelarus 🕮 40
Stop AIDS Chicago 🕮 249
Stop AIDS Projekt Berlin 🕮 110
Sussex County AIDS Committee 🕮 233
Swindon Project for AIDS Counselling & Education 🕮 94
TAP 🕮 *See* AIDS Project
Terrence Higgins Trust 🕮 82
Tidewater AIDS Crisis Task Force 🕮 348
Tijuana AIDS / SIDA Organization 🕮 149
Toledo Wellness Group 🕮 322
Topeka AIDS Project 🕮 258
Triad Health Project 🕮 315
U.S. Conference of Mayors 🕮 234
University of North Carolina - Wilmington 🕮 316
Upper Manhattan Task Force on AIDS 🕮 303
Utah AIDS Foundation 🕮 345
Vaincre le SIDA 🕮 103
Valley AIDS Information Network 🕮 325
Valley AIDS Network 🕮 348
Vermont AIDS Council 🕮 346
Victorian AIDS Council 🕮 32
VLS 🕮 *See* Vaincre le SIDA
Wagga Wagga AIDS Task Force 🕮 27
Wake County Department of Health 🕮 315
Waldo-Knox AIDS Coalition 🕮 261
West Alabama AIDS Outreach 🕮 192
West Glamorgan AIDS Project 🕮 359
Western AIDS Alliance/Cairde 🕮 137
Western Australian AIDS Council 🕮 33
Western North Carolina AIDS Project 🕮 313
Winnebago Health Department 🕮 355
Yellowstone AIDS Project 🕮 285
YHESSI 🕮 333
YMCA 🕮 170
York Area AIDS Coalition 🕮 333
Yorkshire Mesmac 🕮 94

Female
Women & AIDS Resource Network 🕮 297
YWCA AIDS Minority Outreach 🕮 261

Gay
AIDS Information Network 🕮 330
AIDS Response Program 🕮 200
AK Schwule 🕮 112
Criticare 🕮 285
Gay Men's Health Project 🕮 77, 88, 295
Southern Gay Health Project 🕮 137
University of Pittsburgh 🕮 331

Lesbian
Bronx Lesbian AIDS Task Force 🕮 303

Lesbian, Gay, Bi, & Transgendered
AIDS Action Baltimore, Inc. 🕮 263
AIDS Action Council of the Australian Capital Territory 🕮 25
AIDS Regina 🕮 64
AIDS Response of the Seacoast 🕮 288
Arizona AIDS Project 🕮 193
Community Health Project 🕮 303
Groupe de Santé d'Antenne Rose 🕮 37
Hetrick-Martin Institute 🕮 303
National Task Force on AIDS Prevention 🕮 213
Outreach of Daytona Beach 🕮 236
Page Initiative 🕮 333
Persad Center, Inc. 🕮 331
Safe Way / Verien für Prävention für Schwule und Bisexuelle Männer 🕮 35
Sapphex Learn 🕮 235
Stuurgroep AIDS Preventie Homo's 🕮 150
Te Roopu Tatautoko 🕮 159

Information

All Sexes & Sexualities
AIDS Library of Philadelphia 🕮 330
AIDS Resource Center 🕮 234
Alternativa Positiva 🕮 167
Center for Disease Control 🕮 188
Centre Regional d'Information & de Prévention du SIDA 🕮 103
CRIPS 🕮 *See* Centre Regional d'Information & de Prévention du SIDA
Rainbow Center 🕮 245
TPA Network 🕮 188

Lesbian, Gay, Bi, & Transgendered
Health Education Resource Organization, Inc. 🕮 263

Jewish

All Sexes & Sexualities
Jewish AIDS Trust 🕮 82

Research

All Sexes & Sexualities
AIDS & Cancer Research Foundation 🕮 197
AIDS Community Research Consortium 🕮 209
American Foundation for AIDS Research 🕮 203, 303
Canadian Foundation for AIDS Research 🕮 41
CANFAR 🕮 *See* Canadian Foundation for AIDS Research
Community Research Initiative of South Florida 🕮 239
Community Research Initiative of Toronto 🕮 56
Duke AIDS Research & Treatment Center 🕮 314
Oklahoma City Foundation for AIDS Research 🕮 323
Wisconsin Community-Based Research Consortium 🕮 355

Gay
San Diego Community Research Group 🕮 211

Student

All Sexes & Sexualities
American College Health Association 🕮 347

Support

All Sexes & Sexualities
AAA 🕮 *See* Alaskan AIDS Assistance Association
Aberdeen HIV/AIDS Gay Support Group 🕮 168
ABS 🕮 *See* Nottingham AIDS Bereavement Support
ACCM 🕮 *See* AIDS Community Care Montréal
ACQC 🕮 *See* AIDS Center of Queens County
ACT-B 🕮 *See* AIDS Committee of Thunder Bay
Actions Prévention SIDA & Aide aux Malades 🕮 103
Affected by AIDS Support Group 🕮 266
Aid for AIDS 🕮 203
Aid for AIDS, Inc. 🕮 350
Aide Fribourgeoise Contre le SIDA / AIDS-Hilfe 🕮 178
Aide Info SIDA 🕮 37
AIDES Alsace 🕮 101, 106
AIDES Anjou 🕮 98
AIDES Aquitaine 🕮 98
AIDES Armor 🕮 99
AIDES Auvergne 🕮 99
AIDES Basse-Normandie 🕮 99
AIDES Bourgogne 🕮 99
AIDES Bretagne 🕮 105
AIDES Champagne-Ardennes 🕮 99, 105
AIDES Côte d'Azur 🕮 102
AIDES Dauphiné-Savoie 🕮 99, 100
AIDES France-Comté 🕮 98
AIDES Languedoc-Nord 🕮 102
AIDES Limousin 🕮 100
AIDES Loire & Haute-Loire 🕮 105
AIDES Lorraine-Nord 🕮 101
AIDES Marseille 🕮 101
AIDES Monpellier Languedoc Mediterannée 🕮 101
AIDES Nord-Pas-de-Calais 🕮 100
AIDES Orléans Region Centre 🕮 102
AIDES Pairs & Ile de France 🕮 103
AIDES Toulouse-Midi-Pyrénées 🕮 106
AIDES—Martinique 🕮 149
AIDS Action Committee of Perth County 🕮 54
AIDS Action Group 🕮 171
AIDS Action Now! 🕮 56
AIDS Advice 🕮 94
AIDS Advisory Office 🕮 166
AIDS Alliance 🕮 138
AIDS Benefit Committee of New Jersey 🕮 289
AIDS Beratung & Betreuung 🕮 125
AIDS Beratung im Gesundheitsamt 🕮 112
AIDS Care 🕮 224
AIDS Center of Queens County 🕮 303
AIDS Centre 🕮 74, 96
AIDS Committe of Grey-Bruce 🕮 53
AIDS Committee 🕮 64
AIDS Committee of Cambridge-Kitchener / Waterloo 🕮 50
AIDS Committee of Etobicoke 🕮 56
AIDS Committee of Guelph & Wellington County 🕮 49
AIDS Committee of Simcoe County 🕮 49
AIDS Committee of Thunder Bay 🕮 54
AIDS Committee of Windsor 🕮 61
AIDS Community Care Montréal 🕮 62
AIDS Council of South Australia 🕮 30
AIDS Council of Tasmania 🕮 31
AIDS Forum 🕮 110
AIDS Help West 🕮 137
AIDS Info 🕮 65
AIDS Information & Counselling Service 🕮 171
AIDS Information Line 🕮 47
AIDS Infostelle Winterthur 🕮 179
AIDS Line 🕮 32
AIDS Network 🕮 237
AIDS Network of Edmonton Society 🕮 43
AIDS Niagara 🕮 54
AIDS P. E. I. 🕮 61
AIDS Project Los Angeles 🕮 203
AIDS Relief 🕮 71
AIDS Saskatoon 🕮 64
AIDS Services Center, Inc. 🕮 191
AIDS Services of Dallas 🕮 340
AIDS Speekuur 🕮 154
AIDS Support Group 🕮 347
AIDS Support Network 🕮 162, 356
AIDS Support Society 🕮 91
AIDS Task Force of Alabama 🕮 191
AIDS Task Group 🕮 25
AIDS Yukon Alliance 🕮 64
AIDS-Beratung 🕮 129, 135, 148
AIDS-Beratung des Gesundheitsamtes Mainz 🕮 126
AIDS-Beratung im Gesundheit Dresden 🕮

114
AIDS-Beratung im Gesundheitsamt Aachen 108
AIDS-Beratungsstelle des Gesundheitsamt 124
AIDS-Beratungsstelle für Kölner Studierende 124
AIDS-Beratungsstelle Niederbayern 131
AIDS-Beratungsstelle Oberfranken 122
AIDS-Beratungsstelle Unterfranken 135
AIDS-Beratungstelle 109, 126
AIDS-Beratung-Stelle der Stadt Frankfurt 117
AIDS-Hilfe 34, 35, 108, 109, 110, 112, 113, 114, 115, 116, 117, 118, 119, 121, 122, 123, 124, 125, 126, 127, 128, 129, 130, 131, 132, 134, 135, 136, 177, 178, 179
AIDS-Info 66
AIDS-Kontor 166
Aiuta AIDS Ticino 179
Alaskan AIDS Assistance Association 192
Albion Street (AIDS) Centre 26
Aled Richards Trust 70
Algoma AIDS Network 54
All Saints AIDS Service Center 209
Ambulatorio de Saude Mental SUD 39
American Civil Liberties Union 330
American Red Cross AIDS Projects 351
Amitié SIDA 102
ANKORS *See* West Kootenay-Boundry AIDS Network, Outreach & Support Society
Anonyme AIDS-Beratungsstralle des Gesundheithauses 128
Antenne SIDA du Valais Romand 179
APLA *See* AIDS Project Los Angeles
APSAM - GPL *See* Actions Prévention SIDA & Aide aux Malades
Arkansas AIDS Foundation 195
Asociacion de Lucha Contra el SIDA 65
Association Française d'Aide aux Séro-Positifs 82
Awhina AIDS Clinic 163
Ayrshire AIDS Awareness Project Support Group 169
B. C. Coalition of People with Disabilities 45
Banque de Sang Cochin 103
Bay Area AIDS Support Service 163
Being Alive 202, 203, 211
Blue Ridge AIDS Support Group 349
Bobby Goldsmith Foundation 24, 26
Body Positive 70, 73, 76, 82, 87, 89, 90, 91, 93, 137, 163, 164, 168
Body Positive Coalition of Manitoba 47
Body Positive Resource Center 239
Brandon AIDS Support, Inc. 47
BRASS *See* Blue Ridge AIDS Support Group
Bureau Local d'Intervention Traitant du SIDA 63
Bureau Régional d'Action SIDA 61
CAC *See* Cornwall AIDS Council
CADAR *See* Chester & District AIDS Relief
CAIRDE 137
Canadian AIDS Society / Société Canadienne du SIDA 41
CARA - Carers for People Living with AIDS 30
CARE Virginia 347
CAST *See* Community AIDS Support Team
Catholic AIDS Link 82
Center One 236
Central Alberta AIDS Network Society 44
Central Oregon AIDS Support Team 324
Central Valley AIDS Team 199, 200
Central Virginia AIDS Services & Education 349
Centre des R. O. S. É. S. de l'Abititbi-Témiscamingue 63
Centre Elisa Centrum 37
Centre SIDA Amitié 63
Chester & District AIDS Relief 71
CHRU de Nîmes 102
Circle of Care 230
Cleveland AIDS Support 88
Comité des Personnes Atteintes du VIH 62
Comité SIDA Aide Montréal 62
Community AIDS Network 91
Community AIDS Support Team 79
Community Care for AIDS-UTMB 342
Community Support Network of New South Wales, Inc. 26
Cornwall AIDS Council 72
Council Physicians AIDS Office 165
CVASE *See* Central Virginia AIDS Services & Education
Davis Clinic 191
DGSS Institut 115
Diablo Valley AIDS Center 198
Dudley HIV & AIDS Support Group 93
Eclipse 220
Edmonton Persons Living with HIV Society 43
El Proyecto Arizona-Sonora 194
Entraide SIDA 39
Essentiel / HIV Anonyme 62
FACTS *See* Fife AIDS Care Through Support
Family & Friends of PWA's Support Network 249
Family Services Woodfield 229
Fife AIDS Care Through Support 168
Fight For Life 240
Fightback Trust 88, 91
Foundation 37
Fredericksburg Area HIV/AIDS Support Services, Inc. 348
Friends From The Heart 328
GAPA *See* Grupo de Apoio a Pacientes de AIDS
Gay Men's Health Crisis 303
Gesundheitsamt AIDS-Beratungsstelle 115
GG & GD 153
Globe Centre 82
Groupe SIDA Genève 178
Groupe SIDA Neuchâtel 178
Grupo de Apoio a Pacientes de AIDS 40
Gwent AIDS Support Group 359
Hamilton AIDS Network 50
Healing Our Spirit 45
Helping People With AIDS 195, 310
Het AIDS Team 35
Hillingdon AIDS Response Trust 87
HIV Care Consortium 354
HIV Network 93
HIV Positive Peer Support Group 161
HIV Resource Consortium 323
HIV Support Group 163
HIV-Arbeitlung der Charité 110
HIV-Kontoret 166
HIV-Plusline 152
HIV-Positiven Treff 112
Hôpital Antoine Beclere 103
Hôpital Henri Mondor 99
HPA *See* Helping People With AIDS
JARG *See* Jersey AIDS Relief Group
Jersey AIDS Relief Group 64
Kali-Shiva Society 47
KARES *See* Kelowna & Area AIDS Resources, Education, & Support
Kelowna & Area AIDS Resources, Education, & Support 44
Kentuckiana People With AIDS Coalition 258, 260
Kingston AIDS Project 50
KIPWAC *See* Kentuckiana People With AIDS Coalition
Klinik HIV Station 114
Klinikum der Johan-Gutenburg Universit_at 126
Kuopion AIDS-Tukikeskus 96
LASS *See* Leicestershire AIDS Support Services
LAVG *See* Lincolnshire AIDS Voluntary Group
Lee County AIDS Outreach 191
Leicestershire AIDS Support Services 79
Lethbridge AIDS Connection Society 44
Lincolnshire AIDS Voluntary Group 79
Living Pens 195
Living Room 318
London East AIDS Network 82
London Lighthouse 82
Low Country Palmetto AIDS Support Services 334
Madison AIDS Support Network 356
MASG *See* Merseyside AIDS Support Group
Merseyside AIDS Support Group 87
MIENS *See* Mouvement d'Information, d'Education, & d'Entraide dans la Lutte Contre Le SIDA
Mobile AIDS Support Services 192
Mouvement d'Information, d'Education, & d'Entraide dans la Lutte Contre Le SIDA 61
National Association of People With AIDS 249
Nelson HIV/AIDS Support Network 162
New Mexico Association of People Living With AIDS 293
New Orleans PWA Coalition 261
New Zealand AIDS Foundation 160
NMPLA *See* New Mexico Association of People Living With AIDS
Noah's Ark 173, 174, 175, 176
Noahs Ark 174
Nottingham AIDS Bereavement Support 89
Nova Scotia PWA Coalition 48
Oasis AIDS Care Centre 82
Ökumenischer Arbeitskreis AIDS 119
Oulu AIDS-Tukikeskes 95
PACT *See* People With AIDS Coalition of Tucson
Paips Essonne 102
Palette Hamburg e. V. im Schantezhof 119
Palmetto AIDS Life Support Services of South Carolina, Inc. 334
PALS *See* Powys AIDS Line Services
PALSS *See* Palmetto AIDS Life Support Services of South Carolina, Inc.
Parry Sound - Muskoka AIDS Committee 51
Peel HIV/AIDS Network 51
PEG *See* Plymouth Eddystone Group
People Living With AIDS 30, 33
People With AIDS Coalition 263
People With AIDS Coalition Houston, Inc. 342
People With AIDS Coalition of Long Island, Inc. 303
People With AIDS Coalition of Tucson 194
People With HIV/AIDS Support Group 314
Persons with AIDS Society of British Columbia 45
Peterborough AIDS Resource Network 54
PHAN *See* Peel HIV/AIDS Network
PLUSS 164
PLWA *See* People Living With AIDS
Plymouth Eddystone Group 73
Positif 141
Positiivi-yhdistys 96
Positiva Gruppen 175
Positive Advocacy 88
Positive People Portsmouth 76
Positive Place 82
Positive Support 89
Positivia Gruppen-Väst 173
Powys AIDS Line Services 359
Prenzelberger AIDS Projekt 110
Prince George AIDS Society 44
Project Lazarus 261
Provincetown Positive PWA Coalition 272
Psychotherapy Center 195
PWA Coalition 246, 344
PWA Coalition Colorado 228
PWA Coalition of Dade County 239
PWA Coalition of Maine 261
PWA Coalition of New York, Inc. 303
PWA Coalition of Palm Beach 243
PWA Coalition of Tampa Bay 242
PWA Support Groups 313
Queensland AIDS Committee 28
Queensland AIDS Council 28, 29
Queensland Positive People 28
Rådgivningskontoret mot AIDS 167
Reach HIV Support Group 94
Refuge 314
Roze Waas 39
Scottish AIDS Monitor 169
Service aux Séro-Positifs 37
Service Spécialisé SIDA Québec 61
SID'Aventure 105
SIDA Centre 92
SOLAS 168
Somerset AIDS Advice 90
South Wales Immune Deficiency Self Help 359
Southeast Counseling Services 320
Städtisches Gesundheitsamt AIDS Beratungstelle 132
Stop AIDS 204
Survivors 82
SWISH *See* South Wales Immune Deficiency Self Help
Syndicat PTT de la Manche CFDT 105
TAGS *See* Torquay AIDS Support Group
Tampa AIDS Network 242
Tampere AIDS-Tukikeskus 95
TAP *See* Tucson AIDS Project, Inc.
Texarkana AIDS Project, Inc. 194
Thames Valley Positive Support 71
Torbay AIDS Group Supporters 73
Toronto People With AIDS Foundation 56
Torquay AIDS Support Group 73
Tours Elisa 2000 106
Treffpunkt Regenbogen 115
Trondheim AIDS og Infeksjonshelsetjenesten 166
Trondheim Helseråd 166
Tucson AIDS Project, Inc. 194
Turun AIDS-Tukikeskus 96
TVPS *See* Thames Valley Positive Support
Venango-Forest AIDS Support 327
Vermont Cares 346
Vermont PWA Coalition 346
Victoria AIDS Respite Care Society 45
Victoria Persons with AIDS Society 47
Voices of Positive Women 56
Washington County AIDS Task Force 195
West Kootenay-Boundry AIDS Network, Outreach & Support Society 44
Whangarei Health HIV/AIDS Coördinator 163
Witte Raven 35, 38, 39
York AIDS Action Ltd. 88
ZASA *See* AIDS-Hilfe

Female

Centre d'Action SIDA Montréal (Femmes) 62
Positive Women's Network 45

Gay

Equinox 221
Ettie Rout Centre 161
Gay Men's Health Project 137
HIV/AIDS Gay Support Group 168
Positive Friends 32
Positive Image 11
Two-Spirited People of the First Nations Native Awareness Project 56
Victorian AIDS Council 32

Heterosexual, Male

Positive Straight Men 56

Lesbian, Gay, Bi, & Transgendered

AIDS Information 154
AIDS Information & Counselling Service 171
AIDS Support Program 323
AIDS-Hilfe 119, 123
Body Positive Groups 65
Community AIDS Council 194
Gayhälsen 173
Helseutvalget for Homofile 164
HIV Groups 65
Hope HIV Support Group 313

Male

HIV-Hjælpen 66
Positivgruppen 66

BALLS

Gay

Ball Club 11

BDSM

All Sexes & Sexualities

A. E. L. 294
A.S.B. Munch 45, 191, 209, 214, 234, 240, 244, 249, 255, 259, 268, 275, 280, 303, 325, 330, 347

Organizations: BDSM

ACS 70
Alternates 351
Arizona Power Exchange 194
Atlanta Power Exchange 245
Backdrop Club 11
Betty Page Social Club 45, 56
Black Orchid 236
Black Rose 347
Black Widow's Web 173
Chandelles 103
Chicagoland Discussion Group 249
Club J & G 39
Club Sunrise 173
Club X 211
CODE *See* Colorado Organization of Dungeon Enthusiasts
Collars 351
Colorado Organization of Dungeon Enthusiasts 228
Contact Centre (S/M) 12
Continental Leather Pride Committee 228
D&S Society of Baltimore 264
D. S. S. G. 242
Denver Leather Association 228
Domination 240
Eroticism through Sensual Conduct, Attitude, & Power Exchange 286
Escape *See* Eroticism through Sensual Conduct, Attitude, & Power Exchange
Eulenspiegel Society 303
Femina Society International 271
Feminine Disciplinary Society 82
Firebirds 357
FM 214
Group with No Name 248, 338
GWNN *See* Group with No Name
Headspace 244
IDPA *See* International Dungeon & Playroom Association
International Dungeon & Playroom Association 12
Kinky Club 95
Kinky Couples 351
LBW *See* Leather Bondage & Whips
Leather / SM / Fetish Community Outreach 12
Leather Bondage & Whips 327
Leather Caucus of Toronto 56
Leather Pride Project 351
Leather Rose Society 340
Leather United - Chicago 249
Lifestyle Explorers Club 238
LINKS 214
LSMA Köln 124
Marci & Friends 295
Megalesia 62
Melbourne Leather Pride Association 32
Menamore Levi / Leather Club 316
Metro Leather Society 278
Michigan Society for Domination & Submission 273
Molotov 119
MSDS *See* Michigan Society for Domination & Submission
National Leather Association 12, 26, 44, 56, 194, 200, 225, 236, 244, 271, 278, 283, 303, 320, 326, 338, 340, 342
New York Metro D&S Singles 297
NLA *See* National Leather Association
OCLA *See* Orange Coast Leather Assembly
Omaha Players Club 285
Orange Coast Leather Assembly 200
People Exchanging Power 240, 244, 247, 329, 337, 338
PEP *See* People Exchanging Power
Petruchio 197
Power Play 345
RCDC *See* Rose City Discussion Club
Rose City Discussion Club 324
S3C3 *See* Sober, Safe, Sane, Consensual Club - Chicago
SAAFE *See* Southern Alberta Association for Fetish / Fantasy Education / Exploration
Sacramento Leather Association 209
Seattle Kink Information Network 351
Service of Mankind Church 199, 230
SKIN *See* Seattle Kink Information Network
SM / Leather / Fetish Community Outreach Project 12
SM-COP *See* SM / Leather / Fetish Community Outreach Project
SMiL Denmark 66
SMil Norge 164
Sober, Safe, Sane, Consensual Club - Chicago 249
Society 232, 265
South Goes Mad 157
South Sound SM Leatherfolk 350
Southern Alberta Association for Fetish / Fantasy Education / Exploration 42
Sydney Leather Pride Association 26
Tacoma Pride in Leather 351
TAPE *See* Triangle Area Power Exchange
TES *See* Eulenspiegel Society
Threshold 206
Thunderbolt Book Club 82
Torture Garden 82
Triangle Area Power Exchange 315
Tri-State Couples Club 331
United Leatherfolk of Connecticut 230
Valkyrie 70
Vancouver Leather Alliance 45
Vereniging Studiegroep Sado-Masochisme 151, 152, 153, 155, 157, 158
VSSM *See* Vereniging Studiegroep Sado-Masochisme
Western Canada Leather / Fetish Clans Council 42
X-Corrigia 56

Bisexual

SM Bisexuals 69

Female

Ace 334
B.A.D. Girls 326
Banshees 351
Bound by Desire 338
Briar Rose 320
Clit Club 303
Club Domentia 214
Cogent Warriors 214
Common Bond 268
Female Trouble 330
Females Investigating Sexual Terrain 264
FIST *See* Females Investigating Sexual Terrain
Knights of Leather 280
Lady O Society 82
Leather WISDOM *See* Leather Women Into Sadism Dominance Obedience & Masochism
Leather Women Into Sadism Dominance Obedience & Masochism 221
Long Island Ravens 296
Northwest Leather Goddesses 351
OL *See* Outer Limits
Outcasts 214
Outer Limits 351
Pervert Scouts 214
Power Circle 221
Re-Enchantment for Women 82
Reno's Leather Underground 287
Shelix 271
Stichting SMet...! 152
Submissive Females 71
Ultra-Sex Alliance 274
Vereniging Studiegroep Sado-Masochisme 150
VSSM *See* Vereniging Studiegroep Sado-Masochisme
Wanda's Wenches 270
Women's SM Group 82
Women's Welcoming Committee 351
WWC *See* Women's Welcoming Committee

Gay

15 Association 214
Adventurers - Sun Coast 241
AG Leder 121
Alameda County Leather Corps 207
Amalgamated American Male 303
Ambassadors 268
A-Men's Club 65
Arbeits Gemeinschaft S/M & Offentlichkeit 129
Argonauts of Wisconsin 356
Arizona Fellowship Committee 194
ASMF Paris 103
ASS *See* Atlanta S&M Solidarity
Atlanta S&M Solidarity 244
Atons of Minneapolis 280
Avatar 204
Baccus - Detroit 275
Bay Area Levi & Leather Society 339
Bear Club U.K. 75
Beer Town Badgers 357
BFLO *See* Buffalo Fetish & Leather Organization
BIG 188
Black Eagle MC 271
Black Fire Association 312
Black Guard 280
Black Hedgehogs Rheinland 115
Black Panther's Club 178
Blackline Interchain 69
Blue Haze 82
Bluegrass C. O. L. T.s 259
Boot Co. 28
Boots 12
Boots & Breeches Club 74
Boston Ducks 270
Bottoms-Up 288
Branding Iron Club 340
Brotherhood of Pain 342
Brothers In Leather 303
BSG 93
Buffalo Fetish & Leather Organization 298
Café Schwarz 135
California B & B Corps 204
CB&V 286
Celestial Krewe de Cuir 214
Cellar 91
Centurions of Columbus 320
Chain of Command 344
Chaps 326
Chest Men of America 249
Chicago Hellfire Club 249
Cincinnati Chaps 318
Clan Masters 103
CLSMC Eagle 113
Club Australia 26
Club Cuir ESMC 101
Club de Cuir Predateurs 63
Club des Cuirassés de Québec 63
Club LL 152
Club Winnipeg 47
CODE *See* Colorado Organization of Dungeon Enthusiasts
Colorado Organization of Dungeon Enthusiasts 226
Colt 45s 342
COMMAND 264
Conductors L/L 337
Copperstate Leathermen Association 194
Cornhaulers L & L Club 256
Cosmic Order of KA 188
Countrymen 275
Cowtown Leathermen 340
D. A. D. S. 253
D.L. 214
Dads & Sons 188
DALLAS *See* Dallas Area Levi / Leather Association
Dallas Area Levi / Leather Association 340
Defenders 214, 228, 234, 238, 268, 303
Desert Leathermen 194
Disciples of de Sade 340
Dragon LC 320
dreizehn 268
DSSM 82
Dungeon Players 340
Durham Alliance Association 52
East Mercia MSC 89
Edge 56
Enigma 249
Esoterica Society 272
Essex Leather 75
Excalibur of Cleveland 318
Fantasy Youth 82
FFA - FGC 236
Firedancers 340, 344
Firekeepers of Indiana 255
FLC *See* Frankfurter Lederclub e. V.
Frankfurter Lederclub e. V. 117
FSC 110
Gay Male SM Activists 303
Gay Raiders 124
GFMC/DC 234
GLSM *See* Gruppe Leder SM
GOAL 303
Golden Gate Guards 214
Grand Rapids Rivermen 276
GRLP 167
Gruppe Leder SM 119
Gryphons 321
GSN 91
HarborMasters 262
Hardcore 125
Hearts of the West 295
Hijos del Sol 294
Icon Detroit 274
Kansas City Pioneers 283
Key West Wreckers LLC 238
Knight Cruisers 259
Knight Hawks of Virginia 348
Knights d'Orleans 261
Knights of Malta MC 287
Knights of Malta of California Clubs, Inc. 206
L & L Society 274
L/SM Round-Up 214
LC Nordwest 113
LC Saar 132
LC Stuttgart e. V. 132
LCH *See* Lederclub Hamburg
Leather & Lace Society 317
Leather Corps 204
Leather Group 168
Leather Knights 268, 340
Leather Men Düsseldorf 115
Leather Scribes 12
Leathermasters International 12
Leathermen 244
Leathermen Yearning for Northern eXcitement 49
Leder Jeans Club Ost 129
Lederclub Dresden 114
Lederclub Hamburg 119
Lederclub HH 119
Lederclub Leipzig 125
Lederfreunde Rhein-Ruhr Essen 116
Levi/Leather Brigade 335
Levi/Leather Plainsmen 64
LFRR *See* Lederfreunde Rhein-Ruhr Essen
Lion Regiment 247
Lion's Roar 214
Living Art Association 209
LJC Ost *See* Leder Jeans Club Ost
Locker Jocks 292
Loge 70 (Schweitz) 177
Lords of Leather 261
Louisville Nightwings 259
LYNX *See* Leathermen Yearning for Northern eXcitement
M & S Connexion 127
MACT *See* Men of All Colors Together
MAFIA *See* Mid-America Fists In Action
Mall City Cruisers 276
Manpower Network 171
Marked Men 25
Masters & Slaves Together 12
Mates 272
Mavericks 188
MCRA *See* MSC Rhône-Alpes
Melbourne Leather Men, Inc. 32
Memphis Leather / Levi Alliance 336
Men of All Colors Together 225
Men of Discipline 303
Mid-America Fists In Action 249
Midlands Communication Network 256
Mike's Men 270
Minnesota Leather Encounter, Inc. 280
MLC *See* Münchner-Löwen Club e. V.
Moonlight Leather Association of the Deaf 211
Mountain Men of Leather 228
MSC Hannover 121
MSC Rhône-Alpes 101
Münchner-Löwen Club e. V. 128
National Leather Association 196, 255,

261
Neue Regel 238
New York Strap & Paddle Association 304
Nimbus 276
NLA *See* National Leather Association
Norsemen 287
Northern California Leather Association of the Deaf 214
Oberons 357
Officers Club 196
Ohio Broncos 318
OMEN 285
Order of the Marquis & Chevalier 277
Oregon Guild Activists of S/M 326
ORGASM 168. *See also* Oregon Guild Activists of S/M
Ottawa Knights 52
Palm Springs Leather Order of the Desert 208
Panther LL, Inc. 244
Pendragons of Birminham 191
Pennsmen 328
Pocono Warriors 293
Post 45
Quälgeister - FSG Berlin e.V. 110
Rangers 319
Reading Railmen 333
Regiment of the Black & Tans 204
Renegades 304
Ringed Men 25
Rocky Mountain Lambda Lions 228
Rogues LLC 349
S & M Club 214
Saint Crispin L/L Fraternity 240
San Francisco God-Damned Independents 214
Sandia Leathermen 294
SandMen 211
Scandinavian Leather Men 66, 164, 173, 175
Seattle Men in Leather 351
Sex Magik Faeries Circle 214
Shipmates of Baltimore, Inc. 264
SigMa 234
Silver Dolphins LLC 339
Silver Spurs of Dallas 340
Silver State Leather Association 287
SKVdC Sekretariat 110
SLM *See* Scandinavian Leather Men
SLMC *See* Sylter Männer Leder Club
SM Gays 69
SMC Dresden 114
SML *See* Seattle Men in Leather
SNC London 82
Somandros 204
Sons of Capone 49
Sons of Satan 214
Spearhead 56
Stallions 319
Steel City Centurions 192
STUDS-30, Inc. 277
Suncoast Leather Club 239
Sundance Cattle Company 342
Sylter Männer Leder Club 135
Tampa Bay Trailblazers 242
Tartarus 284
TDA - Atlanta 244
Temple of Hecate 318
Tennessee Leather Tribe 336
Texas Renegade Club 342
Three Rivers Leather Club, Inc. 331
Thüringer Lederclub 116
TLC *See* Thüringer Lederclub
Tower City Corps 319
Tradesmen, Inc. 314
Tri-State TCC 331
Trusted Servants 214
Tsarus 336
Tucson Arizona Levi/Leathermen 194
Tucson Knight Owls 194
Unicorns of Madison 356
Universal Brotherhood of Leatherlords 194
Ursine Group 257
Vagevuur 12
Vancouver Activists in SM 45
VASM *See* Vancouver Activists in SM
Vision SM Club 32
Vulcan LL 320
Wasatch Leathermen 345
Wings MC 337
Winnipeg Leather/Levi Club 47
Wisconsin Leathermen's Association 357
Wolf Pack S&M 274

Heterosexual

Alice Kerr Sutherland Society 91
Essemian Press 199
Gyncrocrat Alliance 284
Hellfire Club 303
Moonglow Dining Club 82
Orb & Scepter 286
Society of Janus 214

Lesbian

DAMES *See* Dykes Against Minority Suppression
Dykes Against Minority Suppression 357
Interchange 210
Lesbian Sex Mafia 303
Portland Power & Trust 326
Tannery Row 210
Women's Leather Network 225

Lesbian, Gay, Bi, & Transgendered

Boston Unified Leather Legion 270
BULL *See* Boston Unified Leather Legion
CLUB Calgary 42
Namibian Leather Corps 149
SM Group 75
SMia 164
Tarheel Leather Club 315
Trident Knights 334

Male

Delta International 12
RAP 204
Ring 201

Competitions (see also Competitions & Conventions: BDSM)

Female

Generic Leather Productions 350
Washington State Ms. Leather 350
WSMLO *See* Washington State Ms. Leather

Gay

Mr. Drummer 214

Male

International Mr. Fantasy 285
Washington State Mr. Leather Organization 351

Pony

All Sexes & Sexualities

Other Pony Club 11

Student

All Sexes & Sexualities

Conversio Virium 304

BEARS

Female

T-Bear Club 340
T-Bears of Boston 271

Gay

AHF-Switchboard 117
Appalachian Bears Club of East Tennessee 336
Arktos 319
Backwoods Bears 358
Bären Hamburg 120
Bären Stuttgart 133
Bartmäner Bären Köln 124
Bartmänner Schweiz, Barbus de Suisse, Barbuti Svizzeri, Barbus Svissers, Beardmen Switzerland 177
BC Bears 45
Bear Buddies Toronto 56
Bear Club Japan 148
Bear Club U. K. 82
Bear History Project 12
Bear Paws of Iowa 257
BearHug - U. K. 82
BearHug Group 214
Bears Down Under 26
Bears International 12
Bears LA 224
Bears Netherlands 154
Bears of Central Florida 240
Bears of Mañana 294
Bears of San Francisco 214
Bears of Southwest Florida 239
Bears of the Old Pueblo 194
Bears on Bikes 331
Bears San Diego 211
Bergenfield Bears 304
Berliner Bären Bartmänner 110
Big Beary Bulky Boys 168
Blackjack Bears of Las Vegas 286
Bluegrass Bears 259
Brew City Bears 357
Brisbears 29
Buddy Bears of Philadelphia 330
Carolina Bear Lodge 313
Chesapeake Bay Bears 347
Chi Town Society 250
CIC *See* AHF-Switchboard
Cincinnati's River Bears 318
Cleveland Bears 321
Coalition of Ursine Brothers 194
Columbus Ursine Brotherhood 320
Confederate Bears 314
Dallas Bears 340
Delaware Valley Bears 330
Desert Bears 194
Dixie Bears 243
Double Trouble Bears 329
Florida Bear Hunters 240
Front Range Bears 228
Gais Nounours 103
Girth & Mirth of LA 197
Gold Coast Bears 236
Golden Gate Connection 198
Golden State Bears 200
Great Lakes Bears 250, 277
Greeley Bears 229
Harbour City Bears 26
Heart of Texas Bears 338
Hirsute Fraternity 214
Hirsute Pursuit 258
Hoosier Bears of Indiana 253
Houston Area Bears 342
Kansas City Cave Bears 283
Kiwi Bears 160
Kubs/Kiwi United Bear Social 160
Las Vegas Bears 286
Last Frontier 192
Lone Star Bears 340
Mid-Michigan Bears 277
MnBears 280
Motor City Bears 278
Music City Bears 337
Nederbears 152
New England Bears 268
New York Bears 304
North Country Bears 279
Northeast Ursamen 232
Northwest Bears 351
Old Fort Bears 254
Omikron 255
Orsi Italiani Girth & Mirth 138
Orsiciliani 145
Ozark Mountain Bears 195
Ozbears Australia Inc. 26
Ozbears of South Australia 31
Pacific Bears California LMC 200
PAWS Social Club 171
Red Earth Bears 323
Renegade Bears 351
Rhode Island Grizzlies 334
River Bears 318
Rock Valley Bears 253
San Francisco Leather Bears 214
Show Me Bears 284
Smokey Mountain Bears 336
South Florida Bears 12
Southern Bears 244
Southern Ontario Bears 56
Teddy Bear Leather Club 347
Tidewater Bears 348
Tri-State Bears 321
Ursus 321
Valley Bears 209
Viking Bears 175
West Florida Growlers 242
West Oz Marsupial Bears And Their Supporters 33
Wombats *See* West Oz Marsupial Bears And Their Supporters

Male

Girth & Mirth 12

BODY SIZE

Gay

Affliated Big Men's Clubs 214
Big Men of Hawaii 247
Bulk Club U.K. 82
Chubbies & Chasers of Cleveland 321
Four B's Club 168
Gentle Giants of Oregon 326
Girth & Mirth 98, 103, 110, 120, 124, 127, 128, 142, 152, 156, 157, 197, 211, 214, 228, 236, 250, 268, 278, 280, 284, 310, 315, 317, 328, 337, 348, 351, 357
Great Triad Men 315
Magnum Club 138
Southwest Men At Large 194
X-Large 177

Lesbian, Gay, Bi, & Transgendered

XXXLNT 239

BONDAGE

All Sexes & Sexualities

Axis 72
Northwest Bondage Club 351

Gay

Foot & Rope Club 188
New Orleans Bondage Club 261
New York Bondage Club 304
PBC 332
Pittsburgh Bondage Club 330
San Francisco Bondage Club 214
Sydney Bondage Club 26
Tampa Bay Bondage Club 238
TCBA *See* Twin Cities Bondage Association
Tightropes 48
Twin Cities Bondage Association 280

CONDOMS

All Sexes & Sexualities

Condom Resource Center 207

COUNSELLING

All Sexes & Sexualities

Identity 82

DADDY / BOY

Gay

boys & Dads Association 49
New York Boys & Dads 304
SCMA 201

FAMILY

All Sexes & Sexualities

AGEDO *See* Assoziazione Genitori di Omosessuali
Assoziazione Genitori di Omosessuali 143, 144, 145
Children of Lesbians & Gays Everywhere 56, 57, 250
COLAGE *See* Children of Lesbians & Gays Everywhere
Contact 103
Eltern Telefon 129
Families & Friends of Lesbians & Gays 76
FFLAG *See* Families & Friends of Lesbians & Gays
Friends & Relatives of Gays 321
FROG *See* Friends & Relatives of Gays
Gay & Lesbian Parents 199
Gay & Lesbian Parents Coalition 265
GLPC—MW *See* Gay & Lesbian Parents Coalition
Lancashire Family & Partners Support 79
Leeds Parent's Friend 94
Manchester Gay Parents Group 75
Parent's Enquiry 82
Parents & Friends of Lesbians & Gays 25, 29, 31, 32, 33, 42, 45, 47, 48, 49, 50, 54, 57, 167, 188, 192, 195, 198, 201, 202, 204, 206, 210, 211, 214, 221, 223, 224, 227, 228, 229, 231, 232, 234, 237, 240, 241, 244, 250, 257, 259, 260, 261, 262, 263, 264, 266, 268, 272, 274, 275, 276,

Organizations: Family

277, 278, 279, 280, 284, 285, 286, 287, 289, 298, 304, 310, 311, 313, 314, 315, 316, 317, 318, 319, 321, 324, 325, 326, 328, 329, 330, 332, 333, 335, 336, 337, 341, 342, 346, 352, 354, 356, 358
Parents of Lesbian & Gay Children 30
Parents of Lesbians & Gays 160
PFLAG *See* Parents & Friends of Lesbians & Gays
Pro Familia Homosexuellenberatung 115, 121
Relatives Group 65
Schwuler Väter 135
Solo Parenting Alliance 352
Tarrant County Parents Group 340

Female

Wives of Bisexual & Married Gay Men 319

Gay

APG *See* Association des Parents & Futures Parents Gais
Association des Parents & Futures Parents Gais 103
BAMH *See* Bisexual & Married Homosexual Men's Support Group
Bisexual & Married Homosexual Men's Support Group 30
Gay Fathers 210, 225, 234, 319
Gay Fathers / Fathers First of Houston 342
Gay Fathers Connection 346
Gay Fathers Group 311
Gay Fathers I 304
Gay Fathers of Greater New York 304
Gay Fathers of Long Island 304
Gay Fathers of Westchester 304
Gay Married Men's Support Group 311
GFW *See* Gay Fathers of Westchester
Schwule Väter 133
Schwüle Väter 116
Schwule Väter Köln 124

Heterosexual

PASTELS 94

Lesbian, Gay, Bi, & Transgendered

Eltern Schwuler Söhne & Lesbischwe Töchter 113
Evansville Gay & Lesbian Parents Coalition 254
GALA *See* Gay & Lesbian Parents Coalition
Gay & Lesbian Parent Coalition 344
Gay & Lesbian Parenting Group of Central Ohio 320
Gay & Lesbian Parents 329
Gay & Lesbian Parents Coalition 283
Gay & Lesbian Parents Coalition International 234, 240
Gay/Lesbian Parents of Dallas 340
GLPCI *See* Gay & Lesbian Parents Coalition International
Langley Outreach 44
Monadnock Area Lesbian / Gay Parents 288
New Hampshire Gay Parents 287
OK To Be Us 57
Our Kids 275
Parent's Enquiry 168
Parents & Friends of Lesbians & Gays 358
Parents d'Enfants Homosexuels 38
PFLAG *See* Parents & Friends of Lesbians & Gays
Schwule Väter & Ehemänner 113

FETISH

Clothing

All Sexes & Sexualities

Boston Rubber Club 268
Club Gum 158
Club Whiplash 82
Cruise Club 70
Events 93
Fantasmatic & Fetish Club 39
Fantastic! 83
Felicity 82
Fetish Street 150
International Mackintosh Society 78
Marquis Masquerade 89
Northern Association of Fantasy Fetishists 94
Repentence 82
Rubber Nipple Club 83
SAFE *See* South Australia Fetish / Fantasy Enthusiasts
Severin's Kiss 83
South Australia Fetish / Fantasy Enthusiasts 30
SSSH 89
Vereniging Studiegroep Sado-Masochisme 150
VSSM *See* Vereniging Studiegroep Sado-Masochisme

Bisexual

Minnesota Leather Den 279

Female

Minnesota Leather Den 279

Gay

Grønn Mann 165
Gummi 69
London Blues 83
M. E. C. *See* Mecs En Caoutchouc
Mecs En Caoutchouc 12, 99
New World Rubber Men 12
Rubber Corps 214
Rubber Men's Club 83
Vulcan America Southern California 204

Heterosexual

Nuit du Desir 37
Nylon Club 99

Dildo

Gay

National Dildo Club 188

Enema

Male

Fraternity of Enema Buddies 12

Foot

All Sexes & Sexualities

Lotus Foot Love Club 298

Gay

Foot Friends 304
Foot Guys 238
Footmen 87
National Foot Network 188
NFN *See* National Foot Network
Whitesox 177

Male

Foot Fraternity 188

Foreskin

All Sexes & Sexualities

Circumcision Resource Center 268

Gay

Glans Naked & Unashamed 234
GNU *See* Glans Naked & Unashamed
National Organization of Restoring Men 198
NORM *See* National Organization of Restoring Men
Uncircumcised Society of America 214
Uncut 214
Uncut Club 204
USA *See* Uncircumcised Society of America

Hair

All Sexes & Sexualities

T. S. C. 92

Gay

BROS 12

Mess

Gay

Club Mud 188
Mud Buddies 211
Mud Maniacs 72
SLOSH *See* Society for Lovers Of Slapstick Happenings
SludgeMaster 343
Society for Lovers Of Slapstick Happenings 69

Rubber

Gay

Stockholm Rubber Men's Club 175

Smoking

All Sexes & Sexualities

Hot Ash 12

Gay

Cigar Studs 202, 344
EBC 210
Smoke Exchange 12
Still Smokin' 45

Uniforms

Gay

American Uniform Association 13, 234, 244, 250
AUA *See* American Uniform Association
CHKK 323
European Uniform Club 39
Fits Like A Glove 13
FLAG *See* Fits Like A Glove
Golden State Peace Officers Association 204
Köln Oliv 124
Military & Police Club International 13
Philadelphia Uniform Patrol 330
Phœnix Uniform Club 214
SLUG *See* South Bay Leather Uniform Group
South Bay Leather Uniform Group 219

Male

Patrol Uniform Club of Texas 344

FISTING

Gay

Cascade Handballers 352
FFA/CAC 234
Red Hankies of San Diego 211
Touch 153
TRUST (FF National Network) 188

HEALTH

All Sexes & Sexualities

abc Leipzig e. V. 125
American Social Health Association 188
ASHA *See* American Social Health Association
Halton Regional Health Department 49
Health Shop 79
LINK 57
Options Clinic 51
Sex Information & Education Council 41, 304
Sexual Assault Centre - Hamilton & Area 50
Sexual Assault Centre of Brantford 57
Sexual Assault Support Centre - Ottawa 52
SIECCAN *See* Sex Information & Education Council
SIECUS *See* Sex Information & Education Council
Thunder Bay District Health Unit 54
Thunder Bay Physical & Sexual Assault Centre 54

Female

Kitchener / Waterloo Sexual Assault Support Centre 50
Sexual Assault/Rape Crisis Centre of Peel 51
Sudbury Sexual Assault Crisis Centre 54

Gay

EROS, The Center for Safe Sex 214
Peel Health Department - Sexual Health Info-Line 57
Sexual Assault Centre for Quinte & District 49

Lesbian, Gay, Bi, & Transgendered

National Lesbian & Gay Health Association 188
Ottawa Physicians for Lesbian & Gay Health 52

HUMAN RIGHTS

All Sexes & Sexualities

Canadian Human Rights Commission 41, 57

LIBRARY

All Sexes & Sexualities

Library Corporation 234
Library of Congress 234
Registrar of Copyrights 234

LITERARY

All Sexes & Sexualities

Book Industry Study Group 304
ISBN Agency 304
No Safeword Writers' Group 352

Lesbian, Gay, Bi, & Transgendered

American Library Association 250
Gay & Lesbian Press Association 223

MASTURBATION

Gay

Berlin Jacks 110
Black Jack 204
Chicago Jacks 250
J's Hangout 304
J/O Enthusiasts 234
Melbourne Wankers 32
MEMMOS *See* Men Enjoying Mutual Masturbation & Oral Sex
Men Enjoying Mutual Masturbation & Oral Sex 356
Santé & Plaisir Gai 101
SPG *See* Santé & Plaisir Gai
T.O.M. 311
Vancouver Jacks 45

Lesbian, Gay, Bi, & Transgendered

Cologne Jacks 124

MOTORCYCLE

All Sexes & Sexualities

Œdipus MC 201

Female

Athena Women's MC 222
Leather & Lace WMC, Inc. 210
Moving Violations 268
Sirens MC 304
Sirens MC San Francisco 215
Two Wheelers Auxiliary Troop 286

Gay

41 South MC 163
ACRA *See* Australian Club Run Association
Aquila MC 196
Arizona Rangers MC 194
Atlantic Motorcycle Coördinating Council 188
Atlantis MC 244
Australian Club Run Association 26
Battalion MC 340
Blackhawk MC 253
BLMSC *See* Bournemouth Leather MSC
Blue Max Cycle Club 284
Blue Max MC 204
Border Riders MC 45, 352
Bournemouth Leather MSC 73
Brothers MC, Inc. 238
California Cyclemen MC 211
California Eagles MC 215
Capital City Riders MC 338
Castaways MC 357
Centaur MC 234
CFLM Austria 35
Challengers International MC 240
City Bikers MC 228
Conquistadors MC 240
Constantines, Inc., of the Bay Area 215
Corps of Rangers 204
Corpus Christi MC 339
Council of Southern California Motorcycle Clubs 202
Crucible MC 332
Cycle Runners MC 215
Cycle/Wheels MC 304
Cycles MC 292
Dallas MC 340
Desert Brotherhood MC 286
Dolphins Motor Club 26
Eagle MC 243
East Anglia Bikers 83
Empire City MC 304
Entre Nous MC 268
European Confederation of Motorcycle Clubs

📖 179
Excelsior MC 📖 304
Excess Motorcycle Club 📖 70
FSMC 📖 101
Gai Moto Club 📖 103
Gateway MC 📖 284
Gay Bikers 📖 89
GBMCC 📖 *See* Gay Bikers
Giffins MC 📖 232
Great Lakes Harley Owners 📖 355
Griffins Motor Club 📖 25
Harley Strokers 📖 326
Hartford Colts, MC 📖 231
Heart of Texas MC 📖 344
Highwaymen MC 📖 44
Highwaymen TNT 📖 234
Houston Council of Clubs 📖 343
IMC 📖 *See* Italia Motor Club Milano
Inter-Bike Denmark 📖 13
International Roadmasters 📖 275
Iron Cross MC 📖 62
Iron Eagles MC 📖 270
Italia Motor Club Milano 📖 143
Jackaroos MC 📖 32
Knights of Malta MC 📖 45, 344, 352
Knights of Malta of California Clubs, Inc. 📖 215
Knights on Iron MC 📖 211
La Madrona 📖 215
Leather Motor Club Torino 📖 144
Leder- & Motorradclub Zürich 📖 179
Limburg Motorclub 📖 157
LMC Vienna 📖 35
LMZ 📖 *See* Leder- & Motorradclub Zürich
LOBOCS MC 📖 202
Manchester Superchain MSC 📖 76
MC Faucon, Inc. 📖 62
MC Nordlicht Hamburg 📖 120
MCF Leather Motor Club Firenze 📖 145
MCLB 📖 *See* Motorradclub LederBären Berlin
Midland Link MSC 📖 93
MLCV 📖 *See* Moto Leather Club Veneto
Mooncussers MC 📖 272
Moto Leather Club Veneto 📖 138
Motorcity Men of Leather 📖 277
Motorcycle Men of Alberta 📖 44
Motorcyclemen of New Mexico 📖 294
Motorradclub LederBären Berlin 📖 110
MS Panther Köln e. V. 📖 124
MS Rotterdam 📖 157
MSC Amsterdam 📖 152
MSC Barcelona 📖 172
MSC Belgium 📖 37
MSC Berlin e.V. 📖 110
MSC Black Angels Köln 📖 108
MSC Finland 📖 95
MSC Hamburg e. V. 📖 120
MSC Iceland 📖 136
MSC London 📖 83
MSC Madrid 📖 172
MSC Rhein-Main, Frankfurt 📖 135
MSC Rote Erde Dortmund 📖 114
MSC Scotland 📖 168
MSC Südwest 📖 117
MSC Suisse Romande 📖 178
MSC Viking 📖 124
Pacific Bears California LMC 📖 215
Pacific Coast MC 📖 204
Pegasus Motorcycle Owners Club 📖 215
Philadelphians MC 📖 330
Pittsburgh Motorcycle Club 📖 332
Potomac MC 📖 234
Rainbow MC 📖 215
Rangers MC 📖 28
Riders MC 📖 268
River City Outlaws 📖 344
Road Riders MC 📖 339
Rochester Rams MC 📖 311
Rocky Mountaineers MC 📖 228
Rodeo Riders 📖 250
Rurals MC 📖 157
Saber MC 📖 237
San Antonio Rough Riders 📖 342
Satyricons MC 📖 286
Satyrs MC 📖 204
Scandinavian Leather Men 📖 174
Severn Links 📖 90
SLM 📖 *See* Scandinavian Leather Men
SMC 📖 *See* Zentralschweizer Schwulen-Motorrad-Club
South Pacific MC 📖 26
Southern Region Motor Club 📖 30
Spartan MC 📖 263
Spartans MC 📖 335
SRMC 📖 *See* Southern Region Motor Club
STARS MC 📖 296
Sunrays MC 📖 237
Sussex Lancers MSC 📖 74
Tejas MC 📖 344
Tennklubben 📖 165
Texas Cadre 📖 338
Texas MC 📖 340
Texas Riders, Inc. 📖 343
Trident 📖 50, 204, 236, 252, 264, 265, 273, 275, 304, 311, 319, 320, 322, 333
Trident International DC Hall, Inc. 📖 265
Unicorn MC 📖 319
Utica Tri's, MC 📖 312
Vanguards MC 📖 330
Vikings MC 📖 268
Warlocks MC 📖 215
Warriors MC 📖 204
Wheels MC 📖 304
Zentralschweizer Schwulen-Motorrad-Club 📖 178

Lesbian
Women's Motorcycle Contingent 📖 215

Lesbian, Gay, Bi, & Transgendered
Mercury Morocycle Club 📖 159
Motorcycle Sports Club 📖 171
Open Road Riders of Chicagoland 📖 250
Riverboat Gamblers Motorcycle Club 📖 337

Male
Iron Guard BC NYC 📖 304

PENIS SIZE

Gay
Nine Plus Club, Inc. 📖 304

Heterosexual, Female
Hung Jury 📖 204

PIERCING

All Sexes & Sexualities
Association of Professional Piercers 📖 215
Canadian Association of Body Arts 📖 41
IPS 📖 175
Stainless Steel Ball 📖 13

Lesbian, Gay, Bi, & Transgendered
Tyger Tyger 📖 83

POLYFIDELITY

All Sexes & Sexualities
Abundant Love Institute 📖 246
Alternatives to Monogamy 📖 253
Beyond Monogamy, Inc. 📖 33
Church of All Worlds 📖 223
Delaware Valley Synergy 📖 328
Erisian Fields Cohousing 📖 325
Family Synergy 📖 198
Family Tree 📖 268
Glendower 📖 283
Group Marriage Alliance 📖 324
Live The Dream 📖 224
Loving Alternatives 📖 254, 333
Potomac Area Lifestyles 📖 264
Potomac Area Polyamory Network 📖 266
Saint Louis Lifestyles 📖 284
South Bay Intinet 📖 223
South Florida Polyamorists 📖 235
Tender Loving Couples 📖 232
Touchpoint Network for the Non-Monogamous 📖 193
Tri-State Polyamory 📖 292

PUBLISHING

All Sexes & Sexualities
Canadian Book Marketing Centre 📖 57
COSMEP 📖 215

Lesbian, Gay, Bi, & Transgendered
Book Marketing Council 📖 83

RESEARCH

Sexuality

All Sexes & Sexualities
Center for Research & Education in Sexuality 📖 215
Kinsey Institute 📖 253
Mariposa Education & Research Foundation 📖 223

Gay
Project Sigma 📖 83

Lesbian, Gay, Bi, & Transgendered
Gay & Lesbian Advocacy Research Project 📖 335
National Council for Research on Women 📖 304
New Era Institute 📖 357
Sexuallberatungsstelle der Abteilung für Sexualforschung 📖 120
VEHN 📖 *See* Verein zur Erforschung der Geschichte der Homosexuellen in Niedersachsen
Verein zur Erforschung der Geschichte der Homosexuellen in Niedersachsen 📖 121
Verein zur Förderung der Erforschung der Geschichte der Homosexuellen in Nordrhein-Westfalen 📖 124

SCAT

Gay
Jack's Number Two 📖 188
Martifoto 📖 13

SEXUAL POLITICS

All Sexes & Sexualities
American Civil Liberties Union 📖 304
Bar Association for Human Rights 📖 188
Committee to Preserve Sexual Liberties 📖 215
Countdown on Spanner 📖 69
Libertarian Alliance 📖 83
Liberty 📖 83
National Campaign for Freedom of Expression 📖 352
National Campaign for Reform of the Obscene Publications Acts 📖 83
Spanner Trust 📖 13
V. V. S. M. 📖 38

Female
Feminists Against Censorship 📖 83
National Organization for Women, Inc. 📖 234

Gay
National Center for Lesbian Rights 📖 188

Lesbian
Lesbian Mother's Defense National Fund 📖 352
National Center for Lesbian Rights 📖 188

Lesbian, Gay, Bi, & Transgendered
Arbeitsgemeinschaft Homosexualität Magnus 📖 129
Coalition for Lesbian & Gay Rights in Ontario 📖 49
Gay & Lesbian Americans 📖 234
Gays & Lesbians Awareness Civil Rights Committee 📖 43
IGLHRC 📖 *See* International Gay & Lesbian Human Rights Commission
International Gay & Lesbian Human Rights Commission 📖 215
Lesbian & Gay Freedom Movement 📖 83
Lesbian & Gay Rights Resource Centre 📖 159
National Gay & Lesbian Task Force 📖 234
Right to Privacy, Inc. 📖 326
Tulsa Oklahomans for Human Rights 📖 324
Virginians for Justice 📖 349

Male
National Organization to Halt the Abuse & Routine Mutilation of Males 📖 215
NOHARMM 📖 *See* National Organization to Halt the Abuse & Routine Mutilation of Males

Transgender
TLC 📖 *See* Transgender Liberation Coalition
Transgender Liberation Coalition 📖 26
Transgender Rights 📖 304

SEXUALITY

All Sexes & Sexualities
519 Church Street Community Centre 📖 57
Brian Coyle Community Center 📖 280
Coalition of Sexuality Organizations 📖 231
EroSpirit Research Institute 📖 207
Film @ Eleven 📖 215
Hush-A-Bye Baby Club 📖 78
INSA 📖 *See* Intersex Society of North America
International Sexual Minorities Information Resource 📖 13
Intersex Society of North America 📖 50
ISMIR 📖 *See* International Sexual Minorities Information Resource
Lavendar & Lace 📖 305
Lesbian & Gay Concerns Network 📖 310
LGCN 📖 *See* Lesbian & Gay Concerns Network
Loft Lesbian & Gay Community Services Center, Inc. 📖 305
Martijn 📖 150
National Coming Out Day 📖 234
National Organization of Circumcision Information Resource Centers 📖 210
National Organization of Sexual Enthusiasts 📖 244
Nederlandse Vereniging voor Sexuele Hervorming 📖 150
New Zealand Prostitutes Collective 📖 160, 163
NOCIRC 📖 *See* National Organization of Circumcision Information Resource Centers
NOSE 📖 *See* National Organization of Sexual Enthusiasts
NSS Seminars, Inc. 📖 196
NVSH 📖 *See* Nederlandse Vereniging voor Sexuele Hervorming
Parents & Friends of Lesbians & Gays 📖 222, 256
PFLAG 📖 *See* Parents & Friends of Lesbians & Gays
QRC 📖 *See* Queer Resource Center
Queer Resource Center 📖 197
Red Rock Mental Health Center 📖 323
Review 📖 253
Sexual Minorities Alligned for Community, Education, & Support 📖 296
Significant Other Support 📖 341
Skinnydippers 📖 312
SM Aces 📖 *See* Sexual Minorities Alligned for Community, Education, & Support
Sunrise Center 📖 198
TAKOTS 📖 *See* Teenage Kids of Ts
Teenage Kids of Ts 📖 226
TGIC 📖 *See* Transgenderists' Independence Club
Transequal 📖 49
Transgenderists' Independence Club 📖 296
Valley Woman Books & Gifts 📖 200
WOBS 📖 *See* Women of the Beaumont Society
Women of the Beaumont Society 📖 83

Bisexual
Adelaide Bisexual Collective 📖 30
Auckland Bisexual Group 📖 160
Australian Bisexual Network 📖 28
BARN 📖 *See* Bisexual Atlanta Resource Center
Bay Area Bisexual Network 📖 215
Bi Chicago 📖 250
Bi Face 📖 45
Bi's R Us 📖 61
Bi? Shy? Why? 📖 356
BiAtlanta 📖 244
BiCentrist Alliance 📖 234
Bi-Lines 📖 320
BiNet 📖 226, 265, 324, 340, 352, 357
Birmingham Bi Women's Group 📖 92
Bisexual Atlanta Resource Center 📖 244
Bisexual Community Resource Center 📖 268
Bisexual Connection 📖 280
Bisexual Resource Centre 📖 168
Bisexual Support Group 📖 219, 357
Bisexual Support Service 📖 202
Bisexual Women of Color Group 📖 304

Organizations: Sexuality

Bisexual Women's Group 333
Bisexual Women's Support Group 319
Bisexuals in Oxford 90
Bisexuellengruppe 113
BiUnity 330
Biversity Boston 268
Bi-Ways 234
Brisbane Bisexual Centre 28
Champaign-Urbana Bisexual Network 248
East Coast Bisexual Network 268
LGB *See* London Bisexual Group
LGBSA *See* Bisexual Women's Group
LNBi *See* Vereniging Landelijk Netwerk voor Bisexualiteit
London Bisexual Group 83
Memphis Bisexual Alliance 337
New York Bisexual Network 305
North East Bi Group 92
Nottingham Women's Bi Group 89
Options Bisexual Group 45
Preston Bisexual Group 79
Queensland Bisexual Network 29
Richmond Area Bisexual Network 349
ROBIN *See* Richmond Area Bisexual Network
SBSN *See* Sydney Bisexual Support Network
Seattle Bisexual Men's Union 352
Seattle Bisexual Women's Network 352
Sheffield Bisexual Women's Group 90
South Australia Bisexual Network 30
Stichting Bisexualiteit Nederland 152
Stichting Werkgroep Biseksualiteit 152, 154
Sydney Bisexual Support Network 26
Toronto Bisexual Network 57
Valdosta State College Gay & Lesbian Association 246
Vereniging Landelijk Netwerk voor Bisexualiteit 150

Female

Boston Bisexual Women's Network 268
Burlington Women's Council 346
Dornrosa - Frauenselbsthilfe e. V. 119
Idaho Women's Network 247
SCWC *See* South Carolina Women's Consortium
South Carolina Women's Consortium 334

Gay

Act-HIV 179
Baltimore Lambda Alliance of the Deaf 264
Bisexual & Married Gay Men 319
Black & White Men Together 239, 250, 255, 259, 264, 268, 275, 304, 314, 315, 319, 320, 322, 332, 337, 340, 357
BWMT *See* Black & White Men Together
Capitol Men's Club 277
Cicolo Di Cultura Omosexxuale Mario Mieli 141
Coming Out / Being Out Group 228
Coming Out Group 26
Evansdale Men's Support Group 256
For'Hommes 98
Frontiers 356
Gamma Line 32
Gay Fathers 26
Gay Men of the Bronx 305
Gay Men's Alliance of Hudson Valley 305
Gay Men's Community Project 326
Gay Men's Support Group 295
Gay Naturists International 13
Gay Skinhead Group 91
Gays South of Lake Street 280
Gays, Lesbian, & Bisexuals of North Bay Area 52
GLB NBA *See* Gays, Lesbian, & Bisexuals of North Bay Area
GNI *See* Gay Naturists International
Hibiscus Coast Men's Support Group 160
Homosexuelle Initiative 35
HOSI *See* Homosexuelle Initiative
J/OE 264
Krewe of Apollo de Lafayette 260
Long Island Gay Men's Group 305
Long Island Gay Men's Social Group 305
Loving Brotherhood 293
Madison Wrestling Club 356
Married Men's Group 314
Men's Coming Out Group 228
Men's Gay & Bisexual Coming Out Group 28
Men's Rap Group 294
Men's Support Group 284
MGM *See* Monadnock Gay Men. *See also* Mutal Gay Mens' Support Group
Midwest Men's Center, Chicago 250
Monadnock Gay Men 288
Mountain Valley Men 287
Mpowerment Project 324
Mutal Gay Mens' Support Group 160
NAMBLA *See* North American Man Boy Love Association
Nederlandse Vereniging voor Sexuele Hervorming 152
Network of Rhode Island 334
North American Man Boy Love Association 215, 305
North Woods Radical Faerie Circle 280
Northland Gay Men's Center 280
Norwich Gay Men's Health Project 88
NVSH *See* Nederlandse Vereniging voor Sexuele Hervorming
Peer Support Program 228
Pink Cross 177
Prevention Auckland 160
SAG *See* Seacoast Gay Men
SAM *See* Social Alternative for Gay Men
SchwIM *See* Schwule Initiative Minden
Schwule Initiative Minden 127
Schwule Väter 128
Seacoast Gay Men 288
Social Alternative for Gay Men 346
Spectrum 162
Uncut Dallas 341

Heterosexual, Female

Tiffany Club Wives' Support Group 273

Lesbian

ALSO *See* Alternative Lifestyle Support Organization
Alternative Lifestyle Support Organization 348
Always On Sunday 291
Ambitious Amazons / Lesbian Center 277
Aurora, A Northland Lesbian Center 279
Between Ourselves 316
Brazos Valley Women's Group 339
Butch / Femme Network 225
CDM 143
Colectivo de Lesbianas Feministas 167
Coordinamento Lesbische Italiano 141
Dawn 347
Dykes Night Out 169
EVE Fund 215
Every Woman's Coming Out Group 228
Feminine Connection 292
GLWA *See* Lesbian Alliance
Insight 357
Lakes - Mountains Coinnection 287
Last Sunday 334
Lavendar Network 325
Lavendar Triangle 322
LCDC *See* Lesbian Community of Delaware County
Lehigh Valley Lesbians 329
Lesbewell 93
Lesbian Alliance 277
Lesbian Centre 45
Lesbian Coalition 160
Lesbian Community of Delaware County 330
Lesbian Connection 226
Lesbian Fun Society 350
Lesbian Line 163
Lesbian Network 30
Lesbian Support 160
Lesbian Support Group 161, 247
Lesbian Support Rap Group 294
MAW *See* Monadnock Area Womyn
Merrimack Valley Lesbians 271
MLC *See* Montana Lesbian Coalition
Momazons 320
Monadnock Area Womyn 288
Montana Lesbian Coalition 285
New York Femmes 305
NH Lambda 287
Northern Voice 287
Open Arms 255
Out & About 288
Out Among Friends 262
Out For Good 262
Sabra Lesbian Coalition 294
SALO *See* Springfield Area Lesbian Outreach
Shades of Lavendar 297
Shared Times 271
Springfield Area Lesbian Outreach 253
Together At Last Lesbians 354
Triangle Interests 330
Tuscaloosa Lesbian Coalition 192
Upstate Women's Community 335
Visibilia 140
West of Boston Lesbians 271
Wishing Well 222
Wobbles *See* West of Boston Lesbians
Women of the Woods 346
Women United of Nevada 286
Women's Studies 280
WOW *See* Women of the Woods
WOW! 314

Lesbian, Gay, Bi, & Transgendered

Aberdeen LesBiGay Society 168
ABOP Homogroep 156
Abva 155
Acceuil Rencontre Information Service 101
Adirondack GALA 311
Affirmations Lesbian & Gay Community Center 275
AGALA *See* Auburn Gay & Lesbian Association
AGG 168
AGT *See* Associazione Gay Ticino
AHO *See* Aktionsgruppe Homosexualität Osnabrück e. V.
AIDS Shelter Coalition of Manitoba 47
Aktionsgruppe Homosexualität Hannover 121
Aktionsgruppe Homosexualität Osnabrück e. V. 130
Albert Lea Lesbian & Gay Outreach 279
Alliance of Cache Valley 345
Alliance of Lesbian & Gay Organizations of Western Virginia 347
Alternate Lifestyle Alliance of Olaca 240
Alternative Lifestyles Fellowship 288
American College Personnel Association 250
Amigo Kerho 56 97
Andere Kant 37
Andersrum 129
Another Side 324
Aoraki Lesbian & Gay Group 163
Arci Gay 138, 139, 140, 141, 142, 143, 144, 145, 146, 147
Arci Gay e Lesbica 140, 144, 145
ARIS *See* Acceuil Rencontre Information Service
Arlington Gay & Lesbian Alliance 347
Armidale Gay Society 25
Aspen Gay & Lesbian Community 226
Association Gais & Lesbiennes à Liège 38
Association of Lesbians & Gays of Ottawa 52
Associazione Gay Ticino 178
ASTA - Schwulen & Lesbenferat 109
Atlanta Gay Center 244
Attika 144
Auburn Gay & Lesbian Association 191
Auckland Gay & Lesbian Community Centre 159
Auckland Gay & Lesbian Trust 160
Automones Schwulenreferat im AStA 118
BAGAL *See* Brattleboro Area Gays & Lesbians
Basta *See* Stichting Trefcentrum HIG - COC
Begegnungs- & Beratungs-Zentrum lebensart e. V. 119
Bendigo Gay Society, Inc. 31
BiSchoF e. V. 118
Black Lesbian & Gay Centre 83
Blenheim Gay / Lesbian Contact 161
Border Area Lesbian & Gay Group 136
BoSchwul 112
Boston Lesbian & Gay Community Center 268
Both Sides Now 246
Brattleboro Area Gays & Lesbians 346
Bridges 304, 328
BU GLASS 47
BULGA *See* Bulgarian Lesbian & Gay Association
Bulgarian Lesbian & Gay Association 40
Bundaberg Gay & Lesbian Support 29
Büro für Gleichgeschlectliche Lebensfragen in Land Brandenburg 131
BVH - Bundesverband Homosexualität e. V. 108
BVH e. V. - Dortmund 114
Caithness Gay, Bisexual, & Lesbian Connexion 168
Capital District Lesbian & Gay Community Center 296
Caritasverband Beratung Homosexueller Männer & AIDS Beratung 126
Center 286, 335
Center for Lesbian & Gay Community Services 337
Central Jersey Alliance of Gay, Lesbian, & Bisexual People 292
Central Vermont Gay Liberation 346
Centre Gai & Lesbien 103
Centro d'Iniziativa Gay 143
Centro de Informacion y Documentacion de las Homosexualidades en Mexico Celectivo Sol, A. C. 149
CGL *See* Centre Gai & Lesbien
Checkpoint 124
Chiltern Mountain Club 268
CIDHOM *See* Centro de Informacion y Documentacion de las Homosexualidades en Mexico Celectivo Sol, A. C.
Clonmel Gay Group 138
Clovis/Portales Common Bond 294
Club 30 171
Club für Gleichgeschlechtilch Liebende e. V. 117
Coalition 335
COC 150, 151, 152, 154, 155, 156, 157, 158, 159
Colectivo Masiorare 149
Combined Forces 322
Coming Our Gruppe 118
Coming Out Collective 283
Communidad Triangulo Rosa 149
Communita Gay della Svizzera Italiana 179
Community Center 247
Community Outreach Program 48
Cronulla Gay Group 26
CTR *See* Communidad Triangulo Rosa
CVGL *See* Central Vermont Gay Liberation
DAG/LC *See* Detroit Area Gay / Lesbian Council
Dallas Gay & Lesbian Alliance 340
Delaware Valley Gay Neighbors 289
Delftse Werkgroep Homosexualiteit 154
DELGO *See* Downeast Lesbian & Gay Organization
Detroit Area Gay / Lesbian Council 275
Digital Queers 215
Dinos 135
Dorchester Gay & Lesbian Alliance 268
Downeast Lesbian & Gay Organization 262
Edinburgh College of Art L&G Society 169
Edinburgh LGB Centre 169
EGG *See* English-Speaking Gay Group
Ehe-Familien-Jungend & Schwulenberatung 122
Elmwood Park / Cottontown Lesbian & Gay Neighborhood Association 335
Emanzipation e. V. 117
English-Speaking Gay Group 36
Eros Center 141

Erotheek 🕮 155
EZS 🕮 See Lesben & Schwulen Zentrum Saar
Fairfax Lesbian & Gay Citizens Association 🕮 348
Felix Halle 🕮 135
First City Network, Inc. 🕮 246
Flamands Roses 🕮 100
Flensburger Initiative & Treffpunkt für Schwule 🕮 117
FLGCA 🕮 See Fairfax Lesbian & Gay Citizens Association
Fliederlich e. V. 🕮 129
Fox Valley Gay Association 🕮 250
Friends Club 🕮 173
Friends North 🕮 278
Fruits of Our Labors 🕮 261
Fürsorger für Homosexuelle im Caritas Verband 🕮 111
G/L/B Support Group 🕮 320
GAB 🕮 See Gay Advice Bureau
GACH 🕮 See Gelders Advies Centrum Homosexualiteit
Gaeilgeori Aerach Aontaithe 🕮 136
GAI 🕮 See Gai Amitié Initiative
Gai Amitié Initiative 🕮 102
GALA 🕮 See Dorchester Gay & Lesbian Alliance. See also Gay & Lesbian Association. See also Hamilton Gay & Lesbian Alliance. See also Stichting Gay & Lesbian Association Amsterdam
GALOHI 🕮 See Gay & Lesbians of Hawaii Island
GALON 🕮 See Gay & Lesbian Outreach Network
GALS 🕮 See Gay & Lesbian Support
GASA 🕮 See Gay Association of South Africa
Gay & Lesbian Alliance 🕮 231, 242, 262, 312
Gay & Lesbian Alliance at Brooklyn College 🕮 297
Gay & Lesbian Alliance in Orange County 🕮 305
Gay & Lesbian Alliance of Central Texas 🕮 345
Gay & Lesbian Alliance of Greater Danbury 🕮 230
Gay & Lesbian Alliance of Syracuse 🕮 312
Gay & Lesbian Alliance of Ventura County 🕮 224
Gay & Lesbian Association 🕮 350
Gay & Lesbian Association of Central Alberta 🕮 44
Gay & Lesbian Association of Durango 🕮 229
Gay & Lesbian Association of Simcoe County 🕮 52
Gay & Lesbian Association, San Joaquin County 🕮 223
Gay & Lesbian Center, Island Empire 🕮 210
Gay & Lesbian Centre 🕮 45, 62
Gay & Lesbian Community 🕮 193
Gay & Lesbian Community Center 🕮 236, 247, 264, 304
Gay & Lesbian Community Center of Chicago 🕮 250
Gay & Lesbian Community Center of Colorado, Inc. 🕮 228
Gay & Lesbian Community Center of Pittsburgh 🕮 332
Gay & Lesbian Community Centre of Edmonton 🕮 43
Gay & Lesbian Community Council of Utah 🕮 345
Gay & Lesbian Community of Howard County 🕮 265
Gay & Lesbian Community Services 🕮 281, 282
Gay & Lesbian Community Services Center 🕮 204
Gay & Lesbian Community Services Center of Orange County 🕮 200
Gay & Lesbian Counselling & Information Service 🕮 29
Gay & Lesbian Counselling Service of New South Wales 🕮 26
Gay & Lesbian Counselling Service of South Australia 🕮 30
Gay & Lesbian Equality Network 🕮 136
Gay & Lesbian Network 🕮 262
Gay & Lesbian Organization of Reading & Allentown 🕮 329
Gay & Lesbian Outreach Network 🕮 324, 325
Gay & Lesbian Resource Center 🕮 221, 256
Gay & Lesbian Resource Center of Ventura County 🕮 224
Gay & Lesbian Services Network 🕮 283
Gay & Lesbian Support 🕮 310
Gay & Lesbian Support Group 🕮 355
Gay & Lesbian Union of Racine / Kenosha 🕮 358
Gay & Lesbian Welfare, Auckland 🕮 159
Gay & Lesbians of Hawaii Island 🕮 246
Gay Advice Bureau 🕮 171, 172
Gay Alliance 🕮 170
Gay Alliance, Genesee Valley 🕮 311
Gay Association Inland Natal 🕮 171
Gay Association of South Africa 🕮 171, 172
Gay Boys on Campus 🕮 161
Gay Capital Events 🕮 152
Gay Club Hawkes Bay 🕮 162
Gay Group Bloemfontein 🕮 171
Gay Information Mississauga 🕮 51
Gay Liberation Forum Baden-Baden 🕮 118
Gay People of Laurel 🕮 265
Gay People Princeton 🕮 292
Gay Positive Buffalo 🕮 298
Gay Service Network 🕮 338
Gay's Innung 🕮 122
Gay, Lesbian, & Bisexual Activities 🕮 279
Gay, Lesbian, & Bisexual Alliance League 🕮 317
Gay, Lesbian, & Bisexual Community Center 🕮 231
Gay, Lesbian, Bisexual Alliance of Goddard 🕮 346
Gay, Lesbians, & Bisexuals of Skagit 🕮 350
Gayline 🕮 29
Gaymen & Lesbians in Brookhaven 🕮 305
Gays & Lesbians Everywhere in Education 🕮 160
Gays & Lesbians of Watertown 🕮 268
Gays, Lesbians, & Bisexuals of Ames 🕮 256
Gaystudenterna 🕮 174
Gelders Advies Centrum Homosexualiteit 🕮 157
Gelsenkirchen Lesben- & Schwulenintiative 🕮 118
GGG 🕮 See Group Gai Guyanais
GGS 🕮 See Gisborne Gay Support
GHEM 🕮 See Groupe Homo pour l'Expression des Minorités
Gisborne Gay Support 🕮 162
GL 🕮 See Club für Gleichgeschlechtilch Liebende e. V.
GL Friendly 🕮 282
GLA-CV 🕮 See Alliance of Cache Valley
GLAD 🕮 170
GLAS 🕮 See Gay & Lesbian Alliance of Syracuse
GLBA 🕮 See Gays, Lesbians, & Bisexuals of Ames. See also Wesleyan Gay, Lesbian, & Bisexual Alliance
GLBC, University of Miami 🕮 239
GLBS 🕮 See Gay, Lesbians, & Bisexuals of Skagit
GLC 🕮 See Gay & Lesbian Community
GLEE 🕮 See Gays & Lesbians Everywhere in Education
GLEN 🕮 See Gay & Lesbian Equality Network
GLIB 🕮 See Gaymen & Lesbians in Brookhaven
GLNCI / North Central Iowa 🕮 257
GLOBAL 🕮 See Gay, Lesbian, & Bisexual Alliance League
GLORA 🕮 See Gay & Lesbian Organization of Reading & Allentown
GLOW 🕮 See Gays & Lesbians of Watertown
GOHL 🕮 See Grupo Orgullo Homosexual de Liberación
GOLBA 🕮 See Greeley Gay, Lesbian, & Bisexual Alliance
Görlitzer Homosexuelleninitiative 🕮 118
Goulburn Valley Gay Group 🕮 32
Governor's Office of Lesbian & Gay Concerns 🕮 295
Greater Cincinnati Gay / Lesbian Coalition 🕮 318
Greater Utica Lambda Fellowship 🕮 312
Greeley Gay, Lesbian, & Bisexual Alliance 🕮 229
Greenwich Lesbian & Gay Centre 🕮 83
Group Gai Guyanais 🕮 106
Groupe Action Gai 🕮 102
Groupe Homo pour l'Expression des Minorités 🕮 100
Grupo Neuróticos Anónimos Gay 🕮 149
Grupo Nueva Generación 🕮 149
Grupo Orgullo Homosexual de Liberación 🕮 149
Guelph Gay, Lesbian, & Bisexual Equality 🕮 50
HAI 🕮 See Homosexuelle Aktion Ilmenau
HALO 🕮 See Homophile Association of London Ontario Inc.
HALT 🕮 See Homosexuelle Alternative
HALU 🕮 See Homosexuelle Arbeitsgruppe Luzern
Hamilton Gay & Lesbian Alliance 🕮 50
Hannchen Mehrzweck Stiftung für Homosexuelle Selbsthilfe 🕮 108
HASG 🕮 See Homosexuelle Arbeitsgruppe Saint Gallen
HASO 🕮 See Homosexuelle Arbeitsgruppe
HAZ 🕮 See Homosexuelle Arbeitsgruppen Zürich
Heh! 🕮 See Homosexuelle Emanzipationsgruppe
HELB 🕮 See Homosexuelle Emanzipationsgruppe
Het Roze Haagje 🕮 156
HIA 🕮 See Homosexuelle Initiative Aalen
HIE 🕮 See Homosexuelle Initiative Essen
HIGH 🕮 See Homosexuelle Interessengruppe Hagen
HIL 🕮 See Homosexuelle Initiative Lübeck
HIMS 🕮 See Homosexuelle Initiative im Märkischen Sauerland
HIN 🕮 See Homosexuelle Initiative Neumünster
HIOB 🕮 See Homosexuelle Informationsgruppe Ortenau / Baden
HIP 🕮 See Homosexuelle Initiative Passau. See also Homosexuelles Integrationsprojekt Potsdam
HOME 🕮 See Homosexuelle Emanzitpation Gruppe
HOME Zentrum 🕮 121
Homo- en Lesbiennegroep Gehoor 🕮 38
Homo- Lesbiennewerking 🕮 38
Homocentrum Laakdal en Omstreken 🕮 39
Homofil Bevegelse 🕮 165, 166
Homofile Bevegelse 🕮 165
Homogroep Uithoorn 🕮 158
Homogroep Wageningen 🕮 159
Homogruppe Thürmsdorf 🕮 134
Homologay 🕮 178
Homophile Association of London Ontario Inc. 🕮 51
Homosaïque 🕮 102
Homosexuelle Aktion Ilmenau 🕮 122
Homosexuelle Alternative 🕮 128
Homosexuelle Arbeitsgruppe 🕮 179
Homosexuelle Arbeitsgruppe Luzern 🕮 178
Homosexuelle Arbeitsgruppe Saint Gallen 🕮 179
Homosexuelle Arbeitsgruppen 🕮 177
Homosexuelle Arbeitsgruppen Zürich 🕮 180
Homosexuelle Emanzipationsgruppe 🕮 111, 121, 122
Homosexuelle Emanzitpation Gruppe 🕮 121
Homosexuelle Informationsgruppe Ortenau / Baden 🕮 125
Homosexuelle Initiative 🕮 34, 35
Homosexuelle Initiative Aalen 🕮 109
Homosexuelle Initiative Essen 🕮 116
Homosexuelle Initiative im Märkischen Sauerland 🕮 126
Homosexuelle Initiative Konstanz 🕮 125
Homosexuelle Initiative Lübeck 🕮 126
Homosexuelle Initiative Neumünster 🕮 129
Homosexuelle Initiative Passau 🕮 131
Homosexuelle Inititivgruppe & Freunde 🕮 112
Homosexuelle Interessengemeinschaft Unterfranken Warum 🕮 123
Homosexuelle Interessengruppe Hagen 🕮 119
Homosexuelle Kultur Duisburg 🕮 115
Homosexuelle Organisation Thurgau 🕮 178
Homosexuelle Selbshilfe 🕮 112
Homosexuelle Selbsthilfe 🕮 134
Homosexuelle Selbsthilfe e. V. 🕮 108
Homosexuellenberatung in Bartaungs- & Seelsorgenzentrum St. Petri 🕮 120
Homosexuelles Integrationsprojekt Potsdam 🕮 131
Homostudies Utrecht 🕮 158
Homosum 🕮 154
Horizons Community Services, Inc. 🕮 250
HOSI 🕮 See Homosexuelle Initiative
HOT 🕮 See Homosexuelle Organisation Thurgau
HSH 🕮 See Aktionsgruppe Homosexualität Hannover
Huch! Schwulen- & Lesben-Zentrum 🕮 123
HUGS East 🕮 See Mentor Center
Human-Nature & Postorder AEV 🕮 156
IGLAB 🕮 See Ithaca Gay & Lesbian Activities Board
IHBa 🕮 See Initiative Homosexualität Bamberg
IHS 🕮 See Initiativgruppe Homosexualität Stuttgart e. V.
IHT 🕮 See Innitiativgruppe Homosexualität Tübingen
ILGA 🕮 See International Lesbian & Gay Association
Infor Homo 🕮 37
Informationszentrum für Männer 🕮 117
Initiative Homosexualität Bamberg 🕮 109
Initiativgruppe Homosexualität Stuttgart e. V. 🕮 133
Inland Northwest Gay People's Alliance 🕮 247
Innitiativgruppe Homosexualität Tübingen 🕮 134
Insel 🕮 122
Instituto Lambda 🕮 172
International Gay & Lesbian Association 🕮 108
International Lesbian & Gay Association 🕮 158
International Wavelength, Inc. 🕮 215
Island Gay Community Centre 🕮 47
Island Lesbian & Gay Association 🕮 272
Ithaca Gay & Lesbian Activities Board 🕮 299
Ithaca Lesbian, Gay, & Bisexual Task Force 🕮 299
Jackson GALA 🕮 358
Jersey Shore Gay & Lesbian Community Center 🕮 289
Jungendnetzwerk Lambda Niedersachsen e. V. 🕮 112
Kalamazoo Gay / Lesbian Center 🕮 276
KCM 🕮 See Schwulen- & Lesbenzentrum Münster
Kentucky Gay & Lesbian Educational Center 🕮 258
Kindred Spirits 🕮 347
Kingston Lesbian, Gay, & Bisexual Association 🕮 50
Klamath Area Lambda Association 🕮 325
Klick, Schwulengruppe Zürich Oberland 🕮 178
Klub A-3 e. V. - Anders als Andere 🕮 126
Klub Einblick e. V. 🕮 132
Kringen 🕮 155, 157
Kringen, Regio Amerfoort 🕮 156
Lambda Alive 🕮 329
Lambda Association of Fayetteville 🕮 315
Lambda Association of Staten Island 🕮 305
Lambda Community Center 🕮 210, 229
Lambda Eastern Oregon Association 🕮 324
Lambda of Northeast Louisiana 🕮 260
Lambda Panhandlers 🕮 355
Lambda Resourcer Center 🕮 191
Lambda Support Group 🕮 322
Lancaster Lambda 🕮 328

Landsforeningen for Bøsser og Lesbiske 📖 65, 66
Landsforeningen for Lesbisk og Homofil Frigjøring 📖 164, 165, 166
Lavendar Heights 📖 305
LBL 📖 See Landsforeningen for Bøsser og Lesbiske
Lebensart e. V. 📖 114
Lehigh Valley Gay & Lesbian Task Force 📖 329
Leicester Lesbian & Gay Communities' Resource Centre 📖 79
Lesben- & Schwuengruppe Emden 📖 116
Lesben & Schwulen Zentrum Saar 📖 132
Lesbian & Gay Advisory Commission 📖 215
Lesbian & Gay Community Center of Greater Cleveland 📖 319
Lesbian & Gay Community Center of New Orleans 📖 261
Lesbian & Gay Community Network of Western Michigan 📖 276
Lesbian & Gay Men's Community Center 📖 211
Lesbian Gay Bi Association 📖 358
Lesbian, Gay, & Bisexual Community Center 📖 239
Lesbian, Gay, & Bisexual Support Group 📖 272
Lesbians & Gay MEn of New Brunswick 📖 291
Lesbische & Schwule Aktiongemeinschaft 📖 34
Lesch-Selbsthilfegruppe Lesben & Schwule 📖 115
Lexington Gay & Lesbian Services Organization 📖 259
Liverpool Bisexual & Married Gays Group 📖 87
LLH 📖 See Landsforeningen for Lesbisk og Homofil Frigjøring
Logos 📖 146
Lorain Lesbian & Gay Center 📖 321
Lothian LGYM 📖 169
Low Country Gay & Lesbian Information Alliance 📖 335
Lubbock Lesbian & Gay Alliance 📖 344
Lüneburger Schwulengruppe & Rosa Telefon 📖 126
Magnus Hirschfeld Centrum 📖 120
Magnus Hirschfeld Zentrum 📖 116
MALAGA 📖 See Mobile Area Lesbian & Gay Assembly
Manawatu Gay Rights Association Inc. 📖 163
Mandamus Society 📖 348
Man-to-Man Gay Information Centre 📖 152
Matlovich Society 📖 262
Mayor's Office for the Lesbian & Gay Community 📖 305
Memphis Gay & Lesbian Center 📖 337
Men Only Selbsthilfzentrum 📖 122
Mentor Center 📖 322
Metrolina Community Service Project 📖 314
MGLTF 📖 See Mississipi Gay & Lesbian Task Force
Middle Tennessee Gay & Lesbian Alliance 📖 336
Mississipi Gay & Lesbian Task Force 📖 282
Mississipi Phœnix Coalition, Inc. 📖 282
Mobile Area Lesbian & Gay Assembly 📖 192
Moray House College L&G Society 📖 169
More Than You Can Count 📖 291
Na Und e. V. 📖 130
Natal Gay Community 📖 171
National Gay & Lesbian Domestic Violence Victims' Network 📖 226
National Lesbian & Gay Federation 📖 136
NCW GALA 📖 See North Central Washington Gay & Lesbian Alliance
Neuer Freundeskreis Homosexueller 📖 123
New Jersey Lesbian & Gay Coalition 📖 289
New York State Division of Human Rights 📖 295
North Central Washington Gay & Lesbian Alliance 📖 354
North Shore Gay & Lesbian Alliance 📖 271
North Suburban Gay Association 📖 250
North West Gay Support 📖 31
North West Pennsylvania G & L Task Force 📖 333
Northern Ohio Coalition, Inc. 📖 319
Northern Virginia Pride, Inc. 📖 347
Northern Wisconsin Lambda Society 📖 358
NOSS 📖 See Núdeo de Orientção em Saude Social
Núdeo de Orientção em Saude Social 📖 39
NUS East of Scotland Area LGB Network 📖 169
Oasis Resources Center 📖 323
Ocean (County) Lesbian-Gay Alliance, Inc. 📖 289
Open Doors 📖 317
Oregon Gay & Lesbian Cultural Resource Center Task Force 📖 324
Organization for Gay Awareness 📖 289
Other Place 📖 137
Out & About 📖 168
Out & About Indiana 📖 253
Outcomers 📖 138
Outreach Rand 📖 171
Oxford Gay & Lesbian Centre 📖 90
Pacific Center 📖 197
PALS 📖 See People of Alternate Lifestyles
Partages 📖 103
Partners Task Force for Gay & Lesbian Couples 📖 188
People of Alternate Lifestyles 📖 53
Perth Lesbian & Gay Group 📖 170
Phi, Alpha, Gamma 📖 223
Philadelphia Lesbian & Gay Task Force 📖 330
Phœnix Rising 📖 326
Pianeta Viola 📖 142
Piedmont Triangle Society 📖 347
Pink Homo 📖 115
Pink Panther 📖 134
Pink Triangle Coalition 📖 328
Pink Triangle Group 📖 148
Poconos Action Lambda Society 📖 327
Point Gai 📖 103
Polk Gay & Lesbian Alliance 📖 238
Priarie Lesbian & Gay Community 📖 281
Pride in Life, Gays & Lesbians of Southeastern New Brunswick 📖 48
Pride, Inc. 📖 285
Prime Timers International 📖 344
Prince William Gay & Lesbian Association 📖 350
PTS 📖 See Piedmont Triangle Society
Q-GLU 📖 See Queens Gay & Lesbians United
Quad-City Society for Sexuality Education 📖 256
Queens Gay & Lesbians United 📖 305
Rådgivningstjenesten for Homofile 📖 166
RAGE 📖 See Rosa Aktionsgruppe Essen
RAGLC 📖 See Rutland Area Gay & Lesbian Connection
Rand Gay Organization 📖 171
Rat & Tat 📖 131
Rat & Tat Zentrum 📖 113
Referat für Schwule & Lesben 📖 131
Regensburger Schwulen & Lesben Initiative 📖 131
RESI 📖 See Regensburger Schwulen & Lesben Initiative
Resource Center 📖 344
RFSL 📖 See Riksförbundet för Sexuellt Likaberättigande
RGO 📖 See Rand Gay Organization
Riksförbundet för Sexuellt Likaberättigande 📖 173, 174, 175, 176
RLGA 📖 See Rockland Lesbian Gay Alliance
Robert Gordon University LGB Society 📖 168
Rockland Lesbian Gay Alliance 📖 305
Romeo & Julius 📖 122
Rosa Aktionsgruppe Essen 📖 116
Rosa Engel-SchwulLesbische Aktion Hamm 📖 120
Rosa Greif-Schwul-Lesbischer AK im Vorpommern e. V. 📖 118
Rosa Gruppe Arnsberg 📖 109
Rosa Hilfe 📖 117
Rosa Hilfe Schwalm-Alsfed 📖 132
Rosa Linse Leipzig 📖 125
Rosa Lüste 📖 135
Rosa Strippe e. V. 📖 112
RosaLinde 📖 127
Rosarote Panthe-Schwul-Lesbische Aktionegemeinschaft Steiermark 📖 34
Rutland Area Gay & Lesbian Connection 📖 346
SAD 📖 152
SAGA 📖 See Sudbury All Gay Alliance
SALGA 📖 See Southern Appalachian Lesbian & Gay Alliance
San Diego North County Gay & Lesbian Association 📖 211
Santa Cruz Lesbian, Gay, & Bisexual Community Center 📖 221
SAS 📖 See Schwule Aktion Südwest
SchAM 📖 See Schwule Aktion Mannheim e. V.
SchMIT-Z 📖 134
SchulZ 📖 See Schwulen- & Lesben-Zentrum
SCHWARM 📖 See Schwule Arbeitsgruppe Minden
Schweizerische Organisation Homosexuellen 📖 180
Schwugs! 📖 See Schwulengruppe Suhl
Schwuguntia - Verein zur Förderung Sozialer & Kulturelle Interessen e. V. 📖 126
Schwul & Lesben in Plauen 📖 131
Schwul in Eisenach 📖 115
Schwul in Paderborn 📖 131
Schwule Aktion Lübeck 📖 126
Schwule Aktion Mannheim e. V. 📖 127
Schwule Aktion Südwest 📖 133
Schwule Akzeptanz Gera 📖 118
Schwule an der Christian Albrecht Universität 📖 123
Schwule Arbeitsgruppe Minden 📖 127
Schwule Coming Out Gruppe 📖 130
Schwule Gruppe Germersheim 📖 118
Schwule Gruppe Oberberg 📖 119
Schwule Gruppe Witten 📖 135
Schwule Gruppe Wupperthal 📖 135
Schwule Hilfe Göttingen 📖 118
Schwule im Westerwald 📖 109
Schwule in der AIDS-Hilfe 📖 109
Schwule Initiativ Gruppe Mülheim And der Ruhr 📖 127
Schwule Initiative 📖 113
Schwule Initiative Gladbeck 📖 118
Schwule Initiative Rheingau 📖 135
Schwule Initiative Siegen 📖 132
Schwule Internationale Berlin e. V. 📖 110
Schwule-Lesbische Unigruppe 📖 177
Schwulen & Lesben Zentrum 📖 112
Schwulen- & Lesben-Zentrum 📖 124
Schwulen- & Lesbenzentrum Münster 📖 128
Schwulen Selbsthilfegruppe 📖 130
Schwulenforum Trier 📖 134
Schwulengruppe Biedenkopf 📖 127
Schwulengruppe Darmstadt 📖 114
Schwulengruppe Düsseldorf 📖 115
Schwulengruppe Elmshorn 📖 116
Schwulengruppe Freudstadt 📖 117
Schwulengruppe HX/HOL 📖 122
Schwulengruppe Limburg / Weilburg 📖 125
Schwulengruppe Marburg 📖 127
Schwulengruppe Suhl 📖 134
Schwulengruppen 📖 116
Schwulengruppen Biedenkopf 📖 111
Schwulenreferat beim AStа der TU 📖 112
Schwulenzentrum Bochum 📖 112
Schwul-Lesbische Initiative Preetz 📖 131
Schwul-lesbische Jungendegruppe 📖 134
Schwül-lesbischer Stammtisch 📖 118
SchwUlm 📖 134
Schwusos 📖 134
SchwuZ-Schwules Zentrum 📖 123
Seksuaalinen Tasavertaisuus ry 📖 95, 96, 97
Selbsthilfegruppe Gießen 📖 118
Serhume 📖 149
Sesquehanna KONTACT 📖 327
SETA 📖 See Seksuaalinen Tasavertaisuus ry
SFHR 📖 175
SIAG 📖 See Schwule Akzeptanz Gera
SidAH 📖 See Schwule in der AIDS-Hilfe
SIGMAR 📖 See Schwule Initiativ Gruppe Mülheim And der Ruhr
SIR 📖 See Schwule Initiative Rheingau
SIS-ters 📖 See Schwule Initiative Siegen
SIW 📖 See Schwule im Westerwald
SLiP 📖 See Schwul & Lesben in Plauen
SLMA 📖 See Solano Lambda Men's Association
SLUG 📖 See Schwule-Lesbische Unigruppe
SNAP 📖 See Southern Nevada Association of Pride
SOH 📖 See Schweizerische Organisation Homosexuellen
Solano Lambda Men's Association 📖 199
Sonoma Bares of the Northwest 📖 350
Sons & Daughters 📖 335
South Bay Lesbian & Gay Community Center 📖 204
South East Alaska Gay & Lesbian Alliance 📖 193
South Shore Gay & Lesbian Alliance 📖 270
Southern Appalachian Lesbian & Gay Alliance 📖 313
Southern Nevada Association of Pride 📖 286
Southern Oregon Lambda Association 📖 324
Southland Social Group 📖 162
Spectrum 📖 210
Stanford Lesbian, Gay, & Bisexual Community Center 📖 222
Stichting Gay & Lesbian Association Amsterdam 📖 152
Stichting Gay Association 📖 157
Stichting Homo Groep Gemert 📖 155
Stichting Trefcentrum HIG - COC 📖 154
Stockholm Gay Center 📖 175
Stonewall Alliance of Chico 📖 198
Sudbury All Gay Alliance 📖 54
Susquehanna Lambda 📖 333
Tabasco 📖 146
TAGALA 📖 See Toledo Area Gay & Lesbian Affiliation
Takoma Park Lesbians & Gays 📖 264
Tauranga Gay Support Group 📖 163
Tayfriend 📖 170
TCC 📖 See Community Center
Teestube Schwuler Treff 📖 123
Terrace Gay Connection 📖 45
Tillamook County GALA 📖 326
Time Out 📖 262
Toledo Area Gay & Lesbian Affiliation 📖 322
Townsville Gay & Lesbian Resource & Information Network 📖 29
TPLAG 📖 See Takoma Park Lesbians & Gays
Triangle Foundation 📖 275
Triangle Lesbian & Gay Alliance 📖 314
Triborough Triangles 📖 267
Tri-Cities Gay & Lesbian Alliance 📖 274
Tri-State Alliance 📖 253
UGON 📖 See United Gay Organization of Namibia
United Gay Organization of Namibia 📖 149
Up The Stairs Community Center 📖 254
Utah Stonewall Center 📖 345
V. I. D. A. 📖 194
Valley Gay Alliance 📖 272
Verein für Lesben & Schwule 📖 119
Verein für Sexuelle Emanzipation e. V. 📖 112, 133
Verein für Sexuelle Gleichberechtigung e. V. 📖 128
Verein zur Verbesserung der Lebenssituation Homosexueller Frauen & Männer e. V. 📖 130
Vereinigung Homosexualität & Gesellschaft e. V. 📖 109
VHG 📖 See Vereinigung Homosexualität & Gesellschaft e. V.
VSE 📖 See Verein für Sexuelle Emanzipation e. V.
Waiheke Island Gay Support Group 📖 160
Welcome Wagon 📖 341
Werkgroep Gehuwde Homo's Lesbiennes en Partners 📖 39
Werkgroep Homofile Achterhoek 📖 154
Wesleyan Gay, Lesbian, & Bisexual Alliance 📖 231
West Suburban Gay Association 📖 252
WHP 📖 157
WHZ 📖 159

Wichita Gay & Lesbian Alliance 258
WIHG 155
Wingspan 195
Winnipeg Gay / Lesbian Resource Centre 47
Winterthur Schwule 179
WISCH See Winterthur Schwule
Worcester County Lesbian & Gay Alliance 273
WüHST See Würzburger Schwulengruppe
Würzburger Schwulengruppe 136
York Area Lambda 333
ZEH See Zentrale Erfassung Homosexuellendiskriminierung
Zentrale Erfassung Homosexuellendiskriminierung 108

Male

BFI Productions 208
Black & White Men Together 283
BWMT See Black & White Men Together
Men's Center 280
Pride & Unity for Male Prostitutes 159, 161, 163
PUMP See Pride & Unity for Male Prostitutes

Transgender

(SPICE) See Wives'/Partners' Concerns
3G See Grampian Gender Group
ABC See Association Beaumont Continental
Adam Society 273
After Surgery Support Exchange for Transexuals 270
AGAPE 340
AGE See Atlanta Gender Exploration
AGO See Alternative Gender-Oriented
Alaskan Tpeople 193
Alternative Gender-Oriented 314
American Transsexual Education Center 188
Androgyny 204
Animas 239
ASSET See After Surgery Support Exchange for Transexuals
Association Beaumont Continental 99
ATEC See American Transsexual Education Center
Atlanta Gender Exploration 244
Austin Second Image 338
Australia TransGenerist Support Association, Inc. 29
AXA 268
Beaumont Society 83
Beaumont Trust 83
Belfast Buttterfly Club 164
Benjamin 175
Berdache Society 192
Born Free 198
Boulton & Park Society 339
Boys Will Be Boys 26, 28, 33
Bridge Club 264
Buffalo Transition Support 298
Carolina Trans-Sensual Alliance 314
Carousel Club of South Australia 30
Carrousel Club, Inc. 29
CD Research Center 258
CDI See Cross Dressers International
Center for Change, Development, & Support 340
Center for Gender Reassignment 348
Central Illinois Gender Association 253
Central Ohio Gender Dysphoria Program 320
Central Wyoming Transgender Support Group 358
Chameleons 30
Chamleon Society 34
CheLSI e. V. 113
Chicago Gender Society 250
CIGA See Central Illinois Gender Association
City Lakes Crossgender Community 280
Clarke Institute of Psychiatry 57
CLCC See City Lakes Crossgender Community
Club MET 62
Club Neues Leben Nova 128
Connecticut Outreach Society 229
Cornbury Society 45
Cross Dressers International 324
Crossdressers & Friends 258
Crosslynx 169
Cross-Port 318
Crossroads 278
Crossroads of Buffalo 298
Crystal Club 322
Desire 324
Diablo Valley Girls 198
Dream Girls 44
Dreamwear Club 96
East Coast FTM Group 271
Eden Society 241
Elaine Barrie Project 32
Elizabeth Club 147
Emerald City 352
Enchanté 241
Enterprise 268
EON See Expressing Our Nature
Erie Sisters 328
Eurofantasia 166
Expressing Our Nature 312
F2M Fraternity 304
FACT 52, 62
Fanny's 83
Fantasia 240
FATE See Foundation for the Advancement of Transgendered People's Society
Fondation Nationale du Transsexualisme 41
Foundation for the Advancement of Transgendered People's Society 45
FPE See Freedom of Personality Expression
FPSG 215
Franjeppot 38
Freedom of Personality Expression 117
Freie Transenstadt Hamburg 120
FTM International 207
FTM Network 76
FTM Nippon 147
GCTC 343
GDANC Support Group 316
GEC See Gender Education Center
Gemini Gender Group 357
Gender Awareness League 204
Gender Centre, Inc. 24
Gender Congruity Center 235
Gender Council of Australia (W. A.), Inc. 33
Gender Dysphoria Program of Orange County, Inc. 220
Gender Dysphoria Support 283
Gender Education Center 280
Gender Expressions 202
Gender Identity Center of Colorado, Inc. 229
Gender Identity Clinic of New England 231
Gender Identity Project for Transsexuals 305
Gender Identity Support Services for Transexuals 266
Gender Mosaic 52
Gender Talk North 288
Gender Trust 83
Genderstichting (Belgian Gender Foundation) 38
Getting Real 273
Girls CD Group 24
Girls Night Out 297
GISST See Gender Identity Support Services for Transexuals
Glass City Sisters 322
Grampian Gender Group 168
Greater New York Gender Alliance 305
Gulf Area Gender Alliance 261
Gulf Coast Transgender Community 343
Hawaii Transgender Outreach 247
HCDA See Helping CDs Anonymous
Helping CDs Anonymous 343
Het Jongensuur 152
IFGE See International Foundation for Gender Education
IGTA See International Gender Transient Affinity
Illusions Social Club 42
Illusions Social Club II 43
Images 232
IME of Western Michigan 276
Innvestments 272
Institute for Psychosexual Health 357
International Foundation for Gender Education 268
International Gender Transient Affinity 77
Iowa Artistry 256
Jennifer & Friends 287
Ladies After Dark 254
Lebensberatung Für Transsexuelle Menschem Im Saarland 132
Leschemins de Trans 38
LGS See Saint Louis Gender Foundation
Liverbirds 87
Louisville Gender Society 259
MAGGIE See Mid-America Gender Group Information Exchange
Maine Gender Resource & Support Service 262
Memphis Trans-Gender Alliance 337
Metropolitan Gender Network 305
MFGE See Minnesota Freedom of Gender Expression
Mid-America Gender Group Information Exchange 284
Minnesota Freedom of Gender Expression 280
Monmouth Ocean Transgender Group 292
Montgomery Medical & Psychological Institute 188, 192, 235
MOTG See Monmouth Ocean Transgender Group
Myriad Network 273
National Gender Dysphoria Organization & Support Group 275
Nederlandse Vereniging Humanits 152, 158
Neutral Corner 211
New Men & Women of Minnesota 280
New York City Gender Alliance 305
New York Girl & Partner 298
New Zealand Gender Dysphoria Foundation 160
NGDO See National Gender Dysphoria Organization & Support Group
Nightlife 270
Northern Concord 76
Northwest Gender Alliance 326
Northwest Michigan Gender Society 277
NWGA See Northwest Gender Alliance
NYCGA See New York City Gender Alliance
NZGDF See New Zealand Gender Dysphoria Foundation
Oasis 329
Outreach Institute of Gender Studies 13
P. I. Group 230
Pacific Center for Human Growth 224
Paradise Club 322
Pathways Counseling Center 357
Phi Pi Epsilon 175
Philadelphia TS Support Group 330
Phœnix Centre 83
Phœnix Project 226
Phœnix Rising 211
Phœnix Society 170
Phœnix Transgender Support 313
Powder Puffs of California 226
PPOC See Powder Puffs of California
Prairie Rose Gender Club 47
PSGV Transgendered Group 209
Rainbow Gender Alliance 219
Rainbow People 195
RCGA See River City Gender Alliance
Recast Educations & Informational Network 341
Reflection House 345
Reflections 270
Renaissance Education Association, Inc. 233, 264, 291, 327, 328, 333
Rennaissance 291
RGA See Rainbow Gender Alliance
River City Gender Alliance 256
Rose 194
Rosenberg Clinic 342
Sacramento Gender Association 210
Saint Louis Gender Foundation 284
Salmacis 325
San Antonio Transexual Support Group 344
San Francisco Gender Information 215
SATRU 172
SATSG See San Antonio Transexual Support Group
Seahorse Society 26, 28, 32, 83
Selbsthilfegruppe 133
Serenity 238
Silent Passage 334
SIS See Swan's Inner Sorority
SISTI See Society for Initiatives & Services in Transgender Issues
Society for Initiatives & Services in Transgender Issues 207, 208
Society for the Second Self 42, 191, 192, 194, 195, 202, 204, 223, 228, 242, 243, 246, 253, 280, 282, 286, 292, 293, 294, 297, 310, 312, 314, 322, 323, 336, 338, 343, 344, 345
Sooner Diversity 323
South Australia Transexual Support 30
South Wales TV/TS Group 359
Starburst 238
Stichting Ede 157
Stichting Nederlands Gender Centrum 151
Stichting Omd 158
Sunday Society 250
Sunshine Club 270
Survivors of Transexuality Anonymous 305
Swan's Inner Sorority 220
TATs See Texas Association of Transexuals
Tayland House 272
TCNE See Tiffany Club of New England, Inc.
Tennessee Vals 337
TEWAHO See Transgender Education, Welfare, & Health Organization
Texas Assocation of Transexuals 339
TGEA See Transgender Educational Association of Greater Washington
Tiffany Club of New England, Inc. 273
TOPPS See Transexual Outreach
Trangender Forum 208
Trans 355
Trans Post-Op Recovery Residence 62
Trans Reality 129
Trans Support 263
Transexual Lesbians & Friends 352
Transexual Menace 332
Transexual Organization Self Help 293
Transexual Outreach 160
Transexual Support Group 332
Transformatie 154
Transgender Education, Welfare, & Health Organization 159
Transgender Educational Association of Greater Washington 347
Transgender Identity Group 357
Transgender Network 310
Transgender Support Group of Baltimore 264
Transgendered Alliance 268
Transidentitas 130
TRANSITAS 116
Transition Support 57
Trans-Net 72
Transpitt 332
TransPORRS See Trans Post-Op Recovery Residence
Trans-Port 326, 327
Transsexuals In Prison 62
Trans-Trap 169
Trans-tukipiste 96
Transupport 263
Transvestites Transexuals Group Minorities Trust 160
Transvision 66
Trasek 95
Travesty/Transsexualle 180
Triad Gender Association 315
Tri-Ess See Society for the Second Self
Tri-State Transgendered Club 265
TS Gesellschaft Hamburg e.V. 120
TS Peer Support Meetings 343

Organizations: Sexuality

TSG 🕮 *See* Transexual Support Group
TSH 🕮 116, 128
TS-Selbsthilfe Gruppe 🕮 179
TSSG 🕮 280
TV Selbsthilfegruppe 🕮 129
TV/TS Support Group 🕮 337
TVS Verein Transvestitin & Arbeitsgruppe TS 🕮 35
Twenty Club 🕮 231
University of Minnesota 🕮 280
Valley Girls 🕮 354
Vancouver General Hospital 🕮 45
Vereniging LKGT&T 🕮 150
Virginia's Secret 🕮 349
Virginia's Sectret 🕮 349
Viva TS - Selbsthilfe München e. V. 🕮 128
Washington - Baltimore Alliance 🕮 234
WATS 🕮 339
WATS Support, Unity, & Pride 🕮 33
WATSUP 🕮 *See* WATS Support, Unity, & Pride
Werkgroep Facet 🕮 155
West Texas Gender Alliance 🕮 338
Wichita Transgender Alliance 🕮 257
Wives'/Partners' Concerns 🕮 195
Xpressions 🕮 57
XX 🕮 *See* Twenty Club
Ye CG Brits 🕮 232
Zenith Foundation 🕮 45

Transvestite

Canadian Crossdressers Club 🕮 57
CD Network 🕮 311
CDI 🕮 *See* Cross Dressers International
CHIC 🕮 *See* Crossdresser Heterosexual Intersocial Club
Club Travestie Extraordinaire 🕮 83
Cross Dressers International 🕮 328
Cross Expressions 🕮 312
Crossdresser Heterosexual Intersocial Club 🕮 202
Cross-Talk 🕮 225
Delta Omega 🕮 341
East Coast Couples Network 🕮 292
ECCN 🕮 *See* East Coast Couples Network
Educational TV Channel 🕮 196
ETVC 🕮 *See* Educational TV Channel
FPE 🕮 *See* Freedom of Personality Expression
Freedom of Personality Expression 🕮 66, 164, 173
Imperial Queens of New York & Long Island 🕮 305
Indiana Crossdressers Society 🕮 253
IXE 🕮 *See* Indiana Crossdressers Society
LIFE 🕮 *See* Long Island Femme Expression
Long Island Femme Expression 🕮 311
Monarch Social Club 🕮 51
Rose's Club 🕮 90
SCHE 🕮 *See* Society of Cross-Dressing Hardware Engineers
Sigma Beta 🕮 323
Society of Cross-Dressing Hardware Engineers 🕮 268
Stichting Reborn 🕮 154
TransEssex 🕮 74
TV Self Help Group 🕮 83
TVV 🕮 122

Disabilities

All Sexes & Sexualities

Outsiders 🕮 13

Education

All Sexes & Sexualities

Holiday Associates 🕮 215

Student

All Sexes & Sexualities

Cal State / Northridge LGBA 🕮 204
Gender Issues Centre 🕮 54
Lesbian & Gay Student Union at the University of Virginia 🕮 347
Olaf Lesbian & Gay Alliance 🕮 281
OLAGA 🕮 *See* Olaf Lesbian & Gay Alliance
Out & About 🕮 31
Queer Community 🕮 256
Radford Alternative Alliance 🕮 348, 349
Society for Human Sexuality 🕮 352
Spectrum 🕮 257
University of Manitoba 🕮 47
University of Toronto Sexual Education & Peer Counselling Centre 🕮 57

Bisexual

Duke GALA 🕮 234

Gay

ALGUQAM 🕮 *See* Association des Lesbiennes & Gaies de l'Université de Québec à Montréal
Association des Lesbiennes & Gaies de l'Université de Québec à Montréal 🕮 62
Delta Lambda Phi Fraternity 🕮 280, 343

Lesbian

Bridges 🕮 348
Lesbian Bisexual Collective 🕮 334
Lesbians at Queens College 🕮 305
University Lesbians 🕮 280
Yalesbians 🕮 231

Lesbian, Gay, Bi, & Transgendered

10% Group 🕮 280
10% Society 🕮 281, 356, 358
10% Society at NMU 🕮 277
Agnes Scott Lesbian & Bisexual Alliance 🕮 244
ALBGS 🕮 *See* Alliance of Lesbian-Bi-Gay Students
Algonquin College Lesbigays 🕮 53
Alliance 🕮 287
Alliance for Bisexual, Lesbian, & Gay Support 🕮 276
Alliance for Sexual Diversity 🕮 263
Alliance of Lesbian, Bi, & Gay Students 🕮 28
Alliance of Lesbian, Gay, & Bisexual Students 🕮 244
Alliance of Lesbian-Bi-Gay Students 🕮 277
ALSO 🕮 *See* Alternative Lifestyles Support Organization
Alternative Lifestyles Support Organization 🕮 288
Alternatives 🕮 349
American College Personnel Association 🕮 264
Andere Fakultät / Schwulen- & Lesbenreferat 🕮 124
Anza Gay & Lesbian Alliance 🕮 220
Association des Gais & Lesbiennes de l'Université de Sherbrooke 🕮 63
AStA-Referat Schwule & Lesben der Universität Paderborn 🕮 131
AStA-Schwulenreferat 🕮 115, 123
AStA-Schwulenreferat der Uni Hamburg 🕮 120
Auckland University Gay Students Association 🕮 160
Autonomes Schwulenreferat 🕮 126
Autonomes Schwulenreferat der Uni Bielefeld 🕮 112
Babson Gay & Lesbian Alliance 🕮 268
Bard Bisexual, Lesbian, & Gay Alliance 🕮 296
Beyond Tolerance Task Force 🕮 334
B-GALA 🕮 *See* Bisexual, Gay, & Lesbian Alliance
BGALA 🕮 *See* Bryn Mawr / Haverford Bisexual, Gay, & Lesbian Alliance
BGALOR 🕮 *See* Bisexuals, Gays, & Lesbians of Ryerson
B-GLAD 🕮 *See* Bisexuals, Gay Men, Lesbians, & Allies for Diversity
BGLAD 🕮 *See* Bisexual, Gays, & Lesbian Association at Dalhousie. *See also* Bisexual, Gays, & Lesbians at Davis
BiGAYLA 🕮 *See* Bisexual, Gay, & Lesbian Alliance at New Paltz
BiGLM 🕮 *See* Bisexual, Gay, & Lesbian Mountaineers
Birmingham University LGB Association 🕮 93
Bisexual, Gay, & Lebian Association of RIT 🕮 311
Bisexual, Gay, & Lesbian Alliance 🕮 320
Bisexual, Gay, & Lesbian Alliance at JHU 🕮 264
Bisexual, Gay, & Lesbian Alliance at New Paltz 🕮 299
Bisexual, Gay, & Lesbian Alliance at Pitt 🕮 332
Bisexual, Gay, & Lesbian Association 🕮 232
Bisexual, Gay, & Lesbian Association, McMaster University 🕮 50
Bisexual, Gay, & Lesbian Awareness 🕮 356
Bisexual, Gay, & Lesbian Mountaineers 🕮 355
Bisexual, Gays, & Lesbian Association at Dalhousie 🕮 48
Bisexual, Gays, & Lesbians at Davis 🕮 199
Bisexual, Lesbian, & Gay Alliance at City College New York 🕮 305
Bisexual, Lesbian, & Gay Alliance at York 🕮 52
Bisexuals, Gay Men, Lesbians, & Allies for Diversity 🕮 313
Bisexuals, Gays, & Lesbians of Ryerson 🕮 57
Bi-The-Way 🕮 273
BLAGA 🕮 *See* Clark University Bisexual, Lesbian, & Gay Alliane
BLGAY 🕮 *See* Bisexual, Lesbian, & Gay Alliance at York
BLOGS 🕮 169
Boalt Hall, UC Berkeley School of Law Lesbian, Gay, & Bisexual Caucus 🕮 197
Boston University Gay, Lesbian, & Bisexual Caucus 🕮 268
Brandeis Triskelion 🕮 268
Bridge 🕮 263
Bryn Mawr / Haverford Bisexual, Gay, & Lesbian Alliance 🕮 328
Bunte Tunte 🕮 135
Campus Queers 🕮 161
Cardozo Gay & Lesbian Law Student Alliance 🕮 305
Carleton University Gay, Lesbian, & Bisexual Centre 🕮 53
Cégep de l'Outaouais 🕮 53
Central Michigan University Lesbian & Gay Alliance 🕮 277
Centre Gai & Lesbien de l'UQAM 🕮 62
Cercle Homosexuel Etudiant de l'ULB 🕮 37
Chameleon 🕮 322
CHE 🕮 *See* Cercle Homosexuel Etudiant de l'ULB
Clark University Bisexual, Lesbian, & Gay Alliane 🕮 273
CMU-Out 🕮 332
Coalition of Lesbian/Gay Student Groups, Inc. 🕮 341
Coalition of Lesbians, Gay, & Friends 🕮 293
College of Staten Island Lesbian, Gay, & Bisexual Alliance 🕮 305
Colorado College Gay & Lesbian Alliance 🕮 227
Columbia Lesbian, Bisexual, & Gay Coalition 🕮 305
Committee in Support of Gay, Lesbian, & Bisexual People 🕮 329
Committee on Homophobia 🕮 57
Concordia Queer Collective 🕮 62
Cornell Gay & Lesbian Alliance 🕮 257
Cornell Lesbian, Gay, & Bisexual Alliance 🕮 299
Courage 🕮 341
CSU Lambda Delta Lambda 🕮 319
Curtin Stonewall Club 🕮 33
CWRU Gay Lesbian Bisexual Alliance 🕮 319
Cypress College Lambda Union 🕮 198
DAGLO 🕮 *See* Dartmouth Gay & Lesbian Organization
Dartmouth Gay & Lesbian Organization 🕮 287
Delta Lambda Phi Fraternity 🕮 210
Denver University Lesbian, Gay, & Bisexual Alliance 🕮 228
Dickinson College Allies 🕮 328
Diversity 🕮 345
Drake University Alternative Lifestyles 🕮 256
EAGL 🕮 *See* Einstein Association of Gays & Lesbians
Earlham Lesbian, Bisexual, & Gay People's Union 🕮 255
East Stroudsburg University GLBSO 🕮 333
Edinboro Gay Organization 🕮 328
Einstein Association of Gays & Lesbians 🕮 305
ELGO 🕮 *See* Emory Lesbian & Gay Organization
Emory Lesbian & Gay Organization 🕮 244
Eros 🕮 231
Esteem 🕮 162
Flinders University Gay Society 🕮 30
Framingham State College Gays, Lesbians, & Friends 🕮 270
Frankfurter Schwule, Automones AStA-Schwulenreferat 🕮 117
FUGS 🕮 *See* Uppsala Gay Studenter
Gage 🕮 103
GALA 🕮 *See* Gay & Lesbian Association of Adelaide University. *See also* Gay & Lesbian Association. *See also* Poughkeepsie Gay & Lesbian Alliance. *See also* Students for Bisexual, Gay, & Lesbian Awareness
GALA 10 🕮 328
GALA of CSULA 🕮 204
GALA TC 🕮 44
Galileo 🕮 29
GALOR 🕮 *See* Gays & Lesbians of Rice
GaLTaS 🕮 *See* Gay & Lesbian Teachers & Students Association, Inc.
GAMIT 🕮 *See* Gays, Lesbians, Bisexuals, & Friends at MIT
Gay & Lesbian & All Student Association 🕮 312
Gay & Lesbian Alliance 🕮 215, 231, 248, 325
Gay & Lesbian Alliance at Southern Oregon State College 🕮 324
Gay & Lesbian Alliance at UNB/STU 🕮 48
Gay & Lesbian Alliance of Eastern Oregon State College 🕮 325
Gay & Lesbian Alliance San Francisco State University 🕮 215
Gay & Lesbian Alliance SUC-Oswego 🕮 310
Gay & Lesbian Association 🕮 171
Gay & Lesbian Association of Adelaide University 🕮 30
Gay & Lesbian Association of Students & Staff 🕮 47
Gay & Lesbian Association of Students at SIU-E 🕮 252
Gay & Lesbian Association UCLA 🕮 204
Gay & Lesbian Community Alliance 🕮 252
Gay & Lesbian Community at UWM 🕮 357
Gay & Lesbian Law Caucus 🕮 332
Gay & Lesbian Liberation of Waterloo 🕮 60
Gay & Lesbian Olin Business School Alliance 🕮 284
Gay & Lesbian Peer Counselling Group 🕮 51
Gay & Lesbian Resource Center 🕮 285
Gay & Lesbian Student Association 🕮 282, 283, 295, 315, 344
Gay & Lesbian Student Society 🕮 171
Gay & Lesbian Student Union 🕮 210, 294, 322, 348
Gay & Lesbian Students Union 🕮 204
Gay & Lesbian Studies Union 🕮 202
Gay & Lesbian Support Group 🕮 276
Gay & Lesbian Teachers & Students Association, Inc. 🕮 27
Gay & Lesbian Union at NYU 🕮 305
Gay & Lesbian Union at Queens College 🕮 305
Gay College Societies 🕮 137
Gay Information & Concerns 🕮 328
Gay Law Students at Hastings 🕮 215
Gay Lesbian Bisexual Alliance at UVM 🕮 346
Gay Lesbian Bisexual Student Support 🕮 358
Gay Lesbian Bisexual Union 🕮 358
Gay Men & Lesbian Alliance 🕮 268
Gay Men's Support Group 🕮 285
Gay Organization for Alternative Lifestyles 🕮 310
Gay Outreach Association for Lowell Students 🕮 271
Gay People's Union 🕮 210
Gay Students Alliance at Baruch College 🕮 305
Gay, Lesbian, & Allied Student Society 🕮 273
Gay, Lesbian, & Bi Student Organization 🕮

282
Gay, Lesbian, & Bisexual Academics, Students & Staff 📖 42
Gay, Lesbian, & Bisexual Aggies 📖 339
Gay, Lesbian, & Bisexual Alliance 📖 192, 298, 354
Gay, Lesbian, & Bisexual Alliance of Kingsborough 📖 298
Gay, Lesbian, & Bisexual Association of Mc Master 📖 50
Gay, Lesbian, & Bisexual Community Alliance 📖 284
Gay, Lesbian, & Bisexual Union 📖 299, 305
Gay, Lesbian, Bisexual, & Friends Association 📖 311
Gay, Lesbian, Or Bisexual Alliance 📖 259
Gay/Lesbian Association of UTA 📖 341
Gaya Mater Studiorum 📖 140
Gays & Lesbians at Andover Newton Theological School 📖 268
Gays & Lesbians at Notre Dame / Saint Mary's College 📖 255
Gays & Lesbians at the University of Saskatoon 📖 64
Gays & Lesbians at U of T 📖 57
Gays & Lesbians of Humber 📖 57
Gays & Lesbians of Rice 📖 343
Gays & Lesbians on Campus 📖 43
Gays, Lesbian, & Bisexuals of UBC 📖 45
Gays, Lesbians, & Bisexuals International 📖 57
Gays, Lesbians, & Bisexuals United 📖 220
Gays, Lesbians, Bisexuals, & Friends 📖 248
Gays, Lesbians, Bisexuals, & Friends at MIT 📖 268
George Brown College Lesbian, Gay, & Bisexual Students 📖 57
Georgetown Pride 📖 234
Georgia Tech's Gay & Lesbian Alliance 📖 244
Gettysburg College Lambda Alliance 📖 328
GLA/EWU 📖 *See* Gay, Lesbian, & Bisexual Alliance
GLABA 📖 *See* Glendon Gay, Lesbian, & Bisexual Alliance
GLAF 📖 *See* Framingham State College Gays, Lesbians, & Friends
GLANTS 📖 *See* Gays & Lesbians at Andover Newton Theological School
Glasgow Caledonian University L&G Society 📖 169
Glasgow University L&G Society 📖 169
GLASS 📖 *See* Gay & Lesbian Association of Students & Staff. *See also* Gay, Lesbian, & Bisexual Academics, Students & Staff
GLBFA 📖 *See* Gay, Lesbian, Bisexual, & Friends Association
GLBSO 📖 *See* Gay, Lesbian, & Bi Student Organization
GLBSU 📖 *See* Gay, Lesbian, & Bisexual Union
Glendon Gay, Lesbian, & Bisexual Alliance 📖 57
GLLOW 📖 *See* Gay & Lesbian Liberation of Waterloo
GLOBAL 📖 *See* Gay & Lesbian Olin Business School Alliance. *See also* Gay, Lesbian, Or Bisexual Alliance
GLOBE 📖 *See* Rhode Island College Gay, Lesbian, or Bisexual Equality Alliance
GLOH 📖 *See* Gays & Lesbians of Humber
GLSA 📖 *See* Gay & Lesbian Resource Center
GLSS 📖 *See* Gay & Lesbian Student Society
GLUS 📖 *See* Gays & Lesbians at the University of Saskatoon
GOAL 📖 *See* Gay Organization for Alternative Lifestyles
GOALS 📖 *See* Gay Outreach Association for Lowell Students
Graduate Gay & Lesbian Alliance 📖 298
Groupe Gai de l'Université de Laval 📖 63
GUSS 📖 *See* Campus Queers
Hampshire College Gay & Bisexual Men's Alliance 📖 267
Harvard Gay & Lesbian Caucus 📖 269
Heriot Watt University LGB Society 📖 169
Hofstra Gay & Lesbian Student Association 📖 305
Homostudies 📖 157, 158
IMRU of Gloucester County College 📖 293
IUPUI Advocate 📖 255
Lambda 📖 282
Lambda Alliance of Gay Men & Lesbians 📖 285
Lambda Club, University of Victoria 📖 47
Lambda Delta Lambda Sorority 📖 204
Lambda Group 📖 255
Lambda Horizon at Virginia Tech 📖 347
Lambda Lesbian & Gay Student Association 📖 305
Lambda Society at Clemson 📖 335
Law Students for Gay & Lesbian Concerns 📖 338
LBGA 📖 *See* Lesbian, Bisexual, Gay Alliance
Leeds University Lesbian, Gay, & Bisexual Society 📖 94
Lehigh University LesBiGay Alliance 📖 329
Lesbian & Gay Alliance 📖 317
Lesbian & Gay Campus Organization 📖 284
Lesbian & Gay Collective of Mount Royal College 📖 43
Lesbian & Gay Convenors 📖 25
Lesbian & Gay Law Student at NYU 📖 305
Lesbian & Gay Resource Center 📖 228
Lesbian & Gay Rights Caucus 📖 322
Lesbian & Gay Student Association 📖 255
Lesbian & Gay Student Group 📖 163
Lesbian & Gay Student Union 📖 345
Lesbian & Gay Students Association 📖 305
Lesbian & Gay Students of the Toronto Board of Education 📖 57
Lesbian & Gay Support Group, Fordham University 📖 305
Lesbian / Gay Academic Union of Greater Cincinnati 📖 318
Lesbian Bisexual Gay Alliance 📖 288
Lesbian Gay Bisexual Alliance 📖 350
Lesbian, Bisexual, & Gay Alliance 📖 226
Lesbian, Bisexual, Gay Alliance 📖 267
Lesbian, Gay, & Bisexual Aliance 📖 265
Lesbian, Gay, & Bisexual Alliance 📖 221, 256, 292, 298, 305, 325, 334
Lesbian, Gay, & Bisexual Alliance at Penn 📖 330
Lesbian, Gay, & Bisexual Alliance at Plattsburgh 📖 310
Lesbian, Gay, & Bisexual Alliance of UMBC 📖 264
Lesbian, Gay, & Bisexual Alliance SUNY Albany 📖 296
Lesbian, Gay, & Bisexual Association 📖 333
Lesbian, Gay, & Bisexual Association at SUNY Postsdam 📖 310
Lesbian, Gay, & Bisexual Caucus 📖 269, 296
Lesbian, Gay, & Bisexual Center 📖 269
Lesbian, Gay, & Bisexual Coalition 📖 252
Lesbian, Gay, & Bisexual Collective of Douglas College 📖 44
Lesbian, Gay, & Bisexual Community at Boston College 📖 269
Lesbian, Gay, & Bisexual Community, Carleton College 📖 281
Lesbian, Gay, & Bisexual Coöperative at Yale 📖 231
Lesbian, Gay, & Bisexual Issues Committee 📖 50
Lesbian, Gay, & Bisexual Organization 📖 211
Lesbian, Gay, & Bisexual Resource Center 📖 280
Lesbian, Gay, & Bisexual Student Alliance 📖 231, 333
Lesbian, Gay, & Bisexual Student Association 📖 278
Lesbian, Gay, & Bisexual Student Union 📖 211, 233, 242
Lesbian, Gay, & Bisexual Student Union of the University of Florida 📖 237
Lesbian, Gay, & Bisexual Students' Association 📖 45
Lesbian, Gay, & Bisexual Union - Kent 📖 321
Lesbian, Gay, & Bisexual Union SUNY 📖 297
Lesbian, Gay, Bisexual Association 📖 200
Lesbians In Law 📖 215
Lesbians, Bisexuals, & Gays of McGill 📖 62
Lesbigais de l'Université de Québec à Hull 📖 61
LesBiGay Services of Kansas 📖 257
Lesbigays Cité Collégiale 📖 53
LesBiGays, Unlimited 📖 352
LGB Awareness League 📖 191
LGBA 📖 *See* Denver University Lesbian, Gay, & Bisexual Alliance. *See also* Lesbian, Gay, & Bisexual Alliance SUNY Albany
LGBIC 📖 *See* Lesbian, Gay, & Bisexual Issues Committee
LGBRC 📖 *See* Lesbian, Gay, & Bisexual Resource Center
LGBSA 📖 *See* Lesbian, Gay, & Bisexual Student Alliance. *See also* Lesbian, Gay, & Bisexual Student Association
LGBU 📖 *See* Lesbian, Gay, & Bisexual Union SUNY
LGBU-Kent 📖 *See* Lesbian, Gay, & Bisexual Union - Kent
LIL 📖 *See* Lesbians In Law
Macalester Gays, Lesbians, & Bisexuals United 📖 280
Macquarie University Gay & Lesbian Association 📖 27
Mary Washington College Gay / Lesbian / Bisexual Student Association 📖 348
Maynooth Gay & Lesbian Society 📖 138
Melbourne University Gay Society 📖 32
MGALA 📖 357
Miami University Gay, Lesbian, & Bisexual Alliance 📖 322
Monash University Gay Collective 📖 32
MTSU Lambda Association 📖 337
MUGALS 📖 *See* Murdoch University Gay & Lesbian Society
Münchner Hochschwule - Schwulenreferat der LMU 📖 128
Murdoch University Gay & Lesbian Society 📖 33
National Gay & Lesbian Task Force Campus Project 📖 234
Network 📖 255
New School Gay, Lesbian, Bisexual Collective 📖 305
Normandale Community College Lesbian & Gay Network 📖 280
North Carolina State Lesbian / Gay Student Union 📖 316
North of Scotland NUS 📖 170
Northwestern University Bisexual, Gay, & Lesbian Alliance 📖 250
Oberlin College Lesbian, Gay, & Bisexual Union 📖 322
OHO 📖 96
Oklahoma University Gay, Lesbian, & Bisexual Alliance 📖 323
OLGSR 📖 *See* Organization for Lesbian & Gay Student Rights
Organization for Lesbian & Gay Student Rights 📖 234
OUT 📖 253, 255
Out On Campus 📖 45, 61
Penn GALA 📖 330
People for Lesbian, Gay, & Bisexual Concerns 📖 248
Pink & Purple 📖 114
Poughkeepsie Gay & Lesbian Alliance 📖 310
Pride at UIC 📖 250
Program for Gay, Lesbian, & Bisexual Concerns 📖 267
Purdue Gay Alliance 📖 255
Queen Margaret College L&G Society 📖 169
Queensboro Community College Lesbian & Gay Male Alliance 📖 305
QUT Campus Queers 📖 28
R. O. S. PO. 📖 143
Regina Students Homophile Society, Inc. 📖 64
Rensselaer Gay, Lesbian, & Bisexual Alliance 📖 296
Rhode Island College Gay, Lesbian, or Bisexual Equality Alliance 📖 334
SAGA 📖 313
Saginaw Valley State College Gay & Lesbian Alliance 📖 278
Saint Andrew's University GaySoc 📖 168
Saint John's University Lesbian, Gay, & Bisexual Alliance 📖 305
SALSA 📖 *See* San Antonio Lambda Students Alliance
Sam Houston GLBA 📖 343
San Antonio Lambda Students Alliance 📖 344
SchLUB 📖 *See* Schwule-Lesbische Unigruppe
SchwBile Referat 📖 115
SchwUL 📖 *See* Schwule an der Univesität Leipzig
Schwule an der Univesität Leipzig 📖 125
Schwule Hannöversche Studenten 📖 121
Schwule Uni Gruppe 📖 123
Schwule-Lesbische Unigruppe 📖 178
Schwulen- & Lesben-Initiative der Universität Dortmund 📖 114
Schwulenreferat 📖 134
Schwulenreferat an den Aachener Hochschulen 📖 109
Schwulenreferat ASta in der FH Fulda 📖 118
Schwulenreferat beim AStA der WW-Uni 📖 129
Schwulenreferat der Bochumer Ruhr-Universität 📖 112
Schwulenreferat Fachhochschule Neiderrhein 📖 125
Schwulenreferat im AStA der Carl von Ossietsky Universität Oldenburg 📖 130
Schwulenreferat im AStA der Christian Albrecht Universität 📖 123
Schwulenreferat im AStA der Fachhochschule 📖 129
Schwulenreferat im AStA der GH Essen 📖 116
Schwulenreferat im SprecherInnenrat der Friedrich-Alexander Universität Erlangen Nürnberg 📖 116
SchWUnG 📖 *See* Schwule Uni Gruppe
Sexual Minority Student Alliance 📖 349
SHS 📖 *See* Schwule Hannöversche Studenten
Smith College Lesbian, Gay, & Bisexual Alliance 📖 272
State University Association of Lesbians & Gays 📖 276
Stirling University LGB Society 📖 167
Stonewall Union of Students 📖 33
Students for Bisexual, Gay, & Lesbian Awareness 📖 337
Syracuse University Gay, Lesbian, Bisexual Student Association 📖 312
Temple Lambda Alliance 📖 330
Ten Percent of U 📖 274
Territory University Gay Society 📖 28
Towson State University Gay & Lesbian Outreach 📖 264
Triangle Club 📖 352
Triangle Coalition 📖 283
Trigon 📖 328
TUGS 📖 *See* Territory University Gay Society
U.C. Alliance of Lesbian, Gay, & Bisexual People 📖 318
UAB G/L Student Union 📖 191
UC Irvine GLBSU 📖 201
Uglesett 📖 165
UK Lambda 📖 259
Unigaie 📖 178
UNIGLOW 📖 *See* University of Northern Iowa Gay & Lesbian Outreach
Union of Lesbians, Gays. & Bisexuals 📖 209
Unitec Gay & Lesbian Support Association 📖 160
United Theological Seminary Lesbian & Gay Caucus 📖 280
University Bi Community 📖 280
University Lesbian, Gay, & Bisexual Alliance 📖 279
University of Alabama Gay & Lesbian Alliance 📖 192
University of Chicago Gay & Lesbian Alliance 📖 250
University of County Cork Gay Society 📖 137
University of Michigan 📖 274
University of Minnesota 📖 280
University of Minnesota Lesbian & Gay Law

Organizations: Sexuality: Student

Students Association 280
University of New South Wales Gay & Lesbian Department 27
University of North Dakota G&L Coalition 317
University of Northern Iowa Gay & Lesbian Outreach 257
University of Ottawa Lesbigays 53
University of South Australia Gay, Lesbian, & Bisexual Association 31
University of South Florida Gay, Lesbian, & Bisexual Coalition 242
University of Sunderland LGB Group 92
University of Teeside LGB Group 88
University Students' Council - GLBi Commissioner 51
Uppsala Gay Studenter 176
URI Gay, Lesbian, & Bisexual Association 334
USUA Bisexual, Gay, & Lesbian Association 195
UWOUT 51
UW-Parkside Gay & Lesbian Organization 358
Vassar Gay People's Alliance 310
West College Gay & Lesbian Student Union 220
West of Scotland Area NUS 169
Western Kentucky University Lambda 258
Wilde Alliance 34
William Mitchell College of Law Gay & Lesbian Association 280
Williams Bisexual, Gay, & Lesbian Union 273
Yale GALA, DC 234
Zart & Heftig 180

Male

Delta Lambda Phi Fraternity 286

Youth

All Sexes & Sexualities

Youthlink - Inner City 58

Gay

Alternative Youth Club - Tri State Area 230
Boy Zone 163
Breakaway - Gay Youth Group 34
Icebreakers 160, 162
Peer Education Project 83

Lesbian

Brooklyn Lesbian Youth Sisters 298
Maui Lesbian/Gay Youth Project 246

Lesbian, Gay, Bi, & Transgendered

Antarius 110
Arci Gay 145
ASPYN *See* Safer Place Youth Network
Bay Area Sexual Minority Youth Network 215
Bisexual, Gay, & Lesbian Youth of New York 306
Coalition for Bisexual, Gay, & Lesbian Youth in Peel 51
Come Out Jungengruppe 112
Community Health Project Outreach to Teens 306
Danbury Area Gay, Lesbian, & Bisexual Youth Group 230
District 202 280
Föreningen BHUS 175
FRAGLY *See* Framingham Regional Alliance of Gay & Lesbian Youth
Framingham Regional Alliance of Gay & Lesbian Youth 270
GALY-NY *See* Gay & Lesbian Youth in New Jersey
Gay & Lesbian Community Center of Colorado, Inc. 228
Gay & Lesbian Teen Task Force 247
Gay & Lesbian Young Adults 341
Gay & Lesbian Youth in New Jersey 289
Gay & Lesbian Youth of Hudson Valley 306
Gay & Lesbian Youth of Seattle 352
Gay & Lesbian Youth Services 298
Gay Switchboard Dublin 137
Gay Youth Alliance 211
Gay Youth Calgary 43
Gay Youth Milwaukee 357
Gay, Lesbian, & Bisexual Teens 237
GLASS 315
Growing Alternative Youth 332
GYM *See* Gay Youth Milwaukee
HATCH *See* Houston Area Teen Coalition of Homosexuals
HAZ *See* Homosexuelle Arbeitsgruppen Zürich
Hetrick-Martin Institute 306
Homosexuelle Arbeitsgruppen Zürich 180
Houston Area Teen Coalition of Homosexuals 343
Houston Institute for the Protection of Youth 343
Howick Gay Youth Group 160
Icebreakers 162, 163
Indianapolis Youth Group 255
Jeunes & Etudiant(e)s Homosexuel(le)s de Tour (JEHT) 103
JUB *See* Jungendberatung Düsseldorf
Jugendgruppe Jackpoint 179
Jugendgruppe Rose 177
Jugendgruppe Space 178
Jugendgruppe WIGWAM 179
Junge Lesben & Schwule im Thurgau 178
Jungendberatung Düsseldorf 115
Jungendnetwerk Lambda e. V. 110
LAMBDA Services Youth OUTreach 341
Lambda Youth & Family Empowerment 215
Lambda Youth Network 198
Lambda Youth Services 312
Lambda-Junge Lesben & Schwule im Freistaat Sachsen e. V. 114
Lesbian & Gay Youth Group 296
Lesbian & Gay Youth of Rochester 311
Lesbian & Gay Youth Ottawa Hull 53
Lesbian & Gay Youth/Calgary 43
Lesbian, Gay, & Bi Youth 46
Lesbian, Gay, & Bisexual Teen Support Group 276
Lesbian, Gay, & Bisexual Youth of Toronto 57
Long Island Gay & Lesbian Youth, Inc. 306
LuST *See* Junge Lesben & Schwule im Thurgau
MAG Jeunes Gais 103
Maison des Homosexualités 104
Max & Moritz Jugendgruppe 133
Mayor's Office for the Lesbian & Gay Community 306
Monadnock Outright 287
National Coalition for Gay, Lesbian, & Bisexual Youth 220
National Gay Youth Network 215
National Youth Advocacy Alliance 338
Oasis 354
Odyssey 354
One-In-Teen Youth Services 337
Ostfreisische Schwulen- & Lesbeninitiative 116
Other Place 137
Out Reach 294
OutFit 313
Outright 263, 314
Outright Vermont 346
Outright Youth in Kingston 50
Outspace Schwul-Lesbische Jungendgruppe 121
OYINK *See* Outright Youth in Kingston
PALS *See* People of Alternate Lifestyles
Parents & Friends of Lesbians & Gays 286
PAYSO *See* Positivity About Youth Sexual Orientation
People of Alternate Lifestyles 195
PFLAG *See* Parents & Friends of Lesbians & Gays
Phœnix Pride Youth Group 320
Pink Triangle Coalition 328
Pink Triangle Youth of Edmonton 43
POLEN 149
Positivity About Youth Sexual Orientation 51
Project 10 62
Qpido 174
Rainbow Youth Trust 160
Respect 162
Safer Place Youth Network 316
SAIM *See* Sufficient As I Am
Sappho & Apoll Schwulen & Lesben-Jungendgruppe 113
Schwule Jungendclique Frankfurt 117
Schwule Jungendgruppe Koblenz 123
Seacost Outright 288
Sexual Minority Youth Assistance League 234
SJK *See* Schwule Jungendgruppe Koblenz
SNHAGLY *See* Southern New Hampshire Gay & Lesbian Youth
Southern New Hampshire Gay & Lesbian Youth 288
Stonewall Youth Group 169
Sufficient As I Am 264
Supporters of Worcester Area Gay & Lesbian Youth 273
Teen Options Clinic 288
Time Out Youth 314
Tir-State Gay / Lesbian Awareness Dialogue Group 287
Twentysomething 306
Ungdomsgruppen for Bøsser og Lesbiske i Sønderjylland 67
Verkeerd Geparkeerd Homojongeren 38
Windfire 276, 278
Young & Gay 32
Young Gay & Lesbian Alliance of Oklahoma City 323
Young Gays 30
Your Turf 329
Youth Outreach Program 204
Youth Rap Group 352

Male

Merrimack Valley Youth Group 288

SHAVING

Gay

Clippers 77, 188
Men Shaving Men 46
Philly Hair Razors 244
We Enjoy Shaving 188

SPANKING

All Sexes & Sexualities

P. M. Club 242

Gay

C. L. E. F. 13
Castigatio 150
Society of Spankers 58

Heterosexual

NESS *See* Northeast Erotic Spanking Society
Northeast Erotic Spanking Society 273
Public Eye 79

Male

Spankclub 36

SPIRITUALITY

All Sexes & Sexualities

Radical Faerie Circle 250

Gay

Radical Faerie Circle 199

Lesbian, Gay, Bi, & Transgendered

Shouts in the Wilderness, Leather Circle of Hope 341

SWINGERS

All Sexes & Sexualities

Forum Society 359
Sterling 271

Heterosexual

New Zealand Swing Club 163

TATTOO

All Sexes & Sexualities

Alliance of Professional Tattooists, Inc. 265
Flesh Canvas 91
Tattoo Club of Great Britain 69

Gay

Canadian Tattoo Association 41
Dutch Tattoo Foundation 152
Friends of the Tattoo Archive 13
Illustrated Men 223
National Tattoo Association 188
T & P Men 13

UNCIRCUMCISION

Male

Uncirc South Australia 30

WATERSPORTS

Gay

Golden Shower Association 306
Golden Shower Buddies 215
Northwest Rainmakers 352
NYPT 13
Rainmakers Club 306
Rubber Sex Groep 152
Water Boys of San Diego 188

WRESTLING

All Sexes & Sexualities

Bay Area Boxing Club 216
Global Wrestling Alliance 13

Gay

Alternative Sports 13
NCWC *See* Northern California Wrestling Club
Northern California Wrestling Club 216
Pacific Northwest Wrestling Association 352
Spartans Wrestling Club 331
Tampa Bay Wrestling Club 241
Wrasslin' Bears 216

Lesbian, Gay, Bi, & Transgendered

Knights Wrestling Club 306
Metro Gay Wrestling Alliance, Inc. 306
MGWA *See* Metro Gay Wrestling Alliance, Inc.
Wrestling Club Of Portland 326

Male

Houston Wrestling Club 343

PERFORMERS

MUSIC

BDSM

All Sexes & Sexualities

Genitorturers 290

PHOTOGRAPHERS

BDSM

All Sexes & Sexualities

Akita, Masami 147
Fux, Andreas 110
Optic Verve 58
Ryan, Janet 283

Lesbian, Gay, Bi, & Transgendered

Ultimate Productions 221

EROTIC

All Sexes & Sexualities

Alexandre, Claude 104
Alper, Barbara 306
Berquet, Gilles 104
Blum, Günter 132
Boudoir Portraits 220
Braun, Etienne 148
Carlos Clarke, Bob 83
Chester, Mark 216
Chevalier, Remy 232
Chouraqui, Robert 101
Couto, Dan 58
Czernich, Peter 132
Del Valle, J. L. 104
Derby, Phil 208
Eichler, Wolfgang 118
Ferron, Michael 152
Gabrielly, Vince 306
Gatewood, Charles 216
Glover, Thomas 306
Gonzales, Efrain 298
Graff, Laura 269
Hamilton, China 91
Housk, Randall 83
Ireland, Chris 27
John, Harald 35
Jones, Jeanette 75
Karo Design 120
Ken Marcus Studio 201
Kert, Kelvin 104
Kloster, Doris 306
L'Hermite, Christian 27
Lemaire, Guy 38

Leslie, David 83
Leurquin, Jacques 39
Marshall, John 87
Morey, Craig 199
Morgan J. Cowin Photography 221
Morrow, David 306
Mourthé, Christophe 104
Mueller, Richard 286
Musson, Victoria 13
Musy, Gerard 104
Rondelle, Gordon 83
Samotowka, Ted 51
Santerineross, John 292
Serieys, Philippe 105
Soyez, Jean-François 37
Steinmeier Photography 250
Stephan Richter Photography 131
Todd Friedman Photography 197
Toko Koschnick, Peter 120
Watson, Trevor 83
Willems, Dany 37
Wolech, Helmut 35
Yamazaki, Shinji 148

Gay

Patrioli, Tony 143

FETISH

All Sexes & Sexualities

Abrams, Steve 250
Boeki, L. 37
Hard Art Design 134
Kâa, Heïdi 36
Kroll, Eric 306
Plakidas, Nicolas 128

Gay

Volanti, Ron 252

SEXUALITY

Transvestite

Girls Like Us, Ltd. 83

PIERCERS

All Sexes & Sexualities

Accent In Ink 328
Alter Ego 286
Anubis Warpus 216
Arbuckle's Tattoo & Piercing Emporium 256
Ars Subcutan 127
Art Accent Tattooing 261
Asgard Body Piercing 13
Attitudes 326
Auroboros 58
Baldo's Piercing Studio 134
Bangcók, Hank 250
Bee's Knees 27
Black Sun Studio 62
Black Universe 66
Blake House Studios 75
Body Accents 254
Body Armour Piercing & Tattooing 169
Body Art Studios 70
Body Aware 188
Body Basics 250
Body Circle Designs 352
Body Designs 296
Body Manipulations 152, 216
Body Piercer 27
Body Piercing by Tee 58
Body Work Productions 319
Bodylink Body Piercing 31
Bodyworks 83
Bound By Design 228
Bravo 242
Cage 208
Chain Link Addiction 319
Chris 250
Claw 211
Cockell, Denis 83
Cold Steel 83
Coyote, Ken 221
Creative Art Collection 148
Dakota Steel, Inc. 222
David 27
Dehaan, Jan 156
Denise Robinson Body Art 53
DEXTRA *See* Denise Robinson Body Art
DK Profashion 66
Exotic Body 210
Extremus Body Arts 283
Fleshworks 316
Forbidden Fruit 333
Freizeitverein Priapos 35
Future Shock 255
Gallina, Raelyn 208
Gauntlet, Inc. 104, 204, 216, 306
Gerd 326
G-Nation 347
Graven Image 209
Hardware, Inc. 294
House of David 79
House of Whacks 250
HTC Body Adornment Studio 194
Inferno 331
Iron City Ink Tattoos 332
Jones, Mark 194
Kellner, Bernhard 121
Lagaipa, Darryn 326
Lasting Impressions 256
Leather Tiger 237, 240, 242
Living Colour Tattoo 53
London Piercing Clinic 83
Long Island Connection 299
Metal Morphosis 84
Meyerson, Adam 272
Moon Mystique 257
Multitek Services 84
Musafar, Fakir 206
Needleworks 93
Next! Body Piercing 46
Nirvana 169
Nomad 33, 216
Obscurities 341
Oslo Piercing Studio 164
Pagan Metal 84
Pat's Tats 312
Perforations 74
Perforations Piercing Studio 234
Piercing Experience 244
Piercing Exquisite 349
Piercing Urge 24, 27
Piercings Unlimited 322
Piercology 320
Pike's Peak Tattoo 227
Planet K 338, 344
Playspace 352
Pleasurable Piercings, Inc. 290
Polymorph Body Art Gallery 27
Precision Body Piercing 208
Primeval Body 204
Professional Body Piercing by Jack 221
Quintessential Transfigurations 43
Red Devil Studios 225
Red Ring Studios 255
Richmond, Gary 326
Rings & Things 74
Rings of Desire 261
Rites of Passage 266
Ritual 294
Rocquet, Olivier 101
Sachs 294
School of Professional Body Piercing 296
Scoville, Rob 294
Shaman Body Piercing 306
Ship to Shore Tattooing & Body Piercing 337
Simpson, Gary 71
Sine Qua Non 294
Skin & Bones 341
Slacker 332
Stainless Steel Body Art 58
Staircase Tattoos 221
Sterling Rose Tattooing & Piercing 316
Suzie Q Pleasure & Pain 116
Tatau Obscur 110
Tattoo World 237
Tattooing & Piercing Studio 152
Tullous, Don 210
Underground Art 337
Urban Tribe 244
Venus Modern Body Arts, Inc. 306
WA Creations 352
Yount, Jack 243
Zoom 338

PRINTERS

ADULT

All Sexes & Sexualities

Breene Lithograph, Inc. 224
Eve Browne Fashions 189
Mindanao Printing Company 280
Mountaintop Design & Typography 229

GENERAL

All Sexes & Sexualities

Academic Bookbinding 280
Adams Press 250
Aprinco Book Manufacturers 54
Banta Company 356
Bawden Printing, Inc. 254
Best Book Manufacturers 58
Book Mart Press 292
Bookcrafters 274
Bookmasters 317
Braun-Brumfield 274
Capital City Press, Inc. 346
Courier Corporation 271
Courier Westford Inc. 273
Crane Duplicating 270
Cushing-Malloy 274
David Printing 198
Delmar Printing & Publishing 314
Delta Lithograph 224
Donihe Graphics, Inc. 336
Edwards Brothers 274
Eerdmans Printing Company 276
Globe Graphics Communications 49
Griffin Printing & Lithograph Co. 200
Griffin Printing/Spilman 210
Harlo Press 275
Hignell Printing Limited 47
Jostens Printing & Publishing 224
Key Press 342
Kimberly Press 221
Kromar Printing 47
Lidec 62
Malloy Lithographing 274
Maple-Vail 333
Maracle Press 52
Matthews, Ingham, & Lake Inc. 49
McLaren Morris & Todd Ltd. 51
McNaughton & Gunn 278
Merril Company 204
Metropole Lithographers 58
Mitchell Press Ltd. 46
Morgan Printing & Publishing 338
Multiprint, Inc. 290
National Reproductions Corporation 277
Norcal Printing 216
Nørhaven A/S 67
Omnipress 356
Our Print Shop 220
Patterson Printing 274
Porcupine's Quill Inc. 49
Port City Press, Inc. 306
Professional Press 313
Publishers Press 345
Quebecor America Book Group 306
R. R. Donnelly & Sons 250
RBW Graphics 51
Rose Printing 242
Scarecrow Press 291
Shear-Davis 274
Thomson-Shore, Inc. 275
Tri-Graphic Printing (Ottawa) Ltd. 53
Van Volumes Limited 272
Viking Press/Banta 279
Walsworth Publishing Company 284
Whitehall Company 239

PROMOTERS

All Sexes & Sexualities

Chain Gang Promotions 84

PUBLIC SPEAKERS

BDSM

All Sexes & Sexualities

Wiseman, Jay 197

GENDER ISSUES

All Sexes & Sexualities

Henkin, William 216

Transgender

Miller, Niela, M.S. Ed., LCSW, LMHC 189

SEXUALITY

All Sexes & Sexualities

Jacques, Trevor 13
Carellas, Barbara 13
Sprinkle, Annie 299

Lesbian, Gay, Bi, & Transgendered

Queen, Carol 216

PUBLISHERS

AUDIO TAPES

BDSM

Male

Skye 277

BOOKS

BDSM

All Sexes & Sexualities

AZZLO 148
Editions Jaybird 37
Eros Publishing 352
Mystic Rose Books 230
SAK Publishing 277
Virtjack Studios 14
WholeSM Publishing Corporation 58

Gay

Dædalus Publishing Company 216

Heterosexual

Fetish Factory Ltd. 14
Marquis Magazine 14
Treville Edition, Ltd. 148

Heterosexual, Male

On Your Knees 278

Lesbian, Gay, Bi, & Transgendered

GLB Publishers 13

Bondage

All Sexes & Sexualities

Shunga Comix 276

Gay

Bondage Book 204

Erotic

All Sexes & Sexualities

Circlet Press 269
Editzioni d'Essai 146
Gates of Heck 349
NBM Publishing 306
Nexus 84
Pure Imagination 14
Tease! 14

Gay

Plastic Cow Productions 198

Lesbian, Gay, Bi, & Transgendered

Artistic Licentiousness 352
Badboy Books 306
Hard Candy Books 306
Richard Kasak Books 306

Fetish

All Sexes & Sexualities

Tim Woodward Publishing Ltd. 84

Heterosexual

Benedickt Taschen Verlag GmbH 124
Editions Astarté 104
Editions Dominique Leroy 104
Editions Vents d'Ouest 100
Futami - Shobo Co., Ltd. 147
Glittering Images 146
Quartet Books Limited 84
Vaar 154

General

All Sexes & Sexualities

Body Art 14
Body Art, Publications Ltd, 14
Crossing Press 14
Para Publishing 221
Picador, Div. of Pan Macmillan 84
Rutgers University Press 291

Medical

All Sexes & Sexualities

Merck Manual 333
Merck Research Laboratories 333

Polyfidelity

All Sexes & Sexualities

Anapol, Deborah, IRC 221

Sexuality

All Sexes & Sexualities

Added Dimensions Publications 208

Publishers: Books: Sexuality

Alamo Square Press 216
Artemis Creations Publishing 14
Barbo Carlson Enterprises 258
Big Breakfast Publishing 320
Down There Press 14
Infantæ Press 352
Penis Power Quarterly 208
Re/Search Publications 15
Rhinocerous Books 306
St. Martin's Press 306
Urania Books 238

Female

Cleis Press 332
Kitchen Table, Women of Color Press 14
Women's Press 58

Gay

Gay Sunshine Press / Leyland Publications 216

Lesbian

Timely Books 336

Lesbian, Gay, Bi, & Transgendered

A. D. Thompson & Co., Publishers 221
Acolyte Press 150
Albino Verlag 108
Alyson Publications, Inc. 269
Arcados-Versand 177
Bottomliners 84
Cahiers Gai-Kitsch-Camp 14
CKC *See* Cahiers Gai-Kitsch-Camp
éditions aubrey walter 69
Edizione Gruppo Abele 139
Gai-Kitsch-Camp (CKC) 14
Gay Men's Press 69
Janssen Verlag 110
JH Press 306
Lesbian & Gay Studies 84
Leyland Publications 216
Masquerade Books 306
Other Way Press 84
Purple Stone Press & Productions 271
Queer Press 58
Queer Words 359
Routledge Press 76, 306
Verlag Rosa Winkel 108

Male

Factor Press 192

Spanking

All Sexes & Sexualities

BoisLine 247
Diamond Distribution 278
Imperia Press 15
Wildfire Club 15

DIRECTORIES

AIDS

All Sexes & Sexualities

AIDS Directory 84
Nam Charitable Trust 84

BDSM

All Sexes & Sexualities

Alternate Sources 14, 15
Amador Communications 15
Black Book 15
Domination Directory International (DDI) 208
Kink, Ink 14, 15
Strictly Speaking Publishing Co. 208

esbian, Gay, Bi, & Transgendered

Womanlink 15

Gay

Black Pages International 15
Blackline Press & Services 15
Spunk 216
Studio Iguana 216

Lesbian, Gay, Bi, & Transgendered

Womanlink 15

Books

All Sexes & Sexualities

Cumulative Book Index 297
H. W. Wilson Company 297
J. Whitaker & Sons 84
K. G. Saur Publishing Company 306
Literary Market Place 306
R. R. Bowker 292

Booksellers

All Sexes & Sexualities

American Booksellers Association 306
National Association of College Stores 322

Fetish

All Sexes & Sexualities

Fetasy Guide 15
Gear, Inc. 15

General

All Sexes & Sexualities

Connexions Annual 41
Connexions Information Sharing Services 41
Sources 42

Libraries

All Sexes & Sexualities

Canadian Library Association 53
McIntyre Media 58

Naturism

All Sexes & Sexualities

Bold Type, Inc. 197

Sexuality

All Sexes & Sexualities

Alternative Lifestyles Directory 15
American Library Association 251
Directory of Gay & Lesbian Community Publications in the United States & Canada 200
Directory of Professional Groups of Gays & Lesbians 251
Leydig Trust 15
Niche Catalog Publications 325
Outposts 336
Planet Sex The Handbook 15
Redwood Empire Agency 200
Winter Publishing, Inc. 15

Bisexual

Bisexual Community Resource Center 269
International Directory of Bisexual Groups 269

Gay

Knight Publishing 204

Lesbian

Calendar of Events 238

Lesbian, Gay, Bi, & Transgendered

Alternative Phone Book 251
American Library Association 251
BJ Ventures 84
Colorado Community Directory 226
Community Yellow Pages 204
DAC Marketing, Inc. 251
Directory of Bookstores Specializing in Gay, Lesbian, & Feminist Books 251
Ferrari Publications 189
Gai Guide 89
Gai Project 89
Gay & Lesbian Periodicals Directory 15
Gay To Z Directory 84
Gay To Z Publishing, Ltd. 84
Gaybook 216
Gayellow Pages 306
Lambda Press 53
Lambda Publications 251
Lavendar Listings 320
Lesbian & Gay Pink Pages, Chicago 251
Long Beach Directory 202
New Vista Publishing 15
Orange County Directory 202
OUT! Resource Guide 251
Palm Springs Directory 202
Pink Pages 49
Places of Interest 189
Q Community Events Calendar 163
Queer Biz Oy 96
Queer Guide - Brighton 74
Renaissance House 306
Stiefel 108
Turkey Media Services 202
Visitors Guide to Gay Britain 84

Transgender

National Shemale Directory 189
Salishon Society 189

Transvestite

JMPG 197

Tattoo

All Sexes & Sexualities

Tattoo Directory 207

DOCUMENTARIES

BDSM

Heterosexual

Since May Productions 293

Sexuality

All Sexes & Sexualities

Cambridge Documentary Films, Inc. 15

Lesbian, Gay, Bi, & Transgendered

Off The Beaten Path 194
Triangle Television, Inc. 160
Voice & Vision Productions 278

FILMS

Sexuality

Female

Feline Films 216

GUIDES

Sexuality

All Sexes & Sexualities

Complete Guide to Internet Sex Resources 15
Cruiser 177
International Sexual Minorities Information Resource 15
ISMIR *See* International Sexual Minorities Information Resource
ISMIR Events Calendar 15
Pointer to Sex Information on the Net 15
PtSIotN *See* Pointer to Sex Information on the Net
Transvestite's Guide 84
WayOut Publishing Company 84

Bisexual

Gay & Lesbian Services Guide 235
Training By Design 235

Gay

Guide 269
Poach Gay Guide 189
Pocket Guide to Hawaii 247

Lesbian, Gay, Bi, & Transgendered

Babilonia Edizione 139
Bent Guide to Gay/Lesbian Canada 42
Berlin & Brandenburg, Sachsen, Sachsen-Anhalt von Hinten 108
Best Guide 150
Bruno Gmünder Verlag 108
City Map Produkties 150
Columbia Fun Maps 306
Companion Publications 189
Damron Address Book 189
Damron Company 189
ECW Press 42
Free Map of Amsterdam 152
Freedom Editions 84
G'Day Guide 24
Guida Gay 139
Guide Gai du Québec 62
Hinnerk 120
Hots Spots 236
HX (Homo Xtra) 307
Larry's Guide to the Ghetto 58
Lifestyle Publishing Inc. 246
London Pink Pathways 54
Odysseus 189
Odysseus International Ltd. 189
Pages 246
Schwule Männer 108
Spartacus 108
This Week Guide 261
Western New York Sentinel 298

Transvestite

Crossdressers InfoGuide 244

INFORMATION

Sexuality

All Sexes & Sexualities

ASPE 139
OutProud! 189
QueerAmerica 189

Lesbian, Gay, Bi, & Transgendered

COC Magazijn 152

MAGAZINES

AIDS

All Sexes & Sexualities

Alerte 97
Art & Understanding 296
Positively Friends 226
PWAlive Publications, Inc. 281

Gay

Positive Times 69
Silveraim Ltd. 69

Lesbian, Gay, Bi, & Transgendered

POZ 307

Alternative

All Sexes & Sexualities

Rip Off Press, Inc. 196

Lesbian, Gay, Bi, & Transgendered

Electronic Gay Community Magazine 189
Land of Awes Information Services 189

Arts

All Sexes & Sexualities

Time Out 84

Female

Women's Review of Books 16

Lesbian, Gay, Bi, & Transgendered

Bruno Gmünder Verlag 108
Euros 108
Evergreen Chronicles 281
HOMologie 151
Omega Literary Arts Magazine 208
OutArt 338

BDSM

All Sexes & Sexualities

Attitude 240
B & D Pleasures 202
Backdrop Club 207
Black Leather In Color (BLIC) 307
BLIC Collective 307
Body Play & Modern Primitives Quarterly 206
Boudoir Noir 59
Chainmail 238
Chaud Business SPRL 37
Checkmate & DungeonMaster 15, 16
Church of Epiphany 207
Common Bonds 207
Contact S. M. 37
Continental Spectator 189
Cruella 73
De Sade's World 307
Demonia 104
Diversity Magazine 44
Divine Press 72
Divinity 72
DM International 352
Domina 84, 307
Dominant Publications 46
Dominantly Yours 189
Executive Imports International 307
Fantasy of Gord 359
Fer Rouge 16
Fetish Network 240
Fundgeon Times 202
Goddess 73
H. G. Publications 359
Halcyon 88
Headpress Magazine 72
Insight Books 206
Katharsis 18
Kink 46
Kinky People Places & Things 352
Leather Journal 16, 17
Lexicon 217
M. J. Production 157
Master's Way 207
QUIM 84

Raging Rhino Productions 📖 238
Rendez-Vous 📖 37
Retro Systems 📖 18
RM Distribution, Ltd. 📖 16
Rogue-Hagen Publications 📖 73
S & L Sales Company 📖 205
S. A. D. E. 📖 172
Sadean 📖 18
Sandmutopia Guardian 📖 307
SB Publishing, Ltd. 📖 92
Schlagzeilen 📖 120
Scorpion 📖 73
Secret Magazine 📖 36
Servant's Quarters 📖 18
Six of the Best Publishing 📖 18
Société Comedit 📖 104
Some Bizarre 📖 92
Sortilège 📖 104
Sublime 📖 157
Telecentral Electronics 📖 15, 16
Twilight 📖 110
TWS Ent. 📖 191
Unleashed 📖 94
Unlimited 📖 94
Utopian Network 📖 307
Villeinage 📖 343
Wild Side 📖 191
Wild Times 📖 205
Women who Administer Punishment (WhAP) 📖 18

Gay

Alternate Publishing Company 📖 16
Bandanna 📖 291
Brush Creek Media 📖 217
Centurion 📖 151
Corporal Contacts 📖 84
Cuir Magazine 📖 225
Desmodus, Inc. 📖 217
Disziplin 📖 110
Drummer 📖 217
Editions du Triangle Rose 📖 18
International Leatherman 📖 217
James Publishing Group, Inc. 📖 251
Kumpel 📖 110
Leather Journal 📖 225
Mach 📖 217
Manifest Reader 📖 16
Mr. SM 📖 66
Orange Press ApS 📖 66
Projet X 📖 18
Red Plaid 📖 251
Sir! 📖 84
ST Publishing 📖 84
Vogel Verlag 📖 110, 111
Z&O 📖 111

Heterosexual

Black Box Productions Ltd. 📖 84
Capitulation 📖 296
Carter Stevens Presents 📖 332
Chained 📖 332
Diamond 📖 253
Dominant & Submissive Pleasure 📖 236
F. A. 📖 104
Fantastic Books Publications 📖 296
Key 📖 70
N. S. P. 📖 18
Passion, Our Leather Soul 📖 253
Pussy Cat 📖 84
Scene 📖 104
Society of O 📖 236
Sussex Mailbox 📖 70
Wanda 📖 18
World of Payne 📖 332

Heterosexual, Male

Mistress Jacqueline Magazine 📖 201
Pacific Force 📖 201
Power Xchange 📖 201
Sapphire 📖 73
Strictly Stories 📖 18
Subculture 📖 18

Hetersexual

Behind The Scene 📖 196

Lesbian

Bad Attitude 📖 269
Brat Attack 📖 216
Brazen Bitch Quarterly (BBQ) 📖 59
Phantasia Productions 📖 269
Pussywhipped! 📖 18
Six of the Best Publishing 📖 18
Venus Infers 📖 217

Lesbian, Gay, Bi, & Transgendered

Alternate Woods Publishing 📖 269
Australian Leather Men (ALM) 📖 24
Bitches With Whips 📖 352
DM International 📖 352
Mastery Magazine 📖 269
Metropolitan Slave 📖 16
Northwind 📖 46
Selective Publishing, Inc. 📖 16

Male

Katharsis 📖 16
Katharsis 📖 16, 20
Mistress 📖 16
Olympia Publishing (UK) Ltd. 📖 16, 18

Bears

Gay

American Bear 📖 228
Big Ad Productions 📖 217
Big Boys & Buddies 📖 75
Big Bull, Inc. 📖 228

Body Size

Heterosexual, Male

Big Time Publications 📖 210
Oakhaus 📖 248
Squish 📖 210
Wilson Barber's Quarterly 📖 248

Bondage

All Sexes & Sexualities

B & D Pleasures 📖 202
Bondage Fantasies 📖 202
Bondage Reader 📖 202

Bisexual

Bi Monthly Bondage 📖 248
Subnormal 📖 248

Gay

Bound & Gagged 📖 18, 19
Outbound Press 📖 18, 19

Heterosexual, Male

Bondage Life 📖 18
Harmony Concepts, Inc. 📖 18

Male

Olympia Publishing (UK) Ltd. 📖 19
Pleasure Bound 📖 19

Corsets

Transvestite

Corset Digest 📖 244

Daddy / Boy

Gay

Daddy Magazine 📖 264
Daddybear 📖 266
Ganymede Press, Inc. 📖 264

Lesbian, Gay, Bi, & Transgendered

Chiron Rising 📖 224
Chiron Rising Publications 📖 224

Erotic

All Sexes & Sexualities

Champagne Productions 📖 19
Continental Spectator 📖 189
Desire 📖 84
General Media Inc. 📖 19
Hightail Publishing 📖 228
Hotshots 📖 211
Libido 📖 19
Libido, Inc. 📖 19
Paramour Magazine 📖 269
Penthouse Variations 📖 19
Red Sky Publishing, Limited 📖 84
Sunshine Publishing Co. 📖 211
TopHat's Calendar of Erotica 📖 19

Gay

Advocate Men 📖 205
All Man 📖 97
All Your Dreams Fulfilled 📖 199
Avenue Services 📖 207
Beau Magazine 📖 19
BlackFire 📖 189
BLK Publishing Co. 📖 189
Blue Nights 📖 313
Blueboy Magazine 📖 307
Bodyshot 📖 19
Brush Creek Media 📖 217
Centaur Magazine 📖 199
Editions SAN 📖 97
Espace MAN 📖 97
First Hand 📖 293
Fraction Presse SARL 📖 97
Gay Obsessions 📖 97
Guys Magazine 📖 293
Handjobs 📖 207
Hommes 📖 97
Honcho 📖 97, 307
Husky Magazine 📖 217
In Touch 📖 207
Jean Paul 📖 97
Jock 📖 307
Machismo 📖 307
Magayzine 📖 19
Mandate 📖 307
Manscape 📖 312
Manshots 📖 312
Mike Arlen's Guys 📖 84
Mirza, Inc. 📖 292
MMG Services Inc. 📖 307
Numbers 📖 307
Obsession 📖 307
Paragon 📖 153
PCP 📖 199
PDA Press, Inc. 📖 355
Playguy 📖 307
PowerPlay 📖 217
Pride Publishing & Typesetting, Inc. 📖 313
Publications Nouvelles 📖 97
Pump It Up! 📖 292
Sportomatic, Ltd. 📖 19
Stars 📖 307
Steam 📖 355
Straight to Hell (The Manhattan Review of Unnatural Acts) 📖 307
Torso 📖 307
Wetherby Studios 📖 84

Heterosexual, Female

Playgirl 📖 307

Heterosexual, Male

Penthouse 📖 307
Penthouse International, Ltd. 📖 307

Lesbian

Black Lace 📖 189
BLK Publishing Co. 📖 189
Girlfriends 📖 217

Lesbian, Gay, Bi, & Transgendered

Babilonia 📖 139
Babilonia Edizione 📖 139
Chicos 📖 172
Gay Italia 📖 139
Marco 📖 139
Studios J. M. R. 📖 172

Fetish

All Sexes & Sexualities

A. M. Publications 📖 326
A. P. M. C. 📖 20
Aggressive Women Magazine 📖 84
B & D Pleasures 📖 202
Batteries Not Includeed 📖 322
Bizarre 📖 200
Black Leather Times 📖 265
Blue Blood 📖 265
BNI 📖 322
CBLT 📖 265
Chatt 📖 59
Chatterly's 📖 59
Club Caprice 📖 133
Delice Garden 📖 38
Disciples of Semiramis 📖 19
DM International 📖 20, 21
Dominique & Rubber Fun 📖 70
Epidermal Intrusions 📖 194
Eagle Press 📖 338
Fetish 📖 225
Fetish Bazaar 📖 202
Fetish Times 📖 19
FLAS 📖 75
Footsy 📖 75
G & M Fashions Ltd. 📖 75
Gear, Inc. 📖 205
Get Kinky 📖 337
In Uniform 📖 326
Kastley GmbH 📖 133
Katharsis 📖 19
Knickers & Upskirts 📖 70
Leather Journal 📖 225
Leg Tease 📖 296
Mang Publishing 📖 19
Maniac 📖 104
Marquis Masquerade 📖 89
Modern Products 📖 337
Necronomicon 📖 73
«O» Magazine 📖 19
Offrande 📖 20
Pagan Metal 📖 84
Pediform 📖 338
Redeemer 📖 84
Redemption Films 📖 84
Rem-mer Ltd. 📖 296
Ritual Magazine 📖 84
Ritual World 📖 84
RM Distribution, Ltd. 📖 19
Rubber Rebel 📖 205
Shiny 📖 75
Skin Two 📖 84
Spartacus 📖 200
Swish Publications Ltd. 📖 84
Taste of Latex 📖 20, 21
Tim Woodward Publishing Ltd. 📖 84
Webeverlag 📖 127
Winter Publishing, Inc. 📖 19
Zeitgeist 📖 84
Zeitgeist International 📖 84

Gay

Brush Creek Media 📖 217
Detonator 📖 84
Foreskin Quarterly 📖 217
Noose Letter 📖 19
Raunch 📖 194
Tom's Ranch 📖 194
Your Ass & My Face 📖 281

Heterosexual

Amber E. 📖 206
Boot Lovers' Digest 📖 19
Crib Sheet 📖 206
Editions Astarté 📖 104
Fetish Factory Ltd. 📖 19, 90
Marquis Magazine 📖 19, 90
Strictly Speaking Publishing Co. 📖 19

Heterosexual, Male

Splosh 📖 74

Male

Hair to Stay 📖 19
SludgeMaster 📖 343
Winter Publishing, Inc. 📖 19

Transvestite

Spartacus 📖 200
Transformation 📖 200

General

All Sexes & Sexualities

Caress Magazine 📖 74
Details 📖 307
Face 📖 84
Write Solution 📖 74

Female

Everywoman 📖 84

Gay

Arena 📖 84

Lesbian, Gay, Bi, & Transgendered

Breakaway Publications Ltd. 📖 85
Rouge Magazine 📖 85

Health

Lesbian, Gay, Bi, & Transgendered

Urban Fitness 📖 201
Urban Publishing, Inc. 📖 201

Literary

All Sexes & Sexualities

Books In Canada 📖 59
Boston Book Review 📖 269
Canadian Review of Books Ltd. 📖 59
Independent Review 📖 25
Library Journal 📖 307
New York Review of Books 📖 307
Publishers Weekly 📖 307

Publishers: Magazines: Literary

Lesbian, Gay, Bi, & Transgendered

Amador Communications 📖 20
Literatussi 📖 120
Porno Pen 📖 20

Penis Size

Gay

Small Etc. 📖 296
Small Gazette 📖 296

Photography

All Sexes & Sexualities

Scenario 📖 91

Piercing

All Sexes & Sexualities

Body Modification Ezine 📖 20
Gauntlet, Inc. 📖 20
In The Flesh 📖 307
OB Enterprises 📖 307
P. A. U. K. 📖 92
Paisano Publications 📖 196
Piercing Fans International Quarterly (PFIQ) 📖 20
Piercing World 📖 92
Savage 📖 196

Polyfidelity

All Sexes & Sexualities

Touchpoint 📖 193

Scat

Gay

Scat Times 📖 20
Winter Publishing, Inc. 📖 20

Sexual Politics

All Sexes & Sexualities

Body Politic 📖 85
Whorezine 📖 217

Female

Heresies 📖 307
Women of Power Magazine 📖 272

Gay

Nummer 📖 135
Nummer Verlag 📖 135

Lesbian, Gay, Bi, & Transgendered

Box 📖 108
Libertarians for Gay & Lesbian Concerns Newsletter 📖 274
Løvetann 📖 164
Maine Progressive 📖 262

Sexuality

All Sexes & Sexualities

ARTpolice Agency 📖 281
Borxan Publications 📖 22
Brush Hill Press 📖 269
Celebrate The Self 📖 192
Disability Rag 📖 259
DM International 📖 353
Eclectic Attitudes 📖 240
EIDOS Magazine 📖 269
Enamored Writer 📖 238
Eros Comix 📖 353
Factor Press 📖 192
Fetish Network 📖 240
Future Sex 📖 217
General Media Inc. 📖 307
Greenery 📖 217
Haworth Press 📖 20, 22
Inciting Desire 📖 221
It's Okay! 📖 54
Journal of Gay & Lesbian Psychotherapy 📖 20
Journal of Gay & Lesbian Social Services 📖 20
Journal of Homosexuality 📖 22
Journal of Sex Research 📖 317
Kundalini Publishing, Inc. 📖 217
Lady Green 📖 217
Man Bag 📖 281
More! Productions 📖 197
Observer 📖 121
Paradise 📖 307
Penthouse Forum 📖 307
Phœnix Counsel, Inc. 📖 54
Phun Ink Press 📖 226
Private Tymes 📖 226
Redemption 📖 22
RGN 📖 22
Rome Gay News 📖 22
Sabazio 📖 22
Slippery When Wet 📖 197
Spunk 📖 205
Tantra Magazine 📖 294
Zoomorph 📖 22

Bisexual

AJA Publishing Corp. 📖 310
Anything That Moves 📖 217
Bisexuality Newsletter 📖 202
Dream Magazine 📖 211
Gibbin Publications 📖 202
Klinger Publications 📖 211
Options Magazine 📖 310
San Francisco Bay Area Bisexual Network 📖 217

Female

At The Crossroads 📖 194
Cauldron 📖 202
Choices Women's Medical Center, Inc. 📖 299
Connexions 📖 197
Female FYI 📖 205
Feminist Bookstore News 📖 217
Feminist Studies 📖 265
Fireweed 📖 59
Girl Jock 📖 217
Herspectives 📖 45
Hikané 📖 270
Iowa Woman Endeavors, Inc. 📖 255
Iowa Woman Magazine 📖 255
Kinesis 📖 46
OISE 📖 59
On Our Backs 📖 217
On The Issues 📖 299
Ozark Feminist Review 📖 195
Radiance, The Magazine For Large Women 📖 22
Resources for Feminist Research 📖 59
Sage 📖 244
Sing Heavenly Muse! 📖 281
Trivia 📖 267
Unforgettable Fire 📖 291
We Are Visible 📖 206
Woman To Woman 📖 195
Womanist 📖 53

Gay

Adonis Atlantic Presse Editions 📖 97
Anderschume / Kontiki 📖 177
Bear Magazine 📖 217
Big Bull, Inc. 📖 228
Brush Creek Media 📖 217
Bulk Male 📖 228
Columbia Publishing Company 📖 264
Cornerstone Publications 📖 160
Dirty 📖 307
Diva 📖 85
Express 📖 160
Gayme Magazine 📖 269
Iniquity 📖 307
Lust 📖 135
Magnus Verlag 📖 108
Malebox 📖 42
Men Into Underwear 📖 358
Military & Police Uniform Association 📖 225
Military & Police Uniform Association Newsletter 📖 225
Millivres Ltd. 📖 85
MJ Enterprises 📖 358
Nummer Verlag 📖 135
OMPO 📖 22
Oral Majority 📖 22
Out & About 📖 217
Paws Magazine 📖 307
PDA Press, Inc. 📖 218
Pink Triangle Press 📖 42
Pulse Magazine 📖 170
TRASH 📖 290
Tribe 📖 264
wilde 📖 218
Winter Publishing, Inc. 📖 22
Zymurgy 📖 269

Lesbian

Alternate Woman 📖 261
Broadsheet Magazine 📖 160
conMOCIÓN 📖 239
Deneuve 📖 217
Dyke Review 📖 217
Dykes, Disability, & Stuff 📖 356
Editions Nitram 📖 42
Friday Night Womyn's Group 📖 239
FRS Enterprises 📖 217
Gazelle 📖 42
Hurricane Alice 📖 281
Informher 📖 239
Lavendar Enterprises 📖 189
Lavendar Life 📖 189
Lesbian Calendar 📖 189
Lesbian Connection 📖 277
Lesbian Ethics 📖 294
Lesbian Information Line 📖 62
Lesbian Interest Press (LIP) 📖 312
Lesbian Network 📖 25
Lesbian News 📖 196
Lonnie Marshall Publications 📖 261
Maize 📖 295
qc Magazine 📖 42
Shamakami 📖 22
Shamakami, Incorporated 📖 22
Sinister Wisdom 📖 197
Sinister Wisdom, Inc. 📖 197
Sorority Magazine 📖 59
TLC Productions 📖 189
Womanlife, Inc. 📖 160

Lesbian, Gay, Bi, & Transgendered

10 Percent 📖 217
Advocate 📖 205
Alamo Square Press 📖 217
Alternatives 📖 205
Amador Communications 📖 20
Amigo/CPC 📖 36
Andere Welt 📖 108
Apolo 📖 149
Association Ibiza 📖 101
Attitude 📖 85
Bad Attitude 📖 85
Black Sheets 📖 20
Blasé Ltd. 📖 85
BLK 📖 189
BLK Publishing Co. 📖 189
Broad Magazine 📖 75
Browning Grace Communications 📖 217
Bruno Gmünder Verlag 📖 108
Burn 📖 24
Campaign 📖 24
Chow Chow Productions 📖 353
Colectivo Sol, A.C. 📖 149
Colorlife! 📖 307
Come Out! 📖 177
Cruise Magazine 📖 278
CTN Magazine 📖 217
Del Otro Lado 📖 149
Don & Adonis 📖 108
Double Face 📖 97
Du & Ich 📖 108
Empathy 📖 335
Fab Magazine 📖 59
Fag Rag 📖 339
Febo Editores, S. A. de C. V. 📖 149
Flamingo 📖 40
Flash 📖 170
Foerster Verlag 📖 108
Forum Homosexualität und Literatur 📖 108
Frighten The Horses 📖 217
Gaie France en Português 📖 167
Gay & Lesbian Advcacy Research Project 📖 335
Gay Club I. L. R. E. S. 📖 167
Gay Media 📖 177
Gay Scotland 📖 169
Gay Times 📖 85
Gayzette 📖 24
Go Info 📖 53
Goldstein Publications 📖 307
Harpies & Quines 📖 169
Heat Seeking Publishing 📖 217
Hermes 📖 149
Holy Titclamps 📖 217
Homo- und Lesbiennejongerenkrant 📖 36
Homosexuelle Initiative 📖 35
HOMOture 📖 217
HOSI 📖 *See* Homosexuelle Initiative
Hothead Paisan 📖 231
Ibiza 📖 101
Icon 📖 59
Infor Homo 📖 36
IQ Magazine 📖 85
Island Lifestyle Magazine 📖 246
Journal Gaie Presence 📖 97
Just Out 📖 324
Kalani Honua, Inc. 📖 246
Kick Publishing Company 📖 275
Kick! Magazine 📖 275
Kiss Contact 📖 40
Lambda Book Report 📖 235
Lambda Edition 📖 108
Lambda Rising, Inc. 📖 235
Lambda-Nachrichten 📖 35
Lawrence Publishing Company (NZ) Ltd. 📖 160
Leine Verlag 📖 108
Lesbian & Gay Pride 📖 22
LGB Guide to Great Britain 📖 22
Liberation Publications Inc. 📖 205
Liberation Publishers 📖 172
Lifestyle Publishing Inc. 📖 246
Loop 📖 46
Magazine Fugues 📖 62
Magazine RG 📖 63
Magnus 📖 108
Magnus Verlag 📖 111
Malchus 📖 347
Männer Aktuell 📖 108
Masquerade Books 📖 307
Masquerade Erotic Newsletter 📖 307
MEGA Scene 📖 208
Metrosource 📖 307
Michael's Thing Magazine 📖 307
Midi Gai Loisirs 📖 101
Millivres Ltd. 📖 85
My Comrade 📖 307
Northern & Shell 📖 85
Open Hands 📖 251
Orange County Blade 📖 201
Orbita Gay Macho 📖 167
Out 📖 307
Out & About 📖 307
Out & About, Inc. 📖 307
Out Publishing, Inc. 📖 307
Out! 📖 160
OUTawa Magazine 📖 53
Outlooks Magazine 📖 279
Outrage 📖 24
Outright 📖 172
Outright! 📖 89
Outspoken 📖 246
Pageprint Limited 📖 169
Phase 📖 85
Pink Power 📖 111
Pink Times 📖 90
Planet 23 Productions 📖 269
Polished Knob 📖 269
Pride Path Magazine 📖 298
PRIDENET 📖 59
PRIDENET, Incorporated 📖 59
Prime 📖 85
Provincetown Advocate 📖 272
qc Magazine 📖 42
Queensland Pride 📖 29
Queer-e 📖 22
Quest Magazine 📖 226
Quest Publications 📖 226
QX 📖 85
Regard 📖 36
Reporter 📖 176
Rome Enterprises, Inc. 📖 278
Scotsgay 📖 169
Screw Magazine 📖 307
Siegessäule 📖 111
Snaxus Productions 📖 339
Teen Fag 📖 353
Tels Quels 📖 36
TRUST, The Handballing Newsletter 📖 218
Virtual Universe Publications Ltd. 📖 85
Voice Magazine 📖 196
Wicked Women 📖 22
Worlander Pty. Ltd. 📖 24
Xtra! 📖 35
¡Y Que! 📖 149
Young Gays Club (YGC) 📖 22
Youth Magazine 📖 235
Zauberflöte 📖 129
Zizo 📖 36

Male
Changing Men 🕮 257
Playboy 🕮 251
Transgender
Feminique 🕮 348
Gender Review 🕮 226
Skyclad Publishing 🕮 22
Transgendered Magazine 🕮 271
Transsexual Voice 🕮 244
Transsisters, The Journal of Transsexual Feminism 🕮 22
TV-TS Confidential 🕮 288
Writer's Etc. 🕮 288
Transvestite
Club TV 🕮 189
Continental Spectator 🕮 189
Creative Design Services 🕮 329, 331
Dragazine 🕮 225
Female Mimics International 🕮 223
He-She Directory 🕮 189
International Transcript / CDS 🕮 331
Ladylike 🕮 329
Leoram, Inc. 🕮 223
Sissy Exposé 🕮 223
Taffeta 🕮 70
TransVamp 🕮 22
TransVamp Publications, Ltd. 🕮 22
TV Connection 🕮 353
Shaving
Gay
Mercury Productions 🕮 339
Smooth Buddies Bulletin 🕮 339
Spanking
Omega Marketing 🕮 77
All Sexes & Sexualities
Awakenings 🕮 278
BB Publications 🕮 278
Cul D'Or 🕮 77
Paddles 🕮 25
Scene One 🕮 223
Shadow Lane 🕮 223
Gay
Report 🕮 85
ST Publishing 🕮 85
Heterosexual
Carter Stevens Presents 🕮 332
CF Publications 🕮 299
Men Under Control 🕮 299
Spanks-A-Lot 🕮 332
Spirituality
All Sexes & Sexualities
McGinley, Robert, Ph.D. 🕮 197
Solitary 🕮 356
Gay
Crucible 🕮 22
Swingers
All Sexes & Sexualities
Loving Alternatives 🕮 212
Omnific Designs West 🕮 212
Watersports
Gay
Gold'n Stream 🕮 22
Winter Publishing, Inc. 🕮 22
Youth
All Sexes & Sexualities
Project X 🕮 307
MAILING LISTS
Female
Lesbian
National Women's Mailing List 🕮 201
General
All Sexes & Sexualities
Resources Mailing Lists 🕮 269
Libraries
All Sexes & Sexualities
Willowood Press 🕮 189
Sexuality
Gay
Malebox Direct Mail Service 🕮 42
Lesbian, Gay, Bi, & Transgendered
Provincetown Purchase Company 🕮 272
Renaissance House 🕮 308
Strubco, Inc. 🕮 308
MISCELLANEOUS
All Sexes & Sexualities
93 S/M Designs 🕮 22
Integrity Indexing 🕮 314
Female
Astarte Shell Press 🕮 263
Spinsters Ink 🕮 281
Gay
Pagan Press 🕮 308
Lesbian
Lavendar Circle Press 🕮 292
Naiad Press, Inc. 🕮 242
Rising Tide Press 🕮 299
Lesbian, Gay, Bi, & Transgendered
Edward-William Publishing Company 🕮 339
Gay Presses of New York 🕮 308
Meikänainen 🕮 96
Womyn's Braille Press, Inc. 🕮 281
Transgender
Reluctant Press 🕮 347
BDSM
All Sexes & Sexualities
Comba-Borel 🕮 85
NEWSLETTERS
Sexual Politics
Transgender
In Your Face 🕮 308
NEWSPAPERS
AIDS
All Sexes & Sexualities
AIDS Treatment News 🕮 218
BDSM
All Sexes & Sexualities
B & D Pleasures 🕮 202, 203
Cuir Underground 🕮 218
Leather Links 🕮 203
Heterosexual
Carter Stevens Presents 🕮 332, 333
Dominant Domain 🕮 308
Dominant Mystique 🕮 308
Female Domination Forever 🕮 332
Female Supremacy 🕮 311
Feminine Illusion 🕮 308
Fetish Video Review 🕮 332
Footprints 🕮 332
La Carnivale 🕮 310
Mistress Cherie's Orchard 🕮 333
New Esoteric Press 🕮 308
S&M News 🕮 333
Thor Publications 🕮 297
Tiffany Enterprises 🕮 311
Whipping Post 🕮 310
Whips 🕮 297
Bondage
Heterosexual
Bondage Times 🕮 311
Tiffany Enterprises 🕮 311
Fetish
All Sexes & Sexualities
B & D Pleasures 🕮 203
Bizzare Erotic Fantasies 🕮 203
In Step 🕮 224
Heterosexual
Fetish World 🕮 308
New Esoteric Press 🕮 308
General
All Sexes & Sexualities
Chicago Tribune 🕮 251
Daily Mail 🕮 85
Feminist Press at The City University of New York 🕮 308
Guardian 🕮 85
Times 🕮 85
Women's Studies Quarterly 🕮 308
Female
Sojourner - The Women's Forum 🕮 269
Literary
All Sexes & Sexualities
Los Angeles Times Book Review 🕮 205
Village Voice 🕮 308
Voice Literary Supplement 🕮 308
Gay
James White Review 🕮 281
Sexuality
All Sexes & Sexualities
Big Ted & Manu 🕮 161
Community News 🕮 235
Faerie Dish Rag (FDR) 🕮 205
Hot & Bothered 🕮 53
Houston Voice 🕮 343
Mailshoppe Inc. 🕮 59
Mountain Top Publishing 🕮 228
North Park Review 🕮 212
Provincetown Magazine 🕮 272
Queer Press, Inc. 🕮 235
River Bend Vision 🕮 256
Rocky Mountain Oyster 🕮 228
Spectator Magazine 🕮 199
Tab International 🕮 59
Tamaki Makaurau 🕮 161
Update 🕮 201
USECA Communications Inc. 🕮 53
Wire 🕮 242
Bisexual
Bi Focus 🕮 331
Bifocal 🕮 281
Female
Colorado Woman News 🕮 228
Defiance 🕮 333
Feminist Voices 🕮 356
Fountain 🕮 236
Hera 🕮 297
Herland Sister Resources, Inc. 🕮 323
Herland Voice 🕮 323
Klondyke Kontact 🕮 193
Labyrinth 🕮 331
Liberation 🕮 30
Life In Out 🕮 322
Minnesota Womens' Press 🕮 281
off our backs 🕮 235
Signals 🕮 293
Sonoma County Women's Voices 🕮 222
Valley Women's Voice 🕮 267
Women's Community Center 🕮 297
Women's Times 🕮 212
WomenWise 🕮 279
Womyn's Press 🕮 325
Gay
Celebrity Circumcision Survey Master List 🕮 201
Frontiers 🕮 225
Gay Gazette 🕮 85
Gesprecks- en Onthaalcentrum u. z. w. 🕮 36
GOC 🕮 *See* Gesprecks- en Onthaalcentrum u. z. w.
H. 🕮 226
Indiana Word 🕮 253
Mavericks 🕮 293
Planet Homo 🕮 225
Quest Publications 🕮 226
RFD 🕮 336
Silveraim Ltd. 🕮 85
Sodomite Invasion Review 🕮 46
Uitkomst 🕮 36
White Crane Newsletter 🕮 218
Word Publications 🕮 253
Lesbian
Aché 🕮 196
Amazon Times 🕮 264
Common Ground 🕮 295
Common Lives, Lesbian Lives 🕮 257
Dimensions 🕮 338
Dinah 🕮 317
Entre Nous Newsletter 🕮 220
Grapevine 🕮 34
Island Lesbian Connection 🕮 246
Kuumba 🕮 189
Ladies Home Companion 🕮 325
Lavendar Express 🕮 289
Lavendar Letter 🕮 328
Lavendar Morning 🕮 276
Lesbian Contradiction 🕮 218
Lesbian Health News 🕮 320
Lesbian Information San Antonio 🕮 344
Lesbian News 🕮 222
Lesbian Resource Center Community News 🕮 353
Lesbian Voices 🕮 287
Lesbian World Newsletter 🕮 319
Lesbians in Colorado 🕮 228
Lestalk 🕮 284
LISA 🕮 *See* Lesbian Information San Antonio
Lite & Lively 🕮 53
Mama Raga 🕮 235
Matrix 🕮 295
New Phazes Newsletter 🕮 227
Radical Chick 🕮 308
Rose Publications 🕮 284
She Bang 🕮 85
Virago 🕮 334
WomanSpace 🕮 344
Womenspace 🕮 286
Womyn's Community Newsletter 🕮 354
Word is Out! 🕮 320
Lesbian, Gay, Bi, & Transgendered
Ace Publishing, Inc. 🕮 194
Adelaide Gay Times 🕮 30
Adelaide GT 🕮 30
Alabama Forum 🕮 191
All Points North 🕮 76
Alliance News 🕮 341
Alliance of Massachusetts Asian Lesbians and Gay Men 🕮 269
Alternate Expressions 🕮 298
Ambush 🕮 260
Amethyst 🕮 297
Angles 🕮 46
Apex 🕮 261
Arkansas Advisor 🕮 195
Au Courant 🕮 327
Awhina 🕮 163
Baltimore Alternative 🕮 264
Baltimore Gay Paper 🕮 264
Bay Area Reporter 🕮 218
Bay Windows 🕮 269
Beacon 🕮 203
Berkshire Alternatives 🕮 273
Best Publishing Group 🕮 151
Between Ourselves 🕮 316
Between The Lines 🕮 273
Beyond 2002 🕮 353
Blikk 🕮 164
BLK Publishing Co. 🕮 189
Blue Ridge Lambda Press 🕮 347
Bluestone Media 🕮 31
Bottom Line 🕮 208
Boyz 🕮 85
Breathing Space 🕮 287
Bromfield Street Educational Foundation 🕮 269
Brother Sister 🕮 32
Capital Q 🕮 27
Capital Xtra! 🕮 53
Center News 🕮 205
Christopher Street 🕮 308
Cleveland For You & Akron Too! 🕮 319
Coming Out Pagan 🕮 265
Common Bond 🕮 294
Community 🕮 296
Community Connections 🕮 313
Community News 🕮 324
Community Pride Reporter 🕮 261
Community Voice 🕮 243
Compass 🕮 205
Concord 🕮 251
Dallas Voice 🕮 341
David Enterprises 🕮 198
David Magazine 🕮 198
De Gay Krant 🕮 151
Diva & Empress Publications, Inc. 🕮 273
Diversity 🕮 247
Dore 🕮 337
Down Town 🕮 108
Down Town Redaktion Nord 🕮 121
Dykespeak 🕮 218
Ecce Queer 🕮 353
Echo Magazine 🕮 194
Edge 🕮 205
Emerald City News 🕮 258
Encounter 🕮 242
Equal Time 🕮 279

Publishers: Newspapers: Sexuality

Etcetera Magazine 244
Exit 97, 172
Facette 115
Fag Rag 269
Family Next Door 208
First 108
For You 256
For You Productions 319
Friendly Voice 241
Front Page 316
Frontera Gay 212
Gay & Lesbian Quarterly 208
Gay & Lesbian Times/Uptown 196
Gay Alaska 192
Gay Anglia 71
Gay Chicago Magazine 251
Gay Community News 246, 269
Gay Community News (GCN) 136
Gay Express 108
Gay GAIA 291
Gay Life 108
Gay Ol' Times 327
Gay People's Chronicle 317
Gay Review 269
Gay Scene 308
Gaybeat 317
Gayly Oklahoman 323
GAYmeinsam 135
Gay-Plus 117
Gaze Magazine 279
Gazette 236
GLSO News 259
Graffitti 354
Hag Rag 357
Hamburger Gay Information 120
Highland Publications, c. c. 172
Identity Newspaper 192
Identity, Inc. 192
Illico 97
Impact 260
IN Newsweekly 269
IN Publications 269
In Step 355
In Step Magazine 282
In The Life 295
Infogai 172
Information Express 349
Jungle Vine 246
Kacmer Publishing Co. 247
Kentucky Word 258
Lambda Publications 251
Las Vegas Bugle 286
Latest Isssue 210
Lavendar Pages 218
Lavendar Prairie News 248
Lavendar Publishing 46
Lavendar Reader 222
Leaping La Crosse News 356
Left of Center 335
Letter 258
Letterhead 258
Maize 281
Masco Communication 190
Melbourne Star Observer 31
Metra 277
Metro Line 231
Michael Sürth Verlag 108
Mississipi Voice 282
Mom Guess What! 210
MX 85
Network for the 10% Plus 289
New Voice 285
New York Native 308
News 320
News of the Columbus Gay & Lesbian Community 320
News-Telegraph 282, 283
Nightlines 251
Nouveau Midwest 318
Now Cleveland 321
Nürnberger Schwulenpost 129
Observer 195
Odyssey Magazine 218
Ohio Word 317
On The Wilde Side 308
Open Hands 235
Our Own Community Press 347
Our Paper 220
Our Times 78
Out 332
Out and About 348, 354
Out Front 228
Out in the Mountains 346
Out Magazine 308
Out of London Limited 85
Out Pages 236
Out! Magazine 294
Outlines 251
OutNow 196
Outwords 298
Parachute 257
Parlee Plus/ Equal Time the News 296
Paz y Liberación 343
Perceptions 64
Personally Speaking 258
Philadelphia Gay News (PGN) 190
Phœnix Press 261
Phœnix Resource 193
Phœnix Rising 218
Piasa Publishing Company 282, 283
Pillar of the Gay, Lesbian, & Bisexual Community 345
Pink Express 162
Pink Paper 85, 312
Pink Triangle Press 46, 53, 59
Planet Homo 239
Playland Magazine 220
Plus Voice 251
Preferred Stock 228
Pride Publishing & Typsetting, Inc. 314
Progress Tribune 335
Proud Out Loud 294
Publicació Degana del Moviment Gai a Catalunya 172
Q Notes 314
Query 336
Record 308
Reno Informer 287
Richmond Pride 349
Rosa Zone 112
San Antonio Marquise 344
San Francisco Bay Times 218
San Francisco Sentinel 218
Sappho's Isle 295
Scoop 236
Scots Scene 169
Seattle Gay News 353
Senior Action in a Gay Environment (S. A. G. E.) 308
Sentury Publications 251
Sierra Voice 281
Silveraim Ltd. 76, 85
Slant 218
Sound Out 350
South Bay Times 220
South Texas Voice 344
Southern Voice 244
Spank 333
Speak Out 353
Star Magazine 208
Stonewall News 308
Stonewall News Spokane 354
Stonewall Union Reports 320
Suburban Network 252
Support Line 237
Sydney Star Observer 27
SYOL Ltd. 297
Tacoma Sounds 354
Tattler 260
Ten Percent 205
Texas Triangle 339
That New Magazine 308
This Month in Mississipi 282
This Week in Saint Louis (TWISL) 247
This Week in Texas (TWT) 338
Thud 85
Times of the Heartland 285
Toledo Area Gay & Lesbian Affiliation 322
Triangle 240
Triangle Journal News 337
Triangle Rising 195
Tulsa News 324
TWIST 353
Ultra Ink, Inc. 251
Update 212
Verlag W.-D. Fritsch 108
Voices Magazine 260
Volumé 298
Washington Blade 235
WAVES 232
Wayves 48
We The People 222
Weekly News 235
Western Express 194
Westside Publishing 33
Windy City Times 251
Wisconsin Light 355
Women Centered News 296
WomenWorks 279
Womyn's Words 241
Word Publications 258, 317
WSO - Westside Observer 33
Xtra! 59
Xtra! West 46
Young Gay/Lesbian Life 353

Male
FFT Publishing 22
Mail2Male 22

Transgender
ADF Editorial Services 168
Boy's Own 85
FTM Network 85
Grace & Lace Letter 282
Tartan Skirt 168

Spanking

Heterosexual
Spanking Times 311
Tiffany Enterprises 311

NEWSWIRE SERVICES

Sexuality

Lesbian, Gay, Bi, & Transgendered
GayNet 294

VIDEOS

BDSM

All Sexes & Sexualities
Beth Tyler Labs 231
M & M Productions 218
West Video 159

Gay
Marathon Films 22
Shotgun Video 218

Heterosexual
AVI Productions 22

Lesbian
O Productions 308

Bears

Male
Girth & Mirth 22

Bondage

All Sexes & Sexualities
Bon Vu Enterprises 198

Gay
Grapik Arts Productions 218
Zeus 205

Heterosexual
Star Maker Video 308

Erotic

All Sexes & Sexualities
FM Concepts 207
Rosebud Productions 225

Gay
Colt Studios 223
Paragon 153

Fetish

All Sexes & Sexualities
Starbright Productions 218

Gay
Bi Coastal Productions 212
BIC *See* Bi Coastal Productions

Heterosexual, Male
Messy Fun 339

Piercing & Tattooing

All Sexes & Sexualities
Flash Video 218

Sexuality

All Sexes & Sexualities
Erotica S. F. 218
Focus International 290

Gay
Avalon Video International 23
Bi Line Productions 205
Bijou Video 190
Campus Studios 225

Spanking

Gay
Control-T Studios 206
Studio-7 199

Heterosexual
Nu-West Productions 220
Redboard Video 218

Heterosexual, Male
Camera Art 23

RADIO

AIDS

Lesbian, Gay, Bi, & Transgendered
4TTT FM 103.9 29
QuAC Voice 29

GENERAL

All Sexes & Sexualities
Access Community Radio AM 810 161
CFUV FM 101.9 47
Offbeat 47
SAFE 161
Spectrum Radio AM 558 85
Stichting M.V.S. FM 106.8, Cable 103.8 153

Female
KBOO Radio FM 90.7 326
KTRU FM 91.7 343
WFHB 254
Womansoul 326
Women's Hour 343

Lesbian, Gay, Bi, & Transgendered
Aliens 153
Alternative Accent 161
G.A.Y, The Radio 85

SEXUALITY

All Sexes & Sexualities
Bread & Roses 326
Gay & Lesbian London 85
GLR *See* Greater London Radio
Greater London Radio 85
WMUA 267
Women's Media Project 267

Gay
Gaytime FM 162
Spectrum 162

Lesbian
Amazon Country 331
KBOO Radio FM 90.7 326
Lavendar Wimmin 308
Lesbian Radio 161
Lesbian Sisters 207
LMT 94.4 FM 104
Overnight Productions FM 90.7 207
Plains FM 96.9 161
WUSB FM 90.1 308
WXPN FM 88.5 331

Lesbian, Gay, Bi, & Transgendered
1008 kHz 25
2NCR-FM 92.9 25
2SER FM 107.3 27
3CR Community Radio, AM 855 kHz 31
3D Radio 93.7 FM 30
4CCCC - FM 89.1 29
6RTR FM 92.1 34
95 BFM 161
Abus de Confiance 99
Access Community Radio AM 810 161
After Hours 343
Air Libre FM 107.6 37
All Out Productions 85
Alternating Currents 318
Altra Faccia della Luna 143
Altro Martedi 143
Antenne Rose 37
Arci Gay 145
Blitz 130
Boy Trouble 163

Bulletin Lambda 🕮 63
CFMU 93.3 FM 🕮 50
CFRU FM 93.3 🕮 61
Chocopot 🕮 36
Christchurch Lesbian Gay Radio Collective 🕮 23
CHRW 94.7 FM 🕮 51
CITR FM 101.9 🕮 46
CIUT 89.5 FM 🕮 59
CKCU FM 93.1 🕮 53
CKMS FM 94.5 🕮 61
CKWR FM 98.7 🕮 61
Coming Out Show 🕮 46
Concerning Gay & Lesbians 🕮 345
Contact FM 89 🕮 162
Co-op Radio FM 102.7 🕮 46
Croque Monsieur 🕮 98
Different Strokes 🕮 162
Different Voice 🕮 50
Effetto Diversita 🕮 141
Emission Gaie Cayenne 🕮 106
Emission Homophobie 🕮 98
Emscher-Lipper Andersrum 🕮 118
Ethos 🕮 34
FG FM 98.2 🕮 104
Fliederfunk 🕮 129
FM 100 🕮 106
FM 100.3 🕮 96
FM 102.1 🕮 29
FM 102.3 🕮 63
FM 103.1 🕮 173
FM 104.2 🕮 115
FM 104.6 🕮 105
FM 105.7, Cable 83.1 🕮 156
FM 106.7, 92.2, 89.5, & 98.7 🕮 65
FM 107.1 & 97.8 🕮 124
FM 88 🕮 176
FM 88.7 🕮 99
FM 89 🕮 98
FM 89.2 🕮 174
FM 89.4 🕮 97
FM 90.7 🕮 32
FM 91.2 🕮 114
FM 92.1 🕮 31
FM 92.2, Cable 106.2 🕮 130
FM 94.1 🕮 98
FM 95.3 🕮 174
FM 95.8 🕮 129
FM 96 🕮 98
FM 96.0, Cable 95.4 🕮 120
FM 96.1 or FM 104.5 🕮 118
FM 96.2 🕮 96
FM 96.8 🕮 98
FM 98.9 🕮 66
FM 99.7 🕮 98
Freedom FM 🕮 85
Freewave Radio 🕮 156
Fréquence 4 FM 99.6 🕮 98
Frequence Gaie 🕮 104
Fresh Fruit 🕮 281
G & T Breakfast Show 🕮 161
Gaiement Vôtre 🕮 97
Gay & Lesbian Independent Broadcasters 🕮 308
Gay Alternative 🕮 337
Gay Broadcasting Collective 🕮 163
Gay FM 🕮 29
Gay II Gay 🕮 92
Gay Radio 🕮 30, 145, 174
Gay Radio Information News Service 🕮 27
Gay Radio Programme 🕮 31
Gay Radio Sibilla FM 103 🕮 143
Gay Spirit 🕮 291
Gay Wave Length 🕮 25
Gaydar Show 🕮 283
Gaydreams Radio 🕮 331
Gaywaves 🕮 25, 27, 29, 31
Gaywire 🕮 59
GLIB 🕮 *See* Gay & Lesbian Independent Broadcasters
Göteborg Gay Radio 🕮 173
Grins 🕮 *See* Gay Radio Information News Service
G-Spot Productions 🕮 74
Heather's Show 🕮 46
Homo laber 🕮 114
Homo Radio 🕮 312
Homophonies 🕮 98
In The Pink, The Girls Own Show 🕮 161
Joy Melbourne 🕮 32
Kanal Gay 🕮 174
KFAI FM 90.3 🕮 281
KNON FM 89.3 🕮 341
KOPN FM 89.5 🕮 283
KPFT FM 90.1 🕮 343
KRCL FM 91 🕮 345
Lambda Weekly Radio 🕮 341
Lesbian & Gay Voices 🕮 343
Lesbian Show 🕮 46
Loud & Queer 🕮 161
Nova Radio FM 101.5 🕮 146
Nowhere To Hide 🕮 61
Onda Gay 🕮 146
Out & About - The Gay Radio Show 🕮 61
Out & Out 🕮 27
Out Loud 🕮 30
Out This Week 🕮 85
Outspoken Productions 🕮 76
Outwaves 🕮 23
Overnight Productions 🕮 205
People Like You 🕮 53
Pink Antenna 🕮 59
Pink Channel 🕮 120
Pride FM 🕮 74
Queer Talk 🕮 237
Radio Active FM 89 🕮 163
Radio Bigoudi 🕮 100
Radio Campus FM 91.4 🕮 100
Radio Centraal FM 101.6 🕮 36
Radio Città Aperta FM 99.8 & 100.1 🕮 146
Radio Dreyeckland 🕮 105
Radio Filzlaus 🕮 35
Radio Gribouille 🕮 98
Radio Lightfire 🕮 120
Radio Onda Rossa FM 93.3 & 93.45 🕮 141
Radio One FM 91 🕮 161
Radio Popolare FM 105.5 & 107.6 🕮 143
Radio Punto Stereo FM 88.5, 103.5 🕮 143
Radio Rosa 🕮 65, 66
Radio SETA 🕮 96
Radio Studio Aperto FM 88.25 🕮 139
Radio Tilla 🕮 124
Radio Toinen linja 🕮 96
Rainbow Radio Network 🕮 51
RDU FM 98.3 🕮 161
Rosa Mickrowelle 🕮 115
Sexual Reality 🕮 28
Southern Gay Dreams 🕮 245
Speaking Out 🕮 54
Stichting Urania 🕮 151
Stockholm Gay Radio 🕮 176
Tea With The Boys 🕮 161
Tendences Gaies 🕮 98
This Way Out 🕮 161, 205
TOPS FM 104.1 🕮 28
Triangle Rose 🕮 98
Un Mercoledi da Leone 🕮 146
WAIF FM 88.3 🕮 318
We Are Everywhere 🕮 61
Wear FM 103.4FM 🕮 92
WEVL FM 90 🕮 337
WFTL Radio 🕮 237
Wiener Warmenradio FM 107.3 🕮 35
Wild G.A.L.S. 🕮 27
Word is OUT! 🕮 311
WRFG 🕮 245
WRPI FM 91.5 🕮 312
WRSU FM 88.7 🕮 291
WUSB FM 🕮 311
WXPN FM 88.5 🕮 331

SCULPTORS
EROTIC
All Sexes & Sexualities

Anthony Wojnowski's Artworks 🕮 23

Gay

Van Velsor, Gary 🕮 23

FETISH
All Sexes & Sexualities

Jim Johnson Surplus 🕮 200

GENERAL
Transgender

Pike, Ben 🕮 206

STORES
ART GALLERIES
All Sexes & Sexualities

Akehurst Gallery 🕮 85
Ditury & David 🕮 308
Dove Art 🕮 212
Erotic Art Museum 🕮 120
Erotics Gallery 🕮 308
Fahey / Klein Art Gallery 🕮 205
Galerie Michel Vidal 🕮 104
Galerie Welker 🕮 122
Galleria Erotica 🕮 124
Gallerie Reygers 🕮 128
Kunstbanett 🕮 124
Kunsthaus Fischinger 🕮 133
La Luz de Jesus 🕮 205
Larmes D'Eros 🕮 104
Museum für Angewandte Kunst 🕮 118
Neikrug Photographica, Ltd. 🕮 308
O'Connor, A Gallery 🕮 59
PPS. Gallery 🕮 111
Rita Dean Gallery 🕮 212
Rycroft Gallery 🕮 220
Tamara Bane Gallery 🕮 205
Todd Kaplan Gallery 🕮 222

Lesbian, Gay, Bi, & Transgendered

Galerie Janssen 🕮 111

BARBER SUPPLIES
All Sexes & Sexualities

Valentine & Son, Inc. 🕮 251

BOOKS
BDSM
All Sexes & Sexualities

Editions Jaybird 🕮 37

General
All

Mags 'R' Us 🕮 308

All Sexes & Sexualities

100th. Monkey Books 🕮 59
A. A. Michael Books 🕮 254
Abbey Books 🕮 73
ABC Buchladen 🕮 123
Aberdeen Bookshop 🕮 162
Agora 🕮 155
Alfi News 🕮 353
Alleycat Books Coöp 🕮 92
Alternatives 🕮 74
American Book Center 🕮 153, 154
Andere Buchhandlung 🕮 131
Androgyne 🕮 63
Aradia Books 🕮 193
Aragon Buchladen 🕮 127
Argos 🕮 38
Ariel Books 🕮 46
Art of Fée 🕮 120
Atlantic News 🕮 48
Atomic Books 🕮 264
Auntie's Bookstore 🕮 354
Author Author 🕮 205, 299
Baileywick Books 🕮 230
Bakker 🕮 156
Barbara's Bookstore 🕮 251
Bargain Books & News Stand 🕮 238
Barnett's Bookstore 🕮 243
Basil's Bookstore 🕮 298
Better Books 🕮 169
Beyond Words Bookshop 🕮 272
Biff's Bookstore 🕮 349
Blackthorn Books 🕮 79
Bloodroot 🕮 229
Bloomsbury Books 🕮 324
Blue Door Bookstore 🕮 212
Blue Heron Books 🕮 238
Blue Star Publications 🕮 88
Bluff Park Rare Books 🕮 203
BMCF Antiquariat 🕮 109
Bob Miller Bookroom 🕮 59
Bobbies Bookshop 🕮 169
Boekhandel Mercurius b.v. 🕮 153
Bold Print 🕮 287
Book Depot 🕮 239
Book Exchange 🕮 73, 93
Book Gallery 🕮 308, 329
Book Hampton 🕮 308
Book Loft 🕮 222
Book Mantle 🕮 46
Book Nook 🕮 239
Book Sale Gallery 🕮 299
Book Soup 🕮 205
Book Stall, Inc 🕮 332
Bookcase 🕮 94
Bookhaven 🕮 231
Bookie Joint 🕮 278
Bookland 🕮 255
Bookland Of Mill Creek 🕮 263
Booklegger 🕮 199
Bookmark 🕮 61
Bookmark Bookstore 🕮 88
Bookmarks 🕮 85
Books & Co. 🕮 321
Books & Company 🕮 218
Books 'n' Books 🕮 43
Books Upstairs 🕮 137
Books, Etc. 🕮 85, 224, 263
Bookscene 🕮 89
Bookshop Santa Cruz 🕮 222
Books-N-Things 🕮 284
Bookstore 🕮 270, 282
Bookstore Ltd. 🕮 206
Bookstore on West 25th. 🕮 319
Bookworm 🕮 73, 90
Borderline Books 🕮 27
Borders Book Shop 🕮 245, 255, 256, 265, 270, 274, 283, 331, 332
Borealis Bookstore 🕮 299
Bottega di Monica e Patrick 🕮 144
Bradley Books 🕮 265
Brookline Booksmith 🕮 269
Broward Adult Books 🕮 237
Brug 🕮 38
Bruna 🕮 153
Brushstrokes 🕮 245
Bücherboom 🕮 120
Bücherkiste 🕮 129
Buchhandlung Berliner Promenade 🕮 132
Buchhandlung Decins 🕮 121
Buchladen am Markt 🕮 130
Buddenbrooks 🕮 269
Bull Durham's News 🕮 314
Bulldog News 🕮 350, 353
By The Books 🕮 200
Cahoots 🕮 345
Cardome 🕮 74
Carl von Ossietsky Buchhandlung 🕮 130
Carmichael's Bookstore 🕮 259
Caroline Street Books 🕮 238
Changing Hands Bookstore 🕮 194
Changing Times Bookstore 🕮 243
Chassman & Bem Booksellers 🕮 346
Chelsea Bookstore 🕮 203
Chelsea Station News 🕮 336
Chimney Sweep Books 🕮 222
Circus of Books 🕮 205, 225
City Lights Bookstore 🕮 218
Clean Well-Lighted Place for Books 🕮 220
Clyde Books 🕮 169
Coalesce Bookstore 🕮 220
Cody's Books 🕮 197
Common Knowledge Books 🕮 59
Community Bookshop 🕮 298
Community Counselling & Consultation, Inc. 🕮 209
Community Newscenter #1 🕮 277
Community Newscenter #4 🕮 274
Community Newscenter / Webster's 🕮 276
Compendium 🕮 85
Conant & Conant Books 🕮 326
Constant Reader Bookshop 🕮 357
Cornerhouse Books 🕮 76
Crazy Wisdom Bookstore 🕮 274
Cutting Edge 🕮 292
Daily Planet News 🕮 284
Darakan 🕮 37
Davis-Kidd Bookseller 🕮 336, 337
Dekker / V. d. Vegt 🕮 157
Different Drummer Bookshop 🕮 201
Disco Book Store 🕮 320
Dodds Bookshop 🕮 203
Domus 🕮 140
Downtown Books & News 🕮 313
Dragonfly Books 🕮 337
Dream Haven Books Uptown 🕮 281
Du Beffroi 🕮 38
Earth Spirit 🕮 292
Earthling Bookstore 🕮 221
Easons 🕮 137
Edward's Books 🕮 331
Either/Or 🕮 205
Emporio del Libro 🕮 147
Entitlement—The Book Company 🕮 48

Stores: Books: General

Etc. 📖 191
Euro X 📖 37
Europa Bookstore 📖 339
Exploded Views Books 📖 207
Fanfare Books 📖 54
Farley's Bookstore 📖 329
Fig Garden Bookstore 📖 200
Flying Lemur Bookstore 📖 321
Food For Thought Alternative Book Store 📖 316
Food For Thought Books 📖 53, 267
Four Corner News 📖 298
Fremont Place Book Company 📖 353
Front Page 📖 43
Frontline Books 📖 23
Gaia Bookstore 📖 197
Galisteo News 📖 295
Giovanni's Room 📖 331
Glasgow University Shop 📖 169
Gleebooks 📖 27
Globe News 📖 205
Goerings' Book Center 📖 237
Golden Braid Books 📖 345
Golden Dawn Books 📖 76
Golden Notebook 📖 313
Golden Thread Booksellers 📖 231
Goldmine Bookshop 📖 162
Grand Mello 📖 142
Grand River Books 📖 275
Granville Book Company 📖 46
Grapevine Books 📖 55
Grass Roots 📖 325
Grassroots Books 📖 257
Green Gables Bookstore 📖 325
Greenleaf Bookshop 📖 70
Greenwood's Bookshoppe 📖 43
Gualala Books 📖 200
Harry Schwartz Bookshop 📖 357
Hartwigs Bookshop 📖 32
Harvard Book Store 📖 269
Haus des Buches Carl Habel GmbH 📖 116
Hawley-Cooke 📖 259
Hayats Magazines & Gifts 📖 345
Hays & Sanders Bookstore 📖 195
Hemetro 📖 329
Hibiscus Books 📖 260
Hijman 📖 154
Hippopotame 📖 129
Hog On Ice 📖 218
Horizon Bookstore 📖 248
Hors Château 📖 38
Houseman's 📖 85
Hugendubel 📖 117
Humboldt Buchhandlung 📖 113
Hungry Head Books 📖 325
Hyde Park News 📖 34
Il Seme 📖 140
Imprints - Booksellers 📖 30
In Other Words 📖 326
In Other Words, Ltd. 📖 73
Indecent Exposure 📖 265
Independence News 📖 314
Independent Bookshop 📖 90
Inner Bookshop 📖 90
Intabooks 📖 85
Internationalist Books 📖 313
Ivy's Bookshop 📖 47
Janus 📖 85
John Smith 📖 169
Joseph-Beth Booksellers 📖 259
JP L'Agora 📖 37
Just Books 📖 164
Kepler's Books 📖 209
Key West Island Bookstore 📖 238
Keyhole Bookshop 📖 27
King's English Bookstore 📖 345
Kramer Books & Afterwords 📖 235
L.U.U. Bookshop 📖 94
La Conchiglia 📖 140
Lamp Bookshop 📖 76
Lance Publications 📖 85
Land in Sight 📖 117
Last Word Newsstand 📖 199
Laughing Horse Books 📖 326
Laughing Moon Bookstore 📖 262
Laurel News Agency 📖 265
Left Bank Books 📖 284, 353
Left Bank Bookstall 📖 251
Liberty Books 📖 206
Librairie d'Albret 📖 98
Librarie La Scarabée D'or 📖 104
Lidéfix 📖 37
Lioness Books 📖 210
Litfass 📖 119
Little Store 📖 272
Living Batch Bookstore 📖 294
Lodestar Books 📖 191
Looking Glass Books 📖 327
Lovejoys 📖 85
Luna Books 📖 235
M. Coy Books 📖 353
Magazine 📖 218
Magni 📖 113
Malaprop's Bookstore 📖 313
Manifest 📖 156
Männertreu 📖 129
Marlow Heights Periodicals 📖 266
McNally Robinson Booksellers 📖 47
Metro News 📖 283
Midland Book Centre 📖 93
Modern Times Bookstore 📖 218
Modernway Books 📖 162
Monroe Avenue Book Bin 📖 325
Montanus Aktuell 📖 113, 118, 119, 120, 122, 123, 126, 127, 128, 130, 132
Mosaic Books 📖 309
Mount Royal College Bookstore 📖 43
Munro's Bookstore 📖 47
Mushroom Bookshop 📖 89
Myrtle Bookstore 📖 273
Mystery Loves Company 📖 264
Mystic Bookshop 📖 51
Nahani 📖 311
Neuer Weg 📖 136
News & Photo Shop 📖 321
News from Nowhere 📖 87
Newsbreak 📖 272
Newsland Bookstore 📖 294
Newsstand 📖 350
Northshire Bookstore 📖 346
Northtown Books 📖 196
Nouvelle 📖 38
October Books 📖 77
Octopus Books 📖 46, 53
Old Wives Tales 📖 218
Once Upon a Time 📖 248
Oriana's Bookcafé 📖 335
Oscar Wilde Memorial Bookstore 📖 309
Oude Mol 📖 157
OUT 📖 *See* Once Upon a Time
Oxford Books 📖 245
Pacific Book House 📖 247
Page One Books 📖 77
Pages 📖 59
Paper Shop 📖 75
Paper Skyscraper 📖 314
Pappy's 📖 260
Pavillion Mall Booksellers 📖 319
Pepper's News Stand 📖 355
Pepperland 📖 37
Perrin & Treggett Booksellers 📖 290
Phambili Books 📖 172
Phœnix Books 📖 283
Phœnix Rising 📖 349
Pic-A-Book 📖 356
Pink List 📖 85
Pipeline Bookshop 📖 85
Pistil Books & News 📖 353
Powell's City of Books 📖 327
Prairie Lights Bookstore 📖 257
Proteus 📖 119
Provincetown Bookshop 📖 272
Public House Bookshop 📖 74
Quest Bookshop 📖 347
R B Books 📖 71
R2B2 Books 📖 46
Rainbow Revolution 📖 356
Ray's Playpen 📖 283
Read All About It 📖 74
Read All Over 📖 242
Reader's Feast 📖 231
Red & Black Books Collective 📖 353
Red Herring Coöp Books 📖 48
Redbook 📖 269, 270
Regenbogen Buchhandlung 📖 130
Regulator Bookshop 📖 315
Renaissance Books 📖 284
Risque's 📖 317
Robin's Books 📖 331
Roode Hand 📖 154
Rooie Rat 📖 151
Rosebud & Fish Community Bookstore 📖 327
Rubyfruit Books 📖 242
Ruward 📖 154
Saint Elmo's Books & Music 📖 332
Scholtens 📖 155
Sec 52 Buchladen & Galerie 📖 177
Serri di Piazza, Arcobaleno 📖 141
Shakespeare & Co. 📖 309
Sheela-Na-Gig 📖 137
Sidney's Newstand 📖 261
Silkwood Books, Inc. 📖 311
Single Step Co-op 📖 78
Small Press Traffic 📖 218
Soho Books 📖 89
Southern Books 📖 162
Stacey's Bookshop 📖 218
Steubenville News 📖 322
Steve's Broadway News 📖 353
Stortford Lodge Bookshop 📖 162
Strathclyde University Union Shop 📖 169
Sundance 📖 253
Sunshine Gifts 📖 209
Sunshine News 📖 284
Sutherland's Books 📖 64
Talking Leaves... Books 📖 298
Tattered Cover Book Store 📖 228
This Ain't The Rosedale Library 📖 59
Three Birds Bookstore 📖 243
Three Lives & Co., Ltd. 📖 309
Tower Books 📖 210
Towne News 📖 333
Tribune 📖 156
Tronsmo Bokhandel 📖 164
Tucholsky Buchladen 📖 130
Twenty-Third Avenue Book 📖 327
Unabridged Books 📖 251
Unicorn Books 📖 270
Universal News Agency 📖 205
University Bookstore 📖 257
University Center Bookstore 📖 285
University of Toronto Bookstore 📖 59, 60
Vacaville Book Co. 📖 199
Vertigo Books 📖 235
Village Green Bookstore 📖 298, 299, 311, 329
Volumes 📖 60
Volumes of Pleasure 📖 220
Vrije Boekhandel 📖 158
W. & G. Foyles 📖 85
W. H. Smith 📖 85
Waking Owl 📖 345
Walden Books 📖 247
Waterstones 📖 76, 86, 137
Way Out West Bookshop 📖 25
Wedge Bookshop 📖 93
Wendell's Magazines 📖 309
West & Wilde Bookshop 📖 169
Westchester News 📖 239
Westminster Books 📖 48
Wildcat Books 📖 200
Windsong Books & Records 📖 199
With The Times 📖 43
Wohlthat'sche Buchhandlung 📖 113, 126
Womansline Books 📖 51
Women's Book Club 📖 86
Wordplay 📖 48
Wordsworth 📖 270
World Book & News 📖 205
World Development Centre 📖 138
World Eye Bookshop 📖 270
World's Biggest Bookstore 📖 60
Worldwide News 📖 311
Young & Welshans Books 📖 276
Zapata 📖 123
Zwart Op Wit 📖 153

Female

Antigone Books 📖 195
Aquarius Books 📖 254
Bluestocking Books 📖 335
Book Woman 📖 339
Charis Books & More 📖 245
ClaireLight 📖 222
Crazy Ladies Bookstore 📖 318
Different World 📖 355
Dreams & Swords 📖 255
Dwelling Place 📖 329
Everyone's Books 📖 346
Fan The Flames 📖 320, 321
Gertrude Stein Memorial Bookshop 📖 332
Her Story 📖 333
Herland Book Café 📖 222
Herland Sister Resources, Inc. 📖 323
Imprints Bookstore 📖 354
Iris Books 📖 237
Judith's Room 📖 308
June Addams Book Shop 📖 248
La Fourmi Ailée 📖 104
La Librairie des Femmes 📖 104
Lady Iris 📖 288
Lammas Women's Books & More 📖 264
Lunaria Feminist Bookstore 📖 272
Mama Bears 📖 208
Meristem 📖 337
My Sisters' Words 📖 312
New Words 📖 269
Out of the Dark 📖 348
Page One 📖 209
Pandora Book Peddlars 📖 292
Pearls Booksellers 📖 203
Prairie Moon 📖 247
Purple Moon 📖 348
Raven in the Grove 📖 208
Room of One's Own 📖 356
Silver Moon 📖 85
Smedley's Bookshop 📖 299
Southern Sisters 📖 313
Stepping Stones 📖 209
Toronto Women's Bookstore 📖 59
Two Sisters Bookshop 📖 220
Woman to Woman Books 📖 43
Woman's Place 📖 345
Woman's Place Bookstore 📖 43
Woman's Prerogative 📖 275
Women In Print 📖 46
Women's Book Store 📖 46
Women's Bookshop 📖 50
Women's Project 📖 196
Women's Therapy Center 📖 331
Xantippe 📖 153

Gay

Agora Bokhandel AB 📖 176
Big & Tall 📖 23
Book Bin East 📖 331
Category Six Books 📖 190
Colt Bookstore 📖 85
Hommes Bookshop 📖 308
Intermale Gay Bookstore 📖 153
Lavendelschwert Buchladen 📖 124
LITFASS Der Buchladen 📖 114
Männerschwarm Buchladen 📖 120
Max & Millian 📖 128
Neuens Co-Op 📖 104
Prinz Eisenherz Buchladen 📖 111
Red River Books 📖 72

Lesbian

Book Garden 📖 228
Crone's Harvest 📖 269
Sisterspirit Bookstore 📖 220
Widdershins Books 📖 327

Lesbian, Gay, Bi, & Transgendered

Abaton Books 📖 227
Adam 📖 111
After Stonewall 📖 53
AfterWords 📖 357
Alaska Women's Bookstore 📖 193
Arbor Moon Alternative Bookstore 📖 285
Arcane Bookshop 📖 33
Baffin Books 📖 96
Bailey/Coy Books 📖 353
Beyond The Closet 📖 353
Boadecia's Books 📖 197
Bookshop 📖 27
Bookstore Named Desire 📖 238
Brother's Touch 📖 281
Bruno's 📖 111
Buchladen 46 📖 112
Chapter One Books 📖 291, 292
Choices Books & Music 📖 221
Chosen Books 📖 278
Christopher Street Bookstore 📖 223
Common Language 📖 274
Crossroads Market & Bookstore 📖 341, 343
Curious Times 📖 341
Different Light 📖 218, 225, 308

Dominion News 🕮 47
Ellie's Garden 🕮 344
Erlkœnig Buchladen 🕮 133
Everywoman Books 🕮 47
Faubourg-Marigny Bookstore 🕮 261
Full Circle Books 🕮 294
Gay's The Word 🕮 70
Gegen den Strich Buchcafé 🕮 115
Get Booked 🕮 286
Glad Day Bookshop 🕮 59, 269
Grapevine Books 🕮 287
GW Miami Beach 🕮 239
Hares & Hyenas 🕮 32
Inklings 🕮 343
Lambda Passages 🕮 239
Lambda Resources 🕮 331
Lambda Rising 🕮 233, 235, 264
Lavendar Books 🕮 205
Lavendar Hearts 🕮 329
Lavender's 🕮 240
Liberty Books 🕮 339
Librairie du Bon Secours 🕮 37
Libreria Babele 🕮 139, 142
Libreria Internazionale Luxemburg 🕮 144
Lifestyle Books 🕮 296
Little Sister's Book & Art Emporium 🕮 46
Lobo After Dark 🕮 341
Lobo Bookstore 🕮 339, 343
Max Images 🕮 348
Mother Kali's Books 🕮 325
Mots à la Bouche 🕮 104
Now Voyager 🕮 272
Obelisk The Bookstore 🕮 212
Opening Books 🕮 192
Oscar Wilde Buchladen 🕮 117
Other Side Bookshop 🕮 137
Ottawa Women's Bookstore 🕮 53
Out & About Books 🕮 241
Out! Books 🕮 74
Out! Bookshop 🕮 160, 161, 163
Outright Books 🕮 349
Outwrite Bookstore & Coffeehouse 🕮 245
Pages Video & More 🕮 284
Pandora Books for Open Minds 🕮 276
People Like Us 🕮 251
People's Books 🕮 357
Pink Pyramid 🕮 318
Pride Agenda Bookshop 🕮 251
Pride Bookstore 🕮 348
Rainbow Books 🕮 55
Rainbow Bookshop 🕮 179
Rainbow Bookstore 🕮 321
Rainbows Ltd. 🕮 192
Rising Moon Books & Beyond 🕮 314
Rosa Rummet 🕮 173, 176
Saint Marks Bookshop 🕮 309
Sisters' & Brothers' Bookstore 🕮 294
Sons & Daughters 🕮 276
Source Bookstore 🕮 232
Spartacus Books 🕮 46
Textures 🕮 344
Tomes & Treasures 🕮 243
Trongate Books 🕮 170
Unicorn Bookstore 🕮 225
Village Bookshop 🕮 76
Visions & Dreams 🕮 258
Vrolijk Boekhandel 🕮 153
White Rabbit Books 🕮 314
White Rabbit Books & Things 🕮 315

Transgender

Lee's Mardi Gras Boutique 🕮 308

CLOTHING

Adult Baby

All Sexes & Sexualities

Cozy Time Adult Baby Wear 🕮 43

Transvestite

Especially for Me 🕮 224

Corsets

All Sexes & Sexualities

Banned 🕮 86

Cowboy

All Sexes & Sexualities

Leatherhead Shop 🕮 259

Fetish

All Sexes & Sexualities

Ad Hoc 🕮 86
Air Transilvania 🕮 138
Amour 🕮 160, 161
Annette K Fashions 🕮 115
Arabesque 🕮 178, 180
Artistes 🕮 104
Atom Age 🕮 86
AZZLO Discipline Co. 🕮 148
Barbarella (Armoury) 🕮 89
Bizarr-Mode 🕮 35
Black Stratsch 🕮 111
Blackstyle 🕮 111
Boutique de Sade 🕮 120
Boutique Highlights 🕮 128
Boutique Minuit 🕮 37
Clingline 🕮 72
Cocoon 🕮 86, 93
Cosmic Wear 🕮 124
Crazy Fashion 🕮 130
Crazy Sexy 🕮 177
Crazy World 🕮 70
Dana 🕮 179
Dark Alley 🕮 289
Desire 🕮 90
Dormann, Ulf 🕮 65
Dream Dresser 🕮 225
Dressed To Kill 🕮 251
Dressing For Pleasure 🕮 291
Dynasty 🕮 147
East of Eden 🕮 86
Eccentric Fashion 🕮 178
E-Garbs 🕮 74
Ellen Schippers Design 🕮 153
Fantasy Fayre 🕮 86
Fashion & Tools 🕮 113, 120
Fashion Cats 🕮 115
Fetische in Leder, Latex, & Lack 🕮 117
Fetish Fetish 🕮 86
Folies de Sade 🕮 37
Forbidden 🕮 76
Galactica 🕮 104
Gwendoline 🕮 37
Hautnah 🕮 111
He & She 🕮 60
Honour 🕮 86
Ian's 🕮 309
Kastley GmbH 🕮 133
Kießling Handelsagentur 🕮 128
Larmes D'Hollywood 🕮 38
Leader Ship 🕮 104
Love & Flash 🕮 121
Lucrezia & De Sade 🕮 32
Massad 🕮 157
MGL Sexy Lingerie 🕮 104
Michelle Fashions 🕮 75
Modern Style 🕮 124
Ms. Charade 🕮 46
Naughty But Nice 🕮 255
Nightstyle Designs 🕮 72
Opera 🕮 178
Pagan Metal 🕮 86
Paradiso Bodyworks 🕮 86
Pillow Talk 🕮 78, 91
Planet Alice 🕮 100
Playmates 🕮 201
Purple Passion 🕮 309
Regalia 🕮 311
Regulation 🕮 86
Religion 🕮 70
Riga 🕮 218
S. W. 3 🕮 121
Schwarze Mode 🕮 111
SCL «O» Fashion 🕮 99
Sexy Cats 🕮 115
She'an'Me Fun Fashions 🕮 86, 87
Shiny Fashion 🕮 122, 132
SIN 🕮 190
Sin-A-Matic 🕮 118
Skin Tight 🕮 53, 151
Skin Two 🕮 86
Subwave Design 🕮 66
Things 🕮 172
Throb 🕮 245
Trashy Lingerie 🕮 205
UZI 🕮 229
Woman's Touch 🕮 291
Worn To Be Wild 🕮 259

Female

Leather & Lace Lingerie 🕮 327
Libido 🕮 86
Mud Honey 🕮 309
Purr…effect 🕮 27
Sh! 🕮 86

Gay

IEM 🕮 *See* International Estetic Men
International Estetic Men 🕮 104
Jeans Mode Trends 🕮 111

Lesbian, Gay, Bi, & Transgendered

Zipper Store 🕮 86

Footwear

All Sexes & Sexualities

Boot Factory 🕮 96
Buzios Mode 🕮 115
First In Schumode 🕮 131
Hiegel, Josef 🕮 128
La Ampurdanesa 🕮 172
Spezial Schuversand 🕮 131
Stiletto Shoes AB 🕮 176
Wholesale Boot Supply 🕮 279

Female

High Heels 🕮 133

Transvestite

Little Shoe Box 🕮 86

Leather

All Sexes & Sexualities

Alley 🕮 251
Avalon Leather 🕮 225
Carline Leathers 🕮 251
Felise Leather 🕮 235
Firefly 🕮 264
Funny Skin 🕮 155
Good Sports 🕮 232
Hide & Sleek 🕮 23
JS Leather 🕮 94
King's Leathers 🕮 236
Leathercraft 🕮 60
Midnight Blue 🕮 245
Night Dreams 🕮 349
Philippe Moda Pelle 🕮 38
Pride Leathers 🕮 311
Source Leather Shop 🕮 199
Sun Leather & Lace 🕮 259
Tom's Boutic 🕮 101
Tschul's 🕮 111
Warlords, Inc. 🕮 245
Wendell's Leather Shop 🕮 219
Worn Out West 🕮 219

Female

Ale Design 🕮 180

Gay

Adler & Schmitt Lederwerkstatt 🕮 119
Erne's Sportlade 🕮 180
Man To Man 🕮 37
Robin & Rik Leathermakers 🕮 153
Skarupe 🕮 120

Lesbian, Gay, Bi, & Transgendered

Image Leather 🕮 218

Lingerie

All Sexes & Sexualities

Agent Provocateur 🕮 23
Foxy Lady 🕮 174
French Addiction 🕮 237

Rubber

All Sexes & Sexualities

Basta Boots 🕮 120
Doc Roc 🕮 86
Fit To Be Tied 🕮 222
House of Whacks 🕮 251
Invincible 🕮 86
James Adult Centre 🕮 89
Kunzmann 🕮 122
Leder-Gummistudio 🕮 118
Modern Armour 🕮 77
Rage Fashions 🕮 93
Rik Production 🕮 120
Rubber & Rivets 🕮 200
Rubber Design Modevertriebsgesellschaft 🕮 123
Sealwear 🕮 73
Stretch 🕮 153
Studio 2 🕮 76
Studio Strak 🕮 32
Syren 🕮 205
Weathervain 🕮 91
Wild Designs 🕮 70
Zweite Haut 🕮 111

Gay

Jox 🕮 111

Sexuality

Transgender

Creative Growth Enterprises 🕮 198
Elizabeth 🕮 147
Fem Fashions, Inc. 🕮 309
Jim Bridges' Boutique 🕮 223
Lingerie by Barbie 🕮 43
Vernon's Specialties, Inc. 🕮 271

Transvestite

Abigail Louise 🕮 70
Another World 🕮 74
Cover Girl Shoes 🕮 86
Ethos 🕮 76
Fantasy Fashions 🕮 225
Foxy Lady 🕮 219
Kentucky Woman 🕮 23
Lee's Mardi Gras Boutique 🕮 309
Tina 🕮 172
Transformation Ltd. 🕮 70, 76, 86, 92, 93
Translucere 🕮 251
Unique Quality Products, Inc. 🕮 309

Sports

Gay

Sports Locker 🕮 86

Uniforms

All Sexes & Sexualities

AAA Police Supply 🕮 270
Advance Uniform Co. 🕮 251
Butler's Uniforms 🕮 219
Code-3 Supply Co. 🕮 205
Dornan Uniforms 🕮 309
F & J Police Equipment, Inc. 🕮 297
Frankel's 🕮 60
Gall's, Inc. 🕮 259
Hyssna 🕮 66
Uniforms, Inc. 🕮 205, 221
VGC Uniforms 🕮 251
WearHouse Uniforms 🕮 200

Wigs

Transgender

Wig Service Shop 🕮 290

EROTICA

BDSM

All Sexes & Sexualities

593 Group 🕮 245
Absolute Leather 🕮 241
Adult Scene Supplies 🕮 94
Aphrodite 🕮 106
Atelier 🕮 124
Atomage 🕮 148
B&B Leatherworks 🕮 43
Black Box 🕮 155
Black Market 🕮 251
Body Worship 🕮 309
Boutique Fancy 🕮 177
Bullock's Leather & Accessories 🕮 205
Caliber 🕮 251
Carpe Diem 🕮 139
Conflicto 🕮 66
Construction Zone 🕮 219
Cramp Leather 🕮 353
Crypt 🕮 196, 212, 226, 353
Crypt On Broadway 🕮 196
D. A. B. 🕮 259
Delta Fashion 🕮 173
Demask 🕮 153
Drondale Limited 🕮 169
Eagle Leather 🕮 25
Essex Intim 🕮 75
Eurotique, Inc. 🕮 243
Exotique 🕮 243
Eyecrusher Leather 🕮 358
Fallen Angel 🕮 237
Fantasy Faire 🕮 287
Fantasy Isle 🕮 230
Fantasy Lingerie 🕮 199
G. D. C. 🕮 153
Gear, Clothing, & Accessories 🕮 348
Hard Labor Leather 🕮 205

Stores: Erotica: BDSM

Hard Line 128
Hellfire Emporium 32
Hot Shop 128
Hubba Hubba 270
Il Bolero 63
Innovations 316
J & S Sports Products 278
Key Largo 86
Kinks 318
Läderverkstan 175
Laurie Lane's Leather World 32
Lazy J Leather 257
Leather by Boots 343
Leather Etc. 219
Leather Harvest 230
Leather Maker 205
Leather Man, Inc. 309
Leather Master 238
Leather Rose 331
Leather Shoppe 294
Leather Underground, Inc. 237
Leather Workshop 74
Leatherworks, Inc. 327
Leder Art & Design 121
Leder Boutique bei Günther 111
Leder Spezial 156
Lock, Stock, & Leather 286
Mack's Leathers 46
Magick & Fetish Shop 205
Male Hide Leathers 252
Marquis de Sade 270
Master Leather 165
Master's Toychest 292
Moose Leather 212
Mr. Chaps Leatherworks 120
MVS 122
My Sin 157
Nima 125
Noir 61
Noir Leather 278
Noose 309
Noose II 309
Northbound Leather Ltd. 60
Occhiolino 144
odd isn't. it? 60
Paradis 66
Paradise Sexy Shop 146
Pleasurable Alternatives 290
Pleasure Place 235
Pleasure Zone 245
Poster Hut 245
Pourquoi Pas? 132
Primitive Leather 272
Px3 252
Radical Leather 27
Renate Buccone 66
RoB 219
S. A. M. Co. 298
S. Wolbrecht 173
Sax Leather 27
Shades of Grey 341
Shock 174
Silverlake Leather 206
SM Bladet / SM Shop 66
Spartacus 206
Stairwell Leathers 43
Stockroom 206
Stormy Leather 219
Studio Blu 146
Submission 247
T.R.'s Leather Rack 348
Taste of Leather 219
Things Medieval 323
Tie Me Down 357
Tino Trevino's Leather Den 309
Trader Tom's Fantasy Depot 237
Walhalla 36, 39
Walter's Leder Boutique 111
Water Hole Custom Leather, Inc. 230
Womyn's Ware 46

Female

Mail & Female 153

Gay

ACME Leather & Toy Co. 318
Boy's Cuir Leather Shop 101
Cornelius Men 128
Cruz Leather Works 66
Expectations 86
Follow Me 128
Horsts Laden 111
H•M - Lederwerk 108
IMRU 321
Innovations 270
Jaguar 219
Leather Post / Taz Men 245
Macho Men's Shop 180
Man Fashion 164
Man Leder Shop 125
Man's World 125
Master Leathers 153
Mike's Custom Leathers 265
Mikes Läder 176
Mister B 23
Mohawk Leather 245
Rack 259
Remedy Versand 120
Secrets Boutique 125
Tailors Unlimited 35
Tiberius ASC 35
Tom of Finland Company Inc. 206
TTBM 104
Warehouse 36
Wayne's LeatheRack 206

Lesbian, Gay, Bi, & Transgendered

Black Moon Leather 198
Christine's Lingerie Inc. 243
Cobra Custom Leather Shop 236
Cuir Plus 63
Doc's Leathers & Harley Davidson Gear 60
Europa 92 139
Expectations 153
Fit 2 A T Leather 229
Harness - Sin City 96
Leather Closet 241
Leather Masters 220
Leather Shop 258
Leather Underground 264
London Leather Cave 86
Mephisto Leather 27
Rochester Custom Leathers 311
Schneiderei Ottokar Fischer 115
Seattle Leather Mercantile 353
Second Skin 261
Tan Ya Hide Ltd. 161
Wrapped 153

Male

Leather Rack 235
Mr. S – Fetters, U.S.A. 219
RoB 86, 153

Transgender

Inclinations 271

Corsets

All Sexes & Sexualities

Romantasy 23

General

All Sexes & Sexualities

1st. Old Store 272
20-20 News 263
321 News & Video 315
609 Novelty 49
95th. Street News 319
99th. Floor 252
Action Books & Video 354
Adam & Eve 25, 331
Adult Books & Cinema 317
Adult Bookstore 262, 285, 290
Adult Education Books 296
Adult Entertainment Center 309
Adult Entrée 258
Adult Pursuits 242
Adult Shop 247, 309
Adult World 290, 312, 331
Adults Etc., Etc. 344
After Dark 43
After Dark Adult Warehouse 43
Aircraft News & Books 231
Airline Books 261
Alabama Adult Books 191
Allies Boulevard Bookstore Downtown 297
Allies Boulevard Bookstore East 297
Alligator News & Books 238
Andromeda 140
Ann Street Adult Entertainment Center 309
Ann Summers 86
Annapolis Road Books 265
Another World 296
Aphro Adult Products 30
Aphrodite/Elle 76
Arc en Ciel 101
Atlantic News Agency 289
Autan X 106
B-1 154, 155, 157
Bank News 319
Bargain Books 284
Batchelor's Library 256
Beate Uhse 117, 121, 123, 126, 130, 133
Best Adult Bookstore 290
Birmingham Adult Books 191
Black Rose 31
Body Language 319
Book Nook, Inc. 264
Book-And 298
Bookends 230
Books, Etc. 219
Boulevard Books 332
Boutique Amour 148
Boutique Carrefour du Sexe Inc. 61, 63
Boutique Demonia 104
Boutique Intim 113
Boutique X 105
Boy Toy 229
Broadway Book & Video 281
Broadway News Center 264
Buchfink 113
Bureau 700 155
Burnet Bookstore 312
Bushido 139
Carousel Books 337
Cerebus 73
Chain Link Addiction 319
Château IV Bookstore 335
Christie's Toy Box 258, 323, 327, 341
Christine Le Duc 153, 154, 155, 156, 157, 158
Cinéma Bleu Inc. 60
City Men Shop & Video 111
City Sex Boutique 133
City Sex Shop 123
Clark's Out of Town News 237
Claudia Sexshop 136
Club X Shop 25 34
Cobra 142
Cocoon 77
Come Again Erotic Emporium 190
Congress Book Shop 263
Continental Books 296
Courageous Books 309
Crimson Phœnix 327
Crypt / North Park Adult Video 196
Cupid's Treasures 252
Cupid's Video Boutique 299
Dacapo Sexladen 134
Daily Globe 43
Danish Book World II 257
Deluxe Book Bargains 299
Denmark Books 248
Desert Adult Books 286
Desiderio 142
Detroit Avenue News 319
Discreet Boutique 47, 64
Dr. Müller's Sex Shop 128, 134
Drake's After Midnight Bookstore 206, 225
Dreams Adult Shop 29
Dundalk News 311
Duo Shop 105
East of Eden 200
Eastern Adult Books 328
Eclectics 283
Elise 155
Elite Adult Books 324
Enigma 105
Eppendorfer 120
Erex 153
Erocenter 173, 174, 175, 176
Erogenous Zone 200
Eros 95, 106, 156, 158, 341
Eros Center 141
Eroshop 98
Erotic Corner 156
Erotic Forum 328
Erotic Shop 112, 130
Erotica Plus 61, 286
Erotik Handlung Copenhagen 134
Erotik Shop 125
Etcetera News 309
Ets Cochon 104
Europa 92 139, 147
Exclusively Adult 327
Exotic Bookstore 321
F Street 197, 198, 199, 212
Fantasy for Adults Only 285
Fantasy House 281
Fantasy Island 331
Fantasy Unlimited 353
Fantasy World 91
Fifth Wheel 288
Filmore News 328
First Amendment 227
Forbidden Fruit 339
Forbidden Fruit Uptown 339
Fort Video & News 315
Fountainview News 343
Fourth Street Bookmart 241
Foxes Adult Books 335
Fun House 154
G & D Merchandise 309
Galesburg Adult Book & Video 252
Gallery Bookstore 256
Garden of Eden 200
Gemini 212
Gents 315
Glove Me Tender 253
Go Up 111
Golden Gate 209, 220
Golden Triangle News 332
Goldies 210
Good Vibrations 197, 219
Grand Opening! 190
Great Northern Books 350
Green Door 342
Hair Club 37
Hamilton Book 310
Hans Gay-O-Theek 158
Hardclub 88 104
Harmony 76
Harris Newsstand 294
Hidden Joy 198
Highland Books 206
Highway 71 News 341
Hobson De Nero 88
Holz Variety / Magazine Rack 358
Hot Love 97
Howell Adult Book Store 290
Hudson Video & News 311
Imperial Books 44
Ingrid's Bookstore 323
Intim Boutique 131
Intim Shop 114
Intimshop 130
It's My Pleasure 327
Jerry's Adult Bookstore 354
Journal 123
Kill City 33
Kooky Shop 74
Kools 121
Kraze 93
Kunomeiden GMBH 117
La Sex Shoppe 193
Land Beyond 27
Leather & Lace 229
Leisure Look 74
Lenny's News 261
Libidos-Erotheek 36, 38
Lifestyles for the 90's 270
Ligne 2 104
Little Denmarks Books 255
LL&SS 97
Love Boutique 206, 223
Love Toy Books 270
Lovecraft 51, 60, 86
Loveworks 260
Mac Mac 73
Magic America 140, 141, 142, 143, 144, 146, 147
Magic Moments 74
Magic Top Video Club 147
Main Attraction 356
Marc's Smokeshop 53
Market Street News 355
Max Wonder 266
Mebray Ltd 75
Midnight Adult Book & Video 212
Midnight Special Books 222

Midwest Adult Bookstore 283
Mike's 126
MMV Erotic Shop 113
Monument Books 335
Ms. Kitty's Adult Shop 285
Multi Sexy Boutique 149
Mustang Books & Videos 224
N. M. A. 74
Naughty 'n Nice 323
Naughty But Nice 52, 355, 357, 358
Nauti Nik Naks 163
New Clinton Book Mart 311
News - Books - Cards 237
News Stand 47
Newsstand Adult Bookshop 226
Nine & A Half Weeks 245
Nitch Novelties 335
North End News 311
North Street Bookshop 297
Nu Haven Books & Video 231
Oasis Bookstore 339
Odyssey Book Store 337
Off Broadway Emporium 256
Omni Adult Bookstore 237
Open Enterprises, Inc. 219
Original Bookstore 241
Orion 113
Our Place 316
Panda Bear 261
Paradise Books 356
Paris Adult Bookstore 262
Parkway Books & Videos 223
Passion Flower 208
Pegasus 316
Pegasus Unusual Books 247
Perez Books 198
Peter's Palace 288
Phœnix Bookstore 259
Phylea 104
Pink Pussy 31
Pink Pussycat Boutique 237, 239, 309
Plain Brown Wrapper II 317
Plato's Bookstore 258
Pleasure 123
Pleasure Chest 225, 252, 309, 331
Pleasure Palace 309
Pleasure Palace I 257
Pleasure Palace II 256
Pleasureland 212, 339
Pleasures Entertainment Centers, Inc. 229
Polyester Books 33
Power of Passion 130
President News 315
Priscilla's 263
Private Pleasures 60
Privaty Shop 142
Puss'N'Boots 337
Quasimode 122
Racine News 358
Ram Bookstore 252
Red Barn Adult Bookstore 289
Red Lantern Books 231
Red Lights Sex Center 95
Regal Mag & Toy Shop 162
Return to Sender 46
Revolt Shop 121
Ritual Shoes 86
Roodhorst 153
RVG-Import Oy 97
Salisbury News Agency 266
Salt City Book & Video 299
Sanford Video & News 316
Santa Rosa Adult Books & Video 222
Sarah's Bare Necessities 198
Savage Gifts & Leather 296
Savoy 76
SBD 172
Scene 22 74
Scene One 94
Séduction 63
Select Books & Video 355
Sex & Gay Shop 121
Sex 42 97
Sex Bazar 113
Sex Center 100
Sex Imtim 113
Sex Market 97
Sex Shop 95, 100, 105, 106, 122, 123, 134
Sex Shop Erotik Kaufhaus 132
Sex World 281
Sexotica 180
Sexy Shop 106, 125
Sexyland 112, 126, 180
Shiwa 109
Shop 28 130
Sign of the Times 86
Silver Fox 247
Silver News 265
Sin City Adult Books 327
Smoke Shop 233
Smorgasmatron! 87
Spanky's 353
Sparta-Shop 126
Springfield Books & Video 272
Stallion Book & Video Centre 76
State Street Arcade 356
State Street Bookstore 311
Stilletto 309
Studio One 336
Sweethearts Adult Bookshop 29
Swingers Bookstore 193
T. B.'s Camelot 258
Taboo Center 174
Taboo Tabou 252
Tad's Total Adult Discount Store 43
Taos Book Shop 295
Tender Moments / The Other You 237
Third Eye Centre 170
Thread City Book & Novelty 232
Times Square Books 311
Tom's Toybox 261
Torrington Video Books 232
Tower Newsstand 271
Toy Box 224
Trail Books 239
Treasure Box Video & News 315
Treasure Chest 263
Treaure Chest II 263
Trixx Adult Cinema & Bookstore 342
Turk Street News & Video 219
Unique News 310
Unisex Adult Bookstore 289
United Book 273
Uptown Bookstore 322
Uptown Novelties 245
Valentine Products 87
Variety Books & Video 355
Vénus 100
Venus Adult Book Shop 28
Versatile Fashions 208
Vibration 34
Video Book & News 232
Videomag Plus 63
Village Book & News 298
Whittier Bookstore 324
WIWA International 125
Worldwide Magazines 275
Wos Markt 123
X Factor 230
Xtasy Down Under Male Emporium 309
Zardoz 122

Female

Amazon Bookstore, Inc. 281
Eve's Garden 309
Femme Erotica 31
Toys in Babeland 353

Gay

Adonis Center 114
All Points North 94
Annares 94
Apollo 128
Backdoor 117
Bear Store 219
Beat 32
Body Works Shop 255
Boîte à Films 98
BS-Laden 180
Buddy 128
Channel Six 113
Choc Monsieur 63
Clone Zone 76, 78, 86, 93
Clone Zone Head Office 86
Connection Garage 111
Défi 105
Delta 63
EJB Enterprises 237
Ero Box 111
Eros Boutique 116
Erotic Shop 128
Escape Bookstore 275
Executive Express 43
Frankies Erotik Shop 121
Frontline 121
Gaiety Burlesk 309
Gay International 165
Gay Pleasures / Gay Treasures 309
Gemini 33
Gerotek 129
Golden Boy 100
Hands 125
Heaven Sent Me 297
In Line Diffusion 140, 143, 144
Kitsch 105
Know How 143
Librairie Erotique 99
Loveland 178
Macho City Shop 180
Magic America 143
Man's BCN 172
Menfriends 161
Miroir des Hommes 106
Mister Mosse's Boy Shop 97
New Man im WOS 130
Numbers 27
Paradise 39
Pleasure Chest 239
Sestienda 172
Sex 10 97
Sex Pool 111
Sexashop 100, 101
Sexbox 111
Spartacus 106
Tass Surtur 176
Tomcat Store 331
Tool Shed 27
Yanko 104

Lesbian, Gay, Bi, & Transgendered

Catalog X 237
Crown Books 219
Cupid's Connection 334
Davy's Erotheek 158
Eros 151
Erotic World 129
Europa 92 139
Fantasies 171
Grownups 329
Man's Pleasurechest 111
Newsland 343
Out! Looks 74
Pink Shop 178
Pleasure 122
Priape 60, 63
Quimby's Queer Store 252
Rosa Blum 118
Salon 219
Triangle World & Leather Palace 276
Upstairs Bookshop 334
V. O. I. C. E. / Den of Pleasure 328
Wilde's 53
Worldwide Adult Bookstore 198

Male

City East Adult Bookstore 32
Magazine Rack 278
Man Shop 115

Transvestite

Fantasyland Products 53

Spanking

All Sexes & Sexualities

Naughty Victorian 263

LEATHERWORK SUPPLIES

General

All Sexes & Sexualities

Berman Leathercraft 270
Capital Findings & Leather 60
Leather Factory 190
Leffler's 33
Tandy Leather Co. 190
Veterans Leather 298
Zack White Leather 316

MEDICAL EQUIPMENT

All Sexes & Sexualities

Alfa Medical 299

MILITARY SURPLUS

All Sexes & Sexualities

A. A. Surplus Sales, Inc. 206
AA Surplus Sales 206
Acme Surplus 208
Action Surplus 325
Adventure 1 170
Army & Navy Stores 71, 72, 93
Army Classics 87
Army Navy Store 241, 273
Army Navy Stores 93
Army Navy Surplus U.S.A. 252
Army Surplus Sales Inc. 245
Army Surplus Stores 161
Army-Navy Store of Tampa, Inc. 243
Belmont Army Surplus 252
Big John's 209
Bordesley Army & Navy Stores 93
Callan Military Surplus 87
Camouflage 46
Command Post, Inc. 243
Drolet's Army Surplus 60
Dugout Ltd. 252
Federal Bargain Stores 309
Fulham Army & Navy Store 87
G. I. Joes 223
GI Joe's Genuine Surplus 271
Government Sales, Inc. 231
Government Surplus 170
Hap's Militaria & Collectibles 241
Harrogate Army & Navy Store 88
Headquarters Military Surplus, Inc. 243
Hercules Outfitters 60
Islington Army & Navy Store 87
Jerry's Army & Navy Store 271
Lawrence Corner 87
Lormer Military Shop 241
Lowson's Army & Navy Store 170
M & J Army Surplus 60
Massachusetts Army Navy Store 270
Melrose Army Navy Store 270
Mr Surplus Army Navy Stores 60
New Cross Army Surplus 76
Omaha Surplus 341
Q & M Stores 93
Romeo Trading Co. Ltd. 87
S O S Army Surplus Ltd. 44
Save-More Sport Store 60
Silvermans Ltd. 87
Stewart's Army Surplus 170
Stoughton Army Navy Center 270
Task Force Surplus Supplies 167
Trader 309
United Army Surplus 252
War & Peace 170
West Lynn Military Surplus 46
Winthrop Army Navy Store 270

PIERCING JEWELRY

All Sexes & Sexualities

Shiny Things 63

SAFER SEX PRODUCTS

All Sexes & Sexualities

Boys Own 88
Brush Away 78
Condomi 37
Condoms Plus 212
Rubber Plantation 76
Sussex Safer Sex Supplies Ltd. 74

Lesbian, Gay, Bi, & Transgendered

Condomania 71

SUPPLIERS

DIAPERS

All Sexes & Sexualities

Briggs Corporation 256
Camp International, Inc. 276
Contenta, Inc. 245
Dripride / Weyerhaeuser 258
Duraline Medical Products 321
Duro-Med Industries, Inc. 290
Edley Enterprises, Inc. 288
First Quality Products, Inc. 299
George Disposables 335
Geri-Care Products 291
Health Tec, Inc. 272
Home Delivery Incontinent Supplies Co., Inc. 283

Suppliers: Diapers

Humanicare International, Inc. 292
Medical Disposables Company 245
Mother's Little Helper Diaper Service 220
Nikky / Natural Baby Co., Inc. 293
Professional Medical Products 335
Support Plus 271
V. Jensen 225
Woodbury Products, Inc. 299

ELECTROLYSIS

Transgender

Roxy's Electrolysis 334

MARKET RESEARCH

All Sexes & Sexualities

Rivendell Marketing Company 190

Lesbian, Gay, Bi, & Transgendered

Overlooked Opinions, Inc. 252

MISCELLANEOUS

All Sexes & Sexualities

Goodfellow Corp. 329

Lesbian, Gay, Bi, & Transgendered

Post Option Business Center 353

Transgender

Genie Trimmers 289
Spencer Gifts 289

NEEDLES & ACUPUNCTURE PRODUCTS

All Sexes & Sexualities

Eastern Currents 222

PHOTOPRINTING

All Sexes & Sexualities

Brent Photographics 90
Magic Color Photo Lab 23
R. L. 230
Venus Photography 281

SAFER SEX PRODUCTS

All Sexes & Sexualities

Bell Croyden, John 87
Mayer Laboratories 208
Rubber Tree 191

Lesbian, Gay, Bi, & Transgendered

Rubberstuffers 87

TRAVEL ARRANGEMENTS

BDSM

All Sexes & Sexualities

Ambassador World Travel 245
Atlas Travel East 266
SunMaster 24

Gay

Travel Keys Tours 210

TATTOOISTS

All Sexes & Sexualities

8-Ball Tattoo 321
Accent Tattoo 348
Ania Metalworks 221
Body Graphics Tattoo 229
Capitol Tattoo 266
Creative Tattoo 274
Deana's Skin Art Studio 241
Dermagraphics 353
Endless Pain Tattoo 121
Everlasting Tattoo 219
Great Southern Tattoo Company 265
Images in Ink 290
Into You 87
Midnight Iguana Tattoing, Inc. 243
Mischief Moon 27
Mum'sTattoo 46
No Hope * No Fear 252
Sacred Heart Tattoos 245
Sign Of The Wolf Tattoo 288
Skin Deep Tattoo 246
Skinprint Tattoo 353, 354
Soma Studios 221
Tattoo Connection 111
Tattoo Factory 290
Tattoo Santa Barbara 221
Tattoo You 353
Urban Primitive 60

TELEVISION

AIDS

All Sexes & Sexualities

HIV Update 252

GENERAL

All Sexes & Sexualities

CNBC Real Personal 290
CS4 Media Today 93
James Whale Show 87
Mike Mansfield TV 87
University of Birmingham 93

MARKETING

All Sexes & Sexualities

Bradley Communications Corporation 329
Radio & TV Interview Report 329

SEXUALITY

All Sexes & Sexualities

Erotica Project 219

Female

Fem TV 343

Gay

Closet Case Show 309
Gay Broadcasting System 310
Out In The Nineties 310

Lesbian

Dyke TV 310
Sang Froid 310

Lesbian, Gay, Bi, & Transgendered

Cable Access Channel 21 321
Cable Access TV 324
Cable TV 219
Cathedral of Hope 341
Channel 11 48
Coming Out 48
Dream Team Productions 177
Electric City 219
Gay Cable Nash 337
Gay Cable Network 310
Gay Fairfax 349
Green & Yellow TV 281
Just For The Record 261
KBDI-TV, Channel 12 229
Lambda Report 229
Milwaukee Gay / Lesbian Cable Network 357
Night Scene 324
Our World Television 212
Pink Elephant 177
Prism 46
Public Access Television 261
Queer Program 357
Queer TV 27
Stonewall Union Lesbian / Gay Pride Report 321
To Tell The Truth Television 341
Triangle Express Productions 203
Triangle Television, Inc. 161
Viacom Cabe, Channel 19 337
Warner Cable Channel 47 357
Yellow On Thursday 357

TRAINING

ÆSTHETICS

Transvestite

La Loge de Thalie 37

BDSM

All Sexes & Sexualities

Cléo Dubois Academy of SM Arts 206
Labyrinth 60
Miss Prim's Muir Reform Academy 24
Miss Tresse's Finishing Academy 24
Vesta, Dianna 240

Lesbian, Gay, Bi, & Transgendered

J. B. Productions 221

Male

Meester Terry's SM Society & School 153

SPIRITUALITY

All Sexes & Sexualities

Body Electric School 208

Index of Kink-Aware Professionals

Affirmations
Columbus, 614 445 8277 319
Arsenault, Raymond, Ph.D.
Andover, 508 475 7171 267
Salem, 603 898 5105 288
Ask Isadora
San Francisco, 415 386 5090 212
Baldwin, Guy, MFCC
Los Angeles, 213 667 9194 203
Baxley, Thom
Chicago, 312 275 0130 248
Bernet, Michael
Brooklyn, 718 284 4162 297
Bettinger, Michael, Ph.D., MFCC
San Francisco, 415 563 6100 213
Columbia Medical Plaza
Vancouver, 206 254 1814 354
Easton, Dossie, MFCC
San Francisco, 415 488 1431 213
Egge, Conrad, Ph.D.
Phœnix, 602 230 2025 193
Fuller, Cheryl, M.A., LCPC
Portland, 207 774 4436 262
General Media Inc.
New York, 212 702 6000 307
Goodhew, John, M.D.
Toronto, 416 461 2200 55
Harrison, James, Ph.D.
Asheville, 704 253 3055 313
Hartzog, Dennis, M.Ed, L.P.C.
Dallas / Fort Worth, 214 559 0688 340
Hawkins, Brenda, Ed.D.
Doraville, 404 986 4247 245
Henkin, William
San Francisco, 415 923 1150 213, 216
Hillis, Raymond, Ph.D.
Tesuque, 505 983 3549 295
Horstman, William, Ph.D.
San Francisco, 415 431 1790 213
Hraca, Kim, M.A., MFCC
Berkeley, 510 601 1859 196, 197
Istar, Arlene, CSW, CAC
Albany, 518 439 9270 295
Istvan, John Emery, M.S., MSW, LCSW
Trumbull, 203 268 8858 Ext. 304 232
Karmen, Mel, Ph.D.
San Diego, 619 296 9442 211
Keith, III, Paul, M.D.
Los Angeles, 213 964 1440 203
Knopf, Norton, Ph.D.
Chicago, 312 363 5011 249
Legacy Counseling Center, Inc.
Dallas / Fort Worth, 214 520 6308 340
Mallon, David, MSW
Long Beach, 310 434 8236 202
Manoogian Psychological Associates
Winston-Salem, 910 765 5636 316
Manoogian, Sam, Ph.D.
Winston-Salem, 910 765 5636 316
Manson, Susan, MS, MFCC
Los Angeles, 213 280 9925 203
Marks, Al, Ph.D.
San Diego, 619 296 6134 211
McConnell, John, Ph.D.
San Diego, 619 296 1216 211
Miller, Wynn, MSW, CSW
New York, 212 989 4641 301
Moser, Charles, Ph.D, M.D.
San Francisco, 415 621 4369 213
Murrell, Pat, MSW, LCSW
Saint Louis, 314 569 5795 282
O'Brien, Terence
Sacramento, 916 979 3515 209
Outreach Institute of Gender Studies
Augusta, 207 621 0858 13
Oxenbury, Jane, M. Ed., C. Psyc.
Calgary, 403 240 2501 42
Patti, Vincent-John, ACSW
New York, 212 473 3623 301
Porter, Theresa, Psy.D.
Meriden, 203 237 8978 231
Power, John, MSW
Chicago, 312 327 9886 249
Rendel, Brian, M.A, NCC
Dowagiac, 616 782 9811 275
Ribakoff, Robin, M.F.C.T.
Encino, 818 957 4065 199
Riley Snow, Wynelle, M.D.
Bristol, 860 582 1178 229
Roach, Barbara, L.C.S.W.
Long Beach, 310 424 1755 202
Ruth, Richard, Ph.D.
Wheaton, 301 933 3072 266
Ryan, Barb, M.S.
Eugene, 541 345 5058 325
Sandler, Karen, D.O.
Los Angeles, 213 931 1463 203
Schochet, Rachel, Ph.D., MFCC
San Francisco, 415 641 1292 213
Snyder, Robert, Ph.D.
Saint Louis, 314 727 9088 284
Summit Consulting Group, Inc
East Greenwich, 401 884 2778 334
Tanner, Mark, M.D.
Atlanta, 404 355 2000 244
Theseus Counseling Services
Augusta, 207 621 0858 262
Boston, 617 868 3157 267
Vanek, Stephen, LMSW-ACP
Dallas / Fort Worth, 214 239 8775 340
Verdantmom
Camarillo, 805 987 3162 197
Walsh, Eileen, M.S.
Pawling, 914 855 5306 295

Index of Advertisers

Alternate Sources 14
Arthur Hamilton, Inc. 10
Bondage Life 18
Bound & Gagged 19
Camera Art 23
Checkmate & DungeonMaster 15
Club Caprice 133
Dædalus Publishing Company 216
Diaper Pail Friends (DPF) 9
DM International 20
DPF Newsletter 9
Editions du Triangle Rose 18
Fetish Network 184, 185
Harmony Concepts, Inc. 18
Heartwood Whips of Passion 201
Kastley GmbH 133
Katharsis 16, 20
Larry Townsend 184
Leather Journal 16, 17
Lifestyle Online 1
Northbound Leather Ltd. 41, 56, 60
Outbound Press 18, 19
Piercology 320
Playspace 352
Projet X 18
SIN 190
Sorority Magazine 59
Taste of Latex 21
Telecentral Electronics 16
Urban Primitive 60
WholeSM Publishing Corporation 58
WPC 8

INSTRUCTIONS

Getting your listing into Alternate Sources is easy. To be included in the next edition or to update your current entry, all you have to do is fill in the blanks on the form to the right. Each of the boxes & check boxes indicates one of the types of information your clients or members want to know. Please spend 5 minutes filling in and returning the form today, and help keep Alternate Sources the most complete global directory of its kind.

To make sure that the category you select is the closest to your organization, we suggest that you check out *all* the categories in the Index by Organization Type, just in case there is one better than the first one that catches your eye. If you need a category that is not listed, please ask us about it. We will try to include it.

When you review the titles in the Index by Organization Type, please note that the word *sexuality* usually refers to an organization based on its users' sexual orientation: e.g. Helpline: Sexuality would be for questions about orientation issues. You fill in which orientation in the Primary Clientele check boxes.

Please use the whole width of the boxes on the right by writing *on top of* the grey lettering. Also, use the other side of this form or a separate piece of paper to include a description of your organization, additional comments, and/or questions. A description of up to twenty words is free. (Please contact us on 416 962 1040 for rates for additional words and display advertising.)

Continued on next page...

Detach along perforations

WE WANT IN! LIST US AS FOLLOWS:

Name (Salutation, First Name, Last Name)

Division / Publication Name

Company / Organization

Mailing Address: Suite / P. O. Box Number

Mailing Address: Street & Number

City

State / Province / County

Postal Code / Zip Code | Country

Telephone | 2nd. Telephone

Facsimile | Cellular Telephone

BBS | Maximum Modem Speed

E-Mail Address

URL: www, ftp, gopher, etc.

Publication Frequency / Year | Annual Subscription & Currency

Organization Type (please see Index by Organization Type for list)

Business Hours & Days

Catalogue Prive & Currency

Languages Spoken

Academic Qualifications (Counsellors Only) ☐KAP

Licence Type & Number (Counsellors Only)

Your clients should tell you that they are at least:

You Are: ☐Local ☐State / Provincial ☐National ☐International

Disabled access: ☐Office ☐Office Needs Help ☐WC ☐WC Needs Help

You Accept: ☐Cash ☐Cheque ☐Visa ☐Master Card ☐Traveller's Cheques ☐Amex ☐Diners Club ☐Money Order ☐Discover ☐Directly From Bank Accounts (Electronic Transfer)

Your *Primary* Clientele (*one* only, please): ☐All sexes & sexualities ☐Bisexual ☐Female ☐Gay Male ☐Heterosexual ☐Heterosexual, Female ☐Heterosexual, Male ☐Lesbian ☐Lesbian, Gay, & Bisexual ☐Male ☐Transgender ☐Transvestite / Cross Dresser

Your Ownership is (please pick *all* applicable boxes): ☐Lesbian, Gay, Bisexual or Trangendered ☐Not Lesbian, Gay, Bisexual, or Trangendered ☐For Profit ☐Not For Profit ☐Do Not List Ownership

Place sufficient postage here

Alternate Sources,
P. O. Box 19591,
55 Bloor Street West,
Toronto, Ontario M4W 3T9
CANADA

Please include your description here (up to 20 words are free).

Detach along perforations

INSTRUCTIONS (CONT.)

For all periodicals, please indicate publication frequency and annual subscription. If you're an organization other than a publisher and you publish a regular newsletter, please put its name in the Division/Publication Name box.

If you are a store and also have a separate mail order department, please have them make a copy of this form and send it to us for a separate listing. This does not apply if you just do a little bit of mail order "on the side." In this case, please put something like "Also mail order" in your description. Mail order businesses are listed as national or international, unless otherwise requested.

If you're a counsellor, please indicate your qualifications and licence number(s) in the boxes provided. If you see and understand the needs of people who enjoy BDSM, per DSM-IV, please indicate that you are a Kink Aware Professional (KAP) by putting a tick mark in the KAP box.

BDSM refers to all the leather / SM / fetish combinations and is used as a catch-all grouping, where appropriate.

NOTE

If your organization has closed down, please send this card to us, giving us the name of the organization as it appears in *Alternate Sources*. That way, we can update the database. Thank you.

ORDER FORM

Send to: Alternate Sources, P. O. Box 19591, 55 Bloor Street West, Toronto, Ontario M4W 3T9. Canada

	PRICE	TAX	SUBTOTAL	QTY.	TOTAL
ALTERNATE SOURCES paperback edition	$34.00Cdn. $24.95U.S. £21.99	P.S.T.(Ontario only) $2.72 per copy G.S.T. (Canada only $2.38 per copy			
ALTERNATE SOURCES CD-ROM standard edition	$79.95Cdn. $59.95U.S. £36.95	P.S.T. (Ontario only) $6.40 per copy G.S.T. (Canada Only) $5.60 per copy			
On The Safe Edge paperback edition	$24.95Cdn. $19.95U.S. £14.99	G.S.T. (Canada Only) $1.76 per copy			
On The Safe Edge hardback edition	$34.95Cdn. $29.95U.S. £21.99	G.S.T. (Canada Only) $1.76 per copy			
Shipping & handling: One book $5Cdn. to Canada, $5 U.S. to U.S., £8 to Europe. More books: $2.50Cdn. to Canada, $2.50 to U.S., £4 to Europe		G.S.T. (Canada Only) $0.35 first, $0.18 others			
				GRAND TOTAL :	

PLEASE SEND TO ME AT:

Name (Salutation, First Name, Last Name)

Mailing Address: Suite / P. O. Box Number

Mailing Address: Street & Number

City

State / Province / County

Postal Code / Zip Code

Country

I AM LEGALLY AN ADULT WHERE I LIVE; SIGNED: ____________________

Detach along perforations

ADVERTISE IN ALTERNATE SOURCES!

Yes! We are interested in advertising in the next edition of Alternate Sources.
Please send us your media kit with rate card

Name (Salutation, First Name, Last Name)

Division / Publication Name

Company / Organization

Mailing Address: Suite / P. O. Box Number

Mailing Address: Street & Number

City

State / Province / County

Postal Code / Zip Code

Country

Telephone

2nd. Telephone

Facsimile

E-Mail Address

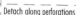

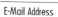

What people are saying about

On The Safe Edge A Manual For SM Play

"The authors have definitely achieved their ambitious goal." "There is a glossary with 88 entries and 14 pages of index, making this very definitely the best reference work of the four [books] for which I have seen the final text...." "*On The Safe Edge* is the only SM how-to-book that is going to work well as a continuing reference book. As a former college professor, text book author, and frequent SM teacher, I can only say to the authors, 'Well done! I look forward to using your book to teach a course.'"
Anthony DeBlase, editor emeritus, *Drummer* magazine; editor, *DungeonMaster*

"...a seminal publication." "*On The Safe Edge* represents a major step forward in S/M writing... [it] can be described as an encyclopædia or textbook [of S/M practices]. However described, its publication is a landmark event for our subculture... No book on S/M has ever been designed to be as accessible as this one... The section on sexually-transmitted diseases [and] drugs... alone are worth the price of the book... *On The Safe Edge* serves our entire community, regardless of sexual orientation... Every S/M library should have this book... buy it as a present for yourself."
Harold E. Cox, Editor, *CheckMate* & *DungeonMaster*

"In the light of prevailing attitudes, a manual such as this ...is a very positive step. Highly recommended."
Skin Two, London, England

"...one of the most comprehensive manuals for sadomasochistic play I have ever seen. Precise and methodical, *On The Safe Edge* should answer any imaginable kinky question. ...it demystifies the practice of SM sexuality and codifies the games in simple language for the average joe and josephine. ...It will lead to a better understanding and acceptance of SM fans and fetishists. It may save lives. It could spice up your marriage. It will mean safer, saner fun...."
R. M. Vaughan, *Books In Canada*

"Book of The Month"
Gay Times Book Service, U.K.

"*On The Safe Edge* sets itself up as a manual on how to play SM safely. What it achieves, however, is the status of *The* Definitive Bible of SM.... Unusually for a manual (even a manual on sex), I found the book completely gripping. It is written in a very friendly and down-to-earth style, and made the process of learning... fun! Put this book on your bookshelf. It is truly invaluable."
Scotsgay, Scotland

"I feel that [*On The Safe Edge*] is the best book about SM to come out this year. It is a must for your collection. When you read it, you'll see why."
Dave Rhodes, publisher and editor, *The Leather Journal*

Detach along perforations

If you have any further questions or comment, please include them here:

Place sufficient postage here

Alternate Sources,
P. O. Box 19591,
55 Bloor Street West,
Toronto, Ontario M4W 3T9
CANADA